PHARMACOLOGICAL BASIS OF NURSING PRACTICE

Julia B. Clark, Ph.D.

Health Scientist Administrator,
National Institutes of Health,
Bethesda, Maryland

Sherry F. Queener, Ph.D.

Professor of Pharmacology,
Indiana University School of Medicine,
Indianapolis, Indiana

Virginia Burke Karb, R.N., Ph.D.

Assistant Professor of Nursing, School of Nursing,
University of North Carolina at Greensboro,
Greensboro, North Carolina

Third Edition

with **64** illustrations

The C. V. Mosby Company

ST. LOUIS • BALTIMORE • PHILADELPHIA • TORONTO   1990

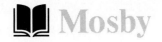

Executive Editor: Don Ladig
Developmental Editor: Robin Carter
Production Editor: Cynthia A. Miller
Production: Editing, Design & Production, Inc.
Book and Cover Design: Gail Morey Hudson

Great care has been used in compiling and checking the information in this book to ensure its accuracy. However, because of changing technology, recent discoveries, research, and individualization of prescriptions according to patient needs, the uses, effects, and dosages of drugs may vary from those given here. Neither the publisher nor the authors shall be responsible for such variations or other inaccuracies. We urge that before you administer any drug you check the manufacturer's dosage recommendations as given in the package insert provided with each product.

THIRD EDITION

The C.V. Mosby Company
11830 Westline Industrial Drive, St. Louis, Missouri 63146

The National Institutes of Health does not necessarily endorse the views expressed in this book.

Library of Congress Cataloging in Publication Data

Freeman, Julia B.
    Pharmacological basis of nursing practice/Julia B. Clark, Sherry
F. Queener, Virginia Burke Karb.—3rd ed.
        p.   cm.
    Includes bibliographical references.
    ISBN 0-8016-6246-X
    1. Pharmacology. 2. Nursing. I. Queener, Sherry F. II. Karb,
Virginia Burke. III.   Title.
    [DNLM: 1. Drug Therapy—nurses' instruction. 2. Pharmacology—
nurses' instruction.   QV 4 F855p]
RM300.F72   1990
615'.1'024613—dc20
DNLM/DLC
for Library of Congress   89-13781
                                                                            CIP

GW/VH/VH 9 8 7 6 5 4 3 2 1

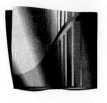

Preface

NEW CONTENT

Pharmacology is a rapidly changing field. The third edition of *Pharmacological Basis of Nursing Practice* contains information on 75 new drugs that have appeared since the second edition was published. We have thoroughly revised the appropriate sections, including the new drugs in tables and integrating the discussion of these agents in the text. All sections of the text have been reviewed and revised to keep up with current knowledge on drug mechanisms and therapeutic uses of agents. The third edition also contains the following new features:

- A unit on **immunopharmacology** composed of two chapters has been contributed by Dr. Stephen M. Hatfield, Immunopharmacologist, Department of Immunology, Pulmonary and Leukotriene Research, Lilly Research Laboratories, Indianapolis, Indiana. Dr. Hatfield is the second contributor to this text, joining Dr. Lynn Roger Willis, Professor of Pharmacology and Medicine, Department of Pharmacology and Toxicology, Indiana University School of Medicine, Indianapolis, Indiana. Dr. Willis has contributed the chapter on over-the-counter drugs to the first, second, and now the third editions.
- **Nursing diagnoses** have been added to the Nursing Process sections wherever they appear throughout the book.
- The Patient Care Implication sections have been subdivided into sections: **Drug Administration** and **Patient and Family Education.** This division is designed to help the student more readily identify and learn these important concepts.
- Throughout the book, there is an increased emphasis on clinically relevant information for the nursing student. **Separate boxes** on geriatric considerations, pediatric considerations, dietary considerations, and drug abuse alerts have been added throughout. Special patient problems are also highlighted in these boxes. Examples of these problems include conditions such as constipation, photosensitivity, and dry mouth.

Pedagogical features retained from previous editions include italicized key terms, chapter end summaries, and study questions. Readings are also included to guide the student who needs to research a specific area in more depth.

FOCUS

This up-to-date, scientifically based text fulfills the three basic requirements of the nursing student studying pharmacology: (1) a clear presentation of the concepts of pharmacology that guide all drug use; (2) a thorough treatment of major classes of drugs, with emphasis on mechanisms of action; and (3) a clear and easily accessible reference on the patient care implications that grow out of an understanding of the pharmacological aspects of specific drugs. This textbook emphasizes the rationale for drug therapy by relating the physiological factors of disease processes to drug mechanisms. Although more thorough in describing the scientific basis of drug action than most textbooks for nursing students, this book carefully reviews pertinent physiological facts so that students can readily see how drugs modify physiological processes.

Students of nursing look forward to pharmacology as one of the important background courses for their professional education, but they often express frustration about trying to remember the large number of drugs they are called on to learn. We have minimized that difficulty by dealing with drug classes first and then by emphasizing the similarities between members of a single drug class. This pedagogical technique of grouping drugs according to mechanism of action is reinforced by the chapter divisions, which are narrower than those of most pharmacology textbooks for nursing students.

ORGANIZATION

The book is divided into twelve sections that represent the grouping we have found to be most effective. However, each chapter within the book is restricted to discrete topics, allowing flexibility for instructors who wish to adapt the textbook to their own curricula. This organization not only allows the instructor to rearrange the order in which material is presented but also gives the students succinct sections to master.

The first ten chapters, which make up Sections I through III, contain introductory material. The goal of these chapters is to provide the background information necessary for discussing drug action and use. The concepts discussed here can be used as a guide for study of the drug classes presented later in the text. It has been our experience as teachers that basic concepts need to be reinforced throughout the study of pharmacology or students will fall out of the habit of organizing material according to these logical precepts. We have, therefore, systematically referred students to these early chapters at logical points throughout the text.

The chapters in Sections IV through XII are organized in a consistent manner. The student is first presented with the physiology and cell biology required as background. When appropriate, disease processes are discussed briefly to explain the aberrant physiological processes involved. Drug classes are presented next, with the mechanisms of action of the particular class discussed first, followed by pharmacokinetics, side effects, toxicity, drug interactions (if appropriate), and special comments on clinical use of the drugs when necessary for clarity. To promote conciseness, we rarely discuss fixed-dosage combination drugs, choosing rather to deal with individual agents. Following the basic material, the appropriate nursing assessment and management are reviewed in a section called *The Nursing Process*. The chapter summary is preceded by *Patient Care Implications*, which presents specialized information required by a nurse for the appropriate administration of the drug and for the proper care, evaluation, and education of the patient. At the end of the chapter, study questions and suggested readings are provided for the student. The readings generally supplement and expand information in the text.

The Nursing Process section in each chapter is a guide for the nursing student in relating knowledge of medications to the overall plan of care for the patient. It is not meant to supplant the use of additional textbooks of nursing or current literature. The focus is almost exclusively on the pharmacological factors rather than on the disease process itself. The Nursing Process section is divided into four parts. The first, Assessment, identifies the types of patients commonly requiring use of the drugs discussed in the chapter. The second part, Nursing Diagnosis, gives examples of appropriate nursing diagnoses. The third part, Management, encompasses the planning and implementation phase of the nursing process. It identifies the type of data

that should be monitored throughout therapy and some of the nursing activities needed to promote the drug activity or to foster patient well-being. Management also contains information on teaching the patient material required for self-management. The fourth part, Evaluation, describes the desired outcome of drug therapy. We anticipate that the beginning practitioner and the nursing student may have difficulty in translating knowledge of a drug action into appropriate nursing interventions. The Nursing Process section leads the student into this translation process. The **Patient Care Implications** section carries this process further—to the level of defining concrete clinical activities.

The specific clinical details of drug use and patient care are purposely separated from the body of the text in the Patient Care Implications section. We believe that this method of presentation enables the student to use the book more efficiently at two levels. First, the student can master the scientific basis of the action of a particular drug. General comments on nursing assessment and management of patients are made in the text and are summarized and brought into focus in The Nursing Process section of the chapter. However, when students enter the clinical setting, they require much more specific information than can be effectively included in the body of the text. We have therefore gathered this information in the Patient Care Implications section, where it is easily accessible and does not interrupt the flow of the discussion on basic principles of drug action. The patient care implications material presupposes that the student is familiar with the drug being discussed. Therefore a person using this section for reference on a completely unfamiliar drug would be well advised *first* to read the appropriate material on the drug in the body of the text.

The specific **organization of chapters** is as follows. Section I begins with two chapters that introduce pharmacology and the principles of pharmacodynamics and pharmacokinetics. These are the only chapters that emphasize the science of pharmacology rather than the pharmacological basis of nursing practice. The chapter on the regulation of the manufacture, sale, and use of drugs is intended to give the student an understanding of the legal aspects concerning medications.

Section II is devoted to material most important for patient care. Chapters on drug administration and calculation of drug dosages prepare the student for the responsibility of administering drugs. The chapters on use of over-the-counter drugs and self-medication and care of the poisoned patient illustrate nursing principles applied to these specialized situations.

Section III is an introduction to neuropharmacology. The principles of neuropharmacology central to so many areas of pharmacology are presented in three short chapters. These chapters are intended to provide an introduction at the first reading and a review at a later reading. Drugs stemming from autonomic pharmacology have applications in so many clinical areas that we have found the most successful approach in our own teaching to be a presentation of autonomic pharmacology first on a theoretical level and later on a systems level.

Section IV is designed to cover those areas of pharmacology that are difficult to define, except that they are systems under cholinergic control. Drugs affecting muscle tone, the eye, and the gastrointestinal tract are discussed in this section.

Section V focuses on those drug classes affecting the cardiovascular and renal systems. The drugs affecting the sympathetic nervous system appear primarily in Chapters 14 and 15, in which circulation and blood pressure are described. From our teaching, we are convinced that it is more rational to present a systems approach to these areas rather than to describe all of cardiovascular pharmacology as variations of adrenergic pharmacology. However, within each chapter we have taken an adrenergic mechanisms approach to the discussion of the cardiovascular disease processes. One chapter is devoted to drug classes affecting the kidney, another to fluids and electrolytes, two chapters to drug classes affecting the heart, and three chapters to drug classes affecting the blood.

Section VI presents drug classes that affect the local mediators, prostaglandins and histamine. This area of pharmacology is rapidly expanding, with several new agents of this type recently appearing on the market. The mechanism of action of aspirin, from its role in pain and fever to its antiinflammatory activity, is first presented and used to introduce the other nonsteroidal, antiinflammatory drugs and drugs used to treat rheumatoid arthritis and gout. The antihistamines are discussed next, followed by a chapter on bronchodilators and drugs used to treat asthma. The latter chapter and the following one on drugs controlling bronchial secretions contain the remaining sympathomimetic drugs not described in detail in the cardiovascular and renal sections.

Section VII is a new unit on immunopharmacology. The first chapter in the section reviews the immune system and the second chapter discusses modulators of immune function. This area of therapeutics is blossoming and the number of drugs has increased to the point that a separate section is warranted.

Section VIII focuses on antimicrobial agents and chemotherapeutic agents. The first chapter of this section introduces the general principles of antimicrobial therapy and explains how these drugs differ from the other agents discussed up to this point. Thereafter, each chapter describes the pharmacology of a major family of antibiotics. Enough microbiology is included to make the clinical uses of each family of drugs obvious. Antifungal, antiviral, and antiparasitic agents are each considered separately, appropriately prefaced by information explaining why these organisms present more therapeutic difficulties than bacteria. The last chapter of the book deals with the many selective poisons used to treat neoplastic diseases. Again, mechanism of drug action is emphasized because an understanding of mechanisms allows the clinical properties of these drugs to be more easily appreciated and puts the nursing procedures into perspective.

Section IX discusses drugs used for treating mental and emotional disorders. Drug abuse is not treated in a separate chapter in this textbook, but the pharmacological basis of drug abuse and its pharmacological treatment are carefully described for each class of drugs. The chapter on sedative-hypnotic and antianxiety drugs also includes a section on alcohol and the treatment of alcoholism. Antipsychotic drugs and antidepressant drugs are presented in separate chapters, since psychoses and depression no longer are held to be the two ends of the same molecular seesaw. We have not emphasized neuroanatomy in discussing any central nervous system processes, having found that this approach does little beyond confusing the student. Instead we have presented central nervous system pharmacology in terms of neurotransmitter mechanisms, another reason for having reviewed the principles of neuropharmacology in an introductory chapter.

Section X presents drugs used to control severe pain. The chapter on the narcotic analgesics highlights how these drugs mimic endogenous substances. The chapter on general anesthetics includes inhalation agents, intravenous agents, and the combinations now used for balanced anesthesia and neuroleptanesthesia. Local anesthetics are discussed with special reference to the routes of administration.

Section XI covers those drugs used for disorders of central muscle control. The spectrum of anticonvulsant drugs is first presented, followed by a chapter that covers the antiparkinsonian drugs and drugs used to treat muscle spasms and spasticity.

Section XII presents drugs that affect the endocrine system. The first chapter in the section describes basic principles that may be applied to all endocrine organs. Subsequent chapters deal with the pharmacology associated with a particular endocrine organ. Sufficient information about endocrine disease states is presented so that students may understand the nursing assessment of these patients. Unlike most texts in pharmacology, this one includes enough information about endocrine testing methods to allow a student to understand the diagnostic procedures patients with many endocrine conditions must undergo. This information again facilitates and complements the material on patient management and teaching.

ACKNOWLEDGMENTS

The production of this textbook has involved several able and experienced members of the editorial staff at The C.V. Mosby Company. We wish to thank Robin Carter, Don Ladig, and Tom Manning, for their special contributions.

Many of our professional colleagues have generously contributed time and expertise in reviewing materials for this book. We especially wish to thank the following people at Indiana University, many of whom critiqued large sections of material for us: Marlene A. Aldo-Benson, M.D., Professor of Medicine; Richard N. Dexter, M.D., Professor of Medicine; Joseph A. DiMicco, Ph.D., Professor of Pharmacology; Bonnie Klank, Pharm.D., Drug Information Specialist; Sandra Morzorati, R.N., Ph.D., Research Assistant in Neurobiology; Donald Niederpruem, Ph.D., Professor of Microbiology and Immunology; Richard Powell, M.D., Professor of Medicine and Biochemistry; Judith A. Richter, Ph.D., Professor of Pharmacology; August M. Watanabe, M.D., Professor of Pharmacology and Medicine; Lynn R. Willis, Ph.D., Reg. Pharm., Professor of Pharmacology and Medicine; Robert Wolen, Ph.D., Associate Professor of Pharmacology; and Thomas M. Wolfe, M.D., Assistant Professor of Anesthesia.

Colleagues at other institutions have also generously contributed time in reviewing materials: Grace Boxer, M.D., Veterans Administration Medical Center, Ann Arbor, Michigan; Marilyn L. Evans, R.N., Ph.D., Associate Professor of Nursing, University of North Carolina at Greensboro School of Nursing; Joseph R. Holtman, Ph.D., Assistant Professor in Pharmacology, U. Kentucky College of Medicine, Lexington, Kentucky; Sandra D. Reed, R.N., M.S.N., Associate Professor of Nursing, University of North Carolina at Greensboro School of Nursing; Jennifer Cooke, R.N., B.S.C.N., Coordinator of Evaluation Systems, Diploma Nurse Program, George Brown College, Toronto, Ontario, Canada; Kaye E. Fox, Ph.D., Associate Professor, The Oregon Health Sciences University, Portland, Oregon; Beth Hoskins, Ph.D., Associate Professor, The University of Mississippi Medical Center, Jackson, Mississippi; Eunice H. Lee, R.N., B.S.C.N., Miss A.J. MacMaster School of Nursing, Moncton, New Brunswick, Canada; Barbara L. MacDermott, M.S., R.N., Associate Professor, College of Nursing, Syracuse University, Syracuse, New York; Byron Noordewier, Ph.D., Assistant Professor, University of North Dakota, Grand Forks, North Dakota; and Gerry White, R.N., Ed.D, Associate Professor, Southern Oregon State College, Ashland, Oregon.

H.R. Besch, Jr., Ph.D., Chairman of the Department of Pharmacology and Toxicology at Indiana University School of Medicine, deserves special mention for the support and help he has given us during the planning, writing, and production of this book. Mrs. Janie Siccardi, Administrative Assistant in the Department of Pharmacology and Toxicology, has greatly aided us in this effort. Thanks also for the support of Patricia A. Chamings, Ph.D., R.N., Dean of the School of Nursing, University of North Carolina at Greensboro School of Nursing. Illustrations in several chapters were rendered by Phil Wilson Artcraft, Sylvia Eidam and Mark Swindle.

We would also like to thank two special colleagues who have lived with the book as long as we have. They are Dr. Stephen W. Queener, Research Scientist, Department of Antibiotic Culture Development, Eli Lilly and Company; and Dr. Kenneth S. Karb, Medical Oncologist, Greensboro, North Carolina.

Julia B. Clark
Sherry F. Queener
Virginia Burke Karb

Contents

I

GENERAL PRINCIPLES OF PHARMACOLOGY

Chapters 1 and 2 cover the principles that govern the action of all drugs in the body. The basic concepts and the terms defined in these chapters recur repeatedly throughout the study of pharmacology. By studying these concepts initially the student is made aware of how to approach the study of individual drugs and how to rationalize the manner in which an individual drug is used clinically.

Chapter 3, *Regulation of the Manufacture, Sale, and Use of Medications,* is intended to place the legal status of modern drugs in perspective. This chapter also introduces the Schedule of Controlled Substances, covers the Drug Efficacy Study Implementation (DESI) rating, and discusses the FDA-assigned pregnancy categories—topics that recur at appropriate places throughout the text. Canadian drug classifications are covered in this chapter and referred to elsewhere in the text.

General Principles of Drug Action

1

Pharmacology is the study of the interaction of chemicals with living organisms to produce biological effects. This text presents those chemicals that produce therapeutically useful effects, chemicals referred to as *drugs*. This chapter reviews the general principles of drug action that form the basis for understanding the action of specific drugs.

PRINCIPLE 1: DRUGS DO NOT CREATE FUNCTIONS BUT MODIFY EXISTING FUNCTIONS WITHIN THE BODY

This principle explains the necessity for understanding the physiology of normal humans and the changes wrought by disease as a background for pharmacology. Drugs must always be considered in terms of the physiological functions they alter in the body. In no case do drugs *create* a function in a tissue or organ. For example, digitalis is a drug used to strengthen the action of the heart. Digitalis produces this effect because the drug alters the existing pattern of ion flow into and out of heart cells; it does not create a new way for the heart to contract. The drug simply alters the natural process.

To emphasize this principle, subsequent chapters on drug families start with a brief description of the normal physiology influenced by that group of drugs.

PRINCIPLE 2: NO DRUG HAS A SINGLE ACTION

The *desired action* of a drug is an expected, predictable response. Ideally, each drug would have the desired effect on one physiological process and produce no other effect. However, all drugs have the potential for altering more than one function in the body. The desired action of the drug is distinguished from all other actions by referring to these unwanted actions as *side effects* or *drug reactions*. Again, digitalis is an example. Digitalis strengthens the failing heart; this is the desired clinical effect of the drug. At the same time, however, digitalis may cause erratic heartbeats. This action is an undesirable side effect.

Predictable reactions arising from the known pharmacological action of a drug account for between 70% and 80% of all drug reactions. For example, barbiturates put a patient to sleep because they depress the central nervous system. However, excessive depression of the central nervous system is lethal, since the brain centers that control breathing will be depressed. Respiratory depression would therefore be an expected toxic reaction when barbiturates are used at doses that allow the drug to accumulate in the body. This type of toxic reaction to excessive amounts of the drug may be distinguished from predictable side effects seen at normal doses of the drug. These predictable side effects are related to the secondary actions of the drug. For example, at normal therapeutic doses barbiturates increase the drug-metabolizing activity of the liver. This ability is unrelated to the therapeutically desired activity of these drugs and, in fact, is the mechanism by which barbiturates cause a number of reactions with other drugs.

Unpredictable reactions to drugs account for between 20% and 30% of all drug reactions. Although experience shows that a certain percentage of the population may be expected to react to a drug in an unusual manner, it is often not possible to predict which individual patient will show the reaction. The unpredictable drug reactions are of two types: idiosyncratic reactions and allergic reactions.

Idiosyncratic reactions are unusual, unexpected reactions to a drug that are most often explained by a genetic difference between the patient and the normal population. For example, a certain small percentage of the population lacks an enzyme called pseudocholinesterase, which is usually found in the bloodstream. Persons lacking this enzyme show no signs of this abnormality until they are exposed to drugs such as succinylcholine. Succinylcholine is a paralyzing agent used before surgery to relax the muscles and allow easy tracheal intubation. In normal persons the drug is very short acting, since it is destroyed by pseudocholinesterase. In persons lacking this enzyme, succinylcholine stays in the bloodstream and the drug is very long acting. These patients require artificial ventilation until the paralyzing effects of succinylcholine wear off, whereas a normal person recovers within a minute or so and requires no assistance. This prolonged reaction to succinylcholine is one example of an idiosyncratic reaction.

Allergic reactions to drugs account for between 6% and 10% of all drug reactions. The allergic reaction may be triggered by the drug in its original form or by a metabolite of the drug formed in the body. Most drugs are not very allergenic, but others are very efficient at stimulating reactions from the immune system.

Drug allergies can be divided into four types, based upon the mechanism of the immune reaction. *Type I* reactions occur soon after exposure and commonly produce *urticaria*, also called *hives*. These raised, irregularly shaped patches on the skin are frequently accompanied by severe itching. Although allergic reactions involving the skin are annoying, in themselves they are not usually serious; this type of reaction can, however, progress to a severe acute allergic reaction that involves the cardiovascular and respiratory systems. This dangerous reaction is called *anaphylaxis* or *anaphylactic shock*. Anaphylaxis is marked by sudden contraction of the bronchiolar muscles and frequently by edema of the mouth and throat. These reactions may completely cut off air flow to the lungs. In addition, blood pressure falls and the patient may go into shock. These violent reactions may occur within a very short time, and aggressive therapy is required to save the patient's life. Few people react to drugs in this way. All the symptoms of type I reactions are caused by immunoglobulins called IgE antibodies, which are released in response to the drug and which prompt target cells to discharge immune modulators such as histamine (Chapter 24). Drugs that are associated with type I reactions include penicillins, cephalosporins, and iodides.

Type II allergic reactions to drugs involve IgM or IgG antibodies, which can trigger lysis of specific blood cells under the appropriate conditions. These delayed reactions are sometimes called *autoimmune responses*. Examples include hemolytic anemia induced by methyldopa and thrombocytopenic purpura induced by quinidine. Procainamide and hydralazine can induce a condition resembling systemic lupus erythematosus.

Type III reactions are frequently described as serum sickness, but symptoms include urticaria, pain in the joints, swollen lymph nodes, and fever. Penicillins, iodides, sulfonamides, and phenytoin can cause this type of delayed reaction, which may involve IgE, IgM, or IgG antibodies.

The *type IV* reaction is contact dermatitis, caused by topical application of drugs.

Any patient can suffer an allergic reaction in response to any drug, but certain drugs are more prone to cause reactions than others. Patients receiving these agents should be closely monitored to detect early signs of allergic responses and thereby be protected from extensive injury.

Allergic reactions do not occur during the first exposure to a drug, since time is required for the immune system to develop the antibodies that cause these reactions. In theory, this fact should aid in predicting which patients are at risk of an allergic reaction; however, documenting prior exposure to a drug is not always easy. Patients do not always know the names of drugs they have received, and they are not always reliable sources of information on prior reactions to drugs. Moreover, persons may be unknowingly exposed to penicillins and certain other antibiotics through food or milk, since these drugs are sometimes used in animal medicine.

PRINCIPLE 3: DRUG ACTION IS DETERMINED BY HOW THE DRUG INTERACTS WITH THE BODY
Drugs Chemically Altering Body Fluids

Drugs produce their actions in one of three ways. First, some drugs alter the chemical properties of a body fluid. Examples are antacids, which enter the stomach and neutralize excess stomach acid. Alteration of the pH of stomach fluid is the only intended action of these drugs. Other examples are drugs that accumulate in the urine and alter the pH of that fluid. By acidifying the urine with ammonium chloride or alkalinizing the urine with sodium bicarbonate, the ion flow in the kidney is altered and drug excretion patterns are changed.

Drugs Chemically Altering Cell Membranes

The second way drugs may act is by nonspecifically interacting with cell membranes. The interaction of the drugs with the cell membrane involves a chemical attraction and is usually based on the lipid nature of the cell membrane and the lipid attraction of the drugs. General anesthetic

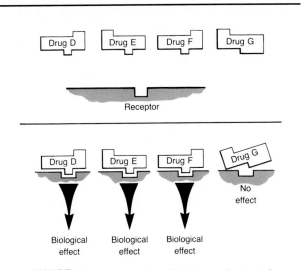

FIGURE 1.1   Lock-and-key fit between drugs and receptors through which they act. Site on the receptor that interacts with a drug has a definite shape. Those drugs that conform to that shape can bind and produce a biological response. In this example only the shape along lower surface of drug molecule is important in determining whether or not the drug will bind to receptor.

gases act in this way (Chapter 45). These agents dissolve in lipid-containing membranes and thereby alter the properties of the cells involved.

Drugs Acting Through Specific Receptors

The third and most common mechanism by which drugs act is through specific *receptors*. The biological activity of many drugs is determined by the ability of the drug to bind to a specific receptor, and in turn the ability to bind to the receptor is determined by the chemical structure of the drug. The interaction of a drug with a specific receptor may be thought of as being analogous to a lock-and-key fit (Figure 1.1). Only drugs and naturally occurring compounds that have a similar shape, that is, chemical structure, may bind to the receptor and produce the biological response (Drugs D and F in Figure 1.1). Only a certain critical portion of the drug is usually involved in binding, not the entire molecule. Therefore drugs that are alike in the critical region but different in other parts of the molecule might also be expected to have biological activity (Drug E in Figure 1.1).

The ability to bind to the receptor and the capability of stimulating an action by the receptor are two different aspects of drug action. The ability to bind to the receptor is known as *affinity*. Drugs with high affinities have a high attraction to the receptor. The capability of stimulating the receptor to some action is called *efficacy*.

When receptors are highly specific and have high affinities for the compounds that bind to them, very low concentrations of these compounds may show biological activity. For example, hormones naturally found in the body act through specific receptors. Some of these hormones are found in the bloodstream at concentrations of less than 1 picomolar, or less than one part per trillion. Nevertheless, these tiny amounts are biologically effective because the hormone is detected and bound by the specific receptor.

Receptors also allow for localization of drug effects to certain tissues. Each tissue or cell type will possess its own unique array of specific receptors. For example, certain cells in the kidney possess specific receptors for antidiuretic hormone. These cells therefore have the capacity to respond to this hormone. Cells in other tissues that lack these receptors are unable to respond to antidiuretic hormone.

Pharmacologists frequently speak of drug receptors. The concept of drug receptors is one of the major concepts in pharmacology. The specific receptors called *drug receptors* are actually natural components of the body intended to respond to some chemical normally present in blood or tissues. For example, there are specific receptors within the brain that respond to morphine and related compounds from the opium poppy, but until 1975 the natural function of these receptors was not known. It is now known that the brain and other tissues contain compounds called enkephalins and endorphins. These natural compounds bind to the so-called morphine receptor and are more potent than morphine in producing analgesia (Chapter 44).

Any compound, either natural or man-made, that binds to a specific receptor and produces a biological effect by stimulating that receptor is called an *agonist*. For example, the hormone norepinephrine binds to specific sites in the heart called beta-1 adrenergic receptors. Stimulation of these receptors causes the heart to beat faster. A synthetic drug called *isoproterenol* acts on the same receptors in the heart and produces the same effects. Both norepinephrine and isoproterenol are therefore called agonists for the beta-1 adrenergic receptor (Chapter 10). Agonists have both affinity for receptors and efficacy, since they cause some action by the receptor.

Some drugs produce their action not by stimulating receptors but by preventing natural substances from stimulating receptors. These drugs are

THE NURSING PROCESS

The concepts presented in this chapter translate logically and directly into the actions required in the nursing process.

Assessment

Assessment is that process through which information is obtained about and from the patient relative to the patient's condition. Assessment involves collecting both subjective and objective data. Subjective data are the information the patient reports to the nurse about present or past complaints. For example, when a patient reports being recently exposed to an infection and currently complains of specific symptoms, such as fever, these bits of information would constitute subjective data. Objective data are obtained directly by the nurse or physician through observation, auscultation, percussion, and palpation. Laboratory data such as blood counts, x-ray films, electrocardiograms, and other tests would also fall under the heading of objective data.

Assessment of a patient requires understanding what physiological systems are altered by the patient's disease. Assessment at this level allows the nurse to put the pharmacological therapy of the disease into the proper perspective.

Potential nursing diagnoses

The nurse analyzes the data obtained from the patient assessment and develops the nursing diagnoses appropriate for that patient. The list of accepted nursing diagnoses is revised regularly, and is published by the North American Nursing Diagnosis Association (NANDA). In relation to drug therapy, there may be *actual*, *potential*, and *possible* nursing diagnoses, as well as *collaborative problems*. For example, a patient begun on sublingual nitroglycerin for control of the pain associated with an attack of angina pectoris may have the nursing diagnosis of "Knowledge deficit related to the correct use and storage of nitroglycerin tablets." A collaborative problem may also be labelled a potential complication, as in "Potential complication: hemorrhage" for the patient on anticoagulant therapy. Nursing diagnoses must always be based on individualized assessment of the patient, so two patients receiving the same drug may not have the same nursing diagnoses. In this book, a few examples of the diagnoses that relate to drug therapy are given, but there may be additional diagnoses appropriate for a patient.

Management

Management is a two-step process involving planning and implementation. Management of a patient arises naturally as a result of understanding the physiological basis of the patient's disease and the physiological processes altered by the drugs prescribed for this patient. Since drugs do not have single actions, this understanding also leads directly to an appreciation of expected side effects of the drug and explains the nursing actions that may be required to aid the effectiveness of the drug. Management also includes a teaching component. Nurses are expected to be able to prepare the patient for the use of the drug on an outpatient basis if necessary.

Evaluation

Evaluation involves determining whether the therapy has achieved the goals established in the planning stage of patient management. For example, knowing the mechanism of action of a drug and the expected effects on various body systems, the nurse may, by continuing assessment, determine if the expected effects are being observed. Evaluation also involves determining that the patient can explain how to take the medication prescribed, why it is being given, and what side effects may be necessary sequelae of drug administration and what side effects may require notifying the nurse or the physician. This phase of evaluation is obviously different for hospitalized patients than for patients in the community.

called *antagonists.* For example, the drug propranolol blocks beta-1 adrenergic receptors and prevents agonists such as norepinephrine from stimulating the receptor normally. Propranolol therefore is classed as an antagonist of the action of norepinephrine. Another example of a drug that acts by antagonizing the action of the normal agonist at the receptor is tubocurarine. At the neuromuscular junction tubocurarine blocks the acetylcholine receptors that are required to maintain muscle tone. In the presence of tubocurarine the natural agonist acetylcholine cannot stimulate the receptors, and muscular paralysis results (Chapter 11). Antagonists have affinity for receptors, but they lack efficacy. When the receptor is occupied by an antagonist, the receptor cannot carry out its normal function.

■ ■ ■

The material presented in this chapter forms the framework on which subsequent specific information about drugs may be placed. For example, as each drug class is studied, the student should first seek to understand the mechanism of action of the drug. Does this drug operate through specific receptors? Does it alter a body fluid or cell membranes? In addition, the student should consider what side effects are likely to occur as a result of the action of the drug in tissues. For example, does the drug affect receptors in more than one organ or tissue? The student should note whether experience has indicated that allergies or idiosyncratic reactions are common with the drug. Finally, the student should consider the balance between the positive effects of the drug and the negative reactions to understand what place the particular drug may have in clinical practice. For example, some very effective drugs have limited clinical use because the side effects are unacceptable for most patients.

With this framework for study, understanding the pharmacology of individual drugs becomes a more rational process and is much more easily accomplished.

SUMMARY

Pharmacology is the study of how chemicals interact with living organisms to produce biological effects in that organism. The chemicals used as drugs do not create functions; they modify existing functions within the body. All drugs have multiple effects. Drugs may produce predictable side effects or may produce unpredictable reactions such as allergies or idiosyncratic responses.

Drugs alter the properties of body fluids, nonspecifically affect cell membrane function, or produce biological effects by interacting with receptors in various tissues. Drugs that bind to receptors and produce the natural response expected from that receptor are called agonists. Drugs that prevent the binding of agonists to receptors are called antagonists.

Understanding drug effects in the body in terms of basic generalized mechanisms allows the health care provider to remember details of drug reactions and toxicity as part of a predictable pattern. This rational approach eliminates the need for rote memorization of repetitious material, since the same information may be common to many drugs of a class.

STUDY QUESTIONS
1. Why is an understanding of physiology basic to an understanding of pharmacology?
2. What is the difference between a drug action and a side effect?
3. What are two major types of unpredictable reactions drugs may produce?
4. What are the four types of allergic reactions drugs may produce?
5. What are the three general mechanisms by which drugs interact with the living organism to produce a biological effect?
6. What is an agonist?
7. What is a drug antagonist?
8. How does affinity differ from efficacy?

SUGGESTED READINGS
Bourne, H.R., and Roberts, J.M.: Drug receptors and pharmacodynamics. In Katzung, B.G., editor: Basic and clinical pharmacology, ed. 4, Norwalk, Conn., 1989, Appleton & Lange.

Bungaard, H.: Drug allergy: chemical and pharmaceutical aspects, Pharm. Int. **1**(5):100, 1980.

Clark, W.G., Brater, D.C., and Johnson, A.R., editors: Drug-receptor interactions. In Goth's medical pharmacology, ed. 12, St. Louis, 1988, Times Mirror/Mosby College Publishing.

Eisenstadt, W.S., and others: Adverse drug reactions: a brief refresher on an ever-present hazard, Postgrad. Med. **74**(3):83, 1983.

Levine, R.R.: How drugs act on the living organism. In Pharmacology: drug actions and reactions, ed. 3, Boston, 1983, Little, Brown & Co.

Levine, R.R.: The scope of pharmacology—definitions. In Pharmacology: drug actions and reactions, ed. 3, Boston, 1983, Little, Brown & Co.

Principles Relating Drug Dose to Drug Action

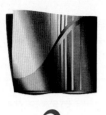

2

Most drugs produce biological effects by interacting with specific receptors at the site of action of the drug. The magnitude of the biological effect produced by a drug is related to the concentration of the drug present at the site of action. Drugs differ not only in their intrinsic ability to produce an effect but also in their ability to penetrate to the site of action and in their rates of removal from that site. *Pharmacokinetics* is the study of how drugs enter the body, reach their site of action, and are removed from the body. *Pharmacodynamics* is the study of drug action at the biochemical and physiological level. Both the pharmacokinetics and the pharmacodynamics of a drug determine how a drug will be administered, how often it will be given, and what a dose will be.

PHARMACOKINETICS

Factors Controlling Drug Absorption by Enteral Routes

In order to be effective systemically, a drug must be present in the blood in a free or available form. For most medications, less than the total amount of administered drug is ultimately available to produce effects on target tissues. *Bioavailability* is a term that describes what proportion of the administered drug is available to produce systemic effects. A drug with low bioavailability is one in which most of the administered dose of the drug is lost or destroyed, never reaching the blood in a form that can be effective. Drugs that are freely and rapidly absorbed have a high bioavailability. The many factors that can influence bioavailability are discussed in the following 3 sections.

Drug dissolution. About 80% of the drugs used in clinical practice are administered orally, primarily because of the ease and convenience of administration by this route. The drug may be given in liquid form, but most often it will be given in a solid form such as a pill, tablet, or capsule (Table 2.1). To achieve this solid form, the drug is usually mixed with other compounds that serve various functions. Starches and other compounds may be added as inert fillers, especially when the actual amount of drug required per dose is too small to be conveniently handled. Adhesive substances called binders may also be added to allow the tablet to hold together after it is compressed in manufacture. Other compounds called disintegrators may be required to allow the tablet to absorb water and to break apart. Lubricants are frequently added to prevent the tablet from sticking to machinery during manufacture. These other additions to the dosage form may make up the bulk of the tablet. The formulation shown in Table 2.2 for tablets containing 100,000 units of potassium penicillin illustrates the use of these agents. In the formulation the active ingredient, potassium penicillin, makes up only 11% of the tablet mass. Stearic acid acts as a lubricant and acacia is a commonly used binder. The other compounds act as fillers and disintegrators.

To be effective the solid dose of a drug must break apart in the gastrointestinal tract and allow the drug to go into solution. Only the dissolved drug is absorbed from the gastrointestinal tract into the blood. Since breakdown of the solid dosage form is the required first step in absorption of the drug, any variability in this process can affect how rapidly and completely the drug is absorbed. The formulation of a tablet or capsule is one important factor that obviously affects dissolution rates. Tablets from different manufacturers that contain the same amount of active ingredient but different types and amounts of inert ingredients may not be identical in clinical action, since each formulation may have different dissolution properties. Tablets may also change with age and conditions of storage. In general, older tablets tend to dry out and become more difficult to disintegrate; hence bioavailability of the drug may be reduced.

Table 2.1   Forms of Medications

Form	Description
Capsules	Solid dosage forms for oral use in which medication is enclosed in gelatin shell that dissolves in stomach or intestine. Gelatin of capsules is colored to aid in product identification. Various manufacturers use distinctive shapes for distinguishing their capsules from those of other companies.
Douche	Aqueous solution used as cleansing or antiseptic agent for part of body or body cavity. Douches are usually sold as powder or liquid concentrate to be dissolved or diluted before use.
Elixirs	Clear fluids designed for oral use and containing primarily water and alcohol with glycerin and sorbitol or another sweetener sometimes added. Alcohol content of these preparations varies.
Glycerites	Solutions of drugs in glycerin; they are primarily for external use. Solution must be at least 50% glycerin.
Patches	The inner surface of the patch contacts the skin and allows transdermal absorption of relatively lipid-soluble drugs. The total amount of drug in the patch is very large, but typically only a small fraction is absorbed.
Pills	Solid dosage forms for oral use in which drug and various vehicles are formed into small globules, ovoids, or oblong shapes. True pills are rarely used; most have been replaced by compressed tablets.
Solution	Liquid preparations, usually in water, containing one or more dissolved compounds. Solutions for oral use may contain flavoring and coloring agents. Solutions for intravenous injection must be sterile and particle free. Other injectable solutions must be sterile. Solutions of certain drugs may also be used externally.
Suppositories	Solid dosage forms to be inserted into body cavity where medication is released as solid melts or dissolves. Suppositories frequently contain cocoa butter (cacao butter or theobroma oil), which is solid at room temperature but liquid at body temperature, or glycerin, polyethylene glycol, or gelatin, which dissolves in secretions from mucous membranes.
Suspension	Finely divided drug particles that are suspended in suitable liquid medium before being injected or taken orally. Suspensions must not be injected intravenously.
Sustained action	Form of medication that is altered so that dissolution is slow and continuous for extended period. Total dosage in sustained action medication is greater than for regular formulations, since drug is not all released at once but over extended period.
Syrups	Medication dissolved in concentrated solution of sugar such as sucrose. Flavors may be added to mask unpleasant taste of certain medications.
Tablets	Solid dosage forms, frequently shaped like disks or cylinders, that contain, in addition to drug, one or more of following ingredients: binder (adhesive substance that allows tablet to stick together), disintegrators (substances promoting tablet dissolution in body fluids), lubricants (required for efficient manufacturing), and fillers (inert ingredients to make tablet size convenient).
Enteric-coated tablets	Solid dosage forms intended for oral use. Medication in tablet form is coated with materials designed not to dissolve in stomach. Coatings do dissolve in intestine, where medication may be absorbed.
Press-coated or layered tablets	Preformed tablet has another layer of material pressed on or around it. This practice allows incompatible ingredients to be separated and causes them to be dissolved at slightly different rates.
Tincture	Alcoholic or water-alcohol solutions of drugs.
Transdermal creams	Relatively lipid-soluble drugs that may be absorbed transdermally. Dosage is usually measured in inches of cream extruded from tube. Protection of the site may be necessary to prevent accidental removal of the cream.
Troches (also called lozenges or pastilles)	Solid dosage forms, frequently shaped like disks or cylinders, that contain drug, flavor, sugar, and mucilage. Troches dissolve or disintegrate in mouth, releasing medication such as antiseptic or anesthetic for action in mouth or throat. Troches dissolve more slowly than tablets.

Table 2.2 Sample Pharmaceutical Formulation for Penicillin (Potassium) Tablets

Ingredient	Amount per tablet (mg)
Potassium penicillin (1595 units/mg)	69
Calcium carbonate	362
Starch	85
Sugar	25
Acacia	78
Stearic acid	3

Contents of the gastrointestinal tract. The presence of food may interfere with dissolution and absorption of certain drugs. However, some drugs are so irritating to the stomach that food may be useful to dilute high local concentrations of the drug. There is considerable variation from person to person in gastric emptying times and, therefore, in the length of time the drug spends in the acid environment of the stomach. In addition, the amount of acid in the stomach varies with the individual and the time of day. The very young and the elderly have less stomach acid than middle-aged persons. Lower acidity may mean less drug is degraded and more is available for absorption.

Chemical properties of the drug. In addition to the physical state of the drug, the chemical nature of the drug determines how satisfactory oral administration will be. First, to pass through the membrane lining the gastrointestinal tract, a drug must be relatively *lipid soluble,* since the membranes themselves contain a high concentration of lipid. Ionic (charged) forms of drugs do not easily pass through these membranes. Many drugs can exist in an ionic state or in an uncharged lipid-soluble state, depending on the chemical environment (pH) in which the drug is found. This environment changes along the gastrointestinal tract, as illustrated in Figure 2.1. The stomach fluid is highly acidic. A drug such as aspirin, which is a weak acid, will be converted from a charged to an uncharged form by the strong acid in the stomach. Since the uncharged form of the drug can readily diffuse through the lipid membranes of the stomach cells, the drug is rapidly absorbed. In contrast, drugs such as penicillins are not stable in the acid

of the stomach, and part of the dose will be destroyed rather than absorbed.

Some drugs that are sensitive to the acid in the stomach may be protected by use of *enteric coatings* on the tablets or capsules (Table 2.1). These coatings are designed to be inert at low (acidic) pH but soluble at higher (alkaline) pH. Therefore the drug passes through the stomach and is released in the intestine. Enteric coatings are also used for drugs that are highly irritating to the gastric mucosa.

The fluids in the small intestine are slightly alkaline. This higher pH favors the absorption of weakly basic drugs, since at this pH range weak bases are uncharged (Figure 2.1). The small intestine also has an enormous surface area for drug absorption, which makes it a major site of absorption. However, some drugs, particularly proteins such as insulin or growth hormone, are destroyed in the small intestine by the action of digestive enzymes from the pancreas.

Drugs that are absorbed from the small intestine are transported by the portal circulation directly to the liver before entering the circulation to the rest of the body, as illustrated in Figure 2.2. The liver metabolizes a significant proportion of certain types of drugs before the drug can enter the general circulation. This process of absorption into the portal circulation with metabolism of the drug in the liver before the drug reaches systemic circulation is called the *first pass phenomenon.* Liver metabolism often inactivates drugs and in this case, the first pass phenomenon lowers the amount of active drug released into the systemic circulation. For example, morphine is very rapidly extracted from the blood and metabolized by the liver; therefore, to achieve the same level of pain relief, it is necessary to administer six times more morphine orally than intramuscularly. In contrast, the related drug codeine is much less affected by the first pass effect; therefore, it takes only 1.67 times more codeine orally than intramuscularly to produce the same degree of pain relief. In these examples, the larger oral doses compensate for the drug lost through inactivation by the liver.

The first pass phenomenon may be avoided by using other routes of administration, such as sublingual (drug dissolved under the tongue), buccal (drug dissolved between the cheek and gum), and rectal routes (Figure 2.2). Drugs administered by these routes are absorbed directly across the mucous membranes and rapidly enter the systemic circulation. The sublingual and buccal routes are useful when a palatable, very lipid-soluble drug is involved. The rectal route is useful, especially when

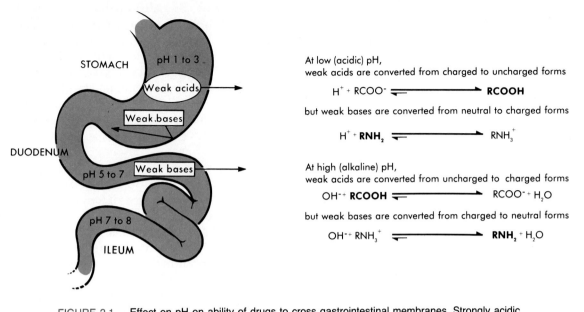

STOMACH   pH 1 to 3

Weak acids

Weak bases

DUODENUM

pH 5 to 7   Weak bases

pH 7 to 8

ILEUM

At low (acidic) pH,
weak acids are converted from charged to uncharged forms

$$H^+ + RCOO^- \rightleftharpoons \textbf{RCOOH}$$

but weak bases are converted from neutral to charged forms

$$H^+ + \textbf{RNH}_2 \rightleftharpoons RNH_3^+$$

At high (alkaline) pH,
weak acids are converted from uncharged to charged forms

$$OH^- + RCOOH \rightleftharpoons RCOO^- + H_2O$$

but weak bases are converted from charged to neutral forms

$$OH^- + RNH_3^+ \rightleftharpoons \textbf{RNH}_2 + H_2O$$

FIGURE 2.1   Effect on pH on ability of drugs to cross gastrointestinal membranes. Strongly acidic environment of the stomach (pH 1 to 3) maintains weak acids in an uncharged form, which is more easily absorbed. Weak bases remain charged in the stomach but are converted to uncharged forms as the pH approaches neutrality (pH 7) or becomes slightly alkaline (pH 7 to 8).

a patient is unconscious. The best physical form for a drug intended for rectal use is a suppository that will melt in the rectum and release the drug for absorption (Table 2.3).

Factors Controlling Drug Absorption by Parenteral Routes

The parenteral routes of drug administration are primarily those that require injection of the drug into the skin, muscle, or blood (Chapter 6). Injection necessarily involves breaking the skin, and sterile technique must be used to prevent bacteria from gaining entry (Table 2.3). Special precautions often must be taken to avoid producing undue tissue damage with irritating drugs. Sometimes these precautions involve preventing the drug from contacting the skin; other drugs require dilution before administration.

Subcutaneous injection (under the skin) is appropriate for drugs that will be used in small volumes and for which slow absorption is desirable. Insulin is an example of such a drug.

Intramuscular injection (into a muscle) is appropriate when larger volumes of a drug must be injected. An example is streptomycin. Absorption from intramuscular sites is faster than from subcutaneous sites, since the muscles are better supplied with blood vessels than is the skin. Absorp-

tion from either subcutaneous or intramuscular sites can be speeded somewhat by applying heat or massage to the site to accelerate blood flow to the area. Absorption can be slowed by decreasing blood flow to the injection site by applying ice packs or by the simultaneous injection of a drug such as epinephrine, which constricts blood vessels.

Drugs intended for intramuscular or subcutaneous injection may be in relatively insoluble forms. Indeed, some drugs are formulated to dissolve slowly and therefore to be absorbed slowly from injection sites. These dosage forms are called *depot* injections.

Intravenous injection (directly into a vein) requires special precautions. Drugs that are to be used intravenously must always be in solution and can contain no particulate matter. Some drugs irritate the veins and cause thrombophlebitis if administered at too high a concentration. Other drugs must be injected slowly to avoid toxic concentrations of the drug reaching the heart or other vital organs. The intravenous route is valuable when drug concentrations must be maintained continuously, but it has the disadvantage that potential harm to the patient is greater by this route than by other routes discussed so far.

Special injection routes may be employed in certain circumstances. For example, local anes-

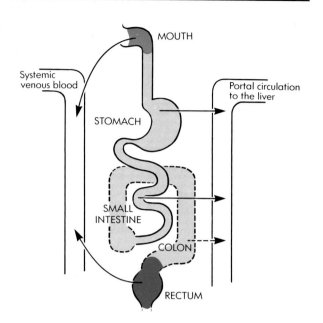

FIGURE 2.2   Two circulatory pathways for materials absorbed from the gastrointestinal tract. Materials absorbed from stomach, small intestine, or colon enter portal circulation, which perfuses the liver before returning to heart. Materials absorbed from these sites are therefore exposed first to the action of liver microsomal enzymes and then are circulated to the rest of the body. In contrast, absorption through membranes lining mouth or rectum deliver the material directly to systemic circulation.

thetics may be injected into the spinal column to produce certain types of anesthesia. In other circumstances drugs may be injected directly into body cavities or joints. These specific routes are employed when conventional routes of injection do not allow high enough drug concentrations to be achieved at the desired site of drug action.

Factors Controlling Drug Persistence in the Blood

Once a drug has entered the blood, its ultimate fate is determined by the chemical properties of the drug and how it is affected by the blood and tissues it contacts. Some drugs are metabolized by enzymes in the blood. An example is succinylcholine, already mentioned in Chapter 1. Drugs that persist in the blood for any length of time are usually bound to proteins in the blood rather than being simply dissolved directly in plasma.

The most important carrier protein is albumin, a protein formed in the liver and released into the blood. Drugs bound to albumin or other carrier proteins remain in the blood, since these proteins as a rule do not diffuse through capillary walls. Drug binding to albumin is a reversible process, and in the blood an equilibrium is established between drug bound to the protein and drug that is free in solution. Only free drug is able to diffuse into tissues, interact with receptors, and produce biological effects. The same proportion of bound and free drug is maintained in the blood at all times. Thus, when free drug leaves the blood, some drug is released from protein binding to reestablish the proper ratio between bound and free drug.

An example of a drug that binds to plasma protein is the anticoagulant dicumarol. In the blood, 99% of this drug is bound to plasma albumin. Therefore only 1% of the blood content of the dicumarol is free to diffuse to its site of action or to its sites of elimination. The net effect of binding to albumin is to create a reservoir of the drug that is released to replenish free drug removed to other sites. In general, drugs that do not bind to plasma albumin remain in the body for shorter periods than do drugs that are tightly bound. A drug such as dicumarol, which is very strongly bound to albumin, remains in the body for up to 3 days. A longer duration of action is thus one characteristic of drugs that are bound to plasma proteins.

Factors Controlling Drug Distribution Throughout the Body

Two of the factors that influence drug distribution have already been mentioned: lipid solubility of the drug and protein binding. A small molecular weight also favors diffusion of the drug through membranes. In general, the smaller and more lipid-soluble a drug, the better able it is to penetrate tissues. This consideration is especially important for drugs that act on organs with a high lipid content, such as the brain. All transport from the blood, however, involves passing through lipid-containing membranes. High concentrations of free drug in the blood and high lipid solubility favor this process.

Factors Controlling Drug Metabolism in the Body

Biotransformation. Biotransformation is the ability of living organisms to modify the chemical structure of drugs. Most drugs are metabolized in the body by the liver, specifically by the *microsomal enzyme* system. These enzymes allow the body to metabolize potentially toxic compounds. Many types of chemical transformations are carried out, but in general these reactions create water-soluble compounds that are more easily eliminated

Table 2.3   Summary of Major Routes for Systemic Administration of Drugs

Route	Description	Advantages	Disadvantages
Oral	Drug swallowed, absorbed from stomach and/or small intestine	1. Convenient 2. Nonsterile procedure 3. Economical	1. Unpleasant taste may cause patient to discontinue medication 2. Irritation to gastric mucosa may induce nausea and vomiting 3. Patient must be conscious 4. Drug may be partly or completely destroyed by digestive juices 5. Absorbed drug enters portal circulation to liver, where drug may be destroyed
Sublingual	Drug dissolved under tongue; absorbed across mucous membranes of mouth	1. Convenient 2. Nonsterile procedure 3. Drug enters general circulation before passing through liver	1. Route is not useful for drugs that taste bad 2. Irritation to oral mucosa may occur 3. Patient must be conscious 4. Only very lipid-soluble drugs are absorbed rapidly enough to be administered by this route
Buccal	Drug dissolved between cheek and gum; absorbed across mucous membrane of mouth	As for sublingual	As for sublingual
Transdermal	Drug absorbed directly through skin	1. Continuous dosage 2. Nonsterile 3. Drug enters general circulation before passing through liver	1. Effective only for lipid-soluble drugs 2. Local irritation can occur 3. Discarded patches may pose danger of poisoning
Rectal	Drug inserted into rectum; absorbed through mucous membranes of rectum	1. May be used in unconscious or vomiting patient 2. Drug enters general circulation before passing through liver	1. Route is inconvenient 2. Drug may irritate rectal mucosa 3. Drug must be made up into suppository
Inhalation	Drug inhaled as gas or aerosol	1. Useful for drugs intended to act directly on lung 2. Useful for drugs that are gases at room temperature and very lipid soluble (i.e., inhalation anesthetics)	1. Absorption across membranes of lung is too slow to be useful for most drugs
Subcutaneous	Drug injected under skin	1. Useful for drugs in soluble or relatively insoluble forms 2. May be used in unconscious or uncooperative patients	1. Sterile procedures are necessary 2. Route produces relatively painful site, and patient may suffer irritation from drug
Intramuscular	Drug injected into muscle mass	1. Relatively rapid absorption, since blood supply is good 2. Useful for drugs in soluble or relatively insoluble forms 3. May be used in unconscious or uncooperative patients	1. Sterile procedures are necessary 2. Minor pain is present on injection for most drugs, but irritation and local reactions may occur
Intravenous	Drug injected directly into vein	1. Allows direct control of blood concentration of drug 2. Most rapid attainment of effective blood levels	1. Sterile procedures are necessary 2. Too rapid injection may produce transient, dangerously high blood concentrations of drug

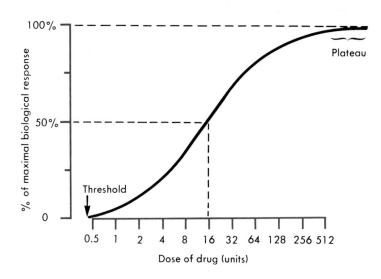

FIGURE 2.3   A log dose-response curve. Percent of maximum biological response is plotted on a linear scale on vertical axis. Dose of the drug is plotted on a logarithmic scale on horizontal axis. Threshold is the dose of drug required to cause a measurable response. Plateau is region of curve where increasing drug dose does not increase the biological response.

from the body by the kidney. These enzymes have two important properties. First, the enzymes are relatively nonspecific. Therefore many drugs may be metabolized by the same enzyme system. Second, the liver has the capacity to synthesize more enzyme in response to being exposed to higher than normal concentrations of certain drugs. This property means that the liver can increase its capacity to destroy a drug over a period of a few days. This increase in microsomal enzyme content in the liver is called *enzyme induction.*

Biotransformation often inactivates drugs, but biotransformation does not always produce inactive products. For example, drugs such as codeine, diazepam, and amitriptyline are all converted by the liver into metabolites that are also active. A few drugs are not active until they are biotransformed by the liver. For example, the anticancer drug cyclophosphamide is inactive, but one of its metabolites produced in the liver is a highly reactive alkylating agent that is effective against cancer cells.

Biotransformation in tissues other than liver. The liver is by far the most important site for biotransformation of drugs, but it is not the only site. For example, systemically administered prostaglandins are destroyed almost instantaneously in the lung. Therefore prostaglandins, which might have use in stimulating uterine contractions, cannot be efficiently administered systemically for this

purpose. The kidney is another important site for biotransformation of certain types of drugs.

Biotransformation may be carried out by bacteria within the colon. This process may limit absorption of the drug from the bowel following oral administration, or it may be a mechanism by which the drug is eliminated from the blood after administration by parenteral routes.

Factors Controlling Drug Elimination from the Body

There are three main routes by which drugs may be eliminated from the body. These routes involve the liver, kidney, and bowel.

Elimination in the feces. The first of these routes involves uptake of the drug by the liver, release into bile, and elimination in the feces. For some drugs, such as erythromycin and certain penicillins, the concentration of drug in the bile may be much higher than its concentration in the blood. Since between 600 ml and 1000 ml of bile is formed each day, this route of elimination may dispose of significant amounts of drug. However, drugs in the bile enter the small intestine, where they may be reabsorbed into the blood, returned to the liver, and again secreted into bile. This secretion and reabsorption process is called *enterohepatic circulation.* Drugs that are extensively reabsorbed from the intestinal tract after biliary secretion obviously persist in the body much longer than drugs that remain in the lumen of the intestine and pass out with the feces. If the reabsorbed drug is in an active form, the duration of action of the drug is prolonged.

Elimination in the urine after metabolism by the liver. The second route of elimination involves the liver and the kidney. Common biotransformations of drug by the liver include formation of glucuronides, hydroxylations, and acetylations. The kidney is also capable of forming glucuronides and sulfates. All of these reactions tend to form more polar compounds, which can be more efficiently excreted by the kidney. For example, a drug such as the antibiotic chloramphenicol normally enters glomerular fluid by passive diffusion but is reabsorbed from the tubules and reenters the blood. In the liver, however, chloramphenicol is transformed into chloramphenicol glucuronide. In this form the drug enters glomerular fluid, cannot be reabsorbed from the tubules, and hence is excreted in the urine.

Various factors may influence the ability of the liver to metabolize drugs. For example, premature infants and neonates have immature livers that are incapable of carrying out certain biotransformations. Therefore these patients may accumulate those drugs that must be metabolized in the liver before they can be excreted by the kidney. Another group of patients who may accumulate drugs normally excreted by this route are those who have suffered hepatic damage, such as that frequently seen in chronic alcoholics.

Elimination in the urine without metabolism by the liver. Some drugs are not extensively metabolized anywhere in the body and are excreted unchanged in the urine. This excretion may take place in one of two ways. Some drugs are excreted by *passive diffusion* into glomerular fluid and are not extensively reabsorbed; hence these drugs enter the urine. Other drugs are *actively secreted* by specific systems in the renal tubule. These active processes lead to more rapid drug elimination and allow much higher urinary concentrations of drug to be achieved. The antibiotic penicillin G is a good example of a drug that is actively secreted by the renal tubule. One half of an intravenous dose of penicillin G can be eliminated in about 20 minutes by active tubular secretion. In contrast, an antibiotic such as tetracycline, which is eliminated primarily by passive diffusion in the kidney, persists in the body for several hours.

Those drugs that are normally eliminated unchanged in the urine will accumulate in the body when there is a loss of kidney function. Patients with kidney disease must frequently have drug dos-

ages lowered to compensate for the reduced ability of the kidney to excrete various substances. Kidney function declines with age even in healthy persons, and elderly patients may show a reduced ability to excrete drugs in their urine. Certain drugs such as aminoglycoside antibiotics are themselves nephrotoxic and may directly damage the kidneys and thereby interfere with their own excretion.

PHARMACODYNAMICS
Dose-Response Curve

The relationship between the dose of drug administered and the response produced is an S-shaped (sigmoid) curve called the *dose-response curve,* as shown in Figure 2.3. This curve is obtained by plotting the observed response (on a linear scale) against the dose of the drug used to elicit that response (on a logarithmic scale). This curve illustrates several important quantitative properties about drugs. First, there is a threshold for each drug-induced response. Doses of drug below that threshold will produce no observable effect. Second, the drug-induced response will reach a plateau rather than increase indefinitely. For example, the drug shown in Figure 2.3 produces its maximum response at a dose of about 512 units. Doubling the dose produces no detectable further effect. Even beginning at lower drug concentrations, doubling the dose still does not double the effect. In this example the 50% maximum response to this drug is produced by a dose of 16 units, but at double that dose (32 units) only about 70%, not 100%, of the maximum response is produced. In summary, the dose-response curve demonstrates that a finite dose is required to see a response and that the intensity of the response produced is not linearly related to the dose.

The dose-response curve in Figure 2.3 shows the effect of a drug on an individual (or average responses from several individuals). The same type of curve is produced when the drug response is instead defined as an all-or-none phenomenon (such as asleep versus awake) and the logarithm of the drug dose is plotted against the percentage of patients who show the drug effect at that given dose. The plateau for this curve will be the drug dose at which all patients respond, and the threshold will be the drug dose below which no patients respond. The recommended therapeutic dose of the drug will be a dose at which most patients respond to the drug. Figure 2.4 shows this second type of dose response curve.

Drugs produce multiple predictable biological effects, and for each of these effects a dose-response curve may be drawn. For example, the drug digi-

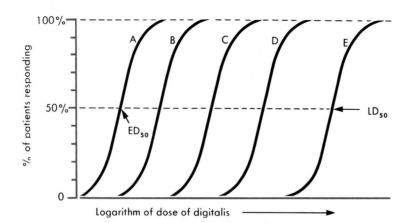

FIGURE 2.4   Log dose-response curves for effects of digitalis. In this example percent of patients responding to digitalis is plotted on vertical axis and dose of digitalis is plotted on logarithmic scale on horizontal axis. Curve A represents strengthened force of contraction of the heart produced by digitalis; curve B measures nausea; curve C measures visual disturbances; curve D measures cardiac arrhythmias; and curve E measures ventricular fibrillation and death. These undesirable effects are all dose-related responses to digitalis.

talis, although increasing the force of contraction of the failing heart, also produces nausea, causes neurological symptoms such as headaches and visual disturbances, induces cardiac arrhythmias, and ultimately triggers ventricular fibrillation. Each of these responses can be plotted as a dose-response curve, as illustrated in Figure 2.4. In comparing the dose-response curves for these other reactions to the curve for the principal therapeutic effect, nausea is seen as an effect observed in a significant number of patients receiving therapeutic doses of digitalis. With increasing doses of the drug, more and more patients will suffer visual disturbances and arrhythmias. At drug concentrations well above normal therapeutic doses, ventricular fibrillation will occur. These predictable drug reactions become an important part of patient care. For digitalis, the visual disturbances are a warning that the concentration of digitalis in the patient is approaching concentrations that can cause cardiac arrhythmias and ventricular fibrillation.

Each drug may be described as relatively safe or relatively dangerous, based on consideration of dose-response curves such as those in Figure 2.4. For example, nausea is frequently associated with the use of digitalis because the doses that produce nausea are only slightly greater than those that increase the force of contraction of the heart. Doses of digitalis that produce more serious reactions are only slightly higher than those that cause nausea. Digitalis, therefore, is a drug with a narrow margin

of safety, and doses must be rigorously controlled and great care must be taken to keep blood levels of the drug within a very narrow range. In contrast, a drug with a wide margin of safety, such as penicillin G, may be given in doses greatly exceeding normal therapeutic doses without much danger of producing direct toxic effects.

Therapeutic index. The relative safety of drugs is also sometimes expressed as the therapeutic index. The therapeutic index (TI) is defined as the ratio of the dose of the drug that is lethal in 50% of the tested population (LD_{50}) to the dose of the drug that is therapeutically effective in 50% of the tested population (ED_{50}), or $TI = LD_{50}/ED_{50}$. Obviously, these figures come from tests conducted in animals. A drug with a high therapeutic index has a wide safety margin; the lethal dose is greatly in excess of the therapeutic dose. A drug with a low therapeutic index is more dangerous for the patient because small increases over normal doses may be sufficient to induce toxic reactions.

Time Course of Drug Action

Drugs may enter the body by a number of routes, but except for the intravenous route, some time will be required for the drug to enter the blood after administration. There is also a delay between the time the drug enters the blood and the time the drug reaches its site of action. If the response to a single dose of a drug is measured as a function of time, the pattern shown in Figure 2.5 is observed.

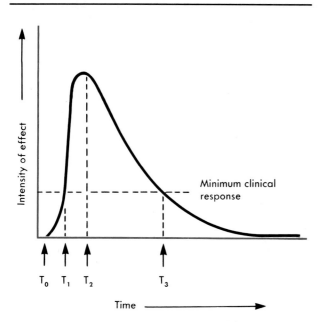

FIGURE 2.5   Time course of action of a single dose of a drug. Drug is administered at T_0. Time interval between T_0 and T_1 represents time of onset of action of the drug. Peak action occurs at T_2. Time interval between T_0 and T_2 represents the time for peak action. At T_3 drug response falls below the minimum required for clinical effectiveness. Time interval between T_1 and T_3 represents duration of action of the drug.

The time for the *onset of drug action* is the time it takes after the drug is administered to reach a concentration that produces a response. As drug continues to be absorbed, higher concentrations of the drug reach the site of action and the response increases. As the drug is being absorbed, it is also subject to the influences that tend to eliminate the drug from the body. Ultimately elimination will dominate, and the actual concentration of the drug in the body will begin to fall. As a result, the response will also begin to diminish. The *time to peak effect* is the time it takes for the drug to reach its highest effective concentration. The *duration of action* of a drug is the time during which the drug is present in a concentration large enough to produce a response and is determined by the rate of absorption and the rate of elimination.

The insulins are a good example of drugs for which an understanding of onset and duration of action is critical to the success of drug therapy. Insulin lowers blood sugar levels, and the peak drug action must be planned to coincide with the absorptive period after meals when blood sugar levels will rise rapidly if no insulin is present. If insulin is injected at the proper dose but at the wrong time, a serious hypoglycemic (low blood sugar) reaction may endanger the patient.

Half-Life of a Drug

The concepts of onset and duration of drug action are also important for understanding the proper timing of administration of drugs that are given repeatedly for a course of therapy. The *drug half-life* or *elimination half-time* is simply how long it takes for elimination processes to reduce the blood concentration of the drug by half. For example, consider a drug like penicillin G. The peak concentration of penicillin in the blood would occur a few moments after the drug is administered intravenously. Thereafter penicillin would be rapidly excreted by the kidney and would disappear from the blood. The length of time required for these processes to decrease the blood concentration of penicillin by 50% is the drug half-life or elimination half-time, which for penicillin G is about 20 minutes. Therefore 20 minutes after the intravenous dose of penicillin, only one half of the initial concentration of the drug would remain in the blood. After 40 minutes only one quarter of the initial concentration would remain, and after 60 minutes only one eighth would remain. During each succeeding 20-minute period the remaining concentration decreases by one half.

For a drug administered by a route where drug absorption is not instantaneous, the elimination processes compete with the absorptive processes, delaying the appearance of peak blood concentrations of the drug. The example shown in Figure 2.6 is for a drug with a half-life of 1 hour. When the drug is given intravenously, the highest concentration is achieved on administration and decreases thereafter because of the elimination processes. When the same dose is given orally, the drug is absorbed relatively slowly so that drug elimination is responsible for lowering the peak drug concentration that can be achieved. Once in general circulation, however, the drug is eliminated in the same way, no matter what the initial route of administration.

Plateau Principle

When a drug is given repeatedly for therapy at fixed dosage intervals, the concentration of drug in the blood reaches a plateau and is maintained at that level until either the dose or the frequency of administration is changed. An example is shown in Figure 2.7, in which a rapidly absorbed drug is administered at fixed intervals. The concentration of the drug in the blood fluctuates around a mean

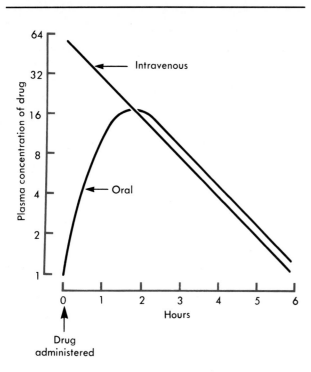

FIGURE 2.6 Absorption and elimination rates for drug administered by oral or intravenous route. Plasma concentration of drug is plotted on a logarithmic scale on the vertical axis.

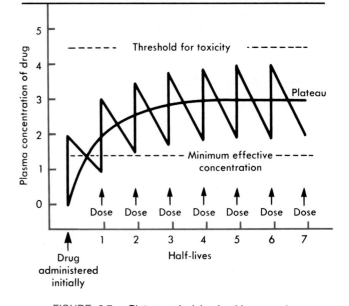

FIGURE 2.7 Plateau principle. In this example drug is administered once every elimination half-time for the drug. Plasma concentration of drug rises and falls as drug doses are rapidly absorbed and slowly eliminated. Drug accumulates over a period of time so that after 4 elimination half-times the average plasma concentration of the drug has reached a steady state. By adjusting the dose, average plasma concentration of drug may be adjusted.

value, which approaches a plateau value after 4 elimination half-times have passed; this happens regardless of the dose or frequency of administration, as long as they are constant. The actual dose of the drug and the frequency of dosage determine what the plateau concentration of drug in the blood is, but they do not determine how long it will take to reach that plateau.

As an example of this plateau principle, consider a patient who is given a drug with a half-life of 24 hours. The patient takes 1 tablet at 8 AM every day. In 4 days the amount of drug being taken in each dose roughly equals the amount of drug being eliminated each day; the plateau has been reached (Figure 2.8, Patient A). In this example this dose is sufficient to produce clinically effective blood levels but is below the level that produces toxicity. On day 6 the patient decides to take 2 tablets instead of 1 tablet each morning. As a result, the mean concentration of the drug in the blood rises, and after 4 days (4 elimination half-times) it reaches a new plateau concentration. At this new higher level some drug toxicity is seen. Therefore the pa-

tient returns to the old dosage schedule of 1 tablet daily. The mean drug concentration returns to the original plateau concentration 4 days later (4 elimination half-times) and is maintained until the dosage amount or intervals change.

Patient B in Figure 2.8 receives the same drug as patient A, but patient B takes 1 tablet every 12 hours instead of once daily. As a result, the plateau concentration of drug in the blood is higher than for patient A. Note, however, that it still takes 4 days (4 elimination half-times) to reach the plateau concentration. After 3 days of therapy patient B mentions some unusual symptoms, which the nurse recognizes as toxic reactions to the drug. On the basis of this report the physician reduces the frequency of drug administration to 1 tablet daily. After 5 days on this dosage schedule the patient complains that the medication effect wears off by the early morning hours. The physician therefore advises the patient to take ½ tablet every 12 hours. This dosage regimen minimizes the fluctuations in drug concentration in the blood; the mean plateau concentration is ultimately the same.

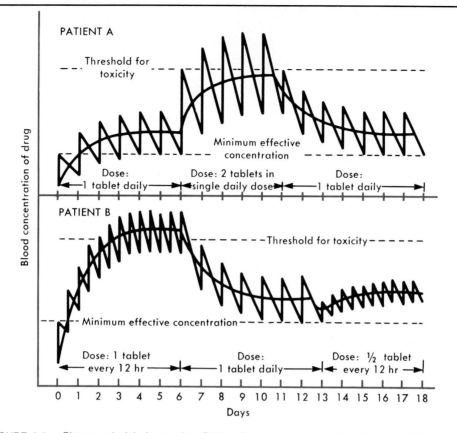

FIGURE 2.8   Plateau principle in practice. Patient A receives a drug with half-time of 24 hours. Increasing dose of the drug from 1 to 2 tablets in a single daily dose increases plateau concentration of the drug. In contrast, patient B illustrates that by dividing the dose (taking ½ tablet every 12 hours rather than 1 tablet once daily) fluctuations in drug concentration are minimized but average concentration is unchanged.

These examples illustrate the importance of maintaining regular dosage schedules and adhering to prescribed doses and dosage intervals. If the total dose of drug administered each drug half-life is held constant, then the average concentration of the drug in the blood stays constant. Timing of the dose (single dose or divided doses) affects the actual peak concentration and the minimal concentration of the drug in the blood. For some drugs, these variations may not be critical, but for many drugs the difference between a safe dose and a toxic dose is not very great.

Monitoring levels of certain drugs in the blood has become a routine part of patient care in many settings. Direct assays for drugs allow physicians to adjust doses to ensure safe and effective blood levels of such drugs as gentamicin, amikacin, digitoxin, and phenytoin, which have a low therapeutic index. The nurse's responsibility in dealing with patients who are being monitored in this way may include drawing blood samples at specific times or adjusting the dosage or timing of doses in response to the physician's instructions.

DRUG INTERACTIONS
Definition of a Drug Interaction

A drug interaction is any modification of the action of one drug by another drug. Drug interactions may either *potentiate* or *diminish* the action of the drugs involved. *Synergism* is a special drug interaction in which the effect of two drugs combined is greater than the effect expected if the individual effects of the two drugs acting independently were added together.

Drug interactions are commonly encountered in clinical practice and are sometimes actively sought as part of a therapeutic program. An excellent example is the treatment of chronic moderate hypertension, which frequently involves several drugs, each amplifying the action of the others to lower the blood pressure.

The negative side of drug interaction is that the therapeutic result expected from a drug can be greatly distorted by the presence of other drugs. This negative side can be diminished when health care personnel are aware of the major drug interactions; are thorough in determining which drugs a patient is taking, including over-the-counter drugs, alcohol, and tobacco; and give careful instruction to the patients about which drugs will interact with their prescribed medication.

Comprehensive lists of drug interactions have been published and may be referred to if necessary when information about rare or unlikely interactions is sought. Clinically important common interactions are discussed with each drug class in this text and are summarized in the Appendix.

Origin of Drug Interactions

Drug interactions may arise when one drug alters the pharmacokinetics of another drug. For example, one drug may alter the dissolution, absorption, protein binding, metabolism, or elimination of another drug. Drug interactions of the pharmacokinetic type are generally one sided, with one drug altering the pharmacokinetics of a second drug without its own pharmacokinetics being altered. The effect of the drug interaction is to change the actual concentration of the second drug in the blood and at its site of action. For instance, if one drug decreases the absorption of a second drug, the actual concentration of the second drug is diminished, and therefore the usual dose will not give the expected result. The same effect is produced if the metabolism or elimination of the second drug is increased by the first drug. Alternatively, if one drug increases the actual concentration of the second drug, the result is potentiation of the second drug. Pharmacokinetic potentiation may arise because one drug increases the absorption or decreases the protein binding, metabolism, or elimination of a second drug, which is therefore present in higher actual concentration than would be anticipated at that dose.

Drug interactions may also arise when one drug alters the pharmacodynamics of a second drug. If two drugs have the same action, drug potentiation will result. An example is seen with the vasodilators, which can lower blood pressure. A vasodilator such as hydralazine might be part of a therapeutic program to control hypertension. Nitroglycerin is

Table 2.4 Oral Administration of Selected Drugs

Drugs normally best taken on an empty stomach with a full glass of water	Drugs normally taken with food to improve absorption
Acetaminophen	Carbamazepine
Aspirin	Cimetidine
Cephalosporins	Griseofulvin†
Erythromycin*	Hydralazine
Isoniazid	Indomethacin*
Penicillins	Lithium
Propantheline	Nitrofurantoin*
Quinidine*	Propranolol
Rifampin	Spironolactone
Sulfonamides	
Tetracyclines*	
Theophylline*	

*Gastric irritation may require taking with food, but absorption is delayed or diminished.
†Take with foods rich in fat for best absorption.

another vasodilator that is taken to relieve angina. Patients who take hydralazine for hypertension and also take nitroglycerin for angina can anticipate a severe hypotensive response to nitroglycerin; they may need to lie down when taking nitroglycerin to avoid fainting.

Drugs that are antagonists often produce pharmacodynamic interactions that diminish the response of both drugs at the usual therapeutic doses. An example is the beta receptor antagonist propranolol, which might be prescribed for a patient with hypertension. If that patient developed asthma, a beta receptor agonist such as isoproterenol would be indicated. Although in this example the therapeutic target for propranolol is the heart and for isoproterenol the therapeutic target is the bronchioles, these drugs would antagonize each other at all organs with beta adrenergic receptors and neither drug would give the desired therapeutic effect. (In fact, propranolol on its own would make the asthma worse and could not be used.)

Alcohol is a frequent cause of pharmacodynamic drug interactions. As a central nervous system depressant, alcohol acts synergistically with the other drug classes that depress the central nervous system: antihistamines, sedative-hypnotics, antianxiety drugs, antidepressants, antipsychotics, general anesthetics, and the narcotic analgesics. At low doses the drowsiness characteristic of these drug classes is exaggerated by alcohol, although at higher doses respiration can be dangerously depressed.

Alcohol may also interact with certain drugs to cause an intense reaction, including flushing of the face, palpitations, rapid heart rate (tachycardia), and low blood pressure (hypotension). This set of symptoms is called the *disulfiram reaction*, named for the chemical first shown to cause the reaction in persons taking alcohol. This reaction is occasionally observed in patients who ingest alcohol while receiving certain antibiotics, the sedative chloral hydrate, oral hypoglycemic agents, as well as other drugs.

Foods may also interact with drugs and alter the effect of therapy, most obviously by altering the absorption of an orally administered drug. A few drugs are better absorbed or tolerated on a full stomach, but most drugs are absorbed more slowly or less completely when taken with food (Table 2.4). A few of these interactions may significantly diminish the clinical usefulness of the drug. For example, the antibiotic tetracycline forms insoluble precipitates with calcium and magnesium in food. This interaction lowers absorption of the drug so that insufficient amounts of the antibiotic enter the blood and therapy fails.

Some food-drug interactions directly antagonize the action of the drug in the body. For example, patients receiving a coumarin anticoagulant may lose the action of the drug if they ingest large amounts of leafy green vegetables and other foods high in vitamin K. Vitamin K directly antagonizes the action of the coumarins.

Conversely, chronic administration of a drug may interfere with normal vitamin metabolism (Table 2.5). For example, long-term use of the antituberculosis drug isoniazid can deplete vitamin B_6 and cause neuritis. This complication can be prevented by administering vitamin B_6 supplement during isoniazid therapy.

Other food-drug interactions may arise when drugs interfere with normal mechanisms for removing noxious compounds from the body. For example, patients receiving monoamine oxidase inhibitors have a diminished ability to metabolize catecholamines and related compounds such as tyramine. When exposed to high concentrations of tyramine from aged cheese, red wine, or other

Table 2.5   Drug Effects on Vitamin Metabolism

Effect	Drugs
Interference with absorption or action of folic acid, which can cause folate deficiency	Aminopterin, antibiotics, anticonvulsants, aspirin, clofibrate, cycloserine, ethanol, methotrexate, oral contraceptives
Depletion of vitamin B_6	Hydralazine, isoniazid, oral contraceptives
Interference with absorption or action of vitamin B_{12}	Aminopterin, antibiotics, anticonvulsants, clofibrate, colchicine, ethanol, oral hypoglycemic agents
Interference with absorption or action of vitamin D	Antacids, anticonvulsants, mineral oil
Interference with synthesis or absorption of vitamin K	Antibiotics, mineral oil

foods, these patients cannot eliminate the tyramine rapidly and the compound may accumulate, causing headache and hypertension.

In addition to foods and medications, environmental chemicals increasingly are being recognized as agents causing significant drug interactions in some patients. For example, polycyclic hydrocarbons in cigarette smoke and the chlorinated hydrocarbons in pesticides are active inducers of liver microsomal enzymes. Persons chronically exposed to these chemicals metabolize drugs such as the antiasthmatic medication theophylline more rapidly than normal. In these persons the blood concentration of theophylline may be lower than desired unless dosage adjustments are made (Chapter 25).

BIOLOGICAL VARIATION

Not all patients respond to a set drug dosage in the same way. Moreover, it is not possible to predict in most cases which patients will be more or less sensitive to a drug than normal. The term *normal* in this context really means average for the population.

Biological variability is based on subtle differences in physiological functions that exist among people. For example, absorption of oral drug doses can be greatly influenced by stomach acidity, gastrointestinal motility, pancreatic function, and gastrointestinal microbiological flora. Yet these parameters vary greatly in normal people. Likewise, people vary in the sensitivity of certain tissues to drugs. This variability may be the result of differences in the numbers of drug receptors, differences in permeability barriers, and many other factors. These factors are all difficult to assess and yet greatly influence the magnitude of drug effects in patients.

In the clinical setting the causes of biological variation are not usually known with any degree of certainty. Patients are observed for the proper response to a drug, and dosages are usually adjusted on the basis of clinical assessment of progress. Although the exact causes of biological variation are not known for an individual patient, some general factors can be delineated that may influence patient responses to medications. These factors include age, sex, overall health status, and genetic background. The most important of these factors are discussed in the following sections.

Effect of Age on Drug Response

The fetus. Developing embryos and fetuses are unintended targets of drugs and chemicals taken by their mothers. The effects of many drugs are benign or at least cannot be proved to be harmful, but a few drugs pose grave risks to the unborn. The degree of damage may be related to dose and length of exposure, but is often also related to the developmental stage of the fetus at the time of exposure. Table 2.6 summarizes potential adverse effects of representative drugs.

Drugs that are absorbed systemically have been categorized by the Food and Drug Administration (FDA) according to the level of risk to the fetus. These FDA Pregnancy Categories are summarized in Table 2.7, along with examples of drugs in each category. Discussions of individual drugs throughout the text will also refer to the FDA Pregnancy Category, when appropriate.

The neonate. Premature infants and neonates may respond to medications quite differently from adults or even older children. Many of these different responses are caused by immaturity of the liver and kidneys in infants. At birth the liver lacks many of the metabolizing enzymes that enable the adult liver to biotransform certain types of compounds. Both microsomal and nonmicrosomal enzyme systems may be reduced. Before these activities increase to normal levels during the first weeks or months of life, the neonate is more vulnerable than the adult to chemicals requiring detoxification in the liver.

The kidney is also less efficient at birth than in adult life. Therefore excretion of many compounds takes longer in the neonate than in an adult. Failure to take into account this reduced excretory capacity in calculating drug dosage can be important when certain drugs are administered to neonates.

The clinical effect of reduced detoxification and excretion in neonates is well illustrated with the antibiotic chloramphenicol. This potentially toxic drug is detoxified in the adult liver by the formation of chloramphenicol glucuronide, a metabolite that is efficiently excreted by adult kidneys. Neonates, unable to form the glucuronide or excrete the drug efficiently, quickly accumulate chloramphenicol and suffer potentially lethal toxicity. This deadly outcome is prevented by reducing the dose of drug administered to take into account the reduced routes of elimination. The result is that less drug is required per kilogram of body weight to maintain effective concentrations of chloramphenicol in neonates than in adults.

The elderly. Elderly patients are also a group especially at risk from many drugs. Several factors may be involved, including altered central nervous system function and reduced renal function. Elderly patients are also more likely to be malnourished and to suffer from chronic diseases for which they may be receiving more than one drug. For these reasons such patients may need special attention in order to detect early signs of drug interactions or drug toxicity related to diminished excretory capacity or altered drug sensitivity.

A good example of the type of drug likely to be most troublesome in elderly patients is an aminoglycoside antibiotic such as gentamicin. The aminoglycosides are excreted almost exclusively by the kidney. Therefore in elderly patients whose normal renal function is significantly lower than that of younger adults, aminoglycosides are excreted at reduced rates. If doses are not carefully reduced to take this effect into account, the aminoglycosides will accumulate. One of the early signs of toxicity may be some loss of hearing or equilibrium. However, loss of hearing or an unstable gait in elderly patients may be mistaken for normal signs of aging. Therefore the older patient may suffer toxicity for a longer time than a younger patient, since in the latter the same signs would be recognized immediately as iatrogenic (caused by a drug).

Genetic Traits

Some drug reactions can be clearly linked to a particular genetic trait that may be more prevalent in certain ethnic groups. For example, the enzyme glucose 6-phosphate dehydrogenase is abundant in the tissues of most people. In red blood cells this

Table 2.6 Adverse Drug Effects During Pregnancy*

Effect of drug	Drugs known to produce the effect in humans
FIRST TRIMESTER EFFECTS ON EMBRYONIC DEVELOPMENT	
Abortion	Isotretinoin, quinine
Multiple anomalies involving cranio-facial development	Dicumarol, ethanol, isotretinoin, methotrexate, paramethadione, phenytoin, quinine, trimethadione
Neural tube defects	Valproate
Goiter	Iodide, methimazole, propylthiouracil
Abnormalities of reproductive organs	Androgens, diethylstilbestrol, estrogens, progestins
Inhibition of growth	Methotrexate, tetracycline, tobacco smoke
SECOND AND THIRD TRIMESTER EFFECTS ON FETAL DEVELOPMENT	
Abortion, mortality	Heroin, isotretinoin, tobacco smoke
Mental retardation	Dicumarol, ethanol
Altered cardiovascular function	Anticholinergic drugs, propranolol, terbutaline
8th cranial nerve damage	Aminoglycoside antibiotics
Hyperbilirubinemia	Nitrofurantoin, sulfonamides
Hemolytic anemia	Nitrofurantoin
Goiter	Iodide, methimazole, propylthiouracil
Abnormalities of reproductive organs	Androgens, diethylstilbestrol, estrogens, progestins
Inhibition of growth	Dicumarol, ethanol, heroin, methotrexate, tetracycline, tobacco smoke
LABOR, DELIVERY, AND PERINATAL PERIOD	
Increased mortality	Tobacco smoking, cocaine abuse
Altered cardiovascular function	Anticholinergic agents, caffeine, heroin, lidocaine, meperidine, propranolol, terbutaline
Gray-baby syndrome	Chloramphenicol
Respiratory depression	Diazepam, meperidine, morphine, phenobarbital, ethanol, tobacco smoking
Respiratory distress	Reserpine
Bleeding	Aspirin, dicumarol, indomethacin
Hypoglycemia	Chlorpropamide, propranolol, tolbutamide
Hyperbilirubinemia	Nitrofurantoin, sulfonamides
Hemolytic anemia	Nitrofurantoin
Hyperirritability	Cocaine abuse

*This list does not include all drugs that affect fetal and neonatal function, but is intended to give representative examples. The nurse should check sources of specific information about individual agents when drugs are administered to pregnant patients.

Table 2.7   FDA Pregnancy Categories

Category	Level of risk with drug exposure	Examples
A	Controlled studies in women fail to demonstrate a risk to the fetus in the first trimester (and there is no evidence of a risk in later trimesters), and the possibility of fetal harm appears remote.	
B	Either animal reproduction studies have not demonstrated a fetal risk but there are no controlled studies in pregnant women, or animal reproduction studies have shown an adverse effect (other than decreased fertility) that was not confirmed in controlled studies on women in the first trimester and there is no evidence of a risk in later trimesters.	Amoxicillin, buspirone, cimetidine, fluoxetine, hydrochlorothiazide, metronidazole, piperacillin
C	Either studies in animals have revealed adverse effects on the fetus and there are no controlled studies in women, or studies in women and animals are not available. Drugs in this category should be given only if the potential benefit justifies the risk to the fetus.	Alteplase, captopril, ciprofloxacin, codeine, enalapril, gentamicin, isoproterenol, lisinopril, morphine, nizatidine, reserpine, tubocurarine
D	There is positive evidence of human fetal risk, but the benefits for pregnant women may be acceptable despite the risk, as in life-threatening diseases for which safer drugs cannot be used or are ineffective. An appropriate statement must appear in the "warnings" section of the labelling of drugs in this category.	Amikacin, midazolam, netilmicin, tobramycin
X	Studies in animals or humans have demonstrated fetal abnormalities or there is evidence of fetal risk based on human experience or both, and the risk of using the drug in pregnant women clearly outweighs any possible benefit. The drug is contraindicated in women who are or may become pregnant. An appropriate statement must appear in the "contraindications" section of the labelling of drugs in this category.	Isotretinoin, lovastatin, methotrexate

enzyme plays a role in generating reduced nicotinamide adenine dinucleotide phosphate (NADPH), a compound required to maintain active hemoglobin. As a result of a genetic alteration, some individuals lack adequate concentrations of this enzyme in their red blood cells. Therefore NADPH is generated slowly. Under normal circumstances this alteration would not be critical. However, if a person with this trait is exposed to chemicals that enhance the conversion of hemoglobin to methemoglobin (a relatively inactive form of hemoglobin), serious problems can arise. Because of the lack of glucose 6-phosphate dehydrogenase, too little NADPH is present to fully reform active hemoglobin. When too much methemoglobin accumulates, the red blood cell is destroyed.

Glucose 6-phosphate dehydrogenase deficiency is important for pharmacology because many drugs accelerate methemoglobin formation. Sulfonamides, antimalarial medications, and analgesic-antipyretic drugs (including aspirin) fall into this category. In a person lacking adequate glucose 6-phosphate dehydrogenase activity, these drugs can cause life-threatening hemolysis (rupture of the red blood cells). The same drugs are relatively innocuous in the vast majority of the population, who possess adequate glucose 6-phosphate dehydrogenase activity.

Certain populations have a high proportion of the gene that causes glucose 6-phosphate dehydrogenase deficiency. For example, 13% of black American males and 20% of black American females may carry this gene. Sardinians also have an incidence of approximately 14%. More than half of the Kurdish Jews tested show glucose 6-phosphate dehydrogenase deficiencies. This genetic difference from the bulk of the American population places patients from these special populations at greater risk for serious reactions with drugs such as those mentioned earlier. When these patients are receiving medications, they should be watched carefully for signs of toxicity.

The rate of drug acetylation in the liver is another genetically determined trait that may affect the incidence of certain drug reactions. Among Americans, both black and white, about half pos-

THE NURSING PROCESS

PHARMACOKINETICS AND PHARMACODYNAMICS

An understanding of pharmacokinetics and pharmacodynamics is involved in the treatment of every patient. Specific drugs may involve consideration of different aspects of pharmacokinetics and pharmacodynamics, but the following presentation outlines in general how these principles may be applied.

Assessment

In the course of assessing the patient, the nurse should ascertain whether any route of administration is inappropriate for the patient. For example, a patient with stomach ulcers might not receive some oral medications. The nurse might also assess which routes of elimination are available in a given patient. For example, the nurse might determine whether the patient has compromised kidney function that would prevent the safe use of many drugs eliminated by the kidney. The nurse might also consider the desired site of action of the drug and consider which drugs would not be able to penetrate to this site because of their distribution properties in the body.

The age of the patient also should guide the nurse in assessment, as should race, culture, and genetic background. For example, the young infant can be expected to have limited ability to metabolize certain drugs and will also be unable to safely receive drugs via certain routes (e.g., injection into the buttocks) because of poorly developed muscle mass or close proximity of nerves that could be damaged. As mentioned earlier, the race or genetic background of the patient may influence the response to medications.

Potential nursing diagnoses

Potential complication: high serum drug levels secondary to acute renal failure.

Potential complication: difficulty in administering prescribed drugs related to burn covering 60% body surface area, and paralytic ileus.

Management

In identifying goals of therapy, the nurse should consider the problem of getting the drug to its site of action at the proper concentration. This consideration would include a knowledge of the proper timing of dosages as well as a knowledge of ways to improve the effectiveness of the drug. For example, the excretion rates of some drugs may be influenced by the pH of the urine. Thus changing the pH of the urine may change the duration of action of a drug and improve the therapeutic effect in the patient. To teach the patient, the nurse should emphasize the appropriate actions the patient might take to maintain drug effectiveness. For example, a patient might be cautioned to avoid antacids with medications if they were known to lower bioavailability of an orally administered drug. Proper timing of doses might be especially emphasized for drugs with short half-lives, whereas the dangers of changing the drug dose without the knowledge of the physician might be emphasized for a drug with a low therapeutic index. Drug interactions might be anticipated and avoided by good patient teaching.

Evaluation

If therapy has not achieved the desired goals, the pharmacokinetics and pharmacodynamics of the drugs being used should be examined as possible causes for the therapeutic failure. Drug interactions may also be involved and should be considered.

sess liver enzyme systems that acetylate drugs and other chemicals slowly, at rates less than half of those of the rest of the population. In contrast, slow acetylation is very rare in Eskimos and persons of Japanese ancestry.

Isoniazid, a drug used to treat tuberculosis, illustrates how the genetically determined ability to acetylate a compound can influence the unwanted reactions that drug produces. Isoniazid is inactivated primarily by acetylation and eliminated by the kidney entirely as metabolites. In slow acetylators the half-life of the drug is about 3 hours, but in rapid acetylators it is only about 1 hour. Liver damage may be more common in rapid acetylators because the concentration of a hepatotoxic acetylated metabolite is high. Slow acetylation may be more closely associated with dose-related toxicity (neuropathy, depression of liver biotransformation enzymes), since the untransformed drug may accumulate in persons with this trait.

SUMMARY

The activity of a drug is related to its ability to reach its site of action and its rate of removal from that site. Enteral administration introduces the drug into the gastrointestinal tract and requires that the drug dissolve and pass through the lipid membranes of cells lining the gastrointestinal tract to enter the blood. Therefore small lipid-soluble drugs are absorbed better than highly ionic (charged) drugs, which are highly water soluble. Drugs adsorbed from the stomach or intestine enter the portal circulation, which exposes a drug to the microsomal enzymes in the liver before the drug enters systemic circulation. In contrast, drugs administered by sublingual, buccal, or rectal routes enter the systemic circulation before reaching the liver. Parenteral routes of administration require injection of the drug into a fluid or tissue. Subcutaneous injection produces slower absorption rates and is suitable for smaller volumes of drug than intramuscular injections.

Drugs are eliminated from the body by three major mechanisms: (1) excretion into the bile, (2) biotransformation of the drug by the liver followed by excretion by the kidney, or (3) excretion of unchanged drug by the kidney. The persistence of a drug in the body is influenced by these elimination processes and by the ability of the drug to enter tissues or be bound by plasma proteins.

The magnitude of the biological effect produced by a drug is related to the amount of drug administered. This relationship is expressed by the dose-response curve. The threshold dose of a drug is the minimum dose required to produce an observable biological effect. Higher doses produce increasing effects until the maximum response is achieved. Doses above those required for maximum drug effects are at best wasteful and increase the incidence of side effects.

When drugs are given repeatedly at fixed dosage intervals, the concentration of drug in the blood reaches a plateau and is maintained at that level until the dose or frequency of dosage is changed. The actual concentration of drug in the blood fluctuates around a mean value. This mean value, or plateau concentration, is achieved after about 4 elimination half-times for the drug. The elimination half-time or drug half-life is the time required for the concentration of drug in the blood to be decreased by half. The dose of a drug influences the plateau concentration of the drug in the blood but does not affect how long it takes for that plateau concentration to be reached. The frequency of drug dosage influences the degree of fluctuation around the mean concentration of that drug in the blood.

When patients receive more than one drug at the same time, the drugs may interact, either diminishing or potentiating the drug response. Drug interactions may arise when one drug alters the dissolution, absorption, protein binding, metabolism, or elimination of another drug. Drug interactions may also occur when drugs either enhance or block the action of other drugs in tissues containing the receptors. Drug interactions frequently involve nonprescription medications and alcohol.

Not all patients respond to a set drug dosage in the same way, primarily because of the biological variability among people. Subtle physiological differences as well as differences in age, sex, health status, and genetic background strongly influence the response to many drugs.

STUDY QUESTIONS

1. Why are pharmacodynamics and pharmacokinetics helpful in understanding the clinical uses of drugs?
2. Describe how a drug in tablet form enters the blood after oral administration. What factors may influence the absorption of this drug?
3. What is the first pass phenomenon? Does the first pass phenomenon affect all routes of administration?
4. What are the advantages and disadvantages of subcutaneous, intramuscular, and intravenous routes of drug administration?
5. How does the binding of drugs to proteins in the blood influence the effect of the drug?

6. What are the microsomal enzymes of the liver, and how do they influence the biological activity of drugs?
7. What is biotransformation?
8. What is enterohepatic circulation?
9. How does glomerular excretion of a drug differ from tubular secretion of a drug in the kidney?
10. What information is expressed in a log dose-response curve?
11. What is the therapeutic index of a drug?
12. What is the onset time for a drug, and how does it differ from the duration of action of a drug?
13. What is the elimination half-time of a drug?
14. What is the plateau principle?
15. How long does it take for a constant average concentration of drug to be achieved if the drug is given at a constant dose and at fixed intervals?
16. What is a drug interaction?
17. Do drug interactions increase or decrease the action of the drugs involved?
18. What are the two major mechanisms by which drug interactions can occur?
19. Which type of drug interaction may actually change the concentration of one of the drugs involved?
20. Which type of drug interaction does not change drug concentrations but does change observed drug responses?
21. Why must biological variability be considered in drug therapy?
22. What are some of the possible reasons for the observed differences in drug response seen among patients?
23. How may smoking, environmental chemical exposure, or dietary patterns influence the response of a patient to a drug?
24. What special consideration may be needed in administering drugs requiring hepatic detoxification to a premature infant?
25. What major organ system involved in drug elimination is likely to have diminished function in normal elderly people? In chronic alcoholics?
26. Why are Afro-Americans, Sardinians, and Kurdish Jews more likely to suffer drug-induced hemolysis than most other American populations?

SUGGESTED READINGS

Pharmacokinetics and drug disposition

Alvares, A.P., and others: Regulation of drug metabolism in man by environmental factors, Drug Metab. Rev. **9**(2):185, 1979.

Brater, D.C.: The pharmacological role of the kidney, Drugs **19**(1):31, 1980.

Carruthers, S.G.: Duration of drug action, Am. Fam. Physician **21**(2):119, 1980.

Dollery, C.T., and others: Contribution of environmental factors to variability in human drug metabolism, Drug Metab. Rev. **9**(2):207, 1979.

Fruncillo, R.J.: Drug disposition in liver disease, Am. Fam. Physician **26**(6):167, 1982.

Fuller, B.B.: Using research in practice: mechanisms of drug tolerance, West. J. Nurs. Res. **4**(1):113, 1982.

Garrett, E.R.: Biological responses and pharmacokinetics, Part 1, Pharm. Int. **1**(6):121, 1980.

Garrett, E.R.: Biological responses and pharmacokinetics. Part 2, Pharm. Int. **1**(7):133, 1980.

Jusko, W.J.: Influence of cigarette smoking on drug metabolism in man, Drug Metab. Rev. **9**(2):221, 1979.

Mayersohn, M.: Clinical pharmacokinetics: applying basic principles to therapy, Drug Ther. **10**(9):79, 1980.

Reidenberg, M.M., and Drayer, D.E.: Drug therapy in renal failure, Ann. Rev. Pharmacol. Toxicol. **20**:45, 1980.

Vesell, E.S.: On the significance of host factors that affect drug disposition, Clin. Pharmacol. Ther. **31**(1):1, 1982.

Weinshilboum, R.M.: Human pharmacogenetics, Fed Proc. **43**(8):2295, 1984.

Drug interactions

Cooper, J.W.: Adverse drug reactions and interactions in a nursing home, Nurs. Homes **36**(4):7, 1987.

D'Arcy, P.F.: Tobacco smoking and drugs: a clinically important interaction? Drug Intell. Clin. Pharm. **18**(4):302, 1984.

Deglin, J.M., and Mandell, H.N.: Drug interactions without anguish, Postgrad. Med. **72**(2):199, 1982.

McInnes, G.T., and Brodie, M.J.: Drug interactions that matter, Drugs **36**:83, 1988.

Sloan, R.W.: Drug interactions, Am. Fam. Physician **27**(2):229, 1983.

Todd, B.: Cigarettes and caffeine in drug interactions, Geriatr. Nurs. **8**(2):97, 1987.

Adverse drug reactions

Eisenstadt, W.S., and others: Adverse drug reactions: a brief refresher on an ever-present hazard, Postgrad. Med. **74**(3):83, 1983.

Fruth, R.: Anaphylaxis and drug reactions: guideline for detection and care, Heart Lung **9**(4):662, 1980.

Drug-food interactions

Carr, C.J.: Food and drug interactions, Ann. Rev. Pharmacol. Toxicol. **22**:19, 1982.

Cerrato, P.L.: When food and drugs collide, RN **50**(4):85, 1987.

Cerrato, P.L.: Drugs and food: when the dangers increase, RN **51**(11):65, 1988.

Giovannitti, C.: Food and drugs: managing the right mix for your patients, Nursing 81 **11**(7):26, 1981.

Hathcock, J.N.: When drugs compromise good nutrition, Drug Therapy **16**(8):71, 1986.

Lamy, P.P.: How your patient's diet can affect drug response, Drug Therapy **10**(8):82, 1980.

Osis, M.: Scheduling drug administration: drug and food interactions, Gerontion **1**(5):8, 1986.

Sriwatanakul, K., and Weintraub, M.: Food-drug interactions: an overlooked clinical problem, Drug Ther. Hosp. **7**(2):62, 1982.

Toothaker, R.D., and Welling, P.G.: Effect of food on drug bio-availability, Annu. Rev. Pharmacol. Toxicol. **20:**173, 1980.

Drugs and the fetus or neonate

Hill, L.M.: Effects of drugs and chemicals on the fetus and new-born, Mayo Clin. Proc. **59**(10):707, 1984.

Nice, F.J.: Can a breast-feeding mother take medication without harming her infant? MCN **14**(1):27, 1989.

Schimmel, M.S., and Rosen, T.S.: Neonatal pharmacology, Resident Staff Physician **29**(9):77, 1983.

Yaffe, S.J.: Prescribing drugs in infants and children: the unique problems, Drug Ther. Hosp. **7**(4):130, 1982.

Drugs and the elderly

Dall, C.E., and others: Promoting effective drug-taking behaviors in the elderly, Nurs. Clin. North Am. **17**(2):283, 1982.

D'Arcy, P.F.: Drug reactions and interactions in the elderly patient, Drug Intell. Clin. Pharm. **16:**925, 1982.

Greenblatt, D.J., Sellers, E.M., and Shader, R.I.: Drug disposition in old age, N. Engl. J. Med. **306**(18):1081, 1982.

Hayes, J.E.: Normal changes in aging and nursing implications of drug therapy, Nurs. Clin. North Am. **17**(2):253, 1982.

Hayter, J.: Why response to medication changes with age, Geriatr. Nurs. **2**(6):411, 1981.

Jarvik, L.F.: A review of drug therapy for elderly patients, Consultant **22**(5):141, 1982.

Lamy, P.P.: The elderly, drugs, and cost control, Drug Intell. Clin. Pharm. **16:**768, 1982.

Matteson, M.A., and McConnell, E.S.: Gerontological nursing: concepts and practice, Philadelphia, 1988, W.B. Saunders.

Nesbitt, B.: Nursing diagnosis in age-related changes, J. Gerontol. Nurs. **14**(7):7, 1988.

Pagliaro, L.A., and Pagliaro, A.M. (editors): Pharmacologic aspects of aging, St. Louis, 1983, The C.V. Mosby Co.

Ramsey, R: Adjusting drug dosages for critically ill elderly patients, Nursing 88 **18**(7):47, 1988.

Sellers, E.M., Frecker, R.C., and Romach, M.K.: Drug metabolism in the elderly: confounding of age, smoking, and ethanol effects, Drug Metab. Rev. **14**(2):225, 1983.

Shaw, P.G.: Common pitfalls in geriatric drug prescribing, Drugs **23:**324, 1982.

Todd, B: Drugs and the elderly: could your patient's confusion be caused by drugs? Geriatric Nurs. **2**(3):219, 1981.

Westfall, L.K., and others: Why the elderly are so vulnerable to drug reactions, RN **50**(11):39, 1987.

CHAPTER

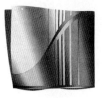

Regulation of the Manufacture, Sale, and Use of Medications

3

Patients receiving medications have always faced certain risks, which include the possibility that (1) the medication will not produce the beneficial effect claimed by those who make and sell the drug, (2) the medication may be directly harmful, and/or (3) the medication may be improperly administered. Modern drug legislation is designed to reduce or to eliminate these risks to patients.

ESTABLISHING THE SAFETY AND EFFICACY OF DRUGS

History of Materia Medica

The earliest form of medical practice involved the use of various natural products that were discovered by trial and error to have certain effects on the body. For example, parts of the poppy plant were known by the ancient Egyptians to relieve pain. This remedy was already ancient when it was recorded in the Ebers papyrus in 1500 BC. Equally ancient is the use of parts of the Ephedra shrub by the Chinese, who called the preparation *ma huang*. In the New World, South American Indians used the bark of the cinchona tree to relieve the symptoms of malaria. Even in more recent times natural products have been introduced for medical practice. For example, in 1785 a British physician named Withering described the use of the leaf of the foxglove plant to relieve edema of a certain type, which had previously resisted all therapy.

Until very recently, natural products such as those just listed were the only medicinal agents, or *materia medica*, available. The most common medications, made from plants or parts of plants, were called botanicals. Some botanicals continue to be used in medical practice, but most have been replaced as chemists have analyzed these crude products and identified active ingredients. The active ingredients are the chemicals found in the crude preparation that are responsible for producing the biological effect of the medicinal agent. For ex-

ample, the poppy plant relieves pain because the plant contains opium. *Ma huang* produces its effects on the heart, lungs, and other organs because it contains ephedrine, an agent that stimulates the sympathetic nervous system. Similarly, it is the quinine in cinchona bark that relieves the symptoms of malaria, and it is the digitalis in foxglove leaves that relieves the edema associated with heart failure.

Identification of the active ingredient in a crude medicinal agent has two benefits. First, the active ingredient may be measured (or assayed) in the crude preparation and the dose adjusted for the content of the active ingredient. For example, the digitalis content of the foxglove leaf may vary from plant to plant. Therefore a dosage based on the amount of the leaf administered may actually contain a variable amount of digitalis and may therefore have variable biological effects. Since the biological activity of a drug is related to the actual dose of the active ingredient, dosages based on the weight of pure digitalis should have a more predictable biological effect.

The second benefit of identifying the active ingredient of a medicinal agent is that the chemical structure and properties of the active drug are revealed. This knowledge can lead to better ways of isolating the active material from natural sources. Digitalis is an example of a drug that is still prepared by extraction from its plant source. Alternatively, once the structure of an active agent is known, chemists may be able to synthesize the material. Ephedrine is an example of a drug now chemically synthesized in a simple, economical process that has replaced the procedure of isolating the drug from plant materials.

Standardization of Medicinal Agents

Recognizing the relationship between drug dose and biological effect produced, most nations

29

of the world have attempted to adopt codes for standardizing the content of medicinal agents. Drugs sold in the United States must comply with the standards established in *The United States Pharmacopeia and the National Formulary*, or the *United States Homeopathic Pharmacopeia*.

The United States Pharmacopeia (USP) contains chemical, physical, and biological information on all active ingredients used in medications. To qualify as a standard, or official, medication, the preparation must conform to the information listed in this source. *The National Formulary* (NF) was originally independent of the USP, but the fourteenth edition, published in 1975, was the last to be published separately. The latest edition, USP XXI and NF XVI, published as a single volume, became official January 1, 1985.

As an example of the type of information found in the USP, we may consider aspirin. The USP classifies aspirin as an antipyretic (fever-reducing)-analgesic (pain-reducing) agent. In the USP, aspirin powder is listed separately from aspirin tablets. A variety of tablet sizes are described, containing amounts of aspirin ranging from 65 to 650 mg (approximately 1 to 10 gr). To meet USP standards, tablets must actually contain between 95% and 105% of the amount of aspirin indicated on the label. For example, an aspirin tablet labeled 500 mg must contain between 475 and 525 mg of aspirin by actual assay. The aspirin used in these tablets must meet the chemical and physical standards listed for that compound in the USP. Although drug doses for adults and children are listed, the USP is less useful for clinical personnel than for persons in pharmaceutical manufacture or pharmacy.

Some drugs used in medical practice cannot be standardized easily by chemical analysis, since the drug preparations are relatively complex mixtures of compounds. Standardization of these products may be obtained by measuring a biological effect. For example, insulin isolated from porcine or bovine pancreas glands is standardized on the basis of the amount of the preparation required to reduce the blood sugar of a test animal a certain amount. Antibiotics may be standardized on the basis of the amount of the preparation required to kill 99.9% of a certain sensitive strain of bacteria in a rigidly controlled laboratory test. Other complex pharmaceutical preparations, such as serums, vaccines, and human blood products, are tested and licensed by the FDA Center for Biologic Evaluation and Research.

Standards for medicinal agents vary somewhat from country to country. There are several phar-macopeias and other references that may apply. In Canada, the current *Compendium of Pharmaceuticals and Specialties* (CPS) indexes agents available in that country and contains monographs on specific drugs. The *British Pharmacopoeia 1988* is the current standard reference for the United Kingdom, but also includes a significant amount of information from the *European Pharmacopoeia*. The *International Pharmacopoeia* is published by the World Health Organization (WHO) and includes drug methods and standardizations for reference use in any country.

The information in these references is often indexed by *generic* or nonproprietary names. The generic name applies to the drug, no matter who manufactures or markets it. The proprietary or *trade* name is the property of a specific drug company. For example, cefuroxime sodium is the nonproprietary name for a specific antibiotic; this single compound is sold under the trade name of Zinacef by Glaxo, Inc., and Kefurox by Eli Lilly & Co.

Government Regulations Concerning Medicinal Agents

Drug manufacturing and sale are regulated by both state and federal agencies. For federal laws to apply, a drug must enter interstate commerce. A drug totally manufactured within a single state and sold only in that state would not be subject to the federal drug laws. Very few drugs fall into this category.

The first effective federal law concerning drugs in the United States was passed in 1906 (Table 3.1). This law was intended to protect citizens from adulterated medicines and from those that contained harmful ingredients but failed to list these ingredients on the label. Each new law passed since that time has been intended to overcome specific problems that have arisen. For example, in the early 1900s a certain patent medicine was advertised as a cure for cancer. The federal government sought to force this company to halt the false advertisement. However, the drug label as it appeared on the bottle was accurate in naming the contents of the medicine. Under the 1906 law, accurate labeling of the contents was all the government could require. When the Sherley Amendment was added in 1912, the federal government gained the ability to control advertising claims as well as the contents of the drug label.

The next major piece of drug legislation, passed in 1938, added the requirement that a drug sold in the United States had to be shown as safe before it could be marketed. Prior to this law a pharmaceu-

THE NURSING PROCESS

CONTROLLED SUBSTANCES

Because of the addictive potential of many controlled substances, legal restraints have been placed on the use of these drugs in medical practice. These regulations as well as the special nature of the drugs add a special burden and responsibility to the nurse.

Assessment

The nurse should take special care to observe whether an individual patient displays signs and symptoms that make the use of the controlled substance appropriate. Nurses should be alert to signs of drug abuse in patients. Patients may have obtained prescriptions from several physicians in order to acquire excessive amounts of controlled substances. The nurse should be alert not only to physical signs of excessive drug use but also to the psychological signs pointing to this problem. For example, a patient who is dependent on drugs obtained under false pretenses may be reluctant to enter the hospital for even the most routine testing, fearing that the drug dependency will be discovered in the closely regulated hospital environment.

Potential nursing diagnoses

Altered bowel elimination: constipation secondary to frequent use of narcotic analgesics

Altered comfort: nausea secondary to narcotic use

Anxiety related to the patient requesting a higher dose or more frequent doses of controlled substances than have been prescribed

Management

In dealing with controlled substances, the nurse has both legal and medical responsibilities. The legal responsibilities include ensuring that controlled substances (schedules II through IV, USA) are kept under lock and key. These substances must be available only to authorized personnel. Records on the use of these substances must be kept so that all of the material is accounted for. Any unauthorized use of controlled substances must be reported to the proper authorities.

The nurse should be aware of the institutional policy on standing orders for controlled substances. For example, for schedule II drugs (USA), the physician's order may require renewal every 48 hours. A nurse who administers the drug after the 48-hour period without obtaining a renewal order is in violation of institutional policy. There are comparable national and institutional restrictions related to Canadian narcotics and schedule G drugs.

Patients receiving controlled substances may express concern about possible drug dependence. The use of the medication should be explained in terms of the patient's own condition, and the patient may be appropriately reassured.

Evaluation

Patient evaluation is at two levels for controlled substances. First, the medical evaluation should be performed as for any other type of drug. The nurse should ascertain if the medication is successfully controlling the signs and symptoms for which it was given. For example, the nurse might evaluate the patient to determine if pain is being adequately relieved in a postsurgery patient receiving morphine. Second, the patient should be evaluated for psychological responses to the addictive drugs. Signs of drug dependence should be noted, as well as excessive fears of addiction. These observations may dictate changes in the therapeutic program.

Table 3.6   Canadian Drug Classification

Classification	Description	Specific substances
NONPRESCRIPTION DRUGS		
Proprietary medicines	Drugs that may be widely purchased for self-treatment of symptoms of minor self-limiting diseases; identified by six-digit code preceded by letters GP	Cough drops, medicated shampoos, minor pain relievers
Over-the-counter drugs	Drugs available through a pharmacy and used on advice of a health professional for control of symptoms of minor self-limiting diseases; identified by six-digit code preceded by letters DIN	Laxatives, cough syrups, cold remedies, sinus preparations, certain vitamins
PRESCRIPTION DRUGS		
Schedule F	Over 200 drugs that may not be used except after professional consultation; identified by symbol Pr on label	Hormones, antibiotics, tranquilizers
Schedule G	Drugs that affect central nervous system (e.g., stimulants, sedatives); identified by symbol C on label	Amphetamines, barbiturates
Narcotics	Drugs used primarily for relief of pain but also possessing significant psychotropic activity; identified by letter N on label	Cannabis (marijuana), cocaine, codeine, morphine, opium, phencyclidine
RESTRICTED DRUGS		
Schedule H	Drugs with no recognized medical use and significant danger of physiological and psychological side effects; available only to institutions for research	Lysergic acid diethylamide (LSD), N, N-diethyltryptamine (DET), N, N-dimethyltryptamine (DMT), 4-methyl-2, 5-dimethoxyamphetamine (STP; DOM)

as well as amounts and dates for all transactions. As in the United States, nurses may be in possession of narcotics or controlled and restricted drugs only when authorized by a physician's order to administer the drug to a patient or when authorized to act as official custodian of drugs for a specific unit of a health care facility. Nurses may, of course, possess these drugs as prescribed by a physician when the nurse is a patient.

Development of New Drugs in Canada

New drugs are evaluated in Canada by a sequence of tests similar to those used in the United States. Promising drugs undergo preclinical testing in three mammalian species, including one nonrodent species, in order to determine threshold doses that produce toxicity or death in these species. The next stage of evaluation is called the clinical pharmacology trial, which is analogous to Phase I trials in the United States. During the clinical pharmacology trial the drug is administered to healthy human volunteers in order to establish the safety of doses that might be required for clinical applications. If the drug proves safe and if manufacturing processes have been developed to allow the production of a pure and uniform preparation

for human use, the manufacturer may apply for permission to distribute the drug to qualified investigators who will test the use of the drug in patients. This stage of testing is analogous to phase II in the United States. Before the drug may be released for general use, extensive documentation must be filed and evaluated concerning the chemical properties of the drug, its formulation, labeling and packaging, as well as all the clinical data on humans and the test data on animals. All new drugs are monitored after they have been placed on the market. Only after extensive information has been accumulated to document the safety of a new drug when used in normal medical practice is the drug released from the controls required by the designation *new drug.*

SUMMARY

The earliest medicinal agents were natural products discovered by trial and error to have certain effects on the body. Most of these crude natural products have now been replaced by preparations containing known amounts of active ingredients. *The United States Pharmacopeia and the National Formulary* and the *United States Homeopathic Pharmacopeia* serve as the reference works establishing the chemical properties, physical properties, and content of medications sold in the United States. Legislation in effect in the United States requires that medicinal agents be accurately labeled and advertised and be safe as well as effective when used as directed. The safety and efficacy of drugs in humans is determined in controlled clinical trials carried out before the drug is released into trade. A drug may not enter clinical trials until extensive toxicity tests in animals have shown that the drug is likely to be safe in human beings.

Drugs that can cause psychological or physical addiction are regulated according to the provisions of the Controlled Substances Act of 1970. Substances are assigned to schedules I through V according to their clinical uses and potential for abuse. Substances assigned to schedule I have a high abuse potential and no accepted clinical uses. At the other extreme, substances assigned to schedule V are medically accepted drugs that have a very limited potential for causing mild physical or psychological dependence. Substances listed in schedule I are illegal to sell or possess in the United States. Those substances in schedule II that do have accepted medical uses are closely regulated throughout manufacture and sale. The appropriate distribution and use of drugs in schedules II through V must be documented by accurately kept records.

Canadian drugs are regulated under the Food and Drugs Act and the Narcotic Control Act. These laws require that drugs be accurately labeled and that they be safe and effective when used as directed. Prescription drugs on schedule G are subject to special restrictions because of their abuse potential. Likewise, narcotics are specially regulated to prevent the unauthorized sale or use of these compounds.

STUDY QUESTIONS

1. What is the "active ingredient" of a medicinal preparation?
2. What advantages are gained by identifying the active ingredient in a crude medicinal preparation?
3. What is the function of the *United States Pharmacopeia* and the *National Formulary?*
4. Outline the steps involved in getting a new drug approved for the United States market.
5. What is a clinical trial?
6. Describe a clinical trial following the *double-blind* design.
7. What is the placebo effect?
8. Suggest two explanations for the placebo effect observed in drug trials.
9. What is the purpose of the informed consent form?
10. What is a treatment IND?
11. What was the purpose of the Drug Efficacy Study Implementation?
12. What are controlled substances?
13. What special precautions are required in handling controlled substances?

SUGGESTED READINGS

Drug regulation

Ballin, J.C.: Regulation and development of new drugs, JAMA **247**:2995, 1982.

Birdsall, C., and others: How safe are generic drugs? Am. J. Nurs. **87**(4):431, 1987.

FDA: Investigational new drug, antibiotic, and biological drug product regulations; treatment use and sale; final rule, Federal Register **52**(99):19466, 1987.

Hayes, A.H., Jr.: Food and drug regulation after 75 years, JAMA **246**:1223, 1981.

Hutt, P.B.: Investigations and reports respecting FDA regulation of new drugs. Part 2, Clin. Pharmacol. Ther. **33**(5):674, 1983.

Investigational new drug regulations, AORN J. **47**(6):1473, 1988.

Jacknowitz, A., and Fischer, R.G.: Inactive ingredients in the pediatric population, Pediatr. Nurs. **13**(2):125, 1987.

McGillick, K.J., and Fernandes, R.: The role of the nurse clinical research associate in testing a new drug, Nurs. Forum **19**(4):379, 1980.

Mullan, P.A.: Winding down the DESI review, Am. Pharm. **21**(2):25, 1981.

Nielsen, J.R.: Handbook of federal drug law, Philadelphia, 1986, Lea and Febiger.

Parks, B.R., Jr.: Orphan drugs . . . pharmaceutical products that may be commercially available in other countries but not in the United States, Pediatr. Nurs. **14**(2):152, 1988.

U.S. Department of Justice: Regulations implementing the comprehensive Drug Abuse Prevention and Control Act of 1970, Federal Register **36**(No. 80):1, April 24, 1971.

Vogel, A.V., Goodwin, J.S., and Goodwin, J.M.: The therapeutics of placebo, Am. Fam. Physician **22**(7):105, 1980.

Wardell, W.M.: New drug development by United States pharmaceutical firms with analyses of trends in the acquisition and origin of drug candidates, 1963-1979, Clin. Pharmacol. Ther. **32**(4):407, 1982.

Weiner, E.E., and Weiner, D.L.: Understanding the use of basic statistics in nursing research, Am. J. Nurs. **83**(5):770, 1983.

Weinstein, S.M.: Use of investigational drugs, NITA (J. of the National Intravenous Therapy Association) **10**(5):336, 1987.

Wertheimer, A.K.: The placebo effect, Pharm. Int. **1**:12, 1980.

Young, F.E., and others: The FDA's new procedures for the use of investigational drugs in treatment, JAMA **259**:2267, 1988.

Current drug information

British Pharmacopoeia 1988, London, Her Majesty's Stationery Office.

Compendium of Pharmaceuticals and Specialties, ed. 28, Canadian Pharmaceutical Association, 1988.

Drug Evaluations, ed. 6, American Medical Association, 1986.

Drug Information, American Hospital Formulary Service, 1989.

Drug Information for the Health Care Provider, ed. 9, United States Pharmacopeial Convention, 1989.

Facts and Comparisons, Facts and Comparisons, Inc., St. Louis, 1989.

FDA Drug Bulletin, published three times a year by the Department of Health and Human Services.

Physician's Desk Reference, ed. 43, Medical Economics Co., 1989.

The International Pharmacopoeia, ed. 3, World Health Organization, 1979.

Nurses and the law

Bergerson, S.R.: More about charting with a jury in mind, Nursing 88 **18**(4):50, 1988.

Gasparis, L., and Noone, J.: How well do you know the legal aspects of nursing? Nursing 87 **17**(4):43, 1987.

Hemelt, M.D., and Mackert, M.E.: Steering clear of legal hazards, Nursing 84 **14**(5):81, 1984.

Luguire, R.: Six common causes of nursing liability, Nursing 88 **18**(11):61, 1988.

Northrop, C.E.: What you don't know can hurt you. Nursing 87 **17**(1):43, 1987.

Northrop, C.E.: Lessons from the law: think before you search, Nursing 87 **17**(7):59, 1987.

Pierce, M.E.: Reporting and following up on medication errors, Nursing 84 **14**(1):77, 1984.

Rabinow, J.: Where you stand in the eyes of the law, Nursing 89 **19**(2):34, 1989.

Smith, C.E.: Patient teaching: it's the law, Nursing 87 **17**(7):67, 1987.

Thomas, C.: States report on NP acts, Nurse Pract. **7**(10):9, 1982.

II

GENERAL PRINCIPLES OF PATIENT CARE

This section is intended to introduce the student to basic nursing activities involved in administering drugs to patients.

Chapter 4, *Over-the-Counter Drugs and Self-Medication*, is included to emphasize the importance of these agents in nursing practice. The legal status of over-the-counter agents, their properties, and drug interactions are discussed. The material is a ready reference for the nurse in assessing the use of nonpresciption medication.

Chapter 5, *Care of the Poisoned Patient*, introduces the study of adverse effects of chemicals, including drugs, on the human organism.

Chapters 6 and 7 focus on the basic nursing activities involved in administering drugs. Chapter 6, *Drug Administration*, presents information and techniques that can assist the nurse in properly administering drugs to provide safe individualized patient care. Chapter 7, *Calculating Drug Dosages*, is designed to help the student achieve proficiency and develop confidence in this basic skill. Drug dosage calculations are presented as a guide to the level of proficiency expected of practicing nurses. Whereas students with good arithmetic skills can readily acquire the ability to solve problems of the level included in this chapter, many students initially experience difficulty because they have forgotten basic rules of arithmetic and algebra. Such students should review these rules before attempting the drug dosage calculations.

CHAPTER

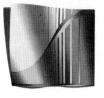

Over-the-Counter Drugs and Self-Medication

4

LEGISLATIVE ORIGIN OF OVER-THE-COUNTER DRUGS

Products intended for the self-medication of a variety of illnesses have been sold in the United States since colonial times. Until the early twentieth century no restrictions governed the contents, potency, purity, safety, efficacy, sale, or advertising of these products, which came to be known as "patent medicines." Consequently, some were of marginal safety and most provided no therapeutic benefit. Most patent medicines were harmless as well as ineffective, but many contained alcohol, narcotics, or other dangerous drugs in unspecified quantities.

Some element of control of the patent medicine industry was achieved with passage of the first Pure Food and Drug Act of 1906 (Chapter 3). This act required that package labels accurately list the ingredients of medicinal products. Any substance present but not listed on the label was deemed an adulterant. A later amendment to the act, the Sherley Amendment (1912), forbade false and fraudulent labeling claims. In 1938, a new Food and Drug Act was enacted. It required proof of safety for all medicinal products. In 1952 the Durham-Humphrey Amendment to the 1938 act specified two categories of drugs: (1) those safe enough for sale without a prescription (over-the-counter, or OTC) and (2) those deemed sufficiently dangerous or unsuitable for self-medication to require sale by prescription only.

Present control of OTC drugs stems from the Kefauver-Harris Amendment of 1962, which required proof of efficacy and lack of teratogenicity in addition to proof of safety. This amendment affected all new drugs introduced after 1962, and all drugs that had entered the market since 1938. For several years after the adoption of this amendment,

This chapter was contributed by Lynn Roger Willis, Ph.D., Professor of Pharmacology and Medicine, Indiana University School of Medicine.

the FDA concentrated primarily on prescription-only drugs in its assessment of efficacy, largely for logistical reasons. In the mid-1970s, however, scrutiny of OTC drugs began. The FDA convened several OTC review panels of experts and assigned them the task of reviewing the various classes of OTC drugs, and assigning each drug to one of the following categories:

Category I: Recognized as safe and effective for the claimed therapeutic indication.

Category II: Not recognized as safe and effective.

Category III: Additional data needed to decide safety and/or effectiveness.

Drugs assigned to category I can be sold. Those in category II cannot. Drugs in category III, if generally recognized as safe, may be marketed while their effectiveness is being evaluated.

Since this review process began, many unsafe or ineffective OTC products have disappeared from the market. Others have undergone labeling changes or have been redesigned. However, since manufacturers are not required to indicate whether the drugs in their products are in category I or III, the effectiveness of all OTC products cannot be assumed simply because their sale is permitted. Some consumer interest groups have objected to the sale of category III drugs, and they have challenged the category I assignment of others. Until the FDA review panels have completed their work to the satisfaction of all concerned, the therapeutic benefit of some OTC drugs will remain questionable.

COMMON PROPERTIES OF OTC MEDICATIONS

Low Doses

A principal concern of today's manufacturers of OTC products is safety. Drug toxicity is dose related, and its risk is reduced when the drug dose is low. Thus most OTC products are provided with

45

THE NURSING PROCESS

OVER-THE-COUNTER DRUGS

Over-the-counter, or nonprescription, drugs will not form a major part of the clinical responsibilities of the practicing nurse. Nevertheless, the nurse is frequently sought as a source of information on these agents. The following presentation is one suggestion for a method of patient counseling about nonprescription medications.

Assessment

Since the patient is involved in self-care, the nurse might assist the individual to clearly state what condition or symptoms are to be treated. For example, if the individual is seeking a medication to treat the symptoms of a cold, the nurse might lead that person to consider exactly what symptoms require treatment. For some persons a cough might be the most outstanding symptom, whereas for others it might be nasal congestion or headache.

Potential nursing diagnosis

Knowledge deficit related to not knowing how to self-medicate for minor health problems

Management

After leading the patient to define exactly what symptoms are to be treated, the nurse might appropriately teach the patient what types of medications are available to treat these symptoms. The nurse might suggest that fixed combinations of ingredients are more difficult to use, since dosages are impossible to regulate for each component of the combination. More control may be gained by using single agents at appropriate doses as necessary for defined symptoms. The nurse should also suggest other sources of information about nonprescription drugs, such as the pharmacist.

Evaluation

Evaluation would be expected to be carried out by the patient involved in self-care. If the patient seeks advice because therapy is unsuccessful, the nurse might lead the patient to consider if the proper medication was administered for the symptom to be controlled and if the right dose was used.

---

low, sometimes less than therapeutic, amounts of active ingredient. Such preparations may serve as little more than placebos, especially for such subjective minor complaints as pain, itch, and sleeplessness. For such indications, proof of product efficacy may be difficult, even when adequate dosage is provided.

Combination of Ingredients

Many OTC products contain several drugs. The drugs may be totally different from one another, or they may be of the same or similar classification. When drugs are taken in combination, adverse interactions between two or more of them may occur. Although the risk of interactions is low for the drugs in a given product, it is not so low when other drugs are taken simultaneously.

OTC products with several ingredients are termed *fixed combination* products; that is, the doses of the drugs in the product are fixed within the tablet or other dosage form and cannot be altered. For example, if a tablet contains 4 mg of antihistamine and 60 mg of decongestant, a patient who needed to increase the antihistamine dosage would also have to take more of the decongestant.

On the other hand, many single-drug OTC products are available. Examples of such products include antihistamines, analgesic-antipyretic drugs, decongestants, cough suppressants, and antifungal drugs. Complete control of drug dosage is possible with single-drug products, and such products can often be purchased less expensively than the heavily advertised combination products.

By understanding the pharmacology of the

drugs in OTC products and the specific needs of the patient, the nurse can advise a rational method of product selection.

MAJOR CLASSES OF OTC DRUGS

The classes of OTC drugs chosen for discussion in this chapter include analgesic drugs, cold and cough remedies, weight control products, and sleeping aids; their component drugs are discussed in other chapters. Also discussed are vitamin C, ophthalmic products, acne treatments, topical anti-infectives and hemorrhoidal products, which are not discussed elsewhere in this text. Finally, several classes of OTC drugs that are discussed in detail in Chapter 11 are not included in this chapter: antacids, antidiarrheals, laxatives, and antiemetics. For an exhaustive review of all OTC drugs, refer to the *Handbook of Nonprescription Drugs*, 8th edition, published by the American Pharmaceutical Association.

Analgesic Drugs

For about 30 years, aspirin and acetaminophen shared the claim of being the most effective OTC analgesic drugs available. In 1984, however, OTC analgesic status was granted to ibuprofen.

Aspirin and ibuprofen are classified as nonsteroidal anti-inflammatory drugs (NSAID). Both inhibit the synthesis of prostaglandins by inhibiting cyclooxygenase, and this action may be related to the mechanism by which they produce analgesia. Acetaminophen is chemically unrelated to either aspirin or ibuprofen. Its mechanism of action seems to differ from that of NSAID, and it can be used by people who cannot tolerate NSAID. The pharmacological actions of these drugs, which are complex, are discussed in detail in Chapter 23. The following discussion focuses on selecting or recommending an OTC analgesic drug for self-medication.

Aspirin and acetaminophen are equally effective at relieving minor aches and pains and reducing fever. Maximum analgesic and antipyretic effectiveness is achieved in most adults with 650 mg of either. Higher doses (as in the "extra-strength" products) provide little, if any, additional relief. Aspirin also relieves the pain and inflammation of arthritic disorders, but acetaminophen does not. The anti-inflammatory effect of aspirin requires higher than usual doses, which should not be taken without medical supervision.

Aspirin produces several side effects. These normally present no problem for individuals who take the drug occasionally, but they may be troublesome to those who take the drug regularly or are particularly sensitive to it. For example, aspirin inhibits platelet aggregation. As little as one 650 mg dose of aspirin may double the bleeding time for several days. Aspirin also irritates the lining of the stomach, sometimes causing pain, discomfort, and, on occasion, bleeding. From 5 to 10 ml of blood may be lost in the stool each day. The bleeding is ordinarily of no consequence with occasional use of the drug, but those who take the drug frequently may develop iron-deficiency anemia. Individuals with a history of peptic ulcer or intestinal bleeding or those who are taking anticoagulant drugs should not take aspirin.

Acetaminophen (Tylenol, Datril, and other brands), on the other hand, is remarkably free of side effects. It does not affect blood clotting mechanisms, nor does it irritate the stomach lining. Rarely, acetaminophen will cause an allergic reaction, often a skin rash. The drug may also damage the liver but only in association with overdosage.

Various dosage forms for aspirin are available, reflecting efforts by manufacturers to overcome some of the problems caused by the drug. To minimize gastric irritation, aspirin is available in buffered, effervescent, and enteric-coated tablets. Timed-release tablets are available for the convenience of persons who must take aspirin regularly. Since aspirin is unstable in aqueous solution, liquid forms are not available. Acetaminophen, on the other hand, is stable in solution and is available in a variety of pleasant-tasting syrups. Both drugs are available in inexpensive but reliable generic forms.

The newest drug in this triad, ibuprofen (Advil, Nuprin), has been available for several years but only by prescription. It is one of several nonsteroidal anti-inflammatory drugs such as indomethacin, naproxen, and sulindac (see Chapter 23). Ibuprofen has been approved for OTC sale largely because it has a wider margin of safety than either aspirin or acetaminophen, especially in cases of overdose. Ibuprofen appears to be more effective for menstrual cramps and is effective against moderate pain that does not respond well to treatment with aspirin or acetaminophen. The recommended OTC dosage of ibuprofen is 200 to 400 mg every 4 hours in persons over the age of 12 years, to a maximum of 1200 mg in 24 hours.

Ibuprofen is recommended for people who cannot tolerate aspirin, but this requires rather narrow interpretation. People who are allergic to aspirin are also likely to be allergic to ibuprofen. Similarly, ibuprofen irritates the gastric mucosa and interferes with platelet function, but the incidence of gastrointestinal bleeding may be less with ibuprofen than with aspirin. The irritation can often be lessened by taking the drug with milk, food, or antacids, but some people will find ibuprofen to be as troublesome as aspirin. For such people, acetaminophen remains the reasonable alternative. No therapeutic advantage is gained by taking any of these drugs together; indeed, aspirin may diminish the effectiveness of ibuprofen.

Probably the most serious hazard associated with the OTC use of ibuprofen is reduced renal blood flow leading to renal failure in some patients. Persons who are taking diuretic drugs for the treatment of hypertension, or who have impaired renal or cardiac function, should not take ibuprofen except under the direction of a physician.

Ibuprofen seems to be superior to aspirin or acetaminophen for relieving certain types of pain, such as that associated with menstrual cramps, muscle strains, and the like. Nevertheless, it is no more effective than aspirin or acetaminophen against most types of mild pain, and is generally more expensive. Consequently, nurses should exercise discretion and judgment when recommending it.

Cold Remedies

Most of the available OTC cold remedies (e.g., Contac, Novahistine, Dristan) contain one or more of the following: a *sympathomimetic drug* to relieve nasal and sinus congestion, an *antihistamine* to dry excessive nasal secretions, and/or an *analgesic drug* to relieve minor aches and pains. Some products contain additional drugs, such as caffeine, one or more vitamins, a laxative, or other substances. A few products contain only a sympathomimetic drug or an antihistamine, but most are sold as combination products.

Sympathomimetic drugs relieve nasal stuffiness and congestion by constricting the blood vessels in swollen nasal membranes, decreasing local blood flow and swelling. When the swelling is relieved, the breathing passages open.

Drugs that are commonly included in OTC cold remedies as decongestants are *phenylephrine, phenylpropanolamine,* and *pseudoephedrine.* These drugs are available in scores of products, and their pharmacological characteristics are discussed in Chapter 14. Of the three, phenylephrine is the least reliable; stomach acid reduces its activity, and its absorption into the blood is often erratic.

For adults, safe and effective decongestant dosages of these drugs are as follows: phenylephrine, 10 mg every 4 hours; phenylpropanolamine, 25 mg every 4 hours; and pseudoephedrine, 60 mg every 4 hours. One half of the adult dose is considered safe and effective for children from ages 6 to 12 years. Children from 2 to 6 years should receive one quarter of the adult dose. Children under 2 years of age should not be given these drugs except on the advice of a physician.

Sympathomimetic drugs can cause stimulation of the central nervous system and vasoconstriction. As a result, side effects of irritability, nervousness, insomnia, headache, and hypertension can occur. Individuals with high blood pressure, thyroid disease, or heart disease are cautioned against taking these drugs unless directed to do so by their physician.

The vasoconstrictive effects of these drugs are intensified in the presence of monoamine oxidase inhibitors (e.g., Marplan, Nardil), which may be prescribed to treat depression (see Chapter 14 for details of this drug interaction) and may cause alarming and dangerous elevations of blood pressure and threat of stroke.

The rationale for including an antihistamine in a product intended to treat the symptoms of the common cold is not based on antagonism of histamine receptors. Unless the cold is associated with conditions of increased histamine release, such as allergic rhinitis, antagonism of histamine receptors will be of no use. (See Chapter 24 for a detailed discussion of antihistamines.) Instead, the justification for including antihistamines in OTC cold remedies rests largely on their anticholinergic action, which reduces the secretion of mucus by the nasal and bronchial mucosa and produces a "drying" effect. This effect, however, is not impressive, especially at approved OTC doses of the antihistamines.

On the other hand, the therapeutic index of antihistamines is high, and little risk of serious toxicity exists for adults. Thus antihistamines may produce relief of mild rhinorrhea in susceptible patients with little risk of adverse effects.

The most prominent side effects of antihistamines are drowsiness and sedation. These effects occur with all OTC antihistamines and at OTC doses. They pose a potentially serious threat to operators of motor vehicles or persons in hazardous occupations. Such persons should not take cold remedies containing antihistamines.

The analgesic-antipyretic ingredients most often found in OTC cold remedies are aspirin and acetaminophen. Several, however, contain salicylamide, which is the amide of salicylic acid. Its analgesic and antipyretic properties are inferior to those of aspirin or acetaminophen, and it is no longer listed in the *United States Pharmacopeia.* Although aspirin and acetaminophen relieve the aches, pains, and feverishness associated with the common cold, one need never purchase a cold remedy that contains either drug. If analgesia is desired, cut-rate, but good quality, aspirin or acetaminophen can be obtained at considerable savings. Indeed, because of their complicated pharmacological characteristics (Chapter 23), aspirin and acetaminophen should be taken only as necessary.

No clear rationale exists for including caffeine, vitamins, laxatives, or other drugs in OTC cold remedies. Caffeine may be included for its mood-stimulating effects, but the dosage necessary for central nervous system (CNS) stimulation is generally higher than that found in the combination cold remedies. Vitamins are necessary only for correction of a vitamin deficiency and, with the possible exception of vitamin C, provide no therapeutic benefits for a cold sufferer. Laxatives, likewise, are of no known value for treatment of a cold.

Vitamin C Preparations

Vitamin C, or ascorbic acid, is necessary for a number of important biochemical reactions in the body, such as synthesis of collagen and adrenal steroids. Collagen provides the supporting framework for tooth, bone, and capillary structures. Vitamin C deficiency manifests itself as scurvy, diminished rate of wound healing, and other conditions.

Ascorbic acid is present in a variety of foods but especially in citrus fruits and vegetables. It is readily absorbed from the intestine and, when taken in recommended minimum daily amounts (60 mg daily in adults), most of it is converted metabolically to oxalate. Little ascorbate appears in the urine. However, when the daily intake of ascorbic acid exceeds 100 mg and the plasma ascorbate concentration exceeds 1.5 mg/dl, ascorbate appears in the urine.

More than 20 years ago, the Nobel laureate, Dr. Linus Pauling, proposed that vitamin C might be effective in treating and preventing the common cold. At that time the proposal was controversial, and it remains so today. Proponents of Dr. Pauling's theory assert that large doses, or megadoses, of ascorbic acid are necessary to saturate the body stores of vitamin C and to buffer the drain on these stores when the cold virus attacks. They recommend a daily intake of 1 to 5 g of vitamin C to prevent, and as much as 15 g per day to treat, a cold.

Many studies have been conducted to test these ideas. Although none have been totally negative, none have shown convincingly that the vitamin alters the severity, occurrence, or duration of the common cold. Megadoses of the vitamin do not saturate tissues any better than the minimum recommended dose.

On the other hand, there are disadvantages to the use of large doses of vitamin C. Diarrhea is a common, though not serious, side effect. In addition, oxalate stones may precipitate in the urinary tract of susceptible individuals, causing serious medical problems. Fortunately, this represents a serious risk only to individuals who have an underlying disorder of oxalate metabolism. Finally, increased urinary excretion of ascorbic acid and the resulting acidification of the urine can alter the rate of excretion of other drugs such as amphetamines, salicylates, and phenobarbital.

Attuned to the controversy surrounding megadose therapy with vitamin C, the nurse is in a position to provide a rational, objective evaluation of its use for patients.

Cough Remedies

A cough may not accompany the common cold, but if it does, it may be either productive or nonproductive. A productive cough removes phlegm from the lower respiratory tract and, unless it becomes nonproductive and excessive, should not be suppressed. A nonproductive cough is generally dry, discomforting, and, because of local irritation caused by the rapid movement of air, may be self-perpetuating. Nonproductive coughs can be safely suppressed and relieved with an OTC cough suppressant (antitussive) drug. Expectorants are also included in many OTC cough remedies. Their antitussive effectiveness is questionable. The detailed pharmacological properties of expectorants and antitussives are discussed in Chapter 26.

Expectorants. The use of expectorants in clinical medicine is controversial. In part, the controversy stems from a lack of objective evidence that expectorant drugs are effective, and partly from confusion concerning the effect expected of an expectorant drug. For some authorities, an expectorant should promote the expulsion of mucus, phlegm, and fluid from the lungs and bronchial passages, that is, enhance the productiveness of a cough. For others, it should relieve a dry, irritating cough by causing the secretion of soothing and protective mucus in the airway. In any case there is little evidence to suggest that expectorant drugs are any better than placebo either for promoting the expulsion of phlegm or relieving a cough.

Guaifenesin recently became the only expectorant approved for use in OTC cough remedies. It stimulates the reflex production of bronchial secretion by irritating the gastric mucosa. In higher dosage, it causes emesis.

Cough suppressants (antitussives). Three cough suppressants have been designated as safe and effective (category I) by the FDA for OTC sale. They are *codeine, dextromethorphan,* and *diphenhydramine.*

Codeine (Chapter 44) suppresses the cough reflex center in the brain. As an opium alkaloid and narcotic drug, it can cause psychological and physical dependence. The liability for dependence is less than that for morphine, however, and it is virtually nonexistent when the drug is used in recommended doses for short periods (10 to 20 mg every 4 to 6 hours). Larger doses may cause nausea, constipation, and drowsiness. The drowsiness is caused by depression of the CNS and is intensified by other CNS depressant drugs (e.g., barbiturates, alcohol, and antihistamines). Codeine should not be taken with any of them. Poisoning with codeine causes respiratory depression.

Abuse of OTC cough preparations that contain codeine has been a problem in the United States, and varying restrictions on their sale have been enacted by state legislatures. These restrictions range from a limit on the quantity that can be purchased by an individual to complete prohibition of sale without a prescription.

Dextromethorphan is a nonnarcotic cough suppressant with approximately the same antitussive potency and efficacy as codeine. As with codeine, dextromethorphan suppresses the cough reflex center in the brain, but it does not cause dependence or respiratory depression. Side effects are uncommon and generally mild, consisting largely of drowsiness and gastrointestinal upset. Overall, dextromethorphan is the best choice for cough suppression.

Diphenhydramine, an antihistamine, is an effective cough suppressant and has only recently been approved for OTC sale. It is not a narcotic drug and therefore does not cause dependence. In adults, the drug suppresses cough at a dosage of 25 mg every 4 hours. Drowsiness commonly occurs at this dosage, however, and may severely limit the usefulness of the drug for many people. Paradoxically, the drug may cause stimulation, not sedation, in small children. It is probably the least useful of the three approved antitussive drugs.

Another opium alkaloid, *noscapine,* has long been considered an effective antitussive drug, but the evidence for this action is old and largely empirical. Consequently, the FDA review panel has assigned the drug to category III, allowing its OTC sale while awaiting additional proof of efficacy. Noscapine, like codeine, suppresses the cough reflex center in the brain, but, unlike codeine, it has no CNS or respiratory depressant actions and

does not cause dependence. The recommended dosage of the drug is 15 to 30 mg every 4 to 6 hours.

Antitussive combinations. Some cough suppressant products consist only of the antitussive drug in a flavored base. Others combine an antitussive drug with an expectorant. Either is suitable for suppressing coughs.

There are several reasons to avoid multidrug "cough and cold formulas" even though they are numerous and heavily promoted by manufacturers. As mentioned earlier, not all coughs should be suppressed. In addition, a cough that accompanies a cold may be caused by irritation of the airway by an annoying trickle of mucus from swollen nasal membranes into the throat (postnasal drip). Stopping the flow of mucus with a decongestant drug should alleviate the cough and eliminate the need for an antitussive drug. On the other hand, if the cough is caused by irritation, low humidity, or "smoker's cough," a decongestant and/or antihistamine will be of no value. A cough suppressant alone should be sufficient.

Decongestant nose drops and sprays. Several sympathomimetic drugs are available over-the-counter as nose drops and sprays for the symptomatic and temporary relief of nasal congestion. These drugs include *phenylephrine, ephedrine,* and *naphazoline,* which are short-acting decongestants, to be used as frequently as every 3 or 4 hours, and *xylometazoline* and *oxymetazoline,* which are long-acting decongestants and are used only 2 or 3 times a day.

Topical decongestants have advantages over the oral decongestants, but there are some serious disadvantages, too. Since the drops and sprays apply the drugs directly to the congested nasal membranes, the onset of action and relief of congestion occur rapidly. In addition, only small amounts of the drugs need be administered, since they are applied locally. Therefore the incidence and severity of systemic side effects (e.g., elevated blood pressure) are reduced.

On the other hand, the intense localized vasoconstriction in the nasal mucosa can cause the phenomenon of rebound congestion, in which the congestion that occurs when the effect of the drug has worn off may be worse than the level that existed in the first place. A vicious cycle can develop in which the user treats the nasal congestion with the cause of that congestion. If unrecognized, this cycle can lead to chronic nasal stuffiness that will no longer respond to the decongestant drugs. Rebound congestion probably cannot be totally avoided when topical decongestants are used, but it can be minimized; and the vicious cycle can be avoided if the drugs are used only sparingly and strictly according to directions.

Sprays are most convenient for adults and older children. Drops are often preferable for use in young children. Topical decongestants should not be given to children under the age of 2 years except as directed by a physician.

Weight Control Products

Obesity is most frequently defined as a condition in which body weight is more than 20% greater than the ideal body weight. It is a complex problem that requires complex treatment. Drug treatment of obesity is of limited value at best. Amphetamines (Chapter 43) have been prescribed for weight control. They, and related drugs, suppress appetite via a central mechanism, but the appetite remains suppressed only as long as sufficient levels of the drug are present in the brain. Unless the overweight person willfully resists the temptation to overeat when hungry, the drug will be of no value. Moreover, tolerance to the appetite-suppressing action of these drugs develops quickly, and they may produce dependence. Amphetamines are not available without a prescription.

Weight loss will occur if caloric use exceeds caloric intake. No available OTC product will enhance the rate at which calories are expended. They can aid only in reducing caloric intake. To that end, it matters little if a dietary aid possesses true pharmacological activity. A placebo can be totally effective in some persons if they consume fewer calories while taking the medication.

The OTC armamentarium for the treatment of obesity for weight control consists principally of *phenylpropranolamine, bulk-producing agents,* and *benzocaine.* Most authorities consider amphetamines to be largely ineffective aids to weight control, and the OTC products even less so. Nevertheless, the FDA has placed these OTC products in category I.

Phenylpropanolamine is structurally related to ephedrine and amphetamine. Its pharmacological characteristics are similar to those of amphetamine; the main difference is that this drug is less potent than amphetamine. Phenylpropanolamine is clearly effective as an appetite suppressant in experimental animals, but its effectiveness in human beings is questionable. The drug has been assigned to category I because in controlled clinical trials human subjects who took the drug lost more weight by the end of the study than did untreated control subjects. The problem with these results, however, is that the weight losses, and the differences between treated and untreated groups in these studies, were small. People who did not receive phenylpropanolamine often lost nearly as much weight as did those who had received the drug.

Amphetaminelike side effects can occur with phenylpropanolamine, although they are generally less intense than those associated with amphetamine. The most common of these side effects are nervousness, insomnia, headache, nausea, and hypertension. Persons with diabetes mellitus, heart disease, hypertension, or thyroid disease should not take phenylpropanolamine, except on the advice of a physician. Persons taking the drug should be aware of its potential for interaction with other adrenergic drugs (Chapter 10). To avoid these side effects and other problems with phenylpropanolamine, the FDA recommends that no more than 75 mg of the drug be taken in any 24-hour period, and for no more than 3 months at a time.

Phenylpropanolamine is potentially harmful. Since 1985, there have been 11 reported instances of cerebral hemorrhage in people who had taken this drug. Ten of the 11 cases involved women, and several apparently occurred after the recommended dosage had been taken.

In recommending a dietary aid containing phenylpropanolamine, the nurse should emphasize the questionable value of the drug alone if caloric intake is not also reduced, the development of tolerance after long-term use of the drug, and the hazards of side effects if the recommended daily dosage is exceeded.

A variety of *bulk producers* are sold as aids to weight reduction. The rationale behind their use stems from their tendency, when taken with one or two glasses of water, to expand and swell in the stomach, thereby producing a feeling of fullness and a loss of appetite. Examples of OTC bulk producers are *methylcellulose, carboxymethylcellulose, agar, psyllium hydrophilic mucilloid,* and *karaya gum.* Unfortunately, the swollen bulk spends little time in the stomach, moving rapidly into the intestine, where it stimulates peristalsis and may exert a laxative effect. Indeed, some bulk producers are also marketed as laxatives and stool softeners (Chapter 13). Bulk producers are probably no more effective at suppressing appetite and caloric intake than is drinking two or three glasses of water before each meal. Yet the FDA has approved bulk producing agents for dietary use.

Several OTC weight control products contain the local anesthetic drug *benzocaine* in tablets or as chewing gum. Presumably, the benzocaine will anesthetize the gastric mucosa or the mucous membranes in the mouth, thereby reducing appetite or removing the pleasurable sensation of taste. To date, there is no conclusive evidence that either effect is helpful in losing weight.

In selecting or recommending an OTC weight control product, the importance of a practical and nutritious diet plan, preferably supervised by a family member, friend, nurse, or physician, cannot be emphasized too strongly. By themselves, the OTC products, being of doubtful effectiveness at best, will certainly not produce weight loss. The success of a weight loss program depends on faithful maintenance of diminished caloric intake.

Sleeping Aids

Insomnia disrupts the restful nights of nearly everyone from time to time. Some people have difficulty falling asleep; others may awaken in the middle of the night and be unable to go back to sleep. The cause of sleep difficulties may be physiological or psychological. In most cases the difficulties are temporary.

A wide variety of common remedies for sleeplessness may be tried. They include warm baths, a dull book, and a glass of warm milk or wine. In severe cases of insomnia the assistance of a physician may be sought, and a powerful sedative-hypnotic drug may be prescribed (Chapter 40). Many people fear the addictive properties of these drugs, but they find little or no relief from simple home remedies. Between these extremes lies the OTC sleep aid.

The FDA has greatly simplified the job of selecting an OTC sleep aid by severely restricting the number of drugs that can be sold as such. Before 1979, OTC sleep aids contained bromides, scopolamine, vitamins, and/or combinations of antihistamines. Since 1979, however, OTC sleep aids may contain an antihistamine alone or an antihistamine in combination with aspirin and/or acetaminophen. The antihistamines that have been approved for use as sleep aids are *pyrilamine maleate* (25 to 50 mg at bedtime), *doxylamine succinate* (25 mg at bedtime), and *diphenhydramine hydrochloride* (25 to 50 mg at bedtime).

The rationale for including an antihistamine in an OTC sleep aid stems from the tendency of the drug to cause drowsiness. This tendency, plus a wide margin of safety, lends credence to marketing claims for the effectiveness of antihistamines in the treatment of occasional insomnia. An analgesic drug is included in some preparations on the assumption that mild nighttime pain may contribute to the sleeplessness.

Clinical comparisons of antihistamines with placebo in sleep laboratories have tended to reinforce the claims of effectiveness, but some authorities remain doubtful.

Product selection in this category of drugs is relatively simple because of the limited number of available active ingredients. Of perhaps more importance from the nursing standpoint is assessment of the cause of the sleeplessness and the actual need for a sleeping aid. If mild pain is keeping someone awake, relief of the pain with aspirin or acetaminophen will often be sufficient to allow sleep to occur. If anxiety is the cause, antihistamine-induced drowsiness may be helpful; but it may also be no more effective than a glass of warm milk or a warm bath, although more expensive. Wise nursing counsel may be the most effective remedy for patients with mild insomnia.

Ophthalmic Products

OTC ophthalmic products are intended only for the symptomatic, short-term relief of mild self-limiting conditions such as "eye fatigue," tearing, "redness," or the itching and stinging associated with allergic or chemical conjunctivitis. The products are sold as *eye washes*, *artificial tears*, and *decongestants*. Conditions involving marked eye pain or blurred vision require attention by a physician.

All OTC ophthalmic products must be clear, odorless, colorless, sterile solutions with a pH and tonicity approximating that of natural tears. They must also contain preservatives to maintain sterility. Sterility cannot be maintained indefinitely, however, and bacterial contamination may be transferred to the eye. Thus cloudy or discolored solutions should be discarded. All ophthalmic products carry an expiration date for the unopened package and a warning that they should be discarded within 3 months of the opening date.

OTC ophthalmic products contain a variety of *nonmedicinal* ingredients. *Tonicity adjusters* (e.g., dextran, glycerin) prevent excessive tearing that can dilute and wash away active ingredients. *Antioxidants* and *stabilizers* (edetic acid, sodium bisulfite or metabisulfite, thiourea, and others) prevent the chemical alteration of the ingredients. *Buffers* (e.g., boric acid, potassium bicarbonate, sodium acetate) maintain the pH of the solution within a range of 6.0 to 8.0. Solutions of higher or lower pH may cause eye irritation. *Wetting agents* (polysorbate 80, poloxamer 282, and others) reduce surface tension. *Preservatives* (e.g., benzalkonium chloride, benzethonium chloride, phenylmercuric nitrate) prevent bacterial growth. *Viscosity-increasing agents* (gelatin, glycerin, lanolin, polyethylene glycol, and others) aid in spreading the solution over the eye.

Decongestant ophthalmic products contain a *sympathomimetic* drug (ephedrine HCl, naphazoline HCl, phenylephrine HCl, or tetrahydrozoline). Local application of one of these drugs to the eye promptly relieves the symptoms of allergic conjunctivitis. By constricting dilated blood vessels in the white of the eye, they also relieve that "bloodshot" look and restore the normal white color to the eyes. Sympathomimetic drugs also stimulate the adrenergic receptors affecting pupillary size and may cause mydriasis. For this reason these products should not be used by persons with narrow-angle glaucoma.

Problems may occur with decongestant ophthalmic products. Rebound congestion can occur by the same mechanism as described for topical nasal decongestants. It can be minimized or avoided by using the medicine only occasionally and strictly according to directions. In addition, the OTC decongestant ophthalmic products will be ineffective if the cause of the symptoms is within the eyeball itself. If bacterial infection is present, the medicine may mask its presence.

Other medicinal agents contained in decongestant and other OTC ophthalmic products include *antipruritics* (antipyrine, camphor, and menthol) and *astringents* (zinc sulfate). Antipruritics produce mild local anesthesia and a cooling sensation. They are considered unsafe because they can mask the presence of foreign abrasive substances in the eye that may damage the cornea. Zinc sulfate is the only acceptable astringent in OTC ophthalmic preparations.

Acne Products

Acne and its treatment. Acne vulgaris is the curse of adolescence, occurring when young people are highly aware of their personal appearance. For them, prevention and treatment of even mild attacks of the disease, with its unsightly pimples and scars, are given high priority.

The pimples and skin eruptions of acne are called *comedones*. They consist of a mixture of sebum, produced by the sebaceous glands of the hair follicles, and epithelial cells shed by the infundibulum of the follicle.

Acne is associated with excessive production of sebum, which impairs the normal washout of infundibular cells that are shed. The cells become compacted and plug the follicle, which then becomes distended with accumulated sebum and cells. The condition is relieved by removal of the plug either by lancing the comedone or by the natural growth of the hair, which brings the plug to the surface. This form of acne, termed *noninflammatory*, is not usually associated with scarring.

Scarring is more likely to occur with the *inflammatory* form of the disease, which is characterized by pustule formation and local inflammation. In this form of the disease comedones do not open at the skin surface to relieve the pressure within the hair follicle. An inflamed follicle may rupture beneath the skin surface and spread sebum, cells, and bacteria to surrounding tissues. Whereas noninflammatory acne can be treated with OTC products, cases of inflammatory acne should be referred to a physician.

Nonmedicinal treatment. External factors may contribute to the development of acne. These factors include personal hygiene, diet, and self-image.

Personal hygiene is important in combating excessive skin oiliness, but there is no evidence that compulsive and vigorous cleansing of the skin is any more effective in preventing acne than is normal washing. Since bacterial infection is not ordinarily associated with acne, the use of antibacterial soaps and antiseptic solutions is neither necessary nor recommended.

The role of diet in acne is controversial. Chocolate has long been condemned as a causative factor, but evidence of a cause-and-effect relationship between chocolate and acne is lacking. Similarly, the evidence does not support the need for dietary restrictions of sweets, nuts, and greasy foods. On the other hand, until a clearer understanding of acne and its cause emerges, individual trial and error with diet, hygiene, and other factors should not be excluded or discouraged.

Noninflammatory acne is treated symptomatically. Treatment consists of (1) removing excess sebum from the skin by washing and (2) promoting the production and turnover of new skin to prevent closure of the pilosebaceous orifices of the hair follicle. The skin should be washed with warm water, mild soap, and a soft washcloth, no more than three times daily. The washing and rubbing will produce some drying and peeling of the skin. Closure of the pilosebaceous orifices can be prevented by the topical application of mildly irritating agents, which will promote desquamation (peeling) and stimulate growth of new skin cells.

Medicinal treatment. The most common OTC

desquamating agents are *sulfur* (2% to 10%), *resorcinol* (1% to 4%), and *salicylic acid* (0.5% to 2%). Resorcinol and salicylic acid often appear in alcoholic solutions that dry quickly and do not leave a visible film. Some products contain all three ingredients.

Dosage forms of these drugs include creams, lotions, gels, and liquids. Ointment bases tend to be greasy and messy. Some soaps include desquamating agents, but this formulation is irrational because rinsing and drying will remove the agents from the skin.

Benzoyl peroxide is a stronger irritant and desquamating agent than are sulfur, resorcinol, or salicylic acid. Used in concentrations of 5% to 10%, it generally produces mild stinging and warming of the skin. For most acne problems benzoyl peroxide is probably no more effective than the milder agents and should be used only after the milder irritants and faithful adherence to a regular schedule of skin washing have been unsuccessful. Benzoyl peroxide is highly irritating and should not come in contact with the eyelids, neck, or lips. Its use should be discontinued if severe and prolonged stinging or irritation occurs.

More serious forms of acne require treatment with medications available only by prescription. Antibiotics may be used topically or orally in low doses. A drug called isotretinoin may be effective in severe cases when the patient is unresponsive to other therapy.

Topical Antiinfective Drugs

Antifungal products. Several common tineal (fungal) infections of the skin generally respond to self-medication with OTC products, although responsiveness depends on several factors. These factors include the strain of fungus, the site of the infection, and the severity and duration of the infection. The microorganisms most often responsible for superficial tinea infections in humans are found in these genera: *Trichophyton, Microsporum, Epidermophyton,* and *Candida.* All but *Candida* infections can be treated with OTC antifungal products (Chapter 36). Moreover, the products are effective only for acute superficial infections. Chronic and extensive infections will respond slowly, if at all, and will often require the attention of a physician. Fungal infections of the toenails or fingernails and those that have penetrated the hair shafts will also generally respond poorly to OTC antifungal products. The nurse should exercise care in selecting or recommending OTC antifungal medications. If the condition involves an apparent tinea infection of the foot (athlete's foot), groin, or

scalp, reasonably rapid results can be expected from OTC products. Suspected fungal infections of other body regions should be referred to a physician.

OTC antifungal preparations include *keratolytic agents, fungistatic agents,* and *fungicides.*

Keratolytic preparations include *selenium sulfide* and *Whitfield's ointment* (Whitfield's ointment contains benzoic acid, 6%, and salicylic acid, 3%). These agents irritate the skin and cause peeling of the superficial layers to expose deeper sites of infection to other antifungal compounds. Selenium sulfide stops cellular growth when it is applied in concentrations of 1% to 2%. It is a common and effective ingredient in antidandruff preparations.

Fungistatic agents include *fatty acids* and *salicylanilide. Sodium propionate* and *undecylenic acid* are fungistatic fatty acids. Sodium propionate is effective in 1% solution and 5% ointment. Undecylenate is effective as the acid (5%) and as the zinc salt (20%). It is commonly employed as an ointment, powder, or spray for the relief of tinea pedis (athlete's foot).

The *fungicidal* drug tolnaftate is effective against the majority of superficial fungal infections except *Candida* species. Tolnaftate is sold in powder, liquid, cream, spray, or gel (all 1%). Relief of itching occurs within several days, but complete suppression of the infection generally requires 2 to 3 weeks of treatment. If the skin is rough and scaly, prior treatment with a keratolytic agent to remove the scale will improve the effectiveness of tolnaftate.

Antibacterial products. OTC antibacterial preparations have been the subject of controversy and review by the FDA. At present, the antibiotic drugs available without a prescription include *bacitracin, neomycin, polymyxin B sulfate, tetracycline hydrochloride, chlortetracycline hydrochloride,* and *oxytetracycline hydrochloride.* The FDA OTC Panel on Antimicrobial Drugs recognizes two classifications of product: skin wound antibiotics and skin wound protectants. The former includes products for the treatment of overt skin infections; the latter refers to products with antibiotics added to prevent the subsequent infection of a wound and the growth of organisms in the product. As of 1979, all OTC antibiotics sold as skin wound antibiotics were classified in category III (i.e., insufficient data to enable determination of safety and/or efficacy). All but neomycin sulfate were classified as safe and effective (category I) for use as skin wound protectants. (These antibiotics are discussed in Chapters 32 and 33.)

When used as directed, the OTC topical antibiotics are generally safe. However, their low concentration in the available products makes their effectiveness against skin wound infections questionable. Bacitracin, neomycin, and polymyxin B sulfate are nephrotoxic if absorbed systemically. With ordinary topical use, such toxicity is rare. Nevertheless, the risk is real and, in view of the questionable topical efficacy of the drugs and their allergenicity, their use is not recommended.

Hemorrhoidal Products

Humans, as the result of environment, heredity, and posture, suffer from a number of painful anorectal disorders, the most prevalent of which is hemorrhoids. Hemorrhoids are varicosities produced by increased pressure in the hemorrhoidal veins. In addition to upright posture itself, hypertension, coughing, pregnancy and labor, physical exertion, straining during defecation, and rectal carcinoma all can contribute to the formation of hemorrhoids. These varicosities, which can occur within or outside the anorectal line, are associated with a variety of symptoms such as itching, burning, inflammation, and swelling. Mild pain and discomfort are common, but bleeding, prolapse of an internal hemorrhoid, and severe chronic pain are symptoms that require the attention of a physician.

OTC products for the treatment of anorectal disorders are intended for the symptomatic relief of pain, itching, and burning. They contain a variety of pharmacological agents, including *local anesthetics, vasoconstrictors, antiseptics, astringents, emollients/lubricants, keratolytics, anticholinergics,* and a variety of miscellaneous agents such as *counterirritants* and *"wound-healing" agents*.

The FDA OTC Panel on Hemorrhoidal Drug Products has ruled on the efficacy of these agents. Antiseptics, "wound healers," and anticholinergics have all been classified as ineffective (category II) in hemorrhoidal products.

Local anesthetics have been judged effective for relief of the itching and burning of hemorrhoids. Of the many local anesthetics available, only two have been shown to be both safe and effective: *benzocaine* (5% to 20%), and *pramoxine HCl* (1%).

Three *vasoconstrictor drugs*—*ephedrine sulfate, epinephrine hydrochloride,* and *phenylephrine hydrochloride*—have been judged effective for the symptomatic relief of hemorrhoidal itching and swelling, although conclusive evidence of effectiveness on swollen hemorrhoidal tissue itself is lacking. Presumably, the vasoconstrictor drugs directly constrict the vascular smooth muscle in the anorectal area.

A variety of *emollients/lubricants (protectants)* have been recommended for use in hemor-

rhoidal preparations. These include *calamine, cocoa butter, cod liver oil, glycerin, mineral oil, petrolatum, shark liver oil,* and *zinc oxide*. All can be administered to the rectum externally and internally except glycerin, which is intended for external use only. Petrolatum may be the most effective of these agents. To be effective, the total protectant concentration of an OTC hemorrhoidal product should be 50%.

Mildly *keratolytic agents,* such as *aluminum chlorhydroxy allantoinate,* have some value in relieving the itching and burning of hemorrhoids. Their usefulness is confined to the external anal tissues, but stronger agents, such as resorcinol and sulfur, are not recommended.

Astringents coagulate skin cell protein, thereby protecting underlying skin cells from dehydration and irritation. *Calamine zinc oxide* and *hamamelis water* (witch hazel), have been judged effective for the relief of hemorrhoidal itching, irritation, and pain. Calamine and zinc oxide may be applied externally and internally to anorectal tissue, whereas hamamelis water is intended for external use only.

Antiseptics are no more effective than washing with soap and water for the prevention of anorectal infections. Indeed, they may adversely alter the normal bacterial flora in that region.

Anticholinergic drugs (e.g., atropine; see Chapter 9) are of dubious value in OTC hemorrhoidal preparations. These drugs are not absorbed through the skin and, if applied to the external anal tissues, do not relieve itching or pain. They can be absorbed across the rectal mucosa, however, and in sufficient dosage can interfere with autonomic nerve function throughout the body. There is no evidence that a local or systemic anticholinergic effect is of any value in the treatment of hemorrhoids.

A *counterirritant drug* distracts from the discomfort of itching, irritation, and pain by stimulating local nerve endings to provide a sensation of warmth, tingling, or coolness. Counterirritation forms the therapeutic basis for the relief of minor muscle aches and pain by OTC remedies that provide "deep-heating" and "penetrating" warmth. In reality, these remedies do not directly affect muscles. Instead, their effects are localized to the skin, where they stimulate local sensory nerve endings. However, since no sensory nerves occur in the rectal mucosa, there is no rational basis for including a counterirritant in an internal hemorrhoidal preparation. A counterirritant may, on the other hand, provide temporary relief of pain and itching if applied externally to the anorectal region. At present, *menthol* is the only recommended counterirritant for external hemorrhoidal preparations. Camphor, oil of turpentine, and hydrastis have been included in various products, but they are considered to be too toxic even for external use or of unproven efficacy.

"Wound-healing agents" include an extract of brewer's yeast, skin respiratory factor (SRF), cod liver oil, and vitamins A and D. No convincing evidence of their effectiveness as wound healers has been found, and until such evidence emerges their value in the treatment of hemorrhoids is questionable.

OTC products for the treatment of hemorrhoids and other mild anorectal disorders are provided in a variety of dosage forms. These include ointments, creams, suppositories, pads, and foams.

Ointments (oil base), *creams* (water soluble), and *gels* are equally effective in delivering active ingredients to the affected areas. Devices such as the "pile pipe," a tube having lateral exit ports, are useful for applying the medication directly into the rectum.

Suppositories are not particularly useful for the treatment of hemorrhoids. They may slip beyond the affected site, releasing their active ingredients in contact with healthy mucosa. In addition, with suppositories the degree of coverage of the affected area may be erratic and cannot be controlled. Finally, because suppositories must melt to release their active ingredients, relief of painful symptoms is delayed.

Foams provide no advantages over ointments and creams; moreover, they are messy.

Personal hygiene and normal bowel habits are important in the successful treatment of hemorrhoids. Many physicians recommend regular sitz baths or soaking with astringent solutions as an adjunct to the use of OTC products for the relief of mild itching and burning sensations. In addition, the diet should be adjusted to avoid either excessively loose or compact stools.

SUMMARY

Over-the-counter (OTC) medications are medicinal agents deemed safe enough for sale without a prescription. The distinction between prescription and OTC drugs was legislated in 1952. OTC medications are evaluated by the Food and Drug Administration and assigned to one of three categories: category I, recognized as safe and effective; category II, not recognized as safe and effective; category III, additional data required to establish safety and/or effectiveness.

OTC medicines often contain low, even subtherapeutic, doses of drugs. Low doses provide some assurance against drug toxicity, but they also limit the number of people who will actually benefit from taking the medicine.

OTC products may also contain several drugs in combination. Combination products provide convenience but have the disadvantage of including drugs that may not be necessary and having doses that cannot be individually controlled. Fixed combinations of drugs also increase the risk of adverse drug interactions.

Cold remedies may contain decongestants, antihistamines, analgesics, and other drugs. Several sympathomimetic drugs are used as nasal decongestants. Antihistamines are more appropriate for the treatment of allergic conditions than for colds. Analgesic drugs are often present in cold remedies in subtherapeutic doses.

Cough remedies consist of expectorants and antitussive drugs. They are appropriate only for the suppression of nonproductive coughs. Expectorants increase secretions in the respiratory tract, but their antitussive effectiveness is questionable. The most effective OTC antitussive drugs are codeine and dextromethorphan. They suppress the reflex cough center in the brain. Codeine is a narcotic drug and has some abuse potential. Dextromethorphan is nonnarcotic and has no abuse potential. Another effective antitussive drug is diphenhydramine, an antihistamine. Because it can cause marked sedation and drowsiness, it is less useful than either of the other two drugs.

OTC weight control products are phenylpropanolamine, bulk-producing agents, and benzocaine. Phenylpropanolamine suppresses appetite in experimental animals, but its effectiveness in humans is questionable. It also produces central nervous system stimulation and high blood pressure if the recommended dosage is exceeded. Bulk-producing agents induce a feeling of fullness and may briefly suppress appetite if taken before meals. Benzocaine is a local anesthetic of unproven effectiveness as an aid to weight control. OTC weight control agents are all of limited effectiveness at best. They are of no help to people who are unwilling or unable to reduce their caloric intake.

OTC sleeping aids contain an antihistaminic drug alone or in combination with an analgesic drug. Antihistamines are effective for the treatment of mild insomnia because they produce drowsiness and sedation. Analgesic drugs are included in some OTC sleep aids because pain may contribute to insomnia in some people.

OTC ophthalmic products include eyewashes, artificial tears, and decongestants. Eyewashes are isotonic buffers. Artificial tears also include a viscosity-increasing agent. Decongestant preparations contain a sympathomimetic drug to reduce redness in the eye or conjunctiva by constricting blood vessels.

OTC acne medications are primarily intended to promote desquamation (peeling), thereby preventing closure of pilosebaceous orifices. This action helps to prevent the formation of comedones (pimples and inflamed, plugged hair follicles). In addition to acne medication, the treatment of non-inflammatory acne includes a program of regular skin washing. The effectiveness of antibacterial or antiseptic soaps for this purpose is doubtful, and their use is not recommended.

Tinea (fungal) infections of the skin can be treated with a variety of OTC products including keratolytic, fungistatic, and fungicidal agents. Keratolytic agents promote peeling of the skin and allow infected lower skin layers to be penetrated by fungistatic or fungicidal medicines.

OTC topical antibiotics have limited usefulness in treating or preventing infections of the skin.

OTC hemorrhoidal products may contain local anesthetics, vasoconstrictors, antiseptics, astringents, emollients/lubricants, keratolytics, anticholinergics, counterirritants, and wound-healing agents. Wound-healing agents are ineffective. Antiseptics and anticholinergic agents are not recommended. Local anesthetics can relieve local itching and burning, as can vasoconstrictors, astringents, emollients, and counterirritants.

STUDY QUESTIONS

1. The present laws that regulate the OTC drug industry have evolved from which law?
2. The Durham-Humphrey Amendment to the 1938 law created two classes of drugs. What are they?
3. What does the Kefauver-Harris amendment to the 1938 law require?
4. FDA review panels on OTC drugs classify the drugs according to three categories. List them.
5. List the advantages and disadvantages of fixed-ratio combination drug products.
6. Name the ingredients of OTC cold remedies.
7. What are the major side effects of antihistaminic drugs?
8. List the OTC expectorant drugs.
9. Name the available OTC cough suppressants.
10. Which drugs are used in OTC products for the treatment of obesity and weight control?
11. Phenylpropanolamine is related to which drugs? What are its side effects?
12. What is the rationale for the use of a bulk-producing agent in a weight control product?
13. What drugs are available in OTC sleep aids?
14. List the classes of ingredients in OTC ophthalmic products.
15. What precautions should be exercised in the use of OTC ophthalmic products?
16. List the commonly available OTC drugs for treatment of acne.
17. OTC antifungal products include which drugs?
18. Distinguish between keratolytic, fungistatic, and fungicidal drugs.
19. Which antibiotics are currently available in OTC preparations?
20. List the ingredients of OTC hemorrhoidal products and describe their actions.

SUGGESTED READINGS

Abcarian, H., and Muldoon, J.P.: When hemorrhoids threaten flare-up, Patient Care **15**(16):16, 1981.

American Pharmaceutical Association: Handbook of Non-Prescription Drugs, ed. 6, Washington, D.C., 1979, The Association.

Benowicz, R.J.: Non-prescription drugs and their side effects, New York, 1977, Grosset & Dunlop.

Hess, P.: Chinese and Hispanic elders and OTC drugs, Geriatr. Nurs. **7**(6):314, 1986.

Hurwitz, S., Kligman, A.M., and Rosenberg, E.W.: How to individualize acne therapy, Patient Care **17**(14):133, 1983.

Johnson, J.E., and Moore, J.: The drug-taking practices of the rural elderly, Appl. Nurs. Res. **1**(3):128, 1988.

Kaufman, J., and others: Over the counter pills that don't work, New York, 1983, Pantheon Books, Inc.

Law, J.: Fatal doses . . . over the counter sales of drugs, Nurs. Times **83**(44):20, 1987.

Lund, M.E.: Over-the-counter overdose, Emerg. Med. **15** (8):177, 1983.

Ries, D.T., and others: Over-the-counter medications: quicksand for the elderly, J. Community Health Nurs. **3**(4):183, 1986.

Shalita, A.R.: A stepped-care approach to treating acne, Mod. Med. **51**(1):90, 1983.

Trainor, P.A.: Over-the-counter drugs: count them in, Geriatr. Nurs. **9**(5):298, 1988.

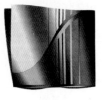

Care of the Poisoned Patient

5

Overview

Toxicology is the study of poisons. A poison is a chemical substance that injures or kills when introduced into the body. There are literally thousands of potential poisons. Drugs, household and industrial chemicals, plants, pesticides, carbon monoxide, and heavy metals are the major agents of poisoning seen in clinical practice.

Poison control centers, located in communities throughout the United States, are usually identified in local telephone books. These centers provide the lay public and health professionals with information on the appropriate first aid and clinical management of suspected poisoning. Large poison control centers may also offer specialized poison treatment and consultation. Educational services such as professional training and poison prevention education for the public may also be offered. In the early 1980s approximately 1.5 million cases were being handled yearly by the poison control centers. About 150,000 of these cases were reported to the Food and Drug Administration, Division of Poison Control. Only about 10,000 of these reported cases required a hospital visit and only 70 cases were fatal. Of cases reported to poison control centers, 60% are typically children under 5 years of age, but only 10% of the deaths occur in this age group. These statistics highlight the tendency of young children to ingest pills, cleaning agents, and plants. Among children under 5 years old, poisoning is the fifth leading cause of death.

The U.S. mortality from poisoning of all types has been reported at approximately 12,000 deaths per year recently. Of these, about half are suicides and half are accidental. Less than 50 deaths per year are considered homicides.

Clinical toxicology is the study of care of the poisoned patient. Poisoning can be acute, subacute, or chronic, depending on the dose, length of exposure, and extent of tissue injury. In this chapter the primary emphasis will be on the acutely poisoned patient. Acute poisoning is usually the immediate and direct result of a single excessive dose. Acute poisoning in children is most commonly caused by the ingestion of plants, drugs, or household products. In adults acute poisoning is often the result of a drug overdose. About 70% of adult drug overdose cases involve a CNS depressant, commonly alcohol (23%) or a benzodiazepine (24%). Alcohol and benzodiazepines greatly potentiate the toxic effects of each other or other CNS depressants.

TOXICODYNAMICS AND TOXICOKINETICS

The general principles of toxicology are those of pharmacology extended to excessive doses. (The principles relating drug dosage to drug action are discussed in Chapter 2). The same factors that control pharmacokinetics and pharmacodynamics also apply to toxicology.

Toxicodynamics describes the harmful effects that a poison produces on the body. The graded dose-response curves described in Chapter 2 relate to toxic effects as well as therapeutic effects. Therefore the symptoms of poisoning reflect the dosage of the poison. Treating the poisoned patient is frequently a complicated matter because the dose of the poison is seldom known with any accuracy and, further, because the identity of the poison itself may not be known. Therefore a thorough assessment of the patient is especially important in cases of poisoning. If the nature of the poison is known, the severity of the symptoms shown by the patient will be important in monitoring the course of treatment. If the nature of the poison is not known, the symptoms become vital in suggesting the nature of the poison. The application of toxicodynamics to the poisoned patient is demonstrated in Table 5.1, which lists symptoms and gives the common poisons that can cause them.

Toxicokinetics deals with the action of a poison in the patient as a function of time. This encompasses the absorption, distribution, localization, biotransformation, and elimination of the poison. The kinetics of a drug overdose, however, is not necessarily that of the therapeutic dose. This is so because a large dose of drug may saturate and overwhelm one or more of the mechanisms controlling absorption, distribution, biotransformation, and elimination of therapeutic concentrations of the drug. Moreover, normal physiological processes, such as heart rate, blood pressure, or respiration, may be compromised and thereby alter the disposition of the drug overdose. In this chapter toxicokinetics is presented as embodying the major steps in the care of the acutely poisoned patient. These steps include nonspecific antidotes to remove poison not yet absorbed, specific antidotes to counteract a few select poisons, and, occasionally, diuresis or dialysis.

CARE OF THE ACUTELY POISONED PATIENT

Nonspecific Antidotes (Table 5.2)

Decontamination. Decontamination is the removal or neutralization of a toxin. If the toxin is on the clothing, skin, or eyes (e.g., insecticide spray), the clothing should be removed and the skin scrubbed well with soap and water. The eyes should be washed with a copious amount of warm water. If the patient has inhaled a noxious gas, that individual should be given fresh air or oxygen to breathe. When a poison or drug overdose has been swallowed, much of it usually remains unabsorbed for some time. In treating poisoned patients, it is common to flush the poison from the gastrointestinal tract. Such techniques as induced vomiting (emesis), gastric lavage, administration of activated charcoal, and catharsis are appropriate to help eliminate a drug overdose that has been swallowed. The dosages for these nonspecific antidotes are listed in Table 5.2.

Emesis and lavage. The stomach is emptied either by emesis or gastric lavage. There are three major points that determine whether vomiting or gastric lavage should be used. First, induction of vomiting is not appropriate when the patient might aspirate the vomitus. Therefore, this method is contraindicated when the patient is lacking normal reflex control of gagging and vomiting and/or is unconscious or having seizures. Second, vomiting

---

┌───┐
⚡ **DRUG ABUSE ALERT: IPECAC**

BACKGROUND

Normally ipecac is administered to induce vomiting in an acute poisoning. Ipecac is readily obtained in a drug store. Chronic administration of ipecac is abuse. This is seen in some child abuse cases and in some cases of eating disorders. In eating disorders, ipecac may be taken to purge ingested food.

PHARMACOLOGY

Ipecac (emetine) is a safe drug for inducing vomiting in emergency home use. Administered chronically, however, ipecac can produce many chronic symptoms. These may not be readily associated with ipecac abuse. Most of these symptoms relate to distorted electrolyte imbalances that arise from continual vomiting and loss of gastric fluids. The active alkaloid of ipecac also has a direct depressive action on heart and skeletal muscle.

HEALTH HAZARDS

Symptoms of continued ipecac administration include chronic diarrhea and vomiting, muscle weakness, colitis, cardiomyopathy, fever, edema, and electrolyte disturbances. Therapy for ipecac abuse is supportive while ipecac is discontinued.
└───┘

is not indicated when the regurgitated material can be damaging to the esophagus or lungs. Such material includes acids, bases, and nonaromatic or nonhalogenated hydrocarbons (oils and solvents). Third, induction of vomiting can take 20 to 30 minutes and therefore should not be used when time is critical.

The emetic of choice is *ipecac syrup*, which will induce vomiting within 30 minutes in 90% of treated patients. With this agent 20% to 60% of the stomach contents can be emptied. *Apomorphine* is another emetic, but it must be prepared at the time of use and it causes respiratory depression. Apomorphine is usually effective within 1 to 15 minutes of administration. Emetics such as salt water (sodium chloride), mustard water, and copper sulfate are considered dangerous and ineffective. When vomiting is induced, the vomitus should be saved for analysis.

Gastric lavage is the preferred method of emptying the stomach in adults. The airway is first protected by an endotracheal tube. Use of a large-bore tube such as an Ewald or Burke tube allows tablets to be retrieved. Gastric lavage is less successful in children because a small-bore tube must be used. Tablets from some drug formulations partially deteriorate and then coalesce in the stomach to form a mass of undissolved drug that is too large

Table 5.1 Physical Symptoms Produced by Common Poisons

Symptoms	Poisoning agent	Symptoms	Poisoning agent
MENTAL/MOTOR		MENTAL/MOTOR—cont'd	
Drowsiness, coma	Acetaminophen		Heavy metals
	Alcohols		Hydrocarbons
	Antihistamines		Sedative-hypnotics
	Carbon monoxide		Tranquilizers
	Insulin		
	Opioids (codeine, others)	CARDIOVASCULAR/RENAL	
	Salicylates	Pulse rate increased	Alcohols
	Scopolamine		Amphetamine
	Sedative-hypnotic drugs		Aspirin
	Tranquilizers		Atropine
	Tricyclic antidepressants		Cocaine
			Parasympatholytics
Excitation, twitch-ing, convulsions	Aminophylline		Sympathomimetics
	Atropine		
	CNS stimulants	Pulse rate de-creased	Digitalis
	Carbon monoxide		Opioids
	Cyanide		Parasympathomimetics
	Local anesthetics		
	Organophosphate insecticides	Hypertension	Amphetamine
	Phenothiazines		Sympathomimetics
Agitation, delirium	Alcohols	Hypotension	Alcohols
	Aminophylline		Aminophylline
	Atropine		Aspirin
	LSD (lysergic acid diethylamide)		Muscarine
	Lead		Nitrates, nitrites
	Marijuana		Opioids
	PCP (phencyclidine)		Sedative-hypnotics
	Physostigmine		Tranquilizers
Paralysis	Botulism	Oliguria, anuria	Carbon tetrachloride
	Heavy metals		Ethylene glycol
			Heavy metals
Ataxia (motor in-coordination)	Alcohols		Methanol
	Anticonvulsants		Mushrooms
	Carbon monoxide		Petroleum distillates
	Hallucinogens		

to be washed out and yet is poorly soluble. Lavage is continued until the return is clear. It should be noted that the first wash is saved for analysis.

Activated charcoal. After emesis or lavage a slurry of activated charcoal may be administered through the lavage tube or a nasogastric tube, or it may be given orally. Because activated charcoal will absorb and inactivate ipecac, it should not be given until after vomiting has occurred. Activated charcoal absorbs a number of drugs and chemicals and thereby prevents their absorption into the body. The charcoal itself, with absorbed chemicals, is eliminated in the feces. Administration of acti-vated charcoal is most effective if given within the first few hours of poisoning. If the poisoning is known to be caused by acetaminophen, activated charcoal should not be given. The antidote for acetaminophen is acetylcysteine, which is ab-sorbed by activated charcoal.

Cathartics. Cathartics are the final common treatment to reduce absorption of poisons from the gastrointestinal tract by hastening their elimina-tion. The preferred cathartics are *sodium sulfate, magnesium sulfate,* or *magnesium citrate.* How-ever, magnesium citrate should not be used after charcoal administration because the citrate can dis-place poisons from charcoal. Oil-based cathartics such as mineral oil and castor oil are not used in

Table 5.1   Physical Symptoms Produced by Common Poisons—cont'd

Symptoms	Poisoning agent	Symptoms	Poisoning agent
ORAL/GASTROINTESTINAL		PUPILLARY—cont'd	
Acetone odor	Acetone Alcohol Salicylates	Constricted pupils	Mushrooms Organophosphate insecticides Opioids
Almond odor	Cyanide	Nystagmus	Sedative-hypnotics
Garlic odor	Arsenic Dimethyl sulfoxide Phosphorus Organophosphate insecticides	DERMATOLOGICAL Jaundiced skin	Arsenic Carbon tetrachloride Mushrooms Naphthalene
Dry mouth	Amphetamine Antihistamines Atropine Opioids Phenothiazines	Flushed skin	Alcohol Antihistamines Anticholinergics
Excessive salivation	Arsenic Corrosives Mercury Mushrooms Organophosphate insecticides	Cherry red skin PULMONARY	Carbon monoxide Cyanide Nitrites
Heavy vomiting	Aminophylline Corrosives Food poisoning Heavy metals Salicylates	Rapid breathing	Amphetamine Carbon monoxide Methanol Petroleum distillates Salicylates
PUPILLARY Dilated pupils	Alcohols Anticholinergics Antihistamines CNS stimulants CNS depressants	Depressed respiration	Alcohol Opioids Sedative-hypnotics Tranquilizers
		Wheezing	Mushrooms Opioids Organophosphate insecticides Petroleum distillates

treating poisoned patients because these oils can speed systemic absorption of some poisons. Cathartics are especially indicated under these circumstances: when enteric-coated tablets have been ingested, when poisoning occurred 1 hour or more previously, or when hydrocarbons have been ingested.

Specific Antidotes (Table 5.3)

A specific antidote is one that directly reverses the toxic action of the poison. In only 5% of poisoning cases is there a specific antidote (see table listing).

Competitive antidotes. A specific antidote may compete at the receptor for the toxin. *Naloxone* displaces narcotics (opioids) at the opioid receptor.

Unlike other opioids, naloxone does not depress the respiratory center; therefore the occupation of the opioid receptor by naloxone protects against respiratory depression. *Oxygen* in high concentration competes with carbon monoxide in binding to hemoglobin to restore oxygenation. *Atropine* blocks the muscarinic receptor from the acetylcholine accumulated in anticholinesterase poisoning.

Chelates. Another category of action of specific antidotes is chelates, compounds that form a nontoxic complex with the toxin. Poisoning by heavy metals in particular is treated with chelates, which form a nontoxic complex with the metal; this complex is quickly eliminated, usually in the urine. Accumulation of the heavy metal is thereby reversed. *Dimercaprol* complexes arsenic, copper,

Table 5.2   Nonspecific Antidotes

Antidote	Trade name	Administration/dosage	Comments
EMETICS			
Ipecac	Ipecac syrup	ORAL, in 8 oz water: *Children 6 mo-1 yr*—10 ml. *Children 1-2 yr*—15 ml. *Adults*—30 ml. Vomiting in 30 min in 90% of patients. May repeat dose after 20-30 min if no vomiting has occurred.	Give only to conscious patients who have gag reflex and are not likely to aspirate vomitus. Do not give when vomitus will itself be injurious (acids, bases, hydrocarbons). Patients should be encouraged to drink water. Water will distend stomach and make it more susceptible to action of ipecac. Walking also helps to induce vomiting. Average return of stomach contents is 20%-60%. Keep vomitus for analysis.
Apomorphine	Apomorphine HCl	SUBCUTANEOUS: *Children*—0.066 mg/kg. *Adults*—0.1 mg/kg.	May cause CNS and respiratory depression or protracted vomiting, which are treated with 0.005 mg/kg naloxone HCl. Keep vomitus for analysis.
GASTRIC LAVAGE			
Water: 0.45% saline 0.9% saline		BY GASTRIC TUBE: *Small children*—10 ml/kg. *Adults*—300 ml.	If patient is in deteriorating condition, unconscious, prone to seizures, or lacking a gag reflex, nasotracheal intubation is necessary before lavage to protect airway. Use large-bore (28-40 French Ewald or Burke orogastric lavacutor) tubing to allow aspiration of tablets. Keep first wash for analysis. Continue washings until return is clear (2-20 L). Administering more than recommended volume will distend stomach and may induce vomiting.
Activated charcoal	Charcoalanti-Dote, Liquid-Antidose	ORAL OR BY GASTRIC TUBE: *Children*—15 to 30 g in 4-8 oz water. *Adults*—25 to 50 g in 8-16 oz water.	Administer as a slurry within first hours of poisoning, after induced vomiting (charcoal will inactivate ipecac) or gastric lavage. Do not use with acetylcysteine in management of acetaminophen poisoning. Do not use magnesium sulfate as cathartic.
CATHARTICS			
Sodium sulfate, 10% solution		ORAL: *Children*—1 to 2 ml/kg. *Adults*—150 to 250 ml.	Preferred cathartic for treating poisoned patients. Contraindicated if patient has heart failure or hypertension.
Magnesium sulfate (Epsom salts), 10% solution		ORAL: *Children*—1 to 2 ml/kg. *Adults*—150 to 250 ml.	Magnesium salts should not be used if patient has renal failure. Citrate should not be used if activated charcoal has been given.
Magnesium citrate, 10% solution		ORAL: *Children*—1 to 2 ml/kg *Adults*—150 to 250 ml	Magnesium salts should not be used if patient has renal failure. Citrate should not be used if activated charcoal has been given.

Table 5.3 Specific Antidotes

Antidote	Poison	Administration/dosage	Comments
Atropine	Anticholinesterase Organophosphates Physostigmine	INTRAVENOUS: *Children*—0.05 mg/kg. *Adults*—0.2 to 2 mg. This is initial dose. Repeat every 20 min until copious secretions are controlled.	Blocks muscarininc receptors to prevent peripheral actions of excessive concentrations of neurotransmitter, acetylocholine. See Chapter 9 for more information on actions of acetylcholine and how atropine blocks actions of acetylcholine. Muscarinic symptoms for whilch atropine is given include nausea, vomiting, diarrhea, sweat, increased bronchial and salivary secretions, and slow heart rate (bradycardia).
Pralidoxime chloride (PAM, PROTOPAM)	Anticholinesterase Organophosphates	Organophosate poisoning: BY INFUSION in 100 ml saline over 15 to 30 min: *Children*—20 to 40 mg/kg. *Adults*—1 to 2 gm. A second dose can be given in 1 hr. Carbamate (neostigmine, pyridostigmine) poisoning. INTRAVENOUS: *Adults*—1 to 2 gm initially, followed by 250 mg every 5 min as necessary to reverse cholinergic crisis.	Reactivates enzyme acetylcholinesterase after inactivation by irreversible anticholinesterases or organophosphates. This allows acetylcholine to be degraded and relieves paralysis (overstimulation) caused by accumulated acetylcholine. Pralidoxime acts mainly outside CNS. In organophosphate poisoning, pralidoxime is given to restore neuromuscular function, especially to relieve paralysis of respiratory muscles. Atropine is given concurrently (see above) to relieve depression of respiratory center and to reverse muscarinic stimulation. In overdose by carbamate anticholinesterases (neostigmine, pyridostigmine and ambenonium, drugs for myasthenia gravis), pralidoxime antagonizes effects of these drugs on neuromuscular junction.
Physostigmine salicylate (Antilirium)	Antimuscarinic anticholinergic	INTRAVENOUS or INTRAMUSCULAR: *Adults*—0.5 to 2 mg. INTRAVENOUS: *Children*—0.5 mg by slow (1 min) infusion. Repeat if needed at 5-10 min intervals until desired effect, or 2 mg total dose, is reached.	Reversible anticholinesterase that increases concentration of acetylcholine at its receptor sites. Reverses both CNS and peripheral anticholinergic effects. Useful for reversing toxic anticholinergic effects due to overdose of atropine and other belladonna alkaloids, tricyclic antidepressants, phenothiazines, and antihistamines. Central anticholinergic effects include anxiety, delirium, disorientation, hallucinations, hyperactivity, seizures, and—in the extreme—coma, medullary paralysis, and death. Peripheral anticholinergic toxic effects include fast heart rate (tachycardia), fever, mydriasis (dilated pupils), vasodilation, urinary retention, decreased secretions, and decreased gastrointestinal motility.
Naloxone (Narcan)	Narcotics (opioids), including pentazocine, propoxyphene, diphenoxylate	INTRAVENOUS: *Adults*—0.4 to 2 mg. Additional doses are repeated at 2-3 min intervals until patient responds or until 10 mg is given. INTRAVENOUS: *Children*—0.01 mg/kg with 0.1 mg/kg as subsequent dose. May also give INTRAMUSCULARLY or SUBCUTANEOUSLY.	Reversible antagonist of opioid receptor. Useful for reversing narcotic depression, including respiratory depression. Naloxone is preferred because it is a pure opioid antagonist and causes no respiratory depression of its own. Naloxone is effective within 2 min and has duration of action of 1-4 hours. Since most opioids have a longer duration of action, effects of naloxone may wear off and patient may relapse, requiring additional naloxone.

Continued.

Table 5.3 Specific Antidotes—cont'd

Antidote	Poison	Administration/dosage	Comments
Ethanol	Methanol Ethylene glycol	INTRAVENOUS: *Adults*—0.6 gm/kg + 7-10 gm over 1 hr; then 10 gm/hr maintenance. *Children*—0.6 gm/kg + 4-5 gm over 1 hr; 5 gm/hr maintenance.	All three alcohols are metabolized by aldehyde dehydrogenase. Ethanol is preferred substrate and thereby blocks metabolism of methanol and ethylene glycol to toxins formaldehyde and formic acid (both alcohols) and oxylate (ethylene glycol). Ethanol is given in additional loading dose to achieve blood level of 100 mg/dl.
Amyl nitrite Sodium nitrite Sodium thiosulfate (Cyanide Antidote Package)	Cyanide	Amyl nitrite: Crush ampule on gauze and have patient inhale vapor. Sodium nitrite: Inject 10 ml of 3% solution after IV line is established. Sodium thiosulfate: Inject 50 ml of 25% solution after administration of sodium nitrite.	Cyanide has almond odor. Toxicity of cyanide is caused by its blockage of enzymes using oxygen in mitochondria (cytochrome oxidase), thereby depressing cellular respiration. Inhibition of cytochrome oxidase depends on binding of cyanide to ferric iron in cytochrome oxidase. Nitrite converts ferrous iron in hemoglobin to ferric iron, producing methemoglobin. This large pool of ferric iron in blood competes with cytochrome oxidase for cyanide, thereby restoring cellular respiration. Thiosulfate accelerates conversion of cyanide to relatively nontoxic thiocyanate, which is readily excreted in urine.
Acetylcysteine (Mucomyst)	Acetaminophen	ORAL: 140 mg/kg as 5% solution mixed with soda, water, or grapefruit juice. Follow with 17 maintenance doses of 70 mg/kg every 4 hr.	Acetylcysteine restores sulfhydryl groups depleted by acetaminophen metabolism. This prevents toxicity to liver produced by metabolites of acetaminophen. Acetylcysteine should not be given with activated charcoal because charcoal absorbs it.
Deferoxamine mesylate (Desferal)	Iron	INTRAMUSCULAR, CONTINUOUS SUBCUTANEOUS, or SLOW INTRAVENOUS: *Adults*—1 gm initially, 0.5 gm at 4 and 8 hr. Further doses if needed, up to 6 gm daily. For IV, do not give at rate greater than 15 mg/kg/hr. Administer IM if possible. *Children*—50 mg/kg IM or IV every 6 hr up to 15 mg/kg/hr by continuous IV. Maximum dosage: 6 gm/24 hr or 2 gm/dose.	Chelates iron and thereby prevents free iron from entering cells and inhibiting chemical reactions. Chelate or iron and deferoxamine is rapidly excreted in urine, removing iron from body.

lead, and mercury. *Penicillamine* is used to complex copper, lead, and mercury (see Chapter 23). *Deferoxamine* is a specific chelate for iron (see Chapter 22). *EDTA* is the chelate used for lead or cadmium intoxication.

Antibodies. In a few instances treatment with specific antibodies to the poison is possible. Antibodies to digoxin are available to counteract toxic levels of this important cardiac drug. These antibodies reverse the cardiac toxicity by complexing the digoxin and lowering the large pool of digoxin that is bound to plasma albumin. The digoxin then is not free to act. Antivenoms are antibodies for certain snake and spider venoms.

Metabolic alterations. Specific antidotes may alter the metabolism of a toxin. *Ethanol* inhibits

Table 5.3   **Specific Antidotes—cont'd**

Antidote	Poison	Administration/dosage	Comments
Dimercaprol (BAL)	Arsenic Gold Mercury Lead	INTRAMUSCULAR: Because dimercaprol is an oil, give deep intramuscularly only. Mild arsenic or gold poisoning: 2.5 mg/kg 4 times daily, 2 days; 2 times, day 3; once daily, 10 days. Severe arsenic or gold poisoning: 3 mg/kg every 4 hr for 2 days, 4 times day 3; twice daily 10 days. Mercury poisoning: 5 mg/kg initially; 2.5 mg/kg 1-2 times daily for 10 days. Acute lead poisoning: 4 mg/kg alone initially, then at 4 hr intervals with calcium disodium edetate (administered at separate site) Maintain for 2-7 days.	Dimercaprol is a sulfhydryl compound that chelates arsenic, gold, and mercury and promotes their excretion in urine. Dimercaprol also reactivates affected sulfhydryl enzymes. Peak plasma concentrations occur 30-60 min after administration. Excretion is complete in 4 hr. Dimercaprol is not very effective for poisoning caused by antimony and bismuth. It is contraindicated in iron, cadmium, and selenium poisoning because chelates are more toxic, expecially to kidney, than metal alone. Alkalinization of urine protects kidney from breakdown of dimercaprol-metal complex in acid urine. Common side effects of dimercaprol are rise in blood pressure with tachycardia (fast heart rate) and burning sensation of lips, mouth, and throat.
Edetate calcium disodium (Calcium Disodium Versenate)	Lead	INTRAVENOUS: 50-75 mg/kg/day in 3-6 doses, each dose administered over at least 1 hr. Can continue for up to 5 days. Wait 2 days before resuming therapy for an additional 5 days. INTRAMUSCULAR: Preferred route for children. Give 35 mg/kg twice daily. After 3-5 days discontinue for 4 or more days.	Calcium bound to EDTA is displaced by lead and resulting chelate is excreted in urine (50% in 1 hr: 95% in 24 hr). EDTA can produce toxic effects, including renal damage and irregularities in cardiac rhythm. Doses must be carefully monitored.
Penicillamine (Cuprimine, Depen, Titratabs)	Copper Lead Zinc Mercury	ORAL: *Adults*—1-1.5 gm daily in 4 divided doses on empty stomach for 1-2 months. *Children*—30-40 mg/kg daily or 600-750 mg/M^2 daily for 1-6 months.	Penicillamine chelates copper, lead, zinc, or mercury, promoting their excretion in urine. Side effects include allergic reactions (principally rashes) and loss of sweet and salt tastes. Severe side effects include bone marrow depression and renal toxicity.

the biotransformation of methanol and ethylene glycol to toxic metabolites, particularly formic acid. *Thiosulfate* enhances the transformation of cyanide to the relatively nontoxic thiocyanate. *Acetylcysteine* restores the sulfhydryl groups of the liver after depletion by acetaminophen metabolism. Sulfhydryl groups protect the liver from toxic metabolites of acetaminophen. *Physostigmine* inhibits acetylcholinesterase, the enzyme that normally degrades acetylcholine. This action allows acetylcholine concentrations to rise at the synapses and compete with anticholinergic drugs blocking these receptors. This reversal by acetylcholine restores function in anticholinergic poisoning by drugs that are either anticholinergic, such as atropine or scopolamine, or have anticholinergic actions, such as antihistamines, tricyclic antidepressants, and antipsychotic drugs. Used as an antidote, *pralidoxime* reactivates acetylcholinesterase after it has been inactivated by an anticholinesterase poi-

THE NURSING PROCESS

POISONING

Assessment

Patients who have been exposed to poisons or have ingested poisons may enter the health care system in any condition, from the child who is alert, oriented, and feeling fine after ingesting a handful of children's vitamins to the patient who requires resuscitation or is comatose and unable to provide any information about the toxic substances. All cases of suspected overdose or poisoning must be treated carefully and thoroughly. Assessment must be complete, but the kind and amount of data that can be obtained in the first few minutes will vary with the immediate condition of the patient. Assessment may include vital signs, blood pressure, complete physical assessment, weight (the dose of many antidotes is based on weight), serum electrolyte levels, liver and renal function studies, blood gases, and electrocardiogram. Equally important in some situations is the patient's history, which may need to be obtained from friends or relatives, and which includes information about the poison(s) ingested (how much, when, what efforts have been tried as treatment) and any relevant preexisting health problems.

Potential nursing diagnoses

Appropriate nursing diagnoses must be developed after the patient assessment. The alert individual who has ingested a small amount of a substance may experience only anxiety related to the situation as a whole, and altered comfort: nausea and vomiting from use of ipecac. A comatose patient may have diagnoses such as ineffective airway clearance related to drug overdose, potential for aspiration, and many potential complications.

The establishment and maintenance of a patent airway and adequate ventilation is always the first priority. What should be done next will vary with the patient's condition. Based on the findings from the assessment, other measures might include supportive care of the unconscious, administration of nonspecific or specific antidotes, and hospitalization for further observation or treatment. Continuous cardiac monitoring may be appropriate, as well as monitoring the vital signs and blood pressure, initiating and maintaining intravenous therapy, measuring intake and output, continued monitoring of appropriate laboratory work (blood gases, liver and renal function studies, serum levels of suspected toxin(s) and/or antidotes), insertion of a nasogastric or orogastric tube for gastric lavage, or induction of vomiting, and so on. The patient and the family should be kept informed of actions being taken and their effect.

Evaluation

Effective treatment for overdose or exposure to toxins occurs when the poisonous substance is eliminated and the patient returns to normal without experiencing side effects associated with the poison or treatment. Sometimes this is easy, such as when the dose of poison is small and relatively nontoxic and treatment has been initiated promptly. Most antidotes will not be administered on an outpatient basis. Before discharge, the patient and the family should be instructed about continuing care or observations that should prompt them to return to the health care facility. If appropriate, instructions about removing toxic substances from the home or workplace should also be given. In some situations referral to the social service department or a community-based nursing care agency may be helpful.

PATIENT CARE IMPLICATIONS

General guidelines for care of patients who have been poisoned

- Assess thoroughly and completely any patient suspected of having ingested a toxic substance, or a toxic amount of a generally nontoxic substance. If the patient's condition obviously requires emergency treatment, the initial assessment may be abbreviated until the patient is stabilized, then further assessment performed. Data in the assessment may include blood pressure and vital signs, neurological examination, level of respiratory effort, presence of cyanosis, breath sounds, electrocardiogram, complete visual inspection, including nose and mouth, blood gases, serum electrolytes, renal and liver function tests, and weight. Obtain a detailed history from the patient and family about the suspected toxic agents, including the amount, how long ago the substance was ingested, efforts made to induce vomiting or dilute the substance, age of the patient, and any coexisting medical problems. Save any samples of the toxic substance, vomitus, or stool; label carefully, and send to the laboratory for analysis.
- Work quickly and efficiently to administer prescribed antagonists or other treatments, but remain calm. Reassure the patient and family that everything possible is being done. Families of children may be especially upset.
- Nurses who work in settings where overdoses or toxic ingestions are commonly seen (e.g., emergency departments, some occupational health settings) should know the following: location of emergency equipment for intubation, assisted ventilation, and resuscitation; telephone number of the nearest poison control center; location of reference guides to emergency treatment of overdoses; location of antidotes, antagonists, and equipment (e.g., lavage tubes) used in that setting, and general procedures to be followed in treating overdose.
- Prevention of overdose is preferable to treatment for overdose; however, preventive health teaching is usually not appropriate during treatment of acute overdose. In working with any patients or families in situations involving drugs or toxic chemicals, general safety measures should be reviewed on a regular schedule. Teaching points to review with patients and families to help prevent accidental ingestion of medicines or toxic household chemicals include: keep medications out of the reach of children, the incompetent, or the confused; keep medications in a locked cabinet; keep household products out of reach of children; keep drugs and chemicals in clearly and correctly labeled containers; use safety latches on cabinets and drawers; never refer to medicines as candy; treat all medicines with respect; use child-proof caps when children are in the environment; use drugs only as prescribed; never double or increase the dose of any drug unless specifically directed to do so by the physician.
- Teach patients never to borrow medications prescribed for another person.
- Ipecac is available in small quantities without a prescription and should be kept in the home (out of the reach of children) for emergency treatment of overdose. However, teach families to call the poison control center before administering ipecac to ascertain that inducing vomiting is appropriate for the ingested substance.
- Teach patients to keep the number of the poison control center handy, near the telephone.
- Instruct patients or families calling for emergency help to bring a sample of the drug or toxic substance, and any vomitus, to the emergency department when they bring the patient.

Ipecac

Drug administration/patient and family education

- Ipecac may be purchased without prescription and may be kept in the home. Do not administer ipecac until directed to do so by the physician and/or poison control center. Any ipecac remaining after a dose has been administered should be discarded. Check expiration dates.
- Drink a full glass of water (8 oz) after taking the ordered dose (1/2 to 1 full glass for a child). A scared child may do better if the water is administered before the ipecac. Avoid milk products.
- Generally, if vomiting does not occur after the first dose, the dose is repeated in about 20 minutes. If vomiting does not occur after the second dose, take the patient to the emergency department.
- Do not give this drug to infants under 6 months of age. Children 6 months to 1 year should be treated in the emergency room.

Continued.

PATIENT CARE IMPLICATIONS — cont'd

Ipecac

Drug administration/patient and family education—cont'd

- If activated charcoal is also prescribed, take the ipecac first, and use the activated charcoal after vomiting has ceased.
- Do not induce vomiting in anyone who is drowsy, as it may predispose to aspiration.
- Save vomitus and send it to the laboratory for analysis.

Apomorphine hydrochloride

Drug administration

- Apomorphine is more effective if the stomach is full. Before administering the dose, have the patient drink a full glass of water (8 oz for an adult, 1/2 to 1 glass for a child). Bouncing a small child gently may also help stimulate vomiting.
- If activated charcoal is also prescribed, administer the apomorphine first, and use the activated charcoal after vomiting has ceased.
- Apomorphine is related to morphine, so it produces many of the same side effects, including drowsiness and CNS depression. As with morphine, the antagonist in the event of overdose is naloxone. Keep naloxone readily available when apomorphine is used. Apomorphine is contraindicated in anyone allergic to morphine.
- Do not administer the solution if its color is green or brown.
- Save vomitus and send it to the laboratory for analysis.

Gastric lavage

Drug administration

- Review the information presented in Table 5.2.
- Follow agency policy and procedure for insertion of an orogastric or nasogastric tube. Insert a large-bore tube to permit tablets or precipitated material to be recovered. It is *absolutely essential* that correct placement of the tube be verified before any fluid is introduced via the tube. Use a syringe to aspirate for stomach contents; auscultate over the stomach as a small amount of air (5 to 10 ml) is injected through the tube. The nurse should hear a popping or gurgling noise as the air is forced into the stomach.
- Place the patient in a sitting or semi-Fowler position during lavage. Slowly inject a large quantity of fluid (300 to 500 ml in an adult),

then slowly aspirate the fluid. Alternate injection and aspiration until the return is clear. Tap water may be used as an irrigant in adults, but 0.9% or 0.45% saline should be used in young children.
- Provide mouth care at the completion of the procedure.

Activated charcoal

Drug administration

- This substance is most effective when administered within 30 minutes of ingestion of the poison.
- The slurry is unattractive. Try putting the mixture into an empty soft-drink can to administer to children. Mix charcoal with water or a small amount of fruit juice. Do not mix with ice cream or milk as these foods will decrease the ability of the charcoal to absorb the toxin.
- Activated charcoal adsorbs ipecac; do not administer these simultaneously.
- Caution patients that activated charcoal may cause feces to turn black.

Cathartics

Drug administration

- See Chapter 13 for additional information about saline cathartics.
- Do not use sodium salts if the patient has a history of heart disease. Do not use magnesium salts if the patient has a history of renal failure. Do not use magnesium sulfate if activated charcoal has been administered.

Atropine

- See Chapter 9 for additional information about atropine.

Pralidoxime chloride

Drug administration

- Review the information presented in Table 5.3.
- Keep a suction machine and intubation equipment readily available when using this drug.
- See Chapter 11 for a discussion of myasthenia gravis. Keep edrophonium, atropine, syringes, and a tourniquet handy when working with patients with myasthenia gravis.
- Monitor patients carefully. Side effects of pralidoxime may mimic effects of ingested substances: dizziness, blurred vision, diplopia, drowsiness, nausea, tachycardia, hyperventilation, and muscle weakness.

PATIENT CARE IMPLICATIONS — cont'd

Physostigmine salicylate

Drug administration

- Review the information presented in Table 5.3.
- Monitor vital signs and blood pressure.
- Treat overdose with atropine, which should be kept at the bedside.
- Since the drug has a short duration of action (30 to 60 minutes), it may be necessary to repeat doses; monitor the patient carefully.
- May be administered intravenously undiluted. Administer at a rate of 1 mg or less over 1 to 3 minutes (adult) or 0.5 mg per minute (child).

Naloxone

Drug administration

- Monitor respirations. Naloxone should promptly increase the respiratory rate and volume. If it does not, the respiratory depression is probably not the result of narcotic overdose, or multiple agents were consumed or injected.
- Keep intubation and resuscitation equipment and drugs readily available when patients manifest respiratory depression.
- Monitor vital signs and blood pressure. Naloxone has a relatively short half-life, and the dose may need to be repeated. Remember that in narcotic addicts this drug may precipitate withdrawal symptoms.
- Monitor neonates carefully. Naloxone may be used to treat neonatal respiratory depression, which may be present if narcotic analgesics were administered in large doses during labor and delivery, or if the mother is a narcotic addict. If the mother is an addict, naloxone will precipitate withdrawal symptoms in the infant.

Ethanol

Drug administration

- Ethanol can be administered intravenously, or via orogastric or nasogastric tube. Orally, a 20% solution is preferred in order to reduce the risk of gastritis, but, if needed, any blended whiskey can be used. If the patient's condition warrants it, oral administration is preferred because the intravenous route is limited to 5% and 10% solutions.
- Monitor blood ethanol levels during therapy.
- Monitor vital signs and blood pressure, and electrocardiogram. When using ethanol for treatment of overdose, keep a suction machine and equipment for intubation and resuscitation at the bedside.

Cyanide antidote package: amyl nitrite, sodium nitrite, sodium triosulfate

Drug administration

- This combination of drugs is recommended for cyanide poisoning and also for treatment of overdose with sodium nitroprusside (see Table 5.3 and Chapter 15).
- Side effects are rare. Monitor vital signs and blood pressure.

Acetylcysteine

Drug administration

- Review Table 5.3 and see Chapter 26.
- Monitor vital signs and blood pressure. Side effects due to acetylcysteine are rare, and include nausea, vomiting, and increase in blood pressure.
- Acetylcysteine has a very bad odor. Try having patient take doses through a straw placed in a cup or container that is tightly capped.

Deferoxamine mesylate

Drug administration

- Monitor blood pressure and vital signs, fluid intake and output, and serum iron levels. Rapid intravenous administration may cause hypotension, tachycardia, erythema, and urticaria. Anaphylactic reactions are rare, but keep epinephrine and intubation and resuscitation equipment handy.
- In acute iron poisoning, treat with deferoxamine as well as lavage and/or induction of emesis, maintain a patent airway, control shock (IV fluids, vasopressors), and correct acidosis (administer sodium bicarbonate or other drugs).
- Intramuscular injection is the preferred parenteral route. Reconstitute powder with 2 ml of sterile water for injection; dissolve all powder before injecting dose.
- After subcutaneous injection, some patients experience a local histamine-like reaction.
- Reserve IV injection for patients exhibiting signs of shock. Reconstitute powder as above, then further dilute with a compatible IV solution. Administer at a rate not exceeding 15 mg/kg/hr.

Patient and Family Education

- Advise patients on long-term therapy to have regular ophthalmic examinations.

Continued.

PATIENT CARE IMPLICATIONS — cont'd

Deferoxamine mesylate

Patient and Family Education—cont'd

- Usually, discontinue chelation therapy during pregnancy. Advise women considering pregnancy to consult their physicians.
- Warn patients that deferoxamine may turn urine red.

Dimercaprol

Drug administration

- Review Table 5.3.
- Monitor vital signs, blood pressure, intake and output.
- Do not administer medicinal iron to patients receiving dimercaprol.
- Avoid skin contact with the drug when preparing doses; wear gloves.
- Keep the urine alkaline to facilitate chelation. Monitor the urine pH.
- For detailed instructions in preparing oil-based suspensions, see Chapter 6.

Patient and family education

- Warn patients that the drug may produce a garlic-like odor to the breath.
- Warn parents that some children have a fever during therapy.

Edetate calcium disodium

Drug administration

- Read orders carefully. Do not confuse edetate calcium disodium used to treat lead poisoning, with edetate disodium, used to treat hypercalcemia.
- Assess urine output before administering. Because the chelate is excreted in the urine, patients with oliguria or renal disease may be unable to tolerate this drug.
- Monitor vital signs, blood pressure, blood urea nitrogen, urinalysis, serum electrolytes, serum creatinine, and intake and output, as well as the electrocardiogram.
- Edetate calcium disodium interferes with the duration of action of zinc insulin preparations. Diabetics who are receiving zinc insulin may need a change in dosage or drug while they are receiving edetate calcium disodium.
- Intramuscular injection is the preferred route of administration in children and in individuals with lead encephalopathy. Procaine may be added to the reconstituted solution to help prevent pain at the injection site.
- Assess the mouth and gums for development of sores. These should subside after drug therapy. Zinc replacement may be necessary between courses of therapy with edetate calcium disodium.

Penicillamine

- Review Table 5.3. Penicillamine is also used to treat rheumatoid arthritis, as discussed in Chapter 23.

---

son. The poison is freed in an inactive form to be eliminated.

Diuresis and Dialysis

Diuresis. Diuresis can be used to hasten elimination of poisons excreted primarily by the kidneys. Diuresis is used when the level of poison in the blood is at a potentially fatal concentration, when the patient is in a coma, and when the patient otherwise has stable cardiovascular, respiratory, and renal function. *Fluid diuresis*, achieved with a potent loop diuretic such as furosemide, increases the glomerular filtration rate and thereby decreases the renal tubular reabsorption of the poison. *Osmotic diuresis* with mannitol or urea prevents reabsorption of the poison in the kidney by creating an osmotic load that effectively flushes the kidney tubule. *Alkalinization* of the urine with sodium bicarbonate enhances the excretion of weak acids such as aspirin and phenobarbital by maintaining them in their ionized form, which is not reabsorbed readily. Similarly, *acidification* of the urine with ammonium chloride or ascorbic acid aids the excretion of weak bases such as amphetamine or phencyclidine by maintaining them in their ionized form, which is not reabsorbed. Diuretics are discussed fully in Chapter 16.

Dialysis. Dialysis is indicated in cases of extreme poisoning or renal failure when the poison is dialyzable. For instance, the anticoagulant warfarin and the cardiac glycoside digitoxin are tightly protein bound in the blood and therefore are not successfully removed by dialysis. *Hemodialysis* is a highly technical and complex procedure in which the blood is shunted from the body and through tubing immersed in physiological buffer. Any chemical present in the blood but not in the buffer diffuses into the buffer because of the concentration gradient. The blood so dialyzed, or "washed," is continuously returned to the body. Salicylate, methanol, and ethylene glycol are especially effectively removed by hemodialysis. *Hemoperfusion* is a relatively new technique in which the blood is pumped from a venous catheter through a column of absorbent material and returned to the patient. Anticoagulation with heparin is necessary to prevent the patient's blood from clotting in the cartridge. Hemoperfusion is effective for high-molecular-weight poisons with poor water solubility because the cartridge has a large surface area for absorption. *Peritoneal dialysis* is the simplest dialysis technique, but, unfortunately, it is the most inefficient in removing the majority of drugs. In peritoneal dialysis physiological buffer is introduced into the abdomen and left there for several hours before being drained and replaced. Because the gastrointestinal tract has a rich blood supply, the blood is dialyzed as it flows through the normal gastrointestinal network.

SUMMARY

Toxicology is the study of poisons. Drugs, household and industrial chemicals, plants, pesticides, carbon monoxide, and heavy metals are the major agents of poisoning seen in clinical practice. In local communities poison control centers provide information on the appropriate first aid for and clinical management of suspected poisoning.

Clinical toxicology is the study of care of the poisoned patient. Poisoning can be acute, subacute, or chronic, depending on the dose, length of exposure, and extent of tissue injury. Acute poisoning is usually the immediate and direct result of a single excessive dose. The principles relating drug dosage to drug action are similar for both pharmacology and toxicology. Toxicodynamics describes the harmful effects of the poison on the body as a function of dose. Since doses of poisons are seldom known with any accuracy, patient assessment is especially important in cases of poisoning. Toxicokinetics encompasses the absorption, distribution, localization, biotransformation, and elimination of the poison.

Nonspecific antidotes are frequently administered in order to remove poison not yet absorbed. If the poison has been swallowed, the stomach may be emptied by inducing vomiting with ipecac. Vomiting is not desirable if the patient might aspirate the vomitus, if the poison is corrosive, or if time is critical. Gastric lavage is the preferred method of emptying the stomach in adults because the tubing used can be large enough to remove undissolved tablets. Activated charcoal will absorb many poisons, preventing their absorption into the body and promoting their excretion in the feces. Cathartics such as sodium sulfate, magnesium sulfate, or magnesium citrate may be administered to hasten the elimination of unabsorbed poisons.

Specific antidotes exist for only about 5% of poisons. A specific antidote directly reverses the toxic action of the poison. Antidotes such as naloxone, oxygen, and atropine compete with the poison for the specific cellular receptor at which the poison is acting. Chelates such as dimercaprol, penicillamine, deferoxamine, and EDTA bind heavy metals and thereby render the metals nontoxic. Antibodies to digoxin and snake venoms specifically complex these poisons. Antidotes such as ethanol, thiosulfate, acetylcysteine, physostigmine, and pralidoxime specifically alter the metabolism of certain poisons to render them less harmful.

Diuresis may be used to hasten the elimination of poisons excreted primarily by the kidneys when the patient is stable but has a potentially fatal concentration of poison in the blood. Alkalinization of the urine with sodium bicarbonate speeds the excretion of drugs that are weak acids, whereas acidification of the urine with ammonium chloride or ascorbic acid aids the excretion of drugs that are weak bases. If the kidneys have failed, dialysis may be used to remove some poisons in critical cases; techniques include hemodialysis, hemoperfusion, and peritoneal dialysis.

STUDY QUESTIONS

1. Define toxicology and clinical toxicology.
2. Determine if your community has a poison control center. What services are offered by this center?
3. What is toxicodynamics? Why is patient assessment so important in treating poisoning?
4. What is toxicokinetics? How does this differ from pharmacokinetics?
5. What is the role of nonspecific antidotes in treatment of acute poisoning?
6. Contrast the uses of emesis and gastric lavage in emptying the stomach. What is the drug of choice for inducing vomiting? Why?
7. When is the administration of activated charcoal indicated? When is it not indicated?
8. What is the role of cathartics in treating acute poisoning? Which drugs are recommended? Why?
9. Describe specific antidotes in each of the fol-

lowing categories: competitive, chelate, antibody, metabolic.

10. When is diuresis indicated in treating acute poisoning? Describe fluid and osmotic diuresis and alkalinization and acidification of the urine and when these processes may be helpful.

11. When is dialysis indicated in treating acute poisoning? Describe hemodialysis, hemoperfusion, and peritoneal dialysis.

SUGGESTED READINGS

Burt, S.D.: Mercury toxicity: an overview, AAOHN J 34(11):543, 1986.

Davis, N.M., and Cohen, M.R.: Today's poisons: how to keep them from killing your patients, Nursing 89 19(1):49, 1989.

DiPalma, J.R.: Human toxicity from rat poisons, Am. Fam. Physician 24:186, 1981.

Drugs, Nursing 90 Books, Springhouse, Pa., 1990, Springhouse, Inc.

Goldfrank, L., Flomenbaum, N., and Weisman, R.S.: General management of the poisoned and overdosed patient, Hosp. Physician 17:24, 1981.

Hanenson, I.B., editor: Quick reference to clinical toxicology, Philadelphia, 1980, J.B. Lippincott Co.

Hathaway, B.K.: Toxicology: an overview, AAOHN J 34(11):518, 1986.

Heller, M.: Overdoses, Am. Fam. Physician 31(4):141, 1985.

Howry, L.B., Bindler, R.M., and Tso, Y.: Pediatric medications, Philadelphia, 1981, J.B. Lippincott Co.

Joubert, D.W.: Use of emetics, adsorbents, and cathartic agents in acute drug overdose, J. Emerg. Nurs. 13(1):49, 1987.

Kaye, S.: Handbook of emergency toxicology, ed. 4, Springfield, Ill., 1980, Charles C Thomas.

Lucy, J.S.: 49 poison plants: what to watch for—what to do, Mod. Med. 49:183, 1981.

Mancini, R.E.: Principles and practices of clinical toxicology, Kalamazoo, Mich., 1983, Upjohn Co.

Miller, M.: Combating caustic substance poisoning, Nursing 87 17(6): 32BB, 1987.

Milstein, M.J., and others: Efficacy of oral N-acetylcysteine in the treatment of acetaminophen overdose. New Engl. J. Med. 319(24):1557, 1988.

Mofenson, H.C., and Caraccia, T.R.: Toxidromes, Compr. Ther. 11(2):46, 1985.

Newton, M., and others: Specific treatments of poisoning by household products and medications, J. Emerg. Nurs. 13(1):16, 1987.

Nielsen, M., and Henry, J.: ABC of poisoning, Brit. Med. J. 289:681, 1984.

Saxena, K.: Acute poisoning: management protocol, Postgrad. Med. 71:67, 1982.

Senanayake, N., and Karalliedde, L.: Neurotoxic effects of organophosphorous insecticides. New Engl. J. Med. 316 (13):761, 1987.

Snyder, D.S.: Digoxin immune Fab ovine, Crit. Care Nurse 8(8):10, 1988.

Thurkauf, G.E.: Acetaminophen overdose, Crit. Care Nurse 7(1):20, 1987.

U.S. Department of Health and Human Services: Bulletin of the National Clearinghouse for Poison Control Centers 25(6), 1981.

Weston, W., III: Childhood poisoning, treating an avoidable disaster, Consultant 23:250, 1983.

Drug Administration

6

At its best, the administration of drugs to patients is an opportunity for the nurse to add to the data base through additional patient assessment, to teach the patient in preparation for self-management of the health condition, to participate in discharge planning with the patient, and to evaluate the effectiveness of the plan of care being implemented by the health care team. At its worst, administration of drugs is a psychomotor task, which, when done carelessly or in haste, can result in errors, inefficient use of time, and possible harm to the patient.

The purpose of this chapter is to present information and techniques that can assist the nurse in providing safe, individualized patient care. For additional information about topics covered in this chapter, see fundamentals of nursing texts, institutional policy and procedure manuals, and the readings at the end of the chapter.

RIGHTS OF DRUG ADMINISTRATION

Traditionally, the teaching of principles of drug administration has centered around the five rights of drug administration (see p. 74): the right drug, via the right route, in the right dose, at the right time, to the right patient. Although at first glance it might seem that these rights should be easy to achieve, the day-to-day practice of nursing requires thoughtful attention to these rights at all times.

The **right drug** suggests not only that the patient receive the drug that was prescribed but also that the patient receive the right drug for the particular health problem. The nurse must pay careful attention to drug orders and medication labels while preparing drugs and be familiar with each patient and the health care problems of that patient. In order to know if a prescribed drug is an appropriate one for a patient, the nurse must know and understand the patient's health problems and be

current in pharmacological knowledge. The rest of this book is devoted to providing basic material about drugs, but in practice the nurse must also regularly consult printed materials as well as other health care professionals for additional information. Some of these sources are discussed in Chapter 7.

In ensuring that the patient receives prescribed medications via the **right route,** the nurse must know well each medication that is administered. The student may have difficulty understanding how or why a nurse could administer a medication via the wrong route, but in a busy nurse's day errors can occur easily. Consider the following situation: An experienced nurse who usually works in the coronary care setting is asked to work for a day in the surgical intensive care unit. The nurse, accustomed to administering morphine intravenously for cardiac pain, administers all parenteral pain medications in the surgical intensive care setting intravenously also (they had been ordered to be given intramuscularly). Fortunately, in this true incident the nurse discovered the errors and reported them, and no harm came to the patients. Errors are discussed in greater detail later in this chapter.

Administering the **right dose** of medication is extremely important. Not only must the nurse double check calculations for mathematical accuracy; the nurse also must ask the question "Is this dose an appropriate one for the size and age of the patient?" This responsibility again emphasizes the need for the nurse to have current knowledge about drugs and their usual dosage ranges. Although the administration of an incorrect dose is serious for any patient, it can be particularly serious in the pediatric patient, for whom prescribed doses are often small. A review of dosage calculations can be found in Chapter 7.

Ensuring that the patient receives drugs at the

right time may be difficult. Often the health care team must weigh the information available about the pharmacokinetics and pharmacodynamics of drugs (discussed in Chapter 2) against the patient's life-style and potential for compliance. In the critical care setting, where one nurse may care for one or two patients, drugs are administered at evenly spaced intervals throughout a 24-hour period. The nurse, although usually very busy, can concentrate on administering medications to a few patients. On a busy general care unit the nurse may have 20 or more patients who must receive drugs, and these patients may be coming and going to the radiology department, therapy, or surgery. In addition, most patients would prefer not to be wakened at night to receive medications. In the home setting it is even easier for the patient to forget a dose or be less careful about intervals between doses. Another factor in the home setting is general life-style. For example, patients who work a night shift and sleep during the day may need help determining the right times to take drugs.

Other factors that influence the right time include whether the patient is receiving multiple drugs, whether a drug can be taken on an empty or full stomach, or whether a prescribed drug can be taken concurrently with other medications. In order to help ensure that patients receive drugs at the right time, the nurse must be knowledgeable about the patient, the health care problems, and the drugs.

Finally, it must be the **right patient** who receives the drug. The nurse must check the patient's identity each time drugs are administered. Not only should the patient be Mr. Smith, but it must be the *right* Mr. Smith. The right patient also means that the right drugs were prescribed for the right patient, and thus the nurse is back to the first of the five rights of drug administration.

PERSONNEL: WHO DOES WHAT?

Many people may be involved in the prescription, preparation, and administration of a drug to a patient. Generally, physicians are the individuals who prescribe drugs. Their authorization to prescribe is granted through licensing and medical practice acts. There are other individuals who do prescribe, including dentists and oral surgeons, osteopaths, podiatrists, nurse practitioners, midwives, and physician's assistants. However, the degree of independence of practice that these and other health care practitioners may exercise varies with laws of the state, province, or nation. This fact introduces the first of many points that the nurse must consider before administering a drug: Who has prescribed the drug, and is that person

---

THE FIVE RIGHTS OF DRUG ADMINISTRATION
The RIGHT drug
The RIGHT route
The RIGHT dose
The RIGHT time
The RIGHT patient

---

recognized to have the legal right to do so in that setting?

In the institutional setting safeguards are often in effect to help prevent unauthorized prescribing of drugs. For example, in order to be granted privileges to practice in an individual hospital, a physician must present appropriate credentials, proof of licensure, and other documents required by that hospital. After a nurse has worked on a nursing unit for several weeks, the physicians will become known to the nurse, which also helps reduce the chance of errors in who may prescribe. Even in the hospital, though, the nurse must be certain of the role of each person on the health care team. For example, in some teaching hospitals it is customary for medical students to have rotations as acting interns (they may have other titles also). These individuals are not yet licensed, yet they may be caring for patients under the supervision of licensed preceptors (physicians). The nurse must be clear about the legal ramifications of administering drugs prescribed by a nonlicensed individual.

In looking for guidance about who may prescribe and whose prescriptions the nurse must administer, the nurse has several sources of information. The first is the nurse practice act (or comparable professional practice act) for that state, province, or country. The second source is the written policies of the employing agency or institution. Finally, nurses must consider their own moral and ethical codes of conduct in deciding whether to administer a specific drug to a patient. The nurse always has the personal right to refuse to administer a medication. For example, a nurse may refuse to give an ordered medication if professional judgment indicates the dose is excessively high. The nurse must notify the physician, and the nurse in charge, of the decision not to administer the medication.

It is important for the nurse to remember that the legal constraints the nurse must consider may have less meaning to the patient. This situation is faced more often in the home setting, where the patient may wish to have the nurse administer a medication or home remedy prescribed or recommended by someone not recognized by the nurse practice act.

Pharmacists, who usually dispense medication, are licensed to do so and are governed by legal statutes. Pharmacies often employ aides or technicians to help in the filling of prescriptions, but these individuals function under the supervision of the registered pharmacist. The pharmacist is an excellent source of information for the nurse or the patient but is often underused in this role.

Who administers drugs varies from state to state and situation to situation. Registered nurses are allowed to administer medications within the legal framework of the nurse practice act. Licensed practical nurses and licensed vocational nurses also have practice acts that regulate the role they play in drug administration. In some areas pharmacists, medication technicians, medical students, emergency medical technicians, or others may administer drugs as employees of an institution or agency. Various students may be permitted to administer drugs in an agency, institution, or other setting if supervised. This includes students in nursing, medical, physician assistant, emergency medical technician, and other educational programs. In the home setting the patient and the family administer drugs.

In summary, the nurse must understand the legal framework establishing who may prescribe, who may dispense, and who may administer drugs.

INSTITUTIONAL POLICIES AND PRACTICES

The nurse practices not only within the legal framework of the practice act but also within the policies and procedures of the employing agency. The nurse is responsible for reading carefully any written information that defines restrictions or expectations of practice within the employing agency structure. Of course, the nurse should not blindly adhere to policy that is in direct conflict with legal guidelines or reasonable ethical and moral standards, but neither should the nurse practice outside the role defined by the agency. Four examples are used here to illustrate this point.

In some agencies verbal orders for drugs may be taken only by registered nurses; students, licensed practical nurses, and others may not take these orders. Some institutions prohibit the nurse from obtaining the patient's informed consent for investigational drugs; this consent may be obtained only by the physician. In other settings the physician alone may administer investigational drugs. A final example is that medication orders written by medical students may be administered only after they are cosigned by a licensed physician. Such policies often develop as an interpretation of the law or to prevent anticipated problems.

A second set of procedures often developed in an agency are a response to previous problems or errors that have occurred. A few examples include: all heparin and insulin doses must be checked by two nurses before they may be administered; any parenteral drugs administered to pediatric patients must be checked by two nurses before being administered; narcotics must be counted at the end of each shift, by two nurses, one from the ending shift and one from the beginning shift.

It is not necessary for the nurse to know exactly why a policy or procedure has developed. It is important for the nurse to practice within policy and procedure guidelines and, if the guidelines need to be changed, to work through the appropriate channels to change them. The beginning nurse may view these do's and don't's as time-consuming, and some probably are not as important as others. However, all were designed to ensure safe patient care. The nurse must remember that sloppy or careless nursing practice has the potential to result in malpractice suits. Failure to adhere to stated policies and procedures may weigh against the nurse in determination of legal liability.

DRUG ADMINISTRATION SYSTEMS

The two major drug administration systems in common use in institutions today are the unit dose system and the stock drug system. In the *unit dose system* each dose of medication is individually wrapped, labeled, and supplied to the patient's unit in sufficient quantity to last 24 hours. On the patient's unit each patient has a designated drawer, box, or container, and the exact number of ordered doses of medications for a 24-hour period are placed in that container by the pharmacy daily. When the nurse prepares to administer a drug, the patient's container is checked for the dose. The labeled medication is taken to the bedside, and after the nurse verifies the patient's identity the dose package is opened, and the nurse administers the dose to the patient. This system has several advantages: the medication remains in a labeled container until the nurse is at the bedside, thus reducing the chance of getting drugs mixed up; patients can be billed by exactly the number of medication doses that are taken; and unauthorized use of medications is decreased. Some disadvantages include increased cost for the pharmacy in setting up this system; the need for additional pharmacists or pharmacy technicians to resupply the patient units each 24 hours and to fill orders for "stat" and new orders; and, often, a need for increased space in the pharmacy for stocking the drugs in the unit dose packages. The system builds in a check on the ordering of medications, as the physician's written order for drugs goes to the pharmacy to be filled, and the pharmacy then stocks the patient's supply. The nurse then checks the drug when administering it. In this way there are at least two opportunities to check the drug and dose for each patient.

In the *stock system* each patient unit is supplied with large-quantity stock containers of the drugs commonly used in that setting or institution. The nurse administering a drug takes the order sheet, Kardex, or medication card to the medication room and prepares the dose of drug from the stock supply, usually putting it into a small medicine cup. The nurse then takes the drug(s), now unlabeled, to the bedside, and after checking the patient's identity administers the prepared drug(s). The advantages to this system are that the pharmacy need not restock the floor stock daily; fewer pharmacy personnel are needed because the calculation and preparation of doses is done by the nurses; "stat" and new orders can be filled immediately because the stock drugs are on the unit. Disadvantages are that the system is usually more time consuming for the nursing staff; billing patients for exact drug use may be difficult; there can be significant waste and inappropriate use of the stock drugs (e.g., nurses and physicians using drugs for their own ailments); and medication errors are more common.

Most institutions use a combination of the two systems. For example, a hospital might supply all nonliquid oral forms in unit dose packages but have the liquid forms in multiple-dose bottles, one bottle per patient. To be effective in any specific institution, the nurse must take time to learn as much as possible about the drug administration system, so that valuable time is not lost in searching the patient unit for a drug that is available only in the pharmacy, or conversely, in calling the pharmacy for a drug available in large quantities on the patient unit.

RECORDING DRUG-RELATED INFORMATION

Recording the administration of drugs is an important responsibility of the nurse. Forms for recording drug administration vary among agencies or institutions, but the following general points usually will apply: the nurse should record that a dose was given as soon after administering the dose as possible. If a dose of medication was omitted, the reason must be noted, usually in the nurses' notes or on the form designated by the agency. Most institutions also require that doses given significantly early or late be accompanied by a notation explaining why. These forms are legal documents, and information recorded on them should be legible and accurate.

There may also be information to be recorded that is related to the route of administration or to the drug itself. A few examples include: the full-minute apical pulse, taken before a cardiotonic is administered; the blood glucose before a "sliding scale" insulin dose is administered; the site of an injection; the location of a topical nitroglycerin preparation. Often such information is recorded directly on the same form for recording that the dose was administered.

Another important kind of information relates to individualized patient care, that is, information related to the assessment, management, or evaluation of a specific patient. To give an example of each, assessment data might include the subjective and objective data that led the nurse to conclude that a "p.r.n." drug was needed: the oral temperature was 102° F., the patient was shivering, and complaining of generalized "achiness." These data lead the nurse to administer aspirin, an available p.r.n. option for that patient. Depending on the forms in use in that institution, such data might be recorded on the nurses' notes or patient progress notes. Information related to the management of a patient might become part of the care plan. An example might be that the patient tolerates physical therapy best when a p.r.n. analgesic is administered 1 hour before the scheduled physical therapy. Another kind of management information relates to the actual techniques of administration. This information might be part of the care plan, or there might be adequate room on the medication record to include this information. An example for a child or some elderly patients is that the patient will take the drug if it is crushed and mixed with a tablespoon of applesauce.

Information related to the patient's response to the medication and the effectiveness of the drug should also be recorded. This may be in the form of subjective or objective data; it would usually be recorded on the nurses' notes or patient progress notes. It is important to remember that most of the forms in the patient's record are legal documents; therefore information recorded on them must be accurate, complete, and signed by the nurse.

MEDICATION ERRORS

All medications are ordered, prepared, and administered with the best intentions. Errors do occur, however, and with surprising frequency.

What Is an Error?

Defining an error is not always easy. It is clear that an error has occurred if a patient receives the wrong drug, if a patient is overmedicated, or if a prescribed drug is omitted. There are many other situations that may or may not be called an error. Consider the following examples: the patient receives tetracycline with a glass of milk (tetracycline should not be administered with milk); a patient in the radiology department receives the 10 AM drugs at noon; through an error in calculation, the patient receives the correct drug at the correct time but in one half the ordered dose.

Some institutions differentiate between an *error* and an *incident*. Others define any deviation from policy and procedure as an error. This variability emphasizes the need for the nurse to know and adhere to the standards of practice defined by the nurse practice act, the policies and procedures of the employing agency and institution, and common sense.

The times at which drugs are administered in a hospital or institution are established by that setting; they are usually part of the policies and procedures. In addition, there is usually a definition of what is meant by administering a drug "on time." For example, a drug to be administered at 10 AM is considered to be on time if administered any time between 9:30 AM and 10:30 AM. The way in which a particular patient unit or entire institution handles deviations from the "half hour before to half hour after" rule does influence whether the time at which a particular drug is administered is called an error. Since the times for q.i.d., b.i.d., and q.d. are set by custom or policy, they also can be readjusted. Another factor that affects the time is the drug itself and how frequently it is ordered. Consider the following situations: A vitamin ordered q.d., customarily given at 10 AM, is accidentally forgotten, and given at 2 PM. Most agencies would not consider this an error and would not notify the physician. Insulin ordered for q.d. is administered at 10 AM instead of before breakfast, when it should be given; this would be an error. Another drug is ordered to be given q.i.d. On a particular unit, that is customarily 10 AM, 2 PM, 6 PM, 10 PM. A nurse misreads the medications record and administers it at 8 AM. Depending on the medication, this may not be considered an error, but the dosage times could be readjusted to 8 AM, 12 noon, 4 PM, 8 PM.

What Are the Causes of Errors?

The rest of this book could be filled with listings of errors that have occurred in the process of administering medications. A few situations involving errors are listed below:

- A drug is ordered for the wrong patient (i.e., written on the wrong patient's chart)
- The wrong dose is ordered
- The correct drug or dose is ordered, but because of poor penmanship the wrong drug or dosage is dispensed
- An error in calculating the dose is made, so the patient receives the wrong dose
- Drugs are given via the wrong route
- The patient's identity is not checked, and the wrong patient receives the drug(s)
- The first person administering a drug fails to record it immediately afterward; a second person, seeing that the drug has not been administered, also does so; the patient has received double doses of everything

What to Do If an Error Occurs

It is the mark of a professional to accept responsibility for one's own actions. First, check the patient. Obtain any subjective or objective data appropriate to the patient's condition. If the patient received the wrong drug or the wrong dose, assess the individual for the effects of the drug. For example, if too large a dose of antihypertensive was administered, take the blood pressure, then put the patient to bed. Notify the nurse in charge and the physician. Fill out any error forms required by the institution. Continue to monitor the patient. Modify personal nursing practice, if needed, to help avoid the error in the future.

Two special points need to be emphasized. The first is that the student or beginning practitioner may lack experience in handling an error or in deciding what is an error. If unsure, the practitioner should always be more conservative rather than less so; that is, always report to the nurse in charge and to the physician any problem associated with drug administration if unsure whether an error has occurred. The second point worth noting is that there are students as well as nurses in practice who want to avoid filling out "incident forms" or "medication error forms" because they think that admitting that an error has occurred will be detrimental to their employment or student status with the institution or agency. Records of errors are very helpful to institutions in trying to develop new policies, procedures, and systems that will reduce the overall incidence of errors. No hospital or agency wants to continue to employ nurses who make re-

---

---

peated errors, especially of a careless nature, but most institutions recognize that anyone can make an occasional error.

How to Avoid Medication Errors

Much of avoiding errors is using and acting on common sense. Read and adhere to institutional policies and procedures; do not try shortcuts. Read each order carefully, asking if this drug makes sense for this patient in this dose. Take the time to look up any drug or dosage that seems questionable. Never assume that the physician was right, the pharmacist was right, or the previous nurse who administered the drugs was right if there is any question.

Be particularly careful in taking verbal or telephone orders because it is easy to misunderstand what is said. The box above outlines the steps to follow in taking a verbal medication order.

Double-check calculations. If still uneasy, have a colleague or the pharmacy double check. If a dose seems incredibly large or small, double check. For example, if the order was for 10 grains of aspirin, but, through an error in recording, it is noted at 100 grains, it would require 20 aspirin tablets, an unusually large dose for a patient. The other extreme: through error, the dose of ferrous sulfate (an iron preparation) for an adult is listed as 30 mg; to administer that dose would require 1/10 tablet, an impossible task. If possible, try to avoid distractions while preparing medications. Leave medications in their labeled containers until at the bedside. Always check the patient's identity carefully. If the patient asks any questions that indicate a possible error, assume the patient is right, and double check. Examples include statements like "That doesn't look like my usual morning pill," "I already took that—Nurse Smith gave it to me earlier today," or "Dr. Jones said I would have a different pill today."

Ask about a history of allergies before administering any new drug. Finally, check each patient within a short period after administering medications.

ADMINISTERING DRUGS TO CHILDREN

Administering drugs to children presents some unique challenges. Not only may the physiological activity of the drug be altered (see Chapter 2), but the child may be unable or unwilling to participate in taking prescribed medications. For the infant and very young child, the doses may be very small, requiring special care in calculation and preparation.

A developmental approach to administering drugs should be used by the nurse who is working with children. An initial plan for drug administration should be based on knowledge about growth and development for different age groups. The child's chronological age may not match the developmental age. After the child becomes known to the nurse and the health care system, careful notation of effective individualized approaches to the child should be recorded in the patient's care plan.

To give an example of a developmental approach, consider a 2-year-old who is to receive an injection and an oral medication. First the nurse should consider available information obtained from assessing the child's general level of functioning, motor ability, interactions with other children, vocabulary, and ability to conceptualize. Then the nurse can consider theories of child development for guidance such as those of Erikson, Freud, and Piaget. The 2-year-old, in Erikson's framework, is in the stage of autonomy versus shame and doubt. Behaviors characteristic of this stage include negativism, difficulty making choices, separation anxiety, and ritual. The child shows pride in performing well, is able to feed self, and has a limited understanding of time.

A few nursing approaches that follow from this include giving simple directions; describing honestly what will occur but not until shortly before administering the medications; asking the child to administer the oral drug (but not asking "Do you want to take your medicine?" because the answer will frequently be "No!"). If possible, the child should be given a choice of beverage to accompany taking of the oral drug, but the choice should be limited (e.g., milk or apple juice). The same pattern should be followed each time drugs are administered. Firmness and consistency are important. The nurse should be prepared with adequate but nonthreatening assistance to restrain the child for the injection. The nurse also needs to give lots of positive feedback when the child cooperates and assists, provide comfort as needed, and encourage family members to do the same. The child of this age often wants to assist or cooperate but needs guidance in how to do so.

It is important to remember that children do vary, and although a developmental approach provides guidance, it does not replace individualized assessment and planning. Children also vary from adults in their ability to understand and accept the intrusive nature of many of the techniques of administration. For example, the young child may be terrified of receiving ear drops because the child cannot see what the nurse is doing to the ears. Injections are not only painful but young children may fear that their insides will come out of the hole created by the needle. The simple measure of applying a bandage over the injection site may be essential to eliminating this fear. These examples may be difficult for the adult caregiver to understand, but adults have learned the ability to reason. Adult patients dislike, even fear, injections also, but they are able to understand that the injection is fast and for their overall benefit. (The developmental approach is discussed in greater detail in the readings listed at the end of this chapter.)

The nurse should also keep in mind that children are usually very concrete in comprehension until reaching their early teens. Thus they have difficulty understanding why an injection in the thigh could help their earache. Children also have trouble understanding time relationships and thinking about long-term consequences. For example, long-term drug therapy for treating a problem such as tuberculosis, seizures, or rheumatic fever may be difficult for the young child to understand.

A few general guidelines related to techniques of administration are helpful. Do not dilute medications in a large volume of liquid or food; if the child does not finish eating all of it, the nurse is left not knowing how much has actually been consumed. Do not disguise medications in a favorite or essential food; the child may be unwilling ever to eat that food again. Do not try to trick the patient into taking medications; be honest but caring in approaching children.

Drawings, simple stories, coloring books, and toys dealing with medications and hospitalization can be useful tools in explaining to preschool and young school-age children what is happening and allowing children to play out their feelings. In a setting where children are frequently treated, the nurse may find it helpful to have available a toy box containing items such as small dolls, medicine cups, and plastic syringes without needles to allow children to "pretend," either before or after medications are administered.

Do not underestimate the ability of the child to understand or adjust to medication administration. At early ages many children can begin to accept responsibility for medication administration, especially for chronic health problems. For example, children 6 to 8 years old can be taught to self-administer insulin correctly.

ADMINISTERING DRUGS TO THE ELDERLY

The elderly patient can also present special problems to the nurse. As mentioned in Chapter 2, the physiological changes that accompany aging will influence the patient's response to medications. In addition, many older patients have accumulated a long list of prescribed drugs, so that the act of taking drugs may consume a large amount of time.

Again, individualized assessment and planning are important in working with the elderly. An important function the nurse can perform is to make certain that all medications ordered for a particular client are still necessary. It sometimes occurs that as side effects to one drug develop, an additional drug is prescribed to treat the side effects. Side effects to the second drug develop, and these are treated by a third drug. Very quickly it may be difficult for the physician, the nurse, and the patient to understand what the drug regimen is designed to do.

Another problem occasionally encountered with the elderly is the use of several health care providers, who may not be communicating with one another about the patient. Thus a patient may have, for example, an ophthalmologist, a cardiologist, a podiatrist, and a urologist, each prescribing treatments and drugs for various problems. This can result in too many drugs being taken, some of which may be antagonistic to each other or contraindicated in the presence of the others.

The nurse caring for the elderly will find that some clients have failing vision and/or hearing.

This can lead to many kinds of errors in self-medication. A similar problem is generalization by members of the health care team. Examples include assuming that confusion or lack of memory is to be expected with aging, with the result that these two symptoms (and others) are overlooked as possible drug side effects or manifestations of drug toxicity.

An elderly patient is still an adult and must be approached as any adult. The elderly individual who has taken many drugs over the years may have established an elaborate ritual associated with taking drugs. It may involve the time of day, the order in which the drugs are taken, the fluid used to swallow drugs, and so on. The nurse may wish to ask the patient about the usual practices before rushing in at 10 AM to quickly administer a handful of drugs. When possible, allowing the patient to continue the usual routine is advisable. The elderly may also be more sensitive to the frequently encountered side effect of nausea. This sensitivity, plus the fact that the patient may have to take a large quantity of drugs, may compound the nausea. It may be necessary to readjust the dosage schedule to spread out the prescribed medications over the course of the day.

An extensive amount of literature outlining problems associated with medication administration and compliance in the elderly is available. The interested reader is referred to the readings at the end of this chapter.

PATIENT EDUCATION AND MEDICATIONS

One of the major goals of nursing care in drug administration is preparation of the patient and the family for return to independent function in the home or community. This means that the patient, when able, will take over the role of self-administration of medications. No one can guarantee that the patient will take a medication exactly as directed and derive the expected benefits of drug therapy. However, careful patient assessment, planning, and teaching by the nurse can help the patient to better understand prescribed medications and how to use them safely.

Attitudes about Medicines

All patients come to the health care system with preexisting ideas and attitudes about medicines—who should take them, whether or not they are generally helpful, the meaning of sickness and health, expectations of the health care team. Additional factors include personally held beliefs, attitudes and opinions of family and friends, religious and cultural beliefs, and influence of the media about certain kinds of medications. Members of the public may not even use the same vocabulary as the health care team. For example, a nurse or physician may use the words *drug, medicine,* or *medication* interchangeably; but these words may have different connotations to the patient.

In order to be successful in preparing the patient for self-management, the nurse must attempt to assess the patient's attitudes about medicines. The nurse can do this formally by asking questions or developing an assessment tool, by remaining attuned to the patient's response to medications in the health care setting, and by attempting to validate these impressions with the patient. The nurse in the hospital or institution is generally "in control" of the medication situation, and the patient can avoid becoming very involved in the self-medication plans. The nurse in the home setting is given many more clues about patient attitudes regarding medication administration. Any plan for teaching patients about drugs will be more successful if it is compatible with the patient's existing beliefs and attitudes. It is possible to change attitudes and beliefs, but this requires careful planning, and it is often very difficult.

General Principles to Teach about All Medications

Regardless of the specific drugs prescribed for a patient, there are some general principles about drugs that patients should be taught. All drugs should be stored out of reach of children and kept in the original labeled containers. Decorative pill boxes are attractive, but many patients fill them with several drugs simultaneously. This practice provides great potential for error and may hasten decomposition of some drugs. Child-proof caps should be used unless the patient's condition makes it impossible for the patient to remain independent with the caps on. Even so, children must be protected from access to drugs. Ideally, all drugs should be kept in a locked container, out of the reach of children.

Medicines should be taken only as ordered. Patients should not "double up" to "catch up" when doses have been missed. They should not share drugs with family or friends. Patients should be warned that altering the dose size does not improve the effect: two is not better than one. If any medication is left after a particular health problem has been treated, it should be discarded. Drugs purchased over the counter should be treated with the same degree of respect as other medications; they are not to be considered less seriously just because

---

SAFE MEDICATION USE: POINTS TO REVIEW WITH ALL PATIENTS

- Take drugs prescribed for you; do not borrow drugs from others or share your own drugs with others.
- Take only the dose prescribed. If you feel the dose is too high or too low, check with the physician before adjusting the dose or frequency of doses.
- When a new drug is prescribed, find out what to do if a dose is missed. Usually, *do not* "double-up" for missed doses. Take a missed dose as soon as it is remembered, unless it is within 2 hours of the next regularly scheduled dose. Resume the regular dose schedule.
- When a new drug is prescribed, find out how to take it in relation to meals or other drugs you may be taking. Some drugs should be taken *with* meals or food, while others should be taken on an *empty stomach*.
- Each time a new drug is prescribed, find out why you are taking it, and what the common side effects are. *Never hesitate* to call the doctor if an unexpected sign or symptom develops; it may be related to the medicines you are taking.
- Store your medicines properly. Usually, this means in a dry place, but not in the bathroom, where there may be steam and moisture, as these may cause medicines to deteriorate and lose strength. Do not mix different pills in the same container, such as a pill box for your pocket or purse. This may cause the medicines to lose their strength, and without labels, you may take the wrong drug by accident.

- Write down the names of the drugs you are taking, and take this list whenever you visit the doctor, nurse, dentist, podiatrist, eye doctor, osteopath, chiropractor, or clinic. Keep all your health care providers informed of all the drugs you are taking, even those you purchase over-the-counter (without a prescription).
- Keep drugs out of the reach of children. Use child-proof caps if there are children in your home. Never refer to medicine as "candy."
- Read the label each time you take a dose of medicine to make sure you are taking the drug you think you are taking; sometimes two different drugs may look alike.
- Wear a medical identification tag, bracelet, or necklace listing chronic health problems, and medication allergies.
- Keep track of your prescription drugs. Try not to run out of them on the weekend or during holiday periods, when it may be difficult to get a prescription refilled. If your drug supply is getting low, call the physician's office. Be prepared to give the nurse the name of the drug and dose, and the name of the pharmacy and pharmacy telephone number where you wish to have the prescription filled.
- Keep the telephone number of the local poison control center near your telephone. Keep ipecac in your home, but out of the reach of children. This drug can be used to make a person vomit if a drug was taken that should not have been. Never use ipecac unless the poison control center or your doctor says you should.

---

they have not been prescribed by a physician or dispensed by a pharmacist.

Patients must be instructed to keep all health care providers informed of all drugs they are taking. Patients taking multiple drugs should keep a list of drugs and dosages, preferably with them at all times, and check it regularly to see if it is current. Patients with chronic conditions or severe allergies should be encouraged to wear a medical identification bracelet or necklace listing the allergy, medical condition, or type of medication used.

All individuals, but especially parents of small children, should keep the number of the local poison control center near the phone in the event of ingestion of or exposure to toxic kinds or amounts of drugs. Children should be taught from the beginning that drugs are not for playing; they are not "candy." This rule applies to all drugs: vitamins, birth control pills, laxatives, and other prescription and nonprescription substances. See the box on Safe Medication Use.

Information about a Specific Drug

In teaching a patient about a specific drug, the nurse must tailor the instructional approach to the needs and abilities of the patient. Careful patient assessment and analysis is the foundation of the teaching plan. Figure 6.1 illustrates a sample drug history that may be helpful in providing data for use in developing a teaching plan. This history could also be incorporated into the general health history done for all patients. It should be shortened or modified as needed.

The patient needs to know the name and dosage of the prescribed drug, why it is being used, and what the anticipated benefits of the drug are. The potential side effects should be discussed in sufficient detail that the patient will be able to list the most frequently encountered side effects. Whether the more serious (sometimes fatal, but also more rare) side effects should be discussed in detail depends on the patient and the situation. All patients and caregivers should be instructed about whom to

Name _____

Age _____ Date _____

Major health problems: _____

_____

Other health problems requiring medications: _____

_____

1. Medications used for major health problems

   These questions are only a guide. The patient's comments may lead the examiner to pursue certain topics in more detail.

   What medicines are you currently taking?

Medicine	Dose	Frequency	Comments

   Are you having problems with any of these medicines? *Go through each medicine, asking the following questions.*

   a. Are you able to take this drug the way it is ordered? What time(s) each day do you take it?
   b. Are you having any side effects? *Use words that the patient can understand, such as "Are there reasons you cannot take this medicine?" or "Are there any problems with taking this medicine?"*
   c. Do you think this drug is helping? *For example, "Is your blood pressure pill helping your blood pressure?"*
   d. If appropriate, ask about cost. *"Some patients find that this medicine is very expensive. Has the cost of this drug been a problem?"*
   e. If appropriate, ask about ability to obtain refills. *"Do you have any problems getting refills for this drug?" "Do you have any problems picking up your refills at the drugstore?"*

   Note anything that might be important in teaching this patient about medications: drugs that should be refrigerated or left at room temperature, dangers of putting drugs in unlabeled containers, importance of storing drugs out of reach of small children, etc.

2. General drug use

   How do you take care of the following problems/conditions? What medicines do you use for them? *"How often do you take the medicine?" "Does it work?" "When did you last take it?"*

   a. Pain: headache, muscle pains, toothaches? *Expand as needed for each patient.*
   b. Gastrointestinal system: constipation, diarrhea, upset stomach, heartburn?
   c. Skin conditions: psoriasis, athlete's foot, dry skin? *Ask about special shampoos and creams.*
   d. Nervous, mental, or emotional disorders: nervousness, being unable to sleep, upset?
   e. Reproductive system: birth control pills, female hormones, menstrual pain, backache?
   f. Nutritional deficiencies: iron, vitamins, bran, yeast, etc.?
   g. Upper respiratory tract, eye, and nose: What do you do for a cold? Cough? Stuffy nose? Sinus problem? Do you take nose drops? Use nasal spray? Eye drops?
   h. Other: special teas, liniments, plasters, soda, drugs made from roots? *Knowledge of local custom is helpful in this category.*

3. General health habits

   a. Do you smoke? How much?
   b. How much whiskey (beer, wine) do you drink? (Response may not be accurate)
   c. How often do you do drugs on a recreational basis? (Response may not be accurate. Remain nonjudgmental.)
   d. Do you follow any special diet (low salt, diabetic, low protein, etc.)? Are you a vegetarian? *In some cases a complete diet history might be warranted.*
   e. Where do you work? What kinds of work have you done in the past? Have you lived anywhere else in the country?
   f. Are you allergic to anything? Are there any medicines you cannot take? Why?
   g. Which immunizations have you received? When did you last have a tetanus shot?

FIGURE 6.1   Sample drug history.

call (e.g., physician, nurse practitioner) if anything unexpected occurs.

If there are any management decisions that the patient must make, the nurse should review these carefully with the patient. Examples include changes in dose strength or frequency, depending on the patient's response to the medication, or home treatment or more frequently encountered side effects. Any measurements that the patient is to make at home should also be practiced by the patient. These include measurements of weight, blood sugar, acetone, and pulse rate.

The patient should be informed of any special considerations related to the taking of the dose itself, such as whether it should be taken on an empty or full stomach, whether milk is to be avoided, or whether taking two particular drugs simultaneously should be avoided. If there is a new drug administration technique involved, the patient must demonstrate how to do this safely and accurately. The nurse should include appropriate general principles related to drug use (see previous discussion).

Finally, the patient should be given information about how and when follow-up will occur and how to call for help or additional information. It is often advisable and helpful to have additional family members present if the instruction is lengthy and complicated. Providing written instructions is a good idea. It also may be helpful to refer the patient to a community-based nursing agency for follow-up in the home setting.

PATIENT COMPLIANCE

Even when the nurse has developed and implemented what seems to be a complete and individualized teaching plan, patient compliance may be poor. The many possible reasons for this include the following:

- The patient or family misunderstood the directions
- Poor vision or hearing leads to errors in understanding or reading labels
- The patient cannot afford the drug
- The patient has no way of getting the prescription refilled
- There are so many medications to take that the patient becomes confused, taking the drugs in incorrect amounts and at wrong times
- The patient cannot manage the new route of administration in the home without help (e.g., self-injection)
- The patient is unable to accept a particular diagnosis (e.g., the teen-ager who does not

---

WAYS TO REDUCE DRUG COSTS

Prescription drugs can be costly. Possible ways to reduce costs for patients include the following:

- Ask the physician if the drug can be prescribed in the generic form.
- Shop around (via telephone) for the "best buy." Pharmacies vary in their prices.
- If the prescription is for a new drug, ask the physician for a few samples, or ask the pharmacist to fill part of the prescription (e.g., to give you 10 tablets of the 100 ordered tablets) until you see if you can take this drug without serious side effects.
- If you must take a drug for an extended period, is there any organization through which you might purchase your drugs at a reduced cost? For example, through the American Association of Retired Persons (AARP), members can buy large quantities of medicines at reduced rates. However, these drugs must be ordered through the mail, so this service is most helpful with drugs that will be needed on a long-term, continuing basis.

---

check blood for sugar in the morning before insulin administration, or who injects insulin too late in the day)
- Side effects that are intolerable occur, and the patient is too embarrassed to mention them to anyone (e.g., sexual impotence)

The nurse who is in the patient's home may find clues to noncompliance: too many pills remain in the bottle at the end of the month, or the patient cannot describe how to take the prescribed medications. In the office or hospital setting it may be less easy for the nurse to find out; only the lack of congruence between objective data and subjective response (e.g., the patient describes taking the antihypertensive, but the blood pressure remains high) may give the nurse a clue. In either case the nurse must use careful nonjudgmental questioning to find out if there is a problem and to help the patient find a way to better manage the health problem (i.e., by taking the drug).

The nurse must be creative in finding ways to help patients. Some frequently tried methods include making a special calendar with items the patient must check off when the dose is taken, or putting the pills into color-coded cups or containers, with each color corresponding to a specific mealtime. The doses of a medication may be prepared for 7 days and left with the patient who has difficulty preparing the dosage form. Pill containers with an alarm are also available; these can be set to go off each time a patient is to take a dose of drug. In other situations compliance can be improved by changing the dose, the time the drug is to be taken, or even the drug itself. Consult the physician. The nurse must learn to remember that patients have the right to choose whether and how they will take their medications; some simply choose to not comply.

TECHNIQUES FOR ADMINISTERING DRUGS BY SPECIFIC ROUTES

In the following section the techniques of administering drugs via the major routes will be discussed. The box on p. 94 lists the steps to be followed in administering any drugs. For more detailed descriptions or additional illustrations, the reader is referred to the sources listed at the end of the chapter.

Oral Route

The most frequently used method of drug administration is the oral route. It is a safe, convenient, and acceptable route for most patients and medications.

After carefully checking and preparing the medication(s) ordered, the nurse identifies the patient, assists the patient to sit upright, if possible, then hands the medication(s) and a glass of water or other preferred liquid to the patient. The patient then puts the pills, tablets, or capsules in the mouth and swallows them with the offered fluid. The patient should drink enough fluid to ensure that the medication reaches the stomach; drugs that lodge in the esophagus can cause irritation and burning and may result in poor absorption. Approximately 4 ounces of fluid is usually sufficient, but the patient should be encouraged to drink more unless the medical condition could be aggravated by a large fluid intake. Patients who are not sitting upright may need additional fluid to help ensure that the medication has reached the stomach.

The nurse must try to ascertain that the medication was actually swallowed and is not being hidden in the patient's mouth. Although this is a rare situation, it does occur, especially with confused individuals or those with certain psychiatric problems. After the patient swallows the drug, the nurse records that the medication has been taken.

Even though the situation described seems straightforward, several factors can influence the administration of oral medications, and the nurse must take them into consideration. The scheduling of medications must reflect whether the drug is best taken on an empty or a full stomach. Another factor is whether a specific liquid should be avoided by the patient. For example, tetracyclines should not be taken with milk.

Patients with multiple chronic health problems (and this includes many elderly clients) may need to take several different drugs simultaneously. The combination of drugs, or the total amount of fluid needed by the patient to swallow the drugs, may be nauseating. If there is reason to believe that the patient may refuse to take all the medications, may tire before all the drugs are taken, or may become too nauseated to take all the drugs, the nurse must try to ensure that the "more necessary" drugs are taken first and the "less necessary" ones are left until last. For example, consider a patient receiving a cardiotonic, an antihypertensive, a diuretic, a potassium replacement, a vitamin, and an iron supplement at 10 AM. It is presumed that all these drugs are necessary for management of the patient's condition. However, the nurse may decide that the cardiotonic, the antihypertensive, the diuretic, and the potassium replacement are of greater priority (more necessary). This is not to suggest that the nurse can simply decide not to administer certain medications but rather that the nurse is frequently required to exercise judgment and make decisions on short notice. A better long-term solution to this multiple drug problem might be to schedule the vitamin and the iron supplement at a time during the day when the patient is taking fewer drugs, and will then have less difficulty in taking all that are ordered.

Many patients have difficulty swallowing whole tablets or capsules. Frequently, the halves of capsules can be separated and the powdered drug poured out. Crushed medications are usually mixed with water or food and then swallowed. Especially with children, it is important to use as little applesauce, or other vehicle, as possible. Otherwise, the child may feel full or refuse the rest of the applesauce; then the nurse has no way of knowing how much of the prescribed dose was actually consumed. See the box on p. 86 for a list of drug forms that should not be crushed.

Children will sometimes take medications wrapped in a "jelly sandwich." Another way to encourage the child is to give the medication in one cup, and follow it with a "chaser" of water, milk, or carbonated beverage in another medication cup; children like the small cups and are not overwhelmed with a large volume of fluid. In choosing a food or fluid to give a child to help disguise or take medications, be careful not to choose items with high sugar content if the medication must be taken on a regular basis because the vehicle may contribute to dental caries. For diabetic children sugar-free vehicles should be used.

Although in some institutions the pharmacy

will, on request, send crushed dosage forms to the nursing unit, it is usually the responsibility of the nurse to crush the medication. There are several ways to do this. Some agencies have pill crushers available in the nursing unit. A mortar and pestle may be used (be sure they are clean before use, and wash away any remaining drug residue and dry them after preparing the dose). It may be possible to place the tablet inside a plastic or paper medication cup, then place a second cup over the pill. Any handy blunt instrument can then be used to crush the tablet between the layers of the cups. Two metal spoons can be nested with the pill between them and used the same way. Regardless of how the drug is crushed, the nurse should be careful to see that all of the powdered drug is brushed into the cup that will be given to the patient.

An alternative to crushing medications is to obtain a liquid form of the drug. Many drugs are available in liquid forms as suspensions or solutions. It is important to make substitutions carefully, often after consulting the physician and pharmacist. For example, a sustained-release form of a drug might be available in tablet form, but the only liquid preparation available may not be a sustained-release form, so dosage frequency might need to be adjusted.

It is generally easy to measure the prescribed dose in a capsule or tablet form, but the liquid preparations require a little more care. If in suspension form, the stock bottle, or unit dose, must be shaken thoroughly before the dose is poured and the medication administered. Inadequate shaking of suspensions can result in the patient receiving a weaker dose from the top of the bottle, then a stronger dose near the bottom of the bottle as the unsuspended particles of drug collect. In the institutional setting medication cups are usually provided for measuring the prescribed dose, unless the drug is supplied in the unit dose from the pharmacy. The medication cup should be placed on a flat surface or held upright at eye level so that the nurse can check that the correct dose has been poured. The base of the meniscus should be at the level of the desired dose (Figure 6.2). For small amounts of liquids or odd quantities, the dose should be measured with a syringe. It is *not* acceptable to "estimate" 2 ml or 12.5 ml of a drug.

In the home setting the patient must frequently use household tablespoons and teaspoons for measuring dosages. If possible, the patient should be encouraged always to use the same spoon, since household spoons are not standardized and switching spoons may result in varying dosages. Liquid forms must frequently be stored in the refrigerator.

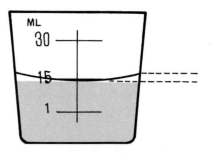

FIGURE 6.2   Reading meniscus. The meniscus is caused by the surface tension of the solution against the walls of the container. The surface tension causes the formation of a concave or hollowed curvature on the surface of the solution. Read the level at the lowest point of the concaved curve.

The availability of a liquid form of a drug does not necessarily ensure patient cooperation in taking the drug. Many liquid forms may be very unpleasant tasting, especially tinctures and elixirs. In the clinical setting the nurse may find a child or elderly adult more willing to take a crushed tablet in food than to take the drug in the liquid form. Some patients may take liquid forms better through a straw placed near the back of the mouth. If the preparation can stain teeth, a straw should be used to ensure that the medication is delivered to the back of the throat, bypassing contact with the teeth. Cutting the straw in half may make it easier for the child to manage.

Another factor influencing oral drug administration is the use or particular property of a drug. For example, Xylocaine Viscous, an oral preparation of lidocaine hydrochloride, is sometimes prescribed to produce relief of oral discomfort in stomatitis; it does this by producing local anesthesia. Using this drug may interfere with swallowing, so it should be taken last if several drugs are being administered simultaneously. A second example is an antitussive, which should usually be taken last because it generally should not be followed with water. Not all oral drugs are to be swallowed. Any drug to be taken via the sublingual or buccal route, for example, should be withheld until the drugs that are to be swallowed have been consumed; then the drug that is to be dissolved should be given.

Regardless of the specific problems and their solutions, the quality of nursing care can be improved, and much time saved, if each nurse records on the patient medication Kardex or care plan anything unique about the administration of medications to each patient.

DRUG FORMS THAT SHOULD *NOT* BE CRUSHED

- Enteric coated tablets
- Sustained release forms. These often have the following suffixes attached to the drug name:
    Dur (as in *duration*)
    SR (Sustained *Release*)
    CR (Controlled or Continuous *Release*)
    SA (Sustained *Action*)
    Contin (*Contin*uous)
- Trade names that imply sustained release: spansules, extentabs, extencaps
- Trade names with the b.i.d. (twice a day) abbreviation in the name, such as Theobid, Lithobid, Cardabid.
- Liquid-containing capsules, although occasionally it may be acceptable to puncture the capsule and squeeze out the contents; consult the pharmacist or manufacturer.

The name alone may not provide enough information. Consult the pharmacist if in doubt. Some forms that look like sustained forms are not, and vice versa. Some capsules containing small, slow-release pellets may be opened, and the pellets sprinkled on applesauce, or gently mixed into liquid or food, but they should not be crushed or dissolved.

Sublingual, Buccal, Troche, Lozenge and Spray Forms

The most frequently prescribed sublingual drugs are the nitrates and nitrites for anginal heart pain. The patient should be instructed to let the tablet dissolve under the tongue. The patient should not drink any fluid while the drug is dissolving. This route of administration may be new to the patient, so care must be taken to ensure that the patient understands how to use drugs taken via this route. Family members can be taught to administer drugs via this route when the patient is unable to do so.

Buccal tablets are designed to be held between the cheek and the gum and allowed to dissolve. The patient should be taught to alternate cheeks with each subsequent dose of medication to minimize the chance for irritation of the mucosa. Any oral irritation should be reported to the physician.

Troches and lozenges should be allowed to dissolve in the mouth. They are usually designed in this drug form to allow for slow release of the drug (i.e., over several minutes).

Another oral form is the sublingual spray. For this dosage form, the patient sprays one or two jets from a small canister into the mouth, under the tongue. The canister delivers a specific dose with each jet.

Administration through Feeding Tubes

Most medications that can be administered orally also can be administered via feeding tubes. Liquid preparations are preferred, but some medications can be finely crushed and mixed with sufficient water to ensure complete passage of the drug to the stomach (see the box on this page for a list of drugs that should not be crushed). Before administering any drug via tube, the nurse must ascertain that the tube is in the correct place. Refer to appropriate texts of nursing fundamentals for details about the care of patients with feeding tubes. If the drugs do not form a solid precipitate, they may be mixed together and administered. Otherwise, the drugs should be administered one at a time, followed by a small amount of water (about 30 ml) to flush the drug through the tube, to help maintain the patency of the tube, and to ensure that subsequent drugs do not precipitate with residue remaining in the tube from an earlier drug. After the final drug is administered, water should again be administered to clear the tube.

PARENTERAL MEDICATIONS: INJECTIONS

The word *parenteral* means outside the intestines, but in common usage it is usually limited to injections. There are many kinds of injections, and they are named by indicating the site at which the medication is deposited. Thus there are intradermal, intramuscular, intravenous, and subcutaneous injections, all of which are encountered by the nurse in everyday practice. Other injection sites used, usually by the physician, include intracardiac (usually reserved for resuscitation efforts), intrathecal (into the subarachnoid space via lumbar or ventricular puncture), and intra-articular (into a joint). The older term *hypodermic* is being replaced gradually by the term *subcutaneous*.

Both advantages and disadvantages are associated with parenteral administration. This route is available for use in patients who are aphagic or not alert or those who lack an adequate gag reflex. It can be used for an uncooperative patient or a child unwilling or unable to take other, usually oral, medications. (If multiple doses are required, intravenous administration is usually preferable for the child because it is less intrusive.) The parenteral route is the only one available for some medications, including insulin and heparin. On the other hand, drugs administered via this route are generally considered irretrievable. In addition, there is a slight chance of infection because the integrity of the skin is broken. Also rare, but possible, is the inadvertent administration into the vascular space. Damage to muscles and nerves can also occur. Injections are also uncomfortable.

As with all medications, the nurse must carefully calculate and prepare the prescribed dose. Many injectable medications are supplied as dry powders and must be reconstituted before administration. Although this sometimes can be done by the pharmacy, frequently the nurse must do this. It is important to carefully read the information supplied by the manufacturer regarding reconstitution of dry medication. There may be restrictions on what fluid(s) may be used for this purpose, or a specific diluent may be supplied by the manufacturer.

Not only must the nurse obtain the appropriate diluent, but the correct amount of diluent must be added to the dry powder. Often beginning practitioners and students find the instructions related to reconstitution difficult to understand. As an example, one form of penicillin states that certain amounts of diluent may be added to the 1,000,000-unit vial to provide the dilutions listed: *Add 9.6 ml, 4.6 ml, or 3.6 ml, to provide 100,000 U, 200,000 U, or 250,000 U per ml respectively*. If the nurse has any question about reconstituting a powder for injection, a colleague or the pharmacy should be consulted.

Once vials of medication have been reconstituted, they should be dated, the time of reconstitution noted, and the concentration labeled. Many institutions also require that the nurse initial the vial and put the patient's name on the vial. Many vials are provided in single-dose concentrations, but in pediatric settings, where the prescribed dose may be quite small, the nurse may be using only a portion of the contents of a medication vial. Reconstituted medications must often be stored in the refrigerator. The nurse should remember to read the label before using stored medications, and observe expiration dates. Many medications may only be used for a short period once they have been reconstituted.

Not all medications for injection are supplied in vials. Many come in small glass ampules, from which a single dose is withdrawn, and the ampule discarded. Other medications are provided in prefilled syringes. The advantages of the prefilled syringes are obvious: they are easy and fast to prepare. However, they are also more expensive to the agency. Most agencies do stock prefilled syringes for narcotics and for selected other situations in which drugs need to be immediately available, such as the emergency drug box or resuscitation cart. There are several manufacturers of prefilled syringes, and the techniques for activating and using the products vary. The nurse should consult the agency or institution for information about devices used in any individual setting.

The choice of syringe and needle to be used for any specific medication depends on the information obtained from assessment of the patient, the route of administration to be used, the characteristics of the fluid to be injected (e.g., waterlike or oil based), and the volume of medication to be delivered. Sample syringe sizes include 1 ml tuberculin and insulin syringes, 2.5 ml syringes, 5 ml, and 10 ml syringes. Larger syringes are often available, but they are rarely used for medication administration via the parenteral route. Tuberculin syringes, marked in 0.01 ml gradations, are the choice when the volume to be administered is small. Insulin syringes are available in 0.5 or 1 ml volumes, although some institutions do stock an insulin syringe with a maximum volume of 25 or 35 units. Tuberculin and insulin syringes should not be substituted for each other.

Needles vary in length and gauge, from 3/8 inch to 3 or more inches in length, and from 14 gauge (large lumen) to 28 gauge (small lumen). Most institutions limit the variety of needles and syringes in stock, so the nurse may have a choice of five syringes and five needle sizes on the nursing unit. The smaller lumen (larger gauge) needles are usually used for intradermal injections. Subcutaneous injections are usually given with a 1/2 or 5/8 inch, 23 or 25 gauge needle. Intramuscular injections are usually given with a 19 or 21 gauge, 1½ to 2 inch needle; occasionally a 16 or 18 gauge needle may be used. See the box on the next page for a discussion of oil-based medications.

After preparing the ordered dose and choosing the appropriate needle and syringe, the nurse goes to the patient's bedside to administer the injection. The nurse first checks the patient's nameband and verifies the patient's identity, draws the curtain or otherwise ensures privacy, explains what is to occur, and assists the patient to assume the necessary position. If it is known that the patient is unable or unwilling to assist in positioning, the nurse should bring adequate assistance to the bedside. Then the nurse should assess the injection site, locate anatomical landmarks, and smoothly administer the injection. The patient should be returned to a comfortable position. The nurse should then record that the medication has been given, noting the location, so that nurses following can

HOW TO PREPARE AN OIL-BASED MEDICINE FOR INTRAMUSCULAR ADMINISTRATION

- Oil-based medicines are released more slowly as it takes the oil longer to be absorbed from the muscle than aqueous solutions. Oil-based medicines should be administered via the IM route only, *never intravenously*.
- Heat the unopened vial or ampule in warm water for several minutes to decrease the viscosity of the oil.
- Roll the vial vigorously between the hands to re-suspend the medication, which is usually an inconspicuous film on the side of the ampule. Resuspension is adequate when no particles of medication remain on the bottom or sides of the vial. Failure to shake or roll the vial sufficiently will result in inaccurate dosage and erratic absorption.
- Draw up the correct dose into a syringe fitted with a large-bore (19 to 21 gauge), 1½ inch needle (for an adult), and administer the dose immediately, before the oil cools.
- Inject the medicine, exerting slow, even pressure on the plunger. Attempting to inject too rapidly can cause pressure to increase within the syringe, and the needle and syringe may separate, causing loss of medication.
- Use large muscle masses, such as the buttock, thigh, or ventrogluteal site. In infants and small children, use the vastus lateralis.
- The oil base can produce palpable lumps because it is absorbed so slowly. Record injection sites, rotate injection sites, and avoid the deltoid muscle.

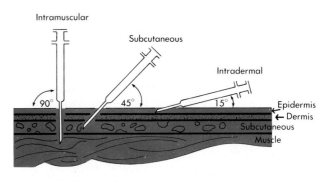

FIGURE 6.3   Comparison of angle of injection and location of deposition of medication for intramuscular, subcutaneous, and intradermal injections.

rotate injection sites. The nurse should carefully dispose of the syringe and needle, according to the procedures of the agency. The nurse should again check the patient to make certain no untoward effects have occurred and to evaluate if the drug is working as anticipated.

Any aspects of the injection that are unique to the patient should be recorded on the medication Kardex or patient care plan to assist other nurses in providing individualized care. More detailed information about drawing up medications, handling equipment, and administering injections can be found in fundamental nursing texts. There is nothing so helpful as practice in learning how to be accurate, efficient, and confident in the administration of injections. The major forms of injections will be discussed briefly in the following section.

Intradermal Injection

An intradermal injection is made just below the epidermis or outer layer of skin (Figure 6.3). It is used for allergy testing and for administration of local anesthetics. Usually a small-bore needle is used, and a small-volume syringe, such as a 1 ml tuberculin syringe. The amount injected is usually small, less than 0.5 ml. The most frequently used sites for allergy testing are the medial surface of the forearm and the back.

In preparation for the injection, the chosen skin surface is cleansed with alcohol; then the surface is allowed to dry or wiped off with a sterile sponge. The skin is held taut with one hand. With the other hand the needle is held bevel up, at a 10- to 15-degree angle, and the skin is gently but smoothly punctured until the bevel is completely under the skin surface. The prescribed amount, or an amount that creates a raised wheal resembling a mosquito bite, is injected. If a wheal is not produced or the site bleeds, it was probably too deep an injection and should be repeated. If several injections are being given in the same site (e.g., on the same forearm), they should be labeled with pen, especially if the reaction is to be checked at 48 hours.

Subcutaneous Injection

Subcutaneous injection is used to place medication below the skin into the subcutaneous layer (Figure 6.3). The volume of a subcutaneous injection is usually less than 1 ml, and usually a 1/2 or 5/8 inch, 23 or 25 gauge needle is used. The needle is inserted at a 45-degree angle, although it may be inserted at a 90-degree angle if the patient has heavy subcutaneous tissue or the nurse has pinched the subcutaneous tissue between thumb and fingers, holding it up from the underlying muscle tissue. The usual injection technique is used: choose the site, cleanse the site with alcohol, let the alcohol

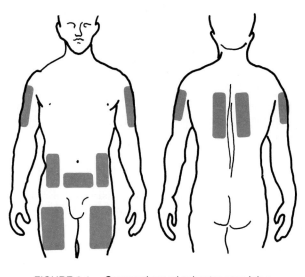

FIGURE 6.4   Commonly used subcutaneous injection sites.

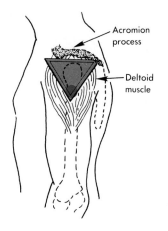

FIGURE 6.5   Deltoid muscle injection site roughly forms an inverted triangle, with the acromium process as the base. The muscle may be visible in well-developed patients.

dry or wipe off with a sterile sponge, hold the skin taut, insert the needle, aspirate for blood, and—if no blood is present—gently but smoothly inject the medication. An alternative technique is to cleanse the skin as described, then gently pinch the subcutaneous tissue between the thumb and the other fingers, and insert the needle, aiming it for the "pocket" created between the subcutaneous tissue being pinched and the tissue below. The two medications most frequently administered via this route are heparin and insulin, and there is continuing controversy about specific aspects of administration of these two drugs. For additional discussion about the administration of these two drugs, consult Chapter 20 (heparin) and Chapter 55 (insulin). The usual sites for subcutaneous injection are illustrated in Figure 6.4.

Intramuscular Injection

Intramuscular injection is probably the method most familiar to students and patients. The majority of people have received medication via this route in the form of antibiotics or immunizations. Because the muscle layer is below the subcutaneous layer of skin, a longer needle is used, usually 1½ inches, often of larger lumen size, such as 19 or 21 gauge. The needle is inserted at a 90-degree angle (Figure 6.3). The choice of needle is influenced by the viscosity of the medication to be injected, the muscle to be used, and the size and age of the patient. A frequent error of beginning students is to choose too short a needle for administration of a medication to a well-nourished adult via a large muscle mass such as the vastus lateralis or dorsogluteal area.

The intramuscular technique is the same as other injection techniques previously outlined. The nurse carefully prepares the ordered medication, takes the syringe to the bedside, checks the nameband and verifies the patient's identity, draws the curtain or otherwise ensures privacy, assists the patient to assume the necessary position, identifies appropriate anatomical landmarks to help define the injection site, cleanses the skin, and then lets it dry. The nurse then holds the skin taut or gently pinches the skin, swiftly inserts the needle at a 90-degree angle, aspirates for blood, and, if no blood is present, gently but smoothly injects the medication. If after withdrawing the needle, there is oozing of a little blood, the nurse applies gentle pressure and may apply a bandage. The patient is repositioned to a comfortable position. The nurse records that the medication has been given, then disposes of needle and syringe as directed by agency policy. Finally, the nurse should check the patient again.

Several muscles are commonly used for intramuscular injections, and these will be discussed briefly below. The *deltoid muscle* is located at the upper arm. It forms a triangular shape, with the base of the triangle along the acromion process and the peak of the triangle ending about one third down the upper arm (Figure 6.5). In the muscular patient (usually male), the deltoid may be clearly

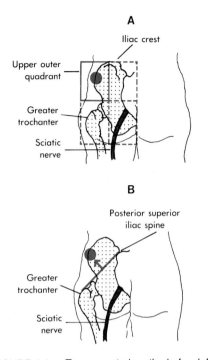

FIGURE 6.6   Two accepted methods for defining the dorsogluteal injection site. In method A, the patient's buttocks can be divided on one side into imaginary quadrants. The center of the upper outer quadrant should be used as the injection site. In method B, the nurse locates by palpation the posterior superior iliac spine and the greater trochanter, then draws an imaginary line between the two. An injection site up and out from that line should be used.

visible. In other patients it may be necessary to palpate it. For several reasons this muscle is seldom used. It is small in children, petite women, the elderly, and many men, so it can accommodate only small amounts of injected fluid (e.g., 1 ml). Bruises or needle marks may be visible, depending on patient clothing, so this may be unacceptable to the patient. The radial nerve is nearby. The advantage of the deltoid muscle is that it is easily accessible.

The *dorsogluteal site* is made up of several gluteal muscles, although the gluteus medius is the muscle used for injections most often. As indicated in Figure 6.6, there are two ways to define this site. The first method *(A)* is to divide the buttocks on one side into imaginary quadrants, and administer the injection in the upper outer quadrant. In the second method *(B)*, the nurse locates the posterior superior iliac spine and the greater trochanter of the femur, then draws an imaginary line between these two. The injection should be given up and out from this line. It is important to have a clear

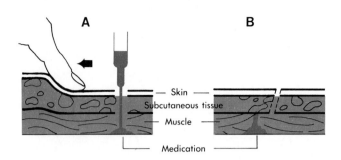

FIGURE 6.7   **A,** In a *Z*-track intramuscular injection, the skin is pulled laterally, then the injection administered. **B,** After the needle is withdrawn, the skin is released. This technique helps prevent the medication from leaking.

view of the area to help define the landmarks. The patient should be lying down, with the toes pointed inward, which helps foster muscle relaxation and thus decreases discomfort. This site should not be used for children under 3 years of age because the muscles are not yet well developed and because of the proximity of the sciatic nerve. In most ambulatory adults the dorsogluteal muscles are well developed and can accommodate an injection volume up to 5 ml if necessary, although any volume over 3 ml may be uncomfortable to the patient.

The *Z-track technique* can be used with any intramuscular injection. However, it was first described for administration of an iron preparation that stains the skin if it leaks out. The dorsogluteal site is most frequently used for injections requiring the Z-track technique. In preparing the drug to be administered, the ordered amount of drug is measured into the syringe; then 0.1 to 0.3 ml of air is drawn up into the syringe; finally, the needle is changed. In administration of drugs via the Z-track method, the skin is pulled taut to one side, causing the layers of skin to "slide" sideways. While the skin is pulled laterally, the needle is inserted and the medication and a small amount of air are injected smoothly and slowly. The nurse pauses for 10 seconds before removing the needle. The needle is withdrawn, and then the skin is allowed to relax (Figure 6.7). This process has the effect of disrupting the track created by the needle, preventing seepage, as well as possible skin discoloration caused by the medication. The site should not be massaged or rubbed.

Both the *vastus lateralis* and the *rectus femoris muscles* are found in the thigh. As shown in Figure 6.8, the two muscles lie side by side. The nurse

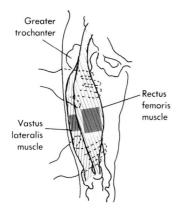

FIGURE 6.8   To define the vastus lateralis muscle injection site and the rectus femoris muscle site, place one hand below the patient's greater trochanter and one hand above the knee. The space between the two hands defines the middle third of the underlying muscle. The rectus femoris is on the anterior thigh; the vastus lateralis is on the lateral thigh.

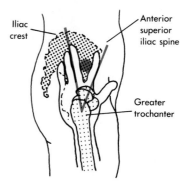

FIGURE 6.9   To locate the ventrogluteal muscle injection site, place the palm of one hand on the greater trochanter of the femur. Make a "V" with the fingers of that hand, with one side running from the greater trochanter to the anterosuperior iliac spine, and the other side running from the greater trochanter to the iliac crest.

places one hand on the patient's upper thigh and one hand on the lower thigh. The area between the nurse's hands should represent the middle third of the thigh and the middle third of the underlying muscle. The vastus lateralis is lateral to midline, whereas the rectus femoris is in the midline. The vastus lateralis is the preferred injection site for children because it is well developed and has few major nerves present that could be injured. This site is also satisfactory for adults. The rectus femoris is most often the muscle chosen by adults who self-administer intramuscular injections because it is easily accessible. The acceptable volume for injection in these sites varies with the age of the patient and the size of the muscle, but up to 5 ml may be administered in one injection to the well-developed adult.

To define the *ventrogluteal muscle,* the nurse creates a "V" between the index finger and the remaining three fingers. The palm is placed on the greater trochanter of the femur, with one side of the "V" extending from the greater trochanter to the iliac crest, and the other side running from the greater trochanter to the anterior superior iliac spine (Figure 6.9). In the adult this muscle may also accommodate up to 5 ml of drug.

Intravenous Injection

The administration of drugs directly into the vascular system via the intravenous route is widely used today for a variety of reasons. If an intravenous infusion line is already in place, IV infusion is easy. Drugs begin to take immediate effect. Side effects caused by intramuscular injection are avoided. On the other hand, errors made via this route can take effect quickly and be serious, even fatal. The possibility of infection with the direct access to the vascular system is also present.

In many settings the technique of venipuncture is done only by members of the "IV team" or comparable group. If no designated team exists, many agencies require special instruction, classes, and supervised practice in venipuncture techniques before nurses are permitted to perform this technique in their usual setting. A general procedure for venipuncture will be outlined below, but it is important to remember that there are many variations in the way the steps are implemented in any specific agency. The student or practitioner is encouraged to become familiar with practices and policies of the agency or institution.

The nurse first inspects the forearms and chooses the venipuncture site. Figure 6.10 illustrates the location of veins commonly used in the forearm. Figure 6.11 illustrates the location of veins on the dorsal aspect of the hand. Other veins, such as those in the feet, are used only if absolutely necessary; their use may require specific physician order in some agencies. The potential problems associated with thrombophlebitis are much more common with lower extremity venipunctures. Scalp veins are used in infants. If the patient is to have repeated venipunctures, the nurse should

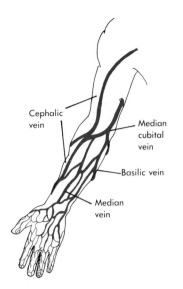

FIGURE 6.10   Veins of the medial aspect of the forearm commonly used for venipuncture.

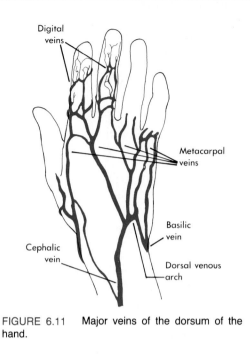

FIGURE 6.11   Major veins of the dorsum of the hand.

choose a distal site rather than a proximal one. The rationale is that with each subsequent venipuncture the site should be moved more proximal, that is, closer to the major vessels of the chest.

After choosing a site and preparing the necessary equipment (needle, intracatheter, heparin well, tubing, blood collection devices, medication), the nurse applies a tourniquet several inches above the expected insertion site. The nurse puts on gloves, palpates the vein to further define its location, then cleanses the skin with alcohol, povidone-iodine solution, or other cleansing substance. The area is allowed to dry, or it is wiped with a sterile sponge. While the nurse uses one hand to stabilize the extremity and the vein, the other hand holds the venipuncture needle bevel up. The insertion site is approached at a slight angle, such as 10 degrees. The skin is punctured, then the vein. The experienced nurse can feel the vein wall being punctured. If blood then appears in the tubing or syringe, the tourniquet is released. The medication is slowly injected into the vein, the blood is drawn, or the infusion device secured to the forearm, depending on the reason for the venipuncture.

In removing any needle or tubing from a vein, the nurse puts on gloves, carefully removes any securing tapes and dressing, places a sterile sponge over the insertion site, and applies gentle pressure; then with the other hand the nurse swiftly withdraws the needle or catheter, pulling straight back from the angle of insertion; then firm pressure is applied for 2 to 5 minutes to prevent bleeding or bruising. A bandage is usually then applied over the insertion site. If medication has been administered, the nurse records this, disposes of any needles and syringes, and again checks the patient. Further elaboration of these techniques can be found in fundamental nursing texts and agency procedure manuals. In addition, the Centers for Disease Control in Atlanta have guidelines for preventing infections in venipuncture and intravenous infusions.

Heparin lock. In some institutions the nurse will administer IV medications via a *heparin well* or *heparin lock*. This device consists of a needle attached to a short length of tubing capped by a piece of resealable rubber. The needle is placed in the vein; then the device is secured to the forearm. Its advantage is that medication can be administered via the intravenous route, but the patient need not be attached to continuous IV infusions or have repeated venipunctures for each dose of medication. Heparin wells are particularly helpful in children needing intravenous medications but not additional fluids; it also permits children to be up and around and not attached to long intravenous tubing.

Heparin may be administered via heparin well, as described in Chapter 20. One method for administering other medications by intermittent infusion via heparin well will be described. The heparin well is inserted and secured, then primed with

1 ml of a solution containing 10 units of heparin per ml. Solutions of 10 units per ml are available in prepackaged syringes or multiple dose vials, or they can be prepared by the pharmacy or the nurse mixing the heparin with normal saline solution to achieve the desired concentration. Each time a drug is administered, the procedure is to (1) cleanse the rubber insertion site with alcohol or other cleansing agent; (2) flush the well with 1 to 2 ml of normal saline solution (this step may be omitted if the drug to be administered is compatible with heparin); (3) administer the prescribed medication via push or infusion; (4) flush the well with 1 to 2 ml of normal saline solution; and (5) administer 1 ml of the solution containing 10 units heparin per ml. The purpose of leaving the heparinized solution in the well is to prevent blood from clotting in the needle. The exact procedure of the individual institution should be followed.

Intravenous tubing. Another way intravenous medications are administered is via tubing in place for the patient who is receiving constant IV fluids. There are at least two variations that should be noted. Frequently the nurse must administer a small amount, usually less than 5 ml, of drug. This is often called "IV push" drug. The nurse, after preparing the drug and verifying the patient's identity, locates an injection site on the IV tubing. The site is cleansed with alcohol or other solution; then 2 ml of normal saline is injected (this step may be omitted if the IV push drug is compatible with the fluids infusing); next the ordered drug is administered, followed again by the saline. The ongoing infusion is then readjusted to provide the ordered rate. Most commercially available IV tubings have check valves, or one-way valves, as part of the tubing. If one is not present, however, the nurse must clamp the tubing above the injection site before administering the drug as outlined above. If there is no check valve, or if the tubing is not clamped, the injected medication will go in the direction of lower pressure, which may be up toward the bag or bottle of fluid instead of down toward the patient. This is to be avoided. The problem with the medication going toward the large bag or bottle of fluid is that the patient does not receive the complete dose of drug until the bag is empty, and drugs administered after that dose may not be compatible with the drug remaining in the fluid line.

The second variation is the administration of a bolus of medication. The drug is prepared and diluted in a larger volume of fluid, at least 50 to 100 ml in adults. It is usually administered over 20 to 60 minutes. This volume can then be administered in several ways. One method is to add the volume to an in-line device such as a burette or

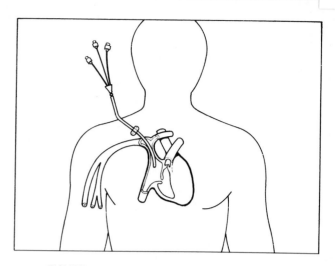

FIGURE 6.12 Triple-lumen central venous catheter in place.

Volutrol. The ongoing fluids are temporarily stopped, the bolus is allowed to infuse, then the ongoing fluids are continued. Another way is to use commercially available infusion tubing that has two ports for hanging IV bags or bottles. These tubing systems have an identified port for attaching the primary fluids and a secondary port for attaching the intermittently administered bolus containing the drugs.

The third variation is to prepare the drug in a small volume of fluid, then attach IV tubing and a needle. The needle is inserted into an identified insertion site on the tubing of the ongoing infusion after the site has been cleansed. The ongoing infusion is clamped off, the bolus containing the drug is allowed to infuse, then the continuous fluids are restarted. The secondary infusion tubing and needle may then be discarded. In order to be effective and efficient, the nurse must become familiar with the equipment and procedures used in the agency.

Central venous catheters and multilumen catheters. Many patients, even those outside of intensive care settings, now have central venous catheters inserted for venous access. The catheters may be inserted into a peripheral vein and threaded into a large vein closer to the heart (a more "central" vein, thus the name "central venous catheter"); or, more commonly, they are inserted by the physician directly into a large central vein, with the insertion site near the clavicle. The distal end of the catheter may be in the subclavian or jugular vein, or the superior vena cava near the junction with the right atrium (Figure 6.12). Once in place, the catheter is sutured to the skin at the insertion site. There are

GENERAL STEPS IN DRUG ADMINISTRATION

1. At the start of the work day, review each patient's record, noting the medical and nursing diagnosis, current problems, relevant laboratory findings, and plan of health care.

2. Compare the physician's original order against the working tools (may be medication Kardex, medication cards, computer printout—whatever is used in that setting to guide the nurse in preparing drugs).
   a. Check for accuracy of transcription:
      Drug name?
      Drug dose?
      Route of administration?
      Frequency of administration?
   b. Check for appropriateness of the order:
      Does this drug make sense for this patient? Is this dose in the usual range for a patient of this age and weight?
   c. Other:
      Have any automatic expiration dates passed?
      Are there new laboratory values to be considered, such as serum levels, culture reports, renal or liver function studies?

3. Look up any new drugs or check any drug information that is unclear.

4. Check the medication supply:
   a. Is stock bottle supply adequate for the shift? If not, reorder from the pharmacy.
   b. Check each patient's drawer to box of drugs. Are the drugs present? Any missing?
   c. Are any "missing" drugs in the refrigerator, on the back of the medication cart, at the bedside? Where else?
   d. Are there sufficient supplies to prepare and administer the drugs (straws, water cups, medication cups, spoons, mortar and pestle, syringes)?

5. Review the specific drugs. Are there any special assessments to be made or data to check before any drug is administered? For example: apical pulse, blood pressure, temperature, urine tests, weight, blood test.
   a. Organize equipment that might be needed.
   b. Make a list if necessary.

6. Check care plans (if not already done) to note personal preferences, previous problems, and nursing care approaches. Make a list of items to remember, such as: applesauce; juices, coffee, crackers, yogurt; "jelly sandwich," ice cream, or other foods to disguise flavors.

7. Just before preparing the drugs, wash hands.

8. The next few steps vary slightly, depending on whether the drugs are prepared in the medication room, as with a stock system, or in the patient's room, with a medication cart and unit dose system. Check the working tool and obtain the medication. Read the label carefully, checking the drug, the dose, and the route of administration.

9. Pour or prepare the dose. If from a stock bottle, read the label again before replacing the bottle. If a unit dose, again, check the label; do not remove the drug from the package.

10. Prepare all the medications for that patient. If preparing medications in the medication room, do the medications for all the patients who are to receive them.

11. Go to the bedside, and identify the patient (if possible, use all three methods):
    a. Call the patient by name. (Be especially careful if there is more than one patient on the unit with the same last name.)
    b. Ask the patient to state his or her full name.
    c. Check the patient identification band. (This may be the only possible way to identify the infant, small child, or confused adult.)

12. Assess the patient.
    a. Note any changes since you last saw the patient.
    b. Obtain any objective data needed before administering the drugs: apical pulse, blood pressure, breath sounds, others.
    c. Obtain any appropriate subjective information.
    d. If the patient is previously unknown to the nurse, or if new drugs are being administered, check on history of allergy.

13. If the data obtained in step 12 were not acceptable, withhold the corresponding drugs. For example, if the apical pulse was 50, do not administer the cardiotonic (use agency policies as guides). Other drugs may be given if the patient's condition is satisfactory.

14. Draw the curtain or otherwise ensure privacy, if needed.

15. Administer the medications, helping the patient as needed. If the medicines are in unit dose packages, they now can be opened. Make certain the patient takes the medication. Do not leave any medications at the bedside unless this is authorized by a physician's order or written institutional policy.

16. Assist the patient to resume a comfortable position.

17. Wash hands.

18. If using a medication cart, and the medication record is kept with the cart, immediately record that the drugs were given. If using a different system, administer all medications, then return to the medication record and record that the drugs were given.

19. Depending on the drug, the patient, and the usual policies and procedures, notify appropriate individuals (e.g., nurse in charge, physician) about doses that were withheld.

20. Record other appropriate information: data obtained during assessment, drugs withheld and why, changes in patient condition.

21. Make appropriate additions to the care plan.

22. Check on patients at appropriate intervals to evaluate the response to the drug therapy.

Drug Administration

In this chapter drug administration has been emphasized. Drug therapy is only a part of total patient care, but for drug therapy to be successful it must be carried out properly. The patient has the right to expect to receive the right drug, in the right dose, at the right time, via the right route of administration.

Assessment

In assessing a patient, the nurse should be answering the question of why this patient might need a particular type of drug. Identifying the reason for medications being prescribed helps the nurse to detect inadvertent errors in which the wrong drug may be administered to a patient.

The nurse should obtain objective and subjective data from the patient to aid in determining the need and effectiveness of drug use. Any patient preferences regarding drug use should be determined and incorporated if possible. Determination of developmental level, especially for children, is necessary to aid in planning nursing care approaches.

Potential nursing diagnoses

Not all patients will have nursing diagnoses as a result of drug therapy. Most patients will have a knowledge deficit about a specific drug at the start of drug therapy. Other diagnoses may develop as the patient develops side effects, is unable to manage self-administration, or has collaborative problems as potential complications.

Management

Implementing the therapeutic plan involves proper administration of the prescribed medication. The nurse may seek information about specific drugs from a variety of sources, including the physician and the pharmacist, and printed materials, such as those discussed in Chapter 7. For a student nurse, the prospect of learning about all the medications to be administered is overwhelming. Once the nurse is in practice, however, repeated administration of medications will facilitate developing a basic understanding of many of the categories of drugs that are frequently used.

Not only must the nurse be knowledgeable about the prescribed medication, but caution must be exercised that the prescribed medication is actually what the patient receives. Thus medications should remain in labeled packages or containers until they are administered.

The patient has a right to receive the medication in the correct dose. Regardless of how drugs are supplied to the patient care unit, the nurse has the responsibility to check labels carefully and to double-check all calculations that must be done. Some nurses have difficulty with the mathematical calculations necessary for determining correct doses. Such nurses should get into the habit of having a colleague verify dosage calculations rather than possibly subjecting the patient to an incorrect dose of medication. The pharmacy may also be of assistance in dosage calculation.

Successful drug therapy may depend on the proper timing of drug doses, as discussed in Chapter 2.

To ensure that the patient receives each drug via the right route of administration, the nurse must know that routes are appropriate for a specific drug and how to administer drugs via that route.

The nurse must develop a sense of suspicion whenever a medication order seems to be out of the ordinary. For example, a dose of medication that seems unusually large or unusually small should be double-checked. When the nurse is at the bedside, if the patient seems hesitant to take the medication, stating that it is new or not what is usually taken, this should suggest to the nurse a need to double-check the physician's orders before insisting that a patient take a medication. Recording that a patient has received a medication should be done as soon as possible after the drug is administered to avoid inadvertent duplicate administration by other members of the health care team.

Continued.

THE NURSING PROCESS — cont'd

Evaluation

The major question to answer during the evaluation period is whether the medication is working as expected. This requires that the nurse know what was expected of the medication, have initial baseline data about the patient, and know what parameters to assess in order to determine if the drug is working as desired and expected. In addition, the nurse must determine if there were any problems associated with the route, time, or dose of medication.

In the process of evaluating a patient, the nurse may discover that a medication error has been made. When this occurs, the procedure followed within the institution for reporting the error should be carried out. The usual procedure involves immediately reassessing the patient and observing the possible effects that have resulted from the incorrect medication or incorrect dose, notifying the physician, and recording the error on appropriate forms (usually provided by the institution). The nurse should not be afraid to report an error. The professional acknowledges when mistakes have been made, placing the well-being of the patient above "saving face." The nurse should seek to learn from the error and modify practice to help ensure that the error will not occur again.

different catheters in use; some example names include the Hickman catheter, the Hickman-Broviac catheter, and the Groshong catheter. The catheters may have one, two, or more ports. They may be used for constant or intermittent infusion; one, two, or all three ports may be in use or not in use at any time, depending on the patients' needs and condition. Some patients are discharged with the catheter in place; before being discharged they must be taught how to clean the catheter and insertion site on a daily basis.

Because the distal end of the catheter is in an area of high blood flow and volume, these catheters permit infusion of large volumes of fluids, and of more irritating fluids and drugs than can be administered via peripheral intravenous lines. There is always a risk of infection or risk of introducing air with the catheters, especially those with multiple ports or openings. Usually, care of the catheter and the insertion site is more rigorous for a centrally placed catheter than for a peripherally placed catheter. For example, cleansing of an injection port on a peripheral catheter may be done with an alcohol swab, whereas the port on a central line may require cleansing with a povidone-iodine solution. Agency procedures should be followed. Also, monitor the patient for signs of infection: fever, redness at the insertion site, and increased white blood cell count.

Care of the ports not in use is important to keep the lumens patent, and agency procedure should be followed. Different types of catheters may require different protocols, but one protocol is outlined here. Change the cap on each port weekly, or when it appears worn. Wear gloves during cap changes, and discard contaminated caps carefully. Irrigate the ports not in use with 2.5 ml of heparinized solution (10 units of heparin/ml) every 12 to 24 hours. Irrigate a port after each intermittent infusion given via that port. If blood is drawn via a port, irrigate the port after the sample is obtained.

Implantable ports. Another form of venous access device is the implantable port, such as the Port-a-Cath. This device is surgically implanted, with the distal end of the catheter inserted into a large central vein. The injection end of the device is implanted subcutaneously, often on the chest wall. The injection end has a self-sealing septum over a small chamber or reservoir, and the tubing extends from the side of the reservoir/chamber to the venous insertion point. The advantage of the system is that once implanted, the port is available for long-term use up to 1 to 2 years. Each time the patient must receive medication, the skin must be punctured with a needle, but there is no daily cleansing procedure as there is with the partially implanted catheters (see above).

To use the device, the nurse puts on sterile gloves, then cleanses the site with a povidone-iodine solution (or as agency protocol directs). With one hand, the nurse palpates and locates the injection end. Once the device is defined and stabilized with one hand, the nurse punctures the skin and septum with a Huber needle attached to a syringe containing sterile saline. Blood is aspirated to help determine patency, then the saline is injected to flush the system. The device may be used to obtain blood samples, administer constant or intermittent infusions, or inject medications. Following use, the device should be flushed with a heparinized solution. Students and nurses working with implanted devices should review the manufacturer's directions and request guidance in using these devices until comfortable with their use and operation.

Drug "pumps." There are now available several devices for slowly injecting a medication, for use by the patient in the home setting. Cancer chemotherapy is the usual reason for using the drug pump. One device is the Auto-Syringe Pump. The device consists of a syringe with a battery attachment for slow injection. It can be used to inject the medication subcutaneously, or can be attached to an implanted infusion port such as the Port-A-Cath, or a partially implanted catheter such as a Hickman catheter. Follow the manufacturer's instructions in preparing and using a drug pump, and have the patient give a return demonstration prior to discharge.

Information about calculation of infusion rates is included in Chapter 7. Additional general guidelines for care of the patient receiving an intravenous infusion are included in Chapter 17.

RECTAL MEDICATIONS

Administering medications via the rectal route is an important alternative for patients who are nauseated or unable to swallow. Drugs administered via this route are usually in the form of suppository or enema.

The procedure for administering medication by enema is the same as for any enema. Usually, the goal is to have the patient retain the medication for as long as possible; therefore a small-volume retention enema will be administered. After preparing the medication and any other necessary equipment, the nurse goes to the bedside, verifies the patient's identity, explains briefly what will be done, then draws the curtain or otherwise ensures privacy. The nurse positions the patient on the left side, places adequate protective covering on the bed, puts on gloves, and lubricates the applicator or tubing tip with water-soluble jelly or lubricant. The patient's buttocks are separated, and the patient is asked to take a deep breath; then the tubing or tip is inserted the desired distance. The medication is administered slowly to avoid stimulation and immediate expulsion. The applicator is withdrawn, and the buttocks are held gently together until the patient's immediate urge to defecate has subsided. The patient's buttocks are washed, and the patient is returned to a comfortable position. The patient should be instructed to try to hold the medication at least 30 minutes (or as indicated by the nature of the medication).

Suppositories are medications that have been mixed with cocoa butter, glycerin, or other substances that allow them to remain solid at room temperature but melt and release the medication when they come in contact with the warm rectal mucosa. Frequently suppositories are stored in the refrigerator to keep them firm. If a suppository is too soft to insert easily, run it under cold water (if foil wrapped) or place it in the refrigerator to help harden it before administering. The general procedure is similar to that for the enema. The nurse wears a finger cot or glove for inserting the suppository, which has been moistened with a water-soluble lubricant. The suppository should be inserted about a finger's distance in the adult, past the anal sphincter. Inserting the suppository blunt end first will help the patient retain the suppository, since the rectal muscles will close gently over the tapered end. If not inserted far enough, it will be uncomfortable to the patient and will be quickly expelled. It may be necessary to place a small gauze pad over the anus to absorb oozing medication after the suppository has been inserted. If the suppository was for the purpose of causing defecation, the patient may defecate as soon as the urge occurs. Unless the medication was prescribed to stimulate defecation, the patient should be cautioned to retain the suppository as long as possible and to report when it is expelled.

VAGINAL MEDICATIONS

Vaginal medications can take the form of douches or irrigations, creams, or suppositories. Occasionally the patient may be able to choose the form she prefers.

Many women are familiar with over-the-counter douche preparations and may feel comfortable with their use. For best effect, douches should be administered with the patient lying down. The tip of the tubing or applicator should be moistened with water or a water-soluble lubricant. The applicator or end of the tubing should be inserted about 2 inches initially, then advanced another 1 to 2 inches as the fluid is allowed to run in by gravity. A fundamentals text offers more complete information about douching.

Vaginal suppositories may be inserted just by pushing in with a finger, or with an applicator supplied by the manufacturer. They may be lubricated with water or a water-soluble lubricant before being administered. It is important that the suppository be placed high in the vaginal vault or it will be quickly expelled.

If the patient is taking a dose once daily, it should be inserted just before the patient goes to sleep, so it will remain in the vaginal vault all night and not drain out or be expelled. If the dose is ordered to be given more than once daily, the patient should remain lying down for a short period after administration of the suppository so that the medication will not be quickly lost. Generally, the patient should be instructed to continue the medication even during the menstrual period and to avoid the use of tampons while taking vaginal medications. It is usually necessary for patients to wear a sanitary napkin during the course of therapy.

Vaginal creams usually come with an applicator supplied by the manufacturer. The same guidelines outlined under vaginal suppositories apply. Creams are generally messier than suppositories and may not be as well accepted by the patient.

SKIN APPLICATIONS

Many medications are applied to the skin, but it is such an easy and commonplace route of administration that the nurse or patient may inadvertently become too casual about them. Some topical preparations, such as emollients for dry skin, may be applied liberally, as needed. Most, however, must be measured and applied as ordered to prevent the patient from receiving too much. The nurse should try to avoid direct contact with the medication to prevent sensitization and to avoid the effects of the medication. The nurse may wear gloves, apply the medication with applicators, gauze, or cotton balls, or make certain that the medication is applied directly from the measuring guide, as is done with topical nitroglycerin preparations (see Chapter 14). Depending on the medication, the nurse must also rotate application sites, and avoid applying the medicine to abrasions, cuts, or other areas where the skin is no longer intact. Finally, some topical preparations require dressings, whereas other do not. If in doubt, the nurse should consult the physician to learn the goals of therapy and the pharmacist to determine the most effective method of administering the drug.

A recent development in topical application is the single-dose, adhesive-backed delivery system. Examples include several types of nitroglycerin preparations, and a scopolamine preparation. The nurse should refer to the manufacturer's literature for guidelines about a specific product because there are differences. Patient instruction sheets which provide illustrations and additional information, are also supplied. Examples of information included will be the preferred location for application of the delivery system, frequency of changing, and whether contact with water while swimming or bathing will affect the delivery system.

EYE MEDICATIONS

Eye medications are usually prepared in the form of drops or ointments. Eye drops are supplied in small volumes, since each dose is only a couple of drops. The nurse and the patient should avoid contaminating the dropper, and each patient in an institutional setting should have a separate bottle of eye drops. Before administering eye drops, the nurse must be certain which eye is to be medicated (if not both). A frequent source of errors is confusion about the abbreviations for left eye (o.s.), right eye (o.d.), and both eyes (o.u.). The patient should be lying down or sitting with the head tilted back. With the hand holding the dropper, the nurse places the hand on the cheek or forehead to stabilize the hand and help prevent injury to the eye. The thumb (or fingers) of the other hand gently pulls down the lower lid; it may be necessary to use a small gauze sponge or cotton ball to help do this and avoid contaminating the eye. The drops are carefully dropped into the lower conjunctival sac, *never* onto the eyeball.

Patients who blink very easily may find this modification of technique helpful when administering eye drops: Place the patient in the supine position, with the head turned to one side, about 45° from midline. The eye to receive the eye drops should be uppermost. With the eye closed, drop the prescribed dose on the inner canthus of the eye. The patient then slowly turns from the side to midline, toward the other side, while blinking. The eyedrops will move via gravity and surface tension into the conjunctival sac.

Eye ointments are applied much the same way as eye drops. A thin line of ointment is applied to the lower conjunctival sac, then the eye is closed and the eyelid gently rubbed to help distribute the dose (Figure 6.13).

A newer drug form available for eye medications is the sustained release-insert, such as the Ocusert Pilo-20 or Pilo-40 systems (manufactured by Alza). This form of pilocarpine was designed for patients with a poor history of compliance and those with conditions that make accurate instillation of eye drops difficult, such as poor vision or arthritis. The insert is placed into the upper or lower conjunctival sac, and the medication is released slowly. Patients should be instructed to make sure that it is in place every morning, since

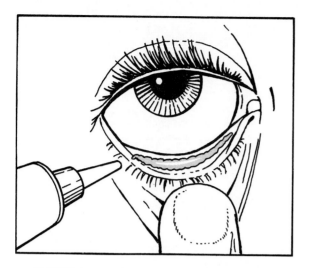

FIGURE 6.13   Administering ophthalmic ointment. To instill the ointment, gently pull the lower lid down as patient looks upward. Squeeze ophthalmic ointment into lower sac. Avoid touching tube to eyelid.

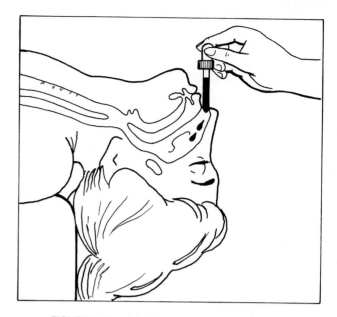

FIGURE 6.14   Administering nose drops. **A,** Gently blow nose. **B,** Open medication and draw up to calibration on dropper. **C,** Instill medication. Have patient remain in position for 2 to 3 minutes. Repeat on other side if necessary.

the unit may fall out at night. The unit is designed to be replaced weekly, but occasionally one will be effective for only a few days before needing replacement. Other drugs may become available in this form or in other new forms. Consult the manufacturer's literature and patient instruction sheet for specific guidelines to new drug forms, both to update personal knowledge and for teaching the patient and family.

Patients should be cautioned to read labels carefully, especially on refilled prescriptions. Only medications labeled for ophthalmic use should be put into the eye. Eye drops should be kept in a safe place, away from other similarly shaped containers. Occasionally patients have inadvertently put glue or other toxic substances in their eyes because they did not read the label or depended on "feel" to select the bottle or tube of medications. Many medications will cause patients to have blurry vision briefly, so patients should not drive or engage in other dangerous activities immediately after using eye medications. Finally, patients should be instructed that the use and misuse of eye medications can have serious consequences, so eye medications should be used only as prescribed.

NOSE DROPS AND SPRAYS

To instill nose drops, have the patient lie down with the head over the edge of the bed (Figure 6.14). Support the patient's head with one hand while instilling the drops with the other. When the pa-

tient's head is in midline, the nose drops will primarily reach the ethmoid and sphenoid sinuses; turning the head toward the side will facilitate having the drops reach the maxillary and frontal sinuses. The patient should remain in this position briefly, then, if possible, bend over into a head-down position to help distribute the drug. The nose should not be blown for at least several minutes so that the medication will not be expelled.

Nose spray requires that the patient inhale via one nostril while occluding the other and squeezing a spray applicator. Remove the applicator from the nares before releasing the pressure to avoid pulling sensitive nasal mucosa to the applicator opening. The head should be upright or tilted slightly back. There are many nose sprays available over the counter, especially the nasal decongestants (Chapter 4). Patients should be cautioned to use these sprays only as needed, for as short a period as possible, and only as directed.

EAR MEDICATIONS

Most ear medications are in the form of drops. The patient should be lying down, affected ear up. The medication should be at body temperature. In the adult or the child over 3 years, pull the top of

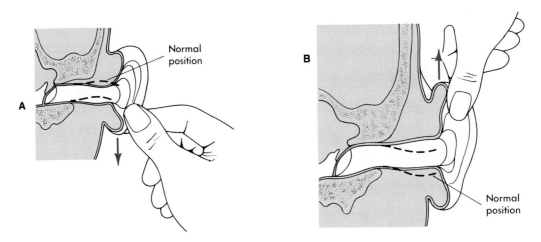

FIGURE 6.15   Straightening the ear canal for administration of ear medication. The patient is lying on his side with the ear up. **A,** For a child under 3, the ear is pulled down and straight back. **B,** For all others, pull the top of the ear up and back.

the ear up and back to straighten the ear canal, then gently drop in the prescribed number of drops. If the patient is a child under 3 years, the ear should be pulled down and straight back (Figure 6.15). The patient should remain with the affected ear up for 10 minutes to allow the medicine to disperse. A medication-soaked cotton ball plug may be gently and loosely placed in the ear to prevent oozing; a dry cotton ball will absorb the medication. If necessary to treat the other ear, the procedure is repeated with the other ear after the 10-minute waiting period.

DRUGS ADMINISTERED VIA ENDOTRACHEAL TUBE

Occasionally, in an emergency situation, it is necessary to administer drugs via endotracheal tube. This route should be used only if necessary, and only if specified by the physician. Drugs typically administered via this route include epinephrine, atropine, and lidocaine. Dilute the prescribed dose in 5 to 10 ml of sterile water and saline. Attach a long needle or soft catheter to the syringe. Auscultate the lungs to verify placement of the endotracheal tube. Keep the patient supine. Hyperventilate the patient with 3 to 5 breaths, remove the ventilator or resuscitation bag, and inject the medication through the endotracheal tube as deeply as the catheter or needle will permit; do not puncture the tube with the needle. Reattach the resuscitation bag or ventilator and hyperventilate the patient again with 3 to 5 breaths. Assess the patient's response to the medication.

INTRAOSSEOUS INFUSIONS

Intraosseous infusion may be used in emergency situations in children when an intravenous infusion cannot be started. In this technique, a special needle is inserted into a large bone, and after verification of placement through aspiration of bone marrow, drugs, fluids, or blood can be infused. Although establishing an intraosseous infusion is easier than starting an intravenous infusion on small children and infants, there are associated potential hazards, including infection. Students or nurses working in agencies where this technique is used should request instruction in its use, and should review carefully the protocol and procedure for intraosseous infusions. For additional information, see the references at the end of this chapter.

OTHER DRUG DELIVERY SYSTEMS

There are other drug delivery systems available for specific drugs or specific purposes, such as pellets for subcutaneous implantation, designed for sustained release of the drug for up to 4 to 6 months. Frequently these are developed in response to a problem in patient compliance with the prescribed dosage regimen, either unwillingness or inability; the latter might occur with limited vision, severe arthritis, or other medical conditions. The nurse faced with a delivery system that is unfamiliar should consult the manufacturer's literature and patient instruction sheet that often accompanies the dosage form.

DRUGS ADMINISTERED VIA INHALATION

There are only a few drugs administered via inhalation, one of the most difficult routes of administration for the nurse to use. For best results this method requires a cooperative patient who can inhale deeply and can manage the psychomotor tasks of using the equipment and preparing the medication. Often, though, the patient is a child and/or anxious or hypoxic because of the condition being treated, such as asthma.

In the hospital or institutional setting, inhalation therapy is fairly common, in the form of oxygen therapy via nasal cannula, nasal catheter, or some form of face mask. Other drugs may also be administered via intermittent positive pressure breathing machines (IPPB). Often there is assistance available in the form of trained respiratory therapists. It is in the outpatient setting, however, where the nurse faces the greatest challenge in ensuring correct use of inhalation therapy.

Several inhalation drug delivery systems are available, such as metered-dose nebulizers, and turbo-inhalers. Each has advantages and disadvantages. The nurse should review carefully the literature supplied by the manufacturer, including the patient instruction sheet. No attempt should be made to teach use of the delivery system if the patient is short of breath or anxious. The nurse should make certain that the patient does a satisfactory return demonstration before concluding that the patient can use the prescribed drug correctly. Patients need to be reminded to keep hand-held nebulizers and other equipment clean to prevent contamination and infection. Patients also must be cautioned to use the product only as ordered, to prevent side effects, drug overdose, and drug dependency.

SUMMARY

The safe administration or drugs to patients requires that the nurse develop practices that ensure the five rights of drug administration: the right drug, via the right route, at the right time, in the right dose, administered to the right patient. Utilizing the nursing process can help the nurse to provide individualized care.

The practice of the nurse is regulated by practice acts, institutional policies and procedures, personal moral and ethical views, and common sense. The nurse in practice should become familiar with the law, as well as with institutional policies and procedures, in order to provide safe, efficient care.

Medication errors occur frequently and for many reasons. The professional nurse remains vigilant in practice to avoid errors but does not hesitate to report errors that do occur. The nurse has the responsibility to question any aspect of a medication order and to refuse to administer a medication if in the nurse's professional judgment it would be harmful to the patient.

Care must be exercised in administering drugs to all patients, but the very young and the elderly present unique problems. To be effective, efficient, and safe, the nurse must incorporate information and theories from physiology, sociology, psychology, normal growth and development, and education, as well as nursing and pharmacology into the development of individualized plans of care for all patients.

The techniques of administering drugs via different routes requires understanding of pharmacology, anatomy, and physiology, as well as familiarity with equipment and the drug administration system in use in any agency. Practice is essential in improving manual skills.

STUDY QUESTIONS

1. What are the five rights of drug administration?
2. In the settings where you practice, who may prescribe drugs? Who prepares them? Who administers them?
3. Describe the differences between a unit dose system and a stock medication system. Which system is used in your practice settings?
4. What is the difference between the nurse practice act, or other legal guideline, and institutional policies and procedures?
5. Give examples of information related to drug administration that might be included on the patient's care plan.
6. In your practice settings, where is information about medications recorded?
7. When the nurse discovers that an error in medication administration has occurred, what should be done?
8. What are some causes of medication errors?
9. How can the theories of Erickson, Freud, or Piaget be used in guiding the nurse in administering medications to children?
10. What are some of the problems encountered in administering drugs to the elderly?
11. Name some general principles related to the safe use of all medications which should be incorporated into patient teaching plans.
12. What kinds of information about drugs should be included in the patient teaching plan?
13. What are the factors that influence patient compliance?

14. For each of the routes of medication administration listed below, answer the following questions:

What are advantages and disadvantages of this route?

Are there considerations unique to the elderly or children with this route of administration?

How is a drug administered via this route?

   a. Oral route: pills, capsules, tablets
   b. Oral route: suspensions, tinctures, elixirs, syrups, solutions
   c. Oral route: sublingual, buccal, troche, and lozenge forms
   d. Oral drugs through feeding tubes
   e. Intradermal injections
   f. Subcutaneous injections
   g. Intramuscular injections
   h. Intravenous injections
   i. Z-track intramuscular injections
   j. Rectal enemas
   k. Rectal suppositories
   l. Vaginal douches
   m. Vaginal creams and suppositories
   n. Skin applications
   o. Eye drops and ointments
   p. Nose drops and sprays
   q. Ear drops
   r. Drugs via inhalation

SUGGESTED READINGS

General sources

Delaney, C.W., and Lauer, M.L.: Intravenous therapy: a guide to quality care, Philadelphia, 1988, J.B. Lippincott.

Horne, M.M., and Swearingen, P.L.: Pocket guide to fluids and electrolytes, St. Louis, 1989, Times Mirror/Mosby College Publishing.

LaRocca, J.C., and Otto, S.E.: Pocket guide to intravenous therapy, St. Louis, 1989, Times Mirror/Mosby College Publishing.

For more information on IV therapy, see the readings at the end of Chapter 17.

The pediatric patient

Axton, S., and Fugate, T.: A protocol for pediatric IV meds, Am. J. Nurs. 87(7):943, 1987.

Bergeson, P.S., Singer, S.A., and Kaplan, A.M.: Intramuscular injections in children, Pediatrics 70(6):944, 1982.

Evans, M.L., and Hansen, B.D.: Administering injections to different-age children, Matern. Child Nurs. J. 6(3):194, 1981.

Evans, M.L., and Hansen, B.D.: A clinical guide to pediatric nursing, ed. 2, New York, 1985, Appleton-Century-Crofts.

Glass, S.M. and Giacola, G.P.: Intravenous drug therapy in premature infants: practical aspects, JOGNN 16(5):310, 1987.

Jerrett, M.D.: Taking the ouch out of injections, Can. Nurse 79(1):24, 1983.

Morrow, J.C.: Simplifying nursing management of pediatric airway and intravenous infusions, J. Emerg. Nurs. 14(2):103, 1988.

Piercy, S.: Children on long-term IV therapy, Nursing 81 11(9):66, 1981.

Sticking little muscles, Emerg. Med. 15(9):185, 1983.

The elderly patient

Bradshaw, S.: Treating yourself . . . improving compliance in the elderly, Nurs. Times 83(6):40, 1987.

Hudson MF: Drugs and the older adult take special care, Nursing 84 14(8):46, 1984.

Matteson, M.A., and McConnell, E.S.: Gerontological nursing: concepts and practice, Philadelphia, 1988, W.B. Saunders.

Ramsey, R.: Adjusting drug dosages for critically ill elderly patients, Nursing 88 18(7):47, 1988.

Ries, D.T., Salerno, E., and Sank, J.: Over-the-counter medications: quicksand for the elderly, J. Comm. Health Nurs. 3(4):183, 1986.

Drug history

Bell, S.K.: Guidelines for taking a complete drug history, Nursing 80 10(3):10, 1980.

Specific drug administration routes or techniques

Arbeiter, J.: The safe way to work with the pharmacy, RN 51(10):91, 1988.

Barrus, D.H., and Danek, G.: Should you irrigate an occluded IV line? Nursing 87 17(3):63, 1987.

Bourne, M.K.: Intraosseous infusion: an innovation of the 1980s? Emerg. Nurs. Rep. 3(5):1, 1988.

Boykoff, S.L., Boxwell, A.O., and Boxwell, J.J.: 6 ways to clear the air from an IV line, Nursing 88 18(2):46, 1988.

Burman, R., and Berkowitz, H.S.: IV bolus: effective, but potentially dangerous, Crit. Care. Nurse 16(1):22, 1986.

Chaplin, G., Shull, H., and Welk, P.C. III: How safe is the air-bubble technique for I.M. injections? Nursing 85 15(9):59, 1985.

Clarke, J., and Cox, E.: Heparinisation of Hickman catheters, Nurs. Times 84(15):51, 1988.

Cunliffe, M.T., and Polomano, R.C.: How to clear catheter clots with urokinase, Nursing 86 16(12):40, 1986.

Fought, S.G.: Venous access in burn injuries, Crit. Care Nurse 8(1):12, 1988.

Francombe, P.: Intravenous filters and phlebitis, Nurs. Times 84(26):34, 1988.

Gever, L.N.: Administering drugs through the skin: the new transdermal route, Nursing 82 12(3):88, 1982.

Giving drugs through an endotracheal tube, Nursing 88 18(4):82, 1988.

Goodman, M.S., and Wickham, R.: Venous access devices: an overview. Oncol. Nurs. Forum 11(5):16, 1984.

Graber, R.F.: Emergency intraosseous infusion, Patient Care 21(11):245, 1987.

Hecker, J.: Improved technique in IV therapy, Nurs. Times 84(34):28, 1988.

Hermann, C.S.: Performing intradermal skin tests the right way, Nursing 83 13(10):50, 1983.

Herring, C.A.: Endotracheal administration of medications, Crit. Care Nurse 8(6):84, 1988.

Holmes, W.: SQ chemotherapy at home, Am. J. Nurs. 85(2):168, 1985.

Hower, D.K.: Using special IV lines at home, Nursing 87 17(7):56, 1987.

Howser, D.M., and Meader, C.D.: Hickman catheter care: developing organized teaching strategies, Cancer Nurs. 10(2):70, 1987.

Instilling eyedrops, Nursing 84 14(3):77, 1984.

Instilling eyedrops in the involuntary blinker, Letter to the Editor, New Engl. J. Med. **318**(4):258, 1988.

Jones, P.M.: Indwelling central venous catheter—related infections and two different procedures of catheter care, Cancer Nurs. **10**(3):123, 1987.

Lenz, C.L.: Make your needle selection right to the point, Nursing 83 **13**(2):50, 1983.

Mazzara, J.T., Parmley, W.W., and Russell, R.O. Jr.: A close look at Swan-Ganz catheters, Patient Care **22**(3):36, 1988.

McConnell E.A.: The subtle art of really good injections, RN **45**:(2):24, 1982.

Meeske, K., and Davidson, L.T.: Teacher's reference on right atrial catheters, J. Pediatr Nurs. **3**(5):351, 1988.

Millam, D.A.: Tips for improving your venipuncture techniques, Nursing 87 **17**(6):46, 1987.

Millam, D.A.: Managing complications of IV therapy, Nursing 88 **18**(3):34, 1988.

Millam, D.A.: Mastering arterial punctures: getting into an artery, Am. J. Nurs. **88**(9):1213, 1988.

Morris, L.L.: Critical care's most versatile tool . . . a multilumen central venous catheter, RN **51**(5):42, 1988.

Newton, G.A.: A better way to chart IV therapy, RN **51**(7):26, 1988.

Peck, K.R., and Altieri, M.: Intraosseous infusions: an old technique with modern applications, Pediatr. Nurs. **14**(4):296, 1988.

Pupo, M.: The Hickman/Broviac catheter: a right atrial catheter, CINA J. **2**(1):16, 1986.

Ramos, L.: Care and management of long-term arterial catheters, Crit. Care Nurse **7**(1):66, 1987.

Sepciale, J.L., and Kaalaas, J.: Infuse-a-port: new path for IV chemotherapy, Nursing 85 **15**(10):40, 1985.

Shepherd, M.J., and Swearington, P.L.: Z-track injections, Am. J. Nurs. **84**(6):746, 1984.

Sohl, L., and Nze, R.: Working with triple-lumen central venous catheters, Nursing 88 **18**(7):50, 1988.

Sumner, J.: Preserving IV power if fluids are restricted, RN **51**(8):26, 1988.

Szunyog, C.L.: Getting I.V. patients ready to go home, RN **50**(10):136, 1987.

Taylor, J.P., and Taylor, J.E.: Vascular access devices: uses and aftercare, J. Emerg. Nurs. **13**(3):160, 1987.

Testerman, E.J.: IV drug administration guidelines: a simplified format, J. Intravenous Nurs. **11**(3):188, 1988.

Tobin, C.R.: The teflon intravenous catheter: incidence of phlebitis and duration of catheter life in the neonatal patient, JOGNN **17**(1):35, 1988.

Todd, B.: Using eyedrops and ointments safely, Geriatr. Nurs. **4**(1):53, 1983.

Todd, B.: Intravenous drug hazards: interactions, adsorption, and inadequate mixing, Geriatr. Nurs. **9**(1):20, 1988.

VanBree, N.S., Hollerbach, A.D., and Brooks, G.P.: Clinical evaluation of three techniques for administering low-dose heparin, Nurs. Res. **23**(1):15, 1984.

Venipuncture made easy—and less painful, Am. J. Nurs. **87**(11):1403, 1987.

Whittaker, N.: Finding the right answer . . . drug calculation, Senior Nurse **6**(6):33, 1987.

Winfrey, A.: Single-dose I.M. injections. How much is too much? Nursing 85 **15**(7):38, 1985.

Wordell, D.C.: Should you crush that tablet? Nursing 88 **18**(1):48, 1988.

Safe drug administration

Clayton, M.: The right way to prevent medication errors, RN **59**(6):30, 1987.

Davis, N.M., and Cohen, M.R.: Learning from mistakes: medication errors to avoid, Nursing 87 **17**(5):84, 1987.

McGovern, K.: 10 golden rules for administering drugs safely, Nursing 88 **18**(8):34, 1988.

Pelletier, L.R., and Poster, E.C.: Method of medication administration: effect on error rates, J. Nurs. Adm. **18**(4):29, 1988.

Poster, E.C., and Pelletier, L.: Primary versus functional medication administration: monitoring and evaluating medication error rates, J. Nurs. Qual. Assur. **2**(2):68, 1988.

Sadler, C.: Improving nursing practice . . . guidelines on safe drug administration, Nurs. Times **83**(46):18, 1987.

CHAPTER

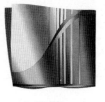

7

Calculation of Drug Dosages

In Chapters 2 and 6 we discussed the various routes by which a drug may be administered and we illustrated the importance of careful control of drug levels in the body. Administering the proper drug dose by the appropriate route is the obvious first step in ensuring that the desired drug concentration will appear in the bloodstream. In this chapter we will consider how to calculate drug dosages.

ROLE OF THE NURSE

The nurse shares moral and legal responsibility with the physician and the pharmacist in administering drugs. In many hospitals the pharmacist calculates and prepares the drug for administration to the patient, based on the physician's order. This practice does not remove legal responsibility from the nurse who actually administers the drug to the patient. It is the nurse who must verify that the correct drug at the proper dose has been prepared (Chapter 6). For this reason the nurse should be familiar with the forms of drugs and be able to recognize common medications.

The nurse's proper role in the clinic may also include questioning a physician's order for a drug when that order seems inappropriate. For example, a drug dose well outside normal clinical dosage ranges might be questioned. It may also be appropriate to question an order for a drug producing toxic reactions if a particular patient might be more susceptible than normal to such reactions. For example, the patient may have complained of stomach distress during hospitalization. That fact might influence the physician to select an enteric-coated drug form, which would be less irritating to the stomach than normal tablets. For this reason it is appropriate for the nurse to call attention to the patient's complaint.

The nurse has access to several sources of information about specific drugs. Manufacturers include specific information related to dosage and toxicity as a package insert with medication. The same information can be found in the *Physician's Desk Reference* (PDR), which also contains a series of color plates showing the dosage forms of specific drugs. The PDR is organized according to drug manufacturer. Other books of similar content are organized according to drug class. One such publication is *Facts and Comparisons*. Another is *USP Drug Information for the Health Care Professional* (USP DI). The USP DI also has a separate volume containing drug information in lay language *(Advice for the Patient)*. Either the PDR, or *Facts and Comparisons,* or the USP DI might be found in the nursing unit or in the pharmacy. Another source of information more likely to be found in a library is the *AMA Drug Evaluations*. This publication not only lists available drugs but also comments on clinical use and toxic reactions. Another useful book is the *Handbook of Drugs for Nursing Practice.* In addition to these publications, numerous drug handbooks or handbooks of therapy are available from several publishers. Some publications, such as the PDR, are published annually, whereas others are published less frequently. Since medical opinion on such subjects as drug toxicity or efficacy can change with increased clinical experience with a drug, it is wise to consult the most recent reference available when questions arise.

READING DRUG ORDERS

Physicians and pharmacists sometimes employ a system of abbreviations in writing orders or prescriptions. These abbreviations are derived from Latin phrases and, although Latin is no longer used in medical communication, their use persists through custom. For this reason the nurse must be familiar with the common abbreviations listed in Table 7.1. Many of the abbreviations designate how

Table 7.1 Abbreviations Encountered in Physicians' Orders and Prescriptions

Abbreviation	Latin phrase	Translation
ad lib.	ad libitum	freely; as much or as often as wanted
aa. (or a̅a̅)	ana	of each
a.c.	ante cibum	before meals
b.i.d.	bis in die	twice daily
c̄	cum	with
gtt.	guttae	drops
h.s.	hora somni	at bedtime
non rep.	non repetatur	do not repeat
o.d.	oculus dexter	right eye
o.s.	oculus sinister	left eye
o.u.	oculus uterque	both eyes
p.c.	post cibum	after meals
p.o.	per os	by mouth
p.r.	per rectum	by rectal route
p.r.n.	pro re nata	according to circumstances
q.s.	quantum sufficit	as much as is necessary
q.d.	quaque die	every day
q.h. q. 4 h	quaque hora	every hour every 4 hours
q.i.d.	quarter in die	four times daily
ss. (or s̄s̄)	semis	one half
stat.	statim	immediately
t.i.d.	ter in die	three times daily

Table 7.2 Systems of Units in Common Use in the United States

System	Unit of mass	Unit of volume
Metric	Gram (Gm)	Liter (L)
Apothecaries'	Grain (gr)	Minims (m)
Household	Pound (lb)	Pint (pt)

Table 7.3 Table of Equivalents within Systems

System	Equivalents
Metric	1.0 Gm = 0.001 kg 1.0 Gm = 1000 mg 1.0 L = 1000 ml
Apothecaries'	1.0 gr = 1/60 dram (dr or L) = 1/480 oz 60 gr = 1 dr 8 dr = 1 oz (or K) 1.0 minim (m) = 1/60 f dr = 1/480 f oz 60 m = 1 f dr (or f L) 8 f dr = 1 f oz (or f K)
Household	1.0 lb = 16 oz 1.0 pt = ½ quart (qt) = ⅛ gallon (gal) 1.0 pt = 16 f oz = 32 tablespoonsful (T) 1.0 T = 3 teaspoonsful (t)

the drug is to be administered. For example, a physician's order might read "Penicillin G 100,000 U q. 3h., p.o." This order would be translated to "100,000 units (U) of penicillin G are to be administered every 3 hours (q. 3h.) by mouth (p.o.)."

Some confusion can be generated by the use of these abbreviations, and the nurse must be certain that the physician's intent is clearly understood. Among the most troublesome are the abbreviations ad lib. and p.r.n. A drug given p.r.n. should be taken at the prescribed interval if the patient requires the drug. For example, a postsurgery patient might have the following order on the chart: "Morphine 10 mg q. 4h., p.r.n.". Every 4 hours the nurse should assess whether the patient requires the morphine for pain relief. If the patient is sleeping or is comfortable, administering the dose may be postponed. According to the drug order, the morphine may be given less frequently than every 4 hours but not more frequently. In contrast, a medication prescribed "ad lib." is given whenever the patient needs it.

The abbreviations discussed here are used as a medical shorthand to save time in communicating between medical personnel. If the use of an abbreviation creates any uncertainty in the mind of the nurse administering the medication, the physician or the pharmacist should be consulted for clarification.

UNITS OF DRUG DOSAGE

In clinical practice, nurses will encounter situations in which they will be called on to translate a physician's order for a certain drug dosage into the proper number of tablets or the proper volume of drug for an individual patient. This section is intended to prepare the student of nursing to handle these problems with skill and confidence.

Before turning to the rather simple arithmetical principles required to solve dosage problems, we must familiarize ourselves with the three systems of units in common use in the United States today. These are the metric system, the apothecaries' system, and the common, household, system (Table 7.2). Within each of these systems we are concerned with the primary units of mass and volume, since all of the problems we will be called on to solve will be expressed in some unit of drug mass and some unit of drug volume.

The primary unit of mass within the metric system is the *gram* (Gm). With prefixes, this unit can be adjusted to express thousan*ds* of grams (1 *kilo*gram = 1000 grams) or thousan*dths* of grams (1 *milli*gram = 0.001 gram). In less common usage are the prefixes *deci* and *centi*, meaning ¹⁄₁₀ and ¹⁄₁₀₀, respectively. The primary unit of volume within the metric system is the liter (L). With prefixes, the liter is commonly divided into thousandths (1 L = 1000 *milli*liters), and less commonly into millionths (1 L = 1,000,000 *micro*liters), or hundredths (1 L = 10 *deci*liters).

The milliliter (ml) is the metric unit equivalent to the unit of gas volume commonly encountered in the clinic, the cubic centimeter (cc).

The primary unit of mass in the apothecaries' system is the grain (gr). It must be remembered that 60 gr constitutes 1 dram and that 8 drams is equivalent to 1 ounce. The primary unit of volume in the apothecaries' system is the minim. The equivalent of 60 minims is 1 fluid dram (f dr); 8 f dr = 1 f oz.

Equivalents within the household system may be familiar from domestic experience. Table 7.3 lists the equivalents for all three systems.

Any of the three systems of units may be used by a physician in ordering drugs. The metric system possesses many advantages in terms of ease of calculation and convenience of units, but use of the older systems still persists in some situations. A nurse may be called on to convert drug doses from one system to another. Unfortunately, the exact equivalents result in awkward and unwieldy values. For example, 1 L = 0.26418 gallons; 1 quart = 0.9643 L; 1 grain = 0.0648 Gm; 1 f oz = 29.57 ml; 1 oz (apothecary) = 31.1 Gm. Obviously these numbers are not convenient in calculations. For this reason certain approximations have been agreed on and these are employed in ordinary circumstances for converting between systems. These conversions are listed in Table 7.4.

Abbreviations for the various units are not entirely standardized in the medical literature. For example, gram may be abbreviated Gm, gm, or g. One set of abbreviations has been adopted for use throughout this book. Table 7.5 summarizes the abbreviations in use for various units.

The apothecaries' system also has some unusual expressions that require explanation. Unlike

Table 7.4 Conversion of Units Between Systems

Apothecaries'	Metric
15 gr	= 1 Gm*
1 dr	= 4 Gm
1 oz	= 32 Gm
15 m	= 1 ml
1 f dr	= 4 ml
1 f oz	= 30 ml†

Household	Metric
1 t	= 5 ml
1 T	= 14 ml
1 pt	= 480 ml (or 500 ml)
1 qt	= 960 ml (or 1000 ml)
1 gal	= 3.84 L (or 4 L)
1 lb (avoirdupois)	= 0.46 kg or 1 kg = 2.2 lb

*Two factors have been used for converting grams to milligrams. The older conversion factor is 65 mg = 1 gr. This factor is the basis for aspirin and acetaminophen formulations (i.e., a 5 gr aspirin tablet contains 325 mg of aspirin). The newer conversion factor agreed on is 60 mg = 1 gr. This new conversion factor is easier to use for drugs, such as morphine, that are frequently administered in small doses (fractions of grains). For example, ¼ gr of morphine equals 15 mg, using the new conversion factor. The student should remember that these factors are simply agreed on for ease of calculation. All the problems presented in this book use the conversion 15 gr = 1000 mg.
†30 ml has been agreed on as the equivalent for 1 f oz, rather than the more exact approximation of 32 ml, since 30 ml is more conveniently and accurately estimated in most clinical glassware.

any other system, apothecaries' units are frequently used with small Roman numerals rather than Arabic numerals. Moreover, in the apothecaries' system the units precede the numeral. For example, 5 gr may be written gr v, gr being the abbreviation for grain and v the Roman numeral for 5. In this system the abbreviation *ss* designates one half. For example, gr iss is translated 1½ gr. Smaller fractions of grains are written out in Arabic numerals. For example, a quarter grain would be written gr ¼.

The nurse in practice deals with solutions of drugs on a daily basis. A *solution* is defined as a given mass of solid substance dissolved in a known volume of fluid (w/v; weight/volume) or as a given volume of a liquid substance dissolved in a known volume of another fluid (v/v; volume/volume). The concentration of a w/v solution is always expressed as units of mass per units of volume. Common concentration units are Gm/ml, Gm/L, mg/ml, gr/m, and dr/f oz. Concentrations are also commonly expressed as percentages, based on the definition of a 1% solution as 1 Gm of solid/100 ml of solution. Proportions are also used as expressions of concentrations. For example, 1:1000 designates a solution containing 1 Gm/1000 ml of solution. Blood levels of certain metabolites are frequently expressed as mg% (mg/100 ml) of solution. Mg/100 ml is equivalent to mg/deciliter, that is, a 1 mg% solution is the same as a 1 mg/deciliter solution.

The relationship between the various expressions of concentration is illustrated in Table 7.6.

CALCULATIONS
Calculating the Strength of Drug Solutions

Calculating the concentration of a drug solution utilizes the following equation:

$$\text{Concentration} = \text{Mass of drug/volume of solution}$$

If you know any two of these quantities, you can solve directly for the third, provided all the quantities are expressed in the same system of units. Therefore, as a first step in the solution of any problem, it is frequently necessary to convert units from one system to another, as we see in example 1.

EXAMPLE 1: *Prepare 1 L of a 5% solution.*
You know:
  1. Volume of solution (1 L)
  2. Concentration (5%)
To solve:
  1. Convert all quantities to the same system of units:

Table 7.5	**Abbreviations for Various Units**	
Unit	Abbreviation used in this text	Other acceptable abbreviations
Gram	Gm	gm, g
Milligram	mg	mgm
Microgram	μg	mcg
Liter	L	l
Milliliter	ml	cc*

*Used for gases only.

$$5\% = 5 \text{ Gm}/100 \text{ ml}; 1 \text{ L} = 1000 \text{ ml}$$

2. Substitute the known quantities into the equation:

$$5 \text{ Gm}/100 \text{ ml} = \text{Mass of drug}/1000 \text{ ml}$$

3. Solve for mass of drug:

$$\text{Mass} = \frac{1000 \text{ ml} \times 5 \text{ Gm}}{100 \text{ ml}} = 50 \text{ Gm}$$

EXAMPLE 2: *What is the strength of a 2 L solution containing 10 Gm of drug?*
You know:
  1. Mass of drug (10 Gm)
  2. Volume of solution (2 L)
To solve:
  Substitute the known quantities into the equation:

$$\text{Concentration} = \frac{10 \text{ Gm}}{2 \text{ L}} =$$
$$\frac{5 \text{ Gm}}{\text{L}} = \frac{0.5 \text{ Gm}}{100 \text{ ml}} = 0.5\% = 1{:}200$$

EXAMPLE 3: *How much of a 2% solution can be prepared with 6 Gm of drug?*
You know:
  1. Concentration (2%)
  2. Mass of drug (6 Gm)
To solve:
  1. Convert all quantities to the same system of units:

$$2\% = \frac{2 \text{ Gm}}{100 \text{ ml}}$$

2. Substitute the known quantities into the equation:

$$2 \text{ Gm}/100 \text{ ml} = 6 \text{ Gm}/\text{Volume of solution}$$

3. Solve for volume of solution:

Table 7.6   Equivalents of Concentration Expressions

%	Ratio	Gm/L	mg/ml	mg/dl	µg/ml
10.0	1:10	100	100	10,000	100,000
1.0	1:100	10	10	1,000	10,000
0.1	1:1000	1.0	1.0	100	1,000
0.01	1:10,000	0.1	0.1	10	100
0.001	1:100,000	0.01	0.01	1.0	10
0.0001	1:1,000,000	0.001	0.001	0.1	1.0

$$\text{Volume} = \frac{6 \text{ Gm} \times 100 \text{ ml}}{2 \text{ Gm}} = 300 \text{ ml}$$

EXAMPLE 4: *Prepare 4 oz of a 0.5% solution from tablets gr v each.*

You know:
1. Volume of solution required (4 oz)
2. Concentration of solution (0.5%)

To solve:
1. Convert all quantities to the same system of units:

$$0.5\% = 0.5 \text{ Gm}/100 \text{ ml}$$

$$4 \text{ oz} = 4 \times 32 \text{ ml} = 128 \text{ ml}$$

$$\text{gr v} = 5 \text{ gr} = 0.333 \text{ Gm}$$

2. Substitute the known quantities in the equation:

$$0.5 \text{ Gm}/100 \text{ ml} = \text{Mass of drug}/128 \text{ ml}$$

3. Solve for mass of drug:

$$\text{Mass} = \frac{128 \text{ ml} \times 0.5 \text{ Gm}}{100 \text{ ml}} = 0.64 \text{ Gm}$$

4. Determine the number of tablets required to total 0.64 Gm:

$$\frac{0.64 \text{ Gm}}{0.33 \text{ Gm/tablet}} = 2 \text{ tablets}$$

As shown, 2 tablets would be dissolved in 4 oz to prepare the desired solution. Note that the conversion was not exact but was very close to a value of 2 and was rounded off. In dealing with scored tablets, one may calculate to the nearest half tablet.

Self-test for proficiency in drug calculations

After thorough study of the previous section, the student should be able to work the following problems. You can check your answers and see the calculations worked out in the answers at the end of this chapter.

SET 1: *Conversions of units and expressions of concentration*
1. A solution is 1/50 gr/m. Express this concentration in the following units:
   a. Gm/L _____
   b. mg/ml _____
   c. % _____
   d. mg% _____
   e. ratio _____
   f. µg/ml _____

SET 2: *Conversion of units used in calculations*
1. The tablets on hand are 0.9 mg each. The order is for gr 1/150. How many tablets should you give?
2. A drug in liquid form contains gr iiss in 1 t. What is the drug concentration in Gm/L?
3. Prepare 3 f oz of a 0.1% solution from tablets gr iss each.
4. How would you prepare 15 gallons of a 1:6000 solution from a powder?
5. The tablets on hand are marked 0.1 mg each. The order is for gr 1/300. How should the nurse proceed?
6. What is the strength of 100 ml of solvent containing gr v?

Calculating the Strength of Diluted Solutions

The examples just given have all dealt with weight/volume problems. In examining volume/volume problems, the basic equation can be modified slightly and the problems solved in much the same way as before. The equation then becomes:

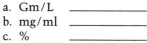

(Concentration of solution) × (Volume of solution) =
(Concentration of stock) × (Volume of stock)

Introduction to Neuropharmacology

8

Overview

Many different classes of drugs, used for a variety of therapeutic purposes, affect the nervous system at some level. Some of these drugs are designed to alter the function of some portion of the nervous system, whereas others alter functions of the nervous system as a side effect. A review of the anatomy and biochemical function of the nervous system is necessary to understand the mechanisms of these drugs and the array of side effects they produce. The purpose of this chapter is to present that review.

The central nervous system includes the brain and spinal cord. The functions of these structures are twofold: first, to monitor, convey, and process signals from sensory receptors throughout the body by way of ascending neuronal pathways; and, second, to sequence information and convey signals to initiate or to modify body actions.

The neurons that relay information from the central nervous system to the rest of the body are called *efferent neurons*. The ascending sensory neurons and the efferent neurons form the *peripheral nervous system*. The peripheral nervous system is subdivided into the *motor nervous system* and the *autonomic nervous system*.

NEUROTRANSMITTERS
Neurotransmitters and Receptors

All neurons use neurotransmitters to contact neurons and other cells. A neurotransmitter is a chemical that is synthesized in the nerve cell and stored inside vesicles (sacs) in the terminal. Most neurons appear to make only one kind of neurotransmitter. When the neuron is stimulated, some of the vesicles merge with the nerve terminal membrane and quantities of neurotransmitter are released. There is a space between the neuron and the cell with which the neuron is communicating.

This space is the *synaptic cleft.* The neurotransmitter molecules diffuse across the synapse and occupy specific *receptors* on the next cell. The function of the receptor is to recognize only one specific neurotransmitter and to initiate a cellular response to that neurotransmitter. The binding of the neurotransmitter to its receptor is reversible. When the neurotransmitter diffuses away from the receptor, the stimulation of the cell is terminated.

Two neurotransmitters, acetylcholine and norepinephrine, are used in the peripheral nervous system. A given class of neurons, however, will use only one of these neurotransmitters. The synthesis and degradation of each neurotransmitter will first be discussed. A description of where each neurotransmitter is found in the peripheral nervous system and the responses produced will follow.

The Neurotransmitter Acetylcholine

Acetylcholine is synthesized in the nerve terminal by the enzyme choline acetylase from choline and an acetate molecule activated by coenzyme A (Figure 8.1). This acetylcholine is packaged in vesicles. On stimulation of the nerve, some of the vesicles release acetylcholine into the synapse, where the acetylcholine diffuses to the opposing membrane and binds at the specific receptors for acetylcholine. In addition, the membrane contains the enzyme acetylcholinesterase, which degrades acetylcholine to acetate and choline. The acetylcholinesterase is very active, and the half-life of the acetylcholine released is only a few milliseconds. Any acetylcholine that diffuses from the synapse into the blood is degraded by nonspecific cholinesterases in the blood or tissues. Thus, when released, acetylcholine produces a response in the next cell by way of the acetylcholine receptor and/or is rapidly degraded by the membrane-bound enzyme acetylcholinesterase or by nonspecific cholinesterases in the blood plasma.

The Neurotransmitter Norepinephrine and the Neurohormone Epinephrine

Norepinephrine is synthesized in the nerve terminal from the amino acid tyrosine (see Figure 8.1). Norepinephrine is a neurotransmitter because it is released from a neuron to act on an adjacent cell. The chromaffin cells of the adrenal medulla also synthesize norepinephrine but convert 80% to 85% of the norepinephrine to epinephrine. These adrenal stores of epinephrine and norepinephrine are released into the blood on stimulation of the adrenal medulla in response to stress. Epinephrine is called a neurohormone because it is released into the blood to produce effects at distant sites.

Most norepinephrine is *not* degraded after release. Instead, norepinephrine is taken back up into the neuron from which it was released and stored again in granules. This process is called *reuptake*. There are two enzymes that can degrade norepinephrine and epinephrine. Monoamine oxidase (MAO) is located in the mitochondria of most cells, including nerve terminals that release norepinephrine. Catechol-O-methyltransferase (COMT) is found in the cytoplasm of most cells. Both MAO and COMT are found in large concentrations in the liver and kidney. Any norepinephrine that diffuses into the blood or any epinephrine in the blood is quickly degraded by the liver and/or kidney. No drugs are used that interfere with COMT, but in later chapters we shall see that drugs which inhibit MAO are used as antidepressant drugs, as an antihypertensive drug, and in the treatment of parkinsonism. Epinephrine and norepinephrine are metabolized to the common product vanillylmandelic acid (VMA). Since VMA is excreted in the urine, the measurement of VMA in collected urine is used as an index of sympathetic activity.

The main features of the peripheral nervous system and its neurotransmitters acetylcholine and norepinephrine will be reviewed as a preparation for discussing drugs that act by modifying neurotransmitter action within the peripheral nervous system. We shall start with the motor nervous system, and then discuss the more complex autonomic nervous system.

MOTOR (SOMATIC) NERVOUS SYSTEM

The motor or somatic nervous system is under both conscious and unconscious control to initiate muscle contraction (Figure 8.2). A motor neuron has a cell body in the spinal cord and contacts a striated muscle at a specialized region, the neuromuscular junction. Motor neurons are found in several cranial nerves and in all spinal nerves. Stimulation of a motor neuron releases acetylcholine at the neuromuscular junction, and the muscle cell reacts to acetylcholine by contracting. Stimulation of a motor neuron may arise as a result of a willed impulse originating in the brain and transmitted to the appropriate neuron in the spinal cord or, unconsciously, as a reflex. A reflex is initiated by sensory input (i.e., heat, touch, pressure, pain), which is transmitted to the spinal cord, then out to the motor neurons without processing by the brain.

AUTONOMIC NERVOUS SYSTEM

Divisions of the Autonomic Nervous System

The role of the autonomic nervous system is to monitor and to control internal body functions such as cardiac output, blood volume, blood composition, blood pressure, and digestive processes, primarily by modifying the tone of tissue smooth muscle and the quantity of tissue secretions (see Figure 8.2). The autonomic nervous system has two distinct efferent divisions, the *parasympathetic (cholinergic) nervous system* and the *sympathetic (adrenergic) nervous system*. Both divisions commonly act on a given organ, but produce opposite responses. This is highlighted in Table 8.1, in which the prominent effects of the two divisions on key tissues are summarized. For example, the parasympathetic division slows the heart rate, whereas the sympathetic division increases the heart rate. This *dual antagonistic innervation* is a hallmark of the autonomic nervous system, allowing full control of organ function according to bodily requirements. This antagonism is a result of two distinct kinds of receptors, adrenergic receptors and cholinergic receptors, coexisting on the same organ. Activation of the cholinergic receptor, in general, produces the opposite cellular response from activation of the adrenergic receptor.

Autonomic Tone

The concept of autonomic tone is also important. Although a minimal but constant release of each neurotransmitter affects each tissue, one branch of the autonomic nervous system is dominant and sets the tone of that tissue to coordinate with other tissues. The sympathetic nervous system provides the dominant tone for the cardiovascular system, so that the magnitude of cardiac and blood pressure responses reflects predominantly the degree of sympathetic tone, which is itself determined and coordinated within the central nervous system. Parasympathetic control of the cardiovascular system is primarily that of a reflex decelerator system to protect against rapid rises in cardiovascular function. On the other hand, parasympathetic tone is coordinated within certain

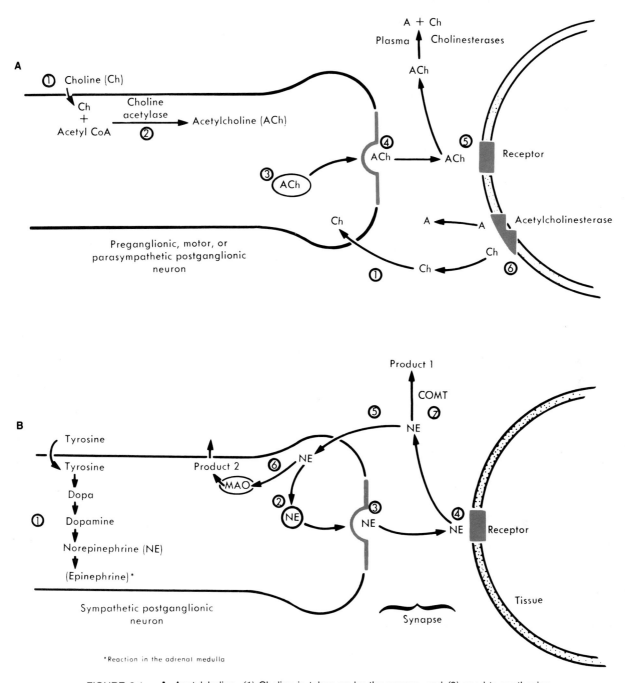

FIGURE 8.1   **A,** Acetylcholine. *(1)* Choline is taken up by the neuron, and *(2)* used to synthesize acetylcholine, which *(3)* is stored in vesicles. On stimulation of the neuron *(4)*, some vesicles merge with the membrane to discharge acetylcholine into the synapse, where acetylcholine diffuses to *(5)* its receptor to activate the cell, or to *(6)* acetylcholinesterase, the enzyme that degrades acetylcholine. Plasma cholinesterases can also degrade acetylcholine. **B,** Norepinephrine. *(1)* Tyrosine is taken into the neuron and in three reactions is modified to norepinephrine, which is *(2)* stored in vesicles. On stimulation of the neuron *(3)*, some vesicles merge with the membrane to discharge norepinephrine into the synapse, where it diffuses to *(4)* its receptor to activate the cell. Most of the norepinephrine is *(5)* taken up by the neuron and reused. Some norepinephrine is degraded by *(6)* the mitochondrial enzyme monoamine oxidase (MAO) or *(7)* the enzyme catechol-O-methyl transferase (COMT) found in most body tissues.

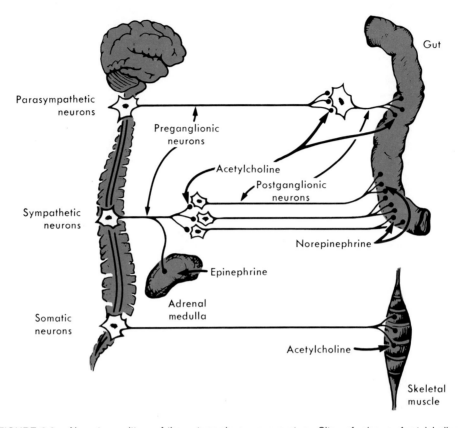

FIGURE 8.2 Neurotransmitters of the autonomic nervous system. Sites of release. Acetylcholine and norepinephrine are released from neurons as indicated on adjacent cells. Epinephrine is released from adrenal medulla into blood to act throughout the body.

brain centers to dominate visual, digestive, and eliminatory functions and to determine the intensity of these responses. The role of the sympathetic nervous system is primarily that of an override system to depress these functions in times of stress.

Preganglionic and Postganglionic Neurons

Each efferent division of the autonomic nervous system is a two-neuron system. The first neuron *(preganglionic neuron)* has its cell body in the brain stem or spinal cord and terminates outside the spinal cord in a special nervous tissue, a ganglion (see Figure 8.2). The first neuron sends a projection out of the spinal cord *(preganglionic fiber)*, which contacts a second neuron *(postganglionic neuron)* within the ganglion. The neurotransmitter for the synapse in the ganglion is acetylcholine. The second neuron has its cell body in a ganglion and by means of a *postganglionic fiber* innervates an internal organ, usually modifying the action of involuntary muscle such as smooth muscle or cardiac muscle.

Role of Acetylcholine, Norepinephrine, and Epinephrine

The most important pharmacological difference between the parasympathetic and sympathetic nervous systems is that the final postganglionic transmitter is different for the two divisions. The preganglionic neurotransmitter at the synapses within the ganglia for both divisions is acetylcholine. However, the parasympathetic nervous system also uses acetylcholine as a postganglionic neurotransmitter. It is for this reason that the parasympathetic nervous system is often called the *cholinergic nervous system.* The sympathetic nervous system uses norepinephrine as the postganglionic transmitter. The sympathetic nervous system has another component, the neurohormone epinephrine. Epinephrine is released from the adrenal medulla as a reaction to stress. The adrenal medulla acts like a postganglionic neuron because it is innervated by a preganglionic fiber and on stimulation releases epinephrine. Epinephrine is carried by the blood throughout the body where epineph-

Table 8.1   Actions of the Autonomic Nervous System

Tissue	Sympathetic (adrenergic) response	Parasympathetic (cholinergic or muscarinic) response
Eye	Dilation (mydriasis)	Constriction (miosis) Accommodation (focus on near objects)
Glands	Increased sweating* Increased salivation (thick, contains proteins)	Increased salivation (copious, watery) Increased tears and secretions of respiratory and gastrointestinal tract
Heart	Increased rate (positive chronotropy) Increased strength of contraction (increased contractility or positive inotropy) Increased conduction velocity through the atrioventricular node (positive dromotropy)	Decreased rate (negative chronotropy) Decreased strength of contraction (negative inotropy) Decreased conduction velocity through the atrioventricular node (negative dromotropy)
Bronchioles	Smooth muscle relaxation (opens airways)	Smooth muscle constriction (restricts airways)
Blood vessels	Dilates vessels in heart and skeletal muscle Constricts vessels in skin, viscera, salivary gland, erectile tissues, kidney	Constricts vessels in heart (not a prominent effect in humans) Dilates vessels in salivary gland and erectile tissues
Gastrointestinal tract 　Smooth muscle 　Sphincters	 Relaxation Contraction	 Contraction Relaxation
Urinary bladder 　Fundus 　Trigone and sphincter	 Relaxation Contraction	 Contraction Relaxation
Uterus	Contraction	
Liver	Glycogenolysis	

*Acetylcholine is the neurotransmitter for this sympathetic response. This is the exception to the rule that norepinephrine is the postganglionic neurotransmitter.

rine not only activates tissue receptors for norepinephrine but also activates additional receptors more specific for epinephrine itself as well. The synonym for the sympathetic nervous system is the *adrenergic nervous system*. The term *adrenergic* comes from the British word for epinephrine, *adrenaline*. (Norepinephrine is called noradrenaline.) The identity of the neurotransmitter at the various sites of the peripheral nervous system is diagrammed in Figure 8.2.

Functional and Anatomical Characteristics of the Autonomic Nervous System

Functional characteristics. Certain characteristics readily distinguish the parasympathetic and sympathetic nervous systems functionally.

These characteristic functions are listed in Table 8.1. The parasympathetic nervous system has dominant control over "regulatory" processes of the body, whereas the sympathetic nervous system provides immediate adaptation for "fight or flight." Indeed, the easiest way to remember the actions of the sympathetic nervous system (and by contrast the parasympathetic nervous system) is to review the "fight or flight" adaptations: the eyes dilate so that vision is improved even in dim light, the bronchioles dilate to let air flow to and from the lungs more readily, the heart beats faster and with greater strength to get blood to muscle, the visceral blood vessels are constricted but muscle blood vessels are dilated so that the increased blood flow can meet demands of cardiac and skeletal muscle for oxygen and nutrients, digestive and excretory processes are slowed, and the liver breaks down stored glycogen to provide glucose for fuel. All of these responses represent actions of the sympathetic nervous system.

Anatomical characteristics. The parasympathetic and the sympathetic nervous systems also differ in their anatomy. The postganglionic neurons of the two systems derive from distinct areas of the spinal cord. The efferent neurons for part of the parasympathetic nervous system arise in the lower area of the brain. These parasympathetic cell bodies include the respiratory and circulatory centers of the medulla, which control cardiovascular and gastrointestinal processes. The remainder of the preganglionic neurons of the parasympathetic nervous system arise from the sacral portion of the spinal cord and allow parasympathetic control of digestive, excretory, and reproductive processes. In contrast, the preganglionic neurons of the sympathetic nervous system all arise in the thoracic and lumbar regions of the spinal cord. Also the number of postganglionic to preganglionic neurons is highly characteristic of each division. In the parasympathetic nervous system each preganglionic neuron contacts one or two postganglionic neurons so that there is discrete neuronal control over organ function. In contrast, the sympathetic nervous system may have 20 or more postganglionic neurons in contact with each preganglionic neuron so that the action on stimulation of preganglionic neurons is diffuse, in keeping with the "alarm" nature of the sympathetic nervous system.

COMMENTS ON THE CENTRAL NERVOUS SYSTEM

The brain and spinal cord are more complex in their neuronal organization than is the peripheral nervous system. This is because information must be processed rather than just transmitted. This processing is accomplished in two ways. First, a given neuron may send out many axonal projections and thereby form synaptic junctions with many different neurons. This arrangement serves to send a flow of information to several areas for further processing. Second, a given neuron can receive information from more than one neuron. Thus dendrites from a given neuron may have synaptic junctions with axons from many neurons. This arrangement serves to collect information from different sources.

Neurotransmitters of the Central Nervous System

An important difference between the central nervous system and the peripheral nervous system is the number of neurotransmitters believed to exist. In addition to acetylcholine and norepinephrine, the central neurotransmitters that will be encountered in discussing central nervous system pharmacology in later chapters include dopamine, serotonin, epinephrine, histamine, gamma aminobutyric acid (GABA), glycine, and enkephalins. Some neurotransmitters, in particular GABA and glycine, are inhibitory rather than excitatory. The neuronal response to these neurotransmitters is to develop a more negative resting potential with a decreased likelihood of firing rather than to depolarize more readily and fire.

Correlations of Function with Neurotransmitters in the Central Nervous System

In the past few years, nerve tracts have been described in the brain and characterized by their neurotransmitter content. These nerve tracts have cell bodies in different areas of the brain to collect information, but the neurons will then converge and form synaptic junctions with many neurons in other regions of the brain. Through surgery or chemical destruction of specific nerve tracts it has been possible to associate control of mental and motor behavior with some of the nerve tracts and their neurotransmitters. Examples include a role for acetylcholine and dopamine in the central coordination of muscle movement (Chapter 35, Central motor control: drugs for parkinsonism and centrally acting skeletal muscle relaxants), a role for dopamine in psychosis (Chapter 28, Antipsychotic drugs), a role for dopamine and serotonin in depression (Chapter 29, Antidepressant drugs), and the role of enkephalins in analgesia (Chapter 31, Narcotic analgesics [opioids]). A current goal in neuropharmacology is to identify how drugs modify behavior through their modification of neurotransmitter synthesis, storage, release, action, and inactivation.

SUMMARY

The actions of the nervous system depend on the release of neurotransmitters to act on specific receptors of the next cell. In the peripheral nervous system the preganglionic neurons of both the sympathetic and parasympathetic nervous system release acetylcholine. Motor neurons also release acetylcholine to stimulate skeletal muscle. The identity of the neurotransmitter differs in the postganglionic neurons: acetylcholine is the neurotransmitter of the parasympathetic or cholinergic nervous system, and norepinephrine is the neurotransmitter of the sympathetic or adrenergic nervous system. In reaction to stress, epinephrine is released by the adrenal medulla to augment and expand the role of the sympathetic nervous system, producing the "fight or flight" adaptations of the body organs.

Body tissues contain distinct receptors for acetylcholine and for norepinephrine. The two neurotransmitters produce opposite tissue responses, and the relative activity of a tissue is controlled by the degree of sympathetic versus parasympathetic activity. The following chapters discuss mechanisms by which drugs either mimic or inhibit the action of the neurotransmitters acetylcholine and norepinephrine. Emphasis will be placed on the receptor populations on which drugs act. This chapter has discussed how each neurotransmitter can potentially act at many tissues. Relatively specific actions, for example, stimulation of the bladder or heart, may be achieved by appropriate doses of selected drugs. However, because it is usually difficult to administer the drug to a single tissue, many predictable side effects are seen resulting from actions in other tissues.

STUDY QUESTIONS

1. What are neurotransmitters?
2. Describe the synthesis, storage, release, and termination of action of acetylcholine and norepinephrine.
3. What are the two divisions of the autonomic nervous system? How are they involved in dual antagonistic innervation and in determining autonomic tone?
4. Describe the neurons of the autonomic nervous system and of the motor nervous system with respect to anatomy and identity of the neurotransmitter used.
5. Describe the "flight or fight" adaptations of the sympathetic nervous system.

SUGGESTED READINGS

Black, I.B.: Stages of neurotransmitter development in autonomic neurons, Science **215**:1198, 1982.

Bunge, R., Johnson, M., and Ross, C.D.: Nature and nurture in development of the autonomic neuron, Science **199:** 1409, 1978.

Cooper, J.R., Bloom, F.E., and Rother, R.H.: The biochemical basis of neuropharmacology, ed. 4, New York, 1982, Oxford University Press, Inc.

Gandhavadi, B.: Autonomic pain. Features and methods of assessment, Postgrad. Med. **71**(1):85, 1982.

Jones, D.G.: Ultrastructural approaches to the organization of central synapses, Am. Scientist, **69**:200, 1981.

Kolata, G.B.: New drugs and the brain, Science **205:**774, 1979.

Langer, S.Z.: Presynaptic receptors and their role in the regulation of transmitter release, Br. J. Pharmacol. **60:**481, 1977.

Snyder, S.H.: Brain peptides as neurotransmitters, Science **209:**976, 1980.

Thal, L.J.: Neurotransmitters and receptors in neurologic disease, Resident Staff Phys. **29**(2):43, 1983.

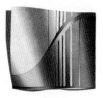

9

Mechanisms of Cholinergic Control

This chapter is intended to be read at two different times during a course in pharmacology. The beginning student should read the chapter for the mechanisms and therapeutic applications but should not be overly concerned with the drugs given as examples. Later, in a course in pharmacology, the student can return to this chapter in order to review the drugs learned by their mechanism of action. The exception is the drug atropine, which is presented in detail in this chapter but not elsewhere.

POPULATIONS OF CHOLINERGIC RECEPTORS AS DEFINED BY DRUG ACTION

In the preceding chapter, three distinct populations of receptors for acetylcholine in the peripheral nervous system were presented: receptors on striated muscle at the neuromuscular junction, receptors on postganglionic neurons within the ganglia, and receptors on other innervated tissues.

Muscarinic Receptors

The distinction among acetylcholine receptors is not just anatomical. Chemical differentiation is made with muscarine, a chemical found in certain mushrooms, which mimics the effects of acetylcholine by slowing the heart rate or stimulating smooth muscle when applied to those tissues. Muscarine produces no effect when applied to skeletal muscles or to ganglia. Muscarine mimics acetylcholine only at the postganglionic receptors. The parasympathetic postganglionic receptors are therefore called *muscarinic* receptors.

As a cholinergic agonist, muscarine is a laboratory tool. It is encountered clinically only as a toxin responsible for acute mushroom poisoning. (There is another kind of mushroom poisoning in which symptoms take several hours to appear.) The symptoms of acute mushroom poisoning appear within an hour or so of ingestion and consist of generalized parasympathetic overstimulation that includes glandular stimulation (sweating, tearing, salivation), an overactive gastrointestinal system (nausea, cramps, diarrhea), cardiovascular symptoms (flushed skin and slow heart rate), constricted pupils, and excessive urination.

Nicotinic Receptors

Nicotine, found in tobacco, is another cholinergic agonist. Nicotine is the laboratory agent that mimics the effects of acetylcholine at the skeletal muscle and ganglionic receptors. Therefore the "nicotinic" receptors are the ganglionic and neuromuscular receptors for acetylcholine. Nicotine is not an effective agonist for acetylcholine at the muscarinic receptors.

DIRECT- AND INDIRECT-ACTING CHOLINOMIMETIC DRUGS

Drugs that mimic the action of acetylcholine act by one of two mechanisms: *directly*, by mimicking acetylcholine (these drugs are chemically related to acetylcholine) or *indirectly*, by inhibiting acetylcholinesterase (these drugs allow acetylcholine to remain intact longer because its degradation is inhibited).

Acetylcholine itself is not commonly used as a therapeutic agent because it produces too many responses and because it is too rapidly degraded in the blood. Rarely, acetylcholine is used topically in eye surgery. Carbachol (Carbacel) and pilocarpine (Pilocar) are examples of direct-acting cholinomimetic drugs used principally in ophthalmology. Bethanechol (Urecholine) is the only direct-acting cholinomimetic drug used systemically.

Table 9.1   Receptor Selectivity of Cholinomimetic Drugs at Therapeutic Doses

Generic and trade names	Muscarinic receptor*	Nicotinic† (neuromuscular) receptor	Therapeutic uses
DIRECT-ACTING			
Bethanechol (Urecholine)	+	0	To stimulate an atonic bladder or intestine
Carbachol (Carbacel and others)	+ [topical]		Miotic (constricts pupil)
Pilocarpine (Pilocar and others)	+ [topical]		Miotic (constricts pupil)
	+ [topical]		
INDIRECT-ACTING: REVERSIBLE INHIBITORS OF ACETYLCHOLINESTERASE			
Ambenonium (Mytelase)	(+)	+	To restore muscle strength in myasthenia gravis
Edrophonium (Tensilon)	(+)	+	To diagnose myasthenia gravis; to differentiate a myasthenic crisis from a cholinergic crisis
Neostigmine (Prostigmin)	+	+	To restore muscle strength in myasthenia gravis
			To stimulate an atonic bladder or intestine
Physostigmine (Eserine)	+ [topical]		Miotic (constricts pupil)
Pyridostigmine (Mestinon)	(+)	+	To restore muscle strength in myasthenia gravis
INDIRECT-ACTING: IRREVERSIBLE INHIBITORS OF ACETYLCHOLINESTERASE			
Demecarium (Humorsol)	+ [topical]	(+) near eye	Miotic (constricts pupil)
Echothiophate (Phospholine)	+ [topical]	(+) near eye	Miotic (constricts pupil)
Isoflurophate (Floropryl)	+ [topical]	(+) near eye	Miotic (constricts pupil)
Pralidoxime (Protopam)	+	+	To reactivate acetylcholinesterase

* +, Stimulation. (+), Stimulation, at high concentrations, of muscles near the eye. 0, No stimulation.
†No drugs are used therapeutically that primarily stimulate nicotine-ganglionic receptors. Stimulation of nicotinic-ganglionic receptors is a toxic effect of cholinomimetic drugs.

Reversible and Irreversible Acetylcholinesterase Inhibitors

The acetylcholinesterase inhibitors can be subdivided into the reversible inhibitors and the irreversible inhibitors. The reversible inhibitors, as the name implies, bind to the enzyme reversibly, and therefore the drug effect wears off as the drug is eliminated from the body, usually in a few hours. Examples of reversible inhibitors of acetylcholinesterase include physostigmine (Eserine), pyridostigmine (Mestinon), and neostigmine (Prostigmin).

The irreversible inhibitors form a permanent covalent bond with acetylcholinesterase, and the enzyme must be completely replaced before the drug effect wears off, a process requiring days to weeks. The most common examples of irreversible acetylcholinesterase inhibitors are the organophosphate compounds, which include potent drugs for constricting the pupil (miotics): demecarium (Humorsol), echothiophate (Phospholine), and isoflurophate (Floropryl); the insecticides parathion and malathion; and several agents developed for chemical warfare. Interestingly, the antidote for poisoning by an irreversible acetylcholinesterase inhibitor is pralidoxime (PAM), which is itself an acetylcho-

linesterase inhibitor. PAM, however, is able to compete with the enzyme for the phosphate group of the inhibitor, thereby eliminating itself and the inhibitor from the enzyme, reversing the "irreversible" inhibition.

THERAPEUTIC USES OF CHOLINOMIMETIC DRUGS

Cholinomimetic drugs are used clinically for three effects in the peripheral nervous system:

1. To restore muscle tone in patients with myasthenia gravis or in surgical patients treated with tubocurarine. This is a nicotinic effect at the neuromuscular junction. The drugs used to increase muscle strength are all acetylcholinesterase inhibitors. Cholinomimetic drugs acting at the neuromuscular junction are discussed in Chapter 11.

2. To constrict the pupil (miosis), a muscarinic effect that is used in ophthalmology. Cholinomimetic drugs administered to act in the eye are described in Chapter 12.

3. To stimulate an atonic bladder or intestine. This is a muscarinic effect. Cholinomimetic drugs affecting the gastrointestinal system are discussed in Chapter 13.

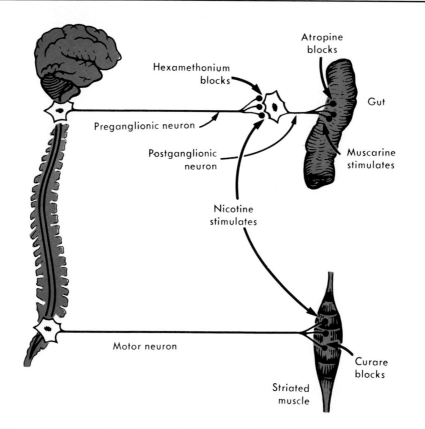

FIGURE 9.1   Acetylcholine is the peripheral neurotransmitter at three receptor populations. Each receptor population is characterized by an agonist and an antagonist as pictured. Muscarine and atropine are the agonist and antagonist of parasympathetic postganglionic (muscarinic) receptors. Nicotine and hexamethonium are the agonist and antagonist of parasympathetic preganglionic (nicotinic) receptors. Nicotine and tubocurarine are the agonist and antagonist of neuromuscular junction (nicotinic) receptors.

Table 9.1 reviews the receptor selectivity of cholinomimetic drugs discussed in detail in other chapters. No clinical use is made of drugs stimulating nicotinic receptors of the ganglia. Ganglia are involved in so many responses as to make their stimulation by drugs clinically useless.

CHOLINERGIC ANTAGONISTS
Anticholinergic Drugs

As illustrated in Figure 9.1, each of the three groups of receptors for acetylcholine is characterized by a drug that blocks the action of acetylcholine at that type of receptor by occupying the receptor and preventing cholinergic action. Since each class of acetylcholine antagonist acts on a discrete receptor population, clinical use of each class of antagonist differs greatly. Table 9.2 reviews receptor selectivity of cholinergic receptor antagonists discussed in detail in other chapters.

Neuromuscular Receptor Antagonists

Tubocurarine primarily blocks the receptors for acetylcholine at the neuromuscular junction and thereby causes muscular relaxation or paralysis. Antagonists of the neuromuscular cholinergic receptor are used chiefly as an adjunct to anesthetics and will be discussed in Chapter 11 (Drugs to control muscle tone).

Ganglionic Receptor Antagonists

The receptors for acetylcholine in the ganglia are blocked by *hexamethonium*, thus blocking transmission for both parasympathetic and sympathetic impulses. Antagonists like hexamethonium lack much specificity in the response produced. Limited use of drugs antagonizing the action of acetylcholine in the ganglia is made in treating severe cases of hypertension. One such drug, trimethaphan, will be discussed in Chapter 15 along with the other antihypertensive drugs.

Table 9.2   Receptor Selectivity of Cholinergic Receptor Antagonists (Anticholinergics) at Therapeutic Doses*

Generic and trade names	Muscarinic receptor	Nicotinic (ganglionic) receptor	Nicotinic (neuromuscular) receptor	Therapeutic uses
Anisotropine	−	0	0	Same as homatropine
Atracurium (Tracrium)	0	0	−	Same as tubocurarine
Atropine	−	0	0	Topical to the eye for mydriasis (dilated pupil) and cycloplegia (paralysis of accommodation); systemic, reduces gastric acid secretion and reduces gastrointestinal motility and tone of the bladder and ureter
Cyclopentolate (Cyclogyl)	− [topical]			Mydriasis and cycloplegia
Gallamine (Flaxedil)	(−)	0	−	Same as tubocurarine
Glycopyrrolate (Robinul)	−	0	0	Same as homatropine methyl-bromide
Homatropine methyl-bromide (Homopin)	−	0	0	To reduce gastrointestinal hyper-motility and gastric acidity
Ipratroprium (Atrovert)	−	0	0	To relax bronchial smooth muscle
Methantheline (Banthine)	−	0	0	Same as homatropine methyl-bromide
Methscopolamine (Pamine)	−	0	0	Same as homatropine methyl-bromide
Metocurine (Metubine)	0	0	−	Same as tubocurarine
Oxyphencyclimine (Daricon)	−	0	0	To control gastrointestinal hyper-motility, gastric acidity, and hyper-motility of the genitourinary and biliary tracts
Pancuronium (Pavulon)	0	0	−	Same as tubocurarine
Propantheline (Pro-Banthine)	−	0	0	Same as oxyphencyclimine
Scopolamine	−	0	0	Same as atropine
Succinylcholine (Anectine)	0	0	−	Depolarizing skeletal muscle relaxant
Trimethaphan (Arfonad)	0	−	0	To lower blood pressure in selected cases of hypertensive crisis
Tropicamide (Mydriacyl)	− [topical]			Mydriasis and cycloplegia
Tubocurarine (Tubarine)	0	(−)	−	Nondepolarizing skeletal muscle relaxant
Vecuronium (Nocuron)	0	0	−	Same as tubocurarine

* −, Inhibition. (−), Inhibition at high concentrations. 0, No inhibition.

Muscarinic Receptor Antagonists

Atropine and *scopolamine* are the prototypes of drugs that block acetylcholine at the muscarinic receptors. These are the parasympathetic, postganglionic receptors for acetylcholine on the heart, smooth muscle, and exocrine glands.

Atropine is an alkaloid originally derived from the leaves of the deadly nightshade or *Atropa belladonna*, which belongs to the potato family. Several other plants also contain atropine and a related drug, scopolamine. These two drugs are often referred to as *belladonna alkaloids*. References to the use of these plants as medicinal agents are found in all ancient medical literature. To this day, atropine remains the most useful and widely versatile of the antimuscarinic drugs.

THERAPEUTIC USES OF MUSCARINIC RECEPTOR ANTAGONISTS

1. To block secretions. Salivation is readily blocked by atropine. Indeed, one classic side effect of atropine is a dry mouth (xerostomia). Secretions in the respiratory tract are also inhibited by atropine. This inhibition of bronchial and salivary secretions is the desired effect when atropine is administered as a preanesthetic agent before surgery. The drying effect of atropine reduces secretions that may be involuntarily aspirated when the patient is drowsy or unconscious.

Atropine and related drugs are moderately effective in depressing gastric acid secretion in patients with peptic ulcers. The role of cholinergic antagonists in treating gastrointestinal disorders is discussed in Chapter 13.

Large doses of atropine and scopolamine dilate the blood vessels in the skin, especially around the face and particularly in children, thus producing a pronounced blushing. The mechanism for this vasodilation is not clear, but since sweating is inhibited by atropine, this flush may represent a mechanism to dissipate heat and a fever may be noted.

2. To depress an overactive gastrointestinal tract. A prominent antimuscarinic effect of atropine is to inhibit the tone and motility of smooth muscle. The gastrointestinal smooth muscle is very sensitive to atropine. Drugs affecting gastrointestinal motility are discussed in Chapter 13.

3. To dilate the eye (mydriasis) and to paralyze accommodation (cycloplegia). Atropine is applied by drops to the eye to block the actions of acetylcholine. The result of this antagonism is dilation of the pupil, since the circular muscles of the iris are relaxed, and blurred vision, since there is paralysis of accommodation. This mydriasis and cycloplegia allow measurements of lens refraction, examination of the retina, and aid in the healing of some infections. Drugs affecting the eye are discussed further in Chapter 12.

Atropine taken orally will also reach the eye. Photophobia (sensitivity to light) as a result of the dilation and blurring of vision (caused by the cycloplegia) are frequent side effects of oral administration of atropine.

4. To increase the heart rate. Atropine is administered to increase the heart rate by antagonizing the acetylcholine released by the vagus nerve at the atrioventricular node of the heart (Chapter 19).

5. To relax bronchial smooth muscle. Ipratropium alleviates bronchospasm, common in many pulmonary diseases.

6. To treat toxicity of cholinergic agents. The most frequent cause of cholinergic toxicity is overexposure to insecticides such as malathion and parathion, which are organic phosphate acetylcholinesterase inhibitors. Atropine will reverse the muscarinic effects (i.e., salivation, tearing, diarrhea, bradycardia) but will not reverse the neuromuscular paralysis. PAM, which regenerates acetylcholinesterase at all sites, is therefore the drug of choice.

7. Side effects may occur in addition to therapeutic effects. The side effects of atropine are extensions of the actions just described. The expected cardiovascular effect is an increase in the heart rate (tachycardia), although a slowing of the heart rate (bradycardia) may be noted with low doses administered intravenously. Dilated pupils and blurred vision are accompanied by an intolerance of the eye to light (photophobia) and, sometimes, eye pain. In addition to a dry mouth and constipation, patients may experience nausea and vomiting. Urinary hesitancy or retention is common. The skin is dry and flushed, and some patients may develop a fever from the inability to dissipate heat through sweating.

Other Uses of Drugs Blocking Muscarinic Receptors

Drugs that are muscacarinic receptor antagonists have other uses unrelated to peripheral muscarinic receptors. Many anticholinergic drugs also have effects in the central nervous system. Some drugs have antitremor activity and are used to relieve certain tremors called *extrapyramidal motor effects* caused by Parkinson's disease, other diseases, and some drugs. Anticholinergic drugs used in the treatment of parkinsonism are discussed in Chapter 35.

Differences in the Central Nervous System Effects of Atropine and Scopolamine

Atropine, particularly in an overdose, produces generalized excitement, which, in the toxic state, may result in hallucinations. In contrast, while scopolamine can produce hallucinations, scopolamine also produces sleepiness, sedation, and amnesia. Scopolamine, unlike atropine, is effective in preventing motion sickness.

SUMMARY

There are three types of receptors for acetylcholine outside the central nervous system. These receptor populations, defined by the drugs muscarine, nicotine, atropine, hexamethonium, and tubocurarine, are as follows:

1. Postganglionic receptors are stimulated by muscarine and blocked by atropine.
2. Ganglionic receptors are stimulated by nicotine and blocked by hexamethonium.
3. Neuromuscular receptors are stimulated by nicotine and blocked by tubocurarine.

The physiological activities associated with these receptor populations are

Muscarinic: Increased glandular secretion, stimulation of the gastrointestinal smooth muscle, vasodilation and slowing of the heart rate, increased urge to urinate, and constriction of the pupils.

Nicotinic (ganglionic): Nonspecific activation of both the sympathetic and parasympathetic nervous systems.

Nicotinic (skeletal muscle): Increased muscle tone and, in excess, fasciculations (rapid, small contractions).

Cholinomimetic drugs may act *directly*, by stimulating receptors for acetylcholine, or *indirectly*, by slowing the degradation of acetylcholine released. This is accomplished by inhibition of the enzyme acetylcholinesterase, which degrades acetylcholine after it is released from the nerve terminal. The indirect-acting cholinomimetic drugs may be subdivided into reversible and irreversible inhibitors.

Therapeutic uses of cholinomimetic drugs are to restore muscle tone (increase muscle strength), to constrict the pupil, and to stimulate an atonic bladder or intestine.

Cholinergic antagonists (anticholinergic drugs) act by blocking a receptor from occupation and activation by acetylcholine.

1. Tubocurarine is the prototype of an antagonist of the neuromuscular nicotinic receptor. The blockade produces muscular relaxation.
2. Hexamethonium is the prototype antagonist of the ganglionic nicotinic receptor. The effects of ganglionic receptor blockage are complex and clinically useful only in reversing severe hypertension.
3. Atropine is the prototype antagonist of the muscarinic receptor. Therapeutic uses of atropine-like drugs (muscarinic antagonists) include
   a. Blocking secretions
   b. Depressing the tone of the gastrointestinal tract
   c. Dilating the pupil and paralyzing accommodation
   d. Raising the heart rate
   e. Counteracting toxicity of cholinergic agents

The classic atropine-like (anticholinergic) effects are dry mouth, blurred vision, photophobia (from dilated pupils), flushed, dry skin, increased heart rate, mental confusion and excitement, constipation, and urinary retention.

Many drug classes other than the anticholinergic drugs have atropine-like side effects. Examples of these drug classes are the antihistamines, the antipsychotic drugs, the monoamine oxidase inhibitors, and the tricyclic antidepressants.

STUDY QUESTIONS

1. What are muscarine and nicotine and how do they relate to receptors for acetylcholine?
2. Contrast the mechanisms of a direct- and an indirect-acting cholinomimetic drug.
3. What three therapeutic uses are made of cholinomimetic drugs?
4. What are the three prototype antagonists and with which receptor population is each associated?
5. List the five actions of atropine that are useful therapeutically.
6. What are "atropine-like" or anticholinergic side effects? List them.

SUGGESTED READINGS

Bebbington, A., and Brimblecombe, R.W.: Muscarinic receptors in the peripheral and central nervous systems, Ad. Drug Res. **2**:143, 1965.

Birdsall, N.J.M., and Hume, E.C.: Biochemical studies on muscarinic acetylcholine receptors, J. Neurochem. **27**:7, 1976.

Ketchum, J.S., and others: Atropine, scopolamine, and ditran: comparative pharmacology and antagonists in man, Psychopharmacologia **28**:121, 1973.

Krnjevic, K.: Central cholinergic pathways, Fed. Proc. **28**:113, 1969.

Rumack, B.H.: Anticholinergic poisoning: treatment with physostigmine, Pediatrics **52**:449, 1973.

Snyder, S.H., and others: Biochemical identification of the mammalian muscarinic cholinergic receptor, Fed. Proc. **34**:1915, 1974.

Steward, D.J.: Anticholinergic premedication for infants and children, Can. Anaesth. Soc. J. **30**(4):325, 1983.

Unna, K.R., and others: Dosage of drugs in infants and children. I. Atropine, Pediatrics **6**:197, 1950.

CHAPTER

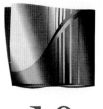

10

Mechanisms of Adrenergic Control

Like Chapter 9, this chapter is intended to be read at the beginning of a course in pharmacology as an introduction and at a later time as a review. When reading as an introduction, the student should pay attention to the mechanisms and the effects associated with these mechanisms. The drugs given as examples and their classification by mechanism will be of interest when the chapter is read at a later time for review.

CATECHOLAMINES AND THEIR RECEPTORS
Naturally Occurring Catecholamines

Dopamine, norepinephrine, and epinephrine are the naturally occurring *catecholamines*, which function as neurotransmitters and neurohormones. Dopamine is derived from the amino acid tyrosine and is the chemical precursor of norepinephrine:

Tyrosine →→ Dopamine →
Norepinephrine → Epinephrine

All three catecholamines are important neurotransmitters in the central nervous system. In the autonomic nervous system, norepinephrine is the sympathetic, postganglionic neurotransmitter, and epinephrine is the neurohormone released from the adrenal medulla in reaction to stress. Dopamine's role in the autonomic nervous system at present is not completely understood.

Classes of Adrenergic Receptors and Adrenergic Responses

The first synthetic catecholamine to be studied was isoproterenol. The existence of two classes of adrenergic receptors was proposed in the late 1940s to explain the different physiological effects elicited by norepinephrine, epinephrine, and isoproter-

enol. *Alpha receptors* are those receptors for which norepinephrine and epinephrine are equally potent, but isoproterenol is less potent. *Beta receptors* are those receptors for which isoproterenol is more potent than or as potent as epinephrine or norepinephrine. Subsequent studies over the years have expanded this classification to include two subtypes in each class: alpha-1, alpha-2, beta-1, and beta-2.

Alpha-1 adrenergic receptors. Alpha-1 receptors account for the primary responses elicited by norepinephrine released from sympathetic postganglionic neurons. Epinephrine is as potent as norepinephrine in stimulating alpha-1 receptors. Physiological effects resulting from stimulation of alpha-1 receptors include the following:

1. Contraction of the radial muscles of the iris. The radial muscles are arranged like the spokes of a wheel so that contraction causes dilation of the pupil (mydriasis). Adrenergic drugs used therapeutically for this effect are discussed in Chapter 12.
2. Constriction of arterioles and veins, which causes an increase in blood pressure. Adrenergic drugs that are used to raise the blood pressure are discussed in Chapter 14.
3. Contraction of smooth muscle sphincters in the stomach, intestine, and bladder.
4. Contraction of the uterus (female) and stimulation of ejaculation (male).
5. Decreased secretions from the pancreas.
6. Breakdown of glycogen in the liver (glycogenolysis) and synthesis of glucose (gluconeogenesis).

No therapeutic use is made of drugs mimicking adrenergic effects listed in items 3 through 6.
Systemic effect of alpha-1 receptor activation.

The general role of the alpha-1 receptor is to stimulate contraction of smooth muscle. The most prominent effect systemically is an increase in blood pressure resulting from the constriction of blood vessels, mainly arterioles. The blood vessels controlled by alpha-1 receptors are those that service the internal organs, mucosal surfaces, and the skin. Blood pressure is in part a reflection of the degree of constriction of these blood vessels, since blood pressure is determined by the cardiac output and the peripheral resistance to blood flow in blood vessels.

Local vasoconstriction. Therapeutic use is made of local vasoconstriction by epinephrine and some other alpha-1 adrenergic receptor agonists (stimulants). Nasal decongestion may be achieved by local application of a vasoconstrictive drug (Chapter 26). Drug absorption from parenteral sites is slowed when a drug is injected with a vasoconstricting agent. Local anesthetics in particular will have a longer duration of action when injected with epinephrine to slow systemic absorption.

Alpha-2 adrenergic receptors. The concept of and experimental proof for a second class of alpha receptors, the alpha-2 receptors, was developed in the 1970s. Alpha-2 receptors were originally found presynaptically on sympathetic neuronal terminals. These presynaptic alpha-2 receptors inhibit the further release of norepinephrine when they are stimulated. The presynaptic alpha-2 receptors therefore function as a negative feedback system to limit the amount of norepinephrine release from the neuron. Alpha-2 receptors are found on platelets where their activation results in platelet aggregation.

Alpha-2 receptors have also been found on the smooth muscle of the blood vessels that determine blood pressure—the resistance vessels. Like alpha-1 receptors, alpha-2 receptors mediate vasoconstriction to increase resistance and thereby increase blood pressure. Current speculation is that the alpha-1 receptors are physically located primarily where sympathetic neurons innervate the blood vessel. Norepinephrine released from the sympathetic postganglionic nerve terminal performs two functions: activation of the alpha-1 receptors on the tissue (usually to elicit smooth muscle contraction); and activation of alpha-2 receptors on the nerve terminal, which inhibits further release of norepinephrine. The alpha-2 receptors on the blood vessel are believed to mediate vasoconstriction to blood-borne dopamine and catecholamines. The therapeutic potential of drugs acting at alpha-2 receptors remains to be developed. The antihypertensive drugs clonidine and methyldopa have been found to stimulate the alpha-2 receptor. This action does not account for their antihypertensive effect, which has been shown to be a result of their activity in the central nervous system.

Beta-1 adrenergic receptor. The beta-1 receptor is stimulated by norepinephrine and by epinephrine, but isoproterenol is a more potent stimulant than either. Physiological responses to activation of beta-1 receptors include the following:

1. Stimulation of the heart. There are three cardiac effects. Activation of the beta-1 receptor in the conducting tissue of the heart speeds the repolarization of the cells. An increase in heart rate (positive chronotropic effect) and an increase in impulse conduction speed (positive dromotropic effect) are the two consequences. Stimulation of the beta-1 receptors in the ventricular muscle increases the force of contraction (positive inotropic response). In Chapter 14 drugs acting on beta-1 receptors that are used for stimulating the heart under certain restricted conditions are presented.

2. Stimulation of the beta-1 receptor of fat tissue stimulates lipolysis, the breakdown of stored fat. The fatty acids that are released can then be used as energy sources by the heart and liver. No therapeutic use is made of drugs mimicking this adrenergic effect.

Beta-2 adrenergic receptor. In contrast to their relative activities on the beta-1 receptors, epinephrine and isoproterenol are equipotent in stimulating beta-2 receptors, whereas norepinephrine is a weak stimulant. Physiological responses to activation of beta-2 receptors include:

1. Dilation of the bronchioles. The relaxation of bronchial smooth muscle decreases airway resistance and makes it easier to breathe. Drugs acting through activation of beta-2 receptors are used to treat patients with restricted airways, primarily caused by asthma or chronic obstructive lung disease. These drugs will be discussed in Chapter 25.

2. Relaxation of uterine smooth muscle. Drugs acting through activation of beta-2 receptors, ritodrine and terbutaline, are used to stop premature labor by relaxing the pregnant uterus. See Chapter 53.

3. Dilation of the blood vessels in the skeletal muscle, brain, and heart. Activation of these beta-2 receptors causes vasodilation and shunts blood to the skeletal muscle, brain, and heart. The drug nylidrin (Arlidin) is used to increase blood flow to these organs (Chapter 14).

4. Breakdown of glycogen in the liver (glycogenolysis) and synthesis of glucose (gluconeogenesis). Note that this is also an alpha-1 adrenergic effect. No therapeutic use is made of this action.

Table 10.1   Receptor Selectivity of Adrenergic Drugs*

Generic and trade names	Alpha receptor	Beta-1 receptor	Beta-2 receptor	CNS	Main therapeutic uses
CATECHOLAMINES					
Dobutamine (Dobutrex)	0	+D	0	0	Fairly specific in increasing cardiac contractility with little increase in heart rate or conductivity
Dopamine (Intropin)	(+)I	(+)I	0	0	At low doses dilates renal arteries by activating dopamine receptors and preventing kidney shutdown in shock
Epinephrine	+D	+D	+	(+)	To treat anaphylactic shock To treat acute asthma attacks To limit systemic absorption of drugs applied for local action
Isoproterenol (Isuprel)	0	+D	+	(+)	Bronchodilator (asthma)
Norepinephrine, levarterenol (Levophed)	+D	+D	0	(+)	To counteract the hypotension of spinal anesthesia
NONCATECHOLAMINES					
Albuterol (Ventolin, Proventil)	0	0	+	0	Bronchodilator
Amphetamine	+I	+I	0	+	To depress appetite To stimulate respiration To counteract narcolepsy
Bitolterol (Tornalate)	0	0	+	0	Bronchodilator
Ephedrine	+I,D	+I,D	+	+	Bronchodilator (asthma) Nasal decongestant To dilate the pupil (mydriasis)
Fenoterol (Berotec)	0	0	+	0	Bronchodilator
Hydroxyamphetamine (Paredrine)	+I	+I	0	0	To dilate the pupil (mydriasis)
Isoetharine (Bronkosol)	0	0	+	0	Bronchodilator
Mephentermine (Wyamine)	+I,D	+I,D	0	+	To counteract the hypotension of spinal anesthesia To depress appetite
Metaproterenol (Alupent, Metaprel)	0	(+)	+	0	Bronchodilator
Metaraminol (Aramine)	+I,D	+I,D	0	0	To counteract the hypotension of spinal anesthesia
Methoxamine (Vasoxyl)	+D	0	0	0	To counteract the hypotension of spinal anesthesia To terminate paroxysmal atrial tachycardia
Naphazoline (Privine)	+	0	0	0	Nasal decongestant

Table 10.1   Receptor Selectivity of Adrenergic Drugs*—cont'd

Generic and trade names	Alpha receptor	Beta-1 receptor	Beta-2 receptor	CNS	Main therapeutic uses
Nylidrin (Arlidin)	0	0	+	0	To stimulate blood flow to heart, brain, and muscles
Oxymetazoline (Afrin)	+	0	0	0	Nasal decongestant
Phenylephrine	+D	0	0	0	Nasal decongestant To terminate paroxysmal atrial tachycardia
Phenylpropanolamine	+I,D	+I,D	+	(+)	Nasal decongestant
Pibuterol (Maxair)	0	0	+	0	Bronchodilator
Prenalterol	0	+	0	0	To increase cardiac output.
Propylhexedrine (Benzedrex)	+	0	0	0	Nasal decongestant
Pseudoephedrine	+I,D	+I,D	+	(+)	Nasal decongestant
Ritodrine (Yutopar)	0	0	+	0	To stop premature labor
Terbutaline (Brethine, Bricanyl)	0	0	+	0	Bronchodilator
Tetrahydrozoline (Tyzine)	+	0	0	0	Nasal decongestant
Tuaminoheptane (Tuamine)	+	0	0	0	Nasal decongestant
Xylometazoline (Otrivin)	+	0	0	0	Nasal decongestant

* +I, Indirectly acting (releases norepinephrine). +D, Directly acts on the receptor. (+), Effect is modest except at high concentration. 0, No effect.

Systemic effects of beta adrenergic receptor activation. The value of the responses to two classes of beta receptors can be appreciated by recalling the "fight or flight" nature of the sympathetic nervous system discussed in Chapter 8. The heart rate and cardiac output increase because epinephrine reinforces the action of norepinephrine on the beta-1 receptors. Blood is shunted to muscle, brain, and heart, where stimulation of beta-2 receptors results in vasodilation, and from the skin and abdominal organs, where stimulation of alpha-1 receptors causes vasoconstriction. Epinephrine also stimulates the liver to break down glycogen to glucose and stimulates the fat cells to break down lipid to fatty acids to provide readily available energy sources for the body.

Table 10.1 reviews the receptor selectivity of these sympathomimetic drugs discussed in detail in other chapters.

Second Messenger Concept and the Beta Receptor

In the 1950s Earl Sutherland began the work of elucidating how epinephrine caused glycogenolysis (breakdown of glycogen to glucose) in the dog liver. He and his colleagues subsequently showed that epinephrine acts by binding to what we now recognize as the beta-2 receptor on the liver cell membrane. When the beta-2 receptor is occupied, there is a structural change that activates the membrane-bound enzyme, adenylate cyclase.

As illustrated in Figure 10.1, this structural change is complex. When occupied, the beta receptor activates a transducer protein called G_s (s, stim-

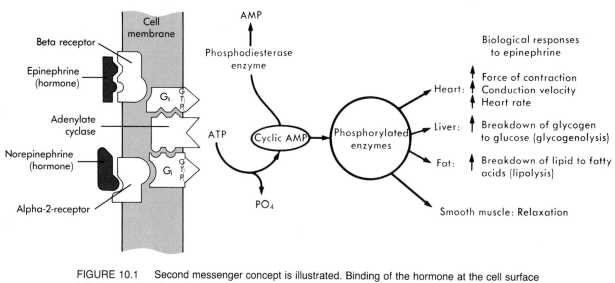

FIGURE 10.1   Second messenger concept is illustrated. Binding of the hormone at the cell surface initiates a series of reactions that modify activity through phosphorylation of key enzymes and thereby modify cellular responses. Cyclic AMP is the *second messenger* because it carries the message that the hormone is at cell surface and translates this message into action by stimulating a phosphorylating enzyme (cyclic AMP dependent protein kinase). Cellular responses to epinephrine characteristic for a given organ are given as examples of biological responses mediated through cyclic AMP.

ulatory protein). G_s then activates adenylate cyclase. The active portion of adenylate cyclase is inside the cell. The enzyme catalyzes the conversion of adenosine triphosphate (ATP) to pyrophosphate (PP) and cyclic adenosine 3′,5′-monophosphate (cyclic AMP). Cyclic AMP is the key to the intracellular action of epinephrine. Epinephrine is the hormone released to signal the cell to act. Cyclic AMP is the "second messenger" that translates the presence of epinephrine at the cell surface to the internal machinery of the cell. Many cyclic AMP molecules are formed as a result of each receptor occupation, amplifying the epinephrine signal. Cyclic AMP produces cellular effects by stimulating other enzymes. The enzymes present in the cell that can be stimulated by cyclic AMP determine the cellular response. In the liver, the response is the breakdown of glycogen. In the heart, the response is an increase in heart rate, force of contraction, and conduction speed. In smooth muscle, the response is relaxation.

Recently it has been shown that the alpha-2 receptor is also linked to the adenylate cyclase. When occupied, the alpha-2 receptor activates a transducer protein called G_i (i, inhibitory protein). G_i then inhibits adenylate cyclase activity. Therefore, the beta receptors (beta-1 and beta-2) and the alpha-2 receptor have opposite effects.

Activation of the alpha-1 receptor is by quite a different mechanism. Activation of the alpha-1 re-

ceptor stimulates the entry of calcium into the cell. The increased cytosolic concentration of calcium changes the activity of certain enzymes. The changes in enzymatic activities account for the actions produced by the activation of the alpha-1 receptor.

Two more features of the cyclic AMP system need to be pointed out. First, epinephrine is not the only hormone that stimulates the formation of cyclic AMP. Most polypeptide hormones, discussed in Chapter 36, are known to work through cyclic AMP. The exceptions are insulin, growth hormone, and prolactin. Each hormone has its specific receptor on its target tissues. This is why each hormone can have tissue-specific actions while using the same second messenger system. Second, cyclic AMP is rapidly degraded by the enzyme phosphodiesterase to 5′-adenosine monophosphate (AMP). A few drugs have been identified that inhibit phosphodiesterase and thereby produce elevated cyclic AMP concentrations. The main drug is theophylline and its dimer, aminophylline. These drugs are used to produce vasodilation in cerebral ischemia and, more importantly, in treating asthma by promoting bronchial dilation (Chapter 25).

Therapeutic Uses and Features of Adrenergic Drugs

The therapeutic use of an adrenergic drug depends on whether it acts on alpha-1, beta-1, or beta-

2 receptors. A variety of drugs have been synthesized that are relatively specific for activating a given receptor type and thereby *directly mimic* some portion of norepinephrine or epinephrine action. Other adrenergic drugs act by a second mechanism of action. These are *indirect-acting* adrenergic drugs, which act by causing the sympathetic, postganglionic neurons to release norepinephrine. This increased amount of norepinephrine activates alpha-1, alpha-2, and beta-1 receptors. Drugs such as amphetamine, ephedrine, and mephentermine also act in the central nervous system, which determines as well as limits their use. The catecholamines are relatively or completely ineffective when taken orally, because they are rapidly destroyed in the gastrointestinal tract or by the liver, whereas many noncatecholamines can be taken orally.

DRUGS INHIBITING ADRENERGIC ACTIVITY

Table 10.2 lists the drugs that interfere with peripheral adrenergic activity and the therapeutic use of these drugs. Several different drug mechanisms interfere with adrenergic activity. These mechanisms include:

1. Blockade of alpha adrenergic receptors
2. Blockade of beta adrenergic receptors
3. Depletion of peripheral neuronal stores of norepinephrine
4. Inhibition of peripheral sympathetic activity through an action in the central nervous system

Each of these mechanisms will be discussed further as to the spectrum of physiological effects produced.

Blockade of Alpha Adrenergic Receptors

Each of the drugs phenoxybenzamine, phentolamine, and prazosin acts selectively to antagonize norepinephrine at the alpha-1 receptors. Infusion of one of these drugs into a person with normal blood pressure produces little change in blood pressure as long as the person is lying down. However, any sudden shift to the upright position causes orthostatic (postural) hypotension because the blockade of the alpha-1 receptors prevents the vasoconstriction necessary to redistribute blood flow. Therefore in orthostatic (postural) hypotension the blood pools in the legs and drains from the head to cause fainting.

Other effects characteristic of blockade of the alpha-1 receptors include a pinpoint pupil (miosis), nasal stuffiness, or, in males, inhibition of ejaculation.

The uses and pharmacokinetics of the alpha-1

receptor antagonists in the treatment of hypertension are discussed in Chapter 15. Terazosin is a specific alpha-2 receptor antagonist in clinical use as an antihypertensive agent.

Blockade of Beta Adrenergic Receptors

Nonselective antagonists. The physiological effects of beta-receptor antagonists can be anticipated by considering the functions of the beta receptors. Blockade of the beta-1 receptors in the heart causes little change in the normal person at rest but limits the increase in cardiac functions normally elicited by exercise and hypertension. Conditions improved by beta-1 receptor blockade include angina and some cardiac arrhythmias. Recently, propranolol, metoprolol, and timolol have been found to be effective treatment for patients with angina to prevent recurrent heart attacks.

Beta-receptor antagonists are also effective in treating hypertension. However, when a beta-receptor antagonist is given with a vasodilator drug, the beta-receptor antagonist inhibits the reflex activation of the heart caused by the drop in blood pressure. For this reason, a beta-receptor antagonist combined with a vasodilator drug is especially effective in treating hypertension. The use of beta-receptor antagonists in the therapy of hypertension is discussed in Chapter 15.

Blockade of beta-2 receptors will limit bronchiole dilation and therefore can severely compromise pulmonary function in patients with asthma. This has led to development of beta-1 selective antagonists (cardioselective antagonists) such as atenolol (Tenormin) and metoprolol (Lopressor).

Propranolol (Inderal) was the first beta-receptor antagonist approved for clinical use in the United States. Propranolol blocks both beta-1 and beta-2 receptors and is used to treat hypertension, angina, and cardiac arrhythmias. In addition, propranolol is an effective prophylactic in the treatment of migraine headaches, although the mechanisms involved are not clear.

Nadolol (Corgard) was introduced in 1980 as a nonselective beta-receptor antagonist for use in treating angina and hypertension. Additional nonselective beta receptor antagonists that have been released for clinical use in the United States include labetolol (Trandate, Vescal) and pindolol (Visken). Labetolol has alpha- and beta-antagonist action.

Timolol (Timoptic), betaxolol (Betoptic), and levobunolol (Betagan) are beta-receptor antagonists that are effective in treating glaucoma, reducing the production of aqueous humor in the eye. They are discussed with other ophthalmic drugs in Chapter 12. Timolol is also used as an antianginal agent.

Table 10.2 Drugs Inhibiting Adrenergic Receptor Activity*

Generic and trade names	Alpha receptor	Beta-1 receptor	Beta-2 receptor	CNS	Main therapeutic uses
ALPHA ADRENERGIC RECEPTOR ANTAGONISTS					
Phenoxybenzamine (Dibenzyline)	−	0	0	0	To treat hypertension secondary to pheocromocytoma To treat vasospastic disorders of the digits (Raynaud's syndrome)
Phentolamine (Regitine)	−	0	0	0	To treat hypertension secondary to pheochromocytoma
Prazosin (Minipress)	−	0	0	0	To treat chronic hypertension
Terazosin (Hytrin)	−	0	0	0	To treat chronic hypertension
BETA ADRENERGIC RECEPTOR ANTAGONISTS					
Acebutolol (Sectral)	0	−	0	0	To treat chronic hypertension
Atenolol (Tenormin)	0	−	0	0	To treat chronic hypertension Prophylactic treatment of angina
Betaxolol (Betoptic)	0	−	0	0	Ophthalmic, to treat glaucoma
Carteolol (Cartrol)	0	−	−	0	To treat chronic hypertension
Esmolol (Brevibloc)	0	−	0	0	To control supraventricular tachycardia
Labetolol (Trandate, Vescal)	−	−	−	0	To treat chronic hypertension Prophylactic treatment of angina
Levobunolol (Betagan)	0	−	−	0	Ophthalmic, to treat glaucoma
Metoprolol (Lopressor)	0	−	0	−	To treat chronic hypertension Prophylactic treatment of angina
Nadolol (Corgard)	0	−	−	−	To treat chronic hypertension Prophylactic treatment of angina
Pindolol (Visken)	0	−	−	−	To treat chronic hypertension Prophylactic treatment of angina
Propranolol (Inderal)	0	−	−	−	To treat chronic hypertension Prophylactic treatment of angina To treat cardiac arrhythmias Prophylactic treatment of migraine
Timolol (Blocadren, Timoptic)	0	−	−	0	To treat chronic hypertension Ophthalmic, to treat glaucoma
DRUGS DEPLETING NEURONAL STORES OF NOREPINEPHRINE					
Guanadrel (Hylorel)	I	I	I	0	To treat severe chronic hypertension
Guanethidine (Ismelin)	I	I	I	0	To treat severe chronic hypertension
Reserpine (Serpasil)	I	I	I	−	To treat chronic hypertension
DRUGS INHIBITING SYMPATHETIC ACTIVITY THROUGH AN ACTION IN CNS					
Methyldopa (Aldomet)	− CNS	0	0	−	To treat chronic hypertension
Clonidine (Catapres)	− CNS	0	0	−	To treat chronic hypertension
Guanabenz (Wytensin)	− CNS	0	0	−	To treat chronic hypertension
Guanfacine (Tenex)	− CNS	0	0	−	To treat chronic hypertension

* − denotes inhibition, 0 denotes no effect, I denotes indirect inhibition resulting from depletion of norepinephrine stores, − CNS denotes a decrease in peripheral sympathetic tone through an action in the CNS.

Depletion of Peripheral Neuronal Stores of Norepinephrine

Guanethidine (Ismelin) and reserpine (Serpasil) are antihypertensive drugs that deplete norepinephrine from peripheral neurons.

Guanethidine is taken up into the postganglionic sympathetic nerve terminals, where it then prevents the release of norepinephrine. After several days the neuronal content of norepinephrine is depleted. Guanadrel is a more recent drug that has the same mechanism.

Reserpine also causes a depletion of norepinephrine stores not only in the periphery but also in the brain. The central action of reserpine is believed to contribute in a major way to the depression of sympathetic tone with this agent.

Reserpine and guanethidine are useful in treating chronic hypertension (Chapter 15) and Raynaud's disease (Chapter 14).

Inhibition of Peripheral Sympathetic Activity through an Action in the Central Nervous System

The central nervous system controls sympathetic activity, although the mechanism of this control is not understood. The preceding section indicated that part of the effect of reserpine is believed to be mediated through an action in the central nervous system. It is now recognized that two other antihypertensive drugs, clonidine (Catapres) and methyldopa (Aldomet), decrease sympathetic tone mainly through an action in the central nervous system. Guanabenz (Wytensin) and guanfacine are more recent antihypertensive drugs that have the same mechanism. The role of these drugs in the treatment of hypertension is described in Chapter 15.

SUMMARY

Effects of adrenergic receptor agonists (stimulants) depend on how selective the drug is for the four classes of adrenergic receptors.

Activation of the alpha-1 receptors causes vasoconstriction, which is seen systemically as a rise in blood pressure. In the eye, pupil dilation (mydriasis) is mediated by activation of alpha-1 receptors. Activation of alpha-2 receptors will appear as a diminution of sympathetic activity, because activation of these presynaptic receptors inhibits the further release of norepinephrine. The characterization of the alpha-2 receptor is recent, and the clinical implications are not yet developed.

Activation of the beta-1 adrenergic receptors increases cardiac activity, whereas activation of beta-2 receptors relaxes the bronchioles. Selective beta-2 adrenergic receptor agonists (stimulants) have been developed for use in treating asthma and other types of reversible bronchiole constriction. The intracellular pathway activated by stimulation of beta receptors is the production of cyclic AMP, a compound that alters the activity of key enzymes. A drug that inhibits the degradation of cyclic AMP will produce the effects characteristic of a beta-adrenergic receptor agonist.

Four mechanisms are described for the inhibition of adrenergic activity. All four mechanisms can be related to drugs effective in treating chronic hypertension. Drugs inhibiting alpha-1 adrenergic receptors would appear to offer the most direct means of lowering blood pressure, but in practice drugs inhibiting the beta-1 adrenergic receptors are clinically more efficacious. In addition to blockade of alpha-1 and beta-1 adrenergic receptors, adrenergic activity can be inhibited by drugs that deplete the norepinephrine stores in the sympathetic postganglionic nerve terminals and by drugs that act in the central nervous system to depress sympathetic activity. These latter two classes of drugs also find primary use as drugs to treat chronic hypertension.

Beta-1 adrenergic receptor antagonists (blockers) are also effective in treating angina and some types of cardiac arrhythmias. Beta-receptor antagonists also limit the production of aqueous humor in the treatment of chronic glaucoma.

STUDY QUESTIONS

1. Which are the three naturally occurring catecholamines and where are they found?
2. What actions are associated with stimulation of the alpha-1 adrenergic receptor? With the stimulation of the alpha-2 adrenergic receptor? With the stimulation of the beta-1 adrenergic receptor? With the stimulation of the beta-2 adrenergic receptor?
3. What does the "second messenger" (cyclic AMP) do?
4. Contrast the mechanism of action of direct-acting and indirect-acting sympathomimetic drugs.
5. What are the four major drug mechanisms that inhibit adrenergic activity? What therapeutic use is made of each of these actions?

SUGGESTED READINGS

Andersson, K.E.: Adrenoreceptors—classification, activation and blockade by drugs, Postgrad. Med. J. **56**(Suppl. 2):7, 1980.

Dickerson, M: Anaphylaxis and anaphylactic shock, Crit. Care Nurse Q. **11**(1):68, 1988.

DiPalma, J.R.: Beta-blocker drug interactions, Am. Fam. Phys. **28**(3):249, 1983.

Hancock, B.G., and Eberhard, N.K.: The pharmacologic management of shock, Crit. Care Nurse Q. **11**(1):19, 1988.

Hirsch, A.M.: Type A behavior pattern and catecholamine excretion during cardiac catheterization, Western J. Nurs. Res. **10**(3):307, 1988.

Jeffries, P.R., and Shelan, S.K.: Cardiogenic shock: current management, Crit. Care Nurse Q. **11**(1):48, 1988.

Johnson, G.P., and Johanson, B.C.: Beta blockers, Am. J. Nurs. **83**(7):1034, 1983.

Jones, S., and Bagg, A.M.: LEAD drugs for cardiac arrest . . . lidocaine, epinephrine, atropine, and dopamine, Nursing 88 **18**(1):34, 1988.

Lowenthal, D.T.: The clinical pharmacology of beta antagonists and centrally-acting alpha agonists, Cardiovas. Rev. Rep **4**(4):481, 1983.

Mitulsky, H.J., and Insel, P.A.: Adrenergic receptors in man, N. Engl. J. Med. **307**(1):18, 1982.

Rice, V.: Understanding shock and how to treat it: drug management, part 3, CINA J. (4):20, 1985.

Vlietstra, R.E.: Beta-adrenergic blockers—choosing among them, Postgrad. Med **76**(3):71, 1984.

Wilkins, M.R., and Kendall, M.H.: Clinical and pharmacological considerations in the use of beta blockers in the geriatric patient, Geriat. Med. Today **2**(9):99, 1983.

Yacone, L.A.: The nurse's guide to cardiovascular drugs, Part 1, RN **51**(8):36, 1988.

Yacone, L.A.: The nurse's guide to cardiovascular drugs, Part 2, RN **51**(9):40, 1988.

IV

DRUGS AFFECTING SYSTEMS UNDER CHOLINERGIC CONTROL

In this section the cholinergic drug classes are presented within the framework of their major therapeutic targets: skeletal muscle, the eye, and the gastrointestinal system. The goal of this section is to present the traditional cholinergic drug classes within a systems setting to allow assessment of the therapeutic role of drugs affecting cholinergic mechanisms relative to drugs acting by other mechanisms.

The drug classes in Chapter 11, *Drugs to Control Muscle Tone*, are the acetylcholinesterase inhibitors and the neuromuscular blocking drugs, so that only cholinergic mechanisms are discussed. The drug classes in Chapter 12, *Drugs Affecting the Eye*, are more diverse, including not only anticholinergic drugs of the atropine type but also adrenergic drugs for pupillary dilation. The discussion of cholinomimetic drugs in treating glaucoma is supplemented by reference to the role of additional drug classes: adrenergics, carbonic anhydrase inhibitors, and osmotic diuretics.

Chapter 13, *Drugs Affecting the Gastrointestinal Tract*, considers several drug classes in addition to cholinergic classes. The role of the cholinergic system is emphasized initially by discussing cholinomimetics to increase and anticholinergics to decrease small intestinal motility. The role of anticholinergic drugs to inhibit stomach acid secretion is discussed, along with the more important roles of antacids to neutralize stomach acid and H_2 receptor antagonists to inhibit stomach acid secretion. Central mechanisms rather than cholinergic mechanisms are cited as the target for drug therapy of nausea and vomiting, which can be considered hyperactivity of the upper gastrointestinal tract. The different roles of antihistamines and the dopamine antagonists are briefly reviewed here but discussed fully in Chapters 24 and 41. Finally, the two major drug classes affecting the large intestine, laxatives and antidiarrheals, are discussed. Cholinergic mechanisms play no role in these drug classes. Antidiarrheals rely chiefly on opiate mechanisms to halt hyperactivity, whereas laxatives provide bulk to stimulate activity.

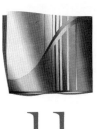

11

Drugs to Control Muscle Tone

Overview

Motor neurons are single neurons originating in the spinal cord and terminating on the muscle. In this chapter, two classes of drugs affecting skeletal muscle that act at the neuromuscular junction to affect the neurotransmitter acetylcholine or its receptor will be discussed. The first class of drugs consists of the *acetylcholinesterase inhibitors,* which are indirect-acting cholinomimetic drugs. These drugs are used to diagnose and to treat myasthenia gravis, a disease of muscular weakness, by increasing the quantity of acetylcholine at the neuromuscular junction to restore muscle contraction. The second class of drugs comprises the *neuromuscular blocking* drugs that occupy the receptors for acetylcholine on muscles and thereby prevent muscle contraction. These drugs are used to produce muscular relaxation for intubation and surgical procedures.

CHARACTERISTICS OF MYASTHENIA GRAVIS

Myasthenia gravis is a disease in which the skeletal muscles quickly show weakness and become fatigued. The muscles most commonly involved are those controlling facial movements, and one early sign of myasthenia gravis is drooping eyelids (ptosis). As the disease progresses, chewing and swallowing become increasingly difficult, and the voice becomes less distinct. Death can result if the intercostal muscles and the diaphragm, muscles essential for breathing, become affected.

The basic defect in myasthenia gravis is a reduction by 70% to 90% in the available receptors for acetylcholine at the neuromuscular junction. This reduction in the number of available receptors appears to be an autoimmune disease brought about by antibodies produced against the receptors. These antibodies block the active site for acetylcholine on the muscle (nicotinic) receptor and also increase

the rate at which the receptors are degraded by the cell. A number of drugs are contraindicated for the patient with myasthenia gravis and are listed in the box on p. 144. These drugs block the neuromuscular receptor to a degree that is not noticeable in a normal person but can dangerously weaken the patient with myasthenia gravis.

ACETYLCHOLINESTERASE INHIBITORS FOR MYASTHENIA GRAVIS (Table 11.1)
Mechanism of Action

Drugs that inhibit the degradation of acetylcholine, acetylcholinesterase inhibitors (anticholinesterases), are the first line of treatment for myasthenia gravis. Acetylcholinesterase inhibitors allow the accumulation of acetylcholine at the neuromuscular junction, and this increase in the concentration of acetylcholine at the neuromuscular junction ensures that available receptors are activated.

The acetylcholinesterase inhibitors used to treat myasthenia gravis are also used to reverse the effects of the competitive neuromuscular blocking drugs used in surgery. This use is discussed in the section on neuromuscular blocking drugs.

Absorption, Distribution, Metabolism, and Excretion

The anticholinesterase drugs used to treat myasthenia gravis are positively charged compounds that are not lipid soluble. These drugs are therefore not readily absorbed orally; the oral dose is 30 times the parenteral dose. The anticholinesterases are metabolized by plasma esterases and by hepatic enzymes to inactive compounds. The drugs and their metabolites are excreted in the urine.

Side Effects

The effective dose must be individualized for each patient. Stress and infection can increase the

---

DRUGS THAT MAY WEAKEN A PATIENT WITH MYASTHENIA GRAVIS

ACTH and glucocorticoids
Anesthetics
   Diethyl ether
   Halothane (Fluothane)
   Lidocaine IV (Xylocaine)
Antiarrhythmics
   Procainamide (Pronestyl)
   Propranolol (Inderal)
   Quinidine
Antibiotics
   Bacitracin (Bacitracin)
   Colistimethate (Coly-Mycin M)
   Colistin (Coly-Mycin S)
   Gentamicin (Garamycin)
   Kanamycin (Kantrex)
   Lincomycin (Lincocin)
   Neomycin (Mycifradin, Neobiotic)
   Netilmicin (Nebcin)
   Paromomycin (Humatin)
   Polymyxin B (Aerosporin, Polymyxin B)
   Streptomycin (Streptomycin)
   Viomycin (Viocin)
Anticonvulsants
   Magnesium sulfate
Antimalarials
   Quinine
Diuretics and other drugs or circumstances promoting hypokalemia (low blood potassium concentration)
Muscle relaxants
   Gallamine (Flaxedil)
   Metocurine (Metubine)
   Pancuronium (Pavulon)
   Succinylcholine (Anectine)
   Tubocurarine
Sedatives, especially those with respiratory depressant effects, such as barbiturates, narcotics, and tranquilizers
Thyroid compound

---

requirement in a given patient. Women in the premenstrual part of their cycle may require higher doses. Very ill patients may become unresponsive to their medication, but temporary reduction or withdrawal of the dose over a 3-day period may restore their responsiveness. Parenteral administration may be required.

Side effects arising from overstimulation of neuromuscular (nicotinic) receptors include muscle cramps, rapid small contractions (fasciculations), and weakness. Acetylcholinesterase inhibitors can also act at sites other than neuromuscular sites. These inhibitors act at muscarinic sites and produce side effects classic for parasympathetic stimulation: excessive salivation, perspiration, abdominal distress, and nausea and vomiting. Patients frequently develop a tolerance to the muscarinic effects of the anticholinesterases.

Anticholinesterase drugs are contraindicated for patients with obstruction of the intestinal or urinary tract. These drugs should be used very cautiously in patients with bronchial asthma. Individuals who are sensitive to bromide should be given neostigmine methylsulfate or ambenonium chloride instead of the more commonly used bromide-containing anticholinesterases.

Specific Drugs

Neostigmine

Neostigmine (Prostigmin) can be used for the diagnosis and treatment of myasthenia gravis. As a diagnostic tool, an intramuscular injection of neostigmine should improve the patient's muscular strength in 10 minutes, and this improvement should last 3 to 4 hours. Neostigmine is also prescribed to relieve the symptoms of myasthenia gravis. Because neostigmine is irregularly absorbed from the gastrointestinal tract, effective drug levels can be difficult to establish with oral administration. Muscarinic side effects, particularly salivation, cramps, and diarrhea, are common enough to limit the long-term use of neostigmine. If neostigmine is used, atropine may also be prescribed to block the muscarinic effects.

Pyridostigmine

Pyridostigmine (Mestinon) is the drug of choice for the treatment of myasthenia gravis. Compared to neostigmine, pyridostigmine is better absorbed from the gastrointestinal tract and longer acting. Adverse effects such as miosis, sweating, salivation, gastrointestinal distress, and slow heart rate are less common with pyridostigmine than with neostigmine.

Ambenonium

Ambenonium (Mytelase) is slightly longer acting than pyridostigmine or neostigmine. Occasionally, patients experience side effects such as jitteriness, headaches, confusion, and dizziness, which are not seen with pyridostigmine or neostigmine. An advantage of ambenonium is that it is not a bromide salt, whereas pyridostigmine and neostigmine are bromide salts. Ambenonium is thus the drug of choice for patients with an allergy to bromides.

Edrophonium

Edrophonium (Tensilon) is a very short-acting acetylcholinesterase inhibitor used as a diagnostic agent. When a new patient with suspected myas-

Table 11.1   Cholinomimetic Drugs for Diagnosis and Treatment of Myasthenia Gravis

Generic name	Trade name*	Administration/dosage	Comments
Ambenonium chloride	Mytelase	ORAL: *Adults*—5 mg 3 or 4 times daily increased every 1 to 2 days as required. *Children*—0.3 mg/kg body weight daily in divided doses, increased gradually if necessary to a maximum of 1.5 mg/kg daily.	Acetylcholinesterase inhibitor. Rapidly absorbed.
Edrophonium chloride	Tensilon Enlon	For diagnosis of myasthenia gravis: INTRAVENOUS: *Adults*—2 mg injected over 15 to 30 sec. If no response, 8 mg is given. May repeat test after 1 hr. *Children:* 2 mg initially as above followed by 5 mg (under 75 lb) or up to 10 mg (over 75 lb).	Very short-acting acetylcholinesterase inhibitor. Diagnosis is positive if muscle strength increases within 3 min (duration, 5 to 10 min).
		To differentiate a myasthenic from a cholinergic crisis: 1 to 2 mg.	A cholinergic crisis if muscle strength decreases (lower medication dose). A patient in cholinergic crisis may require ventilatory assistance after edrophonium injection.
Neostigmine bromide	Prostigmin bromide	ORAL: *Adults*—15 mg every 3 to 4 hr initially, then adjust upward as required. *Children*—begin with 2 mg/kg body weight daily in divided doses.	Acetylcholinesterase inhibitor. High incidence of side effects.
Neostigmine methylsulfate	Prostigmin methylsulfate	INTRAMUSCULAR: *Adults*—0.022 mg/kg body weight (atropine, IM, 0.011 mg/kg may be given to control muscarinic side effects). *Children*—0.01 to 0.04 mg/kg body weight (with 0.01 mg/kg atropine, IM)	Injectable form for diagnosis of myasthenia gravis
Pyridostigmine bromide	Mestinon	ORAL: *Adults*—60 to 120 mg every 3 or 4 hr initially, increased as necessary. *Children*—7 mg/kg in divided doses as required.	Acetylcholinesterase inhibitor; drug of choice for controlling muscular weakness of myasthenia gravis.
	Regonol	INTRAMUSCULAR, INTRAVENOUS: *Adults*—1/30 of oral dose. *Newborn infants of myasthenic mothers*—0.05 to 0.15 mg/kg body weight.	

*These drugs are all available in Canada and United States.

thenia gravis is given 2 mg of edrophonium IV, an increase in muscle strength should be seen in 1 to 3 minutes. If no response is seen, another 4 to 10 mg of edrophonium is given over the next 2 minutes and muscle strength is again tested. If no increase in muscle strength is seen with this higher dose, the muscle weakness is caused by something other than myasthenia gravis. Patients receiving injections of edrophonium commonly show a drop in blood pressure and feel faint, dizzy, and flushed.

A second diagnostic use for edrophonium is to aid in deciding what to do when a patient under treatment for myasthenia gravis becomes weaker. The problem is to identify whether the patient is suffering from an overdose of medication (cholinergic crisis) or increasing severity of the disease (myasthenic crisis). An injection of edrophonium will make the patient in cholinergic crisis temporarily worse (negative Tensilon test) but will temporarily improve the patient in myasthenic crisis (positive Tensilon test).

NEUROMUSCULAR BLOCKING DRUGS
(Table 11.2)

Mechanism of Action

Neuromuscular blocking drugs produce complete muscle relaxation by binding to the receptor for acetylcholine at the neuromuscular junction. The nondepolarizing or competitive blockers bind to the receptor without initiating depolarization of the muscle membrane. The depolarizing drug also binds to the receptor for acetylcholine but does

Table 11.2   Neuromuscular Blocking Drugs

Generic name	Trade name	Administration/dosage	Comments
NONDEPOLARIZING (COMPETITIVE) DRUGS			
Atracurium	Tracrium	INTRAVENOUS: *Adults*—0.3 to 0.6 mg/kg body weight; subsequent doses, 0.05 to 0.1 mg/kg.	Not affected by renal or hepatic impairment. Relatively free of cardiovascular side effects. Doses given are for use with nitrous oxide. Other inhalation anesthetics may require smaller doses.
Gallamine triethiodide	Flaxedil* Triethiodide	INTRAVENOUS: *Adults*—1 to 1.5 mg/kg body weight. Supplemental doses, 0.3 to 1.2 mg/kg. *Children*—2.5 mg/kg initially with 0.3 to 1.2 mg/kg supplemental doses. *Newborns*—up to 1 month of age, 0.25 to 0.75 mg/kg initially, with 0.1 to 0.5 mg/kg supplemental doses.	May cause increased heart rate. Not for use in patients in renal failure. Doses given are for use with nitrous oxide. Other inhalation anesthetics may require smaller doses.
Metocurine iodide	Metubine*	INTRAVENOUS: *Adults*—0.1 to 0.3 mg/kg body weight. Supplemental doses, 0.02 to 0.03 mg/kg.	See tubocurarine chloride. Doses given are for use with nitrous oxide. Other inhalation anesthetics may require smaller doses. Not for use in patients with renal failure.
Pancuronium bromide	Pavulon*	INTRAVENOUS: *Adults and children*—0.04 to 0.1 mg/kg body weight initially with 0.01 to 0.02 mg/kg supplemental doses. Newborns may be very sensitive; use a test dose of 0.02 mg.	Does not cause hypotension. May stimulate heart rate and cardiac output. Doses given are for use with nitrous oxide. Other inhalation anesthetics may require smaller doses.
Tubocurarine chloride (curare)	Tubarine† Tubocurarine chloride*	INTRAVENOUS: *Adults and children*—0.2 to 0.4 mg/kg body weight initially. Supplemental doses, 0.04 to 0.2 mg/kg. Diagnosis of myasthenia gravis: $\frac{1}{15}$ to $\frac{1}{5}$ of above dose.	Intravenous injection should be slow (1 to 1½ min). Do not combine with alkaline intravenous barbiturate solutions. Doses given are for use with nitrous oxide. Other inhalation anesthetics may require smaller doses.
Vecuronium	Norcuron	INTRAVENOUS: *Adults*—0.07 to 0.14 mg/kg body weight for intubation; 0.04 to 0.1 mg/kg initially, followed by 0.015 to 0.02 mg/kg as needed for surgery.	Related to pancuronium but shorter (by one third to one half) in duration. Relatively free of cardiovascular side effects. Doses given are for use with nitrous oxide. Other inhalation anesthetics may require smaller doses.
DEPOLARIZING DRUGS			
Succinylcholine chloride	Anectine* Quelicin* Sucostrin Sux-Cert	INTRAVENOUS: *Adults*—0.6 to 1.1 mg/kg body weight initially. Continuous infusion, 0.1% or 0.2% solution at a rate of 0.5 to 10 mg/min. *Children*—1.1 mg/kg body weight initially with 0.3 to 0.6 mg/kg supplemental doses. *Newborns*—2 mg/kg. Continuous infusion is not recommended for children and newborns.	Duration is only 5 min because of hydrolysis by plasma cholinesterase. This enzyme is missing genetically in some patients, and a prolonged action is seen. May cause cardiac arrhythmias. Doses given are for use with nitrous oxide. Other inhalation anesthetics require smaller doses.
CHOLINESTERASE INHIBITOR			
Hexafluorenium	Mylaxene	INTRAVENOUS: *Adults*—0.1 to 0.3 mg/kg body weight, followed in 2 to 3 min by 0.3 to 0.5 mg/kg succinylcholine. Muscle relaxation lasts 20 to 30 min. For longer procedures, additional succinylcholine, 0.25 mg/kg, is given at 15 to 30 min intervals.	Used with succinylcholine to prolong the action of succinylcholine and to prevent the muscle fasciculations produced by succinylcholine.

*Available in Canada and United States.
†Available in Canada only.

THE NURSING PROCESS

DRUGS USED IN MYASTHENIA GRAVIS

Assessment

Patients requiring acetylcholinesterase inhibitors are those in whom the diagnosis of myasthenia gravis is either confirmed or suspected. The patient may come to the hospital with a wide range of symptoms from mild ptosis (drooping eyelids) and easy fatigability to acute muscular weakness. A total body assessment should be done. The nurse should monitor not only the temperature, pulse, respiration, and blood pressure but also vital capacity, ability to swallow, muscle strength (all of which are impaired in myasthenia gravis), and the degree of ptosis. The nurse should assess the patient's condition for any additional medical problems that may coexist and influence treatment.

Potential nursing diagnoses

Potential ineffective airway clearance related to medication dosage adjustments
Potential impaired swallowing related to inadequate doses of acetylcholinesterase inhibitors
Anxiety related to frequent swings between myasthenic and cholinergic crises, and apparent inability to obtain adequate drug control of myasthenia gravis

Management

The treatment of the patient with myasthenia gravis can be complex and sometimes tricky. It is beyond the scope of this book to discuss all aspects of treatment; consult an appropriate textbook of nursing. The nurse should continue to monitor signs of myasthenia gravis including the ptosis, ability to swallow, vital capacity, and overall muscle strength as well as the vital signs. Medications should be administered exactly on time. A suction machine should be at the bedside if the patient displays any signs of being unable to swallow secretions adequately. Drugs that should be at the bedside include edrophonium, pyridostigmine, atropine, and neostigmine, along with syringes. In addition, equipment for intubation should be readily available if the patient's condition warrants it. The nurse should begin teaching the patient and family about the management of myasthenia gravis in the home setting. If appropriate, the patient can be referred to other members of the health care team for physical therapy or social service, or to the local visiting nurse association.

Evaluation

It is not possible to cure or halt the progression of myasthenia gravis. Successful drug therapy aids the patient to maintain as normal a life-style as possible. With this disease, perhaps more than with many other diseases, patient compliance and understanding are essential to good control of the symptoms. Before discharge the patient should be able to explain how and why the medication should be taken, the signs and symptoms that indicate overdose and underdose with medications, the symptoms that would require notification of the physician, other measures that should be employed to assist in managing the disease (such as the use of a nonelectric alarm clock to awaken the patient for nighttime doses of medication), and medications that should be avoided. For more specific information, see the patient care implications section at the end of this chapter.

---

cause depolarization of the muscle membrane. Since the depolarizing drug does not readily dissociate from the receptor, the depolarization persists. Larger doses of the depolarizing drug also desensitize the receptor to restimulation. Both types of blockade, nondepolarizing and depolarizing, re-sult in muscle paralysis. The two types of neuromuscular blocking drugs can be differentiated by the response to an injection of a drug such as edrophonium, which inhibits the degradation of acetylcholine by acetylcholinesterase. As the concentration of acetylcholine rises in the neuromuscular

THE NURSING PROCESS

NEUROMUSCULAR BLOCKING AGENTS

Assessment

Patients receiving neuromuscular blocking drugs will be those undergoing anesthesia, patients having certain diagnostic studies in which brief muscle relaxation is necessary for the completion of the study, some patients who are "bucking" ventilators, and patients undergoing electroconvulsive therapy. The nurse should determine the pulse, respiratory rate, and blood pressure of these patients. A thorough patient assessment should be done, focusing on the major problems being treated and what diagnostic or therapeutic procedure is to be carried out. The neuromuscular blocking agents usually are used for such a brief period of time that under normal circumstances there are no appropriate laboratory tests that should be monitored.

Potential nursing diagnoses

Ineffective airway clearance related to drug effect
Anxiety related to inability to swallow, ineffective airway clearance, and weakness

Management

Because neuromuscular blocking agents paralyze the patient completely, management includes rapid assessment of the respiratory system and assisted ventilation for the patient when necessary. Before a neuromuscular blocking agent is used, equipment for intubation and suctioning should be at the bedside. The nurse should observe the rate, quality, and depth of respirations and ventilate the patient as needed. If the drugs are being administered by constant infusion, an infusion monitoring device should be used. Remember that neuromuscular blockade agents, when used alone, do not produce anesthesia; medicate the patient for pain if necessary. The nurse should position the patient carefully and check to see that instruments and bed linens are not causing unnecessary pressure on any areas of the patient's body. After the drug has been used, it may take minutes to hours for the effect of the neuromuscular blocking agents to wear off. During this period of time it is important to assess the ability of the patient to breathe unassisted, to cough, and to handle secretions. Patients should be positioned on their sides and the side rails should be kept up. The patient should not be left unattended until it is certain that the patient can adequately cough, handle secretions, and call for help.

Evaluation

These agents are considered successful if they produce sufficient muscle relaxation to allow the procedure or activity to proceed. These are all short-acting drugs, and they are not appropriately prescribed for use outside a hospital setting. For additional specific information, see the patient care implications section at the end of the chapter.

---

junction, a nondepolarizing drug will be displaced and muscle tone will be regained. The depolarizing drug will not be displaced.

Therapeutic Uses

Because neuromuscular blockers can produce complete paralysis, they are administered only to an anesthetized patient. Assisted ventilation should be available for the short-acting succinylcholine and is mandatory when administering the longer-acting neuromuscular blockers. The skele-

tal muscle relaxants do not inhibit pain in any way. The major use of the neuromuscular blocking drugs is to provide muscle relaxation during surgery, particularly relaxation of the abdominal muscles, without using deep general anesthesia, which would relax abdominal muscles by depressing the spinal cord. The neuromuscular blockers are also used with light anesthesia to allow a tube to be passed down easily to the trachea (endotracheal intubation), to relieve spasm of the larynx, to prevent convulsive muscle spasms during electroconvulsive therapy for depression, and to allow breathing to be controlled totally by a respirator (controlled ventilation) during surgery.

Nondepolarizing Drugs
Tubocurarine (curare)

Tubocurarine was originally isolated as the active principle of the South American arrow poison. An animal hit with an arrow containing curare would fall paralyzed a short time later.

Uses. The main uses of tubocurarine are to produce muscle relaxation during surgery or electroconvulsive shock therapy, to reduce muscle spasm in tetanus, and to allow controlled ventilation. Administration is by slow (60 to 90 seconds) intravenous injection. Maximal paralysis occurs within 5 minutes and persists for 60 minutes (range: 25 to 90 minutes). The progression of paralysis begins with the eyelids, then the face, the extremities, and finally the diaphragm, resulting in the cessation of spontaneous breathing. The recovery from neuromuscular blockade can be assisted by injecting edrophonium, neostigmine, or pyridostigmine to increase the amount of acetylcholine at the neuromuscular junction.

Excretion. About 40% of tubocurarine is excreted unchanged in the urine. Patients with renal failure or acidosis will excrete tubocurarine less rapidly and require a smaller dose.

Side effects. Tubocurarine can cause release of histamine, which causes hypotension or bronchospasm (Chapter 24). Hypotension can arise from ganglionic blockade by tubocurarine. Tubocurarine does not cross the placenta or blood-brain barrier.

Drug interactions. Many drugs potentiate the action of tubocurarine, including the anesthetics halothane, ether, methoxyflurane, and enflurane. Many antibiotics potentiate the action of tubocurarine, including the aminoglycosides and the polymyxins (see Chapter 33), bacitracin, lincomycin, and clindamycin. Other drugs that potentiate the action of tubocurarine are the antiarrhythmic drugs, quinidine, the ganglionic blocker drugs, trimethaphan, and magnesium sulfate. Since patients with myasthenia gravis have an exaggerated response to tubocurarine, very small doses of tubocurarine can be used to diagnose myasthenia gravis if tests with edrophonium or neostigmine are inconclusive.

Metocurine (dimethyl tubocurarine) iodide (Metubine)

Metocurine iodide, a semisynthetic derivative of tubocurarine, is 2 to 3 times as potent as tubocurarine but otherwise similar. Metocurine is excreted unchanged in the urine and should not be used in patients with kidney failure.

Gallamine triethiodide (Flaxedil)

Gallamine triethiodide is a synthetic drug similar in action to tubocurarine but with a shorter duration of action. Gallamine does not cause histamine release or ganglionic blockade. The major side effect of gallamine is an increase in heart rate (tachycardia), which is seen a few minutes after injection and which then declines. Gallamine is excreted unchanged in the urine and should not be used in patients with kidney failure.

Pancuronium bromide (Pavulon)

Pancuronium bromide has a faster onset of action than tubocurarine, although the duration of action is similar. Pancuronium does not cause the histamine release or ganglionic blockade characteristic of tubocurarine. Heart rate, cardiac output, and atrial pressure are increased by pancuronium, effects that may be desired in cardiac surgery. Pancuronium is excreted in urine, and doses must be decreased for patients with renal failure.

Atracurium (Tracrium)

Atracurium is a nondepolarizing muscle relaxant. It is shorter in duration than tubocurarine, producing adequate relaxation for 15 to 20 minutes. Atracurium is inactivated by hydrolysis. At usual doses, atracurium does not produce cardiovascular side effects.

Vecuronium (Norcuron)

Vecuronium is a nondepolarizing muscle relaxant that is chemically related to pancuronium. Vecuronium is shorter acting than pancuronium, and the effects of vecuronium are not cumulative with repeated administration. Unlike tubocurarine, the cardiovascular side effects arising from ganglionic or vagal blockade, interference with norepinephrine reuptake, or release of histamine are minimal with vecuronium. The intensity and duration of action of vecuronium are significantly affected by liver damage and modestly affected by renal failure.

Depolarizing Neuromuscular Blocking Drug
Succinylcholine chloride (Anectine and others)

Succinylcholine chloride has the briefest duration of action (5 minutes) of the neuromuscular blocking drugs, because plasma cholinesterases readily degrade succinylcholine. Longer action requires continuous infusion of succinylcholine, but

PATIENT CARE IMPLICATIONS

Drugs for the diagnosis and treatment of myasthenia gravis

Drug administration

- Assess patients for signs of myasthenic crisis (that is, inadequately treated myasthenia gravis): positive Tensilon test; increased blood pressure and pulse; difficulty chewing, swallowing, and coughing; bladder and bowel incontinence; increasing ptosis; difficulty breathing; cyanosis. Differentiate symptoms of myasthenic crisis from those of cholinergic crisis (that is, overtreated myasthenia gravis): negative Tensilon test; abdominal cramps, diarrhea; fasciculations; nausea, vomiting; blurred vision. The following may be seen in either myasthenic or cholinergic crisis: generalized weakness; increased salivation, tearing, and bronchial secretions; general feeling of apprehension; restlessness; difficulty breathing. Keep a suction machine at the bedside.
- Keep edrophonium, pyridostigmine, atropine, neostigmine, and syringes, and a tourniquet at the patient's bedside or together in a convenient place on the patient care unit for rapid treatment of a myasthenic or cholinergic crisis.

- Assess the patient's ability to swallow before preparing an ordered oral dose of acetylcholinesterase inhibitor. If the ability to swallow is deteriorating, it may be necessary to administer a parenteral dose of medication. Ideally, the physician will have written orders for both oral and parenteral doses of acetylcholinesterase inhibitors so valuable time is not lost in trying to call the physician for a medication order if the patient can no longer safely swallow.
- Schedule off-unit diagnostic studies and therapies carefully for the patient with myasthenia gravis so that medication times for acetylcholinesterase inhibitors are not delayed while the nurse waits for the patient to return to the unit. If the patient is not on the unit when a medication is due, take the dose of medication to the patient.
- Regularly assess blood pressure, pulse, vital capacity, presence and degree of ptosis, muscle strength, and ability to swallow as indicators of adequate drug control.
- When neostigmine is used as an antidote for tubocurarine, administer via slow IV push. Continue appropriate ventilatory support until the patient is breathing well unassisted.

---

care must then be taken to avoid desensitizing the muscle. The duration of action is increased by drugs that inhibit cholinesterases. Some patients have abnormal plasma cholinesterases that do not readily degrade succinylcholine. In these patients, the action of succinylcholine will be very prolonged. Conditions that elevate plasma potassium concentration, such as burns, tetanus, massive trauma, or brain or spinal cord injury will prolong the action of succinylcholine.

Uses. The short duration of action makes succinylcholine a drug of choice for such procedures as endoscopy, terminating laryngospasm, endotracheal intubation, orthopedic procedures, and electroconvulsive shock therapy.

Side effects. Children are not as sensitive to succinylcholine on a weight basis as adults, and require higher doses. Children are more apt to show side effects of succinylcholine resulting from parasympathetic stimulation: slow heart rate (brady-

cardia) and cardiac arrhythmias. Succinylcholine does not cross the blood-brain barrier or the placenta.

Succinylcholine initially causes rapid but small contractions of the muscles (fasciculations) before the muscles are paralyzed. This is believed to be the cause of the stiffness and soreness experienced by many patients 12 to 24 hours after they have received succinylcholine. Succinylcholine will also transiently raise intraocular pressure and must be administered before surgery to the eye begins.

Plasma Cholinesterase Inhibitor

Hexafluorenium bromide (Mylaxen)

Hexafluorenium inhibits the activity of plasma cholinesterase. Since this enzyme hydrolyzes and inactivates succinylcholine, the duration of neuromuscular blockade produced by succinylcholine can be prolonged by the concurrent admin-

PATIENT CARE IMPLICATIONS — cont'd

If the pulse is less than 80 beats per minute, administer atropine before the neostigmine.

- For constant infusion of acetylcholinesterase inhibitors, use a volume control device and microdrip tubing to titrate the dose accurately. Monitor respiratory and cardiovascular status.
- For additional information about the nursing management of patients with myasthenia gravis, consult current nursing literature.

Patient and family education

- Teach patients and families about the signs and symptoms of myasthenia gravis, myasthenic crisis, and overdose with acetylcholinesterase inhibitors.
- Other points to teach the patient and family include: Take medications as ordered, when ordered. Forgetting, omitting, or doubling a dose of medication may cause the patient's condition to deteriorate.
- No medication, whether prescription or over-the-counter, should ever be taken without the approval of the physician. In addition, give the patient a list of drugs known to be contraindicated in patients with myasthenia gravis (see text).
- Suggest that patients plan a medication schedule that includes taking doses of acetylcholinesterase inhibitors 30 to 60 minutes before meals to increase strength for chewing and swallowing.
- Take acetylcholinesterase inhibitors with milk or snack to reduce gastric irritation.
- Use a reliable, nonelectric alarm clock to waken the patient for early morning or nighttime doses of medication.
- Keep careful watch on supplies of drugs on hand, and refill prescriptions before they run out.
- Reinforce to patients and families the need to seek medical assistance immediately if the patient's condition seems to be deteriorating.
- Encourage patients to wear a medical identification tag or bracelet, and to carry with them a list of the names and doses of medication being taken.
- For additional information, refer patients and families to local, state, or national myasthenia gravis support groups.

Neuromuscular blocking agents

Drug administration

- Monitor blood pressure, pulse, respirations; auscultate lungs. Monitor arterial blood gases and electrocardiogram.
- Use these drugs only in settings where personnel and equipment are available to provide immediate intubation of the patient. Keep a suction machine, oxygen, mechanical ventilator, or resuscitation bag and resuscitation equipment and drugs handy.
- Remember that these drugs cause paralysis but not anesthesia. Unless patients are also anesthetized, they can still hear, feel, and see, if the eyelids are opened. Remember to remain professional in discussions within the patients' hearing, to talk to patients about sounds in the environment and anticipated nursing care activities, and to use television and/or radio judiciously. Arrange for times when the patient can sleep uninterrupted.
- If the patient is not anesthetized, take care to avoid rough handling, to position the patient in a comfortable position, to offer backrubs if possible, and to medicate for pain if appropriate.
- Keep the reversing agent or antagonist readily available.
- When administering these drugs via constant infusion, a microdrip tubing set and an infusion controlling device should be used.
- Consult the manufacturer's literature for specific guidelines regarding calculation of dosage. In many institutions, induction with a neuromuscular blocking agent must be done by the anesthesiologist or nurse anesthetist; follow agency guidelines.
- When discontinuing therapy with a neuromuscular blocking agent, do not leave the patient unattended until sufficient muscle tone has returned so the patient can breathe, handle secretions, and call for assistance if needed (either verbally or by using the call bell). In infants, assess for the ability to hold the eyelids open or to hold up the legs. Keep the side rails up and the call bell within reach.
- These drugs are not used for home management. Keep the patient and family informed of the patient's condition.

istration of hexafluorenium. In addition, the muscle fasciculations produced by succinylcholine are markedly reduced or eliminated, which in turn reduces the pain often associated with the use of succinylcholine. The duration of action of hexafluorenium is 20 to 30 minutes.

SUMMARY

Acetylcholine is the neurotransmitter at the neuromuscular junction. Acetylcholinesterase inhibitors increase the amount of acetylcholine in the neuromuscular junction. This effect is used therapeutically to restore muscle strength in patients with myasthenia gravis or to terminate the action of nondepolarizing neuromuscular blocking drugs after surgery.

Neuromuscular blocking drugs produce muscle relaxation by preventing acetylcholine from stimulating the neuromuscular receptor. These drugs may themselves cause an initial stimulation with subsequent paralysis (depolarizing drugs), as shown by succinylcholine, or the drug may cause paralysis only (nondepolarizing drugs), as shown by tubocurarine.

Neuromuscular blockers are used to produce muscle relaxation during surgery, intubation, or electroconvulsive shock therapy.

STUDY QUESTIONS

1. Contrast the mechanisms by which the acetylcholinesterase inhibitors (anticholinesterases) increase activation of the neuromuscular junction and the neuromuscular blockers inhibit activation at the neuromuscular junction.
2. List the muscarinic side effects of neostigmine and pyridostigmine. Which drug can be used as an antidote for neostigmine?
3. Describe two diagnostic uses of edrophonium.
4. Contrast the mechanism of the depolarizing and the nondepolarizing neuromuscular blocking drugs. How does edrophonium distinguish between these actions?
5. List the nondepolarizing neuromuscular blocking drugs.
6. List the depolarizing neuromuscular blocking drugs.
7. List the uses of tubocurarine.
8. What genetic alteration do some patients have that prolongs the action of succinylcholine?

SUGGESTED READINGS

Booij, L.H.D.: Neuromuscular blockade, Curr. Rev. Nurse Anes. **10**(1):3, 1987.

Brumback, R.A.: The neuromuscular junction. Part I. Physiology and the effects of drugs and toxins, Am. Fam. Physician **23**(1):88, 1981.

Brumback, R.A.: The neuromuscular junction. Part II. Myasthenia gravis, Am. Fam. Physician **34**(2):126, 1981.

Bruton-Maree, N.: Neuromuscular blocking drugs, J. Neurosc. Nurs. **21**(3):198, 1989.

Conner, C.S.: Atracurium and vecuronium: two unique neuromuscular blocking agents, Drug Intell. Clin. Pharm. **18**:714, 1978.

Drachman, D.B., and others: Myasthenic antibodies cross-link acetylcholine receptors to accelerate degradation, N. Engl. J. Med. **298**:1116, 1978.

Yungbluth, J., and others: Recovery characteristics following antagonism of vercuronium with edrophonium, neostigmine, or pyridostigmine, AANA Journal **56**(2):127, 1988.

CHAPTER

Drugs Affecting the Eye

12

ROLE OF THE AUTONOMIC NERVOUS SYSTEM

The autonomic nervous system plays a major role in controlling the amount of light entering the eye and in focusing images. The amount of light penetrating the eye is controlled by the size of the pigmented iris, which contains two sets of muscles: the sphincter muscles and the dilator muscles. The sphincter muscles are circular muscles with muscarinic receptors innervated by the parasympathetic nervous system. As diagrammed in Figure 12.1, the pupil is constricted when the sphincter muscles contract so that only a small surface on the eye passes light. The dilator muscles contain alpha receptors innervated by the sympathetic nervous system. *Miosis* is the term that refers to a constricted pupil and is achieved primarily by stimulating the muscarinic receptors of the sphincter muscles. *Mydriasis* is the term that refers to a dilated pupil and is achieved either by blocking the muscarinic receptors of the sphincter muscles or by stimulating the alpha receptors of the dilator muscles.

The cornea and the lens determine the focus of images onto the retina. The cornea accomplishes the coarse focusing, but the fine focusing for sharp images and near vision is accomplished by the lens. The shape of the lens is controlled by muscarinic receptors of the parasympathetic nervous system. As diagrammed in Figure 12.1, the accommodation for near vision requires the contraction of ciliary muscles to change the shape of the lens. Ligaments normally pull the lens to keep it relatively flat. The contraction of the ciliary muscles relaxes the ligaments so that the lens becomes rounder as required for near vision. *Cycloplegia* refers to the paralysis of the ciliary muscles by drugs that block muscarinic receptors. Cycloplegia causes blurred

vision, because the shape of the lens can no longer be adjusted for near vision.

ANTICHOLINERGIC DRUGS FOR MYDRIASIS AND CYCLOPLEGIA
(Table 12.1)
Actions

Classic anticholinergic actions include dilated pupils (mydriasis) and blurred vision (cycloplegia). Accurate measurement of lens refraction requires both of these anticholinergic actions. The relaxation of sphincter and ciliary muscles when anticholinergic drugs are instilled into the eye hastens healing of inflammatory conditions, especially after surgery of the eye. Atropine, scopolamine, and homatropine are used for this type of treatment.

Side Effects

Anticholinergic drugs used ophthalmically are applied directly to the eye. Systemic reactions may nevertheless occur when the drug is absorbed into the body, particularly with atropine. These systemic reactions are those associated with anticholinergic effects: a dry mouth and dry skin, fever, thirst, confusion, and hyperactivity. Children are the most prone to systemic toxicity from ophthalmic drugs.

Specific Drugs
Atropine

Atropine is the drug of choice for use in children because atropine is potent and long-acting and children have a very active accommodation. Mydriasis may last 12 days, although accommodation usually returns in 6 days. Since atropine is applied for 3 days, children should be carefully watched for systemic reactions and application

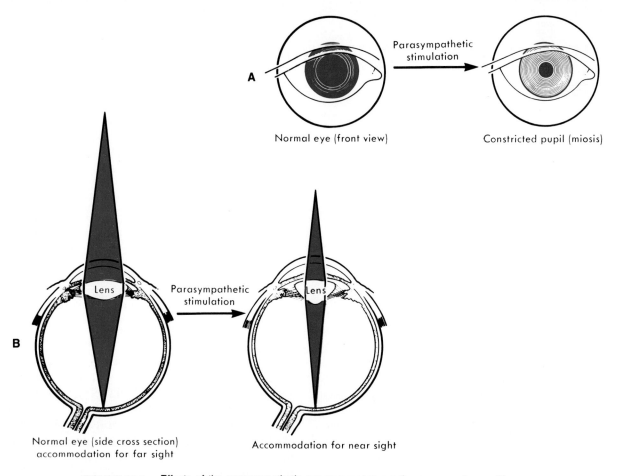

FIGURE 12.1   Effects of the parasympathetic nervous system on the eye are shown. These are mediated through muscarinic receptors. **A,** Pupil is made smaller because circular muscles contract. **B,** Accommodation is made by contracting muscles to thicken lens.

discontinued if any reactions appear. Atropine has been reported to cause a contact dermatitis of the eyelids.

Scopolamine

Scopolamine is used like atropine, but cycloplegia lasts for only 3 days instead of 6 days.

Homatropine

Homatropine is applied 2 or 3 times at 10-minute intervals to produce mydriasis and cycloplegia, which are achieved in 60 minutes. Recovery may take 2 days.

Cyclopentolate (Cyclogyl) and tropicamide (Mydricyl)

Cyclopentolate and tropicamide are rapidly acting mydriatic and cycloplegic drugs. Cyclopentolate is effective in 25 to 75 minutes and accom-

modation returns in 6 to 24 hours. Tropicamide is effective in 20 to 35 minutes, and accommodation returns in 2 to 6 hours. Systemic reactions have been reported with cyclopentolate but not with tropicamide.

ADRENERGIC DRUGS FOR MYDRIASIS
(Table 12.1)

The adrenergic drugs phenylephrine and hydroxyamphetamine are used as mydriatics when only the interior structures of the eye are to be examined and cycloplegia is not required.

Phenylephrine (Neo-Synephrine and others)

Phenylephrine acts on the alpha receptors of the dilator muscles to produce mydriasis. Dilation is maximal in 60 to 90 minutes, and recovery occurs in 6 hours. Cyclomydril is a combination of cyclo-

Table 12.1   Drugs for Mydriasis and Cycloplegia

Drug	Trade name	Administration/dosage	Comments
ANTICHOLINERGIC DRUGS FOR MYDRIASIS AND CYCLOPLEGIA			
Atropine sulfate	Atropine Sulfate* Atropisol* Isopto Atropine* Minims Atropine† Others	Topical solutions, 0.5% to 3%. *Adults*—1 drop of 1% to 3% solution to each eye. Frequency of administration depends on the condition being treated. *Children*—1 drop of 0.125 to 0.5% solution (under 8 yr) or 0.25 to 1% solution (over 8 yr) 3 times daily for 3 days before and once on the morning of the day refraction is measured. Duration: 6 days.	*Children*—refraction measurements. *Adults*—to relax eye muscles during surgery or treatment of eye inflammation. For adults, to aid in eye surgery or treatment of eye inflammation.
Cyclopentolate hydrochloride	AK-Pentolate* Cyclogyl* I-Pentolate* Minims Cyclopentolate† Pentolair*	Topical solutions, 0.5%, 1%, and 2%. *Adults*—1 drop of solution in each eye, repeated after 5 min. Darker irises or children require the stronger solutions. *Children*—1 drop of solution in eye, repeated after 10 min. Onset: 25 to 75 min. Duration: 6 to 24 hr.	To aid in measuring refraction.
Homatropine hydrobromide	AK-Homatropine* Isopto Homatropine* Homatrocel I-Homatrine* Minims Homatropine†	Topical solutions, 2% and 5%. *Adults*—for refraction 1 drop of 5% solution every 10 min 2 or 3 times. Duration: 2 days.	To aid in refraction measurements in adults. To aid in treating mild eye inflammation.
Scopolamine hydrobromide	Isopto Hyoscine Hydro-bromide	Topical solutions, 0.2% to 0.3%. *Adults*—1 drop of solution or ointment to each eye, 1 or more times daily depending on the condition being treated. *Children*—1 drop of 0.2% to 0.25% solution or ointment twice daily for 2 days before refraction measurement. Duration: 3 days.	For children, to measure refraction. For adults, to treat eye inflammation.
Tropicamide	I-Picamide Mydriacyl* Minims Tropicamide† Tropicadyl	Topical solutions, 0.5% and 1%. 1 drop in each eye, repeated in 5 min. Onset: 20 to 35 min. Duration: 2 to 6 hr	To aid in measuring refraction.
ADRENERGIC DRUGS FOR MYDRIASIS ONLY			
Hydroxyam-phetamine hy-drobromide	Paredrine	Topical use, 1 drop of a 1% solution.	Maximum mydriasis in 45 to 60 min. Recovery in 6 hr.
Phenylephrine hydrochloride	Minims Phenylephrine† Mydfrin Neo-Synephrine Hydro-chloride* Others	Topical use, 1 drop of a 2.5% solution.	Maximum mydriasis in 60 to 90 min. Recovery in 6 hr.

*Available in Canada and United States.
†Available in Canada only.

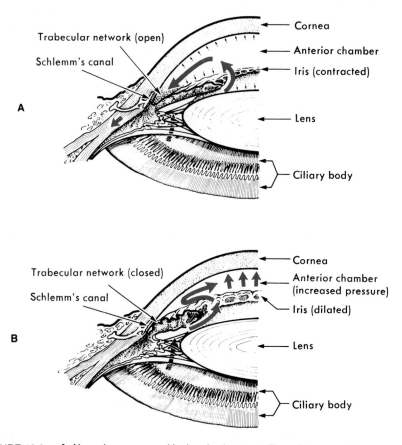

FIGURE 12.2 **A,** Normal eye or eye with chronic glaucoma. Flow of aqueous humor is shown from the ciliary body and around iris. Aqueous humor is normally absorbed into the body through trabecular network into Schlemm's canal. In chronic glaucoma, aqueous humor accumulates because trabecular network degenerates. **B,** Eye in acute glaucoma. Flow of aqueous humor is stopped because iris has blocked trabecular network and Schlemm's canal. Aqueous humor can accumulate quickly to cause a marked rise in ocular pressure that may damage optic nerve.

pentolate and phenylephrine used when maximal dilation is required.

Hydroxyamphetamine (Paredrine)

Hydroxyamphetamine is an indirect-acting alpha adrenergic drug that acts by releasing neuronal stores of norepinephrine. Dilation is maximal in 45 to 60 minutes, and recovery is in 6 hours.

GLAUCOMA AND DRUG THERAPY
Characteristics of Glaucoma

Glaucoma is the increase in intraocular pressure as a result of fluid accumulation between the lens and the cornea. The space between the lens and cornea is filled with *aqueous humor.* Aqueous humor is a protein-poor fluid formed by the ciliary body. As indicated in Figure 12.2, this fluid is normally reabsorbed through the trabecular spaces into Schlemm's canal in a special region of the cornea called the *anterior chamber.* If the aqueous humor cannot be reabsorbed through the anterior chamber, the fluid accumulates and intraocular pressure increases. If the intraocular pressure is not relieved, the optic nerve will become damaged, resulting in blindness.

Chronic (open-angle) glaucoma is the more common form of glaucoma and is very gradual in its onset. The defect is a slow degeneration of the anterior chamber so that the uptake of aqueous humor is impaired (Figure 12.2).

The initial treatment for chronic glaucoma is usually the application of a weak cholinomimetic drug to cause constriction of the pupil (miosis). The therapeutic effectiveness is a result of the spread of the trabecular spaces of the anterior chamber when the sphincter muscles contact. The larger area allows improved uptake of the aqueous humor, which relieves intraocular pressure.

The adrenergic drug epinephrine is the alternative drug to initiate therapy or the next drug added when the miotic drug alone is inadequate. Epinephrine stimulates both alpha and beta receptors, and in the eye, stimulation of alpha receptors reduces resistance to the outflow of aqueous humor, while stimulation of the beta receptors decreases production of aqueous humor.

The adrenergic beta-blocking drug timolol may also be used initially to treat chronic glaucoma or may be applied in addition to the miotic and epinephrine. The mechanism by which blockade of the beta receptors of the eye decreases intraocular pressure is not clear, particularly since stimulation of the beta receptor also causes reduction of intraocular pressure.

The drugs discussed so far are all applied directly to the eye. In resistant cases of glaucoma, systemic drugs are added. A carbonic anhydrase inhibitor is the next drug added because, aside from being weak diuretics, carbonic anhydrase inhibitors are also effective in decreasing the production of aqueous humor.

Osmotic agents such as glycerin, isosorbide, urea, or mannitol provide an immediate but short-term reduction in intraocular pressure by drawing fluid from the eyeball to the hyperosmotic blood.

Acute (closed-angle) glaucoma is characterized by the iris bulging up to shut off access of the aqueous humor to the anterior chamber, as shown in Figure 12.2. This creates an emergency because the build-up of intraocular pressure may become severe rapidly, damaging the optic nerve and causing blindness. Emergency treatment consists of a cholinomimetic drug, a carbonic anhydrase inhibitor, epinephrine, and an osmotic diuretic. This drug regimen provides transient treatment while the patient is being prepared for eye surgery in which the iris is cut to allow fluid access to the anterior chamber once again.

Cholinomimetic (Miotic) Drugs to Treat Glaucoma (Table 12.2)

Pilocarpine (Pilocar and others)

Pilocarpine is the drug of choice for chronic and acute glaucoma. It is a direct-acting cholinomimetic that is active 15 to 30 minutes after application and which lasts 4 to 8 hours. Since pilocarpine is the weakest of the cholinomimetic drugs used, it is the least likely to produce side effects, although it must be applied more frequently. The Ocusert system has been devised to overcome the need for frequent application of pi-

locarpine. The system is placed in the upper or lower cul-de-sac of the eye. Pilocarpine is contained in a reservoir between two membranes and is released over a period of 1 week. The drawbacks include the occasional sudden leakage of pilocarpine, the migration of the system over the cornea, and the unrealized loss of the system from the eye.

Carbachol (Carbacel and others)

Carbachol is also a direct-acting cholinomimetic agent. It is more potent and slightly longer acting than pilocarpine.

Physostigmine (Eserine)

Physostigmine is a short-acting acetylcholinesterase inhibitor that is occasionally used in place of pilocarpine or carbachol in the treatment of chronic glaucoma.

Physostigmine is poorly tolerated with prolonged treatment, because it commonly causes conjunctivitis and allergic reactions. The ointment may cause depigmentation of the eyelids in black persons.

Demecarium (Humorsol), echothiophate (Phospholine), and isoflurophate (Floropryl)

These three potent acetylcholinesterase inhibitors are used to treat chronic glaucoma not responsive to the combination of a weak miotic, epinephrine, and timolol. The effect of these acetylcholinesterase inhibitors is not seen for about 24 hours, but a single application is effective for 12 to 72 hours. Unfortunately, side effects are frequent with these potent miotics. They can cause congestion in the blood vessels of the ciliary body, resulting in a rise in the intraocular pressure. For this reason, they are seldom used to treat acute glaucoma. Spasms may be produced in the muscles of the eyelid as well as the eye itself, resulting in twitching of the eyelids or eyebrows, ocular pain, and headaches.

Additional Drugs to Treat Glaucoma (Table 12.2)

Epinephrine (Glaucon and others)

Epinephrine stimulates both alpha- and beta-adrenergic receptors to increase uptake of aqueous humor and to decrease production of aqueous humor, respectively. When applied directly to the eye in the treatment of chronic glaucoma, epinephrine produces a fall in intraocular pressure that lasts 12 to 24 hours. Mydriasis is transient. Epinephrine may be used as the initial therapy for glaucoma in

Table 12.2 Drugs to Treat Glaucoma

Generic name	Trade name	Administration/dosage	Comments
CHOLINOMIMETIC DRUGS (WEAK MIOTICS)			
Carbachol	Isopto Carbachol* Mistura-C	TOPICAL: 1 drop 0.75% to 3% solution every 8 hr. Onset: 15 to 30 min.	Direct-acting cholinomimetic; miotic, for treating chronic glaucoma.
Physostigmine salicylate Physostigmine sulfate	Isopto Eserine Eserine Sulfate	TOPICAL: 1 drop of 0.25% to 1% every 4 to 6 hr. Ointment for night use primarily. Onset: 30 min.	Acetylcholinesterase inhibitor; miotic for chronic glaucoma; conjunctivitis and allergic reactions common if use is prolonged.
Pilocarpine hydrochloride	Isopto Carpine* Pilocar Various others	TOPICAL: 1 drop, 1% to 2% every 6 to 8 hr. Onset: 15 to 30 min.	Direct-acting cholinomimetic; miotic; drug of choice for treating glaucoma, acute and chronic.
Pilocarpine nitrate	P.V. Carpine Liquifilm* Minims Pilocarpine†	TOPICAL: 1 drop, 1% to 2% every 6 to 8 hr. Onset: 15 to 30 min.	Direct-acting cholinomimetic; miotic; drug of choice for treating glaucoma, acute and chronic.
CHOLINOMIMETIC DRUGS (STRONG MIOTICS)			
Demecarium bromide	Humorsol	TOPICAL: 1 drop 0.125% to 0.25% solution every 12 to 48 hr. Onset: 12 hr.	Irreversible acetylcholinesterase inhibitor; potent miotic for resistant chronic glaucoma. Cataracts can develop with long-term administration.
Echothiophate iodide	Phospholine Iodide†	TOPICAL: 1 drop 0.03% to 0.06% every 12 to 48 hr. Onset: 12 hr.	Same as for demecarium.
Isofluorophate	Floropryl	TOPICAL: ¼ in strip of 0.025% ointment every 12 to 72 hr. Onset: 12 hr.	Same as for demecarium.
ADRENERGIC DRUGS			
Apraclonidine hydrochloride	Iopidine	1 hour before laser surgery instill 1 drop in affected eye; Repeat immediately before surgery.	To control or prevent acute, transient spikes in intraocular pressure following laser surgery for glaucoma.
Dipivefrin	Propine*	TOPICAL: 1 drop into conjunctival sac every 12 hr for glaucoma.	Converted to epinephrine by the esterases in the cornea and anterior chamber.
Epinephryl bitartrate	Epitrate*	TOPICAL: 1 drop of a 0.25% to 2.0% solution one or two times daily.	Persons with darkly pigmented irises may require a higher concentration of solution.
Epinephrine borate	Epinal* Eppy	Same as epinephrine bitartrate	
Epinephrine hydrochloride	Epifrin* Glaucon*	Same as epinephrine bitartrate.	

*Available in Canada and United States.
†Available in Canada only.

Table 12.2   Drugs to Treat Glaucoma—cont'd

Generic name	Trade name	Administration/dosage	Comments
BETA BLOCKERS			
Betaxolol hydrochloride	Betoptic	TOPICAL: 1 drop of a 0.5% solution twice daily.	A cardioselective (beta-1) beta-adrenergic antagonist developed for use in glaucoma.
Levobunolol	Betagan	TOPICAL: 1 drop of a 0.5% solution once or twice daily.	A nonselective beta-adrenergic antagonist.
Timolol maleate	Timoptic	TOPICAL: 1 drop of 0.25% solution twice daily. If not sufficient, a 0.5% solution is used.	A nonselective beta-adrenergic antagonist.
CARBONIC ANHYDRASE INHIBITORS			
Acetazolamide	Acetazolam† AK-Bol Apo-Acetazol-amide† Diamox* Novozolamide†	ORAL: *Adults*—250 mg every 6 hr. *Children*—10 to 15 mg/kg body weight daily in divided doses. Timed-release capsules are taken every 12 to 24 hr but may not be as effective.	A weak diuretic.
Acetazolamide sodium	Diamox, Parenteral*	INTRAVENOUS, INTRAMUSCULAR: *Adults*—500 mg repeated in 2 to 4 hr if necessary. *Children:* 5 to 10 mg/kg body weight every 6 hr.	
Dichlorphenamide	Daranide	ORAL: *Adults*—50 to 200 mg every 6 to 8 hr.	
Methazolamide	Neptazane	ORAL: *Adults*—25 to 100 mg every 8 hr.	
OSMOTIC AGENTS			
Glycerin	Glyrol Osmoglyn	ORAL: *Adults and children*—1 to 1.5 Gm/kg body weight as a 50% or 75% solution once or twice daily.	May flavor with instant coffee or lemon juice to increase palatability. May chill with chipped ice. May cause hyperglycemia in diabetic patients.
Isosorbide	Ismotic	ORAL: *Adults*—1.5 Gm/kg body weight up to 4 times daily.	May chill with chipped ice.
Mannitol	Osmitrol*	INTRAVENOUS: *Adults and children*—0.5 to 2 Gm/kg body weight as a 20% solution infused over 30 to 60 min.	May discontinue when intraocular pressure is decreased even though the full dose has not been given.
Urea	Ureaphil	INTRAVENOUS: *Adults*—0.5 to 2 Gm/kg body weight as a 30% solution infused at 60 drops/min. *Children*—0.5 to 1.5 Gm/kg body weight of a 30% solution infused over 30 min.	Infuse carefully. Patients with hereditary fructose intolerance should not be given urea made up in invert sugar.

*Available in Canada and United States.
†Available in Canada only.

THE NURSING PROCESS

TREATMENT OF EYE CONDITIONS

Assessment

Patients requiring treatment of eye conditions often have no externally visible signs of their condition. A thorough patient assessment should be done, especially of symptoms related to the eye. The nurse should check peripheral vision and test visual acuity using a Snellen chart or asking the patient to read something during the examination process. The patient should be questioned about recent difficulties in driving or ambulating at home; such difficulties might include tripping or bumping into objects. The nurse should examine the eyes closely for any signs of infection, exudate, excessive tearing or dryness, or any other deviation from normal.

Potential nursing diagnoses

Potential for injury related to impaired vision secondary to the specific eye problem
Altered home maintenance management related to insufficient knowledge about eye medications, their use, or their instillation

Management

The drugs discussed in this chapter are used for purposes of assisting in further evaluation of eye problems or in treating glaucoma. Other medications for the eye include antibiotics, glucocorticoids, and lubricants. Before receiving any eye medications for the first time, the patient should be warned about effects that will occur, particularly those related to vision. Blurred vision, photophobia, and other eye symptoms can be frightening to a patient when they occur without warning. In addition, the nurse should teach the patient about possible systemic side effects that may occur.

Evaluation

Drugs used to assist in diagnostic evaluation of the eye are considered successful if they aid in the examination desired without producing local or systemic side effects. Drugs used to treat glaucoma are considered successful if the intraocular pressure is lowered to within safe limits. Before any patient taking eye medications is discharged, it is important that the patient be able to explain why the drug is being used, to demonstrate how to administer the drug correctly, to explain the local and systemic side effects that might occur as a result of drug therapy, to explain what signs and symptoms should prompt the patient to contact the physician, and, particularly in the case of glaucoma, to explain the need for continuing therapy as ordered. For additional specific information, see the patient care implications section at the end of the chapter.

---

young patients, who may suffer spasms of the ciliary muscles controlling accommodation if a miotic is used, and in elderly patients with cataracts, whose vision is compromised by small pupils. Highly pigmented eyes are more resistant to epinephrine than lightly pigmented eyes.

Side effects. Epinephrine can cause a browache and can irritate the eyes. With prolonged use, epinephrine can cause swelling of the eyelids and bloodshot eyes. Symptoms of systemic absorption of epinephrine include a fast heart rate (tachycardia), high blood pressure, headache, sweating, and tremors.

Dipivefrin hydrochloride (Propine)

Dipivefrin (dipivalyl epinephrine) is a prodrug that is itself inactive but is converted to epinephrine by esterases in the cornea and anterior chamber of the eye. Dipivefrin is more lipid soluble than epinephrine and therefore concentrates in the eye more readily than epinephrine.

Apraclonidine (Iopidine)

Apraclonidine is a new drug that prevents acute, transient spikes in intraocular pressure following laser surgery for glaucoma. Apraclonidine

PATIENT CARE IMPLICATIONS

General guidelines in use of eye medications
Drug administration

- Wash hands carefully before administering eye medications to avoid contaminating the patient's eye or the applicator. Wash hands after administering eye medications to rinse off medication residue that might accidentally be rubbed into the nurse's own eye.
- Use a separate bottle or tube of medication for each patient to avoid accidental cross-contamination; wash hands between patients.
- Place ordered dose of eye medication in the lower conjunctival sac and never directly onto the cornea. Avoid touching any part of the eye with the dropper or applicator. For additional information see Chapter 6.
- To prevent overflow of medication into nasal and pharyngeal passages, and thus reduce systemic absorption, occlude or teach the patient to occlude the nasolacrimal duct with one finger for 1 to 2 minutes after instilling the medication.
- When two or more eye medications are to be administered, wait at least 3 minutes between drugs. Administer drops or liquid preparations prior to ointments. Administer glucocorticoid preparations before other drugs. If in doubt, consult the physician.
- Use atropine and the belladonna alkaloids cautiously in elderly patients, as these drugs may precipitate an attack of acute glaucoma.
- Monitor the pulse of patients receiving beta blockers, and teach patients to do the same. If the pulse is below 50 to 60 in an adult, withhold the next dose of medication and notify the physician. Reassess whether the patient is occluding the nasolacrimal duct correctly after administration of each dose.
- Use one drop of a 1% or 2% epinephrine solution to reverse the redness caused by potent acetylcholinesterase inhibitors; consult the physician.
- Use pralidoxime (PAM), 0.1 to 0.2 ml of a 5% solution to reverse the action of the irreversible acetylcholinesterase inhibitors. PAM must be injected subconjunctivally to be effective in the eye (Chapter 9).
- Glycerin may cause hyperglycemia. Monitor blood glucose levels, especially in diabetics.
- See Chapter 16 for additional information about carbonic anhydrase inhibitors.

Patient and family education

- Teach patient how to instill medication correctly, and supervise instillation until the patient is safe and comfortable with it (see above and Chapter 6).
- Teach patient to read labels carefully to ensure administration of correct drug and correct strength.
- Remind patient to keep these drugs out of the reach of children.
- Warn patient to avoid driving or operating hazardous equipment if vision is blurred. Tell adults that they may be unable to drive home following eye examinations during which medications to dilate the pupil (mydriatics) or drugs to paralyze the ciliary muscle (cycloplegics) were used; a friend or family member should drive until the effects of the medication wear off.
- If photophobia occurs, instruct patient to wear sunglasses and avoid bright lights. Tell patient not to wear sunglasses after dusk.
- Instruct patient to administer missed doses as soon as they are remembered, unless within 1 to 2 hours of the next dose. Tell patient not to "double up" for missed doses.
- If headache occurs after doses of glycerin, tell patient to lie down after taking dose.
- To make dose of glycerin or isosorbide more palatable, chill dose over crushed ice. Try flavoring glycerin with instant coffee or lemon juice.
- Teach patient with glaucoma that this eye condition cannot be cured, only controlled. Reinforce the importance of using medications to treat glaucoma as prescribed, and not to discontinue these medications without consulting the physician.
- Drugs used to treat glaucoma may cause pain and blurred vision, especially when therapy is begun. Tell patient that this may diminish with time. Tell patient to try cold compresses to relieve painful eye spasm.
- In infants, atropine eye drops may contribute to abdominal distension. Teach caregivers to keep a record of bowel movements of infants. In the health care setting, auscultate bowel sounds of infants and children receiving atropine eye drops.

Continued.

PATIENT CARE IMPLICATIONS — cont'd

- Warn patient to report the development of any eye irritation.
- Teach patient using eye gel to store the gel at room temperature or in the refrigerator, but avoid freezing it. Discard unused gel kept at room temperature after 8 weeks. After each use, wipe the tip of the tube with tissue and replace the cap tightly.
- Soft contact lenses may absorb certain eye medications, or preservatives in eye medications may discolor the contact lenses. Tell patient wearing contact lenses to question the physician carefully about special precautions which should be observed when eye medications are prescribed.

Sustained-release forms

- Teach patient to review carefully the instruction sheet provided by the manufacturer. The eye system is inserted into the upper or lower cul-de-sac of the eye, and the drug is released slowly; it should need to be replaced only weekly. Tell patient to check each morning and evening to make sure the system is still in place. If the unit seems not to be working, is damaged, or is releasing too much medication, remove it and insert a new one. Because there may be vision changes in the first few hours after the eye system is inserted, teach patient to replace it at night before bed.
- Teach patient to store the eye system in the refrigerator, but avoid freezing it.

---

is administered 1 hour before surgery and again just before surgery begins. Apraclonidine is an alpha-adrenergic agonist that acts by reducing intraocular aqueous formation. Side effects can include upper lid elevation, conjuctival blanching, and mydriasis.

Beta blockers

Beta-adrenergic receptor blockers are effective in lowering intraocular pressure. In many patients, however, the drugs lose effectiveness with time. Although there are many beta blockers, only three have proved suitable for ophthalmic use: betaxolol (Betoptic), levobunol (Betagan), and timolol (Timoptic). Most beta blockers produce corneal anesthesia, which leads to corneal damage. The major advantage of beta blockers is that neither pupil size nor reactivity to light is altered. There may be some irritation and blurred vision at the start of therapy, but these effects usually disappear.

Side effects. Betaxolol, levobunolol, and timolol may produce systemic effects after absorption into the circulation. The most common effects are a decrease in heart rate (bradycardia) and a fall in blood pressure, effects expected with a drug that blocks beta-1 adrenergic receptors. Bronchospasm resulting from blockade of the beta-2 adrenergic receptors has also been reported. Since betaxolol is selective for beta-1 receptors, this drug is preferred for patients with pulmonary problems. Betaxolol is also reported to be associated with less severe systemic cardiac effects.

Carbonic anhydrase inhibitors

Carbonic anhydrase inhibitors to treat glaucoma include *acetazolamide (Diamox), dichlorphenamide (Daranide, Oratrol)*, and *methazolamide (Neptazane)*. Although carbonic anhydrase inhibitors are weak diuretics, the effective action in treating glaucoma is to decrease the formation of aqueous humor. A fall in intraocular pressure is seen only in those individuals with elevated ocular pressure (glaucoma). The fall in intraocular pressure is negligible in individuals with normal ocular pressure.

The carbonic anhydrase inhibitors are taken orally and are maximally effective in 2 hours. The duration of action is 6 to 12 hours. Carbonic anhydrase inhibitors may be added to glaucoma therapy when the combination of a weak miotic, epinephrine, and timolol does not adequately lower the intraocular pressure of chronic glaucoma. Carbonic anhydrase inhibitors are also used with a miotic and epinephrine to lower intraocular pressure in acute (closed-angle) glaucoma.

Side effects. Carbonic anhydrase inhibitors have a number of unpleasant side effects including a loss of appetite, gastrointestinal upset, and a general feeling of lethargy and depression. A tingling sensation (paresthesia) in the fingers, toes, and face is common. Carbonic anhydrase inhibitors commonly produce a slight hypokalemia early in treatment; thus caution should be used in treating patients who are receiving digitalis.

Osmotic agents

Osmotic agents include glycerin (Glyrol, Osmoglyn), isosorbide (Ismotic), mannitol (Osmitrol), and urea (Ureaphil, Urevert). These are used for the short-term treatment only to lower the intraocular pressure of glaucoma before surgery or as an emergency treatment of acute (closed-angle) glaucoma. Glycerin and isosorbide are administered orally; whereas mannitol and urea are administered intravenously.

Glycerin. Glycerin is effective in lowering intraocular pressure 60 minutes after ingestion, and the effect lasts 5 hours. Since glycerin is metabolized, it does not cause a diuresis; however, glycerin can cause hyperglycemia in a patient who has diabetes. A headache, nausea, and vomiting are additional side effects of glycerin.

Isosorbide. Isosorbide is sometimes used in the emergency treatment of acute (closed-angle) glaucoma. Isosorbide does produce diuresis but otherwise has few side effects.

Mannitol. Mannitol is effective in lowering intraocular pressure in 30 to 60 minutes, and the effect lasts for 6 to 8 hours. Mannitol produces a pronounced diuresis, and it also will often cause a headache, nausea and vomiting, and dehydration.

Urea. Urea is less satisfactory than mannitol because urea can penetrate the eye and cause a rebound increase in intraocular pressure when the systemic osmotic effect is over, 8 to 12 hours after administration. Urea is also highly irritating on injection.

SUMMARY

Miosis refers to constricted pupils and is achieved with instillation of certain cholinomimetic drugs.

Mydriasis refers to a dilated pupil and is achieved with instillation of certain anticholinergic drugs that also paralyze the muscles of accommodation (cycloplegia). Mydriasis is produced without cycloplegia by sympathomimetic drugs acting at alpha adrenergic receptors.

Glaucoma refers to a condition in which there is a build-up of aqueous humor behind the cornea such that the pressure may damage the optic nerve if not relieved. Drainage of aqueous humor is achieved by instillation of drugs that decrease the production of aqueous humor and/or increase the uptake of aqueous humor.

STUDY QUESTIONS

1. Define miosis, mydriasis, and cycloplegia.
2. What are the anticholinergic actions in the eye? How are these actions medically useful?
3. Which anticholinergic drugs are used in the eye?
4. What action is mediated by the alpha adrenergic receptor in the eye? Which drugs are used for this effect?
5. Describe glaucoma and the role of aqueous humor.
6. Differentiate between chronic and acute glaucoma.
7. What role do cholinomimetic drugs play in the treatment of glaucoma? Which drugs are used?
8. What role do drugs acting at adrenergic receptors play in the treatment of glaucoma? Describe the actions of epinephrine and timolol.
9. What role do carbonic anhydrase inhibitors and osmotic agents play in the treatment of glaucoma?

SUGGESTED READINGS

Adler, A.G., and others: Systemic effects of eye drops, Arch. Intern. **142**(12):2293, 1982.

Boyd-Monk, H.: Screening for glaucoma, Nursing 79 **9**(8):42, 1979.

Jindra, L.F.: Open-angle glaucoma: diagnosis and management, Hosp. Pract. **18**(10):114C, 1983.

Katz, I.M., and Soll, D.B.: Beta blockers and glaucoma. Am. Fam. Physician **21**(4):150, 1980.

Oppeneer, J.E., and Vervoren, T.M.: Gerontological pharmacology: a resource for health practitioners, St. Louis, 1983, C.V. Mosby Co.

Quail, C., and Waddleton, C.: Treating the glaucomas, Nurses' Drug Alert **4**(9):93, 1980.

Resler, M.M., and Tumulty, G.: Glaucoma update, Am. J. Nurs. **83**(5):752, 1983.

Todd, B.: Using eye drops and ointments safely, Geriat. Nurs. **4**(1):53, 1983.

Wong, E.K., Wang, S., and Leopold, I.H.: How ophthalmic drugs can fool you, RN **43**(3):36, 1980.

Drugs Affecting the Gastrointestinal Tract

13

The gastrointestinal system processes food and water and eliminates undigestible material. The parasympathetic (cholinergic) nervous system acts as a major stimulant of the digestive processes by increasing both digestive secretions and the tone and motility of the smooth muscle of the stomach and intestines. The sympathetic (adrenergic) nervous system plays a minor role in the digestive processes. Although the parasympathetic nervous system acts on all parts of the digestive tract, current research is uncovering a complex system in which activities in each segment of the digestive tract are further regulated by a variety of peptide hormones, prostaglandins, and the biogenic amines histamine and serotonin. At the present time the roles of only a few of these factors are well characterized. This chapter focuses on specific conditions affecting the gastrointestinal tract for which there are pharmacological interventions.

Tone and Motility of the Small Intestine

Drugs affecting the activity of the parasympathetic nervous system in the gastrointestinal tract are presently used mainly to modify the tone and motility of the smooth muscle layers of the intestinal tract.

DRUGS TO INCREASE GASTROINTESTINAL TONE AND MOTILITY (Table 13.1)

Cholinomimetic drugs play a minor role in the treatment of gastrointestinal disorders. Occasionally, bethanecol or neostigmine is administered to stimulate an atonic intestine or bladder. Metoclopramide is a newer drug that stimulates the gastrointestinal tract, but it is not a cholinomimetic drug.

Bethanechol (Urecholine)

Bethanechol is the only direct-acting cholinomimetic drug with sufficient tissue specificity to be administered systemically. At therapeutic doses, bethanechol is relatively specific for the urinary and gastrointestinal tracts. This stimulation is useful for situations in which the bladder or intestine has lost its tone, such as after childbirth, surgery, or other abdominal trauma.

Side effects of bethanechol are those expected from muscarinic stimulation: salivation, flushing of the skin, sweating, diarrhea, nausea and belching, and abdominal cramps.

Bethanechol should never be administered if there is any mechanical obstruction of the gastrointestinal or urinary tract, such as stones or adhesions, because the hypermotility caused by the drug could lead to rupture of the tissue in the presence of an obstruction. Also, bethanechol is never administered intravenously or intramuscularly because the rate of absorption is so fast that toxic plasma concentrations of the drug are reached, resulting in possible heart block or a severe drop in blood pressure. Bethanechol may be administered subcutaneously if the oral route is not effective.

Neostigmine (Prostigmin)

Neostigmine is a reversible acetylcholinesterase inhibitor that is prescribed for its muscarinic as well as its neuromuscular effects (Chapter 11). Neostigmine may be given subcutaneously or intramuscularly in place of bethanechol to restore bladder or intestinal tone. If urination does not oc-

Table 13.1 Cholinergic Drugs Affecting Gastrointestinal Motility and Secretion

Generic name	Trade name	Administration/dosage	Comments
DRUGS TO INCREASE TONE AND MOTILITY			
Bethanechol chloride	Urecholine* Duvoid Myotonachol	ORAL: *Adults*—10 to 30 mg every 6 to 8 hr. SUBCUTANEOUS: *Adults*—2.5 to 5 mg every 6 to 8 hr; maximum, 10 mg/day. Never give IV or IM Onset: 30 min.	Direct-acting cholinomimetic; stimulates atonic bladder, gastrointestinal tract.
Metoclopramide	Reglan	INTRAVENOUS: *Adults*—10 mg injected over 1 to 2 min. *Children under 6 yr*—0.1 mg/kg body weight. *Children 6 to 14 yr*—2.5 to 5.0 mg/kg. ORAL: *Adults*—10 mg 4 times daily, 30 min before bedtime. *Children under 6 yr*—0.1 mg/kg as a single dose. *Children 6 to 16 yr*—0.5 mg/kg daily in 3 divided doses.	Dopamine antagonist; hastens gastric emptying in diabetic gastroparesis and after barium administration.
Neostigmine methylsulfate	Prostigmin methylsulfate*	SUBCUTANEOUS, INTRAMUSCULAR: *Adults*—0.25 to 0.5 mg every 3 to 4 hr to stimulate bladder or gastrointestinal tract. Onset: 10 to 20 min.	Acetylcholinesterase inhibitor; stimulates atonic bladder, gastrointestinal tract.
ANTICHOLINERGIC DRUGS—ANTISPASMODIC DRUGS: TO DECREASE TONE AND MOTILITY			
Belladonna alkaloids (uncharged)			
Atropine sulfate		ORAL, SUBCUTANEOUS: *Adults*—0.3 to 1.2 mg every 4 to 6 hr. SUBCUTANEOUS: *Children*—0.01 mg/kg every 4 to 6 hr.	Reduces gastrointestinal motility and gastric acid secretion. Also reduces the tone of the bladder and ureter.
Belladonna extract		ORAL: *Adults*—15 mg every 8 hr.	As above. Atropine is the active ingredient.
Belladonna fluid extract		ORAL: *Adults*—0.06 ml every 8 hr.	As above. Atropine is the active ingredient.
Belladonna leaf		ORAL: *Adults*—30 to 200 mg.	As above. Atropine is the active ingredient.
Belladonna tincture		ORAL: *Adults*—0.6 to 1 ml every 6 to 8 hr. *Children*—0.03 ml/kg in 3 or 4 divided doses.	As above. Atropine is the active ingredient.
Hyoscyamine hydrobromide (L-isomer of atropine)		ORAL, INTRAMUSCULAR, SUBCUTANEOUS, INTRAVENOUS: *Adults*—0.25 mg every 6 to 8 hr.	As above. Atropine is the active ingredient.
Hyoscyamine sulfate	Anaspaz Levsin	ORAL: *Adults*—0.125 to 0.25 mg every 4 to 6 hr. *Children*—2 to 10 yr, ½ adult dosage; under 2 yr, ¼ adult dosage. INTRAMUSCULAR, SUBCUTANEOUS, INTRAVENOUS: *Adults*—0.25 to 0.5 mg every 4 to 6 hr.	As above. Atropine is the active ingredient.
Scopolamine butylbromide	Buscopan†	ORAL: *Adults*—10 to 20 mg 3 or 4 times daily. INTRAMUSCULAR, INTRAVENOUS, SUBCUTANEOUS: *Adults*—10 to 20 mg 3 or 4 times daily.	Elderly are more sensitive to scopolamine.

*Available in Canada and United States.
†Available in Canada only.

Continued.

Table 13.1 Cholinergic Drugs Affecting Gastrointestinal Motility and Secretion—cont'd

Generic name	Trade name	Administration/dosage	Comments
Scopolamine hydrobromide		INTRAMUSCULAR, INTRAVENOUS, SUBCUTANEOUS: *Adults*—0.3 to 0.6 mg as a single dose.	Elderly are more sensitive to scopolamine.
Charged derivatives of atropine			
Homatropine methylbromide	Ru-Spas No. 2 Sed-Ten SE	ORAL: *Adults*—2.5 to 10 mg every 6 hr. *Children*—3 to 6 mg every 6 hr. *Infants*—0.3 mg dissolved in water every 4 hr.	To reduce gastrointestinal hypermotility and gastric acidity.
Methscopolamine bromide	Pamine	ORAL: *Adults*—2.5 to 5 mg every 6 hr. *Children*—0.2 mg/kg every 6 hr. INTRAMUSCULAR, SUBCUTANEOUS: *Adults*—0.25 to 1 mg every 6 to 8 hr. Onset: 1 hr.	To reduce gastrointestinal hypermotility and gastric acidity.
Synthetic substitutes for atropine			
Anisotropine methylbromide	Valpin	ORAL: *Adults*—50 mg 3 times daily. Onset: 1 hr.	To treat gastrointestinal spasms and to control gastric acid secretion.
Clidinium bromide	Quarzan	ORAL: *Adults*—2.5 to 5 mg 3 or 4 times daily before meals and at bedtime. Reduce dosage to 2.5 mg 3 times daily before meals for elderly patients.	To control gastric acidity and hypermotility.
Glycopyrrolate	Robinul*	ORAL: 1 to 2 mg 3 times daily initially, then 1 to 2 mg 2 times daily for maintenance. Onset: 1 hr. INTRAMUSCULAR, SUBCUTANEOUS, INTRAVENOUS: 0.1 to 0.2 mg every 4 hr. Onset: 10 min.	To treat gastrointestinal hypermotility and control gastric acidity.
Hexocyclium methylsulfate	Tral Film tabs	ORAL: *Adults*—25 mg 4 times daily before meals and at bedtime. May be taken twice daily in combined release capsules.	To control gastric acidity and hypermotility.
Isopropamide iodide	Darbid*	ORAL: *Adults and children over 12 yr:* 5 mg every 12 hr, may increase to 10 mg every 12 hr for severe symptoms.	To control gastric acidity and hypermotility.
Mepenzolate bromide	Cantil	ORAL: *Adults*—25 mg 4 times daily. Increase to 50 mg if necessary.	

cur within 1 hour, the patient should be catheterized.

Metoclopramide (Reglan)

Metoclopramide is a dopamine antagonist, not a cholinomimetic drug. However, it sensitizes the gastrointestinal tissues to the action of acetylcholine, and this action is abolished by anticholinergic drugs. Metoclopramide stimulates motility of the upper gastrointestinal tract without stimulating gastric, biliary, or pancreatic secretions. The tone and amplitude of gastric contractions are increased

Table 13.1   Cholinergic Drugs Affecting Gastrointestinal Motility and Secretion—cont'd

Generic name	Trade name	Administration/dosage	Comments
Methantheline bromide	Banthine	ORAL: *Adults*—50 to 100 mg every 6 hr initially; reduce by ½ for maintenance. *Children*—6 mg/kg daily in 4 doses. Onset: 30 min. INTRAMUSCULAR: *Adults*—50 mg every 6 hr. *Children*—6 mg/kg daily in 4 doses. Onset: 30 min.	Used like atropine.
Oxyphencyclimine hydrochloride	Daricon	ORAL: 10 mg 2 times daily; can be increased to 50 mg if tolerated.	To treat gastric acidity or hypermotility of the gastrointestinal, genitourinary, or biliary tract.
Oxyphenonium bromide	Antrenyl	ORAL: *Adults*—10 mg 4 times daily. Use 5 mg for elderly patients.	To control gastric acidity and hypermotility.
Propantheline bromide	Norpanth Pro-Banthine* Propanthel*	ORAL: *Adults*—15 mg 3 times daily plus 30 mg at bedtime or 30 mg timed-release every 8 to 12 hr. *Children*—1.5 mg/kg daily every 6 hr. INTRAMUSCULAR or INTRAVENOUS: *Adults*—30 mg every 6 hr.	To control gastric acidity and hypermotility of gastrointestinal, genitourinary, and biliary tracts.
Tridihexethyl chloride	Pathilon	ORAL: 25 mg 3 times daily before meals and 50 mg at bedtime. Timed-release, 75 mg every 6 to 12 hr. INTRAMUSCULAR, SUBCUTANEOUS, INTRAVENOUS: *Adults*—10 to 20 mg every 6 hr.	To control gastric acidity and hypermotility of the gastrointestinal tract.
Antispasmodic drugs			
Dicyclomine hydrochloride	Antispas Bentyl Bentylol† Cyclobee†	ORAL or INTRAMUSCULAR: *Adults*—10 to 20 mg 3 or 4 times daily. *Children*—10 mg 3 or 4 times daily. *Infants*—5 mg 3 or 4 times daily.	To control hypermotility of the colon.
Pirenzepine	Gastrozepin†	ORAL: *Adults*—50 mg 2 times daily. May be increased to 3 times daily if needed.	A new antimuscarinic that is relatively specific for the gastrointestinal tract.

as is peristalsis of the small intestine, so that gastric emptying and intestinal transit times are increased. These actions are useful in treating diabetic gastroparesis, a condition in which stomach tone is lost and contents are not emptied readily into the intestine. Metoclopramide is also used to facilitate intubation of the small intestine for biopsy and to stimulate gastric emptying and intestinal transit of barium in radiologic examinations.

Side effects of metoclopramide include restlessness, drowsiness, fatigue, and lassitude in about 10% of patients. Sedation is enhanced with the concurrent use of alcohol, tranquilizers, sleeping medications, or narcotic analgesics. Metoclopramide is contraindicated in patients who have mechanical obstruction, perforation, or possible hemorrhage of the gastrointestinal tract. An increase in gastrointestinal motility poses danger for such patients.

Anticholinergic drugs and narcotic analgesics inhibit gastrointestinal tone and thereby antagonize the action of metoclopramide.

THE NURSING PROCESS

DRUGS TO INCREASE TONE AND MOTILITY

Assessment

Patients requiring drugs to increase tone and motility are those who have had recent trauma or surgery and have resultant atonic intestines or bladder, have diabetic gastroparesis, or in whom barium has been used for radiologic examination. A thorough patient assessment should be done, especially to rule out any obstruction of the bladder or intestine. The nurse should assess the vital signs, check for the presence of bowel sounds, check the fluid intake and output, and palpate the bladder for distention. If a urinary catheter is in place, the nurse should ascertain that it is patent.

Potential nursing diagnoses

Altered comfort related to abdominal cramps or diarrhea

Diarrhea related to drug action/side effect

Management

Because both bethanechol and neostigmine are potent, the nurse should anticipate remaining at the bedside for at least 15 minutes after the drug is administered to observe the patient for side effects. Side effects will usually occur with bethanechol, especially if given via the subcutaneous route. The known drug antidote, atropine, should be readily available before the drug is administered. After the drug is administered, the nurse should monitor the vital signs and measure any fluid or solid output that results from the administration of the medication. If side effects become serious, the nurse should notify the physician and/or consider administering atropine (0.6 mg). If administering metoclopramide intravenously, the nurse should remain at the bedside; oral administration produces much slower effects.

Evaluation

These drugs are considered effective if they increase intestinal tone and/or bladder tone, enhancing the patient's ability to defecate or urinate. In some patients only one or two doses are necessary, after which the patient's body is able to maintain motility unaided. Other patients will require continuous use of these drugs on an outpatient basis. Before a patient is discharged for self-management, the patient should be able to explain how to take the drug correctly, the anticipated effects of the drug, the side effects that may occur and what to do about them, and which symptoms should prompt the patient to seek medical attention. For additional specific information, see the patient care implications section at the end of this chapter.

ANTICHOLINERGIC AND ANTISPASMODIC DRUGS TO DECREASE TONE AND MOTILITY
(Table 13.1)

Anticholinergic drugs (drugs that block muscarinic receptors) inhibit gastric acid secretion and depress gastrointestinal motility. These actions are useful in treating a peptic ulcer or in treating hyperactive bowel disorders.

Table 13.1 lists atropine and its derivatives as well as the synthetic anticholinergic drugs that are used to depress gastric acid secretion in treating peptic ulcers. Homatropine and the synthetic drugs are charged compounds that do not cross the blood-brain barrier to act in the central nervous system. Oxyphencyclimine is an uncharged synthetic compound and is the exception.

Common side effects of anticholinergic drugs are the classic anticholinergic effects described for atropine: dry mouth, photophobia due to dilated pupils (mydriasis), blurred vision (cycloplegia), fast heart rate (tachycardia), constipation, and acute urinary retention. In fact, patients are not getting a dose large enough to suppress acid secretion if they do not have a dry mouth.

Toxic doses of the uncharged anticholinergic

THE NURSING PROCESS

DRUGS TO DECREASE TONE AND MOTILITY

Assessment

The drugs described in this section are used in selected patients who have problems related to excessive intestinal motility or peptic ulcer. A generalized patient assessment should be done with attention to the following points: the vital signs, any subjective patient complaints, the frequency and character of stools, and a check for the presence of occult blood in the stool.

Potential nursing diagnoses

Colonic constipation related to drug side effects

Altered oral mucous membranes related to dry mouth produced as a drug side effect

Management

These drugs are usually used in conjunction with dietary management and other therapies to decrease gastric acid or the symptoms associated with hyperactive bowel disease. The nurse should continue to monitor the patient's subjective complaints and vital signs and to observe the patient for the presence of side effects. The anticholinergic drugs and related compounds should produce side effects if administered in effective dosages. The nurse should assist the patient in finding ways to deal with unpleasant side effects, for instance, sucking on hard candy for treatment of dry mouth. The intake and output of solids and liquids should be checked and the patient questioned about constipation. The nurse should look for central nervous system effects such as restlessness, tremor, or irritability, since these symptoms may indicate a need to reduce the drug dose.

Evaluation

These drugs are effective if the patient complains of fewer symptoms and/or the signs of ulcer disease disappear. Before discharge, patients should be able to explain why and how to take the medications ordered, which side effects will probably occur, possible ways to treat these side effects, which symptoms would warrant notification of the physician, and how to perform any related therapies that have been prescribed, such as dietary manipulation for treatment of ulcer disease. For additional specific information, see the patient care implications section at the end of this chapter.

---

drugs atropine (and its L-isomer, hyoscyamine) and oxyphencyclimine reach the central nervous system and produce central nervous system stimulation: restlessness, tremor, irritability, delirium, or hallucinations. Toxic doses of the charged anticholinergic drugs that do not reach the central nervous system cause ganglionic blockade (usually seen as orthostatic hypotension) or neuromuscular blockade. Death can result from respiratory arrest secondary to neuromuscular blockade.

Table 13.1 also lists drugs that were found to have antispasmodic but not anticholinergic effects. These drugs relax the smooth muscle of the gastrointestinal tract and are used to treat hyperactivity or spasm of the intestine. Side effects of these drugs are not as prominent as those reported for the anticholinergic drugs. Side effects reported include constipation or diarrhea, rash, euphoria, dizziness, drowsiness, headache, nausea, and weakness.

Activity of the Upper Gastrointestinal Tract

STOMACH ACID: DRUGS TO TREAT ULCERS (Table 13.2)

Ulcers and Stomach Acid

An ulcer is the loss of the skin or mucosal tissue that provides the protective layer of cells normally surrounding an organ. In the gastrointestinal system, an ulcer (peptic ulcer) occurs in the esophagus,

---

PATIENT PROBLEM: DRY MOUTH (XEROSTOMIA)

THE PROBLEM:

Drugs produce an excessively dry mouth. This may cause discomfort, trauma to the mouth, bad breath, and potential for injury to the oral mucosa.

SIGNS AND SYMPTOMS:

Dry oral mucous membranes, bad breath, mouth feels dry and sticky.

MEASURES TO DECREASE PATIENT DISCOMFORT:

- thorough, regular oral hygiene, with teeth brushing
- rinse mouth with a pleasant tasting rinse or normal saline (dissolve 1 tsp of salt in a pint of water)
- sip water frequently
- suck on a sugarless hard candy or chew sugarless gum
- avoid drying mouthwashes (those containing alcohol)
- avoid lemon-glycerin swabs for oral hygiene
- keep lips moist with lip moisturizer
- keep environmental air moist with a humidifier
- consider using a commercially available saliva substitute

---

the stomach, or the duodenum as a consequence of the destruction of the mucosal barrier to expose the underlying tissue to stomach acid and to the anatomy of the stomach or in the regulation of stomach secretions. The goal in treating an ulcer is to depress or to neutralize stomach acid to allow the ulcer to heal and to prevent the recurrence of the ulcer.

It is important for patients with esophageal or duodenal ulcers to learn that the conditions causing the ulcer will always be present and only preventive therapy will decrease the incidence of recurrence. An esophageal ulcer results when there is reflux of stomach acid up into the esophagus because of a defective esophageal sphincter. An ulcer in the duodenum results from an overactive secretion of acid in the stomach to the point that the stomach contents cannot be neutralized in the duodenum. The acidic contents then damage the duodenal mucosa. Stomach ulcers are most frequently caused by a tumor, but a nonmalignant cause of stomach ulcers is the reflux of duodenal contents back into the stomach because of a faulty pyloric sphincter. The duodenal contents contain bile acids that disrupt the mucosal barrier normally protecting the stomach from acid and pepsin.

The factors controlling the secretion of hydro-

chloric acid by the parietal cells of the stomach are diagrammed in Figure 13.1. The neurotransmitter acetylcholine (released from a branch of the vagus nerve), the hormone gastrin, and histamine all stimulate the secretion of acid. The role of the hydrochloric acid is to aid in breakdown of connective tissue in food, to activate pepsinogen to pepsin (which degrades protein), and to kill any bacteria ingested in the food. The acidic digest leaves the stomach to enter the duodenum. This movement of digested food lessens stomach distention and thereby removes a stimulus for the release of gastrin and for vagal activity. In response to acidity, the duodenum releases secretin, a hormone that stimulates the release of bicarbonate and digestive enzymes from the pancreas. Secretin also depresses the release of hydrochloric acid by the parietal cells and depresses the motility of the stomach. The bicarbonate released by the pancreas neutralizes the acidity of the partially digested food as it enters the duodenum. This neutralization is also necessary for the digestive enzymes in the intestine to be active.

Drug Treatment of Ulcers

In past years ulcers were treated with antacids and anticholinergic drugs; today, these drugs play a secondary role. The introduction of the H_2 receptor antagonists and the mucosal protective agents has dramatically improved the treatment of ulcers.

Antacids (Table 13.2)

Antacids are weak bases that can be ingested to neutralize the hydrochloric acid secreted by the stomach.

Sodium bicarbonate (baking soda) reacts with hydrochloric acid to yield water and carbon dioxide. Carbon dioxide is a gas and causes the belching frequently associated with the ingestion of sodium bicarbonate. Sodium bicarbonate is the only antacid commonly used that is readily absorbed from the gastrointestinal tract. Taken in excess, sodium bicarbonate also makes the blood slightly alkaline, and in turn the urine becomes alkaline. Excess bicarbonate will stimulate the stomach to secrete more acid (rebound hypersecretion). This hypersecretion can persist after the bicarbonate has been absorbed. For these reasons, sodium bicarbonate is not an antacid of choice when prolonged therapy is required.

Nonsystemic antacids include *alkaline salts of aluminum, magnesium,* and *calcium,* which neutralize acid but are not readily absorbed into the bloodstream. The aluminum and calcium salts tend to cause constipation, whereas magnesium salts tend to have a laxative effect. For this reason, most

Table 13.2   Drugs to Treat an Ulcer*

Generic name	Trade name	Administration/dosage	Comments
ANTACIDS			
Aluminum hydroxide gel	Alterna GEL Amphojel†	ORAL: *Adults*—5 to 30 ml up to 40 ml every 30 min if pain is severe.	Constipating. Long-term use may cause hypophosphatemia. Complexes with tetracycline and can interfere with the absorption of warfarin, digoxin, quinine, and quinidine.
Aluminum carbonate gel	Basaljel	ORAL: *Adults*—5 to 20 ml or 2 capsules every 2 hr up to 12 times daily.	See aluminum hydroxide gel.
Dihydroxyaluminum aminoacetate	Robalate†	ORAL: *Adults*—0.5 to 2 Gm 4 times daily.	Constipating.
Dihydroxyaluminum sodium carbonate	Rolaids	ORAL: *Adults*—1 to 2 tablets 4 times daily.	Constipating in large doses.
Calcium carbonate	Dicarbosil Titralac Tums	ORAL: *Adults*—1 to 4 Gm 1 and 3 hr after meals and at bedtime. Tablets should be chewed before swallowing.	Can be used hourly to keep acid neutralized but some patients will become hypercalcemic. Constipating.
Magnesium carbonate Magnesium hydroxide Magnesium oxide Magnesium phosphate Magnesium trisilicate	Milk of Magnesia		These magnesium salts are laxatives. Must be taken with an aluminum or calcium antacid to maintain normal stool consistency.
H₂ RECEPTOR ANTAGONISTS			
Cimetidine	Tagamet†	ORAL: *Adults*—300 mg with meals and at bedtime until ulcer is healed (3 to 6 wk); then 300 mg at bedtime to inhibit nocturnal secretion.	Administer with meals, because food slows the absorption and prolongs the action of cimetidine. Administer at least 1 hr after antacids or metoclopramide, which reduce the absorption of cimetidine if taken concurrently.
Cimetidine hydrochloride	Tagamet Hydrochloride†	INTRAVENOUS: *Adults*—1 to 4 mg/kg/hr or 300 mg diluted and infused over 15 to 20 min. INTRAMUSCULAR: *Adults*—300 mg every 6 hr. ORAL, INTRAVENOUS: *Children*—20 to 40 mg/kg in divided doses.	Switch to oral doses when ulcer bleeding has stopped.
Famotidine	Pepcid	ORAL: *Adults*—40 mg daily at bedtime, or in 2 divided doses. INTRAVENOUS: *Adults*—20 mg every 12 hr.	Longer acting than cimetidine.
Nizatidine	Axid	ORAL: *Adults*—300 mg daily at bedtime to heal the ulcer, then 150 mg daily to prevent recurrence.	Longer acting than cimetidine.
Ranitidine hydrochloride	Zantac	ORAL: *Adults*—150 mg every 12 hr. INTRAMUSCULAR/SLOW INTRAVENOUS: *Adults*—50 mg every 6 to 8 hr. Maximum daily dose is 400 mg.	Longer acting than cimetidine

*See also Table 13.1, anticholinergic-antispasmodic drugs.
†Available in Canada and United States.
‡Available in Canada only.

Continued.

Table 13.2 Drugs to Treat an Ulcer—cont'd

Generic name	Trade name	Administration/dosage	Comments
MUCOSAL PROTECTIVE AGENTS			
Misoprostol	Cytotec	ORAL: *Adults*—100 to 200 µg 4 times daily at meals and bedtime.	To protect against ulcers from non-steroidal antiinflammatory drugs used for arthritis. Also effective for healing peptic ulcer.
Sucralfate	Carafate Sulcrate‡	ORAL: *Adults*—1 Gm 4 times daily. Take 1 hr before meals and 1 hr before bedtime.	If antacids are prescribed for the relief of pain, they should not be taken 30 min before or after sucralfate.

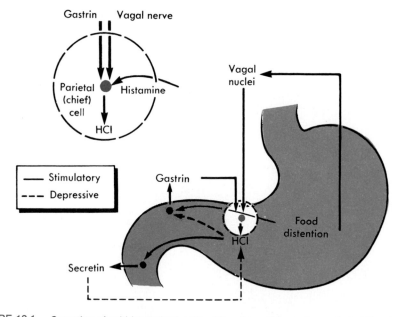

FIGURE 13.1   Secretion of acid by parietal cells of the stomach is under control of the duodenally released hormone, gastrin; the parasympathetic nervous system, via the neurotransmitter acetylcholine; and histamine. Histamine is the most effective stimulant of gastric acid secretion. Note that acid secretion is discontinued when food reaches duodenum, where hydrochloric acid *(HCl)* inhibits gastrin release and stimulates secretin release, and distention of the stomach is lessened, decreasing vagal stimulation.

antacids are a combination of a magnesium salt or hydroxide and an aluminum or calcium salt or hydroxide. Nonsystemic antacids are most effective when taken on an hourly basis. This regimen neutralizes acid without causing the rebound secretion of acid.

The nonsystemic antacids are available as liquids or chewable tablets. The most common side effect is diarrhea or constipation even with a combination antacid. The patient must then add additional antacid: more aluminum or calcium antacid to correct diarrhea or more magnesium antacid to correct constipation. Antacids can impede the absorption of drugs, most notably tetracyclines (antibiotics), digoxin (a cardiac glycoside), and quinidine (a cardiac antiarrhythmic drug).

Anticholinergic drugs (Table 13.1)

Anticholinergic drugs used to treat an ulcer are those already discussed with antispasmodic drugs.

THE NURSING PROCESS

DRUGS IN THE TREATMENT OF ULCER DISEASE

Assessment

Patients with diagnosed or suspected ulcer disease may come to the hospital with a wide variety of symptoms. The presenting picture may range from the patient who is asymptomatic to the patient who is critically ill from excessive blood loss from a large gastric ulcer. The presenting condition will guide the examiner in the focus of the assessment. In addition to a baseline total patient assessment, the nurse should assess the vital signs, the level of consciousness, and the character or quality of any emesis or stool, including the presence of occult blood. Fluid balance is monitored by the fluid intake and output. The nurse should question the patient about possible relevant history, such as recent alcohol intake or previous ulcer disease. Appropriate laboratory tests include a hematocrit and hemoglobin determination.

Potential nursing diagnoses

Altered thought processes related to drug side effect (H_2 antagonists)

Altered health maintenance related to complicated dosing regimens when patient is taking several different drugs

Management

The goal of treating an ulcer is to stop blood loss and to promote the healing of the ulcerated area. The management will in part be based on the severity of the presenting picture. Nursing care includes continued monitoring of the vital signs, the fluid intake and output, the level of consciousness, and the character of any emesis or stool. Appropriate laboratory findings such as the hematocrit, hemoglobin, and serum electrolyte measurements are continually monitored. When the patient's condition is stable, appropriate diagnostic studies, such as upper gastrointestinal x-ray films or endoscopy, may be done. Dietary restrictions to limit the amount of such irritants as coffee, alcohol, and spices may be imposed, and the frequency of meals may be increased with an emphasis on inclusion of milk and milk-related products. Antacids and/or an antihistamine such as cimetidine are often ordered prophylactically for patients who fall into categories associated with frequent ulceration. Examples of such patients include those with head injury, those requiring intensive care for any major surgical or medical problem, and those receiving high-dose glucocorticoid therapy.

Evaluation

These drugs are considered successful if they promote the healing of the ulcer without the patient experiencing side effects resulting from the drug therapy. Before discharge, the patient should be able to explain why the drugs have been ordered; how to take them correctly; how to treat side effects that may occur, such as constipation or diarrhea associated with antacid therapy; which side effects should be reported to the physician; and how to implement dietary or other restrictions prescribed by the physician.

For additional specific information, see the patient care implications section at the end of this chapter.

Anticholinergic drugs are taken before meals so they can then depress the secretion of acid that occurs on eating. Anticholinergic drugs should not be taken with antacids, because the antacids will slow the absorption of the anticholinergic drugs. Moreover, the administration of an antacid with an anticholinergic drug is not rational; the acid will already have been released in response to the meal and neutralized by the antacid, making the anticholinergic drugs useless.

Pirenzepine (Gastrozepin) is a selective anticholinergic drug that inhibits gastric acid secretion without blocking smooth muscle action and without causing an increased heart rate. Pirenzepine is available in Canada but is not available in the United States.

Antihistamines (Table 13.2)

Cimetidine (Tagamet) was released in 1977, the first of a new class of drugs, the H_2 histamine receptor antagonists. These drugs act specifically to block the H_2 histamine receptors that control the basal and stimulated secretion of hydrochloric acid by the parietal cells (Figure 13.1). (The H_1 receptors are blocked by the antihistamines discussed in Chapter 24.) Many investigators believe that both gastrin and acetylcholine act through histamine to cause the release of hydrochloric acid, because the H_2 antagonists are so effective in decreasing acid secretion stimulated by pentagastrin (an active analog of gastrin) or bethanechol (an agonist of acetylcholine), as well as by food, insulin, and caffeine.

Because H_2 antagonists dramatically decrease stomach acid, these drugs are effective in alleviating many conditions in which stomach acid impedes therapy, including the following:

1. Duodenal ulcer. A duodenal ulcer usually heals within 8 weeks of therapy with H_2 antagonists, but maintenance therapy is necessary to prevent recurrences.
2. Gastric ulcer. H_2 antagonists increase the healing rate of gastric ulcers. Long-term therapy is moderately effective in preventing recurrences.
3. Reflux esophagitis. H_2 antagonists tend to reduce the frequency of symptoms. Long-term therapy may afford sustained improvement.
4. Zollinger-Ellison syndrome. A tumor secretes excessive gastrin that stimulates excessive acid production. H_2 antagonists depress this acid production.
5. Gastrointestinal hemorrhage. Stomach acid intensifies inflammation of the stomach, worsening the hemorrhaging.
6. Pancreatic insufficiency. Digestive enzymes must be administered orally. Without H_2 antagonists, stomach acid inactivates most of the administered enzymes.

Side effects. H_2 antagonists have been remarkably free of general side effects. Central nervous system effects include mental confusion, agitation, and hallucinations; these symptoms are reversible when the drug is discontinued. The CNS effects are more frequent in patients with liver and/or renal disease.

Cimetidine (Tagamet) is well absorbed and has a duration of action of about 4 hours. The standard dosage schedule has been four times daily, but recent studies have indicated that higher doses can be given less frequently and still be effective. Cimetidine is metabolized by the liver and excreted through the kidneys. The dosage must be reduced for patients with impaired kidney function. Cimetidine can cause gynecomastia (breast enlargement) in men and breast tenderness in women owing to a weak antiandrogenic effect.

Famotidine (Pepcid), nizadepine (Axid), and ranitidine (Zantac) can be administered once a day. These drugs are partially metabolized by the liver and excreted by the kidneys. The dosage must be reduced for patients with impaired kidney function. Antacids reduce their absorption. Neither famotidine nor nizadepine nor ranitidine has the antiandrogen activity characteristic of cimetidine that causes gynecomastia in men and breast tenderness in women. None of these drugs interfere with drug metabolism by the liver.

Mucosal Protective Agents (Table 13.2)

Sucralfate (Carafate) is a complex of sulfated sucrose and aluminum hydroxide that is changed by stomach acid into a viscous material that binds to proteins in ulcerated tissue. This appears to protect the ulcer from the destructive action of the digestive enzyme pepsin. Sucralfate is used in the initial treatment (first 1 to 2 months) of a duodenal ulcer. Sucralfate does not neutralize stomach acid nor does it inhibit acid secretion. It should be given alone 30 to 60 minutes before mealtime so that it can be activated by stomach acid and coat the ulcer. Sucralfate will bind digoxin and tetracycline, so these drugs should be taken at a different time of day.

Misoprostol (Cytotec) is an ester of prostaglandin E_1 and represents a new drug class for treating ulcers. Prostaglandin E_1 is normally synthesized in the stomach, where it acts to block gastric acid secretion. The nonsteroidal antiinflammatory drugs (NSAIDs), including aspirin, inhibit the synthesis of naturally occurring prostaglandin E_1 when they dissolve in the stomach. For this reason, bleeding from gastric ulcers is a significant problem with long-term use of NSAIDs. A major market for misoprostol is those patients with arthritis who must take NSAIDs to relieve the inflammation and pain of arthritis. Misoprostol will replace the prostaglandin E_1 that is not produced in the stomach when NSAIDs are present. With the protection of misoprostol, excess acid secretion will be blocked and therefore stomach mucosa protected. Misoprostol may also be used to treat duodenal and peptic ulcers.

Side effects. Only minor effects such as diarrhea, mild nausea, abdominal discomfort, and dizziness are occasionally reported. Serious side effects are bleeding and abortion in pregnant women, an action expected of a prostaglandin E_1 analog. In one study there was bleeding in 50% of pregnant women and a 7% incidence of abortion. Therefore, misoprostol is contraindicated for pregnant women and should be used cautiously by women of childbearing age.

Omeprazole (Losec) is another new drug having a different mechanism. Omeprazole directly inhibits the hydrogen ion pump in the parietal cells of the stomach. Gastric acid secretion can be completely blocked. Omeprazole has not caused toxicity with long-term use. At this writing omeprazole is available only for compassionate use in those patients with the Zollinger-Ellison syndrome. Dosages are adjusted from 20 mg once a day to 120 mg three times a day to keep basic output low. Omeprazole is also a powerful antiulcer agent.

CENTRAL CONTROL: DRUGS AFFECTING VOMITING (EMESIS)
(Table 13.3)

Origin of Nausea and Vomiting

Vomiting (emesis) is an involuntary act of regurgitating the contents of the stomach and is coordinated by an area in the medulla called the *vomiting center.* Nausea is the unpleasant sensation that usually precedes vomiting. Input from three major neural sites can stimulate the vomiting center. The first input is that controlled by the higher central nervous system functions, with vomiting being secondary to emotion, pain, or disequilibrium (motion sickness). The second pathway is that arising from peripheral stimuli, with vomiting being secondary to injury or disease of a body tissue or organ. In particular, irritation of the mucosa of the gastrointestinal tract or bowel or biliary distention stimulates the vomiting center by way of the autonomic neurons carrying information to the central nervous system (afferent neurons). A third pathway is from the chemoreceptor trigger zone, a medullary center sensitive to stimulation by circulating drugs and toxins.

Nonmedicinal Treatments of Nausea and Vomiting

Nausea and vomiting are not necessarily treated with drugs. For instance, the nausea and vomiting of pregnancy is best treated by having the patient sip water or tea and eat small meals, because antiemetic drugs have been shown to cause fetal abnormalities in experimental animals. Many drugs cause nausea and vomiting as side effects because they act directly on the chemoreceptor trigger zone. Examples of such drugs include levodopa, digitalis, opiates (narcotic analgesics), and aminophylline. The effective treatment is to lower the dose of the offending drug or to increase the dose slowly.

Drugs may also irritate the gastric mucosa to cause a reflex stimulation of nausea and vomiting. Aspirin is an example of an irritant drug. The effective treatment is to take the drug with a large volume of liquid or with a meal to dilute the drug.

Drug Therapy for Nausea and Vomiting

Drugs currently used to prevent nausea and vomiting are listed by drug class in Table 13.3. These drugs include antagonists of histamine, acetylcholine, and dopamine, as well as drugs whose actions are not yet determined. The choice of an antiemetic is determined by the cause of the nausea and vomiting. Drugs for treating nausea and vomiting are most effective when administered before nausea and vomiting have begun rather than after. For instance, the drugs effective in treating motion sickness or vertigo are effective when taken about 30 minutes before traveling is begun, but are relatively ineffective if taken after motion sickness has started. The drugs for treating the nausea and vomiting of chemotherapy or radiation therapy are most effective when taken 30 to 60 minutes before the therapy is begun.

Motion sickness and vertigo are most effectively treated prophylactically with certain of the antihistamines or the anticholinergic drug scopolamine. The action of these drugs is not clear. Presumably they reduce the stimulation of receptors in the labyrinth from which signals governing the sense of equilibrium arise.

The effective drugs for reducing the vomiting from chemotherapy and radiation therapy of cancer are those which act at the chemoreceptor trigger zone and are antagonists of dopamine, the major neurotransmitter of the chemoreceptor trigger zone. Most of these dopamine antagonists are drugs that are used as antipsychotic drugs (Chapter 41). These drugs include chlorpromazine (Thorazine), droperidol (Inapsine), fluphenazine (Prolixin), haloperidol (Haldol), perphenazine (Trilafon), prochlorperazine (Compazine), promazine (Sparine), thiethylperazine (Torecan), and triflupromazine (Vesprin). These drugs are also effective in controlling postoperative vomiting, although they are not effective in preventing motion sickness.

The cannabinoids are new additions to antiemetic therapy for cancer chemotherapy. Patients

Table 13.3 Drugs to Control Vomiting

Generic name	Trade name	Administration/dosage	Comments
ANTICHOLINERGIC DRUGS			
Scopolamine	Transderm Scop Transderm-V†	TOPICAL: *Adults*—1 adhesive unit is placed behind the ear several hours before travel. Duration is 72 hr.	Sustained release of scopolamine protects most patients from motion sickness while greatly reducing anticholinergic side effects (blurred vision, sensitivity to light, dry mouth, and drowsiness).
Scopolamine hydrobromide		ORAL, SUBCUTANEOUS: *Adults*—0.6 to 1.0 mg. *Children*—0.006 mg/kg body weight.	One of the most effective drugs in preventing motion sickness, but side effects (dry mouth, drowsiness) limit its use.
ANTIHISTAMINIC DRUGS			
Buclizine hydrochloride	Bucladin-S	ORAL: *Adults*—50 mg 30 min before traveling and 4 to 6 hr later. For vertigo, 50 mg 2 times daily.	Effective for preventing motion sickness.
Cyclizine hydrochloride; cyclizine lactate	Marezine Marzin†	ORAL: *Adults*—50 mg 30 min before traveling and 4 to 6 hr later; maximum, 300 mg daily. *Children*—6 to 10 yr, 3 mg/kg body weight divided into 3 doses daily.	Effective for preventing motion sickness and vertigo
Dimenhydrinate	Dramamine* Gravol† Others	INTRAMUSCULAR: *Adults*—50 mg as needed. *Children*—5 mg/kg body weight divided into 4 doses daily; maximum, 300 mg daily. INTRAVENOUS: *Adults*—50 mg diluted in 10 mg saline solution, injected over 2 min. ORAL: *Adults*—50 to 100 mg every 4 hr. *Children*—5 mg/kg body weight divided into 4 doses; maximum, 150 mg daily. RECTAL: *Adults*—100 mg 1 to 2 times daily.	Effective for preventing vertigo, motion sickness, and the nausea and vomiting of pregnancy. Also causes drowsiness.
Diphenhydramine hydrochloride	Benadryl Hydrochloride*	DEEP INTRAMUSCULAR: *Adults*—10 mg, increased to 20 to 50 mg every 2 to 3 hr if needed; maximum, 400 mg daily. *Children*—5 mg/kg body weight divided into 4 doses; maximum, 300 mg daily. INTRAVENOUS: *Adults*—same as deep intramuscular. ORAL: *Adults*—50 mg 30 min before traveling, then 50 mg before each meal. *Children*—5 mg/kg body weight divided into 4 doses; maximum, 300 mg daily.	Causes sedation. Effective for preventing vertigo, motion sickness, and the nausea and vomiting of pregnancy.
Hydroxyzine hydrochloride	Isaject Vistaril	INTRAMUSCULAR: *Adults*—25 to 100 mg. *Children*—1 mg/kg body weight.	An antianxiety drug. Effective for preventing motion sickness and postoperative nausea and vomiting.

*Available in Canada and United States.
†Available in Canada only.

Table 13.3   Drugs to Control Vomiting—cont'd

Generic name	Trade name	Administration/dosage	Comments
Hydroxyzine pamoate	Vistaril	ORAL: *Adults*—25 to 100 mg 3 to 4 times daily. *Children*—over 6 yr, 50 to 100 mg daily divided into 4 doses; under 6 yr, 50 mg daily divided into 4 doses.	
Meclizine hydrochloride	Antivert* Bonine†	ORAL *Adults*—25 to 50 mg once daily, taken 60 min or longer before traveling; 25 to 100 mg daily in divided doses for vertigo or radiation sickness.	Effective for preventing motion sickness, vertigo, and the nausea and vomiting of radiation therapy. Longer acting than most antihistamines.
Promethazine hydrochloride	Phenergan* Remsed	INTRAMUSCULAR, RECTAL: *Adults*—25 mg, then 12.5 to 25 mg as needed every 4 to 6 hr. *Children*—under 12 yr, no more than half the adult dose. ORAL: *Adults*—25 mg 2 times daily. *Children*—12.5 to 25 mg twice daily.	Effective for preventing motion sickness and vertigo and postoperative nausea and vomiting.
ANTIDOPAMINERGIC DRUGS			
Chlorpromazine hydrochloride	Thorazine	RECTAL: *Adults*—50 to 100 mg every 6 to 8 hr. *Children*—1 mg/kg body weight every 6 to 8 hr. INTRAMUSCULAR: *Adults*—25 mg, then 25 to 50 mg every 3 to 4 hours to stop vomiting. *Children*—0.5 mg/kg body weight every 6 to 8 hr; maximum, 40 mg (up to 5 yr or 50 lb), 75 mg (5 to 12 yr or 50 to 100 lb) daily. ORAL: *Adults*—10 to 25 mg every 4 to 6 hr. *Children*—0.5 mg/kg body weight every 4 to 6 hr.	Watch for hypotension with initial injection. Effective for postoperative nausea and vomiting and that caused by toxins, radiation therapy, or chemotherapy. May cause considerable drowsiness.
Fluphenazine hydrochloride	Prolixin	INTRAMUSCULAR: *Adults*—1.25 mg every 6 to 8 hr as needed.	Effective for postoperative nausea and vomiting and that caused by toxins, radiation, therapy, or chemotherapy.
Haloperidol	Haldol*	INTRAMUSCULAR, ORAL: *Adults*—1, 2, or 5 mg every 12 hr as needed.	Effective for postoperative nausea and vomiting and that caused by toxins, radiation therapy, or chemotherapy.
Perphenazine	Trilafon*	ORAL: *Adults*—8 to 24 mg daily in 2 or more divided doses. INTRAMUSCULAR: *Adults*—5 mg daily.	Effective for postoperative nausea and vomiting and that caused by toxins, radiation therapy, or chemotherapy.
Prochlorperazine	Compazine	RECTAL: *Adults*—25 mg 2 times daily. *Children*—over 10 kg, 0.4 mg/kg body weight daily divided into 3 to 4 doses.	Effective for postoperative nausea and vomiting and that caused by toxins, radiation therapy, or chemotherapy.

*Available in Canada and United States.

Continued.

Table 13.3 Drugs to Control Vomiting—cont'd

Generic name	Trade name	Administration/dosage	Comments
Prochlorperazine edisylate	Compazine	DEEP INTRAMUSCULAR: *Adults*—5 to 10 mg every 3 to 4 hr; maximum, 40 mg daily. *Children*—over 10 kg, 0.2 mg/kg body weight daily.	
Prochlorperazine maleate	Compazine	ORAL: *Adults*—5 to 10 mg every 3 to 4 hr; maximum, 40 mg daily. *Children*—over 10 kg, 0.2 mg/kg body weight daily.	
Promazine hydrochloride	Sparine*	ORAL: *Adults*—25 to 50 mg every 4 to 6 hr as needed. INTRAMUSCULAR: *Adults*—50 mg.	Effective for postoperatve nausea and vomiting and that caused by toxins, radiation therapy, or chemotherapy. Watch for hypotension after intramuscular injection. Sedation and anticholinergic effects common.
Triflupromazine hydro-chloride	Vesprin	ORAL: *Adults*—20 to 30 mg daily. *Children*—0.2 mg/kg body weight divided into 3 doses; maximum daily dose, 10 mg. INTRAMUSCULAR: *Adults*—5 to 15 mg every 4 hr as needed; maximum daily dose, 60 mg. *Elderly*—2.5 to 15 mg daily. *Children*—0.2 to 0.25 mg/kg body weight; maximum daily dose, 10 mg.	Effective for postoperative nausea and vomiting and that caused by toxins, radiation therapy, or chemotherapy.
CANNABINOIDS			
Dronabinol	Marinol	ORAL: *Adults*—5 to 7.5 mg/M^2 every 3 to 4 hr. Begin 4 to 12 hr before chemotherapy and continue 8 to 24 hr after. Dose may be increased by 2.5 mg/M^2 if necessary.	Dronabinol is delta-9-tetrahydrocannabinol, the major active ingredient in marijuana. A particularly effective antiemetic when combined with a phenothiazine. A Schedule II drug.
Nabilone	Cesamet	ORAL: *Adults*—1 mg twice daily, increasing to 2 mg twice daily if necessary.	An especially effective antiemetic for cisplatin chemotherapy.
MISCELLANEOUS DRUGS			
Benzquinamide hydro-chloride	Emete-Con	INTRAMUSCULAR: *Adults*—0.5 to 1 mg/kg body weight at least 15 min before chemotherapy or emergence from anesthesia. Repeat in 1 hr, then every 3 to 4 hr as required. INTRAVENOUS: *Adults*—0.2 to 0.4 mg/kg body weight diluted in 5% dextrose, sodium chloride injection, or lactated Ringer's injection and administered over 1 to 3 min. Additional doses are given IM.	A rapidly acting antiemetic with a short duration of action. Effective in controlling postoperative nausea and vomiting. Acts by inhibiting the chemoreceptor trigger zone.

*Available in Canada and United States.

Table 13.3 Drugs to Control Vomiting—cont'd

Generic name	Trade name	Administration/dosage	Comments
Diphenidol hydrochloride	Vontrol*	ORAL: *Adults*—25 to 50 mg 4 times daily. *Children*—over 6 mo and 12 kg, 5 mg/kg body weight daily divided into 4 doses.	Acts on vestibular apparatus to prevent vertigo after surgery on the middle ear. Effective for postoperative nausea and vomiting caused by toxins, radiation therapy, or chemotherapy.
Domperidone	Motilium†	ORAL: *Adults*—10 mg 4 times/day 15 to 30 min before meals and at bedtime. *Children*—1 drop (0.3 mg)/kg of 1% solution 3 times daily 15 to 30 min before meals and at bedtime if necessary. Oral doses may be doubled if no improvement in two weeks.	Acts peripherally to enhance stomach peristalsis and to prevent the loss of tone associated with vomiting. Effective in preventing the nausea and vomiting that occur after eating in patients with gastroenteritis.
Metoclopramide	Emex† Reglan* Maloxon Maxeran† Reclomide Reglan*	INTRAVENOUS: *Adults*—10 to 20 mg, administered over 2 min. *Children*—up to 6 yr, 0.1 mg/kg body weight; 6 to 14 yr, 2.5 to 5 mg. ORAL: *Adults*—5 to 10 mg 3 times daily 15 to 30 min before meals.	Acts centrally to block stimulation of the chemoreceptor trigger zone and peripherally to enhance gastrointestinal tone. High-dose therapy seems to be effective in reducing nausea and vomiting due to cisplatin therapy.
Trimethobenzamide hydrochloride	Tigan*	INTRAMUSCULAR: *Adults*—200 mg 3 to 4 times daily. For preventing postoperative nausea and vomiting, give 1 dose before or during surgery and another 3 hr after surgery. ORAL: *Adults*—250 mg 3 to 4 times daily. *Children*—15 mg/kg body weight divided into 3 to 4 doses or 100 to 200 mg divided into 3 or 4 doses.	Relieves nausea and vomiting of radiation therapy, in the immediate postoperative period, and in gastroenteritis.

*Available in Canada and United States.
†Available in Canada only.

who smoked marijuana before receiving cancer chemotherapy reported a decreased incidence of nausea and vomiting. Research revealed that the active ingredients, cannabinoids, appeared to depress the chemoreceptor trigger zone. Dronabinol (Marinol) is the major active substance in marijuana and appears to be an especially effective antiemetic when combined with a phenothiazine. Nabilone (Cesamet) is another active cannabinoid. It appears to be especially effective for relieving the nausea from low-dose cisplatin therapy.

There are a few additional drugs that have antiemetic action. Diphenidol (Vontrol) acts on the aural vestibular apparatus. Benzquinamide (Emetecon) and trimethobenzamide (Tigan) inhibit stimulation of the chemoreceptor trigger zone. Domperidone acts peripherally to prevent the loss of gastrointestinal tone, which is an early step in vomiting. Metoclopramide (Reglan) also stimulates the gastrointestinal system, an effect that counteracts the loss of tone in vomiting. In addition, metoclopramide acts at the chemoreceptor trigger zone to prevent vomiting. The active compound in marijuana, Δ^9-tetrahydrocannabinol (THC), is being tested for its reputed superior antiemetic effect in cancer chemotherapy.

THE NURSING PROCESS

DRUGS TO TREAT NAUSEA AND VOMITING

Assessment

Patients may develop nausea with associated vomiting from a variety of causes, including reaction to general anesthesia, reaction to other drugs, motion sickness, viral and bacterial infections, or other medical problems such as intestinal obstruction. After doing a total patient assessment, the nurse should focus on the patient's vital signs, assess the character and quantity of any emesis, listen for the presence of bowel sounds, obtain a brief neurological examination, and measure the fluid intake and output. Relevant history to be obtained from the patient might include such things as precipitating factors, exposure to recent infectious processes, and recent changes in diet or recent medications that have been taken.

Potential nursing diagnoses

Altered thought processes related to drowsiness produced as a drug side effect

Potential for injury related to impaired vision related to drug side effect (e.g., scopolamine)

Management

Drugs used to treat nausea and vomiting provide only symptomatic relief; they do not treat the actual cause of the nausea. During the management phase, attempts will be made to treat the underlying condition and/or diagnose causative agents. Antiemetics will be used for relief of symptoms. The nurse should continue to monitor the vital signs and the fluid intake and output and should assess the subjective complaints of the patient related to nausea and vomiting. The patient should be observed for side effects, although these are usually not severe when these drugs are used in their usual doses. Central nervous system depression, hypotension, and dry mouth are seen frequently. Reducing odors of food and other substances from the patient's environment, limiting intake to clear liquids, and providing back rubs or cool washcloths applied to the forehead are measures that may aid patient comfort.

Evaluation

Because these drugs only treat symptoms, their success is measured by a reduction in the subjective complaint of nausea and by less vomiting. Often the condition causing the nausea and vomiting is self-limiting, and with time the need for antiemetics will decrease. When discharged with an antiemetic drug, the patient should be able to explain why and how to take the drug, what the frequency of drug administration should be, the anticipated side effects of the medication, and what should be done if nausea and vomiting are unrelieved by the medication.

For additional specific information, see the patient care implications section at the end of the chapter.

Side Effects and Drug Interactions of Antiemetic Drugs

The side effects of antiemetic drugs are those characteristic of the drug class. All of the drugs used as antiemetics cause drowsiness. Scopolamine also causes the usual anticholinergic side effects of blurred vision, dilated pupils, and dry mouth. Because of these anticholinergic effects, antihistamines are more frequently prescribed to prevent motion sickness than is scopolamine in spite of the superior effectiveness of scopolamine.

Occasionally extrapyramidal symptoms are seen with the dopamine antagonists. Extrapyramidal symptoms are disorders of motor control associated with too little dopamine in a certain area of the brain. The side effects of the dopamine antagonists are more fully discussed in Chapter 41.

The major drug interaction of antiemetics is a

synergistic depression with drugs depressing the central nervous system, particularly when respiratory depression is involved. For instance, vomiting secondary to alcohol intoxication or ingestion of narcotic analgesics can be relieved with a dopamine antagonist, but the resultant respiratory depression makes this treatment undesirable.

Activity of the Large Intestine

DRUGS TO CONTROL DIARRHEA
(Table 13.4)

About 8 liters of fluid travel through the intestines of the average adult in 24 hours. Water ingested in food or drink accounts for about 2 liters, and secretions (salivary, gastric, biliary, and pancreatic) account for about 6 liters. Since only 100 to 200 ml of water is normally excreted daily in feces, the intestines are very efficient in reabsorbing water and electrolytes.

Definition

Diarrhea has no precise definition but rather refers to bowel movements that are frequent (more than three per day), fluid (unformed stools), or large (greater than 200 Gm per day). Acute diarrhea lasts for hours or days, whereas chronic diarrhea lasts more than 3 to 4 weeks. Chronic diarrhea requires a thorough examination to establish a cause, which can then be specifically treated. Acute diarrhea rarely requires treatment beyond avoidance of food and adequate liquid intake.

Replacement Therapy for Diarrhea

The primary treatment of diarrhea is to replace lost fluids and electrolytes. The presence of glucose is required for the intestinal absorption of water and electrolytes, so mild dehydration can be treated with carbonated drinks (which add glucose and bicarbonate) and broths or clear soups (which add sodium and chloride). Infants and the elderly can become seriously dehydrated if an adequate intake of glucose and salts is not maintained to replace the fluid and electrolytes lost. Commercially available drinks for replacement of glucose and electrolytes include Gatorade and Lytren. A similar drink can be made at home with ½ teaspoon of corn syrup or honey and a pinch of table salt added to 1 cup (8 oz) of fruit juice (to provide potassium), alternating with a drink made by adding ¼ teaspoon of baking soda (sodium bicarbonate to 1 cup [8 oz] of water). A simpler drink is made with the following recipe: 1 teaspoon table salt, 1 teaspoon baking soda, and 4 teaspoons of sugar in a quart of boiled water. This latter recipe does not provide needed potassium, however, and if possible ½ teaspoon of potassium chloride should be added to a quart of the solution.

Drug Therapy for Diarrhea (Table 13.4)

The most effective nonspecific antidiarrheal agents are the opioids, which decrease the tone of the small and large intestines in a manner that slows the transit of material. The longitudinal contractions propelling the contents (peristalsis) are inhibited by the opioids, but the circular contractions which cause the segmental activity that mixes the intestinal contents are stimulated by the opioids. The treatment of diarrhea with opioids is nonspecific, and when diarrhea is caused by poisons, infections, or bacterial toxins, opioids can make the condition worse by delaying the elimination of these agents. Opioids that are used to control diarrhea include *opium tincture, paregoric, codeine,* and *diphenoxylate (Lomotil).* The effective antidiarrheal dose is lower than that which can cause

Table 13.4 Drugs to Control Diarrhea

Generic name	Trade name	Administration/dosage	Comments
OPIOIDS AND RELATED DRUGS			
Codeine phosphate; codeine sulfate		ORAL: *Adults and children over 12 yr*—15 to 60 mg every 4 to 8 hr as needed. INTRAMUSCULAR: *Adults and children over 12 yr*—15 to 30 mg every 2 to 4 hr.	A Schedule II drug.
Diphenoxylate hydrochloride with atropine	Colonil Lomotil* Lofene Various others	ORAL: *Adults*—5 mg 3 to 4 times daily. *Children*—8 to 12 yr; 10 mg daily in 5 divided doses; 5 to 8 yr, 8 mg daily in 4 divided doses; 2 to 5 yr, 6 mg daily in 3 divided doses.	A Schedule V drug.
Loperamide	Imodium	ORAL: *Adults*—4 mg initially, then 2 mg with each diarrheal episode, up to 16 mg daily.	Also available as a nonprescription drug. FDA Pregnancy Category B.
Opium tincture		ORAL: 0.6 ml 4 times daily. Maximum single dose is 1 ml. Maximum daily dose is 6 ml.	A Schedule II drug.
Paregoric		ORAL: *Adults*—5 to 10 ml 1 to 4 times daily. *Children*—0.25 to 0.5 ml/kg 1 to 4 times daily.	A Schedule III drug.
BISMUTH SALTS			
Bismuth subsalicylate	Pepto-Bismol	ORAL: *Adults*—30 ml. *Children*—10 to 14 yr, 20 ml; 6 to 10 yr, 10 ml; 3 to 6 yr, 5 ml.	A nonprescription drug. Effective for "traveler's" diarrhea. May turn stools gray-black.

*Available in Canada and United States.

euphoria or analgesia. Toxic doses produce respiratory depression, which can be reversed with a narcotic antagonist.

Opium tincture

Opium tincture is a 10% solution of opium containing 10 mg/ml morphine. The antidiarrheal dose of opium tincture is measured in drops (usually 6 to 20 drops), and such a dose does not usually produce either euphoria or analgesia.

Paregoric

Paregoric (camphorated opium tincture) contains only 0.4 mg/ml morphine and is administered by the teaspoonful. Paregoric has an unpleasant taste.

Codeine

The drug codeine can be given orally, or it can be administered intramuscularly.

Diphenoxylate (Colonil, Lomotil)

Diphenoxylate is an opioid that has a lower potential than codeine or opium tincture for causing drug dependence. Diphenoxylate is combined with atropine to diminish abdominal cramping while reducing the loss of water and electrolytes.

Loperamide (Imodium)

Loperamide is a relatively new antidiarrheal drug that acts to depress both longitudinal and circular contractions of the intestinal smooth muscles and to decrease the release of acetylcholine. This is a broader spectrum of actions on the intestine than is seen with opioids. Loperamide is structurally related to diphenoxylate, but it has no effects on the CNS and does not appear to produce physical dependence. Originally available as a Schedule V drug, loperamide is now available over-the-counter. Loperamide is concentrated by the liver and ex-

THE NURSING PROCESS

DRUGS TO CONTROL DIARRHEA

Assessment

Diarrhea may have a variety of causes, including viral and bacterial infections, response to various medications, and physiological diseases of the colon. The nurse should do a thorough patient assessment. Specific points include monitoring the vital signs and the intake and output of solids and liquids, auscultating bowel sounds, and checking the character and quantity of diarrhea. Appropriate laboratory studies related to diarrhea include culturing a stool specimen and testing stools for ova and parasites and the presence of occult blood. The nurse should question the patient about recent exposure to new water or dietary sources, recent exposure to infectious agents, and any new medications that have been started recently.

Potential nursing diagnoses

Altered thought processes related to drowsiness produced as a drug side effect

Colonic constipation related to drug side effects

Management

The treatment of diarrhea is directed at providing symptomatic relief for the patient and at identifying the cause of the diarrhea and treating the cause. The nurse should continue to monitor the vital signs and the intake and output of liquid, and should observe the frequency and character of any additional stools. If laboratory work has indicated a possible specific cause for diarrhea, treatment of this causative agent should be started. Limiting the diet to clear fluids may help to limit diarrhea. In cases in which diarrhea is the result of milk intolerance or other dietary causes, the patient is referred to the dietician for appropriate instruction about prescribed dietary restrictions. The nurse should observe the patient for side effects resulting from the medications, in particular, constipation and sedation. If diarrhea is severe or persists, the serum electrolyte concentrations should be monitored and replacement fluids provided as necessary.

Evaluation

These drugs are considered effective if the frequency of bowel movements is decreased to the patient's normal range. In addition, there should be no side effects such as constipation resulting from drug therapy. Before discharge the patient should be able to explain when and how to take the medication prescribed, symptoms that may indicate too high a dose, and what to do if the drugs do not relieve the symptoms.

For more specific information, see the patient care implications section at the end of the chapter.

---

creted into the bile. Its use is contraindicated in the presence of liver disease.

Bismuth salts

In addition to opioids that depress intestinal motility, many agents have been used as antidiarrheal drugs in the belief that they absorb toxins and thus remove the cause of diarrhea. Of these, only bismuth salts have been proven effective.

Bismuth subsalicylate (Pepto-Bismol) is effective in controlling "traveler's" diarrhea, apparently by binding the bacterial toxins. Bismuth causes the feces to become black, which should not be taken as an indication of blood in the feces. Use in infants or the elderly may produce feces that cannot be expelled (impacted feces).

DRUGS TO RELIEVE CONSTIPATION: LAXATIVES
Origin of Constipation

The major muscular activity of the large intestine is a contraction of circular smooth muscle, which decreases the diameter to segment and knead the fecal mass without moving it along.

THE NURSING PROCESS

DRUGS TO RELIEVE CONSTIPATION

Assessment

Constipation may occur for various reasons, including enforced bed rest, concomitant use of medications such as narcotic analgesics or drugs with anticholinergic action, recent surgery, dehydration, and improper use of drugs used to treat diarrhea. The nurse should do a thorough patient assessment with attention to the vital signs, the fluid intake and output, and the presence of bowel sounds. A digital rectal examination is performed if appropriate to determine the presence of impacted stools. Additional helpful data might include any previous history of constipation and its treatment, the patient's perception of what constipation is, and any recent change in life-style, diet, or medications that might promote constipation.

Potential nursing diagnoses

Diarrhea related to drug side effects

Impaired perianal skin integrity related to diarrhea

Management

The actual treatment of constipation is usually relatively simple. If the problem is a persistent one, it is important to rule out serious causes such as cancer. In addition to stimulating the intestine to produce a bowel movement, it is important to begin teaching the patient about other factors that influence the frequency of stools. The patient can be taught the importance of adequate fluid intake and physical activity. The patient should also be instructed that certain foods and juices tend to cause bulk in the stool and produce gastrointestinal stimulation. The treatment of a complaint of constipation may be different from the final drug program prescribed for the patient for management of chronic constipation at home.

Evaluation

These drugs are considered effective if they either produce a bowel movement within 12 to 24 hours or allow the patient to have bowel movements unaided on a regular basis. Before a patient is discharged to home, it is important that the patient be able to explain how to take the medications ordered and what the desired effects of the medications are, since some cause a laxative effect whereas others keep the stool soft; the patient should also know what to do if the prescribed therapy is no longer effective for treatment of constipation.

For further specific information, see the patient care implications section at the end of this chapter.

About 2 liters of water are removed from the fecal mass in the large intestine. Bulk in the large intestine stimulates stretch receptors to cause a reflex peristalsis, which moves the fecal mass forward. Periodically, usually three to four times daily, strong propulsive contractions occur spontaneously to move the fecal mass through the large intestine. The strongest movements usually occur after the first meal of the day, and the perception of the need to defecate follows the filling of the rectum. The relaxation of the external anal sphincter is a voluntary act, as are the straining move-

---

DIETARY CONSIDERATION: FIBER

Adequate amounts of dietary fiber may help prevent constipation and colon diseases, may help maintain blood glucose levels, and lower blood cholesterol levels. Good dietary sources of fiber include: fruits and vegetables, especially raw, unpeeled or with edible seeds, whole grains and whole grain products: bread, cereals, pastas, bran, oats, peas, beans, lentils.

Table 13.5 Drugs to Relieve Constipation

Generic name	Trade name	Administration/dosage	Comments
BULK-FORMING AGENTS			
Karaya gum		ORAL: 5 to 10 Gm daily, taken with water.	Nonprescription.
Methylcellulose; carboxymethyl cellulose	Cologel Hydrolose	ORAL: *Adults*—4 to 6 Gm daily. *Children*—over 6 yr, 1 to 1.5 Gm daily.	Nonprescription.
Plantago (psyllium) seed		ORAL: *Adults*—2.5 to 30 Gm daily. *Children*—over 6 yr, 1.25-15 Gm daily. Add to water and drink rapidly.	Nonprescription.
Polycarbophil	Mitrolan	ORAL: *Adults*—4 to 6 Gm daily. *Children*—6 to 12 yr, 1.5 to 3 Gm daily; 2 to 5 yr, 1 to 1.5 Gm daily; to 2 yr, 0.5 to 1 Gm daily.	Nonprescription.
Psyllium hydrocolloid Psyllium hydrophilic mucilloid	Effersyllium Konsyl L.A. Formula Metamucil* Modane Bulk	ORAL: *Adults*—1 round teaspoonful (7 Gm) or 1 packet. Add to a glass of water and drink rapidly and then follow with a second glass of water. Repeat 1 to 2 times daily if necessary.	Nonprescription.
STIMULANT (IRRITANT) CATHARTICS			
Bisacodyl	Biscolax* Dulcolax* Various others	ORAL: *Adults*—10 mg. Up to 30 mg may be given to clear gastrointestinal tract. *Children*—over 6 yr, 5 mg. RECTAL: *Adults and children over 2 yr*—10 mg. *Children under 2 yr*—5 mg.	Initial response in 6 to 12 hr. Nonprescription. Do not take within 60 min of milk or antacids. Rectal administration effective in 15 min.
Cascara sagrada	Bileo-Secrin Cas-Evac	ORAL: *Adults*—200 to 400 mg of extract, 0.5 to 1.5 ml of fluid extract, or 5 ml of aromatic extract.	Nonprescription. One of the mildest of the stimulant cathartics.
Castor oil		ORAL: *Adults*—15 to 60 ml. *Children*—over 2 yr, 5 to 15 ml; under 2 yr, 1 to 5 ml.	Castor oil is degraded to ricinoleic acid, which is the active drug. Nonprescription.
Castor oil, emulsified	Neoloid	ORAL: *Adults*—30 to 60 ml. *Children*—over 2 yr, 7.5 to 30 ml; under 2 yr, 2.5 to 7.5 ml.	Nonprescription. This emulsion is mint flavored. Turns alkaline urine pink.
Glycerin suppositories		RECTAL: *Adults*—3 Gm. *Children*—under 6 yr, 1 to 1.5 Gm.	Nonprescription. Effective in 15 to 30 min.
Phenolphthalein	Chocolax Ex-lax Feen-A-Mint Phenolax Various others	ORAL: *Adults*—30 to 270 mg daily. *Children*—over 6 yr, 30 to 60 mg daily; 2 to 6 yr, 15 to 20 mg daily.	Nonprescription. Turns alkaline urine pink.
Senna concentrate	Senokot suppositories	RECTAL: *Adults*—1 suppository. *Children*—over 60 lb, ½ suppository.	
Senna pod	Senokot Various others	ORAL: *Adults*—twice daily give 1 to 2 teaspoonfuls (granules), 2 to 3 teaspoonfuls (syrup), or 2 to 4 tablets. *Children, pregnant or postpartum women, or geriatric patients*—½ adult dose. *Children*—1 mo to 1 yr, 1.25 to 2.5 ml (syrup).	Nonprescription. Not all preparations are recommended for children.

*Available in Canada and United States.

Continued.

Table 13.5 Drugs to Relieve Constipation—cont'd

Generic name	Trade name	Administration/dosage	Comments
Senna, whole leaf		ORAL: *Adults*—0.5 to 2 Gm or 2 ml of senna fluid extract. *Children*—6 to 12 yr, ½ adult dose; 2 to 5 yr, ¼ adult dose; under 2 yr, ⅓ adult dose.	Nonprescription.
Sennosides A and B	Glysennid	ORAL: *Adults*—12 to 24 mg at bedtime. *Children*—over 10 yr. same as adult; 6 to 10 yr, 12 mg at bedtime.	Nonprescription.
SALINE CATHARTICS			
Magnesium citrate		ORAL: *Adults*—1 glassful (about 240 ml). *Children*—0.5 ml/kg body weight.	Nonprescription.
Magnesium hydroxide	Milk of Magnesia	ORAL: *Adults*—10 to 15 ml (concentrated) or 15 to 30 ml (regular). *Children*—0.5 ml (regular)/kg body weight.	Nonprescription.
Magnesium sulfate	Epsom salt	ORAL: *Adults*—15 Gm in a glass of water. *Children*—0.25 Gm/kg.	Nonprescription.
Monosodium phosphate	Sal Hepatica	ORAL: *Adults*—5 to 20 ml with water.	Nonprescription.
Sodium phosphate		ORAL: *Adults*—4 Gm in a glass of warm water. *Children*—0.25 Gm/kg.	Nonprescription.
Sodium phosphate with biphosphate	Phospho-Soda	ORAL: *Adults*—20 to 40 ml in a glass of cold water. *Children*—5 to 15 ml.	Nonprescription.
LUBRICANTS			
Mineral oil	Agoral, Plain Kondremul Plain* Neo-Cultol Petrogalar Plain	ORAL: *Adults*—15 to 30 ml at bedtime.	Nonprescription. To ease strain of passing hard stools. Should not be used regularly because the fat-soluble vitamins (A, D, E, and K) are not absorbed. Response in 1 to 3 days.
FECAL SOFTENERS			
Docusate calcium	Surfak	ORAL: *Adults*—50 to 360 mg daily. *Children*—50 to 150 mg daily.	Nonprescription.
Docusate sodium	Colace Comfolax D-S-S Various others	ORAL: *Adults*—50 to 360 mg. *Children*—6 to 12 yr, 40 to 120 mg; 3 to 6 yr, 20 to 60 mg; under 3 yr, 10 to 40 mg.	Nonprescription.
MISCELLANEOUS			
Lactulose	Cephulac* Chronulac*	ORAL: *Adults*—15 to 30 ml, increased to 60 ml per day if necessary (15 ml = 10 Gm).	Nonprescription. Works by an osmotic effect in 1 to 3 days.

*Available in Canada and United States.

ments to expel the feces. The pattern of defecation described implies that defecation is a regular morning event, but the timing of defecation is highly individual and may occur more or less frequently. A normal bowel movement refers to whatever pattern of defecation results in readily passed feces for a given individual. Constipation arises when the frequency of bowel movements decreases and defecation yields hard stools that are difficult to pass.

Classes of Laxatives (Table 13.5)

Laxative, cathartic, and *purgative* are all terms describing agents that act on the large intestine (colon, bowel) to promote defecation, but these terms have evolved to represent different degrees of action. A laxative produces soft stools with a minimal incidence of abdominal cramping. A cathartic produces a soft to fluid stool and may also cause abdominal cramping. A purgative produces a watery stool and violent cramping to such an extent that shock and hemorrhaging may result. Purgatives are no longer used in medical practice, and only some cathartics, also called stimulant cathartics, are commonly used.

Table 13.5 lists the drugs used as laxatives. Traditionally, laxatives are classified as (1) bulk-forming, (2) stimulant (irritant) cathartic, (3) saline (osmotic) cathartic, (4) wetting agent (softener), and (5) lubricant. Laxatives are indicated for those with true constipation. Causes of constipation include poor bowel habits, narcotic analgesics, drugs with anticholinergic side effects, and the loss of intestinal muscle tone because of surgery, bed rest, or age. Laxatives are also indicated when straining is painful or risky, such as in women with episiotomies and patients with hemorrhoids, hernias, or aneurysms. Laxatives are also used to clean out the large intestine before surgery or examination. With the exception of mineral oil, laxatives act by providing a greater bulk to the fecal mass, primarily by keeping water in the large intestine. The large, hydrated fecal mass can fill the rectum to stimulate defecation, and defecation is accomplished with minimal irritation or strain.

Bulk-forming laxatives

This class of laxatives includes bran, methylcellulose, polycarbophil, and psyllium hydrophilic mucilloid. These laxatives act by retaining water so that the stool remains large and soft. Bulk-forming laxatives provide what should be a part of good nutrition. It is generally felt that people in the developed countries eat a diet that contains too little fiber and favors the formation of small, hard stools. The inclusion of bran, whole grain products, and fibrous fruits and vegetables in the diet promotes the formation of large, soft stools that readily stimulate the large intestine and the rectum.

In a person who does not regularly use laxatives, bulk-forming laxatives will be effective in 12 to 24 hours. Bulk-forming laxatives can also relieve a mild water diarrhea by absorbing water to produce a soft stool.

Stimulant (irritant) cathartics

Stimulant cathartics include cascara, danthron, senna, phenolphthalein, bisacodyl, castor oil, and glycerin. These drugs usually form a soft to fluid stool in 6 to 12 hours. Stimulant cathartics were believed to act only by directly stimulating the motility of the large intestine; however, newer research has indicated that these drugs also inhibit the reabsorption of water in the large intestine.

The stimulant cathartics are the most abused laxatives. When a stimulant cathartic is used for more than 1 week, the large intestine loses its tone and becomes less responsive to any stimulation. Continued use of a stimulant cathartic can produce a diarrhea severe enough to cause dehydration and to lower blood concentrations of sodium and potassium.

Cascara and *senna* are extracted from plants. Cascara is the milder and senna the more potent of these laxatives. They should not be used by mothers breast-feeding infants, since these laxatives are excreted in the milk. Senna and cascara color an acid urine yellow-brown and an alkaline urine red.

Phenolphthalein is found in many over-the-counter laxative preparations. Phenolphthalein enters the enterohepatic circulation and may be effective for several days. In an alkaline urine, phenolphthalein is pink.

Bisacodyl is a synthetic compound that is available both as a suppository and as a tablet. As a suppository, bisacodyl is effective in 15 minutes. As a tablet, bisacodyl is effective in 6 hours. Since bisacodyl irritates the stomach, the tablet is coated to dissolve only in the intestine. This enteric-coated tablet should not be taken within 1 hour of ingestion of such things as milk or antacids, which neutralize stomach acid. Bisacodyl is often used to clear the large intestine for proctoscopic or coloscopic examination.

Castor oil is an old remedy for constipation and is still used medically. Castor oil is the most potent of the stimulant cathartics, producing a watery stool in 2 to 6 hours, which thoroughly removes gas and feces from the intestine. Castor oil has an unpleasant taste that is best disguised by chilling it and administering it with fruit juice.

Glycerin is used only as a suppository. It acts by stimulating the rectum as well as by attracting water to increase bulk and is effective in 15 to 30 minutes.

Saline (osmotic) cathartics

Saline cathartics are poorly absorbed salts of magnesium or sodium: magnesium carbonate, oxide, citrate, hydroxide, or sulfate; sodium phosphate or sulfate; and potassium, sodium tartrate. The concentrated solutions of these salts attract water osmotically into the lumen of the large intestine, and the resulting bulk stimulates peristalsis. Saline cathartics empty the bowel in 2 to 6 hours.

Patients with poor kidney function should not use saline cathartics because these patients cannot excrete the extra salt load from the small fraction of the salt that is absorbed systemically.

Wetting agents (stool softeners)

Wetting agents are detergents that inhibit the absorption of water so that the fecal mass remains large and soft. This class of laxatives is indicated when the objective is to avoid straining to pass the stools. Such laxatives include *dioctyl sodium sulfosuccinate (docusate sodium)* and *dioctyl calcium sulfosuccinate (docusate calcium)*.

Lubricant

The only lubricant laxative still used is *mineral oil,* which is indigestible and acts to soften the feces, thus easing the strain of passing the stools and lessening the irritation to hemorrhoids. Long-term use of mineral oil interferes with the absorption of the fat-soluble vitamins A, D, E, and K. Mineral oil can cause a lipid pneumonia if accidentally aspirated. The wetting agents are regarded as superior to mineral oil in softening the stools for easy passage.

Miscellaneous

Lactulose is a synthetic disaccharide that is not hydrolyzed by intestinal enzymes and is not absorbed. Instead, lactulose is degraded by bacteria in the colon to short-chain organic acids that are not absorbed and act as osmotic agents. The net effect is a moderate fluid accumulation in the colon and the formation of a soft stool. Lactulose may ini-

PATIENT CARE IMPLICATIONS

Cholinomimetics: bethanechol and neostigmine

Drug administration

- Have atropine sulfate (0.5 to 1.0 mg) on hand to counteract excessive cholinergic side effects when administering the cholinomimetics subcutaneously.
- Check doses carefully. The oral dose of bethanechol may be as high as 50 mg, while the subcutaneous dose should not exceed 5 mg.
- Remain at the bedside of patients for the first 10 minutes after administering subcutaneous bethanechol to assess for side effects.
- The physician may order a test dose of one half or less of the usual dose to check for patient response. Monitor the vital signs.
- Check the pulse before administering neostigmine. Notify the physician if the rate is below 80, and withhold the dose pending physician approval. For additional information about neostigmine, see Chapter 11.

Patient and family education

- Teach patients to take oral doses of bethanechol on an empty stomach, 1 hour before or 2 hours after eating.
- If a dose is missed, tell patients to take the missed dose if within 1 to 2 hours of the scheduled time. If close to the next dosing time, omit the missed dose and resume the usual dosing schedule. Do not "double up" for missed doses.
- Remind patients to keep these and all medications out of the reach of children.

Metoclopramide

Drug administration

- Administer undiluted IV doses over 1 to 2 minutes. May be diluted in 50 ml of solution and administered slowly, over at least 15 minutes. When given in conjunction with cancer chemotherapy, give doses 30 minutes before chemotherapy is begun. A second dose may be given in 2 hours and a third dose in 3 hours. For this use, the dose may be as high as 2 mg/kg body weight.

Patient and family education

- Take oral doses 30 minutes before meals; doses may also be taken at bedtime.
- This drug may produce extrapyramidal reactions (see Table 41.2). Instruct the patient to report any unusual side effects, especially protrusion of the tongue, puffing of the cheeks, chewing movements, and involuntary movements of any body parts.
- Teach patients to avoid drinking or operating hazardous equipment until the effects of the medication can be evaluated.
- Tell patients to avoid alcohol while taking this drug, as well as any drug which may depress the central nervous system, such as sleeping medications, tranquilizers, narcotic analgesics, or other drugs which make the patient sleepy.

Anticholinergic and antispasmodic drugs

Drug administration

- Use cautiously in patients with prostatic hypertrophy, pyloric obstruction, obstruction of the bladder neck, or serious cardiac disease. Assess for preexisting glaucoma, as anticholinergics may precipitate an attack of acute angle-closure glaucoma.
- Assess for urinary retention, especially in elderly men with preexisting prostatic hypertrophy. Monitor intake and output. Instruct the patient to report inability to void, increasing difficulty in initiating urination, or a sensation of incomplete bladder emptying. Instruct the patient to void prior to taking each dose.
- Monitor the pulse before administering doses. Withhold dose if pulse exceeds 90 to 100 in an adult. Administer with caution in patients with a history of heart disease characterized by tachycardia.
- Auscultate bowel sounds.
- Treat overdose with neostigmine.

Continued.

PATIENT CARE IMPLICATIONS — cont'd

- Administer IM doses into a large muscle mass such as the dorsogluteal site or rectus femoris muscle in adults, or the vastus lateralis muscle in infants and small children. Use careful technique; aspirate before administering dose to avoid inadvertent IV administration.
- Tincture of belladonna may be prescribed by number of drops. Dilute the dose in 15 to 30 ml of water before administering.
- Keep a record of bowel movements.
- If photophobia occurs, dim room lights.
- If drowsiness or disorientation develops, supervise ambulation, keep siderails up, use night lights.

Patient and family education

- Take doses before meals and at bedtime unless a timed-release form is used. If antacids are also prescribed, take doses 30 minutes before or 2 hours after antacid doses.
- Teach patients that constipation is a common side effect. Instruct the patient to increase the daily fluid intake to at least 3000 ml, to increase dietary intake of fruits and fiber, and to get regular exercise. Tell the patient to keep a record of bowel movements, and if a bowel movement has not occurred in 3 days, to consult the physician. Teach the patient to avoid cathartics or laxatives unless instructed to use specific ones by the physician, as they may be contraindicated in certain medical conditions requiring anticholinergics.
- Caution patients to avoid driving or operating hazardous equipment until the effects of the medication can be evaluated; drowsiness and blurred vision may occur.
- Tell patients to wear sunglasses and avoid bright sunlight if photophobia develops.
- Teach patients to suck on sugarless hard candy or to chew gum to relieve dry mouth. Refer patients to the pharmacist for commercially available saliva substitutes.
- Instruct patients to be careful regarding strenuous activities on warm days, as these drugs inhibit the ability of the body to perspire. Tell the patient to take frequent rest periods to cool off. Teach patients that atropine may produce a fever, especially in children.

- As these drugs often produce annoying side effects when taken in therapeutic doses, patient compliance may be poor. Provide emotional support as needed; teach patients the importance of taking drugs as prescribed.
- Reinforce to patients the importance of keeping all drugs out of the reach of children.
- If combination products are prescribed, review side effects of each drug with the patient.

Drugs to treat ulcers: antacids

Patient and family education

- Avoid administering antacids with tetracyclines, digoxin, or quinidine. Review with patients their complete list of medications, and work out with them a suitable schedule for home drug administration that prevents the antacids from interfering with absorption of any other drugs. Try to schedule antacids ½ hour before or 1 hour after sucralfate; try to schedule H_2 histamine receptor antagonists 1 hour before or 1 hour after antacids.
- Remind patients to chew antacid tablets, not swallow them whole.
- Tell patients to take a small amount of water after doses of antacid liquid to ensure that the antacid dose is carried to the stomach.
- Tell patients to alternate aluminum or calcium salts with magnesium salts to prevent diarrhea or constipation, unless a specific antacid is ordered. Also instruct patients to increase fluid intake to 2500 to 3000 ml per day and increase dietary intake of fruits and fiber to prevent constipation. Note that patients in renal failure should not increase fluid intake, and may require concomitant stool softeners.
- Teach patients to read labels carefully. Antacids vary in their strength, acid-neutralizing ability, sodium content, and in whether other drugs may be included in the formulation. Frequently included drugs are magaldrate, another antacid, and simethicone, an antigas drug.
- Teach patients taking aluminum carbonate or aluminum hydroxide products for hyperphosphatemia not to substitute other antacids. Doses of antacids used to bind phosphate are often administered with meals. Re-

PATIENT CARE IMPLICATIONS — cont'd

fer patients to a dietician for instruction in a low-phosphate diet if indicated.

- Antacids used to treat ulcers are often administered 1 and 3 hours after meals and at bedtime; review prescription orders with patients.

- Teach patients taking antacids to prevent kidney stones by increasing daily fluid intake to 3000 ml.

- Instruct patients requiring sodium restriction for heart disease or other health problems to avoid antacids high in sodium; consult the physician or pharmacist. Example sodium-free products include: Advanced Formula Di-Gel, Calcitrel, Magaldrate, Mi-acid; other preparations are very low in sodium. Example products relatively high in sodium include Gaviscon-2 chewable tablets (36.8 mg), Gas-is-gon (50.6 mg), and Rolaids (53 mg).

- Teach patients to use antacids as prescribed, and avoid frequent self-medication with over-the-counter products unless advised to do so by a physician.

Antihistamines: Cimetidine

Drug administration

- For direct IV injection, dilute 300 mg in at least 20 ml of normal saline. Administer at a rate of 300 mg or less over 2 minutes.

- For intermittent IV infusion, dilute 300 mg of drug in 100 ml of compatible IV solution. Do not add to continuously infusing fluids. Administer over 15 to 20 minutes.

- Warn the patient that there may be discomfort associated with IM administration.

- Read labels carefully. Prefilled syringes are intended for IM use or for diluting for intermittent infusion. Prefilled syringes are *not* for direct IV injection.

- This drug is incompatible with many other drugs for infusion. Do not add other drugs to infusions or cimetidine.

- Usually, administer once-daily doses before bedtime, twice-daily doses in the morning and at bedtime, and more frequent doses with meals and at bedtime.

- If antacids and/or metoclopramide are also ordered, they should be administered 1 hour before or 1 hour after the cimetidine dose.

- The action of many drugs (including aminophylline, caffeine, anticoagulants, and some heart medications) may be potentiated when the patient is also receiving cimetidine, because cimetidine is metabolized by the liver and excreted through the kidney. Assess patients carefully for drug side effects, and monitor appropriate laboratory tests carefully as dosages of other drugs may need adjustment.

- Monitor level of consciousness, blood pressure and pulse, intake and output, and complete blood count. Assess for skin changes and gynecomastia.

Antihistamines: Famotidine, nizadepine, and ranitidine

Drug administration

- Famotidine may be taken concurrently with antacids if necessary.

- For direct IV use of famotidine, dilute 20 mg with 5 to 10 ml of compatible solution, and administer over at least 2 minutes.

- For intermittent infusion of famotidine, dilute 20 mg in 100 ml of compatible solution, and administer dose over 15 to 30 minutes.

- For direct IV use of ranitidine, dilute 50 mg with 20 ml of compatible IV solution, and administer over at least 5 minutes.

- For intermittent infusion of ranitidine, dilute 50 mg in 50 to 100 ml of compatible IV solution, and administer over 15 to 20 minutes.

- Be alert when administering ranitidine IV, as too rapid administration has been associated with bradycardia, tachycardia, and PVCs. Monitor pulse and blood pressure.

- Monitor level of consciousness, blood pressure and pulse, assess for constipation or diarrhea, monitor complete blood count. With famotidine, monitor BUN, serum creatinine, and urinalysis.

Patient and family education (antihistamines)

- Review the side effects associated with the prescribed drug, and instruct patients to report the development of these side effects to the physician.

- Review all prescribed medications with the patient, and help the patient develop a dosing schedule that is consistent with the goals of therapy and possible drug interactions.

Continued.

PATIENT CARE IMPLICATIONS — cont'd

- Warn patients to avoid alcohol and avoid smoking, especially after the final dose of the day, while taking these drugs.

- Emphasize the importance of all aspects of therapy, which may include dietary modification, other drugs, and limiting caffeine intake.

- Warn patients to avoid the use of over-the-counter preparations while taking any of these antihistamines.

Misoprostol

Drug administration/patient and family education

- Question female patients about possible pregnancy before administering first dose. Ascertain that women of childbearing age are informed of the possible side effect of bleeding and abortion before administering first dose.

- Instruct patients to report any new sign or symptom. As more experience is accumulated with this group of drugs, additional information about side effects may be available.

Sucralfate

Drug administration/patient and family education

- Instruct patients to take antacids one half hour before or 1 hour after sucralfate.

- For best effect, instruct patient to take sucralfate with water on an empty stomach, 1 hour before meals and at bedtime.

- Review all medications prescribed, and develop a dosing schedule that is suitable considering known drug interactions. Cimetidine, digoxin, phenytoin, tetracyclines, and fat-soluble vitamins should be taken at a different time of day than sucralfate.

- Instruct patients to keep a record of bowel movements. If constipation develops, teach patients to increase daily intake of fluids to 2500 to 3000 ml, increase level of activity, and increase dietary intake of fruit and fiber. If the patient is taking antacids, changing the brand of antacid may also help; consult the physician.

Antiemetics

Drug administration

- Measure emesis as part of fluid intake and output.

- IV *benzquinamide* has been associated with an increase in blood pressure and cardiac arrhythmias. The IM route is preferred. Monitor the blood pressure and pulse, and administer IV doses slowly.

- Avoid IM use of *trimethobenzamide* in children.

- Use antiemetics with caution in children who may be suffering from Reye's syndrome. This syndrome is characterized by an abrupt onset of persistent severe vomiting, lethargy, irrational behavior, progressive encephalopathy, convulsions, coma, and death.

- Be alert to patient response to the cannabinoids, as some patients may hesitate to use drugs derived from marijuana. Inform patients that psychological or physical dependence is unlikely at therapeutic doses and with short-term use of these drugs.

- Since the gelatin capsule form of *dronabinol* contains sesame seed oil, check for allergy to this oil before administering first dose.

- The antihistamines are discussed in detail in Chapter 24.

- The antidopaminergic drugs are discussed in detail in Chapter 41.

Patient and family education

- Review the side effects of these drugs with the patient. Warn the patient to use antiemetics only as prescribed, and not to self-medicate with leftover doses. The use of these drugs in pregnant women is contraindicated unless the benefit outweighs the risk.

- Warn patients to avoid drinking or operating hazardous equipment when taking antiemetics, as sedation and drowsiness are common.

- Teach patients to avoid other drugs which may depress the central nervous system while they are using antiemetics. These drugs include alcohol, tranquilizers, sleeping medications, narcotic analgesics.

- For treatment of motion sickness, suggest that the patient ride in the front seat of the car if possible, and should face forward, not backward. Take prophylactic drugs 1 to 2 hours before beginning the trip rather than waiting until nausea develops.

- For sustained-release, transdermal drugs, emphasize the importance of reading the instructional leaflet provided by the manufacturer. Instruct the patient to wash hands before applying the device, and afterward. The disc is usually applied behind the ear, in front of the hairline. Avoid cut or denuded skin. Replace every 3 days or as directed by the physician. If the disc falls off, apply a new one. Apply the disc 4 hours before beginning a trip.

- For dry mouth, suggest the patient chew sugarless gum or suck hard candy. Provide frequent mouth care, but avoid drying, alcohol-containing mouthwashes, or lemon and glycerin swabs.

- For the person who is NPO (nothing by mouth), or who has vomited, again provide frequent mouth care. Suggest that the patient suck ice chips; consult the physician for the patient NPO.

- Keep the environment free of odors. Keep food out of sight of the nauseated person. Try clear liquids in small amounts before progressing to a more complete diet.

- If dry eyes are a problem, suggest that the patient use artificial tears on a regular basis; consult the physician.

- Warn the patient that IM antiemetics often produce burning at the injection site.

- Remind patients to keep these and all drugs out of the reach of children.

Drugs to control diarrhea

Drug administration

- Assess patients with diarrhea for history of recent travel, especially international, recent antibiotic use, recent cancer chemotherapy, and recent work with children in day care centers or other settings where harmful microorganisms are easily spread.

- Monitor intake and output, daily weight, skin turgor, level of consciousness, blood pressure and pulse. Monitor serum electrolytes.

- Dilute *opium tincture* in 15 to 30 ml to ensure that the patient receives the entire dose.

- Codeine is discussed in greater detail in Chapter 44.

- *Paregoric* is unpleasant to the taste. Many patients find combination drugs such as Parepectolin more palatable. (Parepectolin 30 ml contains paregoric 2.7 ml, pectin 162 mg, and kaolin 5.5 Gm. Note that combination drugs subject the patient to additional ingredients that may or may not be helpful.)

- Theoretically, addiction to *diphenoxylate* is possible. Overdose with this drug resembles an overdose with a narcotic analgesic and is treated in a similar manner (Chapter 44).

- Diphenoxylate preparations contain a small amount of atropine. A single dose of these preparations would cause few side effects due to the atropine, but the accumulated dose following a day or two of treatment might cause problems. Review the side effects of and contraindications to atropine use.

Patient and family education

- Review side effects with the patient. Note that loperamide is now available over-the-counter, but patients should be cautioned that side effects may be associated with excessive or long-term use.

- Encourage the patient to keep a record of bowel movements. After several days of treatment for diarrhea, the patient may become constipated.

- Teach patients with diarrhea to switch to a clear liquid diet, and increase daily intake to 3000 ml, but avoid full-strength fruit juices. If the patient can afford it, commercially available electrolyte solutions or products such as Gatorade may be helpful.

- Many cases of diarrhea are self-limiting. Teach patients to consult the physician if any of the following occur: diarrhea persists longer than 3 to 5 days; prescribed antidiarrhea medications are not affording relief; stools are especially foul-smelling or contain flecks of blood or large amounts of mucus; or the patient is unable to take in sufficient replacement fluids. Review symptoms of hypokalemia: muscle weakness, fatigue, anorexia, vomiting, drowsiness, irritability, and eventually coma and death. Review symptoms of hypochloremia: hypertonic muscles, tetany, and depressed respiration.

- Caution patients to avoid the use of alcohol.

- Tell patients to avoid driving or operating hazardous equipment if drowsiness develops. This may be dose related.

- Remind patients to keep the perianal area clean to avoid anal irritation, and to wash

Continued.

PATIENT CARE IMPLICATIONS — cont'd

hands carefully after defecating, to avoid spreading infectious organisms.

Drugs to relieve constipation

Drug administration

- Keep a record of bowel movements on all institutionalized, immobilized, or incapacitated patients. Prevention, early detection, and treatment of constipation are much easier and less time-consuming than treatment of severe constipation or impaction.

- Assess bowel sounds before administering any drug to relieve constipation. If bowel sounds are absent, withhold drug dose and notify the physician.

- Read orders and labels carefully. Many of these drugs have similar names. Be alert to the action of each component drug in combination products. For example, Colace contains the stool softener docusate sodium, while Peri-Colace contains docusate as well as casanthranol, a mild stimulant laxative.

- Bulk-forming agents are also sometimes prescribed to treat diarrhea, especially diarrhea associated with tube feedings. If given through a feeding tube, dilute with sufficient fluid to prevent clogging of the tube, and flush the tube with water after administration. Large-bore tubes are probably better suited to administration of these agents.

- Castor oil will not mix with a water-based diluent. Add a small amount of baking soda (less than one-fourth teaspoon) immediately before administering to cause the mixture to fizz, and the castor oil will be partially suspended in the juice for a minute or two. The patient may find it easier to drink this way. In an institution, the routine use of baking soda for this purpose must be cleared by the pharmacy or physician.

- Monitor the serum electrolytes of patients receiving lactulose, especially elderly patients.

- Lactulose is also used to treat elevated serum ammonia levels.

Patient and family education

- Teach patients that a daily bowel movement is not necessary for normal bowel function. Review with parents the inadvisability of encouraging laxative dependence in small children.

- To help keep a regular bowel schedule, teach patients to increase daily fluid intake to 2500 to 3000 ml. Be specific: if necessary, suggest that the patient drink a full (8 oz) glass of water before each meal, and a full glass with each meal.

- Instruct patients to increase daily dietary intake of bran in cereals and other foods; fruits and vegetables, fruit juices, or foods known by the patient to be stimulating to defecation (e.g., hot chocolate or coffee).

- Encourage patients to take regular exercise to aid in bowel regularity.

- Remind patients to use laxatives only as directed. Many laxatives are available without prescription. They may be misused or abused by patients who do not understand that increasing dependence on these drugs can develop with regular use.

- Review with patients using laxatives in preparation for gastrointestinal tract diagnostic procedures the importance of following the prescribed regimen. The major reason that many studies of the GI tract are poor in quality or need to be repeated is that the preparation of the gut or colon was inadequate.

- Tell women who are pregnant or lactating that drugs to relieve constipation should be used only under the direction of a physician.

- Teach patients that changes in bowel habits should be thoroughly evaluated by a physician.

- Special points about *bulk-forming* laxatives: Stir the prescribed dose into an 8 oz glass of fluid and drink the mixture while the drug is still suspended in the liquid. For best results, follow the first glass with a second full glass of water. Never take these drugs dry as they can cause obstruction. Swallow pills whole and do not chew them. Usually, use these agents regularly, 1 to 3 times daily, to promote regular defecation.

- Special points about *stimulant (irritant) cathartics*: Take daily doses at bedtime to promote regular defecation in the morning. Swallow enteric-coated preparations, such as bisacodyl, whole and do not chew them. Do not take bisacodyl preparations within 60 minutes of milk or antacids. Castor oil has

PATIENT CARE IMPLICATIONS—cont'd

an unpleasant taste. Before administering castor oil, assess whether the patient would like it mixed with fruit juice. Some patients prefer to take the castor oil "straight" with the juice as a follow-up so the taste of the juice is not ruined by the medication.

- Teach patients that keeping suppositories in the refrigerator will make them firmer and easier to insert.

- Note in Table 13.5 that many of these drugs change the color of urine. Forewarn patients about these changes.

- Special points about *saline cathartics:* Chill magnesium citrate before drinking to make it more palatable. Drink the entire prescribed amount at once for best results. Teach patients on a sodium-restricted diet to avoid saline cathartics. The saline cathartics are often used to eliminate parasites after anti-helminthic therapy because the trophozoites are not destroyed and can be examined in the laboratory.

- Special points about *mineral oil:* Warn patients that when mineral oil is used on a regular basis there may be leakage of the oil and/or fecal material from the anus. The oil will stain clothing. Suggest that the patient wear a perianal pad or incontinence shield to protect clothing and sheets. The regular use of mineral oil is associated with increased incidence of lipid pneumonia, especially in the elderly. Encourage patients always to sit upright when taking this medication. For long-term treatment of constipation, drugs other than mineral oil are preferred. Do not use mineral oil, or any oil-based substance, to lubricate the nose or mouth of immobilized patients, as they may inadvertently aspirate small amounts.

- Special points about *fecal softeners:* Explain the action of these drugs to patients. Many patients misunderstand their function, and expect defecation to occur a few hours following a single dose of fecal softener, just as it might occur after a stimulant-type drug. For best results, use fecal softeners on a daily, regular basis, as prescribed.

- Caution diabetic patients to monitor blood glucose levels carefully when taking *lactulose*, as the drug contains high concentrations of lactose and galactose.

- Warn patients taking *lactulose* that flatulence and abdominal cramps are common initially, but subside with continued therapy.

---

tially produce gas and cramps. Lactulose has been shown to reduce the incidence of fecal impaction in the elderly. However, elderly patients should have serum electrolytes monitored after treatment for more than 6 months.

SUMMARY

Tone and motility of the small intestine are stimulated by cholinomimetic drugs and inhibited by anticholinergic and antispasmodic drugs.

Stomach acid is neutralized by antacids and its secretion is inhibited by anticholinergic drugs and the H_2-histamine receptor antagonists.

Vomiting is best controlled prophylactically. Antihistamines and scopolamine are most effective for preventing motion sickness. Antidopaminergic drugs are most effective for preventing vomiting from chemotherapy and radiation therapy.

Diarrhea refers to bowel movements that are frequent, watery, and/or large. Lost fluids must be replaced, and, if appropriate, certain drugs can be given. Opioids act to decrease tone and motility of the intestine. Bismuth salts can absorb toxins and other irritants that cause diarrhea.

Constipation refers to bowel movements that are infrequent and difficult to pass. Laxatives promote defecation and are used to relieve constipation or to clean out the large intestine for examination. Classes of laxatives include bulk-forming, stimulant (irritant), saline (osmotic), wetting agent (softener), and lubricant. Chronic use of stimulant or saline laxatives can irritate the large intestine to the point that it becomes inactive. Chronic use of the lubricant mineral oil can create a deficiency of the fat-soluble vitamins A, D, E, and K.

STUDY QUESTIONS

1. What actions do cholinomimetic drugs have on the gastrointestinal tract? Name two cholinomimetic drugs that are used for their activity on the gastrointestinal tract.

2. What actions do anticholinergic drugs have on the gastrointestinal tract?
3. What three factors stimulate the secretion of stomach acid?
4. How do ulcers arise? What does the location of the ulcer indicate?
5. What do antacids do?
6. Name the major side effects of sodium bicarbonate, aluminum and calcium alkaline salts, and magnesium alkaline salts.
7. Why does cimetidine inhibit gastric acid secretion, whereas other commonly used antihistamines do not?
8. What are the three major pathways stimulating vomiting?
9. What are some nonmedicinal treatments of nausea and vomiting?
10. Describe the major differences in the effectiveness of the antihistamines versus the antidopaminergic drugs for types of nausea and vomiting.
11. What is diarrhea? Why is fluid and electrolyte replacement important?
12. What drugs are effective in treating diarrhea? What is their mechanism of action?
13. List the five classes of laxatives. How do they differ in the time for a laxative effect to be produced and in the type of stool produced?
14. Why is the continued use of the stimulant (irritant) cathartics of little help in establishing regular bowel habits?

SUGGESTED READINGS

Baines, M.: Nausea and vomiting in the patient with advanced cancer, part 2, J. Pain Symptom Managem. 3(2):81, 1988.

Baloh, R.W.: The dizzy patient, Postgrad. Med. 73(5):317, 1983.

Brucker, M.C.: Management of common minor discomforts in pregnancy: managing gastrointestinal problems in pregnancy part 3, J Nurse Midwife 33(2):67, 1988.

Clement, D.J., and Meyer, G.W.: Peptic ulcer disease—part I, Pract. Gastroenterol. 7(2):52, 1983.

Clement, D.J., and Meyer, G.W.: Peptic ulcer disease—part II, Pract. Gastroenterol. 7(3):36, 1983.

DiGregorio, G.J., and Fruncillo, R.H.: Antiemetics, Am. Fam. Physician 26(1):200, 1982.

DiPalma, J.R.: Drugs for nausea and vomiting of pregnancy, Am. Fam. Physician 28(4):272, 1983.

DuPont, H.L., and others: Prevention of travelers' diarrhea by the tablet formulation of bismuth subsalicylate, JAMA 257(10):1347, 1987.

Dupont, H.L., Edelman, R., and Kimmey, M.: Infectious diarrhea from A to Z, Patient Care 21(18):98, 1987.

Elliot, D.L., Watts, W.J., and Girard, D.E.: Constipation, Postgrad. Med. 74(2):143, 1983.

Enck, R.E.: Nausea control in hospice care, Caring 7(8):43, 1988.

Evreux, M.: Sucralfate versus alginate/antacid in the treatment of peptic esophagitis, Am. J. Med. 83(Suppl 3B):48, 1987.

Farmer, R.G.: Ten questions physicians most often ask about diarrhea, Consultant 21(5):23, 1981.

Graham, D.Y., Agrawal, N.M., and Rother, S.H.: Prevention of NSAID-induced gastric ulcer with misoprostol: Multicentre, double-blind, placebo-controlled trial, Lancet, December 3:1277, 1988.

Grant, M.: Nausea, vomiting, and anorexia . . . cancer treatment, Semin. Oncol. Nurs. 3(4):277, 1987.

Howry, L.B., Bindler, R.M., and Tso, Y.: Pediatric medications, Philadelphia, 1981, J.B. Lippincott.

Johnson, P.C., and others: Comparison of loperamide with bismuth subsalicylate for the treatment of acute travelers' diarrhea, JAMA 255(6):757, 1986.

Kallman, H.: Constipation in the elderly, Am. Fam. Physician 27(1):179, 1983.

Karb, V.B.: GI drugs: histamine antagonists, sucralfate and metoclopramide, J. Neurosci. Nurs., 20(3):201, 1988.

Lauritsen, K. and others: Effect of omeprazole and cimetidine on duodenal ulcer, New Engl. J. Med. 312(15):958, 1985.

Litwack, K., and Parnass, S.: Practical points in the management of postoperative nausea and vomiting, J. Post. Anesth. Nurs. 3(4):275, 1988.

Lovan, W.D.: Motion sickness, Am. Fam. Physician 28(6):117, 1984.

McKay, S., and Mahan, C.: Modifying the stomach contents of laboring women: why and how, success and risks, Birth 15(4):213, 1988.

Nanzo, M.: Dronabinol and nabilone easy cancer chemotherapy, Nursing 88 18(8):81, 1988.

Opencer, J.E., and Vervoren, T.M.: Gerontological pharmacology: a resource for health practitioners, St. Louis, 1983, The C.V. Mosby Co.

Peura, D.A., and Freston, J.W.: Evolving perspectives on parenteral H_2-receptor antagonist therapy, Am. J. Med. 83(Suppl 6A):1, 1987.

Rogers, A.I.: Answers to questions on diarrhea, Hosp. Med. 19(2):267, 1983.

Rosal-Grief, V.L.F.: Drug-induced dyskinesias, Am. J. Nurs. 82(1):66, 1982.

Rosenberg, J.M., and Kirschenbaum, H.L.: What to watch for with antacids, RN 45(9):54, 1982.

Sager, D.P., and Bomar, S.K.: Quick reference to intravenous drugs, Philadelphia, 1983, J.B. Lippincott.

Stevens, M.H.: The patient with vertigo: what to look for? how to treat? Modern Med. 51(5):108, 1983.

Stratton, J.W., and MacKeigan, J.M.: Treating constipation, Am. Fam. Physician 25(6):139, 1982.

Texter, Jr., E.C.: Famotidine: clinical applications of a new H_2-receptor antagonist, Am. J. Med. 81(Suppl 4B):1, 1986.

Wilson, D.E.: Antisecretory and mucosal protective actions of misoprostol: potential role in the treatment of peptic ulcer disease, Am. J. Med. 83(Suppl 1A):2, 1987.

Wolfe, M.M., and Soll, A.H.: The physiology of gastric acid secretion, New Engl. J. Med. 319(26):1707, 1988.

Zell, S., Carmichael, J.M., and Reddy, A.N.: Rational approach to long term use of H_2-receptor antagonists, Am. J. Med. 82:796, 1987.

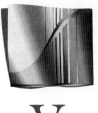

V

DRUGS AFFECTING THE CARDIOVASCULAR AND RENAL SYSTEMS

This section is divided into three groups: drugs affecting circulation and blood pressure (Chapters 14 through 17), drugs affecting the heart (Chapters 18 and 19), and drugs affecting the blood (Chapters 20, 21, and 22).

In Chapters 14 and 15, which cover the pharmacological aspects of circulation and blood pressure, the student will find drugs with the adrenergic mechanisms discussed in Chapter 10 as well as direct-acting vasodilators. Chapter 14 covers the sympathomimetic amines and their use as acute agents to maintain circulation and/or blood pressure. The vasodilators used principally to treat angina and those used chiefly to treat impaired peripheral vascular circulation are discussed. The chapter also presents the use of beta-adrenergic blockers and calcium channel blockers as antianginal drugs. Antihypertensive drugs are presented in Chapter 15 according to their mechanism of action. The importance of planned drug interaction in the treatment of chronic hypertension is reviewed in the chapter summary.

Chapters 16 through 22 are each devoted to a given area of therapeutics for which the pharmacological factors are distinctly focused on a physiological process. Here the chapter titles indicate the traditional scheme of presentation: diuretics, fluids and electrolytes, cardiac glycosides, antiarrhythmic drugs, drugs affecting blood clotting, drugs to lower blood lipids, and drugs to treat nutritional anemias.

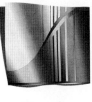

Drugs to Improve Circulation: Sympathomimetics for Shock and Vasodilators for Angina and Peripheral Vascular Disease

14

This chapter covers drugs used primarily to improve circulation: sympathomimetic drugs and selected vasodilators. Because beta blockers and calcium channel blockers have gained widespread use in the treatment of angina, these drug classes are also discussed.

Sympathomimetic drugs restore functions mediated through adrenergic receptors. These drugs are used primarily in the treatment of shock, a condition of poor tissue perfusion in which selective adjustment of cardiac or vascular function may prevent shock from becoming irreversible and progressing to death.

Vasodilators improve blood flow by increasing the size of the blood vessels. Vasodilation has been used in treating angina and peripheral vascular disease. Although some of the activity of vasodilators may be related to alpha or beta adrenergic receptors, most vasodilators work by a mechanism not well understood. As an understanding of these diseases progresses, the role of vasodilators is being reevaluated. Vasodilators used primarily as antihypertensive agents are discussed in Chapter 15.

Sympathomimetic Amines

DIRECT-ACTING SYMPATHOMIMETIC AMINES

Cardiovascular Actions

The rate of blood flow through a tissue is determined by the size of the blood vessels and the arteriovenous blood pressure differential across the tissue. The systolic blood pressure reflects the cardiac output, whereas the diastolic blood pressure reflects the resistance of the tissue vessels to flow. As discussed in Chapter 10, the sympathetic nervous system plays a major role in controlling cardiovascular function. Stimulation of the alpha adrenergic receptors of blood vessels causes vasoconstriction. On a systemic level, this vasoconstriction shows up as a higher blood pressure. Stimulation of the cardiac beta-1 receptors increases heart rate and force of contraction, resulting in an increased cardiac output. Stimulation of the beta-2 receptors, found primarily in the blood vessels of the skeletal muscle, causes vasodilation. Only in unusual circumstances, however, does systemic stimulation of the beta-2 receptors decrease blood pressure.

The net change in cardiovascular function produced by direct-acting sympathomimetic drugs depends on the degree of activity at the three adrenergic receptor subtypes.

Uses in Shock

Shock is a disruption of circulation. Frequently, the blood pressure is too low to force blood through vital tissues. Poor perfusion of the brain results in confusion or coma; poor perfusion of the kidney results in low urine output (less than 30 ml per hour); and poor perfusion of the skin makes the skin cold and clammy. In shock, the body has already activated the sympathetic nervous system to increase blood pressure. Fluid replacement or fluid addition is often the first choice in treating shock to overcome the decrease in the circulating volume caused by the constriction of the peripheral blood vessels. Selected use of direct-acting sympathomimetic amines is made in treating certain types of shock, raising blood pressure by increasing peripheral resistance (activation of alpha-1 adrenergic receptors) and/or by increasing cardiac output (activation of beta-1 adrenergic receptors).

Specific Drugs (Table 14.1)

Levarterenol (Norepinephrine, Levophed)

Mechanism of action. Norepinephrine, the neurotransmitter of the sympathetic nervous system,

Table 14.1 Sympathomimetic Drugs Used to Treat Hypotension and Shock

Generic name	Trade name	Administration/dosage	Comments
Dobutamine hydrochloride	Dobutrex*	INTRAVENOUS: *Adults*—2.5 to 10 µg/kg/min. A 12.5 to 25 mg/ml solution is made up and used.	To stimulate cardiac contractility in cardiogenic shock.
Dopamine hydrochloride	Intropin* Revimine†	INTRAVENOUS: *Adults*—1 ampule (40 mg of the chloride salt in 5 ml) is diluted in 250 ml (800 µg/ml) or 500 ml (400 µg/ml) of solution. Initial intravenous infusion is 2 to 5 µg/kg/min. Onset: 5 min. Duration: 10 min.	To maintain renal blood flow in shock with mild cardiac stimulation.
Epinephrine hydrochloride	Adrenalin chloride* EpiPenn Sus-Phrine	INTRAMUSCULAR, SUBCUTANEOUS, INTRAVENOUS: *Adults*—0.5 ml of a 1:1000 solution IM or SC followed by 0.25 to 0.5 ml of a 1:10,000 solution IV every 5 to 15 min. *Children*—0.3 ml of a 1:1000 solution IM. May be repeated every 15 min for 1 hr if necessary. Onset: minutes. Duration: 1 to 4 hr.	To treat anaphylactic shock.
Isoproterenol hydrochloride	Isuprel hydrochloride*	INTRAVENOUS: *Adults*—1 to 2 mg (5 to 10 ml) diluted in 5% dextrose and infused at a rate of 1 to 10 µg/min. Onset: minutes. Duration: 1 to 2 hr.	To stimulate cardiac contractility.
Levarterenol (norepinephrine) bitartrate	Levophed bitartrate*	INTRAVENOUS: *Adults*—2 to 8 ml of a 0.2% solution in 500 ml 5% dextrose and given by continuous infusion for desired response. Onset: immediate. Duration: minutes.	To maintain blood pressure in life-threatening situations.

*Available in Canada and United States.
†Available in Canada.

Table 14.1   Sympathomimetic Drugs Used to Treat Hypotension and Shock—cont'd

Generic name	Trade name	Administration/dosage	Comments
Mephentermine sulfate	Wyamine sulfate	INTRAVENOUS: *Adults*—600 mg to 1 Grn is diluted in 1 L 5% dextrose and given by continuous infusion to maintain pressure. Onset: immediate. Duration: 30 to 45 min.	To maintain arterial blood pressure during spinal, epidural, or general anesthesia.
Metaraminol bitartrate	Aramine	INTRAMUSCULAR, INTRAVENOUS: *Adults*—2 to 5 mg as a single intravenous injection or 200 to 500 mg diluted in 1 L 5% dextrose given by continuous infusion to maintain pressure. Alternatively, 5 to 10 mg given IM. Onset: 1 to 2 min. Duration: 20 to 60 min.	To maintain pressure during spinal, epidural, or general anesthesia.
Methoxamine hydrochloride	Vasoxyl*	INTRAMUSCULAR, INTRAVENOUS: *Adults*—5 to 20 mg in a single intramuscular dose or 2 to 5 mg given slowly IV. Onset: immediate. Duration: 60 min.	To maintain pressure during spinal and general anesthesia. To control hypotension after ganglionic blockade.
Phenylephrine hydrochloride	Neo-Synephrine hydrochloride*	ORAL, INTRAMUSCULAR, SUBCUTANEOUS, INTRAVENOUS: *Adults*—1 to 10 mg IM or SC; 0.25 to 0.5 mg given IV or 10 mg in 500 ml 5% dextrose infused slowly; 20 mg 3 times per day orally for orthostatic hypotension. Onset: minutes. Duration: 1 to 2 hr.	To maintain pressure during general and spinal anesthesia. To treat orthostatic hypotension and paroxysmal atrial tachycardia.

*Available in Canada and United States.

is a potent agonist of the alpha-1 and beta-1 adrenergic receptors when administered as the drug levarterenol. Levarterenol has relatively little effect on the beta-2 adrenergic receptors.

Levarterenol produces a potent peripheral vasoconstriction and inotropic response. Blood flow is shifted from the skin, visceral and renal vessels (where blood vessels are constricted) to the heart and brain (where blood vessels do not have alpha receptors). On administration, levarterenol initially raises blood pressure dramatically. The increase is quickly great enough to stimulate the baroreceptors in the aorta, thereby triggering reflex stimulation of the vagus nerve, a physiological pro-

THE NURSING PROCESS

SYMPATHOMIMETIC DRUGS

Assessment

Sympathomimetics are used primarily to treat shock. There are many causes for shock, including trauma, blood loss, burns, overwhelming sepsis, cardiac failure (cardiogenic shock), anaphylaxis, and extreme reactions to some drugs. The patient in shock appears pale, with clammy skin. The blood pressure is usually low or may even be absent: the pulse rate may be increased and thready. If alert, the patient may complain of fear of impending doom and may be anxious. The respiratory rate may be increased. Assessment should begin with a thorough patient examination. If the shock is of acute onset, the assessment needs to be rapid and must focus on the most important areas quickly. The nurse should assess the pulse, respirations, blood pressure, and level of consciousness. The patient should be observed and examined for obvious causes of the shock. The nurse should obtain and assess appropriate laboratory work, examples of which might be arterial blood gas concentrations, serum electrolyte concentrations, hematocrit and hemoglobin values, additional blood counts, and blood sugar concentrations.

Potential nursing diagnoses

Cardiac output altered: decreased (This may result in several collaborative problems, such as cardiac dysrhythmias and hypoxia.)

Altered tissue perfusion

Collaborative problems: fluid overload, metabolic acidosis, hypertension, fluid/electrolyte imbalance

Management

The treatment of shock usually begins while data collection continues. Vasopressors used to increase and maintain the blood pressure may be ordered immediately. An infusion control device and a microdrip infusion set should be used, if possible, for intravenous administration. The nurse should monitor the vital signs frequently, as often as every 5 minutes. Replacement fluids and blood are given if ordered. The fluid intake and output are checked and a Foley catheter inserted if needed. The level of consciousness is monitored and the patient attached to a cardiac monitor if necessary. Appropriate emergency care equipment, such as a suction machine and resuscitation equipment, should be readily available. The nurse should remain with the patient and maintain a calm external appearance. Additional data that might identify the underlying process causing the shock should be obtained and the patient observed for side effects, whether the result of shock or the medications being administered. For example, decreased perfusion of the kidneys resulting in decreased urinary output may be the result of shock itself or may be the result of side effects of the drugs being used. In addition to the physiological side effects of the medications, the nurse should look for symptoms such as fear and anxiety that may result from either the shock process or the drugs being administered. The patient and family should be kept informed of what is being done. Finally, the patient should be moved to an acute care setting as soon as the patient is stable. For further information about the treatment of shock and its causes, see appropriate textbooks of nursing.

---

cess called *reflex bradycardia* (slow heart rate). This results because stimulation of the vagus nerve releases acetylcholine. Since acetylcholine slows the heart, this vagal stimulation counteracts the direct stimulation of the heart by levarterenol. The net result of administering levarterenol is therefore an increase in blood pressure with a modest and variable change in heart rate but very strong contractions of the heart.

Administration and fate. Levarterenol is inef-

THE NURSING PROCESS—cont'd

Evaluation

Drugs to treat shock are considered successful if the blood pressure is maintained to provide adequate tissue perfusion. However, successful treatment of shock involves more than maintenance of blood pressure; there should also be successful treatment of the underlying condition and prevention of side effects resulting from the shock process or from the drugs that were used to treat the patient. Only a few vasopressors are used in self-management situations; most are used only in the acute care setting for the patient in shock. An example of a situation in which a patient would be prescribed a vasopressor for home use might be that of a patient with a long history of serious allergic reactions for whom the physician might prescribe epinephrine to be used in certain emergency situations. Before any patient on a vasopressor is discharged, the patient should be able to explain when the medication should be used and how to use it, to demonstrate the correct administration of the medication, and to explain the side effects that occur resulting from the medication; the patient also should know when emergency assistance should be sought. For further specific guidelines, see the patient care implications section at the end of the chapter.

fective when taken orally, being rapidly degraded in the stomach. This drug is administered intravenously, and if it does infiltrate the infusion site, the alpha adrenergic receptor antagonist phentolamine must be infiltrated in the area to counteract the profound vasoconstriction that may lead to tissue ischemia.

Levarterenol is rapidly inactivated by the liver. Like native norepinephrine, levarterenol is taken up and stored in sympathetic neurons identical to the native norepinephrine.

Side effects. Anxiety and a slow, forceful heartbeat are common side effects on administration of levarterenol. Some patients may develop a transient hypertension that is evidenced by a severe headache.

Uses and contraindications. Levarterenol is used to restore blood pressure in acute hypotensive states but only after blood volume has been restored. In the absence of adequate blood volume, tissue perfusion is inadequate after vasoconstriction by levarterenol in spite of increased blood pressure. Kidney perfusion in particular is poor. Levarterenol provides a temporary treatment when the brain or heart is compromised in shock. Levarterenol may be used immediately after cardiac arrest has been terminated to restore and maintain blood pressure.

Levarterenol is contraindicated for patients who have vascular thrombosis because the resulting vasoconstriction could cause tissue death. Levarterenol should not be used to raise blood pressure in patients anesthetized with a drug that sensitizes the heart to catecholamine-induced arrhythmias (Chapter 45).

Drug interactions. Administration of levarterenol to a patient taking an antidepressant drug (either a monoamine oxidase inhibitor or a tricyclic antidepressant) may cause a severe hypertensive response, since these drugs interfere with the degradation and reuptake, respectively, of norepinephrine. A persistent hypertensive response may be elicited if levarterenol is administered after an oxytocic drug during labor.

Epinephrine

Mechanism of action. Epinephrine is a potent agonist of the beta-1 receptors of the heart, increasing heart rate and force of contraction. This cardiac stimulation is achieved with an increase in the oxygen demand of the heart, which may not be tolerable in cardiac disease. Epinephrine also stimulates alpha receptors to cause vasoconstriction, particularly of the vessels in the skin, mucosa, kidney, and visceral organs. Epinephrine also stimulates beta-2 receptors, which alter blood flow because beta-2 receptors mediate vasodilation in the blood vessels in skeletal muscle. The overall response to intravenous administration of epinephrine is a marked increase in heart rate and force of contraction with little or no increase in blood pressure.

Administration and fate. Epinephrine is not active when given orally because it is rapidly inactivated by the gastric mucosa. Epinephrine is administered intramuscularly or subcutaneously. Epinephrine may be inhaled from a nebulizer for relief of bronchospasm. Intravenous administration of epinephrine must be done very slowly and cannot be done using one of the epinephrine suspensions. Intracardiac injection of epinephrine is a last step in attempting cardiac resuscitation when other measures have failed.

Epinephrine is rapidly degraded by the monoamine oxidase and catechol-O-methyltransferase of the liver and kidney. Epinephrine is unstable in alkaline solutions and when exposed to light or air. Pink or brown solutions should not be used.

Side effects. Fear and anxiety are side effects of epinephrine arising from stimulation of the central nervous system. Other side effects include a throbbing headache, dizziness, and pallor caused by vasoconstriction. Stimulation of skeletal muscle causes tremor and weakness, and stimulation of the heart causes palpitation. These effects are usually transient. Hyperthyroid and hypertensive patients are prone to an exaggerated hypertensive response to epinephrine. Cerebral hemorrhage and cardiac arrhythmias are serious reactions to epinephrine.

Uses and contraindications. Epinephrine, administered as soon as possible, is the drug of choice for treating anaphylactic shock. Anaphylactic shock is the result of massive histamine release caused by an allergic reaction and must be promptly treated. Histamine causes profound vasodilation and bronchial constriction. Epinephrine opposes the actions of histamine: epinephrine produces vasoconstriction, raising the blood pressure, and relaxes the bronchioles, restoring breathing. Epinephrine quickly reverses the edema of the larynx and the bronchospasm of anaphylactic shock.

Epinephrine may be administered systemically or by inhalation for relief of bronchospasm resulting from asthma or allergic reactions. Because epinephrine causes vasoconstriction, it is applied topically as a hemostatic agent. Epinephrine injection prolongs the action of local anesthetics by slowing their systemic absorption.

Epinephrine is contraindicated for patients under a general anesthetic that sensitizes the heart to catecholamines. Neither should patients with narrow-angle glaucoma receive epinephrine, nor should women in labor. Epinephrine must be used with extreme care in patients with cardiac arrhythmias, cardiovascular disease, hypertension, or hyperthyroidism. The hyperglycemic, hypoinsulinemic effects of epinephrine will interrupt control of diabetes mellitus.

Drug interactions. Epinephrine should not be administered simultaneously with isoproterenol because the combination can cause cardiac arrhythmias. Cardiac effects of epinephrine are also potentiated by tricyclic antidepressants, antihistamines, thyroxine, digitalis, and mercurial diuretics. A hypertensive response to epinephrine may be seen in patients receiving a monoamine oxidase inhibitor or oxytocin.

Isoproterenol (Isuprel)

Mechanism of action. Isoproterenol is a synthetic catecholamine that stimulates beta-1 and beta-2 adrenergic receptors but has little activity on alpha adrenergic receptors. Isoproterenol will therefore stimulate heart rate and cardiac output. At sufficient doses of isoproterenol, blood pressure will fall because activation of the beta-2 receptors of the blood vessels in skeletal muscle will shunt blood to the muscles and lower peripheral resistance. Smooth muscle, particularly the bronchial and gastrointestinal smooth muscle, is relaxed by isoproterenol. Isoproterenol is effective in treating bronchospasm when administered by inhalation.

Administration and fate. Isoproterenol is not very effective orally. Absorption from a sublingual site is unreliable. Isoproterenol may be given effectively subcutaneously, intramuscularly, or intravenously. The catechol-O-methyltransferase of the liver and other tissues is the major enzyme for degrading isoproterenol.

Side effects. Side effects of isoproterenol include palpitation, tachycardia (fast heart rate), headache, and flushing of the face. Sweating and mild tremors, nervousness, dizziness, and nausea may be experienced.

Uses. The principal use of isoproterenol is as a bronchodilator (see Chapter 25). Isoproterenol is infrequently used as a cardiac stimulant in heart block and in cardiogenic shock secondary to a myocardial infarction or septicemia.

Contraindications and drug interactions. Patients taking digitalis or otherwise disposed toward cardiac arrhythmias should not receive isoproterenol. Isoproterenol should not be administered with epinephrine because together they can induce severe cardiac arrhythmias.

Dopamine (Intropin)

Mechanism of action. Dopamine is a naturally occurring catecholamine capable of acting at alpha and beta adrenergic receptors as well as at its own specific dopaminergic receptors. Appropriate doses of this catecholamine can be selected such that cardiac output is increased while heart rate and mean blood pressure remain unchanged. The unusual and highly desirable property of dopamine is that renal blood flow is directly stimulated at these same doses. Renal function may therefore be maintained in patients being treated for shock as long as supportive therapy maintains adequate blood volume.

Administration and fate. Dopamine must be administered by constant intravenous infusion. Dopamine is rapidly taken up and stored or destroyed by tissues. The infusion rate must be meticulously adjusted to achieve the desired therapeutic results.

Side effects. Dopamine can cause tachycardia (fast heart rate), palpitation, nausea and vomiting, angina, headache, hypertension, and vasoconstriction. A reduction or discontinuance of dopamine infusion is usually sufficient to reverse side effects because dopamine has such a short plasma half-life. Leakage of dopamine around the infusion site must be avoided, but if extravasation does occur, the alpha adrenergic receptor antagonist phentolamine should be infused into the area to reverse vasoconstriction. Untreated extravasation can cause tissue death and sloughing.

Uses. Dopamine is the most widely used sympathomimetic amine for treating shock. The action of dopamine may be controlled by the rate of infusion. Dopamine is used primarily as a renal vasodilator to prevent renal failure in shock and secondarily to increase cardiac output. At low doses (0.5 to 2 μg/kg/min), dopamine acts exclusively on dopamine receptors in the renal arterioles to cause vasodilation. At higher doses (1 to 10 μg/kg/min), dopamine acts at cardiac beta-1 receptors to stimulate cardiac contractility. The beta-1 receptors controlling heart rate and the alpha receptors on blood pressure are not activated. At doses above these, dopamine causes the release of norepinephrine, thereby increasing heart rate and blood pressure.

Contraindications and drug interactions. Like the other sympathomimetic amines, dopamine is contraindicated for patients predisposed to cardiac arrhythmias. Dopamine is not stable in alkaline solutions and should not be made up in a sodium bicarbonate solution. Patients medicated with a monoamine oxidase inhibitor require a reduced dosage of dopamine. Tricyclic antidepressants potentiate the hypertensive action of dopamine. Dopamine should not be administered to women in labor receiving an oxytocic drug because a severe persistent hypertension may be produced. Patients receiving one of the general anesthetics that sensitize the heart to catecholamines may develop arrhythmias if dopamine is administered. Since dopamine dilates renal arteries, the action of diuretic drugs is potentiated.

Dobutamine (Dobutrex)

Mechanisms of action. Dobutamine, like dopamine, at low doses will selectively increase the contractility of the heart without increasing the heart rate. Dobutamine neither stimulates the dopamine receptors of the kidney blood vessels nor releases norepinephrine. At high doses, dobutamine does increase heart rate and conduction velocity (beta-1 adrenergic receptor) and stimulates beta-2 adrenergic receptors.

Administration and fate. Dobutamine has a plasma half-life of about 2 minutes and must be administered by continuous intravenous infusion. Dobutamine is rapidly metabolized to inactive compounds in the liver.

Side effects. Increased heart rate and blood pressure are the most frequent side effects and can be reversed by lowering the infusion rate. Palpitations, shortness of breath, angina, nausea, and headache are infrequent side effects of dobutamine.

Uses. Dobutamine improves cardiac output in patients with congestive heart failure with little effect on heart rate or systolic blood pressure.

Contraindications and drug interactions. Dobutamine is contraindicated for patients in whom the increased force of contraction would be dangerous, as in idiopathic hypertrophic subaortic stenosis. Drugs that may sensitize the heart to the inotropic effects of dobutamine include hydrocarbon inhalation anesthetics and the reserpine antihypertensives. Dobutamine may block the effectiveness of the beta adrenergic blockers and several other antihypertensive agents: guanadrel, guanethidine, and nitroprusside.

Methoxamine (Vasoxyl)

Methoxamine acts selectively to stimulate alpha adrenergic receptors. Methoxamine, which is administered intravenously or intramuscularly, increases blood pressure for 60 to 90 minutes. This vasopressor action is used to treat the hypotension of anesthesia during surgery, primarily for spinal anesthesia when the patient is conscious and aware of the unpleasant effects of hypotension. The increased blood pressure in a patient with normal blood pressure will cause a reflex slowing of the heart rate (reflex bradycardia). Use of this action is made in terminating episodes of paroxysmal supraventricular tachycardia.

Side effects of methoxamine include sustained hypertension with a severe headache. Goose flesh (pilomotor erection), desire to urinate, and vomiting are occasional side effects.

Like the other sympathomimetic vasopressors, methoxamine should be used with caution in patients with heart disease or hypertension and is potentiated in patients receiving oxytocic drugs, monoamine oxidase inhibitors, tricyclic antidepressants, or those patients under general anesthesia of the type that sensitizes the heart to catecholamines.

Phenylephrine (Isophrin, Neo-Synephrine)

Phenylephrine acts selectively to stimulate alpha adrenergic receptors. Phenylephrine is shorter in duration (20 to 50 minutes) than methoxamine, but otherwise the description of methoxamine and its uses, side effects, and drug interactions can be applied to phenylephrine.

Phenylephrine is used mainly as a nasal decongestant (Chapter 26); it is also used to dilate the pupil (Chapter 12). These actions result from stimulation of alpha adrenergic receptors.

INDIRECT-ACTING SYMPATHOMIMETIC AMINES

Mechanism and Uses

Indirect-acting sympathomimetic drugs cause the release of norepinephrine from sympathetic neurons. The norepinephrine so released accounts for the activity of the drug. Like methoxamine, the selective alpha adrenergic receptor agonist, the indirect-acting sympathomimetic amines are used primarily in treating the hypotension of spinal anesthesia. During spinal anesthesia, the sympathetic ganglia lying near the spinal cord may be affected, thereby disrupting sympathetic control of blood pressure. This is usually not to a degree that is life-threatening, but the sensation is unpleasant to the conscious patient. The indirect-acting sympathomimetic amines act directly on the postganglionic nerve terminals to release norepinephrine and restore blood pressure.

Specific Drugs (Table 14.1)

Ephedrine

Mechanism of action. Ephedrine is the prototype of the indirect-acting sympathomimetic amines, although ephedrine can be shown to have direct sympathomimetic actions at alpha and beta adrenergic receptors. Ephedrine, which has been isolated from several plants, has been used in Chinese medicine for 2000 years. The major use of ephedrine is as a bronchodilator (Chapter 25). Ephedrine, seldom used as a vasopressor, is not included in Table 14.1. The vasopressor response to ephedrine is primarily a result of cardiac stimula-

tion, increasing blood pressure through an increase in cardiac output.

Administration. Ephedrine is active administered orally, subcutaneously, intramuscularly, or intravenously for 4 to 6 hours.

Side effects. Ephedrine is a potent stimulant of the central nervous system, and this stimulation is the major side effect. Insomnia, agitation, euphoria, and confusion may be noted. Delirium and hallucinations can occur at high doses. As with other sympathomimetic drugs, headache, palpitation, nausea and vomiting, and difficulty in voiding may be side effects. Repeated administration of ephedrine decreases the effectiveness of the drug. This rapidly developing tolerance (tachyphylaxis) results from the depletion of stored norepinephrine.

Contraindications and drug interactions. Ephedrine should be used cautiously in patients with hypertension, hyperthyroidism, diabetes mellitus, or in males with prostate obstruction. The vasopressor response to ephedrine is potentiated by monoamine oxidase inhibitors, tricyclic antidepressants, and oxytocic drugs. Cardiac arrhythmias may be precipitated by ephedrine in the presence of digitalis or one of the general anesthetics that sensitize the heart to catecholamines.

Metaraminol (Aramine)

Metaraminol has both direct alpha adrenergic agonist activity and an indirect sympathomimetic activity. Metaraminol can deplete norepinephrine stores on repeated administration to cause tachyphylaxis.

Metaraminol is administered intravenously, intramuscularly, or subcutaneously, with the onset of action being 1 to 2 minutes, 10 minutes, and 15 to 20 minutes, respectively. The activity persists for 20 to 60 minutes. Larger doses are administered by intravenous infusion, and care must be taken to avoid leakage of the drug at the infusion site. Metaraminol produces a rise in diastolic and systolic blood pressure, but heart rate is usually decreased as a result of reflex bradycardia. The force of contraction of the heart is increased. Metaraminol is used clinically only to treat certain acute hypotensive states, as in spinal anesthesia.

Metaraminol does not have any pronounced central nervous system effects. Otherwise side effects, contraindications, and drug interactions are identical to those described for ephedrine.

Mephentermine (Wyamine)

Mephentermine is an indirect-acting sympathomimetic drug. The major effect of mephentermine is an increased blood pressure resulting from increased cardiac output and peripheral vasoconstriction. The effects of mephentermine persist for 30 to 60 minutes after subcutaneous administration and continue for up to 4 hours after intramuscular administration. Mephentermine can also be administered as a single intravenous dose. Mephentermine does not cause the tissue irritation characteristic of most vasopressor drugs.

Side effects of mephentermine are minimal and include drowsiness, weeping, incoherence, and, occasionally, convulsions. Contraindications and drug interactions are those described for other vasopressor drugs.

Vasodilator Drugs

DRUG THERAPY FOR ANGINA
Nature of Angina

Blood circulation to the heart. The heart has a very high requirement for oxygen and nutrients. These needs are met by the coronary circulation (Figure 14.1) because the heart muscle cannot use the blood pumped through its chambers. The right and left coronary arteries originate at the aorta as it leaves the heart. The left coronary artery divides into the circumflex branch and the anterior descending branch. The three major vessels of the heart are thus the right coronary artery, circumflex coronary branch of the left coronary artery, and the anterior descending branch of the left coronary artery. These vessels divide and subdivide to the capillaries that finally service the individual cardiac cells. Ordinarily, the heart receives an adequate supply of blood through these coronary vessels.

Angina pectoris. Angina pectoris, which literally means a choking of the chest, is the result of a temporary insufficiency of oxygen to the heart. The heart has a large requirement for oxygen and normally extracts maximum amounts of oxygen from the coronary circulation. The increased oxygen demands of the heart associated with increased work are normally met by increased coronary blood flow.

In about 1 of 50 American adults the coronary arteries become narrowed by fatty deposits that develop just underneath the inner lining of the vessel. This condition is called *coronary atherosclerosis.* The flow of blood in affected vessels is reduced, and the dependent heart muscle no longer receives an adequate blood supply. As the atherosclerosis worsens, the vascular system in the heart compensates by developing additional blood vessels (collateral circulation) to bypass the affected vessel. If a large

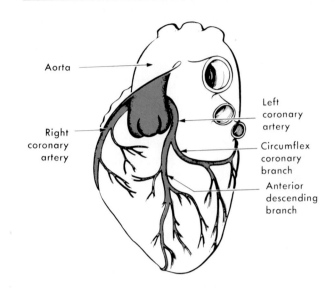

FIGURE 14.1   Coronary arteries. The three major coronary arteries are the right coronary artery and two branches of the left coronary artery: the circumflex coronary branch and the anterior descending branch. These arteries supply blood for heart muscle. Occlusion of one or more of these arteries can cause angina.

enough area of the heart muscle does not receive sufficient oxygen, pain results.

Anginal pain is a sudden, severe, and pressing pain that begins behind the breast bone and radiates up to the left shoulder and arm. Often this pain initially may be a feeling of acute chest discomfort; it also may be felt in the neck, jaw, teeth, arms or elbows, areas to which cardiac pain is physiologically referred. The pain gradually wears off when the person stops and rests. Drugs that increase the heart rate, decrease blood flow to the heart, or cause fluid retention may precipitate anginal episodes. Drugs shown to increase anginal attacks include bromocriptine, diazoxide, digitalis, dobutamine, dopamine, ergotamine, fluorouracil, hydralazine, indomethacin, minoxidil, nifedipine, prazosin, propranolol, thyroid hormone, and tolazoline.

Classic angina is often called *stable angina* or *exertional angina.* In classic angina the large coronary arteries are obstructed by atherosclerosis to the point that blood flow cannot increase to supply more oxygen required by increased work. Coronary atherosclerosis is the most common cause of angina.

Variant angina (Prinzmetal's angina) has a different origin than classic angina. Variant angina is caused by spasms of the large coronary arteries that result in obstruction of blood flow. These coronary spasms have no relationship to exercise and may occur at rest. Variant angina frequently has a daily rhythm, with episodes being more common in the morning. However, most patients with variant angina also have coronary atherosclerosis; in these patients anginal pain may also occur with exertion.

Unstable angina refers to angina that has a changing intensity. Pain comes at decreasing levels of exertion and often at rest. Patients who progress to unstable angina are the most likely to have a heart attack and should be medically reviewed immediately.

Therapeutic options. The treatment of angina depends on the recognition that the supply of oxygen to the heart does not meet the demand. Chronically, the demand for oxygen can be decreased by altering secondary factors that are known to affect the heart adversely. These factors include smoking, excess weight, hypertension, arrhythmias, anxiety, anemia, and lack of regular exercise. The major risk factors for the progression of atherosclerosis are cigarette smoking, hypertension, and high serum cholesterol levels. There is evidence that alteration of these risk factors in patients with angina secondary to coronary atherosclerosis does prolong life.

When angina is severe because of coronary atherosclerosis, *coronary artery bypass surgery* may be indicated. In this type of surgery one or more of the main coronary vessels is bypassed with a graft from the aorta to the lower end of the vessel. Replacement of vessels severely narrowed by atherosclerosis greatly improves coronary blood flow. About 70% of patients have no further angina, and another 20% have markedly reduced angina. A nonsurgical procedure for opening a coronary artery narrowed by atherosclerosis is *percutaneous transluminal coronary angioplasty (PTCA)*. A balloon catheter is inserted into the narrowed area. The balloon is inflated and the vessel is widened. The PTCA procedure is most effective in patients with severe angina who have only one coronary artery severely narrowed. This is usually the left coronary artery servicing the more worked left ventricle.

The pharmacological treatment of angina pectoris rests with three classes of drugs. The nitrates and nitrites primarily offer acute relief of angina. The beta adrenergic blocking drugs offer long-term relief in classic angina. The calcium channel blocking drugs are especially effective in relieving the coronary spasms of variant angina. These three drug classes are discussed in detail in the following section.

Nitrates and Nitrites (Table 14.2)

Mechanism of action. The nitrates and nitrites were originally believed to dilate the coronary blood vessels, thereby increasing blood flow in the heart. It is now understood that most patients with angina have atherosclerosis of the coronary vessels and that atherosclerotic vessels cannot dilate. Furthermore, insufficient oxygen (ischemia) is itself a potent vasodilator; thus the coronary vessels are already dilated during an anginal attack. The nitrates and nitrites act to dilate arterioles and veins in the periphery thereby lowering blood pressure. The reduced blood pressure means that the work of the heart is greatly reduced. This reduced workload lowers the oxygen demand of the heart. The nitrates and nitrites, particularly nitroglycerin, are the mainstay of antianginal medication. The nitrates and nitrites are most effectively used as needed to relieve an acute anginal attack. Patients who understand the factors that precipitate their own anginal attacks can take these medications prophylactically just before those activities.

Administration and fate. The organic nitrates will rapidly relieve anginal attacks when administered sublingually. These organic nitrates include nitroglycerin, isosorbide dinitrate, and erythrityl tetranitrate. All these drugs produce a general vasodilation by acting directly on blood vessels. The side effects of sublingual nitrates are also a result of the generalized vasodilation. These side effects include flushing, headache, and dizziness. The flushing is a result of the vasodilation in the "blush" area of the neck and face. The headache is a result of the pressure imposed by dilated blood vessels in the brain. The incidence of headaches decreases 2 to 3 weeks after initial therapy. The dizziness is the result of the generalized hypotension. The patient should sit or lie down to avoid fainting after taking one of these drugs. Indeed, if the hypotension is severe enough, a reflex increase in heart rate may occur. This will increase the cardiac work and make the pain worse.

The organic nitrates are frequently administered orally in large doses to provide prophylactic treatment for angina. Large doses are required because organic nitrates are rapidly degraded by the liver. However, when large doses of nitrates are given frequently, tolerance rapidly develops, reducing the duration of relief experienced. Studies are underway to determine whether intermittent or pulsed therapy might be best for prophylaxis. The degree of tolerance that is developed to nitrates seems to decrease with intermittent therapy.

Table 14.2   Drugs Prescribed for Relief of Angina Pectoris

Generic name	Trade name	Administration/dosage	Comments
NITRATES AND NITRITES			
Amyl nitrite	Amyl Nitrite	INHALATION: 0.18 to 0.3 ml. Onset: immediate. Duration: 5 min.	Relief of acute angina attacks. Glass pearls are crushed and the volatile liquid inhaled. Odor is unpleasant. Headache, orthostatic hypotension, and reflex stimulation of the heart usually occur.
Erythrityl tetranitrate	Cardilate*	SUBLINGUAL: 5 mg 3 times daily. ORAL, CHEWABLE: 10 mg 3 times daily. If required, the dose may be increased every 2 to 3 days up to 30 mg 3 times daily. Onset: 5 min for sublingual or chewable; 30 min for oral. Duration: 4 hr.	Prophylactic treatment to prevent anginal attacks. Hypotension, headaches, and tolerance to nitrates are possible side effects.
Isosorbide dinitrate	Iso-Bid Isordil* Isotrate Sorbitrate Various others	SUBLINGUAL: 2.5 to 5 mg. CHEWABLE: 5 to 10 mg. Onset: 2 to 5 min. Duration: 1 to 2 hr. ORAL: 5 to 30 mg 4 times daily. Timed-release forms, 40 mg 2 to 4 times daily. Onset: 15 to 30 min. Duration: 4 to 6 hr.	Relief of acute angina attacks. "Possibly effective" prophylactically, especially if taken in anticipation of a stressful situation. Hypotension is the side effect limiting the dose. "Possibly effective" as prophylactic treatment to prevent anginal attacks. Headache can be severe. Tolerance to nitrates may develop.
Nitroglycerin	Nitroglycerin Nitrostat	SUBLINGUAL: Tablets of 0.15 to 0.3 mg initially, up to 0.6 mg as required in individual patients. Individual dosages may be repeated at 5 min intervals, up to 3 tablets in 15 min. Peak action: 3 min. Duration: 10 min.	Direct-acting vasodilator. Drug of choice for angina pectoris. Take at the onset of acute anginal episodes or in anticipation of an episode, as before exercise or sex. Storage containers should be kept cool to prevent disintegration and airtight to prevent volatilization.
	Nitrolingual*	SUBLINGUAL: *Adults*—1 or 2 metered doses (400 μg/dose) on or under the tongue. Repeat at 5 min interval for relief of anginal attack.	A sublingual spray. Should afford relief after a total of 3 doses in a 15 min period.
	Niong Nitrong* Nitronet Klavikordal	ORAL, SUSTAINED-RELEASE: 2.5 to 6.5 mg every 8 to 12 hr. Onset: slow variable. Duration: 8 to 12 hr.	A prophylactic administration of nitroglycerin. Effectiveness of this mode of therapy is not established. Tolerance to nitrates may develop.

*Available in Canada and United States.
†Available in Canada only.

Continued

Table 14.2   Drugs Prescribed for Relief of Angina Pectoris—cont'd

Generic name	Trade name	Administration/dosage	Comments
NITRATES AND NITRITES			
Nitroglycerin—cont'd	Nitrogard* Nitrogard SR*	BUCCAL: 1 mg 3 times daily. May increase to 2 mg. Kept in mouth for several hours. May increase to 4 times daily or add extra for acute prophylaxis, but no more than every 2 hr.	Nitroglycerin is released from a polymer base over several hours to achieve a long duration of action.
Nitroglycerin ointment, 2%	Nitro-Bid* Nitrol* Nitrong*	TOPICAL: Initially 1 inch is spread over an area of skin. This is increased by half-inch increments as required. Absorption is improved by covering the area with plastic. Onset: 30 to 60 min. Duration: up to 3 hr.	A prophylactic administration of nitroglycerin. Effectiveness of this mode of therapy is not established. An excessive dose may cause a violent headache. Area of administration will be irritated and should be rotated. On terminating treatment, the area and frequency of administration should be reduced gradually over 4 to 6 weeks to prevent withdrawal reactions.
	Nitrodisc Nitro-Dur Transderm-Nitro	TOPICAL: Apply to a site free of hair. Do not apply to hands or feet. Change daily to a new site.	Nitroglycerin is impregnated into a polymer bound to an adhesive bandage. Drug is absorbed through the skin over 24 hours.
Pentaerythritol tetranitrate	Peritrate* Pentylan Naptrate	ORAL: Initially 10 to 20 mg 4 times daily. If required, dosage may be adjusted up to 40 mg 4 times daily. Onset: 30 min. Duration: 4 to 5 hr.	"Possibly effective" as prophylactic treatment for angina pectoris. Hypotension, headaches, and tolerance to nitrates are possible side effects. Tablets are taken 30 min before meals or 1 hr after and at bedtime. Taken on an empty stomach.
	Duotrate Pentritol Peritrate SA*	SUSTAINED RELEASE: 30 to 80 mg twice a day. Onset: 30 to 60 min. Duration: 12 hr.	"Possibly effective" as prophylactic treatment for angina pectoris. Hypotension, headaches, and tolerance to nitrates are possible side effects. Tablets are taken 30 min before meals or 1 hr after and at bedtime. Taken on an empty stomach.
BETA ADRENERGIC BLOCKING DRUGS FOR ANGINA			
Atenolol	Tenormin*	ORAL: 100 to 200 mg once daily.	Cardioselective. Little hepatic metabolism. Duration is increased in patients with severely impaired renal function.
Metoprolol	Apo-Metoprolol† Betaloc† Lopressor* Novometoprol	ORAL: 50 mg 3 or 4 times daily. For prophylaxis after a myocardial infarction: 100 mg twice daily.	Cardioselective. Extensive first-pass metabolism. Bioavailability is increased by food.
Nadolol	Corgard*	ORAL: Initially 40 mg daily. May increase dose by 40 to 80 mg every 3 to 7 days. Usual final dose is 80 to 240 mg, administering once a day.	Nonselective. Not metabolized and mainly excreted in the urine. Dosage interval is increased in patients with renal impairment.

*Available in Canada and United States.
†Available in Canada only.

Table 14.2   Drugs Prescribed for Relief of Angina Pectoris—cont'd

Generic name	Trade name	Administration/dosage	Comments
BETA ADRENERGIC BLOCKING DRUGS FOR ANGINA—cont'd			
Propranolol	Inderal*	ORAL: 10 to 20 mg 3 or 4 times daily. Increase as required. Final dose is usually 160 to 240 mg daily, in four doses. Some patients can take twice a day.	Nonselective. Well absorbed. Extensive first-pass metabolism.
Timolol	Apo-Timol† Blocadren	ORAL: 10 to 30 mg twice daily. Prophylaxis for myocardial infarction is 10 mg twice daily.	Nonselective. Well absorbed. Extensive first-pass metabolism.
CALCIUM CHANNEL BLOCKING DRUGS			
Diltiazem	Cardizem	ORAL: 60 mg every 6 hr.	Well absorbed. Continue nitrate therapy.
Nicardipine	Cardene	ORAL: *Adults*—20 mg 3 times daily, adjusted for need and tolerance.	New calcium channel blocker for treating angina and hypertension.
Nifedipine	Procardia Adalat* Apo-Nifed†	ORAL: Initially 10 mg 3 times daily. If required, increase dose every 3 to 7 days. Maximum dosage is 180 mg daily.	Well absorbed. Completely metabolized. Continue nitrate therapy. More selective for smooth muscle than for cardiac muscle.
Verapamil	Calan Isoptin*	ORAL: 240 to 480 mg daily in 3 or 4 divided doses.	Well absorbed. Extensive first-pass metabolism. In patients with cirrhosis, half-life is increased and dose should be lowered by 70%. Continue nitrate therapy.

*Available in Canada and United States.
†Available in Canada only.

Specific Nitrates and Nitrites

Nitroglycerin

Nitroglycerin is considered the drug of choice for angina. When nitroglycerin is taken sublingually, its effect begins in 30 seconds, is maximal in 3 minutes, and lasts for about 10 minutes. A drawback to nitroglycerin is that it decomposes when exposed to light or heat. Nitroglycerin can also volatilize from the tablets, which therefore must be kept in airtight containers. It should be noted that nitroglycerin will sting when placed under the tongue, and this can be used as an indication that the drug is still present.

Several dosage forms for nitroglycerin have become available. A variation of the sublingual form is nitroglycerin lingual aerosol, which allows the drug to be sprayed, in a metered form, on or under the tongue. The aerosol is a substitute for the sublingual tablets in the acute relief of an anginal attack. Extended release buccal forms are intended for prophylactic use. Extended release capsules and tablets have up to 10 times the sublingual dose. These are swallowed and are effective for 8 to 12 hours. Nitroglycerin is very lipid soluble and probably enters the body from the gastrointestinal tract through the lymphatics rather than the portal blood.

Another route of administration for nitroglycerin is through the skin. A measured amount of nitroglycerin ointment is spread on a nonhairy part of the body and held in place with plastic wrap taped over the area. This route of administration is said to produce relief for up to 3 hours. Nitroglycerin is also available impregnated in a polymer bonded to an adhesive bandage. This disc is applied to the skin and nitroglycerin is absorbed through the skin (transdermally) over 24 hours. The unit should be applied to a site free of hair, and the bandage should be placed at a new site each time to avoid irritation.

Nitroglycerin is administered intravenously in acute heart failure. Nitroglycerin can reduce the myocardial ischemia that results when the left side of the heart is failing. Because blood is not being pumped out effectively, pressure builds in the left ventricle. Pulmonary edema results since that is where the blood backs up. Nitroglycerin is an effective dilator of the coronary arteries and therefore allows more oxygenated blood to reach the troubled heart muscle. The heart is able to perform better, and the symptoms of acute heart failure are relieved.

Amyl nitrite

Amyl nitrite is the only nitrite used to treat angina. It is a volatile liquid packaged in an easily crushed vial with a woven cover and is self-administered by inhalation. Amyl nitrite is effective 30 seconds after inhalation and lasts for 3 to 5 minutes. Amyl nitrite has an unpleasant odor, is expensive, and is conspicuous to use. The side effects of headache, orthostatic hypotension, and reflex tachycardia can be pronounced. For these reasons amyl nitrite is seldom used. The "rush" felt when amyl nitrite is inhaled has caused this drug to be abused.

Erythrityl tetranitrate

Erythrityl tetranitrate is the longest-acting of the sublingual or chewable organic nitrates. This drug becomes effective in 5 minutes, and its effects last for 4 hours. This is a long duration compared to nitroglycerin or even isosorbide dinitrate, and

therefore erythrityl tetranitrate is better for prophylactic use than for relief of acute attacks. Erythrityl tetranitrate is also available for oral administration.

Isosorbide dinitrate

Isosorbide dinitrate is another organic nitrate that can be taken sublingually or chewed. It is effective in 2 to 5 minutes and can act for 1 to 2 hours.

Pentaerythritol tetranitrate

Pentaerythritol tetranitrate has not been proved effective for the prophylactic treatment of angina.

Beta Adrenergic Blocking Drugs
(Table 14.2)

Mechanism of action. Beta adrenergic blocking drugs decrease the oxygen requirements of the heart by reducing the workload of the heart. Blocking the beta-1 adrenergic receptors of the heart decreases the heart rate and the force of contraction, and a decrease in blood pressure follows. These actions also benefit coronary circulation by decreasing the resistance in the coronary circulation. However, beta adrenergic blocking drugs are not vasodilators.

As discussed in Chapter 10, there are two subclasses of beta receptors: beta-1 and beta-2. The cardiac selective beta adrenergic blocking drugs are relatively selective for the beta-1 receptors. However, this selectivity is diminished at higher doses. There is no evidence that any particular beta adrenergic blocking drug is better than another in the management of angina. Patients with asthma, diabetes, or peripheral vascular disease are better able to tolerate the selective beta-1 adrenergic blocking drugs. The development of new beta adrenergic blocking drugs has been explosive. Beta-1 selective drugs include acebutolol, atenolol, and metoprolol. Nonselective drugs include oxprenolol, pindolol, propranolol, nadolol, sotalol, and timolol.

Administration. Beta adrenergic blocking drugs have become widely used in the management of classic angina. A beta adrenergic blocking drug is commonly prescribed as prophylactic therapy, and nitroglycerin is prescribed for anginal attacks. Long-term therapy reduces the frequency of anginal pain and decreases the requirements for nitroglycerin. The effective dose is highly individual for each patient. One index of dosage is the decrease in resting heart rate. In patients who have severe angina, enough medication may be given to lower the resting pulse to 50 to 60 beats per minute. If gastro-

THE NURSING PROCESS

ANTIANGINAL DRUGS

Assessment

Patients with angina pectoris have a primary single complaint: chest pain. In the majority of patients pain is associated with exertion, exposure to cold, stress, eating a heavy meal, or other activities; a few patients have no associated cause. The nurse should obtain a thorough patient assessment, focusing on the subjective and objective signs. The pulse, respiration, blood pressure, and level of consciousness should be determined. The history relevant to the onset and duration of the pain should be taken, with questions asked about previous similar episodes and treatments. A detailed description of the nature and location of the pain should be obtained with an electrocardiogram and appropriate laboratory work, including serum enzyme concentrations. The degree of patient distress and previous history of cardiac problems will also determine the amount and focus of assessment. When there is doubt as to the cause of chest pain, the usual practice is to treat the patient as if a myocardial infarction had occurred.

Nursing diagnoses

Potential altered health maintenance related to insufficient knowledge about prescribed antianginal drugs

Potential for injury related to orthostatic hypotension secondary to vasodilator therapy

Management

Once the diagnosis of angina pectoris is made and a myocardial infarction is ruled out, the treatment is with one or more of the nitrates or nitrites, with a beta adrenergic antagonist, or with a calcium channel blocking drug, and the patient is observed and monitored for additional angina attacks. Instruction is begun about the prescribed drugs, and the patient and family are aided in identifying stresses that may precipitate attacks and in planning possible ways to decrease or alleviate these stresses. Additional measures that may be prescribed include losing weight, stopping smoking, controlling blood pressure, and exercising regularly. Appropriate referrals may be to such members of the health care team as the dietitian, the local heart association, or the visiting nurse association. For additional information about the treatment of patients with angina pectoris and other forms of heart disease, see appropriate textbooks of nursing.

Evaluation

The drugs used to treat angina are successful if the pain is relieved and the patient experiences no side effects resulting from drug therapy. The drugs do not halt the progression of disease. Before discharge, the patient should be able to explain when and how to take the medications prescribed, to describe the side effects resulting from the drugs and how to treat them, and to explain what to do if drug therapy does not relieve the symptoms, how to correctly store the medication, and how to test for its continued effectiveness. In addition, the patient should be able to explain adequately why and how other therapies should be implemented, including weight loss, exercises, stopping smoking, and the treatment of hypertension or other medical problems. Finally, for some patients it may be appropriate to evaluate whether the family or close friends are able to explain how to administer a medication (e.g., sublingual nitroglycerin) if the patient were to be unable to do it. For additional specific guidelines, see the patient care implications section at the end of this chapter.

intestinal side effects such as nausea, cramping, or diarrhea occur, taking the drug with meals may lessen these symptoms.

Side effects and contraindications. The most common side effects of beta adrenergic blockers are fatigue and mental lassitude. Depression, nightmares, and psychosis are more severe CNS side effects sometimes seen. Peripheral vasoconstriction may cause cold hands or feet. Sexual dysfunction, including impotence, is a side effect, especially of propranolol and timolol. Beta adrenergic blocking drugs are contraindicated for patients with severely impaired heart or circulatory function (e.g., congestive heart failure, heart block, severe sinus bradycardia, and Raynaud's phenomenon). It is important to note that withdrawal of beta adrenergic blocking drugs should be gradual. Sudden withdrawal can lead to unstable angina, a myocardial infarction, or even sudden death.

Adverse effects of beta adrenergic blocking drugs include bronchospasm, hypoglycemia, and impairment of peripheral circulation. The bronchospasm arises from blockade of the beta-2 receptors of the bronchi. Hypoglycemia results from the inhibition of glycogen breakdown, a process normally stimulated by epinephrine and norepinephrine. Dilation of peripheral blood vessels is mediated by beta-2 receptors. These adverse effects are less common with the beta-1 selective adrenergic blocking drugs.

Beta adrenergic blocking drugs after acute myocardial infarction. Several studies have shown that administration of a beta adrenergic blocking drug after a heart attack reduces the incidence of sudden death by as much as 40%. In addition to reducing the workload of the heart, other actions of beta adrenergic blocking drugs such as the antiarrhythmic and antiplatelet functions may be important.

Specific beta adrenergic blocking drugs. There are now many beta-blockers on the market. Those that have been specifically approved for use as antianginal agents are atenolol, metoprolol, nadolol, and propranolol. Metoprolol, propranolol, and timolol have been approved for prophylaxis against myocardial reinfarction.

Atenolol (Tenormin). Atenolol is a long-acting, cardioselective beta adrenergic blocker. Poorly absorbed from the gastrointestinal tract, the drug is not metabolized but excreted unchanged in the urine. The time between doses must be increased in patients with impaired renal function.

Metoprolol (Lopressor, Betaloc). Metoprolol is a short-acting, cardioselective beta adrenergic blocker. It is well absorbed from the gastrointestinal tract and readily metabolized by the liver.

Nadolol (Corgard). Nadolol is a long-acting, nonselective beta adrenergic blocker. It is not well absorbed from the gastrointestinal tract and up to one fourth of the dose may be excreted in the feces. Absorbed drug is excreted unchanged in the urine. Patients with renal failure should be given the drug less frequently.

Propranolol (Inderal). Propranolol, a nonselective beta adrenergic blocker, is the oldest of the clinically used beta adrenergic blocking drugs. It is well absorbed orally, but it is readily metabolized by the liver.

Timolol (Blocadren, Apo-Timol). Timolol is a short-acting nonselective beta adrenergic blocker. It is well absorbed from the gastrointestinal tract and metabolized by the liver.

Calcium Channel Blocking Drugs
(Table 14.2)

Mechanism of action. Calcium channel blocking drugs, also called calcium antagonists or calcium entry blockers, are a class of drugs currently used in the treatment of angina, certain arrhythmias (Chapter 19), and hypertension (Chapter 15). Skeletal muscle has extensive stores of calcium in the sarcoplasmic reticulum, but both cardiac muscle and vascular smooth muscle lack these stores and must depend on the influx of extracellular calcium for the maintenance of contraction, or tone. The calcium activates the contractile mechanism and must be removed for relaxation. The calcium channel blockers interfere with the initial influx of calcium through specific calcium channels on the cell surface. The calcium channel blockers decrease the oxygen requirements of the heart through several actions. They reduce peripheral vascular resistance by a systemic vasodilation. This means that the workload of the heart is decreased. Calcium channel blockers dilate the coronary vessels by inhibiting contractility of coronary smooth muscle. This action is especially important for relief from variant angina, in which coronary spasm prevents blood flow. The calcium channel blockers also reduce the cardiac contractility (negative inotropy), which decreases the oxygen requirement of the heart. These agents increase coronary blood flow through coronary vasodilation more selectively than they inhibit cardiac contractility. Without this selective preference, the calcium channel blockers would not be clinically useful because they would overly compromise cardiac function. The various drugs of this class differ in the degree of selectivity in coronary vasodilation versus decreased cardiac contractility.

Side effects. In general, the side effects of calcium channel blockers are mild. Headaches and constipation are the most common ones. Since the calcium channel blockers are a recent class of drugs, their medical use is being investigated. These drugs are especially indicated for relief of the coronary spasm of variant angina. However, it is becoming clear that there is a varying degree of coronary spasm even in classic angina. Patients with asthma, diabetes, and peripheral vascular disease, who cannot tolerate beta adrenergic blockers, can benefit from calcium channel blockers.

Drug interactions. There are several important interactions of calcium channel blockers with other drugs. Beta-blockers and calcium channel blockers, if given concurrently, may cause cardiac problems. These problems include a conduction block or arrhythmias and hypotension. Diltiazem and verapamil may inhibit the liver metabolism of several drugs, including carbamazepine, cyclosporine, quinidine, theophylline, and valproate. This may allow these drugs to reach toxic levels in the body. Digitalis glycosides may also accumulate in the presence of calcium channel blockers, resulting in excessive slowing of the heart or a heart block. Disopyramide depresses the force of the heartbeat (negative inotropic effect) and should not be administered within 48 hours of a calcium channel blocker.

Specific calcium channel blocking drugs. Three calcium channel blocking drugs have recently been approved and are used in the treatment of angina and hypertension: verapamil (Calan, Isoptin), diltiazem (Cardizem), and nifedipine (Aldalat, Procardia). In addition, nicardipine (Cardene) has been approved and isradipine (DynaCirc) and nitrendipine (Baypress) are expected to be released shortly. Nimodipine (Nimotop) has been approved for treating cerebral vasospasm.

Verapamil (Calan, Isoptin). Verapamil depresses the atrioventricular node (negative chronotropy and negative dromotropy), an action that makes it a useful antiarrhythmic drug (Chapter 19). A slowing of the heart rate (bradycardia) is common. Verapamil does not cause a pronounced decrease in blood pressure, and therefore reflex sympathetic activity to stimulate the heart is minimal. The slowing of the heart rate and the decrease in blood pressure reduce the oxygen requirements of the heart. Verapamil increases coronary blood flow, which increases the oxygen available to the heart.

Although verapamil is readily absorbed, it is rapidly metabolized by the liver. It must be taken three or four times a day. In the blood, verapamil is 90% bound to albumin. Verapamil is generally well tolerated, with constipation being the most common side effect. Verapamil is contraindicated for patients with atrioventricular conduction disturbances or congestive heart failure.

Nifedipine (Adalat, Procardia). Nifedipine is a potent coronary and peripheral vasodilator. The cardiodepressant effect is minor because nifedipine does not depress the sinoatrial or atrioventricular nodes and because reflex sympathetic activity caused by hypotension counteracts its negative inotropic effect. However, if nifedipine is combined with a beta adrenergic blocking drug, there is risk of severe hypotension and heart failure.

Nifedipine is well absorbed orally. It is completely metabolized before excretion in the urine. The side effects most frequently reported are secondary to peripheral vasodilation: headaches, hypotension, flushing, tingling in the extremities, and edema.

Diltiazem (Cardiazem). Diltiazem produces cardiac effects similar to those of verapamil. The incidence of dizziness, headache, and hypotension is less with diltiazem than with nifedipine and verapamil.

Diltiazem is well absorbed orally and metabolized. Only 35% of metabolites is excreted in the urine. The remainder is excreted in the feces.

PERIPHERAL VASCULAR DISEASE AND VASODILATOR DRUGS
Vasospastic Disorders

Blood flow to the arms and legs, particularly the hands and feet, can be limited by peripheral vascular disease. Basically, the blood vessels may be narrowed by arteriosclerosis or by spasm of the vessels (vasospasm). If the vessel narrowing is a result of arteriosclerosis, vasodilator drugs will be of little value. Vasodilator drugs may worsen the condition because vessels narrowed by arteriosclerosis will not dilate; adjacent vessels will dilate and shunt the blood away from the occluded area. The occluded vessel therefore has its blood flow reduced, not increased, by vasodilator drugs. On the other hand, if the narrowing of the vessel is a result of vasospasm, drugs will be of benefit.

Raynaud's disease is the classic vasospastic disease in which primarily the fingers and toes are affected. In Raynaud's disease the blood vessels of the digits are readily thrown into spasm by cold or emotion, and turn blue or white. Warming restores blood flow. Currently, the most successful drug treatment of Raynaud's disease is reported with two drugs that have been used to treat hypertension: reserpine and guanethidine. These drugs interfere with sympathetic innervation. Reserpine depresses sympathetic tone by depleting stored norepinephrine in the neurons. Guanethidine acts at the sympathetic neuron by blocking the release of norepinephrine as well as depleting norepinephrine stores. These drugs and their side effects are discussed fully in Chapter 15.

Unfortunately, a large number of "vasodilator" drugs advertised for treating peripheral vascular spasm are of doubtful clinical value. These drugs include cyclandelate, isoxsuprine, niacin, nylidrin, papaverine, and tolazoline.

Impaired Cerebral Blood Flow

Vasodilator drugs are sometimes prescribed to improve blood flow in the brain, particularly in elderly patients with arteriosclerosis of cerebral vessels who have suffered strokes or show signs of mental impairment. The problem is cerebral ischemia: insufficient oxygen to areas of the brain. Controlled medical trials are showing that this drug therapy is of little value. There is some medical opinion that vasodilator drugs may make the situation worse by shunting blood away from the unreactive, damaged vessels to areas with adequate blood flow already, as described for peripheral vascular insufficiency resulting from arteriosclerosis. Cyclandelate, ergot mesylates, and papaverine are sometimes prescribed to improve cerebral blood flow. There is no evidence that these drugs alter the progression of cerebral arteriosclerosis. They may improve some symptoms on a short-term basis.

Specific Drugs (Table 14.3)

Cyclandelate (Cyclospasmol)

Cyclandelate acts directly on vascular smooth muscle to cause relaxation. In the laboratory, cyclandelate is a more effective vasodilator than papaverine, but the clinical effectiveness of cyclandelate is considered doubtful. Side effects include belching and heartburn, flushing, headache, weakness, and an increased heart rate.

Ergot mesylates (Hydergine)

Ergot mesylates produce vasodilation in contrast to the ergot alkaloids, which produce vasoconstriction (Chapter 53). Ergot mesylates are of definite value in treating brain disease secondary to hypertension, but the benefit is related to the fall in blood pressure. These alkaloids act centrally to reduce vascular tone and slow heart rate. They act peripherally to block alpha adrenergic receptors. These alkaloids are available in a sublingual dosage form. Sublingual irritation, nausea, and gastrointestinal upset are the side effects. The dihydrogenated ergot alkaloids can markedly reduce heart rate

through their central effect of lowering sympathetic tone.

Isoxsuprine (Vasodilan, Vasoprine)

Isoxsuprine was originally thought to stimulate beta receptors, but its vasodilating action is not blocked by drugs that are antagonists of the beta receptors. Clinical tests have not demonstrated any usefulness for isoxsuprine. Side effects include flushing, hypotension, dizziness, an increased heart rate, and, occasionally, a rash.

Nicotinyl alcohol (Ronigen, Rycotin)

Nicotinyl alcohol has been used as a vasodilator but without good evidence of clinical effectiveness. This drug causes a pronounced flushing, postural (orthostatic) hypotension, and gastrointestinal upset. It can also cause a rash.

Nimodipine (Nimotop)

Nimodipine is a calcium channel blocker approved to treat cerebral vasospasm following subarachnoid hemorrhage. This action alleviates the cerebral ischemia that can follow a stroke, and, by maintaining blood flow, protects the brain from deterioration. This use of a calcium channel blocker is seen as the beginning of a new therapeutic approach for the treatment of various neurologic disorders. Those for neurologic use cross the blood-brain barrier.

Nylidrin (Arlidin)

Nylidrin is the classic example of a drug that stimulates blood flow in muscle. The rationale is to stimulate the beta receptors of the blood vessels to produce vasodilation. However, muscle blood vessels, not the blood vessels of the skin, have beta receptors, so the approach is of little value in vasospastic disorders of the digits. The beta-blocking drug propranolol does not entirely reverse this stimulation, so nylidrin is believed to also act directly on smooth muscle. Side effects attributed to nylidrin include trembling, nervousness, weakness, dizziness, palpitations, and nausea and vomiting.

Papaverine (various trade names)

Papaverine relaxes smooth muscle. In large doses papaverine also depresses cardiac muscle, slowing conduction and prolonging the refractory period. Papaverine has long been used as a smooth muscle relaxant for ischemia of the brain, periphery, or heart. As with the other vasodilator drugs, there is little good evidence that papaverine improves peripheral vascular circulation. Side effects

Table 14.3   Drugs Prescribed for Vasodilation

Generic name	Trade name	Administration/dosage	Comments
Cyclandelate	Cyclospasmol*	ORAL: 300 to 400 mg 4 times daily. Can be decreased gradually to 100 to 200 mg 4 times daily.	A direct vasodilator for use in vasospastic disorders. May cause gastrointestinal disturbances.
Ergot mesylates	Hydergine*	SUBLINGUAL, ORAL: 1 mg 3 times daily.	Can cause marked bradycardia. Relieves symptoms in hypertensive brain disease by lowering blood pressure.
Isoxsuprine	Vasodilan* Vasoprine	ORAL: 10 to 20 mg 3 to 4 times daily. INTRAMUSCULAR: 5 to 10 mg 2 to 3 times daily.	A direct-acting vasodilator. No proved use.
Nicotinyl alcohol	Roniacol† Ronigen Rycotin	ORAL: 50 to 100 mg 3 times daily. TIMED-RELEASE: 300 to 400 mg every 12 hr.	A direct vasodilator that causes pronounced blushing. Gastrointestinal disturbances, tingling sensation, and rashes are side effects. Use has not been proved effective for any vasospastic disorders.
Nimodipine	Nimotop	ORAL: Adults—60 mg every 4 hr, beginning within 4 days after the subarachnoid hemorrhage and continuing for 21 days.	Calcium channel blocker for treatment of cerebral vasospasm following subarachnoid hemorrhage.
Nylidrin hydrochloride	Arlidin* PMS Nylidrin†	ORAL: 3 to 12 mg 3 to 4 times daily.	Stimulates beta adrenergic receptors and also directly dilates vessels. May cause dizziness, tachycardia, and hypotension.
Papaverine hydrochloride	Many trade names	ORAL: 100 to 300 mg, 3 to 5 times daily. TIMED-RELEASE: 150 mg every 12 hr. Can give up to 150 mg every 8 hr or 300 mg every 12 hr. INTRAVENOUS: 30 to 120 mg, over 1 to 2 min. INTRAMUSCULAR: 30 to 120 mg.	Depresses heart. Relaxes smooth muscle directly, particularly of the large blood vessels. Use is to relieve smooth muscle spasm in vascular disease or colic, but its effectiveness has not been proven.
Pentoxifylline	Trental*	ORAL: 400 mg 3 times daily, with meals.	Not a vasodilator. Reduces blood viscosity and improves red blood cell flexibility to improve blood flow.
Tolazoline hydrochloride	Priscoline*	TIMED-RELEASE: 80 mg every 12 hr. INTRAMUSCULAR, SUBCUTANEOUS, INTRAVENOUS: 10 to 50 mg 4 times daily.	A direct-acting vasodilator. May relieve vasospastic disorders.

*Available in Canada and United States.
†Available in Canada.

of papaverine can include flushing of the face, malaise, gastrointestinal upset, and headache. Other reported side effects include excess perspiration, loss of appetite, increased heart rate, and increased depth of respiration. Rarely, a hypersensitivity reaction involving the liver is seen. Symptoms of the liver damage may include jaundice, eosinophilia, and altered results of liver function tests.

Tolazoline (Priscoline)

Tolazoline is an alpha adrenergic antagonist that has an additional direct vasodilating effect. In theory, a drug that blocks the action of norepi-

THE NURSING PROCESS

VASODILATOR THERAPY IN PERIPHERAL VASCULAR DISEASE

Assessment

Patients with signs and symptoms of decreased peripheral blood flow come to the hospital with a variety of symptoms, some of which may be decreased or absent peripheral pulses, complaints of decreased or altered sensation in the extremities, ulcers on the extremities, poor healing of local injuries, absence of hair on the feet and toes, coolness to touch of the extremities, and change in color of the extremities. Patients with reduced cerebral blood flow may have a history of recent or old stroke, transient ischemic attacks, fluctuation in the level of consciousness, confusion, or other signs of decreased cerebral blood flow. A complete patient assessment should be done, and a complete history about onset and course of vascular disease should be obtained. The nurse should assess the blood pressure and pulses, including peripheral pulses, and should make observations relative to the signs just described. Any deviation from normal should be recorded. A mental status examination should also be done.

Nursing diagnoses

Potential for injury related to orthostatic hypotension secondary to drug therapy
Alteration in comfort: headache secondary to vasodilator therapy
Alteration in comfort: nausea secondary to drug therapy

Management

Vasodilators are used to treat the symptoms and prevent recurrences resulting from altered or decreased perfusion. The nurse should monitor the presenting signs and symptoms, especially blood pressure and pulses, and look for drug side effects. If leg ulcers or other problems associated with vascular disease are present, treatment of these should be carried out. In addition to instruction on the medications, the nurse should begin teaching the patient about prevention of trauma to areas with decreased perfusion. Other therapies would include treatment of other medical problems, a prescribed exercise program, weight loss, and restriction of certain activities. An individualized plan of care should be devised by the health care team.

Evaluation

It is difficult to measure the effectiveness of these drugs. They do not alter the course of vascular disease, and it is often difficult to ascertain that they played a role in alleviation of symptoms. Before discharge, the patient should be able to explain when and how to take the ordered medications, the side effects that might occur, and the situations that would require notification of the physician. If other therapies have been prescribed, the patient should be able to explain how to carry out the prescribed regimen. If the patient is going home and will continue to treat manifestations of peripheral vascular disease, the patient should be able to demonstrate how to carry out the prescribed therapies, such as warm soaks or heat that might be applied to ulcers on the legs. For more specific guidelines, see the patient care implications section at the end of this chapter.

---

nephrine at the alpha receptors of the blood vessels should be helpful, but in practice, alpha adrenergic antagonists are not very effective in relieving or preventing vasospasm. Tolazoline is not very effective by itself but will potentiate the action of other drugs. Side effects are frequent with tolazo-line therapy and include headache, nausea, chills, flushing, tingling of the skin, especially the scalp, and gastrointestinal disturbances. Occasionally, irregular heart function is noticed; an arrhythmia or a pounding heart is the most common cardiac symptom.

PATIENT CARE IMPLICATIONS

Sympathomimetic drugs

Drug administration

For safe care of the patient requiring intravenous sympathomimetic drugs for the treatment of shock or hypotension:

- Use a microdrip IV administration set to regulate the drug dose more accurately. Use an electronic IV monitor or regulator to accurately control the rate of fluid and drug administration.
- Monitor the blood pressure and pulse every 2 to 5 minutes until the blood pressure and rate of drug administration are stable, then every 15 minutes. Do not leave the patient unattended.
- Monitor the mean arterial pressure, pulmonary capillary wedge pressure (PCWP), central venous pressure (CVP), or other available indicators of hemodynamic response. Monitor the electrocardiogram.
- Monitor intake, output, and urinary output. Monitor urinary output every 30 to 60 minutes.
- Read drug labels carefully, as some drug forms are not indicated for IV administration. Do not administer any drug intravenously if sediment or discoloration is visible.
- Do not mix two or more drugs in a syringe or in IV solutions. If in doubt, consult the pharmacist.
- Observe patient for development of hypertensive crisis. If it does occur, slow or stop vasopressor drugs, notify physician, and administer specific drug antidotes or phentolamine, an adrenergic blocking drug, as ordered.
- Exercise care to avoid extravasation of these drugs. All of these drugs cause vasoconstriction, and levarterenol or dopamine can cause tissue necrosis or sloughing. For this reason, administer these drugs through a central venous catheter if possible. In the event of extravasation, the physician may order the site of injury infiltrated with a solution of 5 to 10 mg of phentolamine diluted in 10 to 15 ml of normal saline solution.
- Many of these preparations contain bisulfites, which can cause an allergic reaction in susceptible individuals. While uncommon in the general population, this reaction may be seen more often in persons with a history of asthma. Symptoms include dizziness, feeling faint, bluish discoloration of the skin, skin rash or hives, swelling of the face, eyelids, or lips, and difficulty breathing. If possible, obtain a history of allergy or previous health problems preceding drug administration. Observe all patients for unexpected drug reactions.
- Keep patients and families informed of the patient's condition. Provide calm reassurance. Note that shock produces a sense of impending doom and a feeling of anxiety. Administration of adrenergic medication may also produce a tachycardia and palpitations, which contribute to a sense of anxiety.

Epinephrine and isoproterenol

Drug administration

- The usual dose of epinephrine in anaphylactic shock is 0.1 to 1.0 ml (0.1 to 1.0 mg) of 1:1000 solution given subcutaneously.
- Avoid administering epinephrine and isoproterenol simultaneously, as they are both cardiac stimulants.
- Monitor the blood sugar in patients receiving epinephrine, as this drug causes hyperglycemia.

Dopamine

Drug administration

- Dilute the concentrate for injection prior to infusion. Follow dilution guidelines for the agency. One protocol states: add 5 ml of concentrate containing 40 mg dopamine per ml (total of 200 mg of dopamine) to 500 ml of compatible IV solution to obtain a final concentration of 400 µg/ml.

Dobutamine

Drug administration

- Dilute the concentrate for injection to a volume of at least 50 ml with a compatible IV solution before administration. The final concentration should be no greater than 5000 µg/ml.
- Solutions that are slightly pink in color may still be used. After mixing with IV solution, use within 24 hours.

Levarterenol (norepinephrine) bitartrate

Drug administration

- Dilute with 5% dextrose injection, with or without sodium chloride prior to use. In the usual dilution, add 4 mg of drug to 1000 ml of 5% dextrose injection for a concentration of 4 µg/ml.

Continued.

PATIENT CARE IMPLICATIONS — cont'd

Metaraminol

Drug administration

- Dilute with 5% dextrose for injection or 0.9% sodium chloride for injection. See manufacturer's directions for further guidelines.

Antianginal drugs

Drug administration

- For patients with chest pain, assess blood pressure and pulse, auscultate lungs and heart; assess intensity, duration, location, and quality of pain; response to medication; presence of diaphoresis; precipitating factors; electrocardiographic changes; subjective and objective degree of patient distress; patient history; other subjective complaints. Remember that chest pain in the person with a history of angina pectoris may have other causes also.
- In the hospital, it is often customary to keep a small supply of nitroglycerin tablets at the bedside of patients with a history of angina pectoris. Instruct the patient to use as needed, but to notify the nurse when tablets are used. Record the frequency of use, as well as a patient assessment, in the nurses' notes. Count and replenish the tablets each shift.
  INTRAVENOUS NITROGLYCERIN
- Consult manufacturer's literature for specific instructions about dilution, dosage, and administration. Use a microdrip infusion set and a volume control or rate-controlling device to prevent overdosage, and to accurately titrate the dose. Nitroglycerin migrates into plastic tubing. Dilutions should be prepared and kept in glass bottles. If standard polyvinyl chloride (PVC) IV tubing must be used, as much as 80% of the drugs is lost into the tubing. If PVC tubing must be used, adjustments in dose must be made. Use tubing supplied by the manufacturer. Monitor the blood pressure, heart rate, electrocardiogram, and pulmonary capillary wedge pressure. Use this drug only in settings where drugs and experienced personnel to treat cardiovascular emergencies are available.

Patient and family education

- Encourage patients to make all recommended life-style changes, including losing weight to reach desirable body weight, lowering cholesterol levels, ceasing smoking, and engaging in a regular exercise program after approval by the physician.
- Assist patients and families to identify activities which trigger anginal attacks, such

as eating a heavy meal, engaging in strenuous physical activities, lifting heavy objects, exposure to cold weather, and sexual activity. Work with the patient to develop ways to decrease the frequency of attacks, or to lessen the likelihood that activities will cause anginal pain to develop.
- Encourage patients to notify the physician if the frequency, intensity, duration, location, or response to antianginal drugs changes.
- Instruct patients to avoid the use of alcohol as it potentiates the hypotensive effects of the nitrates and nitrites.
- Remind patients to keep all health care providers informed of all drugs being used, as drugs such as diuretics, antihypertensives, central nervous system depressants, narcotics, and sedatives may potentiate the hypotensive effects of the antianginal drugs.
- Teach patients to maintain regular contact with the primary health care provider, and not to stop drug therapy without medical consultation.
- If headache regularly occurs when antianginal drugs are taken, it may indicate too high a dosage. For some patients it may be necessary to use mild analgesics with antianginal therapy; consult the physician.

Nitrates and nitrites

Patient and family education

- If syncope (fainting), dizziness, or hypotension occurs with nitrate or nitrite use, instruct the patient to lie down before taking the prescribed dose of medication.
- Ascertain that the patient can correctly use sublingual drug forms prior to discharging the patient. This may be a new dosage form for the patient. In addition, teach the family how to place a dose under the patient's tongue in the event the patient cannot do it. Tell the patient not to eat, drink, chew tobacco, or smoke while the dose is dissolving.
- For chewable tablets, teach the patient to chew the tablet well, then hold it in the mouth for at least 2 minutes before swallowing. Do not drink, smoke, eat, or chew tobacco while using this form.
- For buccal extended-release tablets, place the dose between the cheek and upper gum, or between the upper lip and gum, and allow it to dissolve over 5 hours. When eating or drinking, place the dose between the upper lip and gum. If the patient wears dentures, place the tablet between the cheek and gum

PATIENT CARE IMPLICATIONS—cont'd

Tell the patient not to use chewing tobacco while using this form. Replace the tablet if it is accidentally swallowed. Tell the patient not to go to sleep with a tablet still in the mouth.

- Review the standard instructions for antianginal agents used to relieve an attack of angina with the patient and family: when chest pain develops, sit down, then use one tablet, letting it dissolve under the tongue or in the cheek, or chew a chewable tablet. If relief is not obtained, repeat the dose in 5 minutes. Repeat again in 5 minutes if needed, for a total of 3 tablets. If the pain persists after 3 tablets, notify the physician or seek medical help. These guidelines may be individualized based on the patient, the patient's condition, and the physician's preference.

- Take oral nitrates and nitrites with meals or snack to reduce gastric irritation.

- Review the ordered drugs carefully with the patient, as well as exactly how and when to take the prescribed drugs, as there are many dosages and drug forms available for these drugs.

- Storage of these drugs: keep drugs out of the reach of children, do not store in the bathroom or near the kitchen sink or other damp areas. Check expiration dates, and replace drugs as needed. For sublingual nitroglycerin, in addition to the above, keep tablets in the original glass container. Once the bottle is opened, remove the cotton and do not replace it. Replace the cap tightly and quickly each time the bottle is opened. Do not put other medicines in the same bottle with the nitroglycerin. When pouring a dose (a tablet), pour one or more tablets into the lid of the bottle, take the dose out, and return remaining tablets to the bottle. Avoid replacing tablets from the palm of the hand into the bottle. To carry a small number of pills, instruct the patient to obtain a small bottle for this purpose from the pharmacist. Do not carry the small bottle too close to the body, as body warmth may cause the pills to lose their strength.

- To prevent an attack of angina, take the prescribed drug before engaging in the activity expected to produce anginal pain. For sublingual or chewable forms, this may be 5 to 10 minutes preceding the activity; for extended-release forms, this may be several hours earlier. For specific patient needs, consult the physician.

- If doses are missed, take the dose as soon as remembered, unless within 2 hours of the next dose (extended-release forms, or isosorbide dinitrate). Do not double up for missed doses.

LINGUAL AEROSOL FORMS

- Review the patient instruction leaflet supplied by the manufacturer. To use, remove the cover. Do not shake the container. Hold the container upright, close to the mouth. Spray one or two sprays (as prescribed by the physician) under the tongue. Close the mouth. Avoid swallowing for a minute or two. This drug may be used like nitroglycerin tablets: when an attack of angina occurs, administer a dose as prescribed. If no relief in 5 minutes, repeat the dose. If no relief in another 5 minutes, repeat the does. If no relief after a total of 3 doses in 15 minutes, seek medical attention or notify the physician. The prescription may be modified for individual patient needs and by physician preference.

TOPICAL TRANSDERMAL FORMS

- Review the patient instruction leaflet supplied by the manufacturer. Do not trim or cut the adhesive patch. Remove the previous patch before applying a new patch. Rotate sites to avoid skin irritation. Apply the patch to an area that is clean and dry, with little or no hair. Avoid scratches, scars, or existing skin irritation. If the patch loosens or falls off, replace it. Side effects are the same as for other antianginal drugs in this group. Transdermal forms should not be used to treat an acute attack of angina.

TOPICAL OINTMENTS

- Review the patient instruction leaflet supplied by the manufacturer. Remove the ointment from a previous dose before applying. Measure the prescribed amount of ointment, using the measuring paper supplied by the manufacturer. Gently spread the ointment over a small area with the measuring paper or small applicator (not the fingertips) about the same size each time. Do not massage the ointment into the skin. Apply to areas with little or no hair. Avoid scratches and scars. Rotate sites to avoid skin irritation. Cover the area with plastic kitchen wrap or other dressing *only* if ordered by the physician. If a dressing is prescribed, it should be used each time the drug is used. If a dose is missed, apply it as soon as remembered, unless it is within 2 hours of the next dose, then follow the usual dosing schedule. Do not use more ointment than ordered, and do not double up for missed doses.

Continued.

PATIENT CARE IMPLICATIONS — cont'd

AMYL NITRATE

- This drug is rarely used for treatment of angina. Teach patient and family to wrap the ampule in a cloth or handkerchief, break the glass ampule within its protective covering, then have the patient inhale several deep breaths.

Beta adrenergic blocking drugs

- See Patient Care Implications in Chapter 15.

Calcium channel blockers

Drug administration

- Assess patients with complaints of chest pain: intensity, duration, location, quality of pain; response to medications; presence of diaphoresis; vital signs, blood pressure and electrocardiographic changes; precipitating factors; patient history; auscultation of heart and lung sounds; and other subjective complaints. Chest pain in the patient with a history of angina pectoris may be due to other causes also.
- In patients taking calcium channel blockers, monitor the blood pressure, pulse, intake and output, and weight. Observe for signs of fluid retention: peripheral edema, subjective complaints of tight shoes and rings, signs of congestive heart failure such as dyspnea on exertion, distended jugular veins, orthopnea, or moist rales on pulmonary auscultation.

Patient and family education

- See the box on p. 237 for a discussion of orthostatic hypotension and the box on p. 187 for a discussion of constipation.
- If appropriate, teach the patient to take and record the pulse daily at home. Instruct the patient to report a change of 10 beats per minute in the resting pulse, or a pulse rate less than 50. Candidates appropriate for this instruction may be those on multiple-drug regimens or those in whom control of side effects has been difficult.
- If appropriate, teach the patient to monitor and record weight on a regular basis. Instruct patients to report a weight gain of greater than 2 lb per day or 5 lb per week. Instruct the patient to report the development of tight rings, shoes, or clothing, or signs of peripheral edema.
- Because of potential drug interactions with other medication, teach patients to keep all health care providers informed of all drugs being used. Tell patients to avoid the use of any over-the-counter preparations unless first cleared by the physician.
- In addition to using these drugs as prescribed, patients may find additional relief by losing weight, stopping smoking, limiting intake of caffeine, avoiding extremes of temperature, and becoming involved in a regular exercise program; consult the physician.
- Emphasize to the patient the importance of taking these drugs as prescribed, and not discontinuing them without consultation with the physician.
- If a dose is missed, teach the patient to take the missed dose as soon as remembered, but not within 2 hours of the next scheduled dose. Do not double up for missed doses.
- Teach patients to report any signs of liver problems: right upper quadrant abdominal pain, jaundice, change in color or consistency of stools, malaise.
- Encourage patients to have regular dental examinations. Review oral hygiene practices, and encourage regular flossing and brushing.

Nifedipine

Drug administration

- To administer sublingually or intrabuccally, puncture the fluid-filled capsule and squeeze the drug into the mouth. The patient may chew the capsule to break it, and direct the contents to the cheek or under the tongue.

Verapamil

Drug administration/patient and family education:

- Teach patients to swallow sustained-release formulations whole, without crushing or chewing. The extended-release tablet may be broken along the scored line.
- Administer IV doses undiluted over at least 2 minutes in the adult, and 3 minutes in the elderly patient. Monitor the electrocardiogram and the blood pressure.

Peripheral vasodilators

Drug administration

- Monitor the blood pressure and pulse when beginning therapy or when changing doses.
- Administer IV doses of papaverine undiluted at a rate of 30 mg or less over 2 minutes. IM injection is preferred. Monitor the electrocardiogram, pulse, respiration, and blood pressure during IV administration and for 1 hour afterward.

PATIENT CARE IMPLICATIONS—cont'd

- Administer IV doses of tolazoline undiluted at a rate of 10 mg or less over 1 minute. May also be diluted and given as an infusion.
- IM doses of isoxsuprine may cause hypotension and tachycardia; monitor the blood pressure and pulse.
- If isoxsuprine is used to prevent labor, monitor intensity, frequency, and duration of uterine contractions. Monitor fetal heart rate at regular intervals.

Patient and family education

- Take doses with meals or antacids to diminish GI symptoms.
- Review box on p. 237 for information about postural hypotension. Hypotension may be potentiated in patients receiving vasodilators who are also receiving other drugs that can cause hypotension, such as diuretics, antihypertensives, central nervous system depressants, narcotics, and sedatives. Instruct patients to keep all health care providers informed of all medications being taken.
- Teach patients to avoid the use of alcohol as it potentiates the hypotensive effects of vasodilators.
- Instruct patients to avoid smoking as it reduces peripheral blood flow.
- Teach patients that time-release formulations must be swallowed whole and not crushed or chewed.
- Encourage patients to lose weight to desirable body weight to help decrease symptoms from peripheral vascular disease.
- Warn patients that nicotinyl alcohol, pentoxyfilline, or papaverine may produce pronounced flushing, which is not harmful.

- Caution patients to avoid driving or operating hazardous equipment if side effects such as dizziness, weakness, drowsiness, or double vision occur.
- Encourage patients to take these drugs as prescribed. Regular, long-term use may be necessary for full benefit to occur.
- Take missed doses as soon as remembered, unless within 2 hours of the next dose. Do not double up for missed doses.
- Papaverine may be used to produce erections in some impotent men. The patient should clean off the base of the penis with alcohol, and inject the prescribed dose into the base of the penis as instructed by the physician. After injection, the patient should massage the penis, and attempt intercourse within 2 hours. Teach the patient to consult the physician if the erection lasts more than 4 hours, the erection is painful, there is bleeding at the injection site that does not stop after pressure is applied, a lump develops where the medication was injected, or the penis is becoming curved.
- Instruct patients taking pentoxyfilline to avoid the use of aspirin or aspirin-containing products while taking this drug.
- Assess patients for hypersensitivity or intolerance to methylxanthines before administering pentoxyfilline. Methylxanthines include caffeine, theophylline, and theobromine, which are the active ingredients in coffee, tea, and chocolate. Pentoxyfilline is contraindicated in persons with intolerance to methylxanthines.

Pentoxifylline (Trental)

Pentoxifylline is a new type of drug for the treatment of peripheral vascular disease. Pentoxifylline increases the flexibility of red blood cells and reduces blood viscosity. These actions improve blood flow through narrowed vessels.

Pentoxifylline is administered as an adjunct to surgery for the treatment of intermittent claudication. Side effects are rare, but include dizziness, headache, nausea, or vomiting. Drug interactions include the potentiation of antihypertensive drugs. Smoking may interfere with the therapeutic action of pentoxifylline since nicotine constricts blood vessels. Toxic symptoms of pentoxifylline include excitement and seizures.

SUMMARY

Sympathomimetic drugs are used in selected situations to improve blood flow in shock. Activation of alpha adrenergic receptors will cause vasoconstriction and increase blood pressure by increasing peripheral vascular resistance. Activation of the beta-1 adrenergic receptors of the heart will increase cardiac output.

Drugs administered primarily to activate alpha adrenergic receptors include the direct-acting sympathomimetics levarterenol (norepinephrine), methoxamine, and phenylephrine, and the indirect-acting sympathomimetics metaraminol and mephentermine.

Epinephrine is used to treat anaphylactic shock because epinephrine not only stimulates alpha receptors to restore blood pressure but also stimulates beta-2 receptors to dilate the bronchioles.

Dopamine is administered at low doses for its unique action to dilate renal arterioles and thereby prevent kidney failure secondary to shock. At intermediate doses, dopamine stimulates the cardiac beta-1 adrenergic receptors to increase cardiac output; at high doses, dopamine is also an indirect-acting sympathomimetic.

Dobutamine is relatively specific at low doses for stimulation of cardiac contractility without stimulation of heart rate, a selective action among cardiac beta-1 receptors. At high doses, dobutamine becomes a nonselective beta adrenergic receptor agonist, stimulating both beta-1 and beta-2 receptors.

Isoproterenol is a nonselective beta adrenergic receptor agonist. Its major use is as a bronchodilator, and its use as a cardiac stimulant is a minor one.

Angina is the pain that results when the oxygen demand of the heart is not met. Nitrates and nitrites, particularly nitroglycerin, offer acute and prophylactic relief. These vasodilators reduce the workload on the heart, which lowers the oxygen demand. In severe cases of angina, the beta adrenergic receptor antagonists may be effective. These drugs decrease the work of the heart by inhibiting sympathetic stimulation of the heart. A new class of drugs, the calcium channel blockers, is proving effective for the treatment of variant angina and may be an alternative to the beta-adrenergic receptor antagonists for some cases of classic angina. The calcium channel blockers inhibit contractility of coronary smooth muscle and also inhibit cardiac contractility.

Several vasodilators are used to treat selected cases of impaired circulation of the digits or brain. The vasodilators used include cyclandelate, the dihydrogenated ergot alkaloids, isoxsuprine, niacin, nylidrin, papaverine, and tolazoline. The therapeutic effectiveness of these drugs is not clear.

STUDY QUESTIONS

1. List the direct-acting sympathomimetic drugs. What is their receptor selectivity and what physiologic actions result?
2. List the indirect-acting sympathomimetic drugs. What is their receptor selectivity and what physiological actions result?
3. Which drug is used to treat anaphylactic shock?
4. Which drug is used as a renal vasodilator?
5. Which drug is used as a selective stimulant of cardiac contractility?
6. Why are sympathomimetic drugs sometimes administered during spinal anesthesia?
7. What is the origin of angina? Describe the differences between classic (exertional) angina, variant angina, and unstable angina.
8. How do the nitrates and nitrites relieve angina?
9. How do the beta adrenergic blocking drugs relieve angina? What are their side effects? For which patients are the cardioselective beta adrenergic blocking drugs especially indicated?
10. How do the calcium channel blocking drugs relieve angina? Why are they especially effective for variant angina?
11. What are two causes of insufficient blood flow to the digits? Which cause is amenable to drug therapy? What role do vasodilators play?
12. List the seven drugs used as vasodilators for improving peripheral circulation. What are some of their common side effects?

SUGGESTED READINGS

Shock

Bowe PL, Stargel WW, and Wagner GS: Sympathomimetic amines in the management of cardiogenic shock, Drug Therapy **5**(10):31, 1980.

Carlson RW, and Weil MH: Axioms on critical care of shock, Hosp Med **17**(10):99, 1981.

Cleary JD: Two inotropic agents: dopamine and dobutamine, Pediatr. Nurs. **14**(5):414, 1988.

DiPalma JR: Vasodilator and inotropic therapy for heart failure, Am Family Phys **31**(6):177, 1985.

Hancock BG, and others: The pharmacologic management of shock, Crit Care Nurse Q **11**(1):19, 1988.

Hill J: Anaphylaxis: diagnosis and emergency care, Hosp Med **17**(10):16, 1981.

Houston MC, Thompson WL, and Robertson D: Shock: diagnosis and management, Ann Intern Med **144**:1433, 1984.

Jeffries PR, and Whelan SK: Cardiogenic shock: current management, Crit Care Nurs Q **11**(1):48, 1988.

Jones S, and Bagg AM: L-E-A-D drugs for cardiac arrest . . . lidocaine, epinephrine, atropine, and dopamine, Nursing **88**(1):34, 1988.

McGraw JP: A graphic solution to the calculation of dopamine and other vasoactive drug dosages, J Emerg Nurs **13**(3):172, 1987.

Rice V: Understanding shock and how to treat it: drug management, Canadian IV Nurs Assoc J **1**(4):20, 1985.

Rimar JM: Shock in infants and children: assessment and treatment, MCN **13**(2):98, 1988.

Angina

Abrams J: A reappraisal of nitrate therapy, JAMA **259**(3):396, 1988.

Beare PG: Calcium entry blockers: actions, use and nursing implications, AAOHN J **35**(6):261, 1987.

Cardin S: Cardiovascular pharmacology: nursing considerations in the administration of verapamil, J Cardiovasc Nurs 2(2):73, 1988.

Deane KW, and Hartshorn JC: Nitrates in the treatment of coronary artery disease, J Cardiovasc Nurs 1(1):81, 1986.

Few BJ: Nifedipine for treatment of premature labor, MCN 12(5):309, 1987.

Goldman L, and others: Costs and effectiveness of routine therapy with long-term beta-adrenergic antagonists after acute myocardial infarction, N Engl J Med 319:152, 1988.

Gruentzig AR, and others: Long-term follow-up after percutaneous transluminal coronary angioplasty: the early Zurich experience, N Engl J Med 316:1127, 1987.

Kent KM: Coronary angioplasty: a decade of experience, N Engl J Med 316:1148, 1987.

Levine R, and Becer NC: Implications, actions and uses of intravenous nitroglycerin, J Emerg Nurs 13(5):301, 1987.

Luchi RJ, and others: Comparison of medical and surgical treatment for unstable angina pectoris, N Engl J Med 316:977, 1987.

May DC, and others: In vivo induction and reversal of nitroglycerin tolerance in human coronary arteries, N Engl J Med 317:805, 1987.

Multicenter Diltiazem Postinfarction Trial Research Group: The effect of diltiazem on mortality and reinfarction after myocardial infarction, N Engl J Med 318:385, 1988.

Miller CL: Medications in angina, Focus Crit Care 15(94):23, 1988.

Nagelhout JJ: AANA Journal Course: advanced scientific concepts. Update for nurse anesthetists—cardiac pharmacology: calcium antagonists, AANA J 56(4):367, 1988.

Packer M, and others: Prevention and reversal of nitrate tolerance in patients with congestive heart failure, N Engl J Med 317:799, 1987.

Parker JO: Nitrate therapy in stable angina pectoris, N Engl J Med 316:1635, 1987.

Schakenbach LH: Prinzmetal's angina: current perceptions and treatments, Crit Care Nurse 7(2):90, 1987.

Schoen RE, Frishman WH, and Shamoon H: Hormonal and metabolic effects of calcium channel antagonists in man, Am J Med 84:492, 1988.

Silber S, and others: Induction and circumvention of nitrate tolerance applying different dosage intervals, Am J Med 83:860, 1987.

Peripheral vascular disease

Baker DE, and Campbell RK: Pentoxifylline: a new agent for intermittent claudication, Drug Intelligence and Clinical Pharmacy 19:345, 1985.

Cheung JY, and others: Calcium and ischemic injury, N Engl J Med 314:1670, 1986.

Grotta JC: Current medical and surgical therapy for cerebrovascular disease, N Engl J Med 317:1505, 1987.

Hartshorn JC, and Deans KW: Pharmacologic treatment of intermittent claudication with special emphasis on pentoxifylline, Cardiovasc Nurs 1(2):65, 1987.

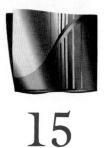

Antihypertensive Drugs

15

HYPERTENSION

Hypertension is generally defined as a resting systolic blood pressure greater than 140 mm Hg or a diastolic blood pressure greater than 90 mm Hg or both in an adult. In the United States it is estimated that this condition may apply to 15% of adults. High blood pressure reflects an increased tone of the arteries and arterioles. Renal, endocrine, or neurogenic diseases are found to be the cause of hypertension in 10% of patients with hypertension. The hypertension in these patients is treated by treating its cause. No primary cause of the hypertension can be found in the remaining 90% of patients with hypertension; this condition of unknown origin is called *essential* hypertension. The patient with hypertension may have no symptoms of this disease but does have an increased risk of stroke, blindness, and heart and renal disease after 10 or more years of sustained high blood pressure that produces vascular and organ damage. The incidence of hypertension is higher in men than in women, higher in blacks than in whites, higher in older than in younger adults, and higher in those with diabetes mellitus, hyperlipidemia, or a family history of hypertension.

FACTORS CONTROLLING BLOOD PRESSURE AND PHARMACOLOGICAL MECHANISMS FOR TREATING HYPERTENSION

The major factors regulating blood pressure are diagrammed in Figure 15.1. These factors center around those influencing the circulating volume through adjustments of body salt and water (renal mechanisms) and those influencing the activity of the heart and blood vessels (cardiovascular mechanisms).

Renal Mechanisms

The kidney plays an important role in maintaining blood pressure through control of the salt and water content of the body (Chapter 16). A decrease in blood pressure stimulates the release of renin from the kidney. Renin release may be partly controlled by beta adrenergic receptors. Renin is a proteolytic enzyme that acts on a protein in the blood to produce the peptide angiotensin I. Angiotensin I is converted to angiotensin II, a small peptide that is a potent vasoconstrictor and therefore increases blood pressure. Angiotensin II also acts on the adrenal cortex to stimulate the secretion of aldosterone. Aldosterone is the mineralocorticoid hormone that acts on the kidney to decrease the excretion of sodium and to increase potassium excretion. The resulting sodium retention expands the plasma and extracellular fluid volumes, which contribute to the elevation of blood pressure.

Cardiovascular Mechanisms

Within the blood vessels, the blood pressure depends on the cardiac output and the resistance to blood flow in the blood vessels. Baroreceptors in the aorta and carotid sinus monitor the blood pressure and send the information to the brain. The brain integrates this information and adjusts the heart rate and resistance of the blood vessels, largely through the sympathetic nervous system, to fine-tune the blood pressure. The vasomotor center in the medulla is a major center in the brain controlling blood pressure. As the neurotransmitter of the sympathetic nervous system, norepinephrine raises blood pressure by stimulating the beta-1 receptors of the heart to increase cardiac output and by stimulating the alpha-1 receptors of the blood vessels, which causes constriction and increases the resistance to blood flow. By contrast, in the

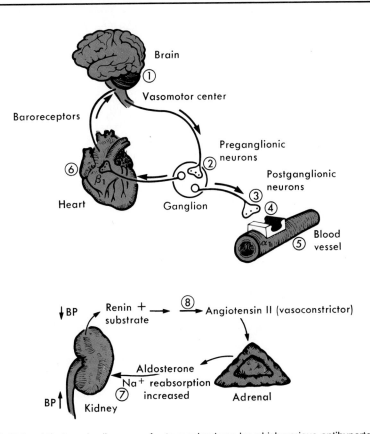

FIGURE 15.1   Numbers in diagram refer to mechanisms by which various antihypertensive drugs appear to act. *(1)* Drugs acting centrally to depress sympathetic tone: clonidine, methyldopa, guanabenz, reserpine. *(2)* Drug blocking ganglionic receptor for acetylcholine: trimethaphan. *(3)* Drugs interfering with norepinephrine synthesis, storage, or release: metyrosine, guanethidine, guanadrel, reserpine, pargyline. *(4)* Drugs (a) blocking alpha adrenergic receptor: prazosin, phenoxybenzamine, phentolamine, labetalol or (b) blocking angiotensin II receptor: saralasin. *(5)* Drugs directly dilating smooth muscle: hydralazine, minoxidil, sodium nitroprusside, diazoxide, calcium channel blockers. *(6)* Drugs decreasing cardiac output: beta adrenergic receptor blockers, calcium channel blockers. *(7)* Drugs blocking sodium reabsorption: diuretics. *(8)* Drugs inhibiting angiotensin II formation: captopril, enalapril.

central nervous system, norepinephrine is the neurotransmitter for nerve tracts that ultimately decrease blood pressure.

Antihypertensive Therapy

There has been an explosion of new drugs for the treatment of hypertension in the past 10 years. Table 15.1 outlines drugs that have a role in the treatment of hypertension. These drugs can be placed into four categories: diuretics, sympathetic depressants, vasodilators, and angiotensin antagonists. The sympathetic depressant drugs encompass several adrenergic mechanisms because adrenergic drugs can lower blood pressure by decreasing the activity of the sympathetic nervous system peripherally or centrally. (Drug mechanisms that modify the activity of the sympathetic nervous system are reviewed in Chapter 9.) Figure 15.1 shows the sites of action of antihypertensive drugs.

Hypertension is commonly treated when the diastolic pressure is greater than 105 mm, which indicates moderate to severe hypertension. If untreated, moderate to severe hypertension is associated with the development of congestive heart failure, renal failure, aneurysms, and strokes. Hypertension with diastolic pressures of 90 to 105 mm is mild hypertension. Mild hypertension is associated with increased morbidity when atherosclerosis is also a factor. A greater incidence of sudden death, usually caused by electrical dysfunction of the heart secondary to poor coronary circulation, or of myocardial infarction, is seen among patients

Table 15.1   Categories of Antihypertensive Drugs

Category	Type	Drugs	Antihypertensive action
Diuretics	Thiazide-type	See Table 16.3	Reduces body salt and water, which decreases arterial blood pressure. May reduce plasma volume. Counteracts the fluid retention caused by certain antihypertensive drugs: methyldopa, reserpine, guanethidine, guandrel, prazosin, hydralyzine, minoxidil, and diazoxide. Enhances the action of most antihypertensive drugs given in long-term therapy.
	Loop	Bumetanide Furosemide Ethacrynic acid	
	Potassium-sparing	Spironolactone Triamterene Amiloride	
Sympathetic depressant drugs	Beta-adrenergic receptor antagonist	Acebutolol Atenolol Carteolol Metoprolol Nadolol Oxprenolol* Penbutolol Pindolol Propranolol Sotalol* Timolol	Reduces cardiac output. Reduces renin release from the kidney. May have a central antihypertensive action. Preferred for individuals with high renin levels, typically young Caucasians. Shown to decrease the incidence of sudden death in patients with a recent heart attack. The cardioselective (beta-1 adrenergic receptors) drugs are acebutolol, atenolol and metoprolol.
	Alpha-adrenergic receptor antagonist	Prazosin Terazosin* Phenoxybenzamine Phentolamine	Blocks the vasoconstrictive action of norepinephrine, thereby decreasing peripheral resistance.
	Alpha and beta adrenergic receptor antagonist	Labetalol	Both alpha and beta receptor antagonistic actions (see above) apply. Alpha receptor antagonist actions predominate. New drug class.
	Centrally acting drug	Clonidine Methyldopa Guanabenz Guanfacine	Inhibits sympathetic outflow from the brain by stimulating alpha receptors in the vasomotor center of the medulla. The result is a decrease in peripheral resistance.
	Centrally and peripherally acting drug	Reserpine	Depletes norepinephrine stores peripherally and centrally, resulting in a decrease in peripheral resistance.
	Ganglionic blocking drug	Trimethaphan Mecamylamine	Blocks the nicotinic receptors of the autonomic ganglia to inhibit both sympathetic and parasympathetic functions. Peripheral resistance is decreased.
	Drug blocking norepinephrine release	Guanethidine Debrisoquine* Guanadrel	Loss of peripheral sympathetic tone decreases peripheral resistance by reducing both cardiac output and peripheral resistance. Used for severe hypertension.

*Available in Canada only.

Table 15.1   Categories of Antihypertensive Drugs—cont'd

Category	Type	Drugs	Antihypertensive action
Sympathetic depressant drugs—cont'd	Drug blocking norepinephrine synthesis	Metyrosine	Decreases peripheral resistance, particularly in presence of a norepinephrine-producing tumor (pheochromocytoma). Rarely used.
	Monoamine oxidase inhibitor	Pargyline	Decreases peripheral resistance. Rarely used because of serious drug-food interactions.
Vasodilators	Arterial vasodilator	Hydralazine Minoxidil Diazoxide	Relaxes arterial smooth muscle to lower peripheral resistance. Used alone, causes rebound tachycardia (increased heart rate) and edema.
	Arterial and venous vasodilator	Nitroprusside	Generalized vasodilation. Useful in hypertensive emergencies.
	Calcium channel blocker	Diltiazem Isradipine Nicardipine Nifedipine Nitrendipine Verapamil	Reduces the tone of blood vessels by reducing intracellular calcium, thereby causing arteriolar dilation and decreased total peripheral resistance.
Angiotensin antagonists	Inhibitor of angiotensin II formation	Captopril Enalapril Lisinopril	Reduces peripheral resistance in individuals with high plasma renin levels.

having both mild hypertension and atherosclerosis. Many physicians reserve treatment of mild hypertension for those patients with significant risk factors for atherosclerosis, such as smoking, high cholesterol values (above 185 mg/dl), high lipid levels, abnormal glucose tolerance test, ECG abnormalities and a family history of atherosclerosis.

In general, drug therapy for hypertension is standard. Yet therapy is changing as more is being learned about hypertension and as new drugs become available. Current therapy is based on a modified *stepped-care approach* in which drugs are added by class until blood pressure is brought under control.

The Joint National Committee on Detection, Evaluation, and Treatment of High Blood Pressure updated and published its recommendations in 1988.

Step 1 is the administration of a single drug from one of four drug classes: diuretics, beta adrenergic blockers, calcium channel blockers, or angiotensin-converting enzyme (ACE) inhibitors. The most common choice is an oral diuretic, usually a thiazide or thiazide-like diuretic. Diuretics are es-

pecially effective as single agents for black hypertensive patients. Diuretics inhibit renal tubular reabsorption, causing diuresis that leads to reduction of body salt and water (extracellular fluid). The loss of extracellular fluid is associated with reduction of arterial blood pressure, but the mechanism of this hypotensive action remains obscure. This hypotensive effect is not seen in normotensive patients. The volume depletion also produces a reduction in plasma volume, although it is not clear that this reduction persists after the first month of therapy. In addition, many antihypertensive drugs cause fluid retention, an action that limits their antihypertensive effect. Diuretics are therefore commonly given with other antihypertensive drugs. Diuretics are discussed in Chapter 16.

Instead of a diuretic, a beta adrenergic receptor blocker may be given as the first drug. Hypertensive individuals with high plasma renin levels are especially responsive to beta adrenergic blockers and rather unresponsive to diuretics. This is because beta adrenergic blockers inhibit the release of renin from the kidney. Unfortunately, renin levels cannot be reliably or readily determined at present. In general, however, white hypertensive patients in the younger age groups have high renin levels, whereas black hypertensive patients in the older age groups have low renin levels. A beta adrenergic blocker is also indicated for patients who have coronary artery disease. Beta blockers have been shown to have a protective effect against sudden death in individuals who have had a heart attack, whereas diuretics may, through a lowering of potassium levels, increase the vulnerability of the compromised heart to sudden failure.

Calcium channel blockers have been added as step 1 drugs. These act by preventing the entry of calcium into the smooth muscle layer of blood vessels. This diminishes the contraction of the blood vessels and results in vasodilation. Calcium channel blockers decrease hypertension without causing reflex sympathetic stimulation or fluid retention. These drugs are especially effective as single agents for older patients and for those with low plasma renin activity.

Angiotensin-converting enzyme (ACE) inhibitors are effective in treating most forms of hypertension and for treating congestive heart failure. The ACE inhibitors are now step 1 drugs. They block the formation of the potent vasoconstrictor, angiotensin II. The antihypertensive response is not associated with an increase in heart rate or cardiac output. The ACE inhibitors seem to be effective as single agents for a wide spectrum of hypertensive patients.

Step 2 therapy is an evaluation of step 1 therapy after 1 to 3 months. If the antihypertensive response is not adequate, one of four actions is taken. First, the patient is evaluated for compliance. Second, the dose of the drug may be increased. Third, the first drug may be discontinued and a new drug started. Fourth, a second drug may be added to the therapeutic regimen. The most common two-drug regimen is the addition of a sympathetic depressant drug to diuretic therapy. The sympathetic drug is commonly a beta adrenergic receptor blocker. However, methyldopa, clonidine, or, occasionally, prazosin or reserpine is an alternative drug used in step 2. The newer drugs guanabenz and guanadrel are also used in step 2.

Step 3 therapy is a further evaluation of step 2 therapy. If the antihypertensive response is still not adequate, a new second drug may be substituted or a third drug may be added. The most common three-drug regimen is the addition of a vasodilator to the antihypertensive therapy. Hydralazine, minoxidil, and prazosin are the vasodilators most frequently used.

Step 4 therapy begins with a careful assessment

of the factors limiting the antihypertensive response. A third or fourth drug may be added.

Patients with essential hypertension may have to take drugs for the rest of their lives to control the condition. Drug therapy can rarely be discontinued after the blood pressure is brought into a normal range. Frequently the drug dosage can be reduced with time. This is important because antihypertensive drugs can produce uncomfortable side effects, whereas the hypertension itself may not produce uncomfortable symptoms, a situation that can make patient compliance with drug therapy difficult. Obesity and high salt intake are factors that aggravate hypertension. If a patient reduces weight and salt intake, drug requirements frequently may also be reduced.

Antihypertensive therapy for special patient populations

Black patients. Hypertension is more prevalent in black Americans. In general, black hypertensive patients respond best to diuretics as monotherapy. ACE inhibitors and beta adrenergic blockers are generally less effective as single agents for black patients than for white patients. However, in combination with diuretics, ACE inhibitors and beta adrenergic blockers are equally effective in white and black hypertensive patients. Other antihypertensive drug classes are equally effective in both racial groups.

Elderly patients. Approximately two thirds of the U.S. population over 65 years of age or older has hypertension. Older patients are more sensitive to diuretics, beta-blockers, and the orthostatic hypotensive effects of other antihypertensive drugs. Calcium channel blockers, beta-blockers, and ACE inhibitors are the most useful drugs for monotherapy in the elderly.

Pregnant patients. Hypertension as a complication of pregnancy is called preeclampsia, and it imposes risk for both the mother and fetus. Diet and bed rest are the first line of treatment, but if high blood pressure persists, methyldopa, hydralazine, and beta-blockers have each proved effective in controlling blood pressure and improving fetal survival. ACE inhibitors and calcium blockers have not yet been proved safe in pregnancy.

DRUGS ALTERING SYMPATHETIC ACTIVITY
Beta Adrenergic Receptor Antagonists
(Table 15.2)

Mechanism of action. Beta adrenergic receptor antagonists are also referred to as beta adrenergic blockers. They have proved to be very effective as

Text continued on p. 235.

Table 15.2 Drugs for Treatment of Chronic Hypertension

Generic name	Trade name	Administration/dosage	Comments
BETA ADRENERGIC RECEPTOR ANTAGONISTS			
Acebutolol hydrochloride	Sectral* Monitan†	ORAL: 400 mg once a day initially. Maintenance dose range: 200 to 1200 mg daily to control hypertension. Do not exceed 800 mg daily in elderly. Reduce dose 50% to 75% for patients with renal failure. FDA Pregnancy Category B.	Cardioselective. Also used as an antiarrhythmic.
Atenolol	Tenormin*	ORAL: 50 mg daily; increase to 100 mg if needed. Reduce dose to 50 mg on alternate days for renal failure. FDA Pregnancy Category C.	Cardioselective. Also used as an antianginal.
Carteolol	Cartrol	ORAL: Adults—2.5 or 5 mg. FDA Pregnancy Category C.	Nonselective.
Metoprolol tartrate	Apo-metaprolol† Betaloc† Lopresor† Lopressor	ORAL: 50 mg 2 times daily. Dosage may be increased to 200 mg daily to control hypertension, maximum 450 mg. FDA Pregnancy Category B.	Cardioselective. Also used as an antianginal and as a prophylaxis against myocardial reinfarction.
Nadolol	Corgard*	ORAL: Adults—40 mg once daily to start. Dosages are increased by 40 to 80 mg every 3 to 7 days until optimum blood pressure control is achieved. The dosage range for maintenance is 80 to 120 mg daily. FDA Pregnancy Category C.	Nonselective. Also used as an antianginal.
Oxprenolol hydrochloride†	Trasicor†	ORAL: Adults—20 mg three times daily initially. Daily dosage may be increased every 2 to 3 weeks by 60 mg to achieve desired response.	Nonselective.
Penbutolol sulfate	Levatol	ORAL: Adults—20 mg once daily.	Nonselective.
Pindolol	Visken*	ORAL: 10 mg twice daily or 5 mg 3 times daily. Dose may be increased in increments of 10 mg/day every 2 to 3 weeks to achieve a satisfactory response. Maximum dose, 60 mg daily. FDA Pregnancy Category B.	Nonselective.
Propranolol hydrochloride	Inderal*	For hypertension: ORAL: 20 mg 3 times daily with a diuretic. Dosage may be increased to 480 mg daily to control hypertension. FDA Pregnancy Category C.	Nonselective. Also used as an antianginal, an antiarrhythmic, as prophylaxis against myocardial reinfarction, as prophylaxis in the treatment of vascular headaches, in the treatment of tremors, and for symptomatic treatment of thyrotoxicosis.

*Available in Canada and United States.
†Available in Canada only.

Continued.

Table 15.2 Drugs for Treatment of Chronic Hypertension—cont'd

Generic name	Trade name	Administration/dosage	Comments
Propranolol hydro-chloride—cont'd		For pheochromocytoma: ORAL: 30 mg 3 times daily with an alpha adrenergic blocking drug to control symptoms from pheochromocytoma. Dosage is increased to 60 mg 3 times daily for 3 days before surgery to remove pheochromocytoma.	Propranolol blocks the beta action on the heart from excess epinephrine produced by a tumor of the adrenal medulla called a pheochromocytoma. An alpha receptor blocking drug must also be used to control the hypertension.
Sotalol hydrochloride†	Sotacor†	ORAL: *Adults*—80 mg two times daily. Daily dosage may be increased by 80 mg every 2 to 3 weeks to achieve desired results.	Nonselective.
Timolol maleate	Apo-Timolol† Blocadren*	ORAL: 10 mg daily initially. Maintenance is 20 to 40 mg daily. Maximum, 60 mg daily in 2 doses. FDA Pregnancy Category B.	Nonselective. Also used as a prophylaxis for myocardial reinfarction and for the treatment of glaucoma.

ALPHA ADRENERGIC RECEPTOR ANTAGONISTS

Phentolamine hydrochloride; phentolamine mesylate	Regitine Rogitine†	ORAL: *Adults*—50 mg every 4 to 6 hr. *Children*—25 mg every 4 to 6 hr. INTRAMUSCULAR, INTRAVENOUS: *Adults*—5 mg. *Children*—1 mg.	Alpha adrenergic blocker. To diagnose hypertension due to pheochromocytoma. To treat a hypertensive crisis secondary to pheochromocytoma, clonidine withdrawal, or tyramine ingestion during monoamine oxidase therapy. To reverse ischemia of levarterenol infiltration.
Phenoxybenzamine hydrochloride	Dibenzyline	ORAL: 10 mg daily. May be increased by 10 mg/day to a maximum dose of 60 mg daily.	Irreversible alpha adrenergic blocker. To treat hypertension secondary to pheochromocytoma. To improve peripheral circulation in Raynaud's disease, ulceration, frostbite, and diabetic gangrene.
Prazosin hydrochloride	Minipress*	ORAL: Initial dosage 2 to 3 mg in divided doses. Dosage may be increased gradually to 20 to 30 mg/day.	Blocks alpha adrenergic receptors and is usually added to a diuretic and a sympathetic depressant, usually a beta blocker.
Terazosin hydrochloride	Hytrin	ORAL: *Adults*—initially, 1 mg daily at bedtime; may increase to 5 mg daily if necessary, in increments. FDA Pregnancy Category C.	Blocks alpha adrenergic receptors and is usually added to a diuretic and sympathetic depressant, usually a beta-blocker.

ALPHA AND BETA ADRENERGIC RECEPTOR ANTAGONIST

Labetalol hydrochloride	Trandate* Normodyne	ORAL: 100 mg twice daily, initially. Maintenance doses are 200 to 800 mg daily for mild to moderate hypertension; 600 to 1200 mg daily for moderately severe hypertension; 1200 to 2400 mg daily for severe hypertension. FDA Pregnancy Category C.	Taken with a diuretic as a step 2 drug. Has a greater effect on standing blood pressure than pure beta adrenergic antagonists. Also has effective vasodilator activity. An injectable preparation is available for hypertensive emergencies. See Table 15.3.

*Available in Canada and United States.
†Available in Canada only.

Table 15.2   Drugs for Treatment of Chronic Hypertension—cont'd

Generic name	Trade name	Administration/dosage	Comments
DRUGS INTERFERING WITH STORAGE AND/OR RELEASE OF NOREPINEPHRINE			
Alseroxylon	Rauwiloid	ORAL: Initial dosage 2 to 4 mg daily; maintenance dosage 2 mg daily.	Active ingredient is reserpine.
Deserpidine	Harmonyl	ORAL: Initial dosage 0.75 to 1 mg daily; maintenance dosage 0.25 mg daily.	Chemically related to reserpine.
Guanadrel	Hylorel	ORAL: 10 mg daily initially, increased daily or less often until desired response is obtained. Maintenance dose is usually 25 to 75 mg daily. May divide the daily dosage. FDA Pregnancy Category B.	More rapidly acting and of shorter duration than guanethidine. Taken with a diuretic. Being tested as a step 2 drug for moderate hypertension. Side effects similar to those of guanethidine but milder.
Guanethidine sulfate	Apo-Guanethidine† Ismelin*	ORAL: *Adults*—initial dosage 12.5 mg daily. Dosage may be increased every 7 days by increments of 12.5 mg to a maximum daily dosage of 100 mg. Further increments of 25 mg to the daily dosage may then be made every week to a maximum of 300 mg daily. *Children*—initial dosage 0.2 mg/kg of body weight daily. Increments of 0.2 mg/kg may then be made of the daily dosage every 7 to 10 days.	Inhibits the release of norepinephrine and eventually depletes neuronal stores of norepinephrine. Used with a diuretic to control severe hypertension. Guanethidine does not enter the central nervous system to cause depression. Common side effects include orthostatic hypotension and diarrhea.
Rauwolfia serpentina	Raudixin Rauval Rauverid Wolfina	ORAL: Initial dosage 200 to 400 mg daily in 1 or 2 doses; maintenance dosage 50 to 300 mg daily in 1 or 2 doses.	Active ingredient is reserpine.
Reserpine	Serpasil* Novoreserpine Reserfia Serpalan	ORAL: *Adults*—initial dosage 0.25 to 0.5 mg daily; maintenance dosage 0.1 to 0.25 mg daily. *Children*—0.25 to 0.5 mg daily.	Depletes norepinephrine stores. Used with a diuretic for the control of essential hypertension. Reserpine is also used to treat the vasospasm of Raynaud's disease (Chapter 14).
CENTRALLY ACTING ANTIHYPERTENSIVE DRUGS THAT INHIBIT ACTIVITY OF SYMPATHETIC NERVOUS SYSTEM			
Clonidine hydrochloride	Catapres* Dixarit†	ORAL: *Adults*—0.1 mg 2 or 3 times daily. Dosage may be increased daily in increments of 0.1 to 0.2 mg. Maintenance doses are commonly 0.2 to 0.8 mg daily and are seldom larger than 2.4 mg daily. Withdrawal symptoms will occur when doses are larger than 1.2 mg daily unless doses are reduced gradually. FDA Pregnancy Category C.	A centrally acting drug reducing sympathetic output. Used with a diuretic for the control of essential hypertension.
	Catapres-TTS	TRANSDERMAL: *Adults*—1 system applied once a week. There are systems delivering 100, 200, or 300 μg/day.	Convenient transdermal patch, changed weekly.

*Available in Canada and United States.
†Available in Canada only.

Continued.

Table 15.2 Drugs for Treatment of Chronic Hypertension—cont'd

Generic name	Trade name	Administration/dosage	Comments
CENTRALLY ACTING ANTIHYPERTENSIVE DRUGS THAT INHIBIT ACTIVITY OF SYMPATHETIC NERVOUS SYSTEM—cont'd			
Guanabenz acetate	Wytensin	ORAL: 4 mg twice daily. May increase gradually to 32 mg twice daily or 64 mg once a day. FDA Pregnancy Category C.	Taken with a diuretic as a step 2 drug. Reduces blood pressure and heart rate. Withdrawal reaction with rebound hypertension may be seen after discontinuing large doses.
Guanfacine	Tenex	ORAL: 0.5 mg twice a day, increased gradually. Maintenance dose is 1 to 3 mg as a single or divided dose. FDA Pregnancy Category B.	Used alone and with a diuretic. Reduces blood pressure and may reduce heart rate. Withdrawal reaction with rebound hypertension may be seen after discontinuing large doses.
Methyldopa	Aldomet*	ORAL: *Adults*—initial dose 250 mg in the morning. After 1 week, the dose may be doubled, with the second 250 mg given at bedtime. Dosage may then be increased to a maximum of 2 Gm daily. *Children*—initial dosage 10 mg/kg body weight divided into 2 to 4 doses. Dosage may be increased gradually after 2 days in increments to a maximum dosage of 65 mg/kg daily.	Acts centrally to depress sympathetic tone. Used with a thiazide diuretic for the control of essential hypertension. An injectable preparation is available for hypertensive emergencies. See Table 15.3.
VASODILATORS			
Direct acting			
Hydralazine hydrochloride	Apresoline* Novo-Hylazin	ORAL: *Adults*—initial dosage to 25 mg 2 or 3 times daily. Dosage may be increased by 10 to 25 mg daily. Maximum dosage, 400 mg in 4 divided doses. *Children*—initial dosage 0.75 mg/kg body weight in 4 divided doses. Dosage may be increased over 3 to 4 weeks to a maximum dosage of 7.5 mg/kg daily.	Usually added to a diuretic and a sympathetic depressant (particularly the beta adrenergic antagonists) for the control of essential hypertension.
Minoxidil	Loniten Minodyl	ORAL: *Adults*—initial dosage 2.5 mg twice daily, increased to 5 mg twice daily after 1 week if needed. Up to 40 mg daily may be given. FDA Pregnancy Category C. *Children*—initial dosage 0.1 to 0.2 mg/kg body weight daily in 2 doses. Increase gradually to 1.4 mg/kg of body weight daily if required.	Usually added to therapy with a diuretic and a beta adrenergic antagonist.
Calcium channel blockers			
Diltiazem hydrochloride	Cardizem	ORAL: *Adults*—initially, 30 mg 3 or 4 times daily, increasing at 1 or 2 day intervals as needed, up to 360 mg daily. FDA Pregnancy Category C.	A good vasodilator. Also used as an antianginal agent.

*Available in Canada and United States.

Table 15.2   Drugs for Treatment of Chronic Hypertension—cont'd

Generic name	Trade name	Administration/dosage	Comments
Calcium channel blockers—cont'd			
Nifedipine	Adalat* Apo-Nifed* Novo-Nifedin* Procardia	ORAL: *Adults*—initially, 10 mg 3 times daily, increasing gradually as needed, to a maximum dose of 180 mg daily. FDA Pregnancy Category C.	A good vasodilator. Does not depress the SA or AV nodes. Also used as an antianginal agent.
Verapamil hydrochloride	Calan Isoptin*	ORAL: *Adults*—initially, 80 mg 3 or 4 times daily. Increase gradually as needed, up to 480 mg daily. FDA Pregnancy Category C.	Depresses the SA and AV nodes. Also used as an antianginal agent, an antiarrhythmic agent, and to treat hypertrophic cardiomyopathy.
Angiotensin converting enzyme inhibitors			
Captopril	Capoten*	ORAL: *Adults*—12.5 mg 3 times daily. May increase up to 25 mg 3 times daily in 1 to 2 weeks. FDA Pregnancy Category C.	May be used alone. Often combined with a diuretic. Also used to treat congestive heart failure.
Enalapril maleate	Vasotec*	ORAL: *Adults*—initially, 5 mg once a day; increase gradually to a maximum of 40 mg daily if needed. FDA Pregnancy Category C.	May be used alone. Often combined with a diuretic. This drug is converted to its active form by the liver.
Lisinopril	Prinivil Zestril	ORAL: *Adults*—initially, 10 mg once a day; increase gradually to a maximum of 40 mg if needed.	May be used alone. Often combined with a diuretic.

*Available in Canada and United States.

antihypertensive drugs. Beta-1 adrenergic receptors are found principally in heart and fat tissue, stimulating heart function and lipolysis, respectively. Beta-2 adrenergic receptors mediate bronchodilation and peripheral vasodilation. The antihypertensive action of beta adrenergic receptor antagonists is not entirely clear, but it appears to result from the decreased cardiac output and from the inhibition of renin production by the kidney. The decreased cardiac output is a result of the inhibition of the beta-1 adrenergic receptors to decrease heart rate, contractility, and automaticity.

One goal in the development of new beta adrenergic blockers has been to develop cardioselective agents, drugs specific for the beta-1 receptor. The adverse side effects associated with blockade of beta-2 receptors include bronchospasm, prolongation of insulin-induced hypoglycemia, and aggravation of peripheral vascular insufficiency. However, the superiority of the cardioselective beta adrenergic blockers for avoiding these complications is not clear.

Another goal in the development of new beta adrenergic blockers has been to find drugs with some intrinsic beta adrenergic activity (partial agonists), as seen in acebutolol, carteolol, oxprenolol, and pindolol. These drugs should produce less cardiac depression and should be safer for patients with compromised cardiac function. The issue of improved safety remains to be proved.

Comparison of beta adrenergic blockers. The available beta adrenergic antagonists do not differ in their antihypertensive effect. However, they do differ in their physiological distribution and metabolism. Dosages of each of the drugs must be individualized for the patient. Some of the drugs must be given two or more times a day, whereas others require only once-a-day administration.

Use as antihypertensive drugs. Beta adrenergic blockers are used as step 2 drugs, added to a diuretic, in long-term antihypertensive therapy. However, there is growing evidence that beta adrenergic blockers are most effective when given as a sole drug to hypertensive patients with high plasma

---

DIETARY CONSIDERATION: SODIUM

Excessive intake of sodium is associated with fluid retention and hypertension in some individuals. The first step in decreasing sodium intake is to stop adding salt to food while cooking or to cooked food during meals. The next step is to eliminate *processed* foods, which contain a large amount of added sodium:

relishes and pickles   potato chips, pretzels
salted popcorn,   canned, frozen, or dehy-
   nuts   drated soup
sauerkraut   bread, rolls, bran, bran
bouillon cubes   flakes
salted crackers   processed cheese,
                                 cheese spreads
canned meat, such as tuna and vienna sausages
salt-cured meat such as bacon, ham, corned
   beef, salt pork, corned beef, luncheon meats,
   frankfurters, sausage
seasonings such as garlic or onion salts, prepared mustard, meat extracts and tenderizers
   such as monosodium glutamate, soy sauce
   and Worcestershire sauce, catsup, and cooking with salt pork or bacon grease
   Teach patients to read food ingredient lists, and to limit or avoid foods containing the following ingredients: salt, baking soda, monosodium glutamate, baking powder, and sodium compounds such as sodium benzoate, sodium citrate, sodium propionate, sodium alginate, sodium sulfite, sodium hydroxide, disodium phosphate, and sodium saccharin.
   As a final step, teach patients to limit or avoid foods naturally high in sodium: milk, eggs, meat (including fish and poultry), cheese, beets and greens, carrots, celery, chard, spinach, kale, and white turnip roots.

---

renin levels. These patients are principally young white patients. Older black hypertensive patients tend to have low plasma renin concentrations and respond better to a diuretic alone or to a diuretic with another type of sympathetic depressant.

Beta adrenergic blockers are especially effective when a step 3 direct-acting vasodilator, such as hydralazine or minoxidil, must be added to the therapy. These vasodilators alone cause a reflex increase in cardiac output because of their marked hypotensive effect. This reflex cardiac stimulation is blocked by the beta adrenergic blockers.

Adverse effects and contraindications. Adverse effects of beta adrenergic blockers are usually mild. The most common side effects are dizziness, fatigue, cool extremities, reduced exercise tolerance, tingling in the fingers or toes, gastrointestinal up-

set, bronchospasm, depression, and sexual dysfunction (impotence in men).

Patients with abnormal cardiovascular function are the most likely to encounter more serious side effects, such as pulmonary edema, hypotension, cardiac failure, and an atrioventricular nodal block.

Beta adrenergic receptor blocking drugs should not be discontinued abruptly because such an action may exacerbate angina, myocardial infarction, or ventricular dysrhythmias. Instead, the dosage should be reduced gradually over 1 to 2 weeks with careful monitoring of the patient for these possible complications.

Beta adrenergic receptor blockers are used with caution in patients whose health status could be worsened by this class of drugs; specific conditions include poor cardiac function, asthma, peripheral vascular disease, and diabetes. Blockade of beta receptors can compromise cardiac function, induce bronchospasm, and inhibit peripheral vasodilation. Hypoglycemia normally elicits the discharge of epinephrine. The effects of this released epinephrine will not be noticed easily in a patient who is taking a beta adrenergic receptor blocking drug. This is an important point for those patients with diabetes mellitus who are taking insulin or an oral hypoglycemic drug.

Other uses. Beta adrenergic blockers are also used in the treatment of angina (Chapter 14) and certain arrhythmias (Chapter 17) and after myocardial infarction. The use of these drugs after myocardial infarction is to prevent sudden death resulting from electrical abnormalities in the recovering heart. Recent studies have specifically shown the efficacy of timolol, propranolol, and metoprolol in reducing the incidence of sudden death after a heart attack.

Specific beta adrenergic blocking drugs

Acebutolol (Monitan, Sectral). Acebutolol is an intermediate-acting, cardioselective beta adrenergic blocker. It is moderately well absorbed when taken orally. Acebutolol is metabolized by the liver, but the drug is mostly excreted unchanged, both in the urine and in the feces through enterohepatic circulation.

Atenolol (Tenormin). Atenolol is a long-acting, cardioselective beta adrenergic blocker. Poorly absorbed from the gastrointestinal tract, the drug is not metabolized but is excreted unchanged in the urine. The time between doses must be increased in patients with impaired renal function.

Carteolol (Cartrol). Carteolol is a new nonselective beta adrenergic blocker.

PATIENT PROBLEM: ORTHOSTATIC HYPOTENSION

THE PROBLEM
The blood pressure drops markedly as the individual moves from lying to sitting or standing.

SIGNS AND SYMPTOMS
Dizziness, light-headedness, weakness, syncope (fainting).

ASSOCIATED OR CONTRIBUTING FACTORS
Long periods of standing; hot weather; hot showers or baths; ingestion of alcohol; exercise, especially when followed by immobility; dehydration.

PATIENT AND FAMILY EDUCATION
- Tighten calf muscles regularly while standing, or take a break to walk around frequently.
- If possible, consider sitting instead of standing at work.
- Reduce the temperature of baths and showers.
- Wear support stockings. In severe cases, tailor-made waist-high stockings may be needed.
- Avoid the use of alcohol.
- Move slowly from lying to sitting. Hold on to something while moving from lying to sitting or standing, to provide support.
- Maintain an adequate fluid intake to avoid dehydration, especially in the summer or if perspiring profusely.
- If severe, consult the physician: a change in drug or dose may be needed.

ADDITIONAL NURSING CARE MEASURES
- Monitor the blood pressure with patient lying, sitting, and standing, to document hypotension; check both arms.
- Supervise ambulation. Instruct patients with marked hypotension to call for assistance when moving from a reclining to a standing position.

Esmolol (Brevibloc). Esmolol is an ultra-short-acting, cardioselective beta blocker. It is administered intravenously for rapid, short-term control of ventricular rate in patients with atrial fibrillation or atrial flutter during surgery or medical emergencies. (See Chapter 19 for discussion of drugs to control cardiac arrhythmias.)

Metoprolol (Lopressor, Betaloc). Metoprolol is a short-acting, cardioselective beta adrenergic blocker. It is well absorbed from the gastrointestinal tract and readily metabolized by the liver.

Nadolol (Corgard). Nadolol is a long-acting, nonselective beta adrenergic blocker. It is not well absorbed from the gastrointestinal tract, and up to one fourth of the dose may be excreted in the feces. Absorbed drug is excreted unchanged in the urine. Patients with renal failure should be given the drug less frequently.

Oxprenolol (Trasicor). Oxprenolol is a short-acting, nonselective beta adrenergic blocker. It is well absorbed and metabolized by the liver. Oxprenolol is available in Canada but not in the United States.

Penbutolol (Levatol). Penbutolol is a new long-acting, nonselective beta adrenergic blocker.

Pindolol (Visken). Pindolol is a short-acting, nonselective beta adrenergic blocker. It is quite well absorbed when taken orally. Pindolol is metabolized by the liver, but about half the dose is excreted unchanged in the urine.

Propranolol (Inderal). Propranolol, a nonselective beta adrenergic blocker, is the oldest of the clinically used beta adrenergic blocking drugs. It is well absorbed orally, but it is readily metabolized by the liver.

Sotalol (Sotacor). Sotalol is a very long-acting nonselective beta adrenergic blocker. It is moderately well absorbed and poorly metabolized by the liver. Most of the drug is excreted unchanged in the urine. Patients with renal failure should be given the drug less frequently. Sotalol is available in Canada but not in the United States.

Timolol (Blocadren, Apo-Timol). Timolol is a short-acting nonselective beta adrenergic blocker. It is well absorbed from the gastrointestinal tract and metabolized by the liver.

Alpha Adrenergic Receptor Antagonists
(Table 15.2)

Prazosin (Minipress) and Terazosin (Hytrin)

Mechanism of action. Prazosin and terazosin are vasodilators. They lower blood pressure by blocking alpha-1 adrenergic receptors. Both arterioles and veins dilate, reducing the total peripheral resistance. Prazosin and terazosin are largely used as second or third drugs in the treatment of hypertension. A diuretic is usually necessary because the alpha-1 adrenergic blockers may cause fluid retention. Prazosin must be taken two or three times daily. Terazosin is taken once daily.

Side effects. The most common side effects are dizziness, light-headedness, palpitations, and fainting due to orthostatic hypotension. Other complaints may include weakness, fatigue, drowsiness, blurred vision, nasal congestion, nausea, edema, and weight gain.

Drug interactions. Because blood pressure is lowered to a degree that can interfere with the perfusion of blood in the heart, attacks of angina may be precipitated by alpha-1 adrenergic blockers. On the other hand, they can interact with nitroglycerin to relieve an anginal attack. However, the blood pressure may be lowered so much that the patient faints. Anti-inflammatory drugs tend to cause fluid retention, and this may be made worse with alpha-1 adrenergic blockers.

Phentolamine (Regitine)

Phentolamine is a short-acting and reversible alpha adrenergic receptor antagonist. The major effects of phentolamine are vasodilation resulting from blockade of alpha-1 adrenergic receptors, and cardiac stimulation believed to be secondary to blockade of the presynaptic alpha-2 adrenergic receptors. (The presynaptic alpha-2 adrenergic receptors are associated with uptake of norepinephrine; see Chapter 10.)

This drug is not well absorbed orally, and intravenous or intramuscular administration is more common.

Phentolamine has specific clinical uses as a vasodilator. One use is to lower blood pressure in patients with a tumor of the adrenal medulla, which secretes large amounts of epinephrine (the tumor is called a pheochromocytoma). Another use is to lower blood pressure in patients who are being treated with a monoamine oxidase (MAO) inhibitor and are suffering from the "cheese reaction," a hypertensive crisis that can be reversed with phentolamine. (See Chapter 29 for a discussion of the "cheese reaction.") A third use is to treat patients being withdrawn from the antihypertensive drug clonidine, who may suffer a temporary hypertensive crisis.

A major use of phentolamine is to infiltrate a site where levarterenol (norepinephrine) or metaraminol has leaked into the tissue surrounding the infusion site. Phentolamine reverses the profound vasoconstriction that can otherwise cause tissue death.

Side effects of the systemic use of phentolamine include hypotension, a fast heart rate (tachycardia) as a reflex response of the body to the hypotension, nasal congestion secondary to the vasodilation, and general gastrointestinal upset.

Phenoxybenzamine (Dibenzyline)

Phenoxybenzamine is an irreversible alpha receptor antagonist with a duration of action lasting several days. The prominent side effect of phenoxybenzamine is postural hypotension, which refers to a fall in blood pressure when rising from a recumbent to a standing position. In a normal person, postural hypotension is not seen because compensatory vasoconstriction redirects blood flow so that blood does not drain from the head to the legs on standing, which would cause fainting. In a person treated with phenoxybenzamine or other drugs that deplete peripheral norepinephrine, the compensatory vasoconstriction is lost. Reflex tachycardia, nasal congestion, and gastrointestinal upset are other common side effects of phenoxybenzamine resulting from its alpha adrenergic antagonist activity.

Phenoxybenzamine is used to control the high blood pressure caused by the elevated plasma levels of epinephrine in patients with the adrenal tumor pheochromocytoma when they are not yet ready for surgical removal of the tumor. Phenoxybenzamine is also used to dilate blood vessels in the skin, as in the treatment of Raynaud's phenomenon, in which there is a prominent neurogenic vasoconstriction of the blood vessels of the skin, particularly in the hands and feet (Chapter 14).

A major source of drug interactions with phenoxybenzamine is overstimulation of beta adrenergic receptors by drugs such as epinephrine that have both alpha and beta adrenergic receptor agonist activity. The blockade of alpha receptors allows beta receptor activation to go unopposed. Tachycardia is exaggerated. The vasodilator activity of drugs (as of the opioids) is exaggerated in the presence of phenoxybenzamine.

Alpha and Beta Adrenergic Receptor Antagonist (Table 15.2)

Labetalol (Trandate, Vescal)

Labetalol has both alpha and beta receptor antagonist activities. It is effective orally, but it does not yet have a clear role in the step therapy of hypertension. The decrease in heart rate is not as pronounced with labetolol as with other beta antagonists. The alpha antagonist effect is more prominent with labetolol than the beta antagonist effects, and a decrease in peripheral resistance is probably the major therapeutic effect.

Labetolol is metabolized by the liver and excreted in the urine. The drug is normally administered twice daily and is best taken with a meal because food increases the bioavailability of this drug.

Orthostatic hypotension may be experienced early in therapy. Other adverse effects noted include gastrointestinal upset, fatigue, nervousness, dry mouth, and tingling of the scalp. Side effects characteristic of other beta adrenergic antagonists are also seen.

Drugs Interfering with the Storage and/or Release of Norepinephrine
(Table 15.2)

Reserpine (Serpasil)

Reserpine and related drugs are often called rauwolfia alkaloids because reserpine was originally isolated from the *Rauwolfia serpentina* bush of India. Reserpine was originally used as an antipsychotic drug but has been replaced by the phenothiazine tranquilizers for this use. Reserpine is effective in lowering blood pressure because it depletes stores of norepinephrine from neurons both in the central and the peripheral nervous systems. The central action produces sedation and tranquilization. The reported incidence of depression with reserpine has varied from 27% to 40%. Occasionally, patients taking reserpine will become severely depressed to the point of attempting suicide. More commonly, patients complain of a lethargic feeling, an increased appetite, and increased dreaming. Nightmares are sometimes a complaint.

Other side effects of reserpine can be related to the decreased sympathetic tone: vasodilation, resulting in a flushed, warm feeling, and nasal congestion. Some side effects of reserpine can be related to the predominant parasympathetic tone when sympathetic tone is depressed: salivation, stomach cramps, and diarrhea. Since reserpine augments gastric acid secretion through the increased parasympathetic tone, it should not be used in patients with a peptic ulcer.

Guanethidine (Ismelin)

Mechanism of action. Guanethidine is a very potent antihypertensive drug that is restricted for use in controlling severe hypertension. This drug enters peripheral sympathetic neurons, being taken into the cell by the same mechanism as for the reuptake of norepinephrine. Inside the neuron, guanethidine blocks norepinephrine release. Guanethidine does not cross the blood-brain barrier and therefore produces no central effects. Because norepinephrine is not available for release from peripheral sympathetic neurons, both the peripheral vascular resistance and the cardiac output are decreased.

Administration and duration. The effects of guanethidine may take 1 to 2 weeks to reach the maximum therapeutic response to a given dosage regimen. Moreover, effects of guanethidine persist for 7 to 10 days after therapy is discontinued.

Side effects. A number of uncomfortable side effects arise from the depletion of peripheral norepinephrine stores. Orthostatic (postural) hypotension, as described for phenoxybenzamine, is a special problem with guanethidine therapy, too. The tone of blood vessels is diminished by guanethidine and, if the patient moves suddenly from a reclining to a standing position, the appropriate vascular changes cannot take place quickly enough for proper blood redistribution. The blood stays in the periphery and drains from the head on standing, resulting in fainting. Patients taking guanethidine must be instructed to change body positions slowly. Other side effects resulting from the depletion of norepinephrine include a slow heart rate (bradycardia) and diarrhea. This diarrhea can be severe and of an explosive nature after meals. In men, failure of erection or ejaculation may arise secondary to the loss of vascular tone. Guanethidine also causes sodium retention; therefore a diuretic is administered concurrently.

Contraindications. Contraindications for guanethidine therapy include the presence of angina, cerebral insufficiency, or coronary artery disease, conditions that are further compromised by the loss of vascular tone.

Drug interactions. A number of drug interactions have been noted for guanethidine. Patients taking guanethidine are supersensitive to administered catecholamines. Patients become less responsive to guanethidine when an indirect-acting adrenergic drug such as amphetamine or ephedrine is taken or when a tricyclic antidepressant drug is taken. These indirect-acting adrenergic drugs release stored norepinephrine from neurons, an action that overcomes the effect of guanethidine to block release of norepinephrine. Tricyclic antidepressants block the uptake of guanethidine into the neuron so that guanethidine cannot reach its site of action.

Guanadrel (Hylorel)

Guanadrel has actions similar to those of guanethidine but with more rapid onset of action and shorter duration of action. The side affects of guanadrel are similar to those of guanethidine but less severe.

Centrally Acting Antihypertensive Drugs that Inhibit the Activity of the Sympathetic Nervous System
(Table 15.2)

Methyldopa (Aldomet)

Methyldopa is taken into sympathetic neurons and metabolized to methylnorepinephrine. Methylnorepinephrine is stored in granules and released on stimulation of the neuron. Methylnorepinephrine is called a *false transmitter*, since it takes the place of norepinephrine. Until recently the antihypertensive effect of methylnorepinephrine was believed to result from the ineffectiveness of methylnorepinephrine as a vasoconstrictor. Recently it has been shown that methylnorepinephrine is a potent vasoconstrictor, so the action of methylnorepinephrine as a false transmitter for peripheral sympathetic neurons does not account for the antihypertensive effects of methyldopa. The effect of methyldopa in the central nervous system to decrease the activity of the sympathetic nervous system is now believed to account for the antihypertensive effect of the drug. Methyldopa decreases sympathetic tone and has a tranquilizing effect on behavior.

Side effects common to methyldopa are related largely to the decrease in central sympathetic activity. Drowsiness is common at the beginning of treatment. Unpleasant sedation, depressed mood, and nightmares are occasional complaints. Tiredness and fatigue may be noted. Peripheral effects include a slow heart rate (bradycardia), diarrhea, dry mouth, and occasional ejaculatory failure in men.

Occasionally, methyldopa causes a false positive Coombs' test. A positive Coombs' test indicates hemolytic anemia, but it is rare for the patient taking methyldopa to have hemolytic anemia in spite of the positive test. Methyldopa may also cause a mild alteration of liver function tests. Methyldopa is therefore not a drug to use for patients who already have impaired liver function, since the drug will interfere with evaluating the course of the disease. This alteration of liver tests ordinarily occurs during the first 6 weeks of therapy, and it is reversed by discontinuing methyldopa.

Clonidine (Catapres)

Clonidine has an antihypertensive effect as a result of its action in the central nervous system. It activates alpha receptors in the vasomotor center of the medulla, an action that inhibits activity of the sympathetic nervous system. Heart rate and cardiac output are decreased and account for the reduction in blood pressure.

Clonidine is commonly used with a diuretic in antihypertensive therapy. New therapeutic uses for clonidine have developed. Clonidine is used in the prophylaxis of vascular headaches and to treat the vasomotor symptoms of menopause. The symptoms of opioid withdrawal and nicotine withdrawal can often be controlled by clonidine. Gilles de la Tourette's syndrome, a condition of severe and multiple tics, is alleviated by clonidine therapy.

Common side effects of clonidine therapy include drowsiness, dry mouth, and constipation. Sudden discontinuance can be dangerous. After discontinuing therapeutic doses for 12 to 48 hours, many patients experience symptoms of a sympathetic rebound: restlessness, insomnia, tremors, increased salivation, and increased heart rate (tachycardia). If clonidine is not reinstated, further symptoms follow: headaches, abdominal pain, and nausea. The most severe reaction is a hypertensive crisis that is best treated in the hospital with a combination of alpha-blocking and beta-blocking drugs: phentolamine and propranolol. To avoid these withdrawal problems, clonidine doses are gradually reduced over a week or more.

Guanabenz (Wytensin)

Guanabenz has a mechanism of action similar to that of clonidine, inhibiting sympathetic activity by activating alpha receptors in the central nervous system. Guanabenz has a long duration of action, 12 to 24 hours, and may require only once-a-day dosage. It is metabolized and excreted in the urine.

The most common side effects are drowsiness, dry mouth, dizziness, weakness, and headache. Withdrawal rebound hypertension can occur if guanabenz is discontinued abruptly.

Vasodilators for Treating Chronic Hypertension (Table 15.2)

Hydralazine (Apresoline)

Hydralazine acts directly on arteriolar smooth muscle to cause relaxation. The mechanism is not known. The drop in arterial blood pressure is great enough to activate the baroreceptors of the aorta. This activation causes a reflex stimulation of the heart, which increases cardiac output and partially compensates for the fall in blood pressure (reflex tachycardia). Hydralazine also causes sodium retention. Because hydralazine causes reflex stimulation of the heart and increases sodium retention, it is most effective in reducing hypertension when added to a diuretic to counteract the sodium retention and a beta adrenergic receptor antagonist (propranolol, nadolol, or metoprolol) to block the reflex stimulation of the heart.

Side effects common to hydralazine include headache, palpitation, loss of appetite, nausea, vomiting, and diarrhea. In the absence of a beta antagonist, hydralazine can cause angina in susceptible individuals as a result of the reflex stimulation of the heart. Hydralazine is not a good drug for a patient with angina, coronary artery disease, or congestive heart failure because of the indirect cardiac effects.

The main problem that has been documented in the past after long-term therapy at high doses of hydralazine is the appearance of a "lupus-like" syndrome. Lupus erythematosus is an autoimmune disease with symptoms of fever, joint pain, chest pain, edema, and circulating antibodies to DNA. The syndrome induced by hydralazine is similar, but it is reversed when the drug is discontinued. The appearance of lupus-like symptoms is infrequent when smaller doses of hydralazine are used in combination with diuretic and sympathetic blocking drug. Patients on hydralazine therapy are monitored for the appearance of the anti-DNA antibodies and lupus erythematosus (LE) cells.

Minoxidil (Loniten)

Minoxidil is a direct-acting vasodilator like hydralazine, but is more potent. This drug must be given with a diuretic to control fluid retention and a beta receptor blocker to prevent reflex tachycardia. A side effect of minoxidil is excessive hairiness, which may develop after a few weeks of treatment. Some patients experience transient nausea, headaches, or fatigue when treatment is started.

Calcium Channel Blockers

Calcium channel blockers are effective in the treatment of angina, arrhythmias, and hypertension. These agents lessen the amount of intracellular calcium in smooth muscle to lower vascular tone, an action that reduces peripheral resistance. Cardiac function is also depressed because of reduced intracellular calcium. The calcium channel blockers each differ in their relative effect on vascular and cardiac tissue.

Side effects of calcium channel blockers are generally mild. Headaches, dizziness, and edema are occasional complaints. The depression of AV nodal conduction may lead to heart block. Beta-adrenergic blockers act synergistically with calcium channel blockers to depress AV conduction and depress cardiac contractility. The digitalis glycosides act additively with the calcium channel blockers to depress AV conduction. These drugs should be used with caution in patients with congestive heart failure.

Diltiazem (Cardiazem) depresses both the sinoatrial (SA) and atrioventricular (AV) nodes but produces little negative inotropic effect (decrease in the strength of the heart beat). Diltiazem is effective in dilating coronary vessels, making it a good antianginal agent. Diltiazem is well absorbed orally and extensively metabolized.

Nicardipine (Cardene) is more selective for vascular smooth muscle than for cardiac muscle. This means that nicardipine is a potent vasodilator and also dilates the coronary vessels with little or no depression of conductivity.

Nifedipine (Procardia, Adalat) is similar to nicardipine in being more selective for smooth muscle than for cardiac muscle.

Verapamil (Calan, Isoptin) depresses the SA and AV nodes, an action that makes it a useful antiarrhythmic drug (Chapter 19). A slowing of the heart rate (bradycardia) is common.

Calcium channel blockers awaiting release at the time of this revision include isradipine (DynaCirc) and nitrendipine (Baypress).

Angiotensin-converting Enzyme (ACE) Inhibitors

The angiotensin-converting enzyme (ACE) inhibitors have rapidly found a role in the treatment of chronic hypertension. Note in Figure 15.1 that angiotensin II is a potent vasoconstrictor. Angiotensin II is formed from angiotensin I by angiotensin converting enzyme. When this enzyme is inhibited, the amount of angiotensin II formed decreases. Another action is an increase in the amounts of the vasodilator peptide, bradykinin. The ACE inhibitors block the degradation of bradykinin. The net effect of ACE inhibitors is to decrease peripheral vascular resistance. This action makes the ACE inhibitors useful in treating congestive heart failure.

ACE inhibitors may be used alone or in combination with beta adrenergic blockers or diuretics for the treatment of chronic hypertension. They are especially useful in treating renovascular hypertension. They are well tolerated and have little, if any, adverse effects on the central nervous system func-

THE NURSING PROCESS

ANTIHYPERTENSIVE DRUGS

Assessment

Patients with a persistent blood pressure exceeding 90 mm Hg diastolic pressure and/or an excessively high systolic pressure may be appropriate candidates for antihypertensive therapy. In some cases the cause of the hypertension may be clearly identified, as in renal disease, but most of the time it is not. Additional baseline data that should be obtained in these patients include weight, usual dietary practices related to salt intake, serum electrolyte concentration, blood urea nitrogen, and measures of renal and cardiovascular function.

Nursing diagnoses

Sexual dysfunction related to drug's side effect: impotence
Noncompliance related to intolerable side effects
Potential complication: severe hypotension

Management

In cases of hypertensive crisis, patients may be admitted to the acute care setting for pharmacological manipulation of the blood pressure. The use of a cardiac monitor, standby availability of a vasopressor agent, and sophisticated vascular monitoring may all be appropriate. In less acute situations, therapy may be started in the hospitalized or ambulatory patient. Parameters to monitor include the blood pressure and other vital signs, fluid intake and output, weight, serum electrolyte concentration, serum and urinary glucose levels, and other laboratory data specific to side effects of individual drugs, for instance, a blood count and liver function studies with methyldopa. Planning should be started for patient self-management at home, including determination by the health care team of other medications such as diuretics or potassium that may be needed, when sodium and/or caloric restrictions are required, and instruction about the potential dangers of hypertension.

Evaluation

Ideally, therapy with antihypertensive drugs will allow the patient's blood pressure to remain below 140/90, and the patient will be free of side effects such as orthostatic hypotension, drowsiness, and impotence (see text). In many, if not most cases, it is not possible to achieve all these goals. The patient should be able to explain the hazards of untreated hypertension, why therapy is necessary, how to take the prescribed medications safely, why additional drugs such as diuretics or potassium may be needed, possible anticipated side effects and what to do about them, how to follow any dietary restrictions prescribed, and what situations warrant calling the physician. If the patient or family is to record weight or blood pressure on a regular basis, the ability to do this correctly should be demonstrated. The patient should be able to state the desired body weight. For more specific guidelines, see the patient care implications section at the end of this chapter.

tion or on carbohydrate or lipid metabolism. Dizziness, a skin rash, swelling, and an increase in serum potassium levels (hyperkalemia) have been reported.

Drug interactions have been reported for the ACE inhibitors. Foods or drugs high in potassium may contribute to hyperkalemia. The hypotensive effect of ACE inhibitors is enhanced by diuretics, alcohol, and beta adrenergic blockers. Nonsteroidal anti-inflammatory drugs (NSAIDS), especially indomethacin, may antagonize the antihypertensive effect of the ACE inhibitors and cause sodium retention leading to edema.

Captopril (Capoten) is rapidly absorbed after oral administration and is effective within 1 hour. About half of the drug is excreted unchanged in the urine.

Enalapril (Vasotec) is a prodrug, designed to be absorbed orally. On absorption, enalapril is deesterified to the active drug, enalaprilat, which is an inhibitor of angiotensin converting enzyme like captopril. However, patients with liver disease may be unable to activate enalapril.

Enalaprilat injection (Vasotec injection) is the active form of enalapril in a dosage form to treat a hypertensive emergency.

Lisinopril (Prinivil, Zestril) has a longer duration of action than captopril or enalapril, with most patients requiring just one daily dose.

DRUGS USED IN HYPERTENSIVE EMERGENCIES

A hypertensive emergency cannot be simply defined. The blood pressure may be severely elevated or only moderately elevated. The important feature is that there is impending end-organ damage, usually of the brain, heart, or eyes. Unstable neurological symptoms suggesting damage to the brain include headache, restlessness, confusion, and even convulsions. Hemorrhaging may be apparent in the eye. Drugs that are currently used to treat hypertension emergencies by rapidly lowering blood pressure are listed in Table 15.3.

Vasodilators (Table 15.3)

Diazoxide (Hyperstat)

Diazoxide acts directly to relax arteriolar smooth muscle. This action lowers blood pressure but does not affect the venous side of circulation. Diazoxide is therefore not useful for those conditions requiring the decreased venous return produced by trimethaphan.

The advantage of diazoxide treatment is that a bolus of the drug can be given intravenously over 30 seconds and will usually be effective in 5 minutes and remain effective for 2 to 12 hours. Blood pressure does not need to be continuously monitored as with trimethaphan treatment. The patient rarely becomes excessively hypotensive. Diazoxide causes retention of sodium and water, which must be treated with a diuretic. Diazoxide also causes hyperglycemia.

Sodium nitroprusside (Nipride)

Sodium nitroprusside acts directly on the smooth muscle of both arterioles and venous vessels. The result is an immediate decrease in blood pressure with no increase in venous return. There are no notable side effects with short-term use of nitroprusside. Blood pressure must be constantly monitored, and the drug is administered by intravenous drip. Nitroprusside is unstable in light, so it should not be used more than 4 hours after it is dissolved. Side effects arise from the use of nitroprusside for several days. Some of it is metabolized to thiocyanate, which can produce ringing in the ears (tinnitus), blurred vision, and hypothyroidism.

Ganglionic Blocking Drug (Table 15.3)

Trimethaphan (Arfonad)

Trimethaphan blocks the receptors for acetylcholine in the ganglia and is a ganglionic blocking drug. Ganglionic blocking drugs inhibit both sympathetic and parasympathetic activity and therefore have limited clinical uses. It is used in treating some hypertension emergencies. Because trimethaphan has a short duration of action, it is administered by continuous intravenous drip, during which blood pressure must be constantly monitored. Side effects result from the inhibition of both sympathetic and parasympathetic tone. Severe hypotension can result from the inhibition of sympathetic tone. Intravenous drip is then discontinued until the blood pressure begins to rise again. Side effects from loss of parasympathetic tone include pupillary dilation, loss of accommodation, drying of mucous surfaces, constipation, and urinary retention.

The disadvantages of trimethaphan therapy are that blood pressure must be carefully followed and that the loss of pupillary reflexes makes it difficult to monitor ongoing neurological damage to the brain, when neurological damage was the presenting set of symptoms. Also trimethaphan can be unpredictable in its effects: patients already on antihypertensive medication or with a reduced blood volume may be unusually sensitive to trimethaphan. Some patients do not respond readily to trimethaphan; others are initially responsive but become unresponsive.

Trimethaphan does decrease venous return of blood and lower cardiac output. These actions are helpful when the patient has a condition such as a dissecting aortic aneurysm, hypertensive encephalopathy, acute left ventricular failure, or cerebral

Text continued on p. 249.

Table 15.3   Drugs Used in Hypertension Emergencies

Generic name	Trade name	Administration/dosage	Comments
Diazoxide	Hyperstat*	INTRAVENOUS: *Adults*—150 mg or 5 mg/kg body weight. *Children*—5 mg/kg body weight. Administered over 30 sec. May be repeated after 30 min.	A direct-acting vasodilator. Acts rapidly (2 to 5 min) and lasts 2 to 12 hr. Increases venous return and cardiac output. Blood pressure fall is rarely excessive, so blood pressure monitoring is not critical.
Enalaprilat	Vasotec	INTRAVENOUS: *Adults*—1.25 mg administered over 5 min every 6 hr. Use 0.625 mg for patients on diuretic therapy or in renal failure.	The angiotensin-converting enzyme inhibitor in its active form for intravenous administration. Clinical response should be seen in 1 hr.
Labetalol	Normodyne Trandate*	INTRAVENOUS: *Adults*—20 mg or 0.25 mg/kg injected over 2 min. Additional injections of 40 to 80 mg may be given in 10 min intervals until blood pressure control is achieved or a total dose of 300 mg has been given. Alternatively, may be infused at a rate of 2 mg/min.	A mixed alpha and beta blocker. Clinical response is seen in about 5 min.
Methyldopa hydrochloride	Aldomet*	INTRAVENOUS: *Adults*—250 to 500 mg in 100 ml 5% dextrose, administered slowly over 30 to 60 min. Maximum dose is 1 Gm in 6 hr. INTRAVENOUS: *Children*—5 to 10 mg/kg in 5% dextrose, administered over 30 to 60 min. Maximum dose is 65 mg/kg body weight or 3 Gm daily.	Centrally acting antihypertensive. Clinical response may take several hours. Duration of action is 10 to 16 hours.
Nitroglycerin	Nitro-Bid* Nitrol Nitrostat* Tridil*	INTRAVENOUS: *Adults*—initially 5 μg/min; increase in 5 μg increments every 3-5 min until a clinical response or 20 μg/min is reached.	Direct-acting vasodilator. Doses are stated for non-PVC intravenous infusion sets. PVC may absorb nitroglycerin. IV nitroglycerin is also used to reduce cardiac load or as an antianginal agent in emergency situations. Effective immediately.
Sodium nitroprusside	Nipride* Nitropress	INTRAVENOUS: Dissolve 50 mg in 500 to 1000 ml of 5% dextrose. Infuse 0.5 to 8 μg/kg/min. Solution must be protected from light and discarded after 4 hr.	A direct-acting vasodilator. Acts rapidly (1 to 2 min). Continuous infusion is necessary to maintain hypotensive effect. Decreased venous return with no change in heart rate. Blood pressure must be carefully monitored and infusion rate adjusted to maintain desired level.
Trimethaphan camsylate	Arfonad*	INTRAVENOUS: Administered as a 0.1% (1 mg/ml) infusion in 5% dextrose. The rate of infusion is begun at 0.5 to 1 mg/min and increased gradually until the blood pressure falls by 20 mm Hg. After several minutes, the rate is again increased until the blood pressure reaches the desired level.	A rapidly acting drug that blocks acetylcholine receptors in the ganglia. Inhibits both sympathetic and parasympathetic nervous systems. Decreases venous return and cardiac output. Blood pressure must be carefully monitored, since the hypotensive effect is variable and unpredictable.

*Available in Canada and United States.

PATIENT CARE IMPLICATIONS

Antihypertensives

Drug administration/patient education

- Encourage the patient to lose weight to reach desirable body weight and to restrict dietary intake of sodium, as these may reduce the need for antihypertensive drug therapy.
- Assess patients thoroughly and thoughtfully on a regular basis. Poor compliance with drug therapy may result in part from the fact that patients may not feel better while on antihypertensives, and may feel worse. Patients may feel reluctant to discuss side effects such as impotence, and may discontinue a drug if this or other side effects occur. In addition, the cost of drug therapy, especially when two or more drugs are required, may be prohibitive.
- Reinforce to patients the need to take these medications as directed, and not to discontinue therapy abruptly or without consulting the physician.
- Work with patients to find a way to help them to remember to take their medicines. Activities such as marking off a calendar when doses are taken or preparing a week's doses at one time may keep the patient more involved and help serve as a reminder.
- Teach patients about orthostatic hypotension, a common side effect of antihypertensive therapy. See box on p. 237.
- Monitor blood pressure and pulse at least every 4 hours when patients are begun on antihypertensive therapy, during periods of dosage adjustment, or when orthostatic hypotension is a problem. Assess the blood pressure with the patient lying, then sitting, then standing; check both arms. For selected patients, it may be necessary to teach a family member to measure and record the blood pressure in the home setting.
- Supervise the ambulation of the hospitalized patient on antihypertensive therapy to guard against injury should the patient become dizzy or faint. Be especially alert with the elderly, who are more sensitive to drug effects.
- Teach patients to keep all health care providers informed of all drugs being used, and to avoid over-the-counter medications unless approved by the physician. The incidence of hypotensive episodes is increased if patients taking antihypertensives take other drugs which may also cause hypotension, including other diuretics, central nervous system depressants, barbiturates, or alcohol.
- Monitor daily weight in the hospitalized patient. Weigh patients under standard conditions: same time, same scales, same amount of clothing. Observe for fluid retention: pitting edema (edema characterized by indentations that remain in the skin for seconds to minutes after pressure has been applied by the examiner's finger), dependent edema, tight rings, shoes, and clothing. Auscultate the lungs to detect pulmonary rales. If possible, instruct patients to monitor and record their weight at home. Report to the physician a weight gain in excess of 2 pounds per day or 5 pounds per week.
- Record intake and output in the hospitalized patient.
- Refer the patient to a dietitian or teach the patient about dietary sodium. See the box on p. 236.
- When patients are taking combination products containing two or more drugs, teach them about each drug in the product, and assess for side effects for each drug. For example, the drug Apresoline contains hydralazine and hydrochlorothiazide; the drug Ser-Ap-Es contains hydralazine, hydrochlorothiazide, and reserpine.
- If a dose is missed, instruct patients to take the dose as soon as remembered, unless within 2 hours of the next dose, then resume the usual dosing schedule. Do not double up for missed doses.
- Caution patients to avoid driving or operating hazardous equipment if sedation or sleepiness occurs.
- Review the box on p. 170 for measures to help patients with dry mouth.
  INTRAVENOUS ANTIHYPERTENSIVE THERAPY
- Monitor blood pressure and pulse every 3 to 5 minutes until stable, then every 15 to 30 minutes.
- Use an electronic infusion monitor and a microdrip infusion set to titrate drug dose more accurately.
- Monitor the electrocardiogram.
- Keep patients in bed for up to 3 hours after drug administration. Keep call bell within reach and siderails up.

Beta adrenergic receptor antagonists

Drug administration

- See general guidelines for antihypertensive drugs.

Continued.

PATIENT CARE IMPLICATIONS — cont'd

- Take the apical pulse for a full minute before administering dose. If the pulse is less than 60 in an adult or 90 to 110 in a child, withhold the dose and notify the physician. Specific guidelines may vary with an individual patient or by physician preference. Be especially alert to bradycardia (low pulse rate) if the patient is also taking a cardiac glycoside.
- Monitor the blood pressure. Review the general guidelines, above.
- Monitor general parameters of cardiovascular function: intake, output, daily weight, serum electrolytes. Because these drugs accumulate in the presence of renal failure, monitor the blood urea nitrogen (BUN).
- Treatment of overdose with beta blockers is symptomatic.
- Bronchospasm occasionally occurs. Observe for signs of respiratory distress, auscultate lung sounds, monitor respiratory rate.
- Assess patients for signs of depression: withdrawal, insomnia, anorexia, lack of interest in personal appearance.
    INTRAVENOUS ESMOLOL
- Dilute according to manufacturer's directions to a concentration of 10 mg/ml. Dosage is individualized, but one regimen specifies a loading dose of 500 µg/kg/min for 1 minute, followed by a maintenance infusion of 50 µg/kg/min for 4 minutes. These may be repeated at regular intervals. Monitor blood pressure, pulse, and electrocardiogram.
    INTRAVENOUS METOPROLOL
- May be given by direct IV push. Administer dose over at least 1 minute. Monitor blood pressure, pulse, and electrocardiogram.
    INTRAVENOUS PROPRANOLOL
- Check dose carefully: IV dose is much smaller than oral dose. May be given undiluted or diluted in 5% dextrose solution. Administer at a rate of 1 mg/minute or more slowly. Monitor blood pressure, pulse, and electrocardiogram.

Patient and family education

- Emphasize the importance of taking these drugs as prescribed for optimal benefit. Caution patients not to discontinue these drugs without consultation with the physician, and to avoid letting prescriptions run out. Reinforce to patients that several weeks of therapy may be needed to gain maximum effects.

- Orthostatic hypotension may be a problem; review the box on p. 237.
- Teach patients to take oral doses with meals or snack to reduce gastric irritation.
- Many side effects can occur with beta blockers. Tell patients to report any unexpected sign or symptom to the physician. Teach patients to report signs of thrombocytopenia: unexplained bruising or bleeding; signs of agranulocytosis: unexplained fever or sore throat.
- Teach diabetic patients that beta blockers may mask the symptoms of hypoglycemia, so patients should monitor blood glucose levels carefully during periods of dosage adjustment or when starting or stopping the drug.
- Tell patients that if drowsiness occurs they should avoid driving or operating hazardous equipment until it wears off. If severe or persistent, notify physician.

Alpha adrenergic receptor antagonists

Drug administration/patient and family education

- See general guidelines for antihypertensives.
- Nasal congestion may be a problem. Inform patients this side effect may decrease with continued use of the prescribed drug. Caution patients to avoid the use of over-the-counter medications to self-treat this annoying side effect.
- Sexual dysfunction is common. Assess tactfully about sexual problems; many patients are reluctant to discuss sexual difficulties. Sexual problems may prompt patients to discontinue medications. Provide emotional support as needed. Remind patients not to discontinue medications without notifying physician.
- Caution patients to avoid driving or operating hazardous equipment until the effects of these medications are known. Dizziness and lethargy may be common.
- For overdose with phenoxybenzamine, place patient supine with head lowered and feet elevated if possible. An abdominal binder and leg bandages may also be used. Epinephrine is contraindicated, but IV norepinephrine (levarterenol) may be helpful.
    INTRAVENOUS PHENTOLAMINE
- Dilute 5 mg with 1 ml of sterile water; may be further diluted. Administer at a rate of 5

PATIENT CARE IMPLICATIONS — cont'd

mg or less over 1 minute. Monitor blood pressure and pulse every 30 seconds, and electrocardiogram. Do not leave patient unattended until stable. Treatment of overdose is with dopamine; do not use epinephrine.

- Prazosin and terazosin are especially prone to cause orthostatic hypotension, particularly when therapy is started and during periods of increasing dosage. See box on p. 237 for a discussion of orthostatic hypotension. Instruct patients to take the first dose, and any increased dosages, at bedtime, and to be especially careful when getting up at night during the first few days of therapy. Warn families about this side effect, so they will not be frightened, and will know that they should lay the patient down.

Alpha and beta adrenergic receptor antagonist: Labetolol

Drug administration/patient and family education

- See general guidelines about antihypertensive therapy, and information about beta adrenergic receptor antagonists.
  INTRAVENOUS LABETOLOL
- May be given undiluted or diluted in most common IV solutions.
- Administer at a rate of 20 mg over at least 2 minutes. Monitor blood pressure and pulse every 5 to 10 minutes until stable. Monitor electrocardiogram. Keep patient supine for several hours following injection, and supervise ambulation.

Reserpine and related drugs

Drug administration/patient and family education

- See general guidelines for antihypertensives.
- Serious mental depression is a side effect. Assess patients carefully for changes in mood or affect; assess for anorexia, insomnia, impotence, withdrawal, and mood swings. Instruct families to report the development of any change in the patient's personality.
- Take doses with meals or snack to reduce gastric irritation.
- Monitor the patient's pulse. Tell the patient to notify the physician if noticeable changes in heart rate occur.
- Emphasize to patients that several weeks of therapy may be necessary to see full drug benefit.

Guanethidine and guanadrel

Drug administration/patient and family education

- See general guidelines of antihypertensives.
- Diarrhea may be severe; see p. 193.
- The drugs may cause hypoglycemia. Instruct diabetics to monitor blood glucose levels closely during the start of therapy and periods of dosage adjustment.
- Dry mouth may occur; see box on p. 170.
- Nasal congestion may be a problem. Caution patients to avoid treatment with over-the-counter products without consulting the physician.

Methyldopa

Drug administration/patient and family education

- See general guidelines about antihypertensives.
- Dry mouth may occur; see box on p. 170.
- Mental depression is a side effect. Assess patients carefully for changes in mood or affect; assess for anorexia, insomnia, impotence, withdrawal, and mood swings. Instruct families to report the development of any change in the patient's personality.
- Diarrhea may occur; see p. 193.
- Nasal congestion may be a problem. Caution patients to avoid treatment with over-the-counter products without consulting the physician.
- Methyldopa may alter liver function tests. Teach patients to report the development of malaise, fever, right upper quadrant abdominal pain, or change in the color or consistency of stools. Monitor liver function tests.
- Tell patients that urine may darken if exposed to the air.
- The *intravenous* form is methyldopate hydrochloride. Dilute dose in 100 to 200 ml of 5% dextrose in water. Administer dose as an infusion over 30 to 60 minutes. Avoid IM or subcutaneous administration.

Clonidine, guanabenz, and guanfacine

Drug administration/patient and family education

- See general guidelines about antihypertensives.
- Dry mouth may occur; see box on p. 170.
- Constipation may occur; see box on p. 187.

Continued.

PATIENT CARE IMPLICATIONS — cont'd

- Emphasize to patients the importance of not discontinuing these drugs abruptly. Teach patients to have prescriptions refilled before the supply on hand runs out. Unreliable patients should not take these drugs. See withdrawal symptoms, in text.
- If an oral dose is missed, take it as soon as remembered, unless within 2 hours of the next dose. Do not double up for missed doses. If two or more doses are missed, notify the physician.
- Clonidine is available in a transdermal form. Review patient instruction leaflet provided by manufacturer with patient. Patient should not cut or trim patch. Remove old patch. Apply to clean, nonhairy area, but avoid areas of skin irritation or scars. Rotate sites. If patch becomes very loose or falls off, replace it with a fresh patch; if only slightly loose, cover with adhesive tape. Replace weekly. If a patch is overdue for replacement by 3 days or more, notify physician; do not apply two patches at once.

Hydralazine

Patient and family education

- See general guidelines about antihypertensives.
- Tell patients to notify the physician if lupus-like symptoms develop; see description in the text.
- Instruct patients to report the development of tingling of fingers or numbness, as this may signal peripheral neuropathy; pyridoxine may be prescribed.
- Suggest that patients take oral doses with food or snack to reduce gastric irritation.

Minoxidil

Patient and family education

- See general guidelines about antihypertensives.
- This drug may cause hypertrichosis (excessive hairiness) after several weeks of therapy. Instruct patients to report this side effect. The hair can be shaved, bleached, or removed depending on the location and severity. Caution patients not to discontinue the medication without contacting the physician.
- The side effect of hypertrichosis led to the development of topical minoxidil (Rogaine), used to stimulate hair growth in men who

are balding. Instruct patients to follow instructions supplied by the manufacturer. Wash hair daily before applying solution, and dry scalp and hair thoroughly. Apply prescribed amount, using supplied applicator. Wash hands to remove any solution left on the hands. Do not use a hair dryer to dry the scalp after drug application. If using it at night, wait at least 30 minutes after applying solution before going to bed. If a dose is missed, apply it as soon as remembered, unless close to time for the next dose; do not double up for missed doses. Tell the patient to report local side effects (e.g., itching, scalp burning, skin irritation) or systemic effects such as dizziness, flushing, headache, tingling of hands or feet, weight gain.
- Instruct the patient to report the development of shortness of breath, increased heart rate, or changes in heart rhythm. Assess for distended jugular veins, pulmonary rales.

Calcium channel blockers

See Patient Care Implications, Chapter 14.

Angiotensin-converting enzyme (ACE) inhibitors

Drug administration: Intravenous enalaprilat

- Check dose; IV dose is much smaller than oral dose. May be given undiluted, or dilute with up to 50 ml of a compatible IV solution (see manufacturer's guidelines). Administer dose over at least 5 minutes. Monitor blood pressure and pulse. Keep patient supine until blood pressure is stable.

Patient and family education

- See general guidelines to antihypertensive drugs.
- Caution patients to avoid excessive amounts of foods high in potassium (see Diet Considerations: Potassium, p. 259). Teach patients to avoid salt substitutes unless approved by the physician, as these often contain large amounts of potassium.
- Tell patients to take captopril on an empty stomach, 1 hour before meals, unless instructed otherwise by the physician.
- If a dose is missed, take it as soon as remembered, unless close to the time for the next dose. Do not double up for missed doses.
- Teach patients to report the development of fever, sore throat, or signs of infection.

PATIENT CARE IMPLICATIONS — cont'd

Drugs used in hypertension emergencies

Drug administration

- Ideally, place the patient in an intensive care unit. Monitor electrocardiogram, blood pressure, pulse, respirations, level of consciousness, intake, urinary output; insertion of a Foley catheter may be necessary.
- These drugs should not be mixed with other drugs in an infusion or a syringe.

INTRAVENOUS DIAZOXIDE

- May be administered quickly, undiluted (e.g., 150 mg over 30 seconds or less), or may be diluted and given as a slow infusion over 20 to 30 minutes. Because it is highly alkaline, avoid intramuscular or subcutaneous injection. Make certain that IV line is patent before administering, and inspect insertion site for irritation or redness. If extravasation occurs, apply ice packs. Treat drug overdose/severe hypotension with a sympathomimetic such as norepinephrine. Monitor the blood glucose as the diazoxide may cause hyperglycemia.

INTRAVENOUS SODIUM NITROPRUSSIDE

- Dilute as directed by manufacturer. Cover prepared infusion with aluminum foil to protect from light. Titrate dose based on physician guidelines and patient response; a typical dose is 3 μg/kg of body weight/min (adults) or 1.4 μg/kg/min (small children).

To treat overdose, discontinue nitroprusside and administer amyl nitrate (Chapter 14) for 15 to 30 seconds every minute until a sodium nitrite solution for intravenous administration can be prepared. Administer a 3% sodium nitrite solution at a rate of 2.5 to 5 ml per minute up to a total dose of 10 to 15 ml. After this, inject sodium thiosulfate intravenously, 12.5 Gm in 50 ml of 5% dextrose in water over a 10 minute period. Monitor the patient carefully throughout. Signs of overdose can reappear for up to several hours, and sodium nitrite and sodium thiosulfate can be repeated at half the dose listed. Monitor thiocyanate levels if the drug is used longer than 72 hours. Use dopamine to correct hypotension.

INTRAVENOUS TRIMETHAPHAN

- Dilute as directed by manufacturer. Titrate dose based on physician guidelines and patient response; a typical dose is 0.5 to 1.0 mg/min. Monitor patient response closely. If blood pressure does not drop with patient in supine position, try lowering the head of the bed, but monitor patient closely for signs of cerebral anoxia; note that the drug produces pupillary dilation so this objective sign may be of little significance. To treat severe hypotension, use phenylephrine or mephentermine, or try dopamine.

---

hemorrhage, since the pressure is removed from the weakened tissue.

SUMMARY

The goal in treating patients with hypertension is to achieve and maintain arterial blood pressure below 140/90 mm Hg, if possible. Weight reduction, salt restriction, and moderation of alcohol consumption are appropriate life-style changes to aid in this objective. In addition, a number of drugs are available that may be used alone or in combination. These drugs have a variety of mechanisms.

Diuretics decrease vascular smooth muscle tone by volume depletion and sodium reduction. Sympathetic blockers include the beta blockers, the centrally acting adrenergic inhibitors, and the peripherally acting adrenergic inhibitors. Beta blockers decrease cardiac output and inhibit renin production by the kidney. Centrally acting adrenergic inhibitors inhibit activity of the sympathetic nervous system through actions in the central nervous system. Peripherally acting adrenergic inhibitors decrease the release of the neurotransmitter thereby preventing vasoconstriction. Vasodilators may act directly on the vascular smooth muscle or may block alpha receptors mediating vasoconstriction on the vascular smooth muscle. Calcium channel blockers act as vasodilators and decrease cardiac load. Angiotensin converting enzyme (ACE) inhibitors block the conversion of angiotensin I to the potent vasoconstrictor, angiotensin II. The antihypertensive drugs in use are listed in Table 15.1 by category.

Unfortunately, the drugs used to control hypertension can also cause annoying side effects. The knowledgeable health professional can offer sympathetic understanding to the patient adjusting to these medications. Gastrointestinal disturbances are common with all of the drugs. The drugs depressing sympathetic tone tend to produce weakness or lethargy and occasionally impotence in men. Vasodilators tend to cause headaches, dizziness, and palpitations.

Hypertensive emergencies are treated with rapidly acting drugs. Diazoxide and sodium nitroprusside, which are vasodilators, or trimethaphan, which is a ganglionic blocking drug, are frequently used in treating hypertensive emergencies. The antihypertensive drugs enalaprilat, labetalol, and methyldopa are available in injectable forms for treating hypertensive emergencies as is the vasodilator nitroglycerin. The alpha adrenergic receptor antagonists phentolamine and phenoxybenzamine are used in selected cases of hypertensive emergency resulting from excessive endogenous norepinephrine.

STUDY QUESTIONS

1. Describe the renal mechanisms controlling blood pressure.
2. Describe the cardiovascular mechanisms controlling blood pressure.
3. Name the beta adrenergic receptor antagonists used as antihypertensive drugs. How does blockade of the beta receptors lower blood pressure? What are the side effects of these drugs?
4. For what situations is phentolamine used as an antihypertensive drug? What is the mechanism of action?
5. How does the action of phenoxybenzamine differ from that of phentolamine?
6. How does the use of prazosin differ from that of phentolamine?
7. List which antihypertensives act by interfering with storage and/or release of norepinephrine.
8. List which antihypertensives act centrally to inhibit sympathetic activity.
9. How do calcium channel blockers decrease hypertension?
10. How do ACE inhibitors work? What are their limiting side effects?
11. List which antihypertensives used in the chronic treatment of hypertension are direct-acting vasodilators.
12. How is saralasin used clinically?
13. Which drug is both an alpha and a beta adrenergic antagonist?
14. List three drugs and their mechanisms of action that are used to control a hypertensive emergency.
15. What is a limiting side effect of reserpine?
16. What is orthostatic hypotension? Which antihypertensive drugs are commonly associated with orthostatic hypotension as a side effect?
17. Which antihypertensive is associated with the synthesis of a false transmitter?
18. What reaction may occur with the sudden discontinuance of clonidine?
19. Describe reflex tachycardia. Which antihypertensive drugs may cause reflex tachycardia?
20. Why is patient compliance with antihypertensive therapy frequently poor?

SUGGESTED READINGS

Abrams WB: Pathophysiology of hypertension in older patients, Am J Med **85**(suppl 3B):7, 1988.

Allinger RL: Folk beliefs about high blood pressure in Hispanic immigrants, West J Nurs Res **10**(5):629, 1988.

Armstrong BA: Protocol: isolated systolic hypertension in the elderly, Nurse Pract **12**(6):18, 1987.

Ashby D: The patient with essential hypertension, J Post Anesth Nurs **2**(3):197, 1987.

Avorn J, Everitt DE, and Weiss S: Increased antidepressant use in patients prescribed beta-blockers, JAMA **255**:357, 1986.

Bartucci MR, and others: Factors associated with adherence in hypertensive patients, ANNA Journal **14**(4):245, 1987.

Ben-Ishay D, Leibel B, and Stessman J: Calcium channel blockers in the management of hypertension in the elderly, Am J Med **81**(suppl 6A):30, 1986.

Blanski L, and others: Esmolol, the first ultra-short-acting intravenous beta blocker for use in critically ill patients, Heart Lung **17**(1):80, 1988.

Breckenridge A: Current controversies in the treatment of hypertension, Am J Med **84**(suppl 1B):36, 1988.

Bulpitt CJ, and Fletcher AE, Importance of well-being to hypertensive patients, Am J Med **84**(suppl 1B):40, 1988.

Byington RP, Curb JD, and Mattson ME: Assessment of double-blindness at the conclusion of the beta-blocker heart attack trial, JAMA **253**:1733, 1985.

Campbell DJ: Circulating and tissue angiotensin systems, J Clin Invest **798**:1, 1987.

Croog SH, and others: The effects of antihypertensive therapy on the quality of life, N Engl J Med **314**:1657, 1986.

Cunningham SG: Nonpharmacologic management of high blood pressure, Cardiovasc Nurs **23**(4):18, 1987.

Curb JD, and others: Long-term surveillance for adverse effects of antihypertensive drugs, JAMA **253**:3263, 1985.

Dalley KA, and Ruksnaitis N: Glucagon: a first-line drug for cardiotoxicity cause by beta blockade, J Emer Nurs **12**(6):387, 1986.

Evans MJ: Tips for taking a child's blood pressure quickly, Nursing 83 **13**(3):61, 1983.

Ferguson RK, and Vlasses PH: Hypertensive emergencies and urgencies, JAMA **255**:1607, 1986.

Fontana SA: Update on high blood pressure: highlights from the 1988 national report, Nurs Pract **13**(2):8, 1988.

Gavras I, and Gavras H: Clinical utility of angiotensin converting enzyme inhibitors in hypertension, Am J Med **81**(suppl 4C):28, 1986.

Gotto AM Jr: Interactions of the major risk factors for coronary heart disease, Am J Med 80(suppl 2A):48, 1986.

Gruchow HW, Sobocinski KA, and Barboriak JJ: Alcohol, nutrient intake, and hypertension in US adults, JAMA 253:1567, 1985.

Jain AK, and others: Clonidine and guanfacine in hypertension, Clin Pharmacol Ther 37:271, 1985.

Katz AM, and others: Cellular actions and pharmacology of the calcium channel blocking drugs, Am J Med 79(suppl 4A):2, 1985.

Koniak-Griffin D, and Didgson J: Severe pregnancy-induced hypertension: postpartum care of the critically ill patient, Heart Lung 1(6):661, 1987.

Kub JP: Ethnicity—an important factor for nurses to consider in caring for hypertensive individuals, West J Nurs Res 8(4):445, 1986.

Kyncl JJ: Pharmacology of terazosin, Am J Med 80(suppl 5B):12, 1986.

Langford HG, and others: Dietary therapy slows the return of hypertension after stopping prolonged medication, JAMA 253:657, 1985.

Laragh JH: Atrial natriuretic hormone, the renin-aldosterone axis, and blood pressure-electrolyte homeostasis, N Engl J Med 313:1330, 1985.

Manzo M: Sodium nitroprusside for hypertensive crisis, Nursing 87 11:98, 1987.

McDonald RH, Jr: The evolution of current hypertension therapy, Am J Med 85(suppl 3B):14, 1988.

McDonald M, Postgrad Med 77:1985, and Grimm RH: Compliance with hypertension treatment.

Miettinen TA, and others: Multifactorial primary prevention of cardiovascular diseases in middle-aged men, JAMA 254:2097, 1985.

Moser M: Historical perspective on the management of hypertension, Am J Med 80(suppl 5B):1, 1986.

Nakagawa-Kogan H, and others: Self-management of hypertension: predictors of success in diastolic blood pressure reduction, Res Nurs Health 11(2):105, 1988.

National High Blood Pressure Education Program: The 1988 report of the joint national committee on detection, evaluation, and treatment of high blood pressure, Arch Intern Med 148:1023, 1988.

Plawecki HM, and others: Compliance and health beliefs in the Black female hypertensive client, J Natl Black Nurses Assoc 2(1):38, 1987.

Powers MJ, and Jalowiec A: Profile of the well-controlled, well-adjusted hypertensive patient, Nurs Res 36(2):106, 1987.

Ray WA, Schaffner W, and Oates JA: Therapeutic choice in the treatment of hypertension, Am J Med 81(suppl 6C):9, 1986.

Smith WM: Epidemiology of hypertension in older patients, Am J Med 85(suppl 3B):2, 1988.

Sowers JR: Managing geriatric hypertension: a brief review, Geriatrics 40:63, 1985.

Streedbeck NW: Beta-adrenoceptor blockade and anesthesia, AANA J 56(4):334, 1988.

Stuart EM, and others: Nonpharmacologic treatment of hypertension: a multiple-risk-factor approach, J Cardiovasc Nurs 1(4):1, 1987.

Trounson LW: Hypertensive crisis, J Post Anesth Nurs 3(2):102, 1988.

Watts RJ: Sexual functioning, health beliefs, and compliance with high blood pressure medications, Nurs Res 31(5):278, 1982.

Weinberger MH: Antihypertensive therapy and lipids, Arch Intern Med 145:1102, 1985.

Wikstrand J, and others: Primary prevention with metoprolol in patients with hypertension, JAMA 259:1976, 1988.

Williams GH: Converting-enzyme inhibitors in the treatment of hypertension, N Engl J Med 319:1517, 1988.

Diuretics

16

Diuretics are drugs that increase urine flow. There are several mechanisms by which drugs can produce this effect, but the clinically important drugs of this class act on the kidney. This chapter reviews pertinent renal physiology and discusses the mechanism of action and clinical properties of diuretic drugs.

FUNCTION OF THE NEPHRON IN SALT AND WATER BALANCE

The functional unit of the kidney is the nephron (Figure 16.1). Glomerular filtration is the first step in the production of urine. Blood is brought into contact with a filtering surface in the glomerulus, where water and small molecules pass into the tubule, leaving behind most proteins and protein-bound small molecules. The remainder of the nephron adjusts the salt and water content of the tubular fluid to achieve *homeostasis,* a balanced condition in which the body retains the salt and water required for proper function and eliminates the excess. For the purpose of understanding diuretic drugs, this discussion will be limited to six ions or molecules: sodium (Na^+), chloride (Cl^-), potassium (K^+), water (H_2O), bicarbonate (HCO_3^-), and organic ions.

Sodium ion sites. Sodium ion freely enters the tubular fluid from the glomerulus so that the fluid entering the proximal convoluted tubule has the same sodium ion content as blood. The proximal convoluted tubule actively removes sodium ion from the tubule. No further sodium ion is removed in the descending limb of Henle's loop, but in the ascending limb sodium ion passively follows chloride ion out of the tubule. In the distal convoluted tubule, sodium ion is removed by two processes. One is an active pump like that in the proximal convoluted tubule. The second one is a pump that exchanges sodium ion for potassium ion so that as

sodium ion is reabsorbed, potassium ion is excreted.

Chloride ion sites. The major site for chloride ion removal from tubular fluid is in the ascending limb of Henle's loop. This active removal of chloride ion draws sodium ion along with it and effectively dilutes the tubular fluid.

Potassium ion sites. Potassium ion is not the primary ion involved in the action of any diuretic drug; these drugs are designed to alter sodium ion excretion patterns. Nevertheless, potassium excretion is altered by some of these agents, and the effects on some patients may be detrimental. Potassium ion may be reabsorbed in the ascending limb of Henle's loop. Secretion of potassium occurs in the distal convoluted tubule, where the ion is exchanged for sodium ion (Figure 16.1).

Water sites. The kidney is the primary site for maintenance of water balance. Water may be recovered from the tubule by diffusion in the proximal convoluted tubule and in the descending limb of Henle's loop. The ascending limb of Henle's loop and the distal convoluted tubule are relatively impermeable to water. Final concentration of the urine is achieved in the collecting duct. Removal of water at this site is regulated by antidiuretic hormone (ADH), which increases permeability of the tissue to water and thereby increases water retention.

Bicarbonate sites. Bicarbonate, which is the main buffer for the blood, freely enters tubular fluid from the glomerulus and must be recovered for the body to maintain proper acid-base balance. Reabsorption of bicarbonate occurs in the proximal convoluted tubule. Reabsorption of bicarbonate is not direct but involves the action of the enzyme carbonic anhydrase. Carbonic anhydrase converts hydrogen ion and bicarbonate ion in the tubular fluid to carbon dioxide and water. Carbon dioxide can

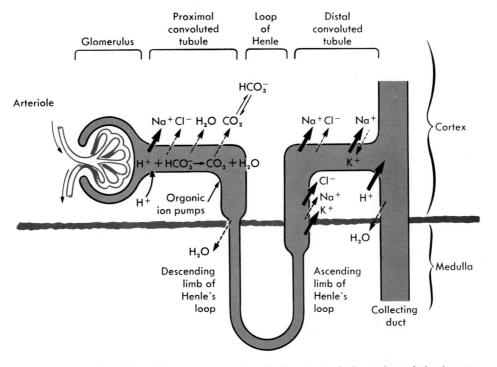

FIGURE 16.1   Sites of secretion and reabsorption of salt and water in the nephron. Active (energy-requiring) processes are designated by bold arrows; passive diffusion is designated by broken arrows.

Table 16.1   Summary of Diuretic Effects on Tubular Transport

Drug	Excretion increased					Excretion blocked		
Loop diuretics	Na⁺	H₂O	K⁺	Cl⁻	—	Uric acid	Li⁺	—
Thiazides and related drugs	Na⁺	H₂O	K⁺	Cl⁻	HCO₃⁻	Uric acid	Li⁺	—
Potassium-sparing diuretics	Na⁺	H₂O	—	—	HCO₃⁻	—	—	K⁺,H⁺
Carbonic anhydrase inhibitors	Na⁺	H₂O	K⁺	—	HCO₃⁻	Uric acid	—	—
Osmotic diuretics	(Na⁺)*	H₂O	(K⁺)*	(Cl⁻)*	—	—	—	—

*Large doses.
NOTE: The effects on ion transport shown are those commonly observed in humans during chronic therapy with normal clinical doses. With prolonged therapy, those ions whose excretion is increased may become depleted from the body, whereas those whose excretion is blocked may accumulate. Lithium ion accumulation is clinically important only for those patients receiving lithium carbonate therapy for mania. Uric acid accumulation is usually important only for those patients predisposed to gout.

freely pass into the tubular epithelial cell and is reabsorbed, whereas bicarbonate ion stays in the tubule. The reabsorbed carbon dioxide is quickly reconverted to bicarbonate within the kidney cell and becomes available to the bloodstream.

Organic ion pumps. The kidney has the capacity to rapidly secrete complex ions such as amino acids and other natural compounds. This process occurs near the proximal convoluted tubule in the cortical portion of the descending limb of Henle's loop. Many drugs, including several diuretics, enter tubular fluid by this mechanism, which is referred to as an organic ion pump. Since some diuretics work only from within the tubule, the action of the drug depends at least in part on the proper function of this active secretion mechanism.

Table 16.2 Summary of Clinical Uses of Diuretic Drugs

Conditions responding to diuretics	Loop diuretics	Thiazides and related compounds	Potassium-sparing diuretics	Carbonic anhydrase inhibitors	Osmotic diuretics
Essential hypertension	+	+	+		
Edema caused by congestive heart failure, renal disease, cirrhosis of the liver	+	+	+		
Pulmonary edema	+				
Diabetes insipidus		+			
Acute mountain sickness				+	
Open-angle glaucoma				+	
Excessive intraocular pressure				+	+
Brain edema					+

Mechanism of diuretic action. The diuretics considered in this chapter achieve their effects by increasing sodium ion excretion. Since water tends to follow sodium ion in the kidney, when sodium ion is excreted, so is water. Several distinct mechanisms for increasing sodium ion excretion exist and all may be understood in terms of the renal physiology just discussed. Specific mechanisms are discussed with the individual drugs and summarized in Table 16.1.

Clinical uses of diuretics. Diuretics are widely used in medicine, not only for their effects on kidneys but also for other actions in the body. For example, these drugs are a mainstay in treating hypertension (Chapter 15). A summary of the range of clinical uses of diuretics is shown in Table 16.2. Specific applications are also discussed with each drug and the clinical properties are summarized in Tables 16.3 to 16.5.

Loop Diuretics

Ethacrynic acid, furosemide, and bumetanide are called loop diuretics because the primary site of their diuretic action is in Henle's loop. These drugs inhibit the active reabsorption of chloride ion in the ascending limb of Henle's loop. Since chloride ion reabsorption is prevented, the passive reabsorption of sodium ion is also blocked. Therefore sodium chloride is retained in the tubule and excreted in the urine, carrying body water with it. Although ordinarily 99.4% of the sodium ion entering the tubule is reabsorbed, under the influence of loop diuretics only 70% to 80% is reabsorbed, along with an equivalent amount of chloride ion. Potassium ion is also excreted in higher than normal amounts in response to these drugs (Table 16.1).

The loop diuretics are the most potent class of diuretics known. The rapid, powerful action of these drugs must be carefully monitored to avoid profound dehydration and salt depletion.

Since loop diuretics promote the loss of excess salt and body water, they are useful agents for controlling edematous states, such as those occurring in congestive heart failure, renal disease, cirrhosis of the liver, lymphedema, nephrotic syndrome, and ascites associated with cirrhosis or malignancies (Table 16.2).

Ethacrynic acid (Table 16.3)

Mechanism of action. Ethacrynic acid has all the actions of the loop diuretics, as described in the preceding section.

Absorption, distribution, and excretion. Ethacrynic acid is well absorbed from the gastrointestinal tract, producing a diuretic effect within 1 hour of administration. The drug is also appropriate for intravenous administration, producing diuresis within 2 to 10 minutes when given by that route. Ethacrynic acid should not be given by intramuscular or subcutaneous injection, since the drug can cause severe pain and irritation at the injection site.

Ethacrynic acid is bound to proteins in the bloodstream, and in the protein-bound form is not available for glomerular filtration. The drug is, however, secreted into the tubule by the organic anion pump in the descending limb of Henle's loop (cortical portion). The effectiveness of ethacrynic acid depends on its being able to enter the tubule, since diuresis is produced from within the tubule.

Table 16.3   Summary of Diuretic Drugs: Loop Diuretics

Generic name	Trade name	Administration/dosage	Diuretic effect		
			Onset	Peak	Duration
Bumetanide	Bumex	ORAL: *Adults*—1 mg each morning; if needed, a second dose may be given 6 to 8 hr later. Usual daily doses are less than 4 mg, except in severe renal failure, when doses may reach 15 mg daily. FDA pregnancy category C.	30 min	1 to 2 hr	4 to 6 hr
		INTRAVENOUS: *Adults*—initially 0.5 to 1 mg to relieve pulmonary edema; repeat dose in 20 min if necessary.	5 to 10 min	15 to 20 min	3 to 4 hr
Ethacrynic acid	Edecrin*	ORAL: *Adults*—50 to 100 mg initially; thereafter 50 to 200 mg daily. FDA pregnancy category C. *Children*—25 mg initially, increasing by 25 mg to maintain.	30 min	1 to 2 hr	6 to 8 hr
		INTRAVENOUS: *Adults*—50 mg. Not recommended for children by this route.	5 to 10 min	15 to 20 min	1 to 3 hr
Furosemide	Lasix* Novosemide† Uritol†	ORAL: *Adults*—20 to 80 mg once or twice daily. FDA pregnancy category C. *Children*—2 mg/kg initially, increasing by 1 or 2 mg/kg after 6 to 8 hr; maximum dose, 6 mg/kg.	30 to 60 min	1 to 2 hr	6 to 8 hr
		INTRAVENOUS: *Adults*—20 to 40 mg once or twice daily. *Children*—1 mg/kg initially, increasing by 1 mg/kg after 2 hr; maximum dose 6 mg/kg.	5 to 10 min	15 to 20 min	1 to 3 hr

*Available in Canada and United States.
†Available in Canada only.

About two thirds of the normal dose of ethacrynic acid is excreted in the kidney, the remainder being eliminated by the liver. In the kidney, ethacrynic acid exists primarily as the free drug and as a complex with cysteine. The cysteine–ethacrynic acid complex formed in the body is many times more effective than the free drug.

Toxicity. The most likely toxic reaction to ethacrynic acid is actually an excess of the action for which the drug is prescribed. Ethacrynic acid is so potent that excessive salt and water loss can occur quickly. Dehydration with reduction in blood volume can precipitate circulatory collapse. Vascular thromboses and emboli may be generated, especially in elderly patients. Electrolyte depletion may be a more gradual process marked by weakness or lethargy, dizziness, leg cramps, anorexia, vomiting, and possibly mental confusion.

Orthostatic hypotension may occur. Patients who tend to rise quickly from a sitting or lying position need to adapt to moving slowly to allow accommodation of blood pressure (see Patient Problem: Orthostatic hypotension, p. 237). The most serious danger is risk of injury from falls.

Ethacrynic acid increases the loss of ions other than sodium and chloride, such as potassium and calcium. Excessive potassium loss impairs proper functioning of the heart, skeletal muscle, kidneys, and other tissues. Many physicians routinely prescribe some form of potassium replacement for their patients receiving ethacrynic acid for prolonged periods. Loss of calcium may rarely be sufficient to produce tetany. Most patients will not require calcium replacement, but serum calcium levels should be observed periodically.

Uric acid excretion is partially blocked by eth-

Table 16.4 Summary of Diuretic Drugs: Thiazide Diuretics and Agents with Similar Mechanisms

			Diuretic effect		
			Onset	Peak	Duration
THIAZIDE DIURETICS					
Bendroflumethia-zide	Naturetin*	ORAL: *Adults*—initially, 5 mg once daily; maintenance, 2.5 to 15 mg once daily or less frequently. *Children*—maximum dosage 0.4 mg/kg daily in 2 doses; reduce dose for maintenance.	1 to 2 hr	6 to 12 hr	18 to 24 hr
Benzthiazide	Aquatag Exna Hydrex	ORAL: *Adults*—50 to 200 mg; once daily for low doses, divide doses over 100 mg daily. FDA pregnancy category B. *Children*—1 to 4 mg/kg daily in 3 doses initially; dose reduced for maintenance.	2 hr	4 to 6 hr	12 to 18 hr
Chlorothiazide	Diuril*	ORAL: *Adults*—0.5 to 1 Gm once or twice daily. *Children*—22 mg/kg daily in 2 doses. *Infants*—under 6 months, 10 to 20 mg/kg daily in 2 divided doses.	2 hr	4 hr	6 to 12 hr
Chlorothiazide so-dium	Diuril (Sodium)	INTRAVENOUS: *Adults*—500 mg twice daily.	15 min	30 min	6 to 12 hr
Cyclothiazide	Anhydron Fluidil	ORAL: *Adults*—1 to 2 mg once daily; maintenance, 1 mg 2 to 4 times weekly. *Children*—initially, 0.02 to 0.04 mg/kg daily; reduce dose for maintenance.	6 hr	7 to 12 hr	18 to 24 hr
Hydrochlorothia-zide	Diuchlor-H† Esidrix* HydroDIURIL* Novohydra- zide† Oretic Thiuretic Urozide†	ORAL: *Adults*—initially, 25 to 200 mg once or twice daily; mainte-nance, 25 to 100 mg daily or less frequently. *Children*—1 to 2 mg/kg daily in 2 doses. *Infants*—un-der 6 mo, up to 3 mg/kg daily.	2 hr	4 hr	6 to 12 hr
Hydroflumethia-zide	Diucardin Saluron	ORAL: *Adults*—50 to 200 mg; once daily for low doses; divided doses over 100 mg daily. FDA pregnancy category D. *Children*—1 mg/kg daily; adjust as needed for mainte-nance.	1 to 2 hr	3 to 4 hr	18 to 24 hr
Methyclothiazide	Aquatensen Duretic† Enduron	ORAL: *Adults*—2.5 to 10 mg once daily. *Children*—0.05 to 0.2 mg/kg daily.	2 hr	6 hr	24 hr
Polythiazide	Renese	ORAL: *Adults*—1 to 4 mg once daily; maintenance, 0.5 to 8 mg daily, according to response. *Chil-dren*—0.02 to 0.08 mg/kg daily.	2 hr	6 hr	36 hr

*Available in Canada and United States.
†Available in Canada only.

Table 16.4   Summary of Diuretic Drugs: Thiazide Diuretics and Agents with Similar Mechanisms—cont'd

Generic name	Trade name	Administration/dosage	Diuretic effect		
			Onset	Peak	Duration
Trichlormethiazide	Metahydrin Naqua	ORAL: *Adults*—1 to 4 mg once daily. FDA pregnancy category B. *Children*—0.07 mg/kg daily in single or divided dose.	2 hr	6 hr	24 hr
NONTHIAZIDE DIURETICS WITH THIAZIDE-LIKE MECHANISMS					
Chlorthalidone	Hygroton* Novothalidone† Thalitone	ORAL: *Adults*—25 to 100 mg after breakfast daily or less frequently. FDA pregnancy category B. *Children*—2 mg/kg once daily for 3 days per week.	2 hr	2 hr	24 to 72 hr
Indapamide	Lozide† Lozol	ORAL: *Adults*—2.5 mg/day taken in the morning; may be increased after a few days to 5 mg/day. FDA pregnancy category B.	1 to 2 hr	2.3 to 3.5 hr	24 to 72 hr
Metolazone	Diulo Mykrox Zaroxolyn*	ORAL: *Adults*—5 to 20 mg once daily. FDA pregnancy category B.	1 hr	2 hr	12 to 24 hr
Quinethazone	Aquamox† Hydromox	ORAL: *Adults*—50 to 100 mg once daily, or 150 to 200 mg alternate days or 3 times weekly.	2 hr	6 hr	18 to 24 hr

*Available in Canada and United States.
†Available in Canada only.

acrynic acid (Table 16.1). Therefore in certain susceptible patients gout may develop. For most patients the increase in serum uric acid produces no symptoms.

Ethacrynic acid has caused gastrointestinal disturbances in a few patients, especially those receiving the drug continually for several months. A sudden, severe, watery diarrhea indicates the drug should be withdrawn. The physician may discontinue the drug permanently if these symptoms arise.

Ethacrynic acid affects ion transport in several body tissues other than the kidney. Altered sodium and potassium transport may be associated with toxicity to certain cells in the inner ear. Transient or permanent deafness has been observed in patients receiving ethacrynic acid, especially those receiving very high doses or those patients with reduced renal function in whom the drug accumulates.

Drug interactions. The potassium-depleting ef-fect of ethacrynic acid makes this drug dangerous for patients receiving digitalis. Lowered potassium content in the tissue predisposes the heart to toxicity from the cardiac glycosides, which may include fatal arrhythmias. Note that corticosteroids are also potassium-depleting agents and may add to the danger of electrolyte imbalance when given with ethacrynic acid.

Ethacrynic acid lowers the renal clearance of lithium, a drug used for the control of manic cycles in manic-depressive psychosis (Table 16.1). Under these conditions lithium may accumulate and severe toxicity may occur. These drugs are ordinarily not given together.

Ethacrynic acid has an antihypertensive action that may be additive with that of other antihypertensive agents. Care is required to prevent excessive hypotension when these drugs are used together.

The ototoxic effect of ethacrynic acid may be potentiated by aminoglycoside antibiotics (Chapter

47), which are themselves ototoxic. Since permanent deafness may result from this combination, it should be avoided if at all possible.

Ethacrynic acid is strongly bound to serum proteins and may therefore displace other drugs from protein-binding sites. The result of this action is to increase the concentration of the free, active form of the displaced drug. The anticoagulant warfarin is known to be displaced in this manner by ethacrynic acid. Higher concentrations of unbound warfarin produce greater anticoagulant effects and may produce toxicity.

Furosemide (Table 16.3)

Mechanism of action. Furosemide has all the actions described previously for the loop diuretics. In addition, at high doses furosemide may occasionally increase bicarbonate excretion, whereas other loop diuretics have little direct effect on such excretion. Furosemide is the loop diuretic most likely to be included in therapy to control hypertension, being used either alone or in combination with other antihypertensive agents.

Absorption, distribution, and excretion. Furosemide is well absorbed from the gastrointestinal tract, producing diuresis within 1 hour. Diuresis occurs within minutes of an intravenous dose. Furosemide can also be administered intramuscularly.

A significant portion of furosemide in the bloodstream is bound to protein. Free drug is filtered in the glomerulus; furosemide also enters the tubular fluid by the organic anion pump. As with ethacrynic acid, it is only the drug within the tubule that is active in producing diuresis. About two thirds of an ingested dose of furosemide is ultimately found in the kidney, with most of the remainder being excreted in the feces. A small amount is metabolized.

Toxicity. Furosemide is capable of producing the same acute dehydration, orthostatic hypotension, salt depletion, and potassium depletion as previously described for ethacrynic acid. Calcium loss and uric acid accumulation also occur with furosemide as for ethacrynic acid.

Various types of dermatitis and occasional blood dyscrasias have been reported. The brisk diuresis produced by furosemide may be associated with urinary bladder spasm, thirst, perspiration, muscle cramps, weakness, and/or dizziness. It also impairs glucose tolerance in some patients, and rarely the drug has precipitated diabetes mellitus.

Gastrointestinal effects and ototoxicity are less common with furosemide than with ethacrynic acid.

Furosemide may produce an allergic interstitial nephritis that can result in reversible renal failure. Lupus erythematosus may be activated by furosemide.

Drug interactions. Furosemide causes potassium depletion to the same extent as ethacrynic acid and for this reason should also be used with great care in patients receiving digitalis or potassium-depleting steroids. Furosemide, like ethacrynic acid, blocks lithium excretion and may lead to toxic lithium accumulation. Its potential may be enhanced by aminoglycoside antibiotics or other ototoxic drugs.

Furosemide may increase the effect of tubocurarine, which can lead to muscle paralysis and paralysis of respiration. For this reason the drug is usually discontinued a few days before surgery, if possible.

Furosemide and salicylates are both secreted by the organic anion pump. Since this pump system has limited capacity, furosemide may block the excretion of salicylates. Clinically, this process may be important for patients receiving high doses of salicylates for rheumatoid diseases. If these patients are also given furosemide, salicylates may accumulate and cause salicylate toxicity.

Bumetanide (Table 16.3)

Mechanism of action. Bumetanide is similar to furosemide in inhibiting the active reabsorption of Cl^- in the ascending limb of Henle's loop. The main difference between bumetanide and other loop diuretics is that bumetanide is much more potent. For example, 1 mg of bumetanide given orally is as effective as approximately 40 mg of furosemide. Like the other loop diuretics, bumetanide is used to control edematous states due to various medical conditions (Table 16.2).

Absorption, distribution, and excretion. Bumetanide is completely absorbed following oral administration. The pharmacokinetics of bumetanide and furosemide are similar (Table 16.3). In the bloodstream bumetanide is almost completely bound to plasma protein. The drug is eliminated by renal mechanisms as well as by other routes. In renal failure the half-life of bumetanide is unchanged, which suggests that these alternative routes of elimination may be highly effective.

Toxicity. Because of its potent diuretic action, bumetanide can cause acute dehydration, orthostatic hypotension, salt depletion, and potassium depletion, just like the other loop diuretics. Azotemia, high uric acid concentration in the blood, and impaired glucose tolerance can also occur.

Ototoxicity, blood dyscrasia, gastrointestinal

distress, and rashes are all possible reactions to bumetanide. Large doses may cause severe muscle pain (myalgia) in patients in renal failure.

Drug interactions. Bumetanide can interact similarly to furosemide. In addition, indomethacin reduces the diuretic action of bumetanide. Since bumetanide is a relatively new drug, more interactions may become evident as additional clinical experience is gained.

Thiazide diuretics (Table 16.4)

Mechanism of action. Thiazide diuretics have multiple effects on the nephron. These diuretics block sodium and chloride reabsorption in the distal convoluted tubule. This action leads to increased excretion of sodium chloride and body water and establishes a new state of salt and water balance in which there is a lower level of body sodium than before the drug was given. In addition to this action, thiazide diuretics also inhibit carbonic anhydrase in the proximal convoluted tubule, thereby elevating the excretion of bicarbonate and an additional increment of sodium. This minor component in the action of thiazide diuretics is lost after a few days. Potassium excretion is also enhanced by the thiazide diuretics, but this effect is not required for diuresis and is usually considered a toxic side effect.

Thiazide diuretics are less potent than ethacrynic acid or furosemide and are more suitable for use in outpatients. The drugs can be used to control edema associated with heart or kidney disease, as well as that due to corticosteroid or estrogen therapy. The use of thiazide diuretics in controlling hypertension is discussed in Chapter 15.

Absorption, distribution, and excretion. Thiazide diuretics are well absorbed from the gastrointestinal tract and may begin to take action in the kidney within 1 hour of ingestion. Peak diuretic action can occur anytime from 2 to 6 hours or more after the oral dose, depending on which individual thiazide preparation is used. The various preparations differ in the timing and duration of diuretic effects (Table 16.4). In general, the longer-acting thiazide diuretics are highly bound to serum proteins. Their long duration of action is related to their slow elimination from these protein-binding sites.

Thiazide diuretics remain primarily in the extracellular water in the body except for the renal concentration. Thiazides are secreted into the renal tubule by the organic anion pump. Most of the dose leaves the body by this route. Some drug, however, is eliminated by the liver, which secretes these drugs into the bile.

Chlorothiazide is available for intravenous dosage. The onset of action is somewhat more rapid by this route, but the duration of effect is not greatly altered from that observed with oral doses. This preparation must never be administered intramuscularly or subcutaneously. Great care should be taken to prevent leakage of the drug into the tissues when it is given intravenously.

Toxicity. Long-term administration of thiazide diuretics can lead to fluid and electrolyte imbalance, which may produce the classic signs: thirst, weakness, lethargy, restlessness, muscle cramps, and fatigue. The electrolyte imbalance most likely to be observed in patients receiving thiazide diuretics is excessive potassium and chloride ion loss. The loss of these ions leads to metabolic alkalosis. Potassium supplements may be required to remedy this situation. Chloride loss alone is usually mild and does not need to be treated.

Calcium excretion is blocked by thiazide diuretics, and increased serum calcium levels may result. The parathyroid glands may also be affected by long-term therapy with these diuretics. Uric acid

Table 16.5   Fixed Combinations Including Diuretic Drugs

Components	Trade names
THIAZIDES WITH POTASSIUM-SPARING DIURETICS	
Hydrochlorothiazide + amiloride	Moduretic
Hydrochlorothiazide + spironolactone	Aldactazide, Spirozide
Hydrochlorothiazide + triamterene	Dyazide, Maxzide
THIAZIDE WITH ACE-INHIBITOR	
Hydrochlorothiazide + captopril	Capozide
Hydrochlorothiazide + enalapril	Vaseretic
Hydrochlorothiazide + lisinopril	Prinzide, Zestoretic
THIAZIDE WITH ALPHA-BLOCKER	
Polythiazide + prazosin	Minizide
THIAZIDE WITH BETA-BLOCKER	
Bendroflumethiazide + nadolol	Corzide
Chlorthalidone + atenolol	Tenoretic
Hydrochlorothiazide + metoprolol	Lopressor HCT
Hydrochlorothiazide + propranolol	Inderide
Hydrochlorothiazide + timolol	Timolide
THIAZIDE WITH CENTRALLY ACTING ANTIHYPERTENSIVE	
Chlorthalidone + clonidine	Combipres
Hydrochlorothiazide + methyldopa	Aldoril
THIAZIDE WITH RAUWOLFIA	
Hydrochlorothiazide + reserpine	Hydropres, Mallopress
Trichlormethiazide + reserpine	Metatensin
THIAZIDE WITH VASODILATOR	
Hydrochlorothiazide + hydralazine	Apresazide, Apresodex
THIAZIDE WITH RAUWOLFIA AND VASODILATOR	
Hydrochlorothiazide + reserpine + hydralazine	Ser-Ap-Ex, Unipres

Includes many commonly used fixed combinations but does not include every available combination.

excretion is also blocked and the increased blood levels may precipitate an attack of gout in susceptible individuals.

Thiazide diuretics have a direct irritative effect on the gastrointestinal tract and may give rise to symptoms ranging from simple nausea and vomiting to constipation, jaundice, and pancreatitis.

Thiazides have a direct effect on the central nervous system. Mild symptoms include dizziness, headache, and paresthesia. At very high concentra-tions such as those found in drug overdose, mental lethargy may progress to coma, although heart function and respiration are not markedly depressed.

Blood dyscrasias and allergic reactions have been observed. Although urticaria or other mild forms of allergy are more common, severe serum sickness and anaphylactic reactions have been noted.

Thiazides cause hypotension by a mechanism

GERIATRIC DRUG ALERT: DIURETIC DRUGS

THE PROBLEM

Elderly patients are often more sensitive to the effects of diuretic drugs than are other adults. For example, loop diuretics and thiazides can cause excessive hypotension and severe electrolyte imbalances. Potassium-sparing diuretics more often cause hyperkalemia in the elderly than in others.

SOLUTIONS

- Dosages of these drugs for the elderly may be lower than for other adults.
- Blood pressure should be carefully monitored.
- Precautions should be taken against orthostatic hypotension.
- Electrolyte balance should be carefully monitored.
- Dietary counseling may be required to maintain potassium balance.

apparently unrelated to their action as diuretics. Some patients may suffer orthostatic hypotension when receiving these drugs. Thiazides occasionally lower glomerular filtration rate when given intravenously. This effect is of little consequence to most patients, although a patient with already reduced renal function may be adversely affected.

Drug interactions. Since thiazide diuretics have intrinsic hypotensive activity, they may potentiate the action of other antihypertensive agents, especially those that act at ganglionic or peripheral adrenergic sites (Chapter 15).

Thiazide diuretics are commonly included in fixed combinations which are marketed primarily for use as antihypertensives. Examples of some of these fixed combinations are listed in Table 16.5.

Potassium loss is enhanced when thiazide diuretics are given with corticosteroids or adrenocorticotropic hormone (ACTH). Hypokalemia (low concentration of potassium in the blood) may render the patient more sensitive to digitalis toxicity.

Thiazides may increase the response to tubocurarine, a muscle relaxant commonly used in surgery. Patients receiving both of these drugs should be carefully observed for signs of excessive tubocurarine activity.

Thiazide diuretics frequently alter the requirement for insulin or other hypoglycemic agents. A diabetic who must receive one of the thiazides should be carefully observed during the first few days of thiazide therapy to prevent loss of diabetes control.

Lithium excretion is blocked by thiazides and other diuretics. The increased danger of lithium toxicity prevents the safe use of both these drugs at once.

Potassium-sparing diuretics (Table 16.6)

Mechanism of action. Potassium-sparing diuretics inhibit the pump mechanism that normally exchanges potassium for sodium in the distal convoluted tubule (Figure 16.1). This pump is under the control of mineralocorticoid hormones, such as aldosterone, which increase sodium retention and promote potassium loss. Aldosterone is present in greater than normal amounts in edematous states resulting from congestive heart failure, nephrotic syndrome, and hepatic cirrhosis.

Spironolactone, one of the potassium-sparing diuretics, competitively blocks the action of aldosterone in the sodium-potassium exchange pump, thereby causing sodium to remain in the tubule and be excreted. Potassium is not pumped into the tubule and so is spared from excretion.

Triamterene, another diuretic of this class, produces the same effects as spironolactone but by a direct mechanism that is not dependent on aldosterone. These properties explain the fact that spironolactone is most effective under circumstances in which aldosterone is elevated, whereas the more rapidly and directly acting triamterene is effective when aldosterone is low, high, or normal.

Amiloride, the newest of the potassium-sparing diuretics, acts in the same way as triamterene.

Since the sodium-potassium pump in the distal convoluted tubule is ordinarily responsible for reabsorbing only a small fraction of the sodium from the tubule, blockade of this pump increases sodium excretion only slightly. This limits the effectiveness of the potassium-sparing diuretics.

Spironolactone is used to control edema in congestive heart failure, cirrhosis of the liver, and nephrotic syndrome. Spironolactone may ameliorate the effects of excessive aldosterone levels in patients suffering from the endocrine disorder hyperaldosteronism. The drug may also be useful in treating hypertension and reversing potassium loss arising from various conditions. Triamterene is used in many of the same situations as spironolactone. Amiloride has uses similar to those of the

Table 16.6 Summary of Diuretic Drugs: Potassium-Sparing Diuretics and Carbonic Anhydrase Inhibitors

Generic name	Trade name	Administration/dosage	Diuretic effect		
			Onset	Peak	Duration
POTASSIUM-SPARING DIURETICS					
Amiloride	Midamor*	ORAL: *Adults*—5 to 10 mg daily as a single dose. FDA pregnancy category B.	Similar to effect of triamterene		
Spironolactone	Aldactone* Novospiroton† Sincomen†	ORAL: *Adults*—25 to 200 mg daily in divided doses. *Children*—3.3 mg/kg daily in divided doses.	Effects build over a period of days		
Triamterene	Dyrenium*	ORAL: *Adults*—25 to 100 mg daily with meals; do not exceed 300 mg daily. *Children*—2 to 4 mg/ kg daily in divided doses.	2 to 4 hr (maximal effect not seen for several days)	6 hr	7 to 9 hr
CARBONIC ANHYDRASE INHIBITORS					
Acetazolamide	Acetazolam† Diamox*	ORAL, INTRAVENOUS: *Adults*—250 to 375 mg once daily; alternate-day therapy may be used.	About 1 hr (oral)	2 to 4 hr (oral)	6 to 12 hr (oral)
Dichlorphen-amide	Daranide	ORAL: *Adults*—initially 100 to 200 mg, then 100 mg every 12 hr until desired effect achieved; maintenance, 25 to 50 mg 1 to 3 times daily.	0.5 to 1 hr	2 to 4 hr	6 to 12 hr
Methazolamide	Neptazane	ORAL: *Adults*—50 to 100 mg 2 or 3 times daily.	2 to 4 hr	6 to 8 hr	10 to 18 hr

*Available in Canada and United States.
†Available in Canada only.

other potassium-sparing diuretics. If amiloride is used in long-term therapy, less sodium excretion and less potassium retention are observed than with other drugs of this class. Amiloride also corrects metabolic alkalosis more effectively than spironolactone or triamterene.

Absorption, distribution, and excretion. Spironolactone is a steroid derivative related in structure to natural mineralocorticoids (Chapter 51). Spironolactone is not highly water soluble, but the drug is formulated using very fine particles to improve absorption from the gastrointestinal tract. Peak therapeutic effects with spironolactone are observed several days after treatment is begun (Table 16.6). This delay is related to the mechanism of action of the drug and is not a result of delay in absorption or other pharmacokinetic properties of the drug.

Spironolactone is extensively metabolized much the same as the natural steroids it chemically resembles. Metabolites of spironolactone appear in the urine and in lesser quantities in the bile.

Triamterene, although not a steroid like spironolactone, is also relatively insoluble in water. Intestinal absorption is somewhat variable but usually satisfactory. Most of the orally administered dose appears in the urine within 24 hours. The drug enters the renal tubule by both glomerular filtration and tubular secretion. Unlike spironolactone, the peak effect of this drug is observed within hours of an oral dose.

Amiloride is excreted primarily by the kidneys. About 60% of an oral dose is recovered unchanged in the urine within 48 hours of administration. Absorption of the drug is impaired if it is taken with food.

Toxicity. Spironolactone, triamterene, and amiloride may cause serum potassium levels to increase dangerously. Patients with impaired renal function or excessively high potassium intake are especially at risk. Fatal cardiac arrhythmias may result.

Spironolactone can cause various endocrine alterations, since the drug chemically resembles not only mineralocorticoids but also androgens and progestins. Females may observe menstrual irregularities, hirsutism, and deepening of the voice. Males may observe gynecomastia (breast development) and have difficulty in achieving or maintaining erection. Symptoms in both sexes are usually reversed when the drug is discontinued.

Spironolactone produces tumors in rats exposed to the drug for long periods. For this reason, its use should be restricted to cases in which the benefit clearly outweighs this risk. Spironolactone should not be used in an attempt to control edema in pregnancy. If the drug is used in lactating women, breast-feeding should be discontinued, since metabolites appear in breast milk.

Triamterene and amiloride may produce a reversible azotemia revealed by an increased blood urea nitrogen (BUN). Gastrointestinal disturbances, skin rashes, and drug fever have been observed in patients receiving spironolactone, triamterene, or amiloride.

Drug interactions. Two potassium-sparing diuretics should not be concomitantly administered, nor should these drugs be administered to a patient receiving potassium supplements or ingesting a diet rich in potassium.

Use of the potassium-sparing diuretics with antihypertensive agents may require reduction in doses of the latter drugs, since spironolactone, triamterene, and amiloride may have additive antihypertensive effects with these agents.

When spironolactone is combined with other diuretics, dosages may have to be reduced. It can prevent distal tubular reabsorption of sodium, making the diuretics that act early in the nephron even more effective. Amiloride given in fixed combination with hydrochlorothiazide is not as effective in preventing hypokalemia as are spironolactone and triamterene.

Spironolactone reduces vascular responsiveness to norepinephrine. This effect may impair maintenance of normal blood pressure in patients under local or general anesthesia.

Carbonic anhydrase inhibitors (Table 16.6)

Mechanism of action. Diuretics that inhibit carbonic anhydrase in the kidney prevent the secretion of hydrogen ion into the renal tubule and the reabsorption of carbon dioxide from the renal tubule. As a result, the excretion of bicarbonate is rapidly increased and the urine becomes alkaline. The diuretic action of these carbonic anhydrase inhibitors arises from the fact that sodium ion accompanies the excreted bicarbonate. However, bicarbonate excretion is much greater than sodium ion excretion, and these drugs are classified as weak diuretics. Moderate amounts of potassium, phosphate, and chloride ion are also lost in the urine. When carbonic anhydrase inhibitors are given over a long period of time, metabolic acidosis may occur. Since metabolic acidosis prevents the action of these diuretics, these drugs are not suitable for long-term continuous administration as diuretics.

Carbonic anhydrase inhibitors are primarily used in the treatment of glaucoma, congestive heart failure, and convulsive disorders.

Absorption, distribution, and excretion. Many carbonic anhydrase inhibitors are chemically related to the sulfonamide antibiotics. These drugs tend to be well absorbed from the gastrointestinal tract. The most widely used drug of this class, acetazolamide, has a plasma half-life of about 2 hours and is concentrated in the kidney. Tissue levels in the kidney may be two to three times the plasma concentration within one-half to two hours of an oral dose. Acetazolamide enters the tubule by the organic anion pump. The drug also inhibits carbonic anhydrase in other tissues.

Acetazolamide and other carbonic anhydrase inhibitors are sometimes given on alternate days rather than continuously (Table 16.6). The intent of this type of therapy is to prevent the kidney from becoming resistant to the action of the drug, that is, to prevent metabolic acidosis. During the day without the drug, the carbonic anhydrase inhibitors are cleared from the body and kidney function returns to its predrug condition. When the drug is readministered on the following day, it is as effective as when first given.

Toxicity. Reactions to these drugs are not very common, especially when they are used in intermittent or short-term therapy. These sulfonamide derivatives are capable of causing a variety of blood dyscrasias, fever, and rash. Drug precipitation in the urine has occurred, causing the formation of stones.

These drugs have direct actions on a number of tissues, including the central nervous system. Paresthesia, nervousness, sedation, lassitude, depression, headaches, vertigo, and other symptoms have been reported.

The conditions of patients already suffering

THE NURSING PROCESS

DIURETIC THERAPY

Assessment

Patients with a variety of medical conditions may require diuretic therapy, including those patients with cardiac, renal, or hepatic insufficiency, hypertension, and other problems characterized by too much retained fluid or poor fluid mobilization. These patients may come to the hospital with such signs and symptoms as edema, congestive heart failure, pulmonary edema, elevated blood pressure, altered level of consciousness, and weight gain. In addition, patients with problems of fluid balance may display serum electrolyte abnormalities. The nurse should perform a total patient assessment, focusing on the presenting signs and symptoms and appropriate laboratory and other objective data that would help further define the nature of the patient's problems.

Nursing diagnoses

Fluid volume deficit related to furosemide therapy as manifested by excessive urine output, decreased skin turgor, and orthostatic hypotension

Potential complication: hypokalemia

Potential sleep pattern disturbance related to nocturia secondary to diuretic therapy

Management

Choice of diuretic depends on the patient's condition, the speed with which fluid needs to be eliminated, available routes of administration, and other drugs the patient may be receiving. The nurse should ascertain what actions are required to aid drug therapy. For example, dietary and fluid restrictions may be required to speed the process of fluid removal and to prevent reaccumulation. Monitoring of fluid intake and output, serum electrolyte levels, blood urea nitrogen, uric acid, body weight, blood pressure, and observing for the appearance of new signs or symptoms may be required with individual patients. The nurse should watch for side effects known to occur with a specific drug, such as ototoxicity with ethacrynic acid. For a patient who is not fully alert or who is immobilized, the insertion of a Foley catheter will decrease the discomfort of using the bedpan and facilitate accurate measurement of urine output. Use of cardiac monitoring may assist in the treatment of critically ill individuals.

Evaluation

Diuretic therapy is effective when excess fluid is lost and blood pressure is maintained, without producing abnormalities in electrolyte status or side effects resulting from the medication. For some patients it is necessary to tolerate minor side effects to achieve required diuresis. The most common electrolyte imbalance, potassium depletion, may be overcome by administering a potassium supplement. As minimum preparation for discharge, the nurse should teach the patient why the medication is necessary, major possible side effects, and symptoms that should be reported to the physician. The nurse should also discuss why additional medications such as potassium supplements may need to be taken and how to monitor the general physical condition relative to diuretic therapy by performing activities such as recording the daily weight, fluid intake and output, and blood pressure. The patient should be able to repeat and to explain the appropriate information. If a restricted diet has been prescribed, the patient should demonstrate an ability to choose menus within the limits of the diet plan.

For specific clinical information about individual agents, the student should refer to the patient care implications section at the end of this chapter.

DRUG ABUSE ALERT: DIURETICS

BACKGROUND

Diuretics may be abused by patients obsessed with weight loss. The acute weight loss produced by diuretics has been exploited by some diet clinics who may initiate the program with a diuretic so that dramatic weight loss will occur early; but this weight loss is short-lived and the earlier weight recurs with rehydration. Such acute weight loss is occasionally exploited in high school and college wrestling programs; the diuretics allow a wrestler to meet a weight limit at weigh-in and the athlete usually attempts to rehydrate before wrestling. Diuretics may also be abused by patients obsessed with excretory functions, who use the drugs to achieve large volumes of urine. Such patients, who may also abuse cathartics, often view this ritualistic drug-taking as purification of the body.

PHARMACOLOGY

Diuretics promote an acute loss of body water and therefore cause an immediate drop in body weight. The amount of diuresis is related to the dose and strength of the drug employed and also related to the patient's water balance.

HEALTH HAZARDS

Long-term use of diuretics can cause severe electrolyte imbalances, especially if patients are not receiving careful counseling on dietary practices. If patients are receiving drugs from more than one physician or from unauthorized sources, follow-up care to monitor for the development of side effects may be lacking. The use of these drugs in weight control is unjustified, especially in healthy young athletes with no preexisting edema.

---

from respiratory acidosis may worsen from these drugs, which tend to produce metabolic acidosis.

Drug interactions. Acetazolamide and other carbonic anhydrase inhibitors produce more marked potassium excretion than sodium excretion. Potassium depletion is therefore likely to occur. This possibility is made even more likely by corticosteroids or ACTH given concomitantly. Digitalis toxicity is increased in the presence of low serum potassium.

Osmotic diuretics

Osmotic diuretics are nonelectrolytes that are filtered by the glomerulus but not significantly reabsorbed or metabolized. Therefore osmotic diuretics enter the renal tubule and are highly concentrated in renal tubular fluid. The high osmolality in the tubule reduces reabsorption of water with the result that urine production is increased. At high doses some increase in sodium excretion is produced, but this is not observed in most clinical circumstances. These drugs are therefore exceptions to the generalization that sodium excretion precedes water excretion during diuretic therapy.

Osmotic diuresis may be used clinically to prevent permanent damage during acute renal failure. The usefulness of osmotic diuresis in these cases frequently depends on maintaining adequate urine volume without altering electrolyte balance. Osmotic diuretics also increase the osmolality of the plasma, which allows reduction of osmotic pressure inside the eye and in the cerebrospinal fluid.

The two agents currently used as osmotic diuretics, mannitol and urea, are usually administered intravenously. Mannitol is the preferred agent in most circumstances.

Toxicity produced by these agents depends on the amount of drug administered and how much the drug affects fluid balance. These drugs are retained within the extracellular space and on intravenous administration can cause an acute expansion of extracellular fluid volume. This volume expansion may be hazardous to a patient with reduced cardiac reserve.

Fluid and electrolyte imbalances may develop, especially if a degree of renal impairment exists. Under these circumstances the diuretics tend to accumulate in the blood and may cause dangerous shifts in salt and water balance. Pulmonary congestion, acidosis, thirst, blurred vision, convulsion, nausea and vomiting, diarrhea, tachycardia, fever, and angina-like pain may be noted occasionally. Local irritation with thrombophlebitis can also occur.

Urea should not be used in a patient with liver failure, since the high levels of urea may place additional demands on liver function.

Organomercurial diuretics

Organomercurial compounds inhibit active chloride ion transport in the ascending limb jof Henle's loop. Chloride excretion therefore increases and causes an increase in the excretion of sodium ion and water, but the effect is self-limiting and the drugs lose effectiveness within days. Organomercurial compounds are irritative to the gastrointestinal tract and are unreliably absorbed by the oral route. For this reason these drugs are usually best administered intramuscularly.

Organomercurial diuretics are seldom used in modern clinical practice, since newer, safer, and more convenient agents have become available.

Text continued on p. 270.

PATIENT CARE IMPLICATIONS

General guidelines for diuretic therapy

- Carefully measure and record intake and output. Report unexpected findings to the physician. For example, oliguria (scanty urine output) or anuria (no urine output) would be unexpected after an increase in a diuretic dose. Patients at home are not usually required to measure intake and output, except in the case of severe kidney or heart disease, but encourage patients to report output that seems to be abnormal.

- Weigh the patient in the acute care setting at least daily. Weigh the patient under standard conditions: same time (usually in the morning), after the patient has voided or the catheter bag is emptied, but before breakfast. Use the same scale each day, and have the patient wear the same amount of clothing. If appropriate to the patient's ability and resources, teach the patient at home how to keep a daily or weekly weight record. Tell the patient to report to the physician a weight gain or loss greater than 2 pounds per day, or five pounds per week, unless otherwise instructed by the physician.

- Monitor the blood pressure regularly. Although all patients receiving diuretic therapy would be expected to experience an initial drop in blood pressure, the elderly, those receiving intravenous diuretics, and those also taking anithypertensives may experience a precipitous fall in blood pressure, and in rare instances go into shock. Other drugs that can cause hypotension, and thus can potentiate hypotension in a patient receiving diuretics, include central nervous system depressants, barbiturates, narcotics, and antihypertensives. Initially, monitor the blood pressure with the patient in both the sitting and lying positions, and compare the measurements from each arm. Review with the patient the symptoms of orthostatic hypotension (see box on p. 237).

- Caution patients to avoid the use of alcohol, as it enchances hypotension.

- To monitor for fluid retention, measure abdominal girth or circumference of one or both legs. To ensure accurate measurement, mark the patient's skin with small ink marks to indicate the correct placement of the tape measure from day to day.

- Check dependent areas daily for the presence of or change in the amount of pitting edema.

In pitting edema, an indentation or depressed area made by the examiner's finger remains visible in the skin for seconds to minutes after the pressure has been released. Dependent areas where this is more likely to occur include the sacral area and the feet and legs.

- Assess for symptoms of dehydration: thirst, decreased skin turgor, nausea, lightheadedness, weakness, increased pulse, oliguria, decreased blood pressure, and elevated hemoglobin, hematocrit, and blood urea nitrogen (BUN) levels.

- Assess for electrolyte abnormalities, and monitor the serum levels of potassium, sodium, calcium, magnesium, and bicarbonate. The signs and symptoms of common electrolyte abnormalities are summarized in Table 17.1.

- Teach the patient the importance of taking potassium supplements, if prescribed, and work with the patient to find a preparation the patient is willing to take (see Chapter 17). Many effervescent preparations are unpalatable. Enteric-coated tablets have been implicated in small bowel ulceration and should not be used. Oral solutions are the preferred form of therapy, but they are often unpleasant tasting. Dilute these solutions in juice or milk to reduce the risk of gastric irritation and to make the taste tolerable. Take potassium with meals to reduce gastric irritation. Encourage hypokalemic patients to increase dietary intake of potassium-rich foods (see box on p. 259).

- Caution patients taking diuretics not to switch to salt substitutes without first consulting the physician. The public is increasingly aware of the need to limit salt intake, and some patients will switch to salt substitutes on their own. Salt substitutes contain a variety of electrolyte salts, and the exact proportions vary from product to product. A patient may inadvertently contribute to electrolyte abnormalities by using a salt substitute. For example, a patient taking a potassium-sparing diuretic may develop hyperkalemia if a salt substitute containing a high portion of potassium salts is used.

- Refer patients as needed to the dietician for instruction about special dietary restrictions, which may include sodium, calories, cholesterol, and other factors.

PATIENT CARE IMPLICATIONS — cont'd

- Teach patients about their need for diuretic therapy, and review the anticipated side effects of the prescribed drug(s). Poor compliance is sometimes a result of patient annoyance caused by frequent and excessive urination. Take diuretics ordered once a day in the morning, and twice daily diuretics in the morning and afternoon, to avoid interrupting sleep to urinate.
- Dehydration and hypovolemia can contribute to thromboembolic disorders. Assess the patient for pain in the chest, calves, and pelvis that might indicate thromboembolism.
- For some patients, intermittent therapy (every other day) will achieve the desired effects, but with fewer side effects.
- Teach patients to take their diuretics as ordered. If a dose is missed, it should be taken as soon as remembered, unless within a few hours of the next dose (varies with the frequency of the dosing schedule), in which case it should be omitted and the regular dosing schedule resumed. Tell patients not to double-up for missed doses.
- Thirst is often a frequent side effect. Review the box Patient Problem: Xerostomia on p. 170.

Loop diuretics

Drug administration

- Review general guidelines for patients receiving diuretics.
- Assess for development of hyponatremia, hypocalcemia, hypokalemia, and hypochloremic alkalosis (see Table 17.1). Monitor serum electrolytes.
- Monitor blood glucose, as these drugs may cause hyperglycemia. Review drug interactions and counsel patients as appropriate.
- Assess patients receiving warfarin and loop diuretics for signs of excessive anticoagulation (see Chapter 20).
- Monitor serum uric acid levels and assess for signs of gout.
- Assess for signs of ototoxicity: tinnitus (ringing in the ears), reduced hearing acuity, and vertigo.
- Question patients about previous allergy to sulfonamides before administering first doses. Observe for allergic response, including development of rashes.

INTRAVENOUS BUMETANIDE

Usually given undiluted, but may be mixed with 5% dextrose in water, 0.9% sodium chloride, and lactated Ringer's solution. Administer dose over 1 to 2 minutes. Following IV use, monitor blood pressure every 15 to 30 minutes until stable, keep siderails up, and supervise ambulation.

INTRAVENOUS ETHACRYNIC ACID

- May be given undiluted, or 50 mg of ethacrynic acid diluted in 50 ml of 5% dextrose in water or 0.9% sodium chloride. Do not mix with other drugs. Do not administer if solution is discolored or contains particulate matter. Administer at a rate of 10 mg or less over 1 minute, or infuse total dose over 30 minutes. Check infusion site carefully: thrombophlebitis is common, and extravasation causes pain and tissue irritation. Following IV use, monitor blood pressure every 15 to 30 minutes until stable, keep siderails up, and supervise ambulation.

INTRAVENOUS FUROSEMIDE

- May be given undiluted, or added to 5% dextrose in water or normal saline. Inspect solution before administering, and do not use if solution is yellow. Do not mix with other drugs. Administer at a rate of 20 mg per 1–2 minutes. Following IV use, monitor blood pressure every 15 to 30 minutes until stable, keep siderails up, and supervise ambulation.

INTRAMUSCULAR FUROSEMIDE

- Intramuscular injection of furosemide may cause transient pain at the injection site.

Patient and family education

- See general guidelines for patient receiving diuretics.
- Potassium supplements are often prescribed concomitantly. As noted in the general guidelines, emphasize the importance of taking these as prescribed, refer to the dietician as needed, and review good dietary sources of potassium. Teach patients that diarrhea, vomiting, and anorexia (loss of appetite), if prolonged or severe, may also cause hypokalemia, and should be reported to the physician. Caution patients also taking a cardiac glycoside to be especially careful to avoid hypokalemia. Review other drug interactions with the patient, as appropriate.
- Caution diabetic patients to monitor blood glucose levels carefully, as hyperglycemia may occur, requiring an adjustment in diet or dose of insulin.

Continued.

PATIENT CARE IMPLICATIONS — cont'd

- Instruct patients to report signs of agranulocytosis (depressed production of white blood cells): unexplained fever, chills, sore throat, or enlarged lymph nodes. This is a rare but serious side effect of drug therapy. See the box Patient Problem: Depressed White Blood Cell Production on p. 599.
- Take oral preparations with meals or just after eating to reduce gastric irritation.
- Warn patients in renal failure that bumetanide may cause myalgia (muscle pain).
- Tell patients to report the development of skin changes, rashes, photosensitivity, nausea, vomiting, or any unexpected sign or symptom. See the box Patient Problem: Photosensitivity on p. 647.

Thiazide diuretics

Drug administration

- See the general guidelines for diuretic therapy.
- Thiazides may cause hypokalemia, hypochloremia, alkalosis, hyponatremia, and hypomagnesemia. Assess for these electrolyte abnormalities, and monitor serum electrolyte levels: see Table 17.1.
- Monitor blood glucose as these drugs may cause hyperglycemia.
- Review drug interactions and counsel patients as appropriate.
- Monitor serum uric acid levels and assess for signs of gout.
- Monitor the serum blood urea nitrogen (BUN) and serum lipid levels.
  PARENTERAL CHLOROTHIAZIDE
- Dilute each vial (0.5 Gm) with at least 18 ml of sterile water. Dilute further if desired with 5% dextrose in water or sodium chloride injection. Do not mix with other drugs or blood products. Administer at a rate of 0.5 Gm or less over 5 minutes. Check insertion site and avoid extravasation as the drug is extremely alkaline. Do not administer IM or subcutaneously.
- The thiazides can cause a paradoxical antidiuretic effect in patients who have diabetes insipidus (Chapter 50).

Patient and family education

- See general guidelines for diuretic therapy.
- Potassium supplements may be prescribed, but patients may be able to prevent hypokalemia by increasing their daily dietary intake of potassium-rich foods (see box on p. 259). If potassium supplements are prescribed, emphasize the importance of taking these as prescribed. Teach patients that diarrhea, vomiting, and anorexia (loss of appetite), if prolonged or severe, can also cause hypokalemia, and should be reported to the physician. Concomitant administration of adrenal corticosteroids may also predispose the patient to hypokalemia.
- Caution diabetic patients to monitor blood glucose levels carefully, as hyperglycemia may occur, requiring an adjustment in diet or dose of insulin.
- Take oral doses with meals to reduce gastric irritation.

Potassium-sparing diuretics

Drug administration

- See general guidelines for diuretic therapy.
- The potassium-sparing diuretics may cause hyperkalemia or hyponatremia. Assess for these electrolyte imbalances and monitor serum electrolyte; see Table 17.1.
- There are many combination products available containing both a potassium-losing diuretic and a potassium-sparing diuretic. The goal of the combination is to promote diuresis while maintaining normal serum potassium levels. Patients receiving combination drugs are potentially at risk for side effects due to any of the component drugs; see Table 16.5. Instruct patients to report the development of any unexpected sign or symptom.
- Monitor blood glucose levels and blood urea nitrogen (BUN).

Patient and family education

- Instruct diabetic patients to monitor blood glucose levels, as these drugs may produce hyperglycemia.
- Take doses with meals or snack to reduce gastric irritation. Spironolactone tablets may be crushed and mixed in syrup or fluid of the patient's choice. The triamterene capsule may be opened and the contents mixed with food or fluid for patients who have difficulty swallowing capsules.
- If patients have been switched to a potassium-sparing diuretic, or a potassium-sparing diuretic is prescribed in addition to a potassium-losing diuretic, impress on them the need to *omit* previous potassium supple-

PATIENT CARE IMPLICATIONS — cont'd

ments that may have been ordered; consult the physician. In addition, the patient should *limit* intake of potassium-rich foods; see box on p. 259.

- Instruct patients to avoid salt substitutes which contain potassium, while taking potassium-sparing diuretics.
- Caution patients taking triamterene that photosensitivity may develop; see Patient Problem: Photosensitivity on p. 647.

Carbonic anhydrase inhibitors

Drug administration

- Review general guidelines for diuretic therapy.
- Monitor serum electrolytes and assess for electrolyte abnormalities, especially metabolic acidosis; see Table 17.1. Intermittent therapy may be used to limit the development of acidosis.
- Read orders carefully: tablets and extended-release capsules are available.
- Review drug interactions and counsel patients as appropriate.
- Monitor serum uric acid levels and blood glucose levels.
- Assess for signs of kidney stone formation: renal colic (severe flank pain), hematuria (blood in the urine), and oliguria.

INTRAVENOUS ACETAZOLAMIDE

- Dilute each 500 mg of acetazolamide with at least 5 ml of sterile water for injection, and administer at a rate of 500 mg over at least 1 minute. May be further diluted with standard IV fluids and administered over 4 to 8 hours. Avoid intramuscular injection as it is very painful.

Patient and family education

- Review guidelines for diuretic therapy.
- Instruct diabetic patients to monitor blood glucose levels; a change in diet or insulin dose may be needed.
- Review expected effects and possible side effects. Instruct patients to report the appearance of any unexpected sign or symptom.
- Instruct patients to avoid driving or operating hazardous equipment if drowsiness, dizziness, lightheadedness, or visual changes occur; notify the physician.
- A metallic taste in the mouth may occur. Sucking sugarless hard candy, chewing sugarless gum, and frequent oral hygiene may help.

- Photosensitivity may occur: see the box Patient Problem: Photosensitivity on p. 647.

Osmotic diuretics

Drug administration/patient and family education

- See the general guidelines for diuretic therapy.
- Monitor serum electrolytes and assess for electrolyte abnormalities; see Table 17.1.
- Assess for signs of circulatory overload: monitor vital signs and blood pressure, intake and output, and daily weight. Assess breath and heart sounds. Assess for signs of pulmonary congestion and/or congestive heart failure: dyspnea, labored respiration, tachypnea, tachycardia, distended neck veins, rales, agitation, fluid retention, and weight gain.
- These drugs are often administered to patients with increased intracranial pressure. Assess level of consciousness and monitor indicators of cerebral function: blood pressure, pulse, intracranial pressure, Glasgow Coma Scale or institutional equivalent.
- Determine with physician the desired daily fluid balance. Infusion rate may be titrated to output. Diuresis may be copious, especially initially; a urinary catheter may be needed. If the urine output falls below 30 to 50 ml per hour, notify the physician.
- Oral fluids may or may not be permitted. Occasional ice chips may be permitted to help relieve thirst.
- If extravasated, osmotic diuretics cause local skin and tissue damage. Before instituting infusion, ascertain that IV is secure and patent, with no signs of redness or infiltration, and that rate of flow is not sluggish. Inspect infusion site regularly. If infiltration is suspected, discontinue infusion and restart in another site.

INTRAVENOUS MANNITOL

- Read order carefully. Mannitol is available in several concentrations. Do not confuse mannitol with mannitol hexanitrate, an antianginal drug. It is not necessary to dilute mannitol. Check ampule or bottle for crystallization, a common problem. If crystals are present, warm the container under running water until crystals dissolve. Let cool to body temperature before administering. Use an inline IV filter for 15%, 20%, and 25% solutions. Do not add to other IV solutions, medications, or blood products. The rate of ad-

Continued.

PATIENT CARE IMPLICATIONS — cont'd

ministration is usually 1 to 2 Gm/kg over 30 to 90 minutes, but is variable.

INTRAVENOUS UREA

■ Urea must be diluted to make a 30% solution (30% solution equals 30 Gm of urea per 100 ml or 300 mg/1 ml). Dilute with 5% or 10% dextrose in water or with 10% invert sugar in water; some manufacturers supply the diluent. (Patients with hereditary fructose intolerance (aldolase deficiency) may have a severe reaction to the invert sugar solution if it is used as a diluent. Symptoms include hypoglycemia, nausea, vomiting, tremors, coma, convulsions.) Infuse at a rate of 4 ml per minute (1200 mg per minute) or slower. Use only fresh solutions and discard any unused portions. Do not mix with blood or other drugs in the same syringe.

■ These drugs are rarely used outside of the acute care setting; keep patient and family informed of the patient's condition.

SUMMARY

Passive diffusion in the glomerulus allows water and small molecules to enter the renal tubule. In the proximal convoluted tubule, bicarbonate ion is reclaimed from the fluid by the action of carbonic anhydrase. Sodium is also actively reabsorbed, bringing along chloride ion and water. Water is removed in the descending limb of Henle's loop, whereas chloride and potassium are actively reabsorbed in the ascending limb of Henle's loop. Active sodium ion reabsorption occurs in the distal convoluted tubule, and potassium is secreted into the tubule. Final water removal from the tubular fluid occurs in the collecting duct. Diuretics increase urine flow by increasing the loss of sodium in the urine, which causes concomitant loss of water.

Ethacrynic acid blocks chloride reabsorption in the ascending limb of Henle's loop, thereby passively blocking sodium reabsorption. This potent diuretic may be given orally or intravenously. Toxicity may involve dehydration, potassium loss, deafness, and gastrointestinal disturbances. Digitalis toxicity may be increased with ethacrynic acid.

Furosemide has the same mechanism of action as ethacrynic acid. Furosemide can be given orally, intravenously, or intramuscularly. Toxicity includes acute dehydration, dermatitis, and blood dyscrasias. Furosemide may increase the toxicity of digitalis and nephrotoxic antibiotics.

Bumetanide has the same mechanism of action as the other loop diuretics, ethacrynic acid and furosemide. Bumetanide is an extremely potent diuretic that may be given orally or intravenously. Toxicity includes reactions common to other loop diuretics. In addition, bumetanide may cause blood dyscrasias, rashes, and gastrointestinal distress.

In patients in renal failure, the drug may cause myalgia.

Thiazide diuretics block sodium and chloride reabsorption in the distal convoluted tubule, increasing salt and water excretion. Thiazide diuretics are primarily oral agents, although chlorothiazide is available for intravenous use. These drugs should not be administered intramuscularly or subcutaneously. They may produce potassium loss and chloride loss, leading to metabolic alkalosis. Thiazides have central nervous system effects, allergic reactions, and hypotensive effects. They frequently alter the requirement for insulin or other hypoglycemic agents in diabetics.

Potassium-sparing diuretics inhibit the sodium-potassium exchange mechanism in the distal convoluted tubule. Spironolactone blocks the action of aldosterone on this exchange mechanism, whereas triamterene and amiloride act independently of aldosterone. These weak diuretics have the advantage that, unlike most of the other diuretics, they do not cause excessive loss of potassium. One possible toxic reaction to these drugs is high concentrations of potassium in the blood. Spironolactone produces tumors in laboratory animals.

Carbonic anhydrase inhibitors prevent the secretion of hydrogen ion into the renal tubule and the reabsorption of bicarbonate. Sodium ion is excreted along with the bicarbonate ion. Potassium excretion is also increased. These drugs ultimately produce metabolic acidosis, which in turn prevents their diuretic action. Carbonic anhydrase inhibitors are used in the treatment of glaucoma, congestive heart failure, and convulsive disorders. These drugs are administered orally and may affect the central nervous system.

Osmotic diuretics cause increased osmotic concentrations within the renal tubule, thereby drawing water from the bloodstream into the tubule. These agents are given intravenously. Mannitol and urea have been used in this manner.

Organomercurial diuretics inhibit chloride ion transport in the ascending limb of Henle's loop. The action of these drugs is short-term only and they must be administered by intramuscular injection. These drugs are rarely used in modern therapy.

STUDY QUESTIONS

1. What is the nephron?
2. What is the function of the glomerulus?
3. What is the renal tubule?
4. Where is sodium reabsorbed from the renal tubule?
5. Where is chloride reabsorbed from the renal tubule?
6. Where is potassium reabsorbed, and where is it secreted in the renal tubule?
7. Which parts of the tubule are most permeable to water?
8. What is the mechanism by which bicarbonate ion is recovered from the tubular fluid? Where does this occur?
9. What is the general mechanism by which all diuretics act?
10. What is the specific mechanism of action of loop diuretics?
11. How may ethacrynic acid be administered?
12. What toxicity is characteristic of ethacrynic acid?
13. What drug interactions occur with ethacrynic acid?
14. How may furosemide be administered?
15. What toxicity is characteristic of furosemide?
16. What drug interactions occur with furosemide?
17. How does bumetanide differ from the other loop diuretics?
18. What is the specific mechanism of action of thiazide diuretics?
19. How may the thiazide diuretics be administered?
20. What toxicity is characteristic of thiazide diuretics?
21. What drug interactions can occur with thiazide diuretics?
22. What is the specific mechanism of action of the potassium-sparing diuretics?
23. How may the potassium-sparing diuretics be administered?
24. What toxicity is associated with the potassium-sparing diuretics?
25. What drug interactions occur with the potassium-sparing diuretics?
26. How do carbonic anhydrase inhibitors produce diuresis?
27. How are carbonic anhydrase inhibitors administered?
28. What toxicity is characteristic of carbonic anhydrase inhibitors?
29. What drug interactions occur with carbonic anhydrase inhibitors?
30. How are the osmotic diuretics administered?
31. What reactions occur with the osmotic diuretics?

SUGGESTED READINGS

Diuretics: a quick review, Nursing 83 **13**(8)64, 1983.

Eilers, M.A.: Pharmacologic therapeutic modalities: osmotic and diuretic agents, Crit. Care Q. **5**(4):44, 1983.

Eknoyan, G.: Diuretic-induced hyperglycemia, Drug Therapy **13**(3):229, 1983.

Gever, L.N.: Thiazide diuretics: minimizing their adverse effects, Nursing 84 **14**(2):72, 1984.

Gever, L.N.: Bumetanide—the latest loop diuretic, Nursing 87 **17**(4):115, 1987

Halstenson, C.E., and Matzke, G.R.: Bumetanide: a new loop diuretic, Drug Intell. Clin. Pharm. **17**(11):786, 1983.

Horne, M.M., and Searingen, P.L.: Pocket guide to fluids and electrolytes, St. Louis, 1989, C.V. Mosby Co.

Karb, V.B.: Electrolyte abnormalities and drugs which commonly cause them, J. Neurosc. Nurs. **21**(2):125, 1989.

Kirschenbaum, H.L., and Rosenberg, J.M.: What to watch out for with thiazides, RN **46**(7):28, 1983.

Lamb, C.: When diuretics affect electrolytes, Patient Care **16**(8):62, 1982.

Lant, A.: Diuretics: Clinical pharmacology and therapeutic use, Drugs **29**: 57, 1985.

Martinez-Maldonado, M., and Benabe, J.E.: Clinical uses of potassium-sparing diuretics, Drug Therapy **18**(3):48, 1988.

Metheny, N.M.: Fluid and electrolyte balance: nursing considerations, Philadelphia, 1987, J.B. Lippincott.

Rosenberg, J.M., and Kirschenbaum, H.L.: What to watch out for with nonthiazides, RN **46**(8):41, 1983.

Weinberger, M.H.: Diuretics and their side effects. Dilemma in treatment of hypertension. Hypertension II (3 pt 2):II 16, 1988.

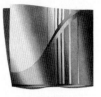

Fluids and Electrolytes

17

Fluids and electrolyte solutions are used in various clinical situations to try to reestablish proper salt and water balance. In the sense that these solutions are returning the body to homeostasis, they may be thought of as drugs. This chapter reviews the general classes of fluids and solutions that are commonly employed in medicine. Although a full discussion of the clinical indications for these solutions is outside the scope of a text in pharmacology, the most important physiological and clinical factors in the use of these solutions are covered.

REGULATION OF SALT AND WATER BALANCE

Fluid Compartments

Water comprises 60% of the weight of an average person. Although water passes easily through most tissues, certain physical and permeability barriers allow the body to be divided into compartments where water content may be independently regulated. For example, in a person who weighs 70 kg there would be 42 liters of water, with 28 liters of that water found inside the cells (Figure 17.1). This water, along with its dissolved solutes, is called *intracellular fluid*. The *interstitial fluid* bathes the outside of the cell and allows it to exchange waste products and receive nutrients. *Plasma* constitutes an important separate fluid compartment similar to interstitial fluid, but it is more accessible to manipulation and testing. *Extracellular fluid* primarily includes interstitial fluid and plasma but also other fluids such as lymph and cerebrospinal fluid.

Composition of Body Fluids

The fluid compartments in the body differ in the concentration of important ions and other sol-

utes. In plasma the major solute is sodium chloride (Figure 17.2). The primary buffers maintaining the pH of blood at 7.4 are bicarbonate (HCO_3^-, 27 mEq/L) and protein (16 mEq/L). Interstitial fluid is similar to plasma except that the protein content is very much reduced.

Inside the cell, high concentrations of both protein and potassium are found, but the sodium ion concentration is much lower. The major buffer for the intracellular fluid is phosphate, shown in Figure 17.2 as PO_4^{-3} but actually present as a mixture of HPO_3^{-2} and $H_2PO_3^{-1}$. Magnesium ion is also a significant constituent of intracellular fluid, serving as an important component of critical enzyme systems.

Movement of Fluid and Electrolytes between Compartments

Water moves freely through the vascular walls separating plasma from interstitial fluid and through the cell membranes separating intracellular fluid from interstitial fluid. Movement of ions and other solutes is rigidly controlled, however, so that optimum concentration differences are maintained between the compartments. The concentrations of these solutes influence the disposition of water among the compartments. In order to understand the distribution of water and the various solutes, it is necessary to recall certain concepts from chemistry and physiology.

Osmosis is the term used to describe the movement of water across a semipermeable membrane (a membrane that selectively limits the passage of some chemicals; for example, a cell membrane is a semipermeable membrane). The direction of movement is determined by the concentration of solutes in the water on either side of the membrane. Water moves toward the solution hav-

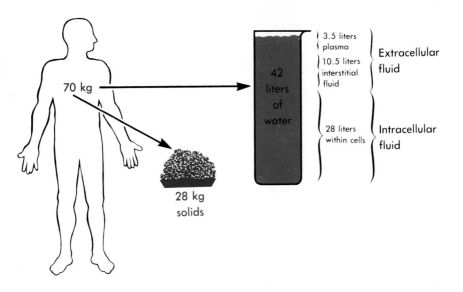

FIGURE 17.1   Distribution of water in the human body. The figure shows the common distribution pattern for males. In females about 50% of the body weight is found as water, but the proportion of intracellular to extracellular fluid is the same as for males.

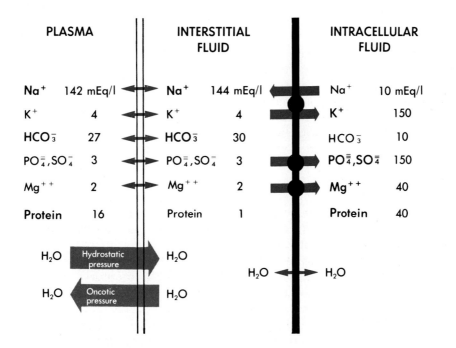

FIGURE 17.2   Movement of water and solutes between body compartments. The double-headed arrows represent simple diffusion; straight arrows represent pressure-regulated processes. Arrows passing through or in contact with circles represent active transport of solutes.

Table 17.1 Common Electrolyte Imbalances

Solute	Normal concentration in plasma	Signs of deficiency	Signs of excess
Sodium ion	136 to 145 mEq/L	Anorexia, nausea, vomiting; increased intracranial pressure; oliguria leading to anuria.	Dry, sticky membranes; fever; weakness and disorientation; oliguria.
Potassium ion	3.5 to 5.0 mEq/L	Muscle weakness; diminished tendon reflexes; paralytic ileus; cardiac arrhythmia.	Nausea and vomiting; muscle weakness; changes in ECG.
Bicarbonate ion	24 to 31 mEq/L (pH 7.35 to 7.45)	Metabolic acidosis (pH <7.35); weakness; deep, rapid breathing (Kussmaul); stupor or unconsciousness.	Metabolic alkalosis (pH >7.45); hypertonicity of muscles; depressed respirations; tetany.
Calcium ion	4.7 to 5.6 mEq/L	Tetany; prolonged QT interval on ECG.	Weakness, fatigue, thirst; nausea, anorexia; muscle cramping.
Magnesium ion	1.3 to 2.3 mEq/L	Flushing, hypertension; neuromuscular irritability.	Nausea, vomiting; diarrhea, colic.

ing the higher concentration. The effect of osmosis is to reduce the difference in concentration of the solutions on either side of a semipermeable membrane.

The movement of water by osmosis across semipermeable membranes creates osmotic pressure. For example, if a solution of sugar is enclosed in a synthetic membrane that allows water but not sugar to pass through the membrane and the sealed sac is submerged in pure water, two things will happen. First, water will enter the sac at a greater rate than it leaves the sac. Second, as water enters the solution-filled sac, pressure inside the sac will increase and oppose the entry of more water. The pressure that would be required to completely prevent the net movement of water into the sac is a measure of the osmotic pressure of the solution.

The osmotic properties of a solution are related to the concentration of solute, but, rather than the mass of the solute, it is the number of particles (ions, atoms, or molecules) that is important. For example, a 0.5 molar solution of glucose contains 90 Gm/L and has a potential osmotic pressure of 9650 mm Hg. In contrast, a 0.5 molar solution of sodium chloride contains 29 Gm/L and has a potential osmotic pressure of 19,300 mm Hg. The greater potential osmotic pressure of the sodium chloride solution results from the ionization of sodium chloride to release two particles for every molecule of salt: a sodium ion

and a chloride ion. Glucose does not ionize, and each molecule of the sugar remains as a single particle.

The main determinant of the osmolarity of the extracellular fluid is the concentration of sodium chloride. Solutions that have the same osmolarity as plasma are called *isotonic*. Isotonic solutions include 5% dextrose and 0.9% NaCl solutions. Hypertonic solutions have an osmolarity above that of plasma (>310 milliosmoles/L); hypotonic solutions have lower osmolarity than plasma.

Oncotic pressure is another important regulator of the movement of water between the plasma and the interstitial fluid. This pressure is generated by the difference in protein concentration between plasma and interstitial fluid. Although most solutes in plasma pass freely through the pores of the vascular walls that separate plasma from interstitial fluid, proteins cannot leave plasma by that route. Since proteins act like any other solute to cause the movement of water, the result of this differential protein concentration is that movement of water from interstitial fluid toward plasma is promoted.

Without a balancing force, oncotic pressure would tend to dilute the protein in plasma and increase pressure in the plasma compartment. Oncotic pressure is balanced, however, by *hydrostatic pressure* generated by the force of contraction of the heart. In the arteriolar vasculature where blood

Table 17.2   Solutions Used for Parenteral Therapy

Solution	IV dosage	Comments
Dextrose in water (2.5%, 5%, 10%, 20%, 25%, 38%, 40%, 50%, 60%, 70%)	Isotonic (5%) 90 to 125 ml/hr usual but may range much higher; doses of hypertonic solutions are individualized for specific purposes.	Isotonic dextrose (D5W) maintains or replaces fluid without altering electrolytes. Hypertonic dextrose is used to prevent brain damage caused by hypoglycemic shock or to supply extra calories to patients unable to handle excess fluid required with 5% dextrose (see Table 17.4).
Dextrose in saline (2.5%, 5%, or 10% dextrose in various combinations with 0.11%, 0.2%, 0.225%, 0.3%, 0.45%, or 0.9% NaCl)	Doses adjusted as needed for specific fluid and electrolyte needs of patient.	Hypotonic solution (2.5% dextrose, 0.45% NaCl) drives fluid from plasma into interstitial space. Isotonic solutions supply calories and replenish salt and water.
Dextrose in saline with potassium chloride (5% or 10% dextrose with 0.2%, 0.225%, 0.33%, or 0.45% NaCl and 0.075%, 0.15%, 0.224%, or 0.3% potassium chloride)	Doses adjusted as needed for specific fluid and electrolyte needs of patient.	This mixture is used to replenish salt and water when potassium replacement is also required. Dosage must be carefully monitored to avoid potassium overload, especially when renal function is compromised.
Dextrose with electrolytes (5% with Electrolyte No. 48, No. 75, Ionosol, Isolyte, Normosol, Plasmalyte; 10% with Ionosol, Isolyte; 38% with Electrolyte pattern T; 50% with Electrolytes pattern A, B, or N)	Refer to specific information supplied with each individual preparation.	These complex mixtures are used in special circumstances to correct massive electrolyte imbalances.
KCl in water (11.25%, 15%, 24%)	Must be diluted before use and administered at rates less than 10 to 15 mEq/hr for minimally depleted patients or up to 40 mEq/hr for severely depleted patients.	As supplied, these solutions are strongly hypertonic (15% = 2000 mEq/L) and must be diluted before administration. Concentrations are commonly 40 to 60 mEq/L.
Lactated Ringer's solution (0.6% NaCl, 0.03% KCl, 0.02% $CaCl_2$, 0.31% Na lactate)	90 to 125 ml/hr commonly employed.	This balanced salt solution supplies, in mEq/L, these ions: Na^+ 130, K^+ 4, Ca^{++} 3.0, Cl^- 109. It is used to maintain or restore fluid and electrolyte balance, especially when mild acidosis is also present. A portion of the lactate present is converted to bicarbonate, which elevates blood pH.
Magnesium sulfate (10%, 50%)	10% solution should be infused at rates less than 1.5 ml/min. More concentrated solution is for intramuscular administration.	This nearly isotonic solution (10%) is used to reverse severe magnesium deficiencies, as maintenance during total parenteral nutrition, and to control convulsions of eclampsia.
NaCl in water (0.45%, 0.9%, 3.0%, 5.0%)	Isotonic (0.9%) and hypotonic (0.45%) 90 to 125 ml/hr but may range much higher for initial therapy; 3% solution up to 80 ml/hr; 5% solution up to 50 ml/hr.	Isotonic saline supplies 154 mEq of Na^+ and 154 mEq of Cl^- per liter. Used to replace sodium and water loss.

Continued.

Table 17.2 Solutions Used for Parenteral Therapy—cont'd

Solution	IV dosage	Comments
Ringer's solution (0.86% NaCl, 0.03% KCl, and 0.033% CaCl$_2$)	90 to 125 ml/hr commonly employed.	This balanced salt solution supplies, in mEq/L, these ions: Na$^+$ 147.5, K$^+$ 4, Ca^{++} 4.5, Cl$^-$ 156. Used to maintain or restore fluid and electrolyte balance. Additional K$^+$ is required to correct severe potassium depletion.
Sodium bicarbonate in water (1.4%)	Doses are calculated to reverse acidosis (individualized for each patient).	Commercially available solutions (4.2%, 7.5%, 8.4%) are hypertonic and must be diluted before use. One liter of 1.4% NaHCO$_3$ contains 167 mEq/L of Na$^+$. This essentially isotonic solution is used to reverse metabolic acidosis.

Table 17.3 Blood, Blood Components, and Blood Substitutes

Preparation	Dosage/administration	Comments
Whole blood	One unit = 450 ± 45 ml blood + 63 ml CPD (citrate-phosphate-dextrose) or CPDA-1 (citrate-phosphate-dextrose-adenine), administered intravenously through a 170 μm filter.	Used to treat patients who have lost more than 20% of their blood volume. Whole blood acts as a volume expander and maintains oxygen transport.
Plasma	Monitored by clinical response to intravenous infusion.	Used as a volume expander when oxygen transport is not seriously impaired.
Albumin, human (5%, 25%) (Albuconn, Albuminar, Albutein, Buminate, Plasbumin)	Adjusted according to need of the patient, but should be less than 250 Gm/48 hr.	Used to expand plasma volume. Normal human serum albumin preparations contain significant amounts of Na$^+$, which may be dangerous for patients on sodium-restricted diets.
Plasma protein fraction (5%) (Plasmanate, Plasma Plex, Plasmatein, Protenate)	*Adults*—1 to 1.5 L of 5% solution infused at 5 to 8 ml/min, adjusted as necessary. *Children*—33 ml/kg infused at 5 to 10 ml/min to correct dehydration.	Used for hypovolemic shock in adults, to correct dehydration in children, and to supply protein to patients with deficiencies. This human plasma protein fraction is 83% albumin, <17% globulin, and <1% gamma globulin.
Dextrans (Dextran 40, Dextran 70, Dextran 75)	Infusion rates may be rapid initially, but total daily dose should not exceed 2 Gm/kg or 20 ml/kg.	Dextran 40 (molecular weight 40,000) has effects that last 2 to 4 hr. Dextran 70 (molecular weight 70,000) and Dextran 75 (molecular weight 75,000) are cleared by the kidney more slowly than Dextran 40; the duration of action of these preparations is about 12 hr. Used for shock.
Hetastarch (6% in 0.9% NaCl) (Hespan)	Rates of infusion for acute hemorrhagic shock are 20 ml/kg/hr or less.	Used as a plasma volume expander in shock or hypovolemia.

Table 17.4 Fluids Used for Total Parenteral Nutrition

Solution	IV dosage	Comments
Hypertonic dextrose (50% or 70%)	Diluted with water or amino acid solutions to initial concentrations of about 12.5%. Longer-term therapy may ultimately require 25% to 30% solutions. Minimum adult requirements for dextrose are about 150 Gm daily. Initial infusion of 1000 to 1200 ml of 12.5% dextrose approximates that requirement; dosage can be gradually increased as needed to meet caloric requirements.	These highly hypertonic solutions must be administered into a central vein with sufficient blood flow to dilute the sugar. Special care is required to maintain aseptic conditions, since these catheters remain in use for prolonged periods. Infusion should be terminated gradually to avoid rebound hypoglycemia.
Crystalline amino acids (Aminess, Aminosyn, BranchAmin, FreAmine III, HepatAmine, NephrAmine, Novamine, ProcalAmine, PenAmin, Travasol, TrophAmine, Veinamine)	May be given at about 1 Gm/kg body weight per day, as needed to prevent protein breakdown and negative nitrogen balance. Solutions contain mixtures of essential and nonessential amino acids. TrophAmine contains taurine, an amino acid required by neonates.	A 3.5% solution is nearly isotonic, supplies 140 cal/L and may be administered via a peripheral vein. Various commercial amino acid solutions include appreciable amounts of sodium as well as other electrolytes.
Intralipid (10%, 20%) Travalmulsion (10%)	May be given by peripheral vein 1 ml/min for 10% or 0.5 ml/min for 20% over 30 min initially as needed to supply calories (20% contains 2000 cal/L) or replace essential fatty acids. This preparation should supply 60% or less of total calories. Dosage should not exceed 2.5 Gm fat/kg body weight daily. Children and infants require lower infusion rates.	Soybean oil 10% or 20% stabilized with egg yolk phospholipids with glycerol to adjust to isotonicity. Major fatty acids contained in Intralipid are linoleic and oleic. Travamulsion contains a full array of essential fatty acids with the major components being similar to those of Intralipid.
Liposyn (10%, 20%)	As for Intralipid.	Safflower oil 10% or 20% stabilized with egg phospholipids. This preparation contains more linoleic acid but much less linolenic acid than Intralipid.

pressure is highest, hydrostatic pressure predominates over oncotic pressure. The result is that in the arteriolar side of the capillaries, water, along with dissolved nutrients and other solutes, moves from the plasma into the interstitial fluid, where it is available to the cells. Pressure on the venous side of the capillaries is lower. This lower venous pressure is not sufficient to fully block the movement of water. Therefore oncotic pressure is the predominant regulator on the venous side of the capillaries and allows the movement of water and solutes, including waste products, back into the plasma compartment.

Diffusion describes the movement of solutes across semipermeable membranes. The direction of movement is toward the less concentrated solution. As with osmosis, the process lowers the difference in concentration between the two solutions. Free diffusion of most ions and solutes takes place between plasma and interstitial fluid, but the cell membrane is not normally permeable to most solutes found in extracellular fluid. Sensitive control of uptake and release of solutes is maintained by *active transport* systems on the cell membrane. For example, the high intracellular concentration of potassium is maintained by the action of Na^+, K^+–ATPase, an active transport system that hydrolyzes a molecule of ATP in order to exchange three sodium ions for two potassium ions. Other active transport systems maintain the high intracellular concentrations of phosphate and magnesium ion.

CLINICAL INDICATIONS FOR FLUID THERAPY

Loss of Extracellular Fluid Volume

Several clinical conditions can cause the loss of both water and solutes from the extracellular fluid compartment. For example, sudden hemorrhage, prolonged vomiting, excessive diarrhea, or

FLUIDS AND ELECTROLYTES

Assessment

A careful visual inspection of each patient is a good starting point in assessing the need for fluids, electrolytes, and nutrition, or in deciding that the patient is overloaded or receiving too much. Observe for edema, especially in dependent areas; check skin turgor, auscultate breath and heart sounds, monitor the vital signs, weight, intake and output. Depending on the patient's known diagnoses, observe for specific electrolyte imbalances. Observe for signs of nutritional deficiency, remembering that weight and intake measures alone are poor indicators. Monitor appropriate laboratory values, including serum electrolytes, BUN, and blood gases.

If the patient is receiving intravenous fluids or nutrition, observe the administration set-up, starting at the level of the patient: check the insertion site, observe for signs of infiltration or infection, check the placement and patency of the tubing, the rate of flow, and the amount of fluid remaining.

Nursing diagnoses

Fluid volume excess related to malnutrition as manifested by edema and low protein levels

Potential complication: hypervolemia

Potential for infection related to long-term total parenteral nutrition

Management

The decision to initiate, terminate, or change the fluid and electrolyte therapy for a specific patient depends on the ongoing and cumulative data base gathered during the assessment phase. In addition, the patient's general condition and response to previous therapy must be taken into consideration. The patient recovering from uncomplicated general surgery may need only 2 to 3 days of maintenance IV therapy, since it is anticipated that the patient will resume general oral intake shortly. Another patient may develop infection, fistulae, or be so generally debilitated that the decision is made to begin total parenteral nutrition in addition to fluid and electrolyte replacement. Keep the patient informed about the goals of therapy. Enlist the help of the patient and family in monitoring the IV, and encourage them to report any unexpected subjective or objective finding. Continue to monitor the parameters identified above. Observe for both the desired and undesired effects of therapy. Label all IV fluids and medications carefully, and monitor their rate of flow.

Evaluation

Therapy with fluids and electrolytes is effective if the desired goals have been achieved without harmful consequences to the patient. For some patients this may mean merely that fluid intake and output were maintained until the patient could again eat and drink. For others, this might mean that nutritional imbalances were corrected, and the patient gained a desired amount of weight. For still other patients, this could mean correction of electrolyte abnormalities that were potentially life threatening.

If the patient is being switched to an oral electrolyte replacement, review with the patient and family how the medication is to be administered, work with the patient to find an acceptable dosage form, review the need to continue the medication as desired, review the side effects, and discuss the situations that should cause the patient to call the physician or nurse (e.g., signs of electrolyte overload). If appropriate, the patient should be taught to measure intake and output or weight at home. The interactions of all the patient's medications should be reviewed. If the patient is to continue hyperalimentation at home, teach the patient and family about the desired goals of therapy, and carefully review the technical tasks associated with the therapy: for example, care of the insertion site, how to change the bottle, and what to do if the line fails to function. Referral to social service and a visiting nurse agency may be helpful. For more specific information, see the patient care guidelines at the end of this chapter.

PEDIATRIC DRUG ALERT: BENZYL ALCOHOL

THE PROBLEM
Benzyl alcohol is a bacteriostatic agent commonly used in solutions of sodium chloride and other drugs. Neonates are especially sensitive to this agent and deaths have occurred when solutions containing benzyl alcohol were used in this age group.

SOLUTIONS
- Avoid administration of bacteriostatic saline (with benzyl alcohol) to newborns
- Do not dilute drug with bacteriostatic saline if the drug is to be used in newborns
- Do not flush IV lines in newborns with bacteriostatic saline

plasma loss through large areas of burned skin may cause the loss of both fluid and salts, but the fluid remaining in the extracellular compartment may stay essentially normal in composition, at least for a time. If the fluid loss is excessive and uncompensated, the patient may enter hypovolemic shock in which the blood volume becomes so depleted that organ perfusion is compromised. The symptoms of this condition include lowered blood pressure, increased heart rate, rapid respiration, restlessness, pale and clammy skin, and decreased urine output. Without adequate perfusion, the kidneys may fail completely. Hypovolemic shock is potentially life-threatening and requires rapid replacement of fluid and electrolytes to restore the proper distribution of volume throughout the body.

In certain conditions extracellular fluid volume may be decreased primarily by water loss. For example, patients who fail to take in adequate water may suffer dehydration. This condition is reasonably common in elderly persons who may have inefficient thirst centers in the brain. Unconscious patients lose between 1000 and 1700 ml of water in insensible perspiration, the breath, and urine each day; this water must be replaced daily in order to avoid dehydration. In certain circumstances violent, watery diarrhea and high-volume renal failure may cause loss of water in excess of salt loss. All of these circumstances may require replacement of lost volume and special attention to restore the proper proportion of solutes in the extracellular fluid.

Fluid deficiency requiring therapy is associated with weight loss in excess of 5% of normal body weight, dry lips and eyes, decreased blood pressure, and depressed central nervous system activity. Skin turgor is also diminished.

Fluid Excess

In certain conditions the extracellular fluid volume is expanded to a degree that may impair cardiovascular functioning, in part by increasing venous pressure. Fluid excess may arise from diseases such as heart failure or renal impairment. These conditions impair the body's ability to eliminate fluid. Alternatively, fluid excess can arise from the improper administration of intravenous fluids. The main route for elimination of excess fluid is through the kidneys. Treatment is aimed at preventing further overload and, if necessary, assisting the kidney by pharmacological means. For example, digitalis given to strengthen the contraction of the heart in a case of heart failure will improve perfusion of the kidneys and assist in mobilizing and eliminating excess fluid. Diuretics will also enhance the production of urine.

Signs of fluid excess include swelling and other indications of excess fluid in subcutaneous tissues (edema), bounding pulse, distension of the jugular vein, difficult or noisy breathing, and warm moist skin.

Electrolyte Imbalances

The proper concentrations of ions and solutes in the extracellular compartment can be disrupted by diseases or medical interventions. The most commonly encountered imbalances are described in the following discussion and in Table 17.1.

Sodium ion. As noted earlier, sodium is the major ion determining the osmolarity of the plasma and interstitial fluid. *Hypernatremia* (excessive sodium ion concentration in the plasma) can arise when a patient has experienced loss of water with retention of salt. Alternatively, hypernatremia may arise when excessive sodium has been administered with fluids or medications. In hypernatremia water moves from the cells into the extracellular fluid in an attempt to reduce the sodium ion concentration and restore equal osmolarity between the fluid compartments. *Hyponatremia* (plasma sodium concentrations less than 130 mEq/L) arises most commonly in patients who are losing water and electrolytes but are receiving water without adequate electrolyte replacement. In an extreme case this condition is called water intoxication. The low sodium ion concentration of the extracellular fluid causes water to move into the cells in an attempt to restore equal osmolarity between the two compartments.

Table 17.5   Intravenous Infusion: Problems, Signs and Symptoms, and Suggested Nursing Actions

Problem	Signs and symptoms	Nursing actions
Pain during infusion	Patient discomfort	Some drugs are irritating via the intravenous route; slow the rate of infusion Warm IV fluids to room temperature before hanging Rule out phlebitis (below)
Occluded infusion	Decreased rate of infusion or no infusion Backup of blood into tubing Possible discomfort	Check to see that clamp is open or electronic device is turned on Inspect tubing for kinks Remove dressing over insertion site (using aseptic technique); check for kinks, remove old dressing, and retape insertion site If fluid level in bag or bottle is low, raise the level of the bag or bottle, or replace it with a full bag or bottle With some infusion devices (e.g., Port-a-Cath) or with multi-lumen central catheters, thrombolytics such as urokinase may be used to dissolve clots occluding IV flow; follow agency policies If all else fails, restart IV
Extravasation (leaking of fluid/drug into tissue surrounding vein; due to tear in vein)	Decreased rate of infusion or no infusion Patient discomfort Puffiness, edema of extremity or insertion site Coolness distal to insertion site No blood return when bag or bottle is lowered below the level of the insertion site	Discontinue IV and restart line at another site Apply warm soaks (follow agency procedure) If drug is known to be caustic (e.g., mechlorethamine), there may be specific measures to carry out, including infiltration of the area with steroids or drug antidote; consult physician or agency policies
Phlebitis (irritation/inflammation of the vein)	Patient discomfort Red streak coursing the arm Site is warm to touch Possible edema	First, slow the rate of infusion, while doing further assessment If phlebitis confirmed, discontinue IV and restart line at another site Apply warm soaks (follow agency procedure)
Septicemia	Fever, chills, symptoms of shock, malaise, hypotension IV insertion site may appear normal Headache, nausea, vomiting	Notify physician Rule out other causes: respiratory tract infection, urinary tract infection, wound infection Discontinue IV, culture catheter tip and fluid (or as agency procedure directs), restart IV line at another site
Fluid overload	"Noisy," rapid respiration, rales Distended neck veins Increased pulse rate, increased blood pressure Patient appears in distress Puffiness, edema of dependent areas Weight gain	Slow infusion to "keep open" rate Notify physician
Embolism	Shortness of breath Chest and shoulder pain Cyanosis Hypotension, weak pulse Loss of consciousness	Place patient on left side, in Trendelenburg position Notify physician Remain with patient, taking vital signs

---

PATIENT PROBLEM: DIARRHEA IN INFANTS

THE PROBLEM

In most cases, diarrhea is mild and self-limiting but infants and young children may be thrown into dangerous states of dehydration and electrolyte imbalance if the diarrhea is severe or prolonged. Hypotension and coma can arise when fluid losses equal 5% of body weight; losses of 10% can cause shock, and death ensues at higher losses.

ASSOCIATED OR CONTRIBUTING FACTORS

In underdeveloped nations, diarrhea is a significant cause of mortality in infants and children, with death resulting from dehydration and electrolyte imbalance. Poor sanitation may expose children and adults to infectious agents that cause diarrhea. Even if the diarrhea is caused by bacterial contamination of food or water, treatment is often successful if salt and water balance are maintained. Intravenous replacement of fluids is expensive, unavailable to many people, and unnecessary in the majority of cases. Aggressive oral replacement with properly balanced solutions is first-line treatment.

SOLUTIONS

- Oral rehydration therapy (ORT) should begin early in the course of the disease
- In the United States, preparations are available under the trade names Lytren, Pedialyte, Rehydralyte, and Resol
- In Canada, Lytren and Pedialyte are available
- In other countries, the World Health Organization (WHO) Diarrheal Disease Control Program supplies ORS-bicarbonate or ORS-citrate in premeasured packets that are mixed with one liter of potable water before use

---

Potassium ion. *Hyperkalemia* (excessive potassium ion concentration in the plasma) causes less osmotic disturbance than does a sodium ion imbalance, but potassium ion imbalances can be life-threatening because cardiac function may be impaired. Potassium-induced cardiac dysfunction appears in the electrocardiogram as depressed ST segments, widened QRS complexes, and peaked T waves. Hyperkalemia may result from massive tissue injury when large numbers of cells die, releasing their high intracellular concentrations of potassium into the extracellular fluid. Renal failure may also cause retention of potassium, as may the potassium-sparing diuretics discussed in Chapter 16. *Hypokalemia* (low potassium ion concentration in the plasma) can result from the use of diuretics such as furosemide, ethacrynic acid, or the thiazides. Poor nutrition or poor gastrointestinal absorption can also result in hypokalemia. Vomiting depletes the body of potassium, along with fluid and other salts. Replacement of potassium is necessary to restore normal function, but the replacement should be spread out over several days to avoid cardiac stress.

Hydrogen ion and bicarbonate ion. The balance of these two ions regulates the pH of the plasma and interstitial fluid. An increase of hydrogen ion over bicarbonate ion lowers the pH of extracellular fluid, causing acidosis. An increase of bicarbonate ion over hydrogen ion causes a rise in pH of the extracellular fluid, or alkalosis.

Acid-base imbalances arise from respiratory or metabolic causes. *Respiratory acidosis* arises when pulmonary ventilation is impaired. Without adequate ventilation, the carbon dioxide concentration in the blood rises. In the blood, carbon dioxide becomes carbonic acid, which lowers blood pH. Pneumonia, pulmonary obstructive disease, and depressed respiration can all produce respiratory acidosis. Therapy is aimed at the underlying disease. *Metabolic acidosis* may arise when excess acid is produced, as in diabetic acidosis, lactic acidosis, starvation, or certain types of poisonings.

Respiratory alkalosis can be induced by hyperventilation, through which excessive amounts of carbon dioxide are lost. *Metabolic alkalosis* arises when excess hydrogen ion is lost, as in prolonged vomiting or nasogastric suctioning. Respiratory alkalosis seldom requires intravenous therapy, but metabolic alkalosis may often be treated with isotonic saline. During metabolic alkalosis, bicarbonate excretion becomes limited by the progressive depletion of sodium. Administering isotonic saline allows the kidney to sacrifice the sodium required to accompany excreted bicarbonate. With this assistance the kidney usually reestablishes acid-base balance.

DIETARY CONSIDERATION: VITAMINS

Vitamins are among the essential nutrients. If the diet is varied and plentiful, vitamin deficiencies are rare. Digestive disorders and certain drugs can interfere with vitamin absorption. Examples of good sources of major vitamins are listed below:

Vitamin	Good dietary sources
A (retinol)	Liver, kidney, fish liver oils, cream, butter, whole milk, whole milk cheese, fortified margarine, skim milk, skim milk products, dark green and deep yellow fruits and vegetables. (contain a precursor of vitamin A)
D	Exposure to sunlight, fortified milk, liver, egg yolk, butter, cream, fish liver oils.
E	Widely distributed in foods, especially wheat germ and vegetables oils
K	Fruits and leafy vegetables cereals, dairy products meat, tomatoes
C (ascorbic acid)	Citrus fruits other fruits and vegetables
B-COMPLEX VITAMINS	
Thiamine	Organ meats, legumes, nuts whole or enriched grain products wheat germ, brewer's yeast
Riboflavin	Milk and milk products organ meats, eggs leafy green vegetables whole or enriched grain products
Niacin	Meats, legumes, nuts, peanut butter whole grain and enriched grain products tryptophan, a niacin precursor, is also found in protein foods of animal origin
Pantothenic acid	Liver, kidney, salmon, egg legumes and peanuts whole grains milk, fruits, vegetables, molasses, yeast
Biotin	Organ meats, egg yolk legumes, nuts, mushrooms
Folic acid	Leafy green vegetables, orange juice liver, peanuts, legumes whole grains, wheat germ
Vitamin B_{12}	Animal protein products only (meat, milk, fish and shellfish, eggs, cheeses)
Pyridoxine	Meat, fish, egg yolks legumes and nuts, potatoes whole grains, wheat germ, yeast prunes and raisins, bananas

FLUID AND ELECTROLYTE SOLUTIONS

Hydrating Solutions

Conditions such as hemorrhage or shock, in which plasma volume is acutely reduced, require replacement of fluid as initial therapy. Replacement of lost fluid volume allows kidney function to be maintained, preventing further development of dangerous electrolyte imbalances. Perfusion of other vital organs is also maintained by this strategy.

Sodium chloride in water. Isotonic saline (Table 17.2, p. 275) is used to replace extracellular fluid volume and to treat sodium depletion and metabolic alkalosis. Dangers associated with the use of isotonic saline include circulatory overload and hypernatremia. Metabolic acidosis may arise when excess chloride ion promotes bicarbonate ion loss in the kidney. Hypokalemia may arise as excess sodium ion forces potassium ion excretion by the kidney. Hypertonic saline solutions should be used in small volumes and administered carefully for the correction of severe hyponatremia.

Ringer's solution and lactated Ringer's solution. These solutions are used to replace fluid, sodium, and other electrolytes (Table 17.2). Often called balanced solutions or maintenance solutions, these preparations are appropriate to replace volume if renal function is not seriously compromised. The potassium found in these solutions cannot be eliminated by the body and may accumulate to dangerous levels unless the kidney is functioning. For this reason renal function must be established before these fluids are administered.

Ringer's solution is appropriate replacement therapy for patients who have lost fluid and electrolytes through the alimentary tract, for burn patients, for postoperative patients, as well as others with dehydration or sodium depletion. Lactated Ringer's solution is most appropriate for patients who, along with other electrolyte imbalances, are also acidotic. The lactate in this solution, being converted to bicarbonate by the liver, ultimately provides stronger basic cations in the blood than do the simple inorganic salt solutions.

Dextrose in water. Dextrose, or glucose, in an isotonic solution (5%) is appropriate for most situations in which rehydration is needed. In addition to the fluid, the solution supplies about 170 calories or 560 kilojoules per liter. Electrolytes are not supplied in this solution. Hypertonic glucose solutions are given slowly to avoid tissue damage. These hypertonic solutions may be used to shift fluid from the interstitial space into the plasma. Isotonic dextrose solutions may be infused through peripheral veins, but hypertonic dextrose solutions should be infused through a central vein to avoid excessive irritation.

Dextrose solutions may have other components added for infusion, but not all additives are compatible. For example, dextrose solutions are never used in the same intravenous line with whole blood because the sugar causes hemolysis (rupture of red blood cells). The pharmacist is a ready source of information about compatibilities of intravenous fluids.

Solutions to Correct Specific Electrolyte Imbalances

Dextrose in saline may be used in hydrating patients and replacing sodium loses. Five percent dextrose in 0.9% saline has about the same properties as normal saline (discussed above). Five percent dextrose in 0.45% saline may be used to shift fluid from plasma into the interstitial space, an action that may cause difficulty for cardiac patients with cardiac, renal, or liver disease who already suffer from edema and poor venous return.

Potassium chloride is often added to intravenous fluids in order to replace potassium lost from the gastrointestinal tract or through the kidney. Replacement must be undertaken carefully to avoid causing hyperkalemia and its dangerous side effects. Dosage is calculated from a knowledge of approximate loss for the individual patient.

Sodium bicarbonate solutions are used occasionally to reverse metabolic acidosis. Isotonic solutions are prepared from hypertonic commercially available stocks that must not be used full strength.

Magnesium sulfate is used to correct severe magnesium deficiencies. The 10% solution is nearly isotonic and may be used intravenously, but the 50% solution is strongly hypertonic and is used intramuscularly.

Plasma Expanders

In hemorrhage or hypovolemic shock, rapid filling of the plasma compartment may be a life-saving measure. This volume replacement may be accomplished in several ways (Table 17.3, p. 276), depending upon the needs of the patient.

Whole blood is appropriate for use in patients who have lost more than 20% of their blood volume. Cross-matching to test for blood group compatibility is required, although O-negative blood can be used as a universal donor until cross-matched blood is available. Whole blood obviously replaces fluid, electrolytes, and oxygen-carrying capacity lost through hemorrhage.

Plasma is a natural cell-free fluid that performs all the functions of whole blood except for oxygen transport. Cross-matching is not required.

Human albumin and plasma protein fraction expand plasma volume by increasing the plasma protein concentration. The resulting increase in plasma oncotic pressure causes water to move from the interstitial space into plasma compartment. The albumin preparation contains appreciable amounts of sodium that may cause problems for certain patients with cardiovascular disease.

Dextran and hetastarch are complex carbohydrate molecules too large to pass out of the capillaries or vascular walls. Therefore these compounds are restricted to the vascular space, generating osmotic forces that cause water to enter the blood vessels, thereby expanding plasma volume.

Text continued on p. 290.

PATIENT CARE IMPLICATIONS

General guidelines for care of patients receiving intravenous fluids and other replacement solutions

- Maintain vigilance whenever working with intravenous fluids (IV fluids) or IV drugs, as the administration of any substance directly into the vascular system has the potential for serious and rapid consequences.

- Inspect the patient receiving IV fluids at least hourly. Assess for correct infusion rate, inspect the bag or bottle, tubing, monitoring devices, and area surrounding insertion site. Assess patient for signs of fluid overload, and observe for any of the common problem associated with IV fluid therapy. See Table 17.5 for a summary of common IV problems and suggested nursing actions.

- Monitor skin turgor, intake and output, weight; inspect dependent areas for edema; monitor vital signs, auscultate heart and lung sounds; and monitor central venous pressure and pulmonary capillary wedge pressure if available.

- Be familiar with agency or institutional policies and procedures regarding IV administration. These policies may specify who may start IVs, who may add electrolyte solutions or drugs to infusions, what the procedures are for routinely changing the tubing or insertion site, redressing central line insertion sites, and so on.

- Use measures to prevent complications of IV administration, in addition to assessing for their development and subsequent treatment. For example, cleanse insertion sites thoroughly prior to initiating IV therapy, and wear sterile gloves when starting IVs. Cleanse injection ports well with alcohol or povidone-iodine solution before puncturing them. Use Luer-Lok connections to prevent accidental pulling apart of IV tubing. Choose insertion sites where catheters are less likely to be dislodged by patient movement, and tape catheters securely. Wear gloves when discontinuing IV catheterization.

- Become familiar with the IV equipment used in the agency. Read the package inserts, and attend inservice programs about new equipment.

- Check infusion rates carefully. Nurses who have difficulty calculating IV drip rates should check calculations with another nurse. If a drip rate seems excessively fast or slow, discuss this with another nurse. Some agencies require that two nurses check the infusion rate for infants and small children. See Chapter 7 for information about calculating IV rates of infusion.

- Inspect IV solutions carefully before using. Do not use solutions that are discolored, are leaking, or that contain particulate matter.

- Choose a needle or catheter, administration set, and tubing length appropriate for the patient and the drug. For example, the larger the diameter of the needle or catheter, the faster the fluid will infuse, but the larger the diameter, the more difficult it may be to insert the needle or catheter into the chosen vein. The higher the fluid reservoir (bag or bottle) above the patient, the faster the rate of infusion; generally, the reservoir should be about 36 inches above the insertion site. The viscosity of the fluid will influence the rate of flow; for example, blood infuses more slowly than normal saline or 5% dextrose solutions. The greater the length of tubing from the fluid reservoir to the patient, the slower the rate of flow. Choose a tubing length long enough to allow for safe movement by the patient but short enough that the tubing will not get tangled in the siderails or significantly restrict flow. Finally, choose an administration set appropriate to the ordered rate of flow. For example, if the rate of flow is 150 ml/hr, the drip rate on a "minidrip" set that delivers 60 gtt/ml would be 150 gtt/min, almost too fast to count. That same rate of administration with a set that delivers 10 gtt/ml would be 25, an easy rate to count. Use a minidrip set for infants or small children, when a patient is on a "keep open" or very slow rate, or when drug dose is measured according to patient response, as when an intravenous drug such as dopamine is adjusted based on the patient's blood pressure.

- Use volume control devices to limit the volume a patient could receive in a specified time period; an example is Buretrol, a volume-control device attached to the IV tubing between the fluid reservoir and the patient. The nurse fills the volume control device with a specified volume of fluid and adjusts the flow rate. The patient can receive only the volume contained in the device, until it is refilled. As an example, consider an infant requiring IV fluids. Even if a 500 ml reservoir bag were to be hung instead of a 1000 ml bag,

PATIENT CARE IMPLICATIONS—cont'd

the danger of fluid overload would be significant if all 500 ml were to infuse rapidly. The nurse could fill the volume control device with the amount ordered for 1 hour—say, 30 ml, for this patient—and adjust the flow rate. Even if all of the fluid in the device were to infuse rapidly, the danger of fluid overload would be much less than with 500 ml. Volume control devices also permit the addition of medications to the fluid in the chamber.

- IV pumps and controllers are widely available today. These electronic devices are helpful in maintaining a constant rate of flow; and, because alarms are incorporated into them, they can warn the nurse when a problem has occurred. The IV pump delivers the IV fluid with pressure, while the IV controller adjusts the rate of fluids infusing via gravity. Become familiar with the devices used in the agency. Electronic devices do not replace careful patient assessment and nursing care, but can assist in managing IV therapy.

- The use of in-line IV filters for all medications and solutions is not universally accepted. Nevertheless, many agencies require them. Become familiar with the advantages of the filters in use in the agency. For example, some filters remove only particulate matter, and some do not have air-eliminating capability. The 0.22 μm filter can remove particulate matter, fungi, bacteria, and air, but it is too small to filter TPN solutions. Tubing for blood administration is equipped with a filter. Fat emulsions cannot be filtered.

- Label all fluid reservoirs as directed by agency procedure. A common way is to place a length of adhesive tape along the side of the bag or bottle next to the volume markers on the container. The correct fluid level per hour is marked on the tape. For example, if 1000 ml of fluid is started at 8:00 am, there should be 900 ml remaining at 9:00, 800 ml at 10:00, and so on. Thus, any nurse on duty can determine at a glance whether the infusion is running properly. If the infusion is not correctly timed, do not try to "catch up" by doubling or increasing the rate for the next hour or two. Assess the situation and, if necessary, restart the infusion at another site. If the solution was infusing too rapidly, slow the rate and assess the patient for signs of fluid overload (see Table 17.5). If the extra volume infused was minimal and the pa-

tient's condition is satisfactory, resume the prescribed rate; if the volume was excessive, or signs of fluid overload were present, maintain the IV at "keep open" rate, and notify the physician.

- Label all intravenous solutions carefully, especially when additives have been included, such as potassium, vitamins, heparin, insulin, other drugs. Record the administration of all IV solutions carefully, just as all medications are recorded.

- See Chapter 6 for additional information about IV administration.

Oral and intravenous potassium

Drug administration

- Potassium chloride (KCl) is probably the most frequently administered electrolyte added to IV fluids. (Most sodium chloride administered is supplied by manufacturers in commonly used concentrations; the KCl is more often added by the nurse or pharmacy).

- Ascertain that the patient has adequate kidney function before administering IV potassium.

- Always dilute KCl before administering it intravenously. Carefully check the dose of potassium chloride before adding it. Carefully label containers to which potassium has been added.

- Monitor the patients electrocardiogram and serum potassium level. See Table 17.1 for signs of common electrolyte imbalances. The classic electrocardiographic changes seen with potassium imbalances are as follows: *hypokalemia*, with ST-segment depression, flattened T waves, presence of U waves, and ventricular dysrhythmias; *hyperkalemia*, with tall, thin T waves, prolonged PR interval, ST depression, widened QRS, and loss of P wave.

- Carefully check the rate of administration of IV potassium. The usual rate is 10 to 15 mEq/hr of a solution containing 40 mEq/L unless the patient is severely potassium depleted.

- To treat hyperkalemia, discontinue potassium replacements (IV or oral), and limit potassium-rich foods (see Dietary Consideration: Potassium on p. 259). Emergency treatment includes IV sodium bicarbonate, calcium gluconate (if not contraindicated by existing cardiac conditions), and IV glucose and insulin (which helps shift potassium into

Continued.

PATIENT CARE IMPLICATIONS—cont'd

the cell). Dialysis may also be used.

- Subacute hyperkalemia is treated with cation exchange resins such as Kayexalate, which exchanges sodium for potassium in the intestine. The effect is not evident for several hours to 1 day after administration. The resin is given orally, via nasogastric tube, or as a retention enema. Adverse effects include hypokalemia, hypocalcemia, anorexia, nausea, vomiting, and constipation. Monitor electrolytes. When the resin is given orally or via nasogastric tube, constipation is common, so a mild laxative may be administered concomitantly. For oral administration, dilute the drug in water, syrup, fruit juice, or soft drink.
- Monitor potassium levels carefully in patients with cardiac conditions, as hypokalemia potentiates the effects of cardiac glycosides.
- Do not administer potassium to patients receiving potassium-sparing diuretics (see Chapter 16).

Patient and family education

- Review with patients the importance of taking potassium preparations as ordered. Some patients with be able to maintain potassium levels through dietary intake of potassium-rich foods; see Dietary Consideration: Potassium on p. 259.
- Work with patients to find an acceptable form of potassium. Oral preparations are often unpalatable or difficult to swallow. Enteric-coated tablets have been implicated in small bowel ulceration and should not be used. Effervescent preparations are often unpalatable, and patients soon stop taking them. Oral solutions work well, but they often have a bitter, salty taste.
- Dilute oral solutions in juice or milk if acceptable to the patient. Avoid tomato juice if the patient is on a low sodium diet.
- Dissolve the soluble powders, granules, or tablets in at least 4 ounces of juice or water; avoid tomato juice if the patient is on a low sodium diet.
- Extended-release tablets should be swallowed whole without being chewed or crushed. (A few may be crushed or broken, but most should not be; check with the pharmacist.)
- Extended-release capsules also should be swallowed whole without being chewed or crushed. (A few may be opened and the contents mixed with food, but not all; check with the pharmacist.)
- Take potassium with meals to reduce gastric irritation.

Magnesium sulfate

Drug administration/patient and family education

- Magnesium sulfate is useful orally as a cathartic (see Chapter 13), and parenterally to treat or prevent hypomagnesemia and as an anticonvulsant, especially in pregnancy-induced hypertension (PIH).
- See Table 17.1 for signs of magnesium imbalances. If magnesium imbalance is suspected, monitor the serum magnesium level.
- Intramuscular administration of magnesium is painful. Use large muscle masses and rotate sites. Inject the drug slowly.
- The goal in treating pregnancy-induced hypertension is to obtain a serum level that will inhibit seizures but will not cause respiratory or cardiac paralysis. Several dosage regimens are followed for this purpose; most are initiated with a loading dose, followed by a maintenance dose. Assess the deep tendon reflexes, respiratory rate, and urinary output. If reflexes become diminished or absent, if the respiratory rate decreases, or if the urinary output falls below 30 to 100 ml/hr, the dose of magnesium sulfate may need to be reduced. Monitor vital signs, intake and output, and serum magnesium levels. Monitor fetal heart sounds. In severe cases, monitor maternal electrocardiogram and attach a fetal monitor to assess infant status. Monitor newborns of mothers who received magnesium sulfate for several hours after delivery for signs of hypermagnesemia (see Table 17.1).
- Administer the 10% solution at a rate of 1.5 ml/min.
- Have available equipment for resuscitation in settings where parenteral magnesium sulfate is administered. Have available calcium gluconate and calcium gluceptate as specific antidotes for magnesium overdose.

Sodium bicarbonate

Drug administration/patient and family education

- Sodium bicarbonate is given orally as an antacid (see Chapter 13), and to alkalinize the urine.

PATIENT CARE IMPLICATIONS—cont'd

- During resuscitation efforts, sodium bicarbonate is administered via direct IV push to help correct metabolic acidosis. It is usually included in the emergency drug box or on the resuscitation cart, packaged in labeled, filled syringes.
- For IV administration the drug is diluted and administered at a rate of 2 to 5 mEq/kg over 4 to 8 hours.
- Signs of overdose are metabolic alkalosis and hypernatremia (see Table 17.1). Monitor serum electrolytes and arterial blood gases.

Calcium

Drug administration/patient and family education

- Calcium compounds are antacids (see Chapter 13).
- Read orders carefully. Intravenous calcium compounds include calcium gluconate, calcium chloride, and calcium gluceptate. When possible, the drug should be warmed to body temperature before being administered. The IV route is preferred in infants, but avoid using a scalp vein, as extravasation may cause tissue necrosis. Monitor ECG during IV administration. Keep patient recumbent for 30 minutes following IV administration; monitor blood pressure and serum calcium levels.
- If IV administration is not possible, calcium gluceptate, calcium gluconate, or a combination of calcium glyderophosphate and calcium lactate may be administered IM. (Do not give calcium *chloride* IM.) Use large muscle masses and rotate injection sites. If greater than 5 ml is to be administered IM to an adult, divide the dose in half and administer via two injections. With children, determine whether the dose should be divided.
- Severe hypocalcemia may manifest as tetany. Chvostek's sign and Trousseau's sign may be positive (see a text on physical assessment). Pad the siderails. Have resuscitation equipment readily available.
- Review with patients taking oral calcium supplements foods that are rich in calcium. See Dietary Consideration: Calcium on p. 806.
- Hypercalcemia is discussed in Chapter 52.

Blood, plasma, albumin, and plasma protein fraction

Drug administration

- Review the general guidelines for care of patients receiving intravenous fluids and other replacement solutions.
- Whole blood is administered via a blood infusion tubing set, which usually contains an in-line filter. The infusion is established, usually with normal saline in the primary line (solutions with dextrose may hemolyze the blood, and solutions containing calcium, as in lactated Ringer's solution, may clot the blood). The blood is then piggy-backed to the priming solution, via the second port in the set. This method helps prevent the blood from clotting toward the end of the infusion; it also allows for maintenance of a patent IV access line, even if infusion of the blood must be stopped, as might happen with an allergic reaction.
- Monitor hematocrit, hemoglobin, intake and output, vital signs.
- Before beginning the transfusion carefully check the patient's identification bracelet and the label on the container of blood. Blood type incompatibility is potentially fatal—death can occur after infusion of as little as 50 to 100 ml. Most institutions provide specific, detailed procedures to ensure that blood is carefully checked beforehand—it is important to follow these procedures. Signs and symptoms of a transfusion reaction include flushing, nausea, hypotension, increased pulse rate, difficulty breathing and tightness in the chest, chills, fever, headache, substernal chest pain, vomiting, and sense of impending doom. In addition, hematological changes may occur, including disseminated intravascular coagulation (DIC), thrombocytopenia, and spontaneous bleeding. If the patient is anesthetized or unconscious, it may be difficult to recognize this reaction.
- After initiating the transfusion, remain with the patient for 10 to 15 minutes, monitoring and recording the vital signs. Thoroughly investigate any unanticipated occurrence; stop the infusion (but maintain a patent IV access line by restarting the priming solution), and notify the physician. Hypersensitivity reac-

Continued.

PATIENT CARE IMPLICATIONS — cont'd

tions include rashes, itching, and the symptoms noted above. Minor reactions can frequently be treated with antihistamines or corticosteroids, but occasionally emergency life support measures, including epinephrine, are needed. Know beforehand where emergency drugs and equipment are kept.

- Febrile reactions usually begin with the first 15 minutes of infusion, but may not begin until 1 to 2 hours later. They are characterized by fever (39.4 to 40° C [103 to 104° F]), chills, headache, and malaise. Again, stop the infusion, notify the physician, and investigate the cause.
- Circulatory overload is more common when whole blood is administered, the patient is elderly or an infant, or the patient has cardiac disease. Monitor vital signs and cardiac and lung sounds, and observe for respiratory difficulty and cough.
- Do not mix any medications with blood. If it is necessary to administer an IV medication via the same IV access line, stop the blood infusion, flush the line with saline, inject the medication, flush the line again with saline, and resume the blood infusion.
- Blood cells are large, so a large-diameter needle or catheter should be used.
- When there is concern about fluid overload and/or large volumes must be transfused, whole blood components may be prescribed, such as packed red cells, platelets, cryoprecipitated factor VIII (for hemophiliacs), and fibrinogen. These products are smaller in volume than whole blood, but are generally administered the same way.
- Complete administration of whole blood within 2 to 4 hours; after this time, the blood may clot. (In extreme emergencies, pressure applied to the bag will afford delivery within 10 minutes or less.)
- Blood products deteriorate rapidly if not stored properly and used promptly. Do not thaw frozen products unless they are to be used. Do not procure blood from the blood bank until the patient is ready for the infusion. Do not leave blood products anywhere in the patient care unit. Check and observe expiration dates of all blood products.
- Plasma, albumin, and plasma protein fraction are derived from blood, and the same general guidelines apply.

Dextran

Drug administration

- Monitor weight, blood pressure and pulse, intake and output. Assess for signs of fluid overload (see p. 280). Monitor hematocrit and hemoglobin, serum protein, and serum protein electrophoresis. Assess for development of bleeding.
- Notify physician if urine output falls below 30 to 50 ml/hr.
- Monitor for signs of allergic reaction, as described above.
- If blood must also be administered, flush tubing thoroughly between blood and dextran infusions, as dextran causes blood to coagulate in tubing.
- Use only clear solutions. If crystallization has occurred, heat bottle in warm water bath until crystals dissolve before administering. If blood is drawn for laboratory tests, note on the requisition that dextran is being administered, as dextran may cause false high serum glucose levels and alterations in other blood tests.

Hetastarch

Drug administration

- Monitor for allergic reactions, as described above. Monitor vital signs. Monitor hematocrit, hemoglobin, plasma proteins, and platelets.
- Assess for signs of bleeding.

Total parenteral nutrition (TPN)

Drug administration/patient and family education

- Review the general guidelines for care of patients receiving intravenous fluids.
- Total parenteral nutrition (TPN), or hyperalimentation, must be administered via a central infusion line for solutions more concentrated than 10% dextrose. The central line is placed by the physician under aseptic technique, as described in Chapter 6.
- Follow aseptic technique when manipulating the TPN infusion. These fluids provide favorable conditions for harmful bacteria—it is essential to prevent infection. Follow agency procedures for maintenance of TPN. They will usually specify how often to dress the insertion site, method for dressing, what

PATIENT CARE IMPLICATIONS — cont'd

agent to use to clean injection sites (e.g., povidone-iodine or alcohol), how often to change tubing, and so on.

- Monitor vital signs, and assess for fluid overload (see p. 280). Monitor temperature every 4 hours in the hospital. Instruct the patient at home to notify the physician if fever develops.
- Hypertonic dextrose, amino acids, and fat emulsions are the mainstay of TPN therapy. The rate of flow, additives (vitamins, minerals, electrolytes) and their concentrations must be ordered specifically by the physician. Most agencies have devised a protocol for monitoring the patient, including the frequency of blood work such as serum electrolytes, albumin, BUN, liver function studies, and blood glucose; the frequency of vitamin and mineral infusions; procedures for culturing the catheter tip and fluid if infection develops; and frequency of weighing patient.
- Do not add medications to the solution or administer medications via the TPN line unless specifically permitted by agency protocol. Usually, if other IV medications are needed, a separate peripheral IV line must be started and maintained.
- Maintain the infusion at a steady rate; usually, an electronic monitoring device will be used. Erratic infusion rates may cause fluctuations in blood glucose levels which will induce hyper- and hypoglycemia. If the infusion stops, or must be discontinued abruptly, standing orders are (at most facilities) to begin a peripheral infusion of dextrose 10% to prevent hypoglycemia. When the need for TPN therapy has resolved, the rate of infusion is gradually slowed to help prevent hypoglycemia.
- Assess the patient for appearance of dry, flaky skin, hair loss, and rashes. These signs may indicate essential fatty acid deficiency or zinc deficiency.
- Prepare TPN solutions in a laminar flow hood, where risk of contamination is low.
- Some patients are suitable candidates for TPN administration at home. Work carefully with patient and family to assess learning needs. Provide reassurance. Ascertain that they are able to manipulate the equipment. Refer the patient to social services agency and to a community-based nursing care service.

Amino acid infusions

Drug administration

- Review the general guidelines for TPN.
- Assess for common side effects: nausea, vomiting, flushing, and a sensation of warmth. Less common are chills, headache, abdominal pain, dizziness, rashes, hyperglycemia, and glycosuria.
- Monitor intake and output, serum electrolytes, magnesium, blood ammonia, phosphate, serum protein, cholesterol, BUN, liver function studies, and blood glucose. Observe for signs of essential fatty acid deficiency (hair loss, dry flaky skin).
- Vitamins, electrolytes, trace elements, heparin, and insulin can be administered via the same IV line, but other medications should not be. Do no premix these drugs with amino acid infusions; administer via a Y-connector.
- Use an IV filter. Infuse at a rate not exceeding 4 mg nitrogen/kg/hr.
- Infuse at a steady rate; use an electronic infusion monitor if available.

Fat emulsions

Drug administraton/patient and family education

- See the general guidelines for intravenous therapy.
- Administer fat emulsions via central or peripheral IV line.
- Read the manufacturer's information supplied with the bottle of fat emulsion.
- Fat emulsion should comprise no more than 60% of the total daily caloric intake.
- Inspect before using. If the emulsion has "cracked" (the oil separated from the other products), it should not be used. Do not shake the emulsion.
- Assess for side effects: thrombophlebitis, vomiting, chest pain, back pain, and allergic reactions.
- Begin the infusion slowly (e.g., 1 ml/min) and observe the patient. If no untoward effect has occurred after 15 to 30 minutes, increase the rate of infusion to the desired rate.
- Monitor serum triglycerides. Fat emulsions can cause hyperlipidemia, which should clear between infusions; if it does not, withhold the next dose and notify the physician.
- Do not filter a fat emulsion. If it is piggybacked into a line incorporating containing

Continued.

PATIENT CARE IMPLICATIONS — cont'd

filter, the fat emulsion must be inserted below the level of the filter (closer to the patient).

Vitamins

Water-soluble vitamins may be administered intravenously, while fat-soluble vitamins are administered via IM injection. Vitamins should be administered only parenterally when oral intake and digestion are compromised. Patients with vitamin deficiencies who are able to eat and digest food should be counseled to increase their dietary intake of vitamin-rich foods. See Dietary Consideration: Vitamins on p. 282.

Intravenous Hyperalimentation

Patients who are unable to take oral foods and fluids require maintenance with intravenous nutrients. Dextrose solutions supply some calories, but since only about 3 L of fluid can be administered daily without overloading the circulatory system, only about 500 calories can be supplied each day from isotonic dextrose solutions. For longer-term therapy, more calories from different sources are required. Total parenteral nutrition is now possible using synthetic amino acids, dextrose, and fat emulsions (Table 17.4, p. 277).

Hypertonic dextrose is required for total parenteral nutrition. Solutions for administration are prepared from 50% or 60% dextrose stock solutions, but as they are administered the concentration of dextrose is only 25% to 30%. This hypertonic solution must be administered via a large central vein, where blood flow is sufficient to dilute the strong sugar solution and prevent tissue damage. A 10% dextrose solution is hypertonic but can be given peripherally without damage to veins.

Amino acids are used in total parenteral nutrition to prevent negative nitrogen balance and the breakdown of protein in the body. Pure amino acid solutions, rather than protein hydrolysates, are preferred. At 3.5% concentrations the amino acid solutions offer about 140 calories per liter, as well as a variety of electrolytes. Extra potassium is often required by patients receiving amino acid solutions, since that element is depleted by amino acid metabolism.

Fat emulsions may be administered intravenously during total parenteral nutrition to prevent essential fatty acid deficiency. Since fats have a high caloric content, these preparations may supply a significant proportion (up to 60%) of the daily caloric requirement.

Vitamin and mineral supplements may need to be added to the total parenteral nutrition fluids. A variety of these preparations exist, allowing individual design of the nutrition program.

SUMMARY

Water comprises 60% of the weight of an average person. It is distributed between intracellular fluid (28 L found inside cells), interstitial fluid (10.5 L surrounding cells), and plasma (3.5 L within blood vessels). Sodium chloride is the major solute determining osmolarity of plasma and interstitial fluid. Oncotic pressure is determined by the protein concentration in the fluid compartment. The high concentration of protein in plasma, relative to interstitial fluid, promotes the movement of water from interstitial fluid toward plasma. Oncotic pressure is balanced by hydrostatic pressure, which promotes movement of fluid and solutes from the plasma into the interstitial space. Active transport systems maintain the concentration differences between intracellular fluids and extracellular fluids.

Loss of extracellular fluid volume through trauma or disease requires replacement with fluid. Sodium, potassium, and bicarbonate levels may also be altered and require readjustment. Isotonic saline (0.9%) is used to replace extracellular fluid volume and to treat sodium depletion and metabolic alkalosis. Ringer's solution replaces not only fluid and sodium but other electrolytes such as potassium. Renal function must be established before potassium is administered. Lactated Ringer's solution is similar to Ringer's solution, but it also corrects or prevents acidosis. Five percent dextrose in water is isotonic and supplies about 170 calories per liter, but it supplies no electrolytes. Plasma expanders include whole blood and plasma, which restore fluids and electrolytes. Other plasma expanders utilize protein or high molecular weight carbohydrates to promote movement of water from the interstitial space into plasma.

Long-term support of patients who cannot eat

or drink may include total parenteral nutrition. Hypertonic glucose is infused via a central vein to minimize tissue damage. Solutions of pure amino acids prevent negative nitrogen balance and fat emulsions supply concentrated calories.

STUDY QUESTIONS

1. What are the three main fluid compartments of the body?
2. What are the major buffers of plasma?
3. What is the major difference in composition between plasma and interstitial fluid?
4. What is osmosis?
5. What solute primarily determines the osmotic strength of plasma?
6. What is oncotic pressure?
7. Does the protein content of plasma cause water to move into or out of blood vessels?
8. What is hydrostatic pressure?
9. Does hydrostatic pressure cause water to move into or out of blood vessels?
10. Why are cells able to maintain high intracellular concentrations of potassium, phosphate, and magnesium?
11. What are causes of loss of extracellular fluid volume?
12. What are signs of dehydration or fluid deficit?
13. What can cause fluid excess or overload?
14. What are signs of fluid overload?
15. What is hypernatremia? Hyponatremia?
16. What is hyperkalemia? Hypokalemia?
17. What is respiratory acidosis? How does it differ from metabolic acidosis?
18. What is respiratory alkalosis? How does it differ from metabolic alkalosis?
19. What are the uses of isotonic saline?
20. What are the dangers associated with saline administration?
21. How do isotonic saline, Ringer's solution, and lactated Ringer's solution differ from one another?
22. What is the primary use for isotonic dextrose?
23. Why must dextrose solutions never be mixed with whole blood for administration?
24. What organ system must be functioning *before* potassium replacement is begun?
25. Why are solutions of large molecular weight proteins or carbohydrates able to expand plasma volume?
26. What special precautions for administration are necessary with hypertonic dextrose for parenteral nutrition?
27. What additional supplement may be required by patients receiving amino acid solution for parenteral nutrition?
28. What is the primary advantage of fat emulsions in parenteral nutrition?

SUGGESTED READINGS

Anthony, C.P., and Thibodeau, G.A.: Fluid and electrolyte balance. In Textbook of anatomy and physiology, ed. 12, St. Louis, 1987, C.V. Mosby Co.

Axton, S.Z., and Fugate, T.: A protocol for pediatric I.V. meds, Am. J. Nurs. 87(7):943a, 1987.

Barrus, D.H., and Danek, G.: Should you irrigate an occluded I.V. line? Nursing 87 17(3):63, 1987.

Barta, M.A.: Correcting electrolyte imbalances, RN 50(2):30, 1987.

Birdsall, C.: Do total nutritional admixtures benefit your patients? Am. J. Nurs. 87(1):14, 1987.

Boykoff, S.L., and others: 6 ways to clear the air from an I.V. line, Nursing 88 18(2):46, 1988.

Burns, C., and Crawfod, M.: A method for rapidly calculating intravenous drip rates, Focus Crit. Care 15(4):46, 1988.

Calloway, C.: When the problem involves magnesium, calcium, or phosphate, RN 50(5):30, 1987.

Cohen, M.R.: Improperly mixed I.V. additives, Nursing 87 17(5):16, 1987.

Cosentino, F.: Preparing your patient for home I.V. therapy, Nursing 88 18(11):87, 1988.

Crudi, and Larkin,: Core curriculum for intravenous nursing, Philadelphia, 1984, J.B. Lippincott.

Cyganski, J.M., Donahue, J.M., and Heaton, J.: The case for the heparin flush, Am. J. Nurs. 87(6):796, 1987.

Davis, J.: A handy guide for TPN, Am. J. Nurs. 88(1):103, 1988.

Delaney, C.W., and Lauer, M.L.: Intravenous therapy. A guide to quality care, Philadelphia, 1988, J.B. Lippincott.

Dunn, D.L., and Lenihan, S.F.: The case for the saline flush, Am. J. Nurs. 87(6):798, 1987.

Fogel, R., O'Brien, J., Kay, B., and Balas, A.: Try this simple order for total parenteral nutrition, Nursing 87 17(3):58, 1987.

Gahart, B.L.: Intravenous medications: a handbook for nurses and other allied health personnel, 5th ed., St. Louis, 1988, C.V. Mosby Co.

Gasparis, L., Murray, E.B., and Ursomanno, P.: I.V. solutions: which one's right for your patient? Nursing 89 19(4):62, 1989.

Gever, L.N.: Administering sodium bicarbonate during a code, Nursing 84 14(1):100, 1984.

Glass, S.M., and Glacola, G.P.: Intravenous therapy in premature infants: practical aspects, JOGNN 16(5):310, 1987.

Hazinski, M.F.: Understanding fluid balance in the seriously ill child, Pediatr. Nurs. 14(3):231, 1988.

Herlihy, B.L., and Herlihy, J.T.: Physiologic role and regulation of potassium, Crit. Care Nurse 7(5):10, 1987.

Horne, M.M., and Swearingen, P.L.: Pocket guide to fluids and electrolytes, St. Louis, 1989, C.V. Mosby Co.

Johndrow, P.D., and Worthington, P.: Making your patient and his family feel at home with T.P.N., Nursing 88 18(10):65, 1988.

Josephson, A., Gombert, M.E., and Sierra, M.F.: The relationship between intravenous fluid contamination and the frequency of tubing replacement, CINA J. 3(2):17, 1987.

La Rocca, J.C., and Otto, S.E.: Pocket guide to intravenous therapy, St. Louis, 1989, C.V. Mosby Co.

Lipman, A.G.: Which drugs may induce hyperkalemia? Mod. Med. 49(8):213, 1981.

Little, R.C., and Ginsburg, J.M.: The physiologic basis for clinical edema, Arch. Intern. Med. 144(8):1661, 1984.

Lowrey, S.J., and Ash, S.R.: Diminishing the risks of I.V. potassium chloride, Nursing 88 **18**(6):64, 1988.

Lunger, D.G.: Potassium supplementation: how and why? Focus Crit. Care **15**(5):56, 1988.

MacKinnon, C.: Total parenteral nutrition for patients with respiratory insufficiency, Intensive Care Nurs. **2**(4):166, 1987.

Managing special patient's fluids and electrolytes, Nursing 88 **18**(1):64, 1988.

Mazzara, J.T., Parmley, W.W., and Russell, R.O., Jr.: A close look at Swan-Ganz catheters, Patient Care **22**(3):36, 1988.

McFadden, E.A., and Zaloga, G.P.: Calcium regulation, Crit. Care Q. **6**(3):12, 1983.

McIntyre, E: Precise measurement of fluid administration in hemodynamic monitoring, Crit. Care Nurse **8**(1):51, 1988.

Meeske, K., and Davidson, L.T.: Teacher's reference on right atrial catheters, J. Pediatr. Nurs. **3**(5):351, 1988.

Metheny, N.M.: Fluid and electrolyte balance: nursing considerations, Philadelphia, 1987, J.B. Lippincott.

Millam, D.A.: Managing complications of I.V. therapy, Nursing 88 **18**(3):34, 1988.

Morris, L.L.: Critical care's most versatile tool . . . a multilumen central venous catheter, RN **51**(5):42, 1988.

Nortridge, J.A.: Calculating I.V. medications with confidence, Nursing 87 **17**(9):55, 1987.

Parenteral and enteral nutrition. In AMA drug evaluations, ed. 6, Philadelphia, 1986, American Medical Association.

Pupo, M.: The Hickman/Broviac catheter: a right atrial catheter, CINA J. **2**(1):16, 1986.

Ramos, L.: Care and management of long-term arterial catheters, Crit. Care Nurse **7**(1):66, 1987.

Replenishers and regulators of water and electrolytes. In AMA drug evaluations, ed. 6, Philadelphia, 1986, American Medical Association.

Ross, A.D., and Angaran, D.M.: Colloids vs crystalloids—a continuing controversy, Drug Intell. Clin. Pharm. **18**(3):202, 1984.

Schwartz, M.W.: Potassium imbalances, Am. J. Nurs. **87**(10):1292, 1987.

Sherman, J.E., and Sherman, R.H.: I.V. therapy that clicks, Nursing 89 **19**(5):50, 1989.

Smith, L.: Reactions to transfusion, Am. J. Nurs. **84**(9):1096, 1984.

Sohl, L., and Nze, R.: Working with triple-lumen central venous catheters, Nursing 88 **18**(7):50, 1988.

Taylor, J.P., and Taylor, J.E.: Vascular access devices: uses and aftercare, J. Emerg. Nurs. **13**(3):160, 1987.

Testerman, E.J.: I.V. drug administration guidelines: a simplified format, J. Intravenous Nurs. **11**(3):188, 1988.

Tobin, C.R.: The teflon intravenous catheter: incidence of phlebitis and duration of catheter life in the neonatal patient, JOGNN **17**(1):35, 1989.

Turco, S.J.: Trends and new developments in recent I.V. delivery systems, CINA J. **2**(1):4, 1986.

Zaloga, G.P., and Chermow, B.: Magnesium metabolism in critical illness, Crit. Care Q. **6**(3):22, 1983.

Cardiotonic Drugs: Cardiac Glycosides and Other Drugs for Congestive Heart Failure

18

FUNCTIONS OF THE HEART
Terms Used to Describe Cardiac Function

To understand the action of drugs on the heart, the student must understand the following terms relating to cardiac physiology.

Automaticity is the property of certain cells in the heart to depolarize spontaneously to initiate a beat (contraction of the whole heart). Normally a heartbeat is initiated in the sinoatrial node (SA node), but any of the conductive fibers of the heart are capable of spontaneously depolarizing and initiating beats and in fact do so in certain types of heart disease.

Depolarization is the process by which cells become less negatively charged than extracellular fluid. Depolarization occurs when sodium rushes into the cell as the first event in the generation of the action potential.

Excitability of a cell or fiber in the heart is defined as a measure of the ease with which that cell may be stimulated to depolarize. Certain drugs increase the excitability of cells, that is, they reduce the energy necessary to depolarize the cell, and some drugs can decrease cell excitability.

Action potential is a term describing a burst of electrical activity in a cell. Frequently described as cell "firing," the process is similar to that involved in the conduction of impulses along a nerve fiber. The cell undergoes rapid depolarization followed by a slower repolarization phase, and in the process it stimulates adjacent cells to do likewise. In the heart the generation of an action potential initiates ionic changes inside the cell which cause the myocardial fibers to contract.

Conduction velocity is defined as the rate at which an electrical impulse is passed through the atrioventricular (AV) node. There is a delay in transmission of the impulse to beat from the atrium to the ventricle produced by the AV node. This delay regulates the temporal separation in atrial and ventricular contractions. *Dromotropic* is a term referring to factors affecting conduction velocity. A positive dromotropic response is an increase in conduction velocity, whereas a negative dromotropic response is a decrease in that velocity.

Rate is defined as the number of beats or ventricular contractions per minute. In normal hearts this is the rate of SA node firing. Bradycardia means a slow heart rate. Tachycardia means a fast heart rate. *Chronotropic* refers to changes in heart rate. Positive chronotropic effects are increases in heart rate; negative chronotropic effects are decreases in the heart rate.

Contractility is measured as the strength of the muscular contraction of the heart. *Inotropic* refers to factors affecting the strength of cardiac contraction. A positive inotropic response is an increase in cardiac contractility. A negative inotropic response is a decrease in cardiac contractility.

Anatomy of the Heart

Conductive tissues of the heart. The heart is formed of muscle similar in many respects to skeletal muscle but different, in that many of the fibers are conductive as well as contractile. This property facilitates rapid conduction of action potentials. The action potentials do not pass directly between the atria and ventricles, however, because these two portions of the heart are insulated from each other by a ring of nonconductive tissue. The independence of the atria and ventricles as contractile units is important in regulating the heartbeat.

Within the heart the impulse to beat normally originates at the SA node, a specialized group of automatic cells in the right atrium (Figure 18.1). Another group of specialized fibers, the AV node, transmits this impulse to the ventricles after an important delay.

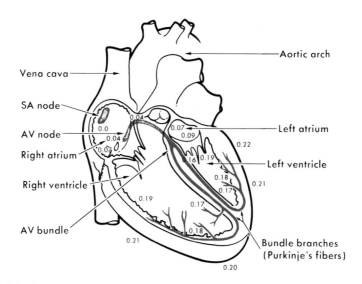

FIGURE 18.1   Transmission of action potentials through the heart. Initiation of a heartbeat occurs at SA node and the action potential is transmitted throughout atria before passing through AV node to ventricles. The numerals designate seconds it takes for impulse to travel from the SA node to the anatomical site designated by the numeral. Note that all parts of the atria have received the impulse within 0.09 second but that transmission to ventricles is delayed during its passage through the AV node so that ventricles do not begin to contract until 0.16 second after SA node firing. This delay allows atria to contract and fill the ventricles before ventricles begin to contract to force blood from the heart.

The heart is innervated by both the sympathetic and parasympathetic branches of the autonomic nervous system (Figure 18.2). The vagus nerve is part of the parasympathetic system; its action is localized in the nodes. Stimulation of the vagus nerve releases acetylcholine, which decreases the rate of depolarization and also makes the cells less excitable. In the SA node these actions decrease the rate of firing and hence reduce heart rate. Stimulation of the vagus nerve also tends to decrease conduction velocity through the AV node. This slowing of conduction velocity increases the temporal separation between contraction of atria and ventricles, and therefore also slows heart rate.

Sympathetic nerve fibers innervate both the atria and the ventricles. Stimulation of the sympathetic nerves releases norepinephrine, which activates the beta-1 adrenergic receptors of the heart. Activation of the beta-1 receptors in the conducting tissue of the heart speeds the repolarization of the cells. An increase in heart rate (positive chronotropic effect) and an increase in conduction velocity (positive dromotropic effect) are the two consequences. Stimulation of the beta-1 adrenergic receptors in the ventricular muscle increases the force of contraction (positive inotropic response).

Regulation of Myocardial Output

Frank-Starling law. The volume of blood that the heart must deliver per second to the arteries varies with stress, exertion, and other factors. How the heart regulates its output to meet these variable demands is described by the *Frank-Starling law* of the heart. This principle of physiology states that the force of muscular contraction is directly related to the stretch of the muscle; the more a muscle is stretched, within mechanical limits, the stronger is its subsequent contraction. With respect to the heart, this principle means that when the ventricles are filled with larger than normal volumes of blood, they contract with greater than normal force to deliver their entire contents to the arteries. Normally blood does not accumulate in the veins, and all the blood coming to the heart is pumped into the arteries.

As the healthy heart responds to acute exercise, the Frank-Starling law applies. The heart increases its force of contraction and hence its output. In addition, sympathetic stimulation increases the

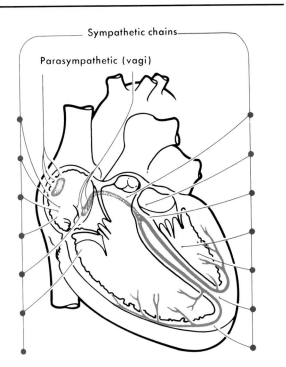

Sympathetic chains

Parasympathetic (vagi)

FIGURE 18.2   Autonomic innervation of the heart.

rate of contraction; this is the second basic mechanism by which the healthy heart increases its output. The peak efficiency of the heart under these conditions is reached at about 150 to 175 beats per minute. Faster rates result in incomplete filling of the ventricles and reduce the overall efficiency of the pump.

To summarize the Frank-Starling law, up to a certain limit the more a muscle fiber is stretched, the greater is its subsequent strength of contraction, but beyond that limit greater stretch actually diminishes the strength of contraction.

Cardiac hypertrophy. If the heart is subjected to chronic demands for increased output, the heart may enlarge. This condition is called *hypertrophy of the myocardium* and may be a normal response to chronic stress. For example, athletes such as long-distance runners and tennis players may have enlarged hearts. In other cases the enlargement of the heart may signal a pathological process. For example, in chronic heart failure the myocardial output gradually falls below the required level resulting from the failure of the myocardium as a pump. As the output falls, the normal regulatory mechanisms come into effect. Hypertrophy of the heart may occur as the body seeks to increase the

efficiency of the pump. Sympathetic stimulation may also be increased to increase the heart rate and hence the output. In many cases, in the absence of acute demands on the heart, these mechanisms will enable a weakened heart to maintain sufficient output. The patient may not complain of symptoms but on examination may have an enlarged heart and high heart rate.

Congestive heart failure. If the mechanisms just described fail and cardiac output falls below venous return, the result is congestive heart failure. The symptoms arise directly as a result of the insufficient cardiac output. The blood pooled in the veins produces increased venous pressure. The excessive venous pressure stretches cardiac muscle fibers beyond their limit and, as predicted by the Frank-Starling law, the strength of contraction falls further. The kidneys do not receive sufficient blood flow to maintain salt and water balance. As a result of these conditions, edema of the lungs and periphery develops as fluid leaks into the tissues from the capillaries. The typical patient in congestive heart failure is therefore short of breath and has a rapid pulse resulting from sympathetic stimulation of the heart, obvious swelling of the hands and feet, and an enlarged heart. All of these acute symptoms may be erased by increasing the cardiac output. It is for this purpose that the drugs discussed in the next section are primarily used.

CARDIOTONIC DRUGS
Cardiac Glycosides

Glycosides are complex steroidlike structures linked to sugar molecules. The drugs discussed in this section are referred to as *cardiac glycosides* because of their potent action on the heart. Many of the clinically useful cardiac glycosides come from species of *Digitalis* (see Table 18.3). The term *digitalis* may refer to a specific drug prepared from the leaf of *Digitalis purpurea*; it may also be used as a generic term to refer to all cardiac glycosides derived from *Digitalis* species.

Actions of cardiac glycosides. The cardiac glycosides are useful in treating congestive heart failure because they directly improve the strength of the heart muscle, elevating cardiac output. Biochemically, these drugs inhibit Na^+, K^+–ATPase and promote accumulation within the heart cells of the calcium necessary for contraction. The result of these actions is increased contractility. As a result of increased contractility, cardiac output is increased, blood flow to the kidneys and periphery is improved, venous pressure falls, and excess fluid begins to be excreted as edema clears. This diuretic

THE NURSING PROCESS

CARDIOTONIC THERAPY

Assessment

Patients who require cardiac glycosides have inadequate cardiac function, manifested in congestive heart failure, pulmonary edema, congenital cardiac defects, cardiac valve abnormalities, or postmyocardial infarction damage. The nurse should obtain baseline data, including the temperature, pulse, respiration and blood pressure, fluid intake and output, weight, serum electrolyte level, blood urea nitrogen, electrocardiogram, and other appropriate laboratory data. The nurse should auscultate the heart and lungs and observe the presence and location of edema, as well as the general condition of the patient. A subjective history of recent dysfunction, such as dyspnea on exertion, shortness of breath, and the need to sleep with the head of the bed elevated is also important.

Nursing diagnoses

Potential altered health maintenance related to insufficient knowledge of cardiac glycoside therapy

Potential complication: electrolyte imbalance/hypokalemia

Management

In some situations the patient will be critically ill when cardiac glycoside therapy is begun, but at other times these drugs may be among a list of several gradually being added to manage a chronic problem. Safe use of the drug involves monitoring the weight, fluid intake and output, electrocardiogram, serum electrolyte level (with specific focus on potassium), blood pressure, and other parameters of cardiovascular function. The nurse should auscultate the heart and lungs when a decrease in fluid in the lungs is anticipated. The nurse should also monitor the pulse when a decrease in the pulse is anticipated, but true bradycardia is often to be avoided. The parameters of the desired goal of therapy should be determined in consultation with the physician. Discharge planning should include determination of the names and dosages of all drugs to be taken, necessary dietary and activity restrictions, and referral to other appropriate departments or agencies such as the dietitian and the public health department for visiting nurse follow-up.

Evaluation

Successful use of cardiac glycosides should lead to weight loss through diuresis, increased cardiac output, decreased pulse, increased feeling of well-being, better tolerance of exertion, and less fluid in the lungs. For safe self-management the patient should be able to explain why and how to take all prescribed medications, any interrelations that may exist (e.g., the need to take potassium supplements if certain diuretics and cardiac glycosides are prescribed together), how to plan meals within prescribed dietary limitations, possible anticipated side effects of each drug, and situations requiring contact with a physician. If appropriate, the patient should know how often to record weight or pulse, be able to demonstrate how to accurately measure the pulse, and know what to do with the data obtained. For more specific guidelines, see the patient care implications section at the end of this chapter.

---

effect of digitalis is secondary to its action on the heart.

Cardiac glycosides are also widely used to control cardiac arrhythmias (Chapter 19).

Administration of cardiac glycosides. Half-lives of the cardiac glycosides may extend to 7 days

(Table 18.1). With repeated equal doses of a drug, the plateau of drug concentration in the blood is not achieved for about four elimination half-times (Chapter 2). Therefore these long half-lives for cardiac glycosides mean that the final desired therapeutic concentration of drug in the blood is not

Table 18.1   Comparison of Pharmacokinetics of Cardiac Glycosides

Drug	Oral absorption	Plasma protein binding	Plasma half-life	Route of excretion
Digoxin	60%-100%*	23%	32-48 hr	Renal
Digitoxin	90%-100%	97%	5-7 days	Hepatic
Deslanoside	Unreliable	25%	33-36 hr	Renal

*Absorption is 60% for tablet form, up to 100% with soft gelatin capsule.

Table 18.2   Time Course of Action of Cardiac Glycoside Preparations

Drug	Route	Onset	Peak	Duration
Digoxin	Oral	1-2 hr	1½-6 hr	2-6 days
	Intravenous	5-30 min	1-4 hr	2-6 days
Digitoxin	Oral	1-4 hr	8-14 hr	14 days
Deslanoside	Intravenous	10-30 min	1-3 hr	2-5 days

achieved for weeks following start of therapy. For many patients such a delay is intolerable. To avoid a long delay in achieving therapeutic concentrations, cardiac glycosides are frequently administered first in a *loading dose*. The loading dose is designed to rapidly raise the concentration in the blood to the therapeutic range. Following the loading dose or doses, a smaller dose is administered on a regular schedule. This smaller dose, called the *maintenance dose*, is designed to maintain the concentration of drug in the therapeutic range. This dose is continued indefinitely, or until some change in the patient's condition requires adjustment of the dose.

The available cardiac glycosides are similar in intrinsic potencies, but they differ markedly in pharmacokinetic properties (Tables 18.1 and 18.2). These properties largely determine the dosage and dosing schedule for the individual preparations (Table 18.3).

Digitoxin (see Table 18.3)

Digitoxin is usually given orally in a dose to produce and to maintain the therapeutic level in plasma of 14 to 26 ng/ml. The dose required to produce the maximum therapeutic effect varies considerably from patient to patient and must be individualized. Digitalizing, or loading, doses would be expected to range from 0.8 to 1.2 mg/day. Since 97% of this drug is reversibly bound to protein in the bloodstream and is inactive, the dose must take into account that only 3% of the dose in the bloodstream is active. Since the half-life of digitoxin is about 6 days, about 10% of the total body store of the drug is excreted each day. The routine daily dose of the drug must compensate for this drug loss. Maintenance doses should be expected in the range of 0.05 to 0.2 mg per day. Consideration of the half-life of the drug is also important when toxicity occurs; toxicity may persist for long periods because the drug is slowly removed from the system.

Digoxin (Table 18.3)

Digoxin is usually given orally in a dose that produces and maintains the therapeutic plasma level of 0.8 to 1.6 ng/ml. Dosage regimens with this drug must also be individualized. Digitalizing doses should be expected to be in the range of 0.75 to 1.25 mg per day. This drug is less highly bound to plasma protein than digitoxin and has a much shorter half-life. The maintenance dose of digoxin must replace the 37% of the total body store of the drug that is lost every day. Maintenance doses

Table 18.3 Summary of Inotropic Agents

Generic name	Trade name	Administration/dosage	Comments
Digitoxin	Crystodigin	ORAL: *Adults*—loading doses may be 0.8 mg followed by 0.2 mg every 6 to 8 hr for 2 or 3 doses (for rapid loading) or 0.2 mg twice daily for 4 days (for slow loading). Maintenance doses range from 0.05 to 0.3 mg daily. FDA Pregnancy Category C. *Children*—Dosage forms are inconvenient for children. Digoxin is more conveniently administered (see below).	Digitoxin is a purified form of the primary active glycoside from *Digitalis purpurea* (purple foxglove). Most patients can be safely started on oral loading doses.
Digoxin	Lanoxin* Novodigoxin†	ORAL (tablets): *Adults*—loading dose initially 0.75 to 1.25 mg divided into two or more doses given at 6 to 8 hr intervals (for rapid loading). Maintenance dose, also used for slow loading, is 0.125 to 0.5 mg daily. FDA Pregnancy Category C. *Children* (elixir)—loading doses that follow should be divided and administered every 6 hr. Premature infants: 0.02 to 0.035 mg/kg. Newborns: 0.025 to 0.035 mg/kg. Infants to 2 yr: 0.035 to 0.06 mg/kg. 2 to 5 yr: 0.03 to 0.04 mg/kg. 5 to 10 yr: 0.02 to 0.035 mg/kg. Over 10 yr: usual adult dose (tablets). Maintenance dose for premature infants is 20% to 30% of loading dose; for all other children, 25% to 35% of loading dose. ORAL (capsule) and INTRAVENOUS: *Adults*—loading dose of 0.25 to 0.5 mg followed by 0.25 mg 2 or 3 more times at 4 to 6 hr intervals. Maintenance dose ranges from 0.125 to 0.5 mg daily. *Children*—loading doses that follow are divided and administered every 6 hr. Premature infants: 0.015 to 0.025 mg/kg. Newborns: 0.02 to 0.03 mg/kg. Infants to 2 yr: 0.03 to 0.05 mg/kg. 2 to 5 yr: 0.025 to 0.035 mg/kg. 5 to 10 yr: 0.015 to 0.03 mg/kg. Over 10 yr: 0.008 to 0.012 mg/kg. Maintenance dose for premature infants is 20% to 30% of oral loading dose; for all other children, 25% to 30% of oral loading dose.	Digoxin is a purified form of an active glycoside from *Digitalis lanata* (white foxglove). Patients started on therapy with the maintenance dose given orally will achieve stable blood concentrations of the drug within 7 days. Bioavailability of digoxin from the tablet is variable and may be as low as 60%. Oral absorption from the solution in a soft gelatin capsule is nearly 100%. Since digoxin is eliminated primarily by the kidneys, dosage may need to be lowered in patients with diminished renal function.
Deslanoside	Cedilanid-D Cedilanid†	INTRAVENOUS: *Adults*—initially 0.8 mg, then repeated at 4 hr. FDA Pregnancy Category C. *Children*—divide the following doses into 2 or 3 portions and administer at 3 or 4 hr intervals. Newborns, 0.022 mg/kg. Infants to 3 yr: 0.025 mg/kg. Over 3 yr: 0.0225 mg/kg. INTRAMUSCULAR: *Adults*—intravenous usually preferred. *Children*—same as for intravenous.	Deslanoside is the desacetyl form of lanatoside C, a glycoside found in *Digitalis lanata* (white foxglove). Deslanoside is used only for emergencies; oral glycosides must be used for maintenance.
Amrinone	Inocor C	INTRAVENOUS: *Adults*—initially, 0.75 mg/kg body weight given slowly over 2 or 3 min. Repeat after 30 min if needed. Maintenance, 0.005 to 0.01 mg/kg/min, according to clinical response.	Patients with atrial flutter may need pretreatment with digitalis to prevent ventricular arrhythmia. Patients need adequate fluid intake to maintain adequate cardiac fluid filling so that response to amrinone is optimal.

*Available in Canada and United States.
†Available in Canada.

Table 18.4   Treatment of Cardiac Glycoside Overdose

Generic name	Trade name	Administration/dosing
Digoxin immune FAB	Digibind	INTRADERMAL: *Adult*—0.1 ml of 0.1 mg/ml solution. Inspect for redness and wheal 20 minutes later. Do not administer full dose if reaction is positive. FDA Pregnancy Category C.
		INTRAVENOUS: *Adult*—give amount equimolar to total amount of digoxin or digitoxin in body. Digoxin immune FAB in a dose of 40 mg binds approximately 0.6 mg of drug. Consult package insert for aid in calculating dosage.

GERIATRIC DRUG ALERT: CARDIAC GLYCOSIDES

THE PROBLEM

Elderly patients receiving cardiac glycosides may have diminished renal or hepatic function and a decreased volume of distribution for cardiac glycosides. As a group they are also more prone to electrolyte imbalances including hypokalemia, which can increase drug toxicity. The appetite suppression due to digoxin can aggravate the problem of poor nutrition in frail, elderly patients.

SOLUTIONS

- Doses must be carefully adjusted and increased slowly to avoid toxicity. Maintenance doses may be lower in geriatric patients than in younger adults
- Watch carefully for signs of electrolyte imbalance
- Instruct the patient in appropriate dietary practices that will minimize risk of electrolyte imbalances

should be expected to be in the range of 0.125 to 0.5 mg per day.

Deslanoside (Table 18.3)

Deslanoside is used only in emergencies when the intravenous route of administration is required. Deslanoside has no role in long-term therapy of congestive heart failure, its only advantage being rapid action when given intravenously. However, it is usually no more rapid in onset of action than digoxin given intravenously. Moreover, adjustment of doses when the patient is switched to oral maintenance therapy is more problematic with deslanoside than with digoxin. For these reasons the drug deslanoside is not widely used.

Toxicity of the cardiac glycosides. There is such a small difference between the therapeutic dose and doses that cause side effects that at one time or another most patients taking cardiac glycosides will experience drug-related difficulties. The symptoms may be neurological, visual, cardiac, or even psychiatric. They often tend to be vague and easily confused with those of congestive heart failure itself.

The neurological or central nervous system effects of cardiac glycosides are now recognized as significant sources of much of the toxicity observed with these drugs. The anorexia, nausea, and vomiting due to these drugs result from stimulation of the chemoreceptor trigger zone in the central nervous system. Weakness, fatigue, fainting, and other neurological symptoms also point to an origin in the central nervous system. Visual disturbances such as dimness of vision, double vision, blind

spots, flashing lights, or altered color vision also occur. Psychiatric disturbances range from mood alterations to psychoses or hallucinations.

The toxic action of cardiac glycosides on the heart may also result partly from central nervous system effects. Whatever the mechanism, the result may be bradycardia (slow heart rate), various arrhythmias that may occasionally induce tachycardia, and ultimately ventricular fibrillation and death (Chapter 19). Patients receiving cardiac glycosides must be checked frequently for heart rate and for the appearance of extra beats or other arrhythmias. It is routine practice in many hospitals to omit the dose if the heart rate is less than 60 beats per minute. Although bradycardia is the most common sign of digitalis-induced arrhythmias, other changes in heart rate are possible. For this reason any change in heart rate or rhythm should be noted and reported.

Because the toxic reactions caused by cardiac glycosides are dose related, they are somewhat predictable (Chapter 2). For this reason many hospitals have developed an assay to measure active cardiac glycosides as an aid in establishing safe doses for individual patients and in diagnosing drug toxicity. These assays are not reliable guides to therapy when the crude cardiac glycoside mixtures are used.

Toxicity of the cardiac glycosides may be increased by the presence of other drugs. For example, potassium-depleting diuretics such as thiazides or loop diuretics (Chapter 16) may predispose a patient to cardiac toxicity, since a low intracellular potassium level increases the likelihood of arrhythmias.

Accidental poisoning of children with preparations of cardiac glycosides is not uncommon. Patients who are around small children should be warned of the potential danger their medicine poses to curious toddlers.

Interest in deriving new inotropic agents that may be administered orally for chronic congestive heart failure has been sparked by the realization that the cardiac glycosides are severely limited in usefulness by their low therapeutic index (Chapter 2).

Treatment of digitalis toxicity. With digoxin or digitoxin overdose, the patient may continue to be at risk during the lengthy period of time required to eliminate these long-acting agents. If symptoms such as arrhythmias or hyperkalemia become life-threatening, digoxin immune FAB (Table 18.4) can be administered to rapidly neutralize free drug. Arrhythmias and electrolyte imbalance can be reversed within 30 minutes. The inotropic effect of the cardiac glycosides persists for several hours longer.

Adrenergic Agents

Stimulation of the beta-1 class of adrenergic receptors in the heart directly increases cardiac contractility by increasing cyclic adenosine monophosphate (cAMP) in heart muscle. The same type of increase in cAMP can be achieved by blocking phosphodiesterase, the enzyme that degrades cAMP. Drugs with these actions may be of value in treating symptoms of acute or chronic congestive heart failure.

Dobutamine (Table 14.1). Dobutamine directly stimulates myocardial beta-1 receptors, but it has little effect on beta-2 receptors and alpha receptors, which predominate in blood vessels. Dobutamine does not activate dopamine receptors in the renal vasculature. The drug has little tendency to increase heart rate or to elevate blood pressure. These properties make it an attractive agent for increasing cardiac output in severely ill patients. A disadvantage of dobutamine is that it must be given intravenously and has a very short duration of action. This drug is therefore appropriate only for acute cardiac decompensation.

Dopamine (Table 14.1). Dopamine directly stimulates myocardial beta-1 receptors but also causes indirect stimulation at this site by releasing norepinephrine from the nerve terminals in the heart.

In addition, dopamine stimulates alpha receptors in blood vessels and dopamine receptors in the renal vasculature. Low doses increase renal blood flow, which may assist in promoting diuresis. Higher doses directly stimulate the heart. Vasoconstriction caused by alpha receptor stimulation appears with the highest doses. Since dopamine can limit cardiac output by these actions in peripheral vessels, the drug is usually selected only for those patients in congestive heart failure complicated by hypotension. Like dobutamine, dopamine must be administered intravenously and has a very short duration of action.

Amrinone (Table 18.3). Amrinone is intended for short-term intravenous use in congestive heart failure when response to other agents has been poor. The drug rapidly increases cardiac output and is additive in its effects with digitalis. The exact mechanism of action of amrinone is not yet completely understood, though the drug is known to inhibit phosphodiesterase. In addition, it has some activity as a vasodilator in the periphery. Milrinone, a chemical relative of amrinone, is under investigation at this writing.

OTHER CLASSES OF DRUGS USED IN CONGESTIVE HEART FAILURE
Diuretics

Diuretics are useful in controlling the pulmonary edema that accompanies severe congestive heart failure. The agent most commonly selected is furosemide, although other diuretics may also be effective (Chapter 16).

In addition to relieving pulmonary edema, a side effect of congestive failure, diuretics may directly improve cardiac function in some patients. In end-stage congestive heart failure, venous pressure is elevated to the point that the heart muscle fibers are excessively stretched during filling of the chambers. Diuretics are said to reduce preload because they lower the pressure forcing blood into the heart chambers. As a result, the muscle fibers are not so abnormally stretched; they are then able to contract with greater power. Therefore contractility of the heart muscle is improved.

The major consideration limiting the use of diuretics in congestive heart failure is the risk of causing electrolyte or fluid imbalances, which may be especially dangerous to the patient in heart failure. Volume depletion or excessive dehydration must be avoided. Patients receiving digitalis should be observed especially carefully to prevent complications arising from the tendency of diuretics to alter potassium concentration in the blood (Chapter 14).

PATIENT CARE IMPLICATIONS

Cardiac glycosides

Drug administration

- Observe patients carefully. Desired effects of therapy include a decrease in pulse rate; slower, less labored respirations, diuresis with accompanying weight reduction; less coughing, less distended neck veins; and better tolerance of exertion. At the same time, observe for signs of toxicity (described in text). Many of these symptoms are seen in older or chronically ill persons, and may not be recognized as drug toxicity. Symptoms include abdominal discomfort, fatigue, confusion, restlessness, anorexia, and nausea and vomiting.

- Take the apical pulse for a full minute before administering a cardiac glycoside. Withhold the dose if the pulse is below 60 in an adult or below 90 to 110 in an infant or small child; notify the physician. Guidelines may vary according to institution or physician.

- To obtain the apical-radial deficit, two nurses take the pulse simultaneously, one counting the radial pulse, the other, the apical pulse. The difference between the pulses is the apical-radial deficit.

- Monitor the serum potassium level as well as other electrolytes. Digitalis toxicity is aggravated in the presence of hypokalemia. If the potassium level is below normal range, notify the physician. Signs of hypokalemia are noted in Table 17.1. Recall that vomiting, chronic diarrhea, nasogastric suctioning, and any state of alkalosis can contribute to hypokalemia, as can administration of potassium-losing diuretics, chronic steroids, amphotericin B, and chronic glucose.

- Monitor serum drug levels when available. Withhold the dose of drug and notify the physician if the serum drug level is higher than the therapeutic range.

- Monitor intake and output, daily weight, vital signs, and heart and lung sounds. Assess for dependent edema in the sacral area and feet and ankles. Assess for jugular venous distention. Use data from central venous or arterial lines if they are available. Monitor the electrocardiogram: the cardiac glycosides can cause prolongation of the P-R interval, S-T segment sagging, any degree of A-V block, and other arrhythmias.

- Read orders and drug labels carefully; do not confuse digoxin with digitoxin.

INTRAVENOUS DIGOXIN

- Monitor the apical pulse, and check serum electrolytes and serum drug level before administering. May be administered undiluted or diluted in 4 ml of sterile water, normal saline, or 5% dextrose for injection; use diluted solution as soon as prepared. Administer each dose over at least 5 minutes. If possible, monitor electrocardiogram during IV administration.

INTRAVENOUS DESLANOSIDE

- Monitor the apical pulse, and check serum electrolytes and serum drug level before administering. May be administered undiluted or diluted in 10 ml sodium chloride injection. Administer at a rate of 0.2 mg or less over 1 minute. If possible, monitor electrocardiogram during IV administration.

Patient and family education

- Review with patients the expected benefits and possible side effects of drug therapy. Review in detail the signs of drug toxicity, especially if the patient is elderly, since the elderly are more sensitive to the effects of the cardiac glycosides.

- Discuss the importance of maintaining an adequate potassium level. Review sources of dietary potassium (see Dietary Consideration: Potassium on p. 259). Patients with heart disease may need instruction in sodium restricted diets, weight reduction diets, and low cholesterol diets; refer to a dietician as needed.

- Review all medications the patient is taking, and emphasize the importance of taking them as prescribed. These may include diuretics, potassium replacements, antihypertensives, and others.

- If appropriate for the patient's ability, resources, and medical condition, teach the patient to monitor and record the apical pulse on a regular basis. It may also be appropriate to teach the patient to measure and record weight on a regular basis. Instruct the patient to report weight gain greater than 2 lb/day or 5 lb/week to the physician.

- Take cardiac glycosides with meals or snack to lessen gastric irritation

- For maintenance therapy, cardiac glycosides are usually taken once a day. Tell the patient that if a dose is missed, to take it as soon as remembered on the day it was missed if

Continued.

PATIENT CARE IMPLICATIONS — cont'd

within 12 hours of the usual time the dose is taken. Do not double up for missed doses; take only one dose a day unless otherwise directed by the physician. Refer patients as needed to community-based nursing care services.

- As always, remind patients to keep these drugs out of reach of children, to keep all health care providers informed of all drugs being taken, and not to self-medicate with over-the-counter drugs without consultation with the physician.
- Suggest that a medical identification tag or bracelet be worn indicating that the patient is taking a cardiac glycoside.

Amrinone

Drug administration

- Review the information about cardiac glycosides, above.
- Monitor the platelet count as well as the parameters noted above.
- Follow the dosage charts supplied by the manufacturer. May be given as a bolus: administer dose over 2 to 3 minutes. May be given as an infusion. Use microdrip infusion tubing and an electronic infusion monitor. Monitor the electrocardiogram and other

data available from central venous or arterial lines.
- At this writing, this drug is used only in acute care settings. Keep patient and family informed of patient's condition.

Digoxin immune FAB

Drug administration

- Review the manufacturer's insert for the latest guidelines.
- Skin testing may be prescribed before the full dose is given (see manufacturer's guidelines). Be prepared to treat an anaphylactic reaction. Patients who are allergic to digoxin immune FAB should not be given the full dose unless absolutely necessary.
- Have available personnel, equipment, and drugs for resuscitation.
- Prepare ordered dose, and administer over 30 minutes, using IV tubing with a 0.22 μm filter, unless cardiac arrest is imminent. May be given as a bolus in that situation. Monitor electrocardiogram and data from central venous and arterial lines as available.
- Monitor serum level of cardiac glycosides and serum electrolytes.
- Keep patient and family informed of the patient's condition.

Vasodilators

Vasodilators reverse the persistent vasoconstriction that arises in late chronic congestive heart failure as a result of long-term compensatory sympathetic nervous system stimulation. Sympathetic nervous system stimulation may be an important driving force for the failing heart, but in the vasculature it constricts vessels, thereby reducing cardiac output and increasing the workload of the heart. Vasodilators reduce the resistance against which the left ventricle must force blood. The result is an increase in cardiac output and a reduction in the workload of the heart.

Several classes of vasodilators are available for use in congestive heart failure. For outpatient therapy, *nitroglycerin* or *isosorbide dinitrate* (Table 14.2) can be employed. Nitroglycerin injection can be used for acute therapy. Alternatively, the related drug *nitroprusside* (Chapter 15) can be used for short-term intravenous therapy in severely ill patients. This agent is often given in conjunction with

an adrenergic agent such as dobutamine or dopamine.

The angiotensin-converting enzyme (ACE) inhibitors *captopril* and *enalapril* (Table 15.2) may also produce vasodilation that is useful in controlling congestive heart failure. These oral agents are used along with diuretics and cardiac glycosides for chronic therapy.

SUMMARY

The pumping action of the heart depends on its ability to contract at the proper time with sufficient strength to force blood from the chambers into the great arteries and thence to the rest of the body. The signal for initiating contraction comes from the SA (sinoatrial) node and spreads to the ventricles through the AV (atrioventricular) node. The frequency of signals from the SA node is lowered by vagus nerve stimulation and increased by sympathetic nerve stimulation. The strength of cardiac contraction is regulated by sympathetic innervation of the ventricles and by the Frank-Starling law.

Cardiac glycosides in use include digoxin, digitoxin, and deslanoside. These drugs increase the strength of contraction of the failing heart by promoting the accumulation of calcium within the heart cells. Deslanoside is an emergency medication suitable only for intravenous use. Both digitoxin and digoxin may be given orally. Digitoxin is very highly bound to plasma protein and is eliminated by the liver. The half-time for its elimination is 5 to 7 days. Digoxin is less tightly bound to plasma proteins, is excreted by the kidney, and has a half-time for elimination of about 36 hours. Both drugs are frequently given at high doses initially, then at lower doses intended to replace the amount of drug that is lost daily through normal elimination processes.

Cardiac glycosides have a very low therapeutic index, producing toxic reactions of increasing severity as serum concentrations rise. As concentrations of digitalis in the bloodstream increase above therapeutic levels, nausea, visual disturbances, central nervous system effects, and cardiac arrhythmias may arise. Bradycardia (excessively slowed heart rate) is a common sign of digitalis toxicity. Pulse rates should be taken before each dose of cardiac glycoside is administered, and the dose may be omitted if heart rates drop below 60 beats per minute.

Other drugs that increase the strength of contraction and may be used in heart failure include dobutamine, dopamine, and ephedrine. These drugs increase the strength of contraction by stimulating beta-1 adrenergic receptors in the heart. Other actions of these drugs arise from varying stimulation of beta-2, alpha, and dopamine receptors. Amrinone increases strength of contraction by mechanisms different from those of other drugs used for heart failure.

Diuretics relieve pulmonary edema associated with congestive heart failure. In addition, these drugs may improve cardiac function by reducing the pressure forcing blood into the heart. As a result, the abnormal stretch of heart muscle fibers is returned to a more normal range and the strength of contraction is increased.

Vasodilators reverse the persistent vasoconstriction that arises in late chronic congestive heart failure as a result of long-term compensatory sympathetic nervous system stimulation. In this way vasodilators increase cardiac output and reduce the workload of the heart.

STUDY QUESTIONS

1. How does heart muscle differ from skeletal muscle?
2. What is the purpose of the ring of nonconductive tissue that separates the atria from the ventricles?
3. Where does the impulse to beat originate in the healthy heart?
4. What structure transmits the impulse to beat from the atria to the ventricles?
5. What is the effect of parasympathetic stimulation on the heart?
6. What is the effect of sympathetic stimulation on the heart?
7. What is the Frank-Starling law of the heart?
8. What symptoms are typical of congestive heart failure?
9. What is digitalis?
10. What is the physiological effect of digitalis on the heart?
11. What is the mechanism of action of digitalis?
12. What is the mechanism by which digitalis produces diuresis in a patient with congestive heart failure?
13. How do digitoxin and digoxin differ in plasma protein binding and route of excretion?
14. Which digitalis preparation has the longest elimination half-time?
15. What is the purpose of the loading dose at the beginning of digitalis therapy?
16. What is the purpose of the maintenance dose in digitalis therapy?
17. Does digitalis have a high or a low therapeutic index?
18. What toxicity is common with digitalis therapy?
19. Why are pulse rates measured *before* administering each prescribed dose of digitalis?
20. What drugs increase the likelihood of digitalis toxicity?
21. What inotropic drugs other than cardiac glycosides are used in congestive heart failure? What is the basis for their action in congestive heart failure?
22. How do diuretics relieve pulmonary congestion in congestive heart failure?
23. How may diuretics improve function in a failing heart?
24. How may vasodilators relieve symptoms of congestive heart failure?

SUGGESTED READINGS

Algeo, S.S., and others: Amrinone: a new therapy for heart failure, Drug Therapy Hosp. **8**(1):81, 1983.

Bachman, J., Bolton, E.D., and Cooke, D.H.: The failing heart, Patient Care **23**(1):132, 1989.

Chatterjee, K.: Digitalis versus newer inotropic agents: which to use, Drug Therapy Hosp. **7**(1):77, 1982.

Curran, C.C., and Mathewson, M.: Use of cardiac glycosides in the critically ill, Crit. Care Nurse 7(6):31, 1987.

Drake, C.E.: Cardiac drug overdose, Am. Fam. Physician 25(1):181, 1982.

Fenster, P.E., and Kern, K.B.: Common drug interactions with digoxin, Drug Therapy 13(2):100, 1983.

Ginsburg, R.: New approaches to CHF: a guide to vasodilator therapy, Mod. Med. 51(11):68, 1983.

Goldberg, P.B.: How do digitalis tolerance and toxicity change with age? Geriatr. Nurs. 1:142, 1980.

Gomez-Arnau, J., and others: Cardiac arrest due to digitalis intoxication with normal serum digoxin levels: effects of hypokalemia, Drug Intell. Clin. Pharm. 16(2):161, 1982.

Heinsimer, J.A., and Lefkowitz, R.J.: The beta-adrenergic receptor in heart failure, Hosp. Pract. 18(11):103, 1983.

Horwitz, L.D.: Congestive heart failure: an overview of drug therapy, Postgrad. Med. 76(2):187, 1984.

Jaffe, M.: Pediatric digoxin administration, DCCN 6(3):136, 1987.

Johnston, G.D.: Clinical and pharmacological considerations in digitalis use in the geriatric patient, Geriatr. Med. Today 2(1):59, 1983.

Konick-McMahan, J.: Jugular vein distention: trouble in the heart's right side, Nursing 89 19(2):100, 1989.

Mathewson, M.A.: New uses for old drugs: vasodilators, Crit. Care Update 9(11):7, 1982.

Mutnick, A.H., Fecitt, S., and Rogers, B.: Update on cardiac drugs: inotropic and chronotropic agents, Nursing 87 17(10):58, 1987.

Parmley, W.W.: To rescue a failing heart, Emerg. Med. 15(5):178, 1983.

Parmley, W.W.: When failure is acute, Emerg. Med. 15(5):180, 1983.

Parmley, W.W.: When failure is chronic, Emerg. Med. 15(5):195, 1983.

Parys, E.V.: Assessing the failing state of the heart, Nursing 87 17(7):42, 1987.

Purcell, J.A., and Holder, C.K.: Cardiomyopathy: understanding the problem . . . supporting cardiac function, Am. J. Nurs. 89(1):57, 1989.

Shocken, D.D.: Congestive heart failure: Dx and Rx in the elderly, Geriatrics 39(11):77, 1984.

Taggart, A.J., and McDevitt, D.G.: Digitalis: its place in modern therapy, Drugs 20:398, 1980.

Yacone, L.A.: The nurses' guide to cardiovascular drugs, RN, Part 1:51(8):36, 1988; Part 2:51(9):40, 1988.

Drugs to Control Cardiac Arrhythmias

19

ELECTROPHYSIOLOGY OF THE HEART

Cardiac arrhythmias are defined as any deviation from the normal rate or pattern of heartbeat. Heart rates that are too slow (bradycardia), too fast (tachycardia), or irregular are all included in this classification. Arrhythmias are also sometimes referred to as *dysrhythmias.*

To understand the pharmacological control of arrhythmias, we must recall the physiological control mechanisms of the heart. The impulse to beat originates in the sinoatrial (SA) node, spreads through the atria causing them to contract, passes through the atrioventricular (AV) node, and finally enters the ventricles and causes contraction of that tissue (Chapter 18).

Normal action potential. Typical action potentials for three types of cardiac tissue are illustrated in Figure 19.1. Atrial and ventricular patterns are quite similar. Both begin with a rapid depolarization, marked by 0 on the curves, which is caused by a rapid rush of sodium ion (Na^+) into the cells. The inside of the cell therefore becomes more positive as the electrical potential shifts from about -90 mV to about $+20$ mV. Shortly thereafter, chloride ion (Cl^-) begins to enter the cardiac cell, so the electrical potential becomes more negative. This phase is marked by 1 on the curve. During the relatively long plateau period, marked phase 2 on the curve, sodium ion and calcium ion (Ca^{++}) slowly enter the cell while potassium ion leaves. As time progresses, the sodium ion and calcium ion stop flowing in but potassium ion continues to flow out (phase 3). During this phase the electrical potential continues to become more negative. In the final phase of the action potential, sodium ion flows out of the cell in exchange for potassium ion, which enters the cell. At the end of this cycle, the cell has returned to the resting potential of about -90 mV and has regained the ability to generate another normal action potential. From the beginning of phase 0 until sometime during the middle of phase 3, atrial or ventricular cells cannot be stimulated to beat again. This span of time is referred to as the *refractory period.* In nodal tissue the refractory period lasts well beyond phase 3 of the action potential.

Automaticity of normal SA nodal cells. The action potential for the SA nodal tissue differs from that of the atrial and ventricular cells in several ways. Most important in terms of cardiac physiology is the gradual depolarization that occurs during phase 4 (Figure 19.1). This ability to gradually shift from a potential of about -70 mV to -50 or -40 mV is what triggers the start of the action potential (phase 0) in these cells. Because of this trait these cells are termed *automatic:* they need no externally applied stimulus to initiate an action potential.

Electrocardiogram (ECG). Measurements of action potentials are performed in laboratories on experimental animals and are very helpful in revealing what happens when a heart beats. However, in the clinical setting, information about the function of a patient's heart is gained from electrocardiogram (ECG) tracings (Figure 19.2). These ECG tracings may be related to action potentials in various parts of the heart. The change in potential marked in Figure 19.2 as P (the P wave) is produced by the initial depolarization of atrial cells (phase 0 on the action potential). Very shortly after this wave of depolarization, the atrium contracts to complete filling of the ventricles. The waves marked Q, R, and S (QRS complex) result from depolarization of the ventricles. Repolarization of the atria occurs at this time but is masked by large changes produced by the ventricles. Ventricular contraction occurs between the QRS complex and the midpoint of the T wave. The T wave is generated by repolarization

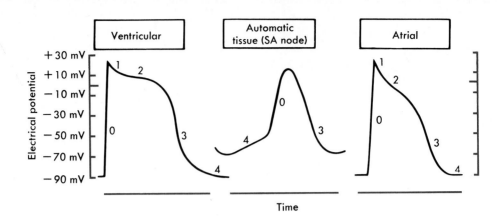

FIGURE 19.1   Typical action potential for three types of cardiac tissues. These action potentials are determined in the laboratory in tissues from experimental animals.

(phases 1 through 3 of the action potential) of the ventricles.

Mechanisms Producing Arrhythmias

Arrhythmias occur because of disorders in the pacing of the heartbeat or disorders in conducting the impulse to beat through the heart tissues, or a combination of these causes.

Disorders in heart pacing are frequently related to changes in the automaticity of the heart. For example, the normal pacemaker of the heart, the SA node, may become overstimulated by the sympathetic nervous system. The catecholamine neurotransmitters for this branch of the nervous system increase the automaticity of the SA node. As a result, phase 4 on the action potential curve is steepened and shortened, phase 0 is triggered more frequently, and the heart beats more rapidly. In contrast, if the vagus nerve is predominant and sympathetic stimulation is removed, the heart rate decreases. This action occurs because acetylcholine from the vagus nerve decreases the automaticity of the SA node.

In addition to these disorders in automaticity at the SA node, the heart may suffer altered rates resulting from *ectopic foci* of automatic cells. These ectopic foci are groups of cells in either the atria or the ventricles that spontaneously beat independently of the SA node. These groups of automatic cells may replace the SA node as the primary pacer for the heart, they may work in combination with the SA node so that the heart responds to both pacemakers, or they may interfere with SA nodal pacing with the result that neither pacing system is effective.

Conduction disorders are primarily of two

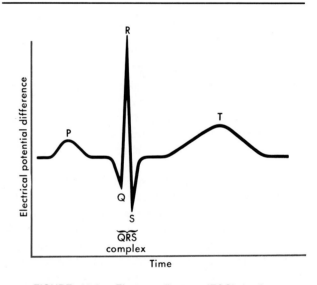

FIGURE 19.2   Electrocardiogram (ECG) tracing showing the patterns typical of normal heart function.

types. One involves an alteration in the conduction time across the AV node. The function of the AV node is to prevent the ventricles from receiving the impulse to beat until the atria have contracted and filled the ventricles (Chapter 18). If the ventricles contract prematurely, ineffective pumping action occurs, since the chambers will be only partially filled. If the delay in transmission through the AV node should become too long, then skipped heartbeats may occur, since the AV node may still be in the refractory period from the last beat when the next impulse arrives from the SA node.

The second type of conduction disorder involves conduction through the contracting tissue. If an area of heart muscle becomes ischemic (oxygen starved) or damaged, it may not only fail to contract but it may also fail to properly conduct an action potential. Ordinarily the action potential spreads across the tissue in a pattern that allows all parts of the tissue to contract at the proper time so that the heart pumps efficiently. The presence of this damaged region alters the pattern of stimulation, and the subsequent contraction may not be rhythmic or effective. Occasionally the damaged area may alter conduction so that a phenomenon called *reentry* occurs. In reentry, the action potential from a single impulse to beat passes more than once through the same group of cells. In the extreme case, reentry may produce a continuous cycle or loop of electrical activity through part of the tissue that prevents the heart from contracting properly.

ANTIARRHYTHMIC DRUGS

The classification system described in Table 19.1 is based on the effects of the drugs on the action potential (Figure 19.1). The main usefulness of the classification system is to demonstrate the mechanistic relatedness of drugs that might otherwise seem unrelated. Even within groups, however, effects of the drugs may differ somewhat. Table 19.2 lists more specifically the actions and reactions generated by each drug.

Antiarrhythmics may have other applications. For example, propranolol, esmolol, and acebutolol block beta-adrenergic receptors (Chapters 10, 15); in the heart this action slows the rate at the SA node and slows conduction through the AV node. The effect at both sites is to slow heart rate. Anticholinergic drugs, such as atropine, may produce the opposite effect by blocking the muscarinic receptors by which the heart responds to vagal nerve stimulation. Calcium-channel blocking drugs such as verapamil primarily change the responses of cells highly dependent upon the so-called slow calcium current (e.g., AV nodal cells or cells in ischemic regions of muscle). Local anesthetics, such as lidocaine and related drugs, alter cardiac cell membranes, and thus change the sodium ion influx that causes phase 0 of the action potential. Table 19.3 lists and describes drugs for controlling arrhythmias.

Class 1-A Antiarrhythmic Drugs (Table 19.1)

Antiarrhythmic drugs of this type depress phase 0 of the action potential (Figure 19.1) and prolong the action potential duration. The effective refractory period is therefore prolonged in atria and ventricles, making the tissue less electrically re-

sponsive. Class 1-A antiarrhythmics are indicated for prophylaxis and treatment of ventricular arrhythmias (premature contractions, tachycardia); quinidine and procainamide may also be used for atrial tachycardia or fibrillation.

Quinidine and procainamide

Quinidine and procainamide have virtually identical mechanisms of action. Both drugs alter calcium distribution within the cardiac cell, thereby decreasing contractility of the heart muscle. Both quinidine and procainamide have atropine-like effects that block the effect of the vagus nerve on the heart. Finally, both drugs alter the membranes of cardiac cells, resulting in a prolonged refractory period. The ability of these drugs to prolong the refractory period of cardiac tissues may explain the ability of the drugs to suppress ectopic foci. The drugs quinidine and procainamide have equipotent membrane effects; however, quinidine has the more potent anticholinergic effect.

Absorption, distribution, excretion. Quinidine sulfate is relatively rapidly absorbed by oral routes. The half-life of quindine in serum is about 6 hours. Quinidine gluconate is somewhat more slowly absorbed orally, and hence slightly longer acting. Quinidine polygalacturonate is reported to be less irritative to the gastrointestinal tract than other forms of quinidine. Quinidine is partially metabolized in liver; up to 50% of a dose may be excreted unchanged in the urine, and the drug may accumulate in patients in renal failure.

Procainamide reaches effective concentrations in the serum (4 to 8 μg/ml) within 1 to 3 hours of an oral dose or within 30 minutes of an intramuscular dose. The half-life of the drug in serum is 3 hours and about half the drug dose is eliminated unchanged in the kidney.

Side effects. The anticholinergic effects of quinidine and procainamide in some ways oppose the direct action of the drugs. The dual effects of quinidine have caused serious complications in the treatment of atrial fibrillation. Although the direct effects of quinidine might be expected to slow the atrial rate, the first observed effect may be an anticholinergic action producing increased conduction through the AV node, with the result that ventricular rates soar dangerously high before quinidine can slow atrial rates.

Toxic effects. The primary difference between quinidine and procainamide is in the toxic effects produced.

Quinidine is commonly associated with gastrointestinal reactions, but the most serious reactions include allergic responses and cardiovascular toxicity. When the drug is given intravenously, hy-

Table 19.1 Classification of Antiarrhythmic Drugs with Indications for Use

Class	Drugs	Effect on action potential	Indications
1-A	Disopyramide Procainamide Quinidine	Depress phase 0; prolong action potential duration	Ventricular and some supraventricular arrhythmias
1-B	Lidocaine Mexiletine Phenytoin Tocainide	Depress phase 0 slightly; may shorten action potential duration	Ventricular arrhythmias
1-C	Encainide Flecainide	Marked depression of phase 0; profound slowing of conduction	Ventricular arrhythmias
II	Acebutolol Esmolol Propranolol	Depress phase 4 depolarization	Supraventricular and other tachyarrhythmias; acebutolol for premature ventricular contractions
III	Amiodarone Bretylium	Prolong phase 3 repolarization	Ventricular tachycardia, ventricular fibrillation
IV	Verapamil	Depress phase 4 depolarization; lengthen phase 1 and 2	Supraventricular tachyarrhythmias

potension may result. Quinidine is an arteriolar and venous dilator. This action may account for the fact that quinidine significantly reduces cardiac output in some patients. At higher doses, usually resulting in blood levels above 8 μg/ml, quinidine may produce ventricular arrhythmias, including ectopic beats, tachycardia, and fibrillation. Quinidine causes a dose-dependent widening of the QRS complex. This effect can be used to monitor its therapeutic activity.

Like quinidine, procainamide may cause gastrointestinal discomfort to patients receiving the medication orally. Procainamide is less completely bound to plasma proteins than is quinidine and therefore less subject to unexpected drug interactions resulting from displacement from plasma protein binding sites (Chapter 2). Allergic and immunological reactions are among the most striking adverse effects of procainamide. With long-term use the drug may produce a syndrome that resembles lupus erythematosus, including symptoms such as arthritis and arthralgia, myalgia, fever, and pericarditis. Direct toxic effects on the heart usually relate to changes in conduction within the heart, especially at the AV nodal tissue and the conducting fibers of the ventricles. These direct toxic effects on the heart are usually produced when blood levels exceed 12 μg/ml. Since normal therapeutic concentrations range from about 4 to

8 μg/ml, it is obvious that this drug, like the other antiarrhythmic drugs, has a very narrow safety margin.

Like quinidine, procainamide widens the QRS complex on the electrocardiogram and lengthens the refractory period.

Disopyramide phosphate

Disopyramide phosphate is similar in action to procainamide and quinidine.

Absorption, distribution, and excretion. Disopyramide is rapidly and almost completely absorbed following oral administration. Biotransformation by the liver produces metabolites with antimuscarinic as well as antiarrhythmic activities. About half of each dose is eliminated unchanged by the kidneys.

Side effects. Ten to 20% of treated patients may experience difficulty in urination, which is an antimuscarinic effect. Up to 10% of patients suffer hypotension (dizziness or fainting), altered heart function (change in rhythm or heart failure), or fluid retention (congestive heart failure). Dry mouth, which is another antimuscarinic effect, is very common but not dangerous.

Toxicity. Overdose causes pronounced widening of the QRS complex and the QT interval of the electrocardiogram. Cardiac arrhythmias may ensue. Apnea, loss of spontaneous respirations and

Text continued on p. 313.

Table 19.2   Mechanism of Action of Antiarrhythmic Drugs

Drug	Predominant mechanism of antiarrhythmic action	Summary of cardiac actions			Adverse reactions
		Conduction velocity	Automaticity	Contractility	
Acebutolol	Relatively selective block-ade of beta-1 receptors in heart increases AV nodal refractory period.	Slowed	Decreased	Decreased	Bradycardia, lowered cardiac output; congestive heart fail-ure; bronchospasm in persons with asthma. FDA Pregnancy Cate-gory B.
Amiodarone	Prolongs action potential duration and refractory pe-riod throughout heart.	Slowed	Decreased	Decreased	Bradycardia; pulmo-nary toxicity; neurotox-icity; hypothyroidism. FDA Pregnancy Cate-gory C.
Atropine	Blocks effects of vagus nerve stimulation.	Hastened	Increased	No change	Dry mouth, cyclople-gia, mydriasis, fever, urinary retention, con-fusion.
Bretylium	Prolongs effective refrac-tory period.	No change	No change or slight increase	No change or slight increase	Bradycardia, hypoten-sion, and precipitation of anginal attacks.
Digoxin	Slows conduction through AV node.	Slowed	Increased at high doses	Increased	Bradycardia, prema-ture ventricular beats, AV nodal tachycardia, anorexia, nausea.
Disopyramide	Suppresses automaticity, especially in ectopic foci, by membrane-stabilizing and anticholinergic effects.	No change or slightly slowed	Decreased	Decreased	Anticholinergic effects: dry mouth, constipa-tion, urinary hesitancy or retention, blurred vi-sion; hypoglycemia. FDA Pregnancy Cate-gory C.
Encainide	Prolongs refractory period in conductive fibers; mark-edly slows conduction in atria.	Slowed	Decreased	No change	New ventricular ar-rhythmias; bradycar-dia; AV block; conges-tive heart failure. FDA Pregnancy Category B.
Esmolol	Cardioselective beta ad-renergic receptor block-ade; increases AV nodal refractory period.	Slowed	Decreased	Decreased	Bradycardia; confu-sion; impaired periph-eral circulation. FDA Pregnancy Category C.
Flecainide	Prolongs refractory period in conductive fibers; mark-edly slows conduction in atria.	Slowed	Decreased	Slightly decreased	New ventricular ar-rhythmias; AV block; bradycardia; conges-tive heart failure. FDA Pregnancy Category C.

Continued.

Table 19.2   Mechanism of Action of Antiarrhythmic Drugs—cont'd

Drug	Predominant mechanism of antiarrhythmic action	Summary of cardiac actions			Adverse reactions
		Conduction velocity	Automaticity	Contractility	
Lidocaine	Increases electrical threshold for ventricular stimulation.	No change	Decreased	No change	Central nervous system effects such as confusion, drowsiness, convulsions. FDA Pregnancy Category B.
Mexiletine	Prolongs refractory period in conductive fibers.	No change	Decreased	No change	Ventricular arrhythmias; shortness of breath; hepatic necrosis. FDA Pregnancy Category C.
Phenytoin	Depresses spontaneous depolarization in ventricular and atrial but not nodal tissue.	No change or slightly hastened	Decreased	No change	Rapid intravenous injection causes severe myocardial toxicity; chronic use produces cerebellar side effects and gingival hyperplasia.
Procainamide	Suppresses automaticity, especially in ectopic foci, by membrane-stabilizing and anticholinergic effects.	Slowed	Decreased	Decreased	Hypotension, decreased cardiac output, ventricular tachycardia, lowered resistance to infection, allergy, gastrointestinal distress; chronic use causes collagen disorders resembling systemic lupus erythematosus. FDA Pregnancy Category C.
Propranolol	Beta adrenergic blockade and membrane-stabilizing effects that increase AV nodal refractory period.	Slowed	Decreased	Decreased	Bradycardia, lowered cardiac output; congestive heart failure; bronchospasm in persons with asthma.
Quinidine	Suppresses automaticity, especially in ectopic foci, by membrane-stabilizing and anticholinergic effects.	Slowed	Decreased	Decreased	Peripheral vasodilation, hypotension, paradoxical ventricular tachycardia, decreased cardiac output, cinchonism, allergy, fever, gastrointestinal distress. FDA Pregnancy Category C.
Tocainide	Increases threshold of excitability in conductive fibers	No change	Decreased	No change	Pulmonary toxicity, allergic reactions, blood dyscrasias. FDA Pregnancy Category C.
Verapamil	Blocks calcium channels and slows conduction through AV node.	Slowed	No change or slightly decreased	Decreased	Hypotension, bradycardia, asystole with intravenous route; gastrointestinal disturbances, light-headedness, headache, nervousness with oral drug. FDA Pregnancy Category C.

Table 19.3 Pharmacological Properties of Drugs Used to Control Cardiac Arrhythmias

Generic name	Trade name	Administration/dosage	Comments
Acebutolol	Monitan† Sectral*	ORAL: *Adults*—200 mg twice daily; adjust according to response.	Mild intrinsic sympathomimetic effect and cardioselectivity both theoretically reduce risk of bronchospasm, hypoglycemia, and impaired peripheral circulation.
Amiodarone	Cordarone*	ORAL: *Adults*—800 mg to 1.6 Gm daily in divided doses for 1 to 3 weeks; reduce dose when control is adequate or side effects occur, 600 to 800 mg daily for 1 month; maintenance, 200 to 400 mg daily. *Children*—10 mg/kg body weight or 800 mg/1.72 M^2 daily for 10 days until control is adequate or side effects occur; reduce to 5 mg/kg or 400 mg/M^2 for several weeks; maintenance, 2.5 mg/kg or 200 mg/M^2, or lowest effective dose.	Very long duration of action (weeks or months) and very slow onset (2 days to 2 months). Amiodarone persists in the body for months after the drug is discontinued.
Atropine		INTRAVENOUS: *Adults*—0.4 to 1 mg every 1 to 2 hr as needed, up to a maximum of 2 mg. *Children*—0.01 to 0.03 mg/kg body weight.	Rapidly effective; excreted by the kidney within 12 hr of administration.
Bretylium tosylate	Bretylol Bretylate†	INTRAMUSCULAR: *Adults*—5 to 10 mg/kg repeated in 1 to 2 hr, then every 6 to 8 hr. One site should receive no more than 5 ml of undiluted drug. INTRAVENOUS: *Adults*—5 to 10 mg/kg repeated every 15 to 30 min to a maximum dose of 30 mg/kg.	Excreted unchanged by the kidneys.
Digoxin	Lanoxin*	ORAL: *Adults*—tablets or elixir, load with 0.5 to 0.75 mg, followed by 0.25 to 0.5 mg every 6 to 8 hr to a total dose of 1 to 1.5 mg; maintain with 0.125 to 0.5 mg daily. *Children*—doses are individualized for age and body weight.	Effective serum level 1 to 2 ng/ml, toxic at 3 ng/ml; excreted by the kidney; elimination half-time about 36 hr. Bioavailability with capsules is higher, so that 0.1 mg dose is equivalent to 0.125 mg in tablets.
Disopyramide	Norpace*	ORAL: *Adults*—100 to 140 mg every 6 hr. Maintenance may use extended release forms 300 mg every 12 hr. *Children*—6 to 30 mg/kg body weight daily divided into 4 doses.	Effective serum level 2 to 4 µg/ml; serum half-life 4 hr; kidneys eliminate 80% of the active drug and metabolites.
Encainide	Enkaid	ORAL: *Adults*—25 mg every 8 hr; after 3 to 5 days may be increased to 35 mg every 8 hr, then 50 mg every 8 hr. Individual dose should not exceed 75 mg.	Rapidly metabolized to active metabolites in liver.
Esmolol	Brevibloc	INTRAVENOUS: *Adults*—0.5 mg/kg body weight in 1 min, then 0.05 mg/kg/min for 4 min. Increase maintenance dose as necessary up to 0.2 mg/kg; use for up to 48 hr.	This very short-acting drug must be given by continuous infusion.

*Available in Canada and United States.
†Available in Canada.

Continued.

Table 19.3   Pharmacological Properties of Drugs Used to Control Cardiac Arrhythmias—cont'd

Generic name	Trade name	Administration/dosage	Comments
Flecainide	Tambocor*	ORAL: *Adults*—100 mg every 12 hr, increasing in increments of 50 mg twice daily every 4 days as needed. Maximum daily dose 400 to 600 mg.	Toxicity increases at plasma concentrations above 0.7 to 1 μg/ml.
Lidocaine	Xylocaine HCl* (for cardiac arrhythmias) Lidocaine* (without preservatives)	INTRAMUSCULAR: *Adults*—emergency use, 4.3 mg/kg, or 3 ml of 10% solution (300 mg). INTRAVENOUS: *Adults*—up to 300 mg in any 1-hour period. *Children*—continuous infusion, 20 to 50 μg/kg body weight/min.	Effective serum level 1 to 5 μg/ml; serum half-life 15 to 20 min; metabolized in liver; toxicity increased by reduced liver blood flow or function.
Mexiletine	Mexitil*	ORAL: *Adults*—200 mg every 8 hr; adjust up or down by 50 to 100 mg per dose every 2 to 3 days. Doses do not exceed 1200 mg daily.	Effective plasma concentrations are 0.5 to 2 μg/ml, but toxicity may be observed even at these levels.
Phenytoin	Dilantin*	INTRAVENOUS: *Adults*—50 to 100 mg given over 10 min. Repeat if necessary at 5 to 15 min intervals. Dose held under 1 Gm, or 15 mg/kg body weight.	Arrhythmias are not official indications for phenytoin, but it has been used for digitalis-induced arrhythmias.
Procainamide	Promine Pronestyl*	ORAL: *Adults*—250 to 500 mg every 3 to 6 hr. *Children*—50 mg/kg daily in 4 to 6 divided doses. INTRAMUSCULAR: *Adults*—250 to 1000 mg every 6 hr. INTRAVENOUS: *Adults*—100 mg over 5 min as needed.	Effective serum level 4 to 8 μg/ml; serum half-life about 3 hr.
Procainamide sustained release	Procan-SR* Pronestyl-SR* Rhythmin	ORAL: *Adults*—50 mg/kg/day divided into 4 doses.	Absorption is variable and may be extremely low in a few patients.
Propranolol	Inderal* Detensol†	ORAL: *Adults*—10 to 30 mg 3 or 4 times daily. *Children*—0.5 to 4 mg/kg daily in 2 to 4 doses. INTRAVENOUS: *Adults*—1 mg each minute up to 30 mg or 0.1 to 0.15 mg/kg administered in increments of 0.5 to 0.75 mg every 1 to 2 min with ECG and blood pressure monitoring. *Children*—0.01 to 0.15 mg/kg over 3 to 5 min with ECG and blood pressure monitoring.	Effective serum level is highly variable; serum half-life 2½ to 4 hr; metabolized in the liver.
Quinidine gluconate	Duraquin Quinaglute* Quinalan Quinate*	ORAL: *Adults*—324 to 660 mg (1 to 2 tablets) 2 or 3 times daily. INTRAMUSCULAR: *Adults*—initially 600 mg; 200 to 400 mg every 4 to 6 hr. INTRAVENOUS: *Adults*—10 mg each minute up to 400 mg with ECG and blood pressure monitoring.	More slowly absorbed than quinidine sulfate.

*Available in Canada and United States.
†Available in Canada.

Table 19.3   Pharmacological Properties of Drugs Used to Control Cardiac Arrhythmias— cont'd

Generic name	Trade name	Administration/dosage	Comments
Quinidine polygalacturonate	Cardioquin*	ORAL: *Adults*—as for quinidine sulfate (1 tablet of 275 mg is equivalent to 200 mg of quinidine sulfate).	Less irritating to gastrointestinal tract than other forms of quinidine.
Quinidine sulfate	Cin-Quin Quinidex Extentabs* Quinora	ORAL: *Adults*—200 to 400 mg 4 times daily. *Children*—6 mg/kg every 4 to 6 hr.	Test dose of 200 mg should be given to test for idosyncratic reactions; effective serum level 3 to 6 µg/ml; serum half-life about 6 hr.
Tocainide	Tonocard*	ORAL: *Adults*—400 mg every 8 hr, adjusted as necessary; maintenance 1200 to 1800 mg daily divided into 3 doses.	Bioavailability is very high and is unaffected by food.
Verapamil	Calan Isoptin	ORAL: *Adults*—240 to 480 mg daily divided into 3 or 4 doses. INTRAVENOUS: *Adults*—initially 5 to 10 mg over 2 to 5 min, repeated if necessary at 30 min. Maintenance with 0.005 mg/kg/min. *Infants to 1 yr*—0.1 to 0.2 mg/kg over 2 min, repeated if necessary at 30 min.	Therapeutic serum levels are 0.08 to 0.3 µg/ml; verapamil is extensively metabolized by the liver.

*Available in Canada and United States.
†Available in Canada.

unconsciousness precede death by cardiovascular collapse.

Class 1-B Antiarrhythmic Drugs (Table 19.1)

Antiarrhythmic drugs of this type slightly depress phase 0 of the action potential (Figure 19.1) and may shorten the action potential duration. As a group, these drugs have much less effect on atria than the class 1-A drugs. Class 1-B antiarrhythmic agents are indicated for ventricular arrhythmias, including those arising from myocardial infarction, cardiac surgery, cardiac catheterization, or digitalis toxicity.

Lidocaine

Lidocaine is a local anesthetic (Chapter 46) that alters sodium ion conduction in heart cells. Its antiarrhythmic action affects ventricular tissue more than atrial or nodal tissues.

Absorption, distribution, excretion. Lidocaine is eliminated primarily by the liver, with over 90% of a dose being rapidly destroyed in that tissue. For this reason the drug is useful primarily when administered as a continuous infusion.

Side effects and toxicity. Lidocaine causes a variety of central nervous system reactions, ranging from muscle twitching and drowsiness to paresthesia, respiratory depression, convulsions, and coma. These reactions may be dose-dependent; CNS reactions are expected when serum concentrations exceed 8 µg/ml. Toxic reactions to lidocaine are more common in patients with reduced hepatic function, since the drug may accumulate in these patients.

In administering lidocaine, it is important to recall that the drug has two separate clinical uses and is packaged differently for each. When intended for use as a local anesthetic, lidocaine is frequently packaged in solution with epinephrine (e.g., Xylocaine [or other trade name] with epinephrine). When used with the local anesthetic, epinephrine acts as a vasoconstrictor to reduce local blood flow and prolong the action of the anesthetic. If lidocaine with epinephrine were inadvertently administered to treat a cardiac arrhythmia, the epinephrine might well trigger a severe arrhythmia by stimulating automaticity of the heart. Lidocaine intended for use in cardiac emergencies is labeled "lidocaine without preservatives" or "Xylocaine for cardiac arrhythmias."

GERIATRIC DRUG ALERT: ANTIARRHYTHMIC DRUGS

THE PROBLEM:

Older patients often respond differently to antiarrhythmic agents than do younger adults. Procainamide and tocainide are more likely to cause dizziness or hypotension in older persons. Amiodarone is more likely to cause ataxias or other neurologic problems in the elderly. They are more sensitive to the antimuscarinic effects (dry mouth, urinary retention) of disopyramide. Clearance of drugs like verapamil, flecainide, or the beta-adrenergic blockers is lower, and these drugs may accumulate. Especially with flecainide, higher serum levels may lead to development of dangerous drug-induced arrhythmias. Older persons may be more susceptible to hypothermia with beta-adrenergic blockers.

SOLUTIONS:

- Lidocaine doses and rates of administration should be cut in half for patients over age 65
- Blood pressure should be carefully monitored
- Be alert to signs of neurological toxicity and ataxia
- Help patients develop strategies to avoid injury from falls if ataxia or dizziness is a problem
- Watch for signs of urinary retention
- Watch for hypothermia in older patients receiving beta-adrenergic drugs

---

Mexiletine

Mexiletine is a recently introduced oral anti-arrhythmic drug. Its mechanism of action is very much like that of parenteral lidocaine, and both drugs have local anesthetic properties. Mexiletine also has anticonvulsant actions.

Absorption, distribution, and excretion. Mexiletine is well absorbed from the gastrointestinal tract, making oral administration practical and effective. The onset of effect is within ½ hour to 2 hours. Excretion is primarily by hepatic metabolism; the half-life of drug in the blood may be doubled in severe hepatic disease but only slightly increased in renal impairment.

Side effects and toxicity. Side effects of mexiletine are generally dose-related, with the incidence increasing when plasma concentrations exceed 2 μg/ml. New ventricular arrhythmias may arise, including premature ventricular contractions and torsade de pointes. Heartburn, nausea, and vomiting usually occur within 2 hours of administration. Agranulocytosis, leukopenia, and thrombocytopenia may cause fever, chills, and unusual bruising or bleeding. CNS effects include dizziness, trembling, nervousness, and unsteady gait. Overdose can cause death due to respiratory failure and asystole.

Phenytoin

Phenytoin, a drug also used as an anticonvulsant (Chapter 34), may alter cardiac function by central nervous system effects. In heart cells, phenytoin changes membrane responsiveness, reducing the possibility for reentry, a process that con-tributes to severe arrhythmias. The major use of phenytoin is in digitalis-induced arrhythmias. Phenytoin is less effective than the other antiarrhythmic drugs for arrhythmias of other types.

Therapeutic, nontoxic levels of phenytoin do not cause significant depression of myocardial contractility. However, the drug is capable of producing dangerous myocardial depression if intravenous administration is too rapid. Bradycardia, hypotension, AV blockade, and cardiac arrest have been observed with venous injection faster than 50 mg per minute. The patient is observed for nausea, dizziness, or drowsiness, which are signs of excessive blood levels of the drug. Chronic use of phenytoin for its antiarrhythmic action is not recommended.

Tocainide

Tocainide, like lidocaine, is an amide-type of local anesthetic. Its action in the heart is very similar to that of lidocaine.

Absorption, distribution, and excretion. Tocainide is completely absorbed orally, whether taken with or without food. The onset of action is within 0.5 to 2 hours and the half-life is about 15 hours. Elimination is nearly equally divided between hepatic metabolism and renal excretion.

Side effects and toxicity. Shaking and trembling signal that maximal doses have been approached. Blisters, peeling skin, or skin rashes may signal a dangerous allergic reaction that can culminate in Stevens-Johnson syndrome. After several weeks of therapy, pulmonary damage can occur, with coughing and shortness of breath. Allergic reactions or pulmonary damage can be fatal.

Class 1-C Antiarrhythmic Drugs (Table 19.1)

Antiarrhythmics drugs of this type markedly depress phase 0 of the action potential (Figure 19.1) and profoundly slow conduction, especially in conductive fibers. Class 1-C antiarrhythmic agents are indicated only for control of life-threatening ventricular arrhythmias.

Encainide

Encainide may have greater effect in ischemic than in normal heart tissue. The drug has little effect on cardiac contractility.

Absorption, distribution, and excretion. Oral absorption is nearly total, with onset of action within 1 to 3 hours. Encainide is eliminated by hepatic metabolism to active metabolites (MODE, ODE). About 90% of the population rapidly form these metabolites while the remaining 10% are slow metabolizers and accumulate little of these metabolites.

Side effects and toxicity. Encainide has been associated with development of new and potentially fatal arrhythmias, especially when daily doses exceed 200 mg. Congestive heart failure, AV blockade, sinus bradycardia, sinus pause, or sinus arrest may occur. Overdose produces widening of QRS, prolongation of the QT interval, AV dissociation, hypotension, bradycardia, asystole, seizures, and finally can cause death.

Flecainide

Flecainide is very similar to encainide, but has local anesthetic action and may decrease contractility of the heart more than encainide.

Absorption, distribution, and excretion. Flecainide is nearly completely absorbed following oral administration with or without food. The major route of elimination is by hepatic metabolism and the drug has a long half-life of approximately 20 hours.

Side effects and toxicity. Flecainide has been associated with development of new and potentially fatal arrhythmias, especially when plasma concentrations exceed 1 μg/ml. Ventricular arrhythmias, congestive heart failure, and AV block are most common.

Class II Antiarrhythmic Drugs (Table 19.1)

Antiarrhythmic drugs of this type are beta-adrenergic receptor blockers that depress phase 4 depolarization of the action potential (Figure 19.1). Acebutolol and esmolol primarily block beta-1 receptors in the heart, but propranolol blocks beta receptors in many tissues.

Acebutolol

Acebutolol is a newer beta-adrenergic blocker that differs from the other two antiarrhythmic drugs of this class by having mild to moderate intrinsic sympathomimetic activity. In theory, blockade with this type of agent would never be complete, which would minimize risk of certain side effects. Acebutolol is used primarily to control premature ventricular contractions.

Absorption, distribution, and excretion. About 70% of an oral dose of acebutolol is absorbed. Metabolism by the liver produces an active metabolite with a longer half-life than that of the parent drug. The peak effect is obtained within 2.5 hours and persists for several hours. Elimination also involves renal excretion.

Side effects and toxicity. Like all beta-adrenergic blockers, acebutolol may cause hypoglycemia, peripheral vasoconstriction, and bronchospasm, but because the blockade is relatively selective for cardiac beta receptors, these effects may in theory be less likely. Overdose may cause slow or irregular heartbeat, dizziness, fainting, difficulty breathing, blue fingernail beds, or seizures.

Esmolol

Esmolol is a recently introduced drug intended for rapid, short-term control of ventricular rates in the face of atrial flutter or fibrillation. It is primarily an emergency medication for perioperative or postoperative use.

Absorption, distribution, and excretion. Esmolol is administered intravenously, is distributed to tissues within 2 minutes, and achieves therapeutic effect within 5 minutes. The duration of effect is only 10 to 20 minutes after the infusion is stopped. The drug is rapidly destroyed by esterases in red blood cells.

Side effects and toxicity. Hypotension is very common in patients receiving esmolol, and may be symptomatic in up to 12% of patients. Reduced peripheral circulation and difficulty breathing may also occur. Overdose may cause slow or irregular heartbeat, dizziness, fainting, difficulty breathing, blue fingernail beds, or seizures.

Propranolol

Propranolol is a beta adrenergic blocking drug (Chapter 10) that decreases contractility in the heart. The drug may decrease cardiac automaticity by blocking the effects of the sympathetic nervous system. The most important antiarrhythmic action of propranolol is to increase the refractory period of the AV node. In addition, the drug has a quini-

THE NURSING PROCESS

ANTIARRHYTHMIC THERAPY

Assessment

Antiarrhythmic therapy is used in patients with cardiac arrhythmias. Diagnosis of the abnormal rhythm is made by use of the electrocardiogram (ECG), although patients may seek medical evaluation with complaints such as "missed beats," "fluttering" in the chest, pounding in the chest, irregular heartbeat (rates), and other subjective complaints. The nurse should perform a thorough cardiovascular assessment to determine the patient baseline, identify possible causes, and determine if other cardiac problems exist.

Nursing diagnoses

Potential altered health maintenance related to insufficient knowledge of the implications of drug therapy

Potential activity intolerance related to fatigue and weakness secondary to drug side effects

Potential complication: cardiac arrhythmias

Management

Treatment of the acute or most serious arrhythmias is usually done in the coronary care unit or other acute care setting, where bedside cardiac monitoring, emergency drugs, and equipment for resuscitation are readily available. For less serious arrhythmias, therapy is begun in the nonacute care setting, although the only accurate way to monitor the effect of the drugs on the rhythm is through cardiac monitoring. After the patient is stabilized and the dose adjusted, cardiac monitoring is needed only intermittently by periodic ECG tracings.

The nurse should ascertain the goal of therapy after consultation with the physician, but in general the goal would be to eliminate a potentially life-threatening arrhythmia and change the patient's arrhythmia to a less serious form or to restore normal sinus rhythm, if possible. The possible goal of therapy will be tempered by the specific arrhythmia displayed, its cause, the general condition of the heart, other physiological problems of the patient, other drugs being used, and the incidence of side effects of therapy. In preparing for discharge, the health care team should decide on the drugs and doses for chronic management, and other treatments that would be appropriate (e.g., dietary restrictions, activity restrictions). During dosage adjustment, the nurse should monitor the vital signs and blood pressure, weight, fluid intake and output, serum electrolyte levels, and laboratory work appropriate for the drug being used. The nurse should also observe the general physical condition of the patient and watch for the appearance of side effects.

Evaluation

Before discharge, it would be desirable to have the patient in a stable cardiac rhythm, either normal sinus rhythm or a nonthreatening arrhythmia. The nurse should evaluate the patient to see if this goal has been met and evaluate for the side effects of therapy. The patient should be able to explain or to demonstrate why and how to take the prescribed drugs, interactions between drugs, how to plan meals within prescribed dietary restrictions, how to manage persistent side effects (e.g., constipation with atropine, hyperglycemia with phenytoin), the signs and symptoms of toxicity, what situations warrant notifying the physician, and what side effects may occur. For more specific information, see the patient care implications section at the end of this chapter.

dine-like membrane effect that slows phase 0 of the action potential.

Propranolol is used for supraventricular arrhythmias, ventricular tachycardias, and drug-induced tachyarrhythmias.

Absorption, distribution, excretion. Propranolol is well absorbed orally, but blood levels are diminished by a substantial first-pass effect (Chapter 2). Elimination is primarily by hepatic mechanisms.

Side effects and toxicity. The most significant dangers of propranolol used as an antiarrhythmic agent result from the beta adrenergic blockade. This effect is especially dangerous in patients with a significant degree of heart failure that has been compensated by increased sympathetic stimulation of the heart. Blockade of these sympathetic influences may produce bradycardia or heart arrest, especially if partial AV block is already present. In addition, propranolol may precipitate severe bronchospasm, since it also blocks the beta receptors in the lung (Chapter 25). This reaction is more common in patients with a history of asthma or allergies.

Of the three beta-adrenergic drugs, propranolol is most likely to cause CNS side effects, such as mental depression, dizziness, drowsiness, insomnia, or weakness.

Class III Antiarrhythmic Drugs (Table 19.1)

Antiarrhythmics of this type primarily prolong phase 3, the repolarization phase, of the action potential (Figure 19.1).

Amiodarone

Amiodarone has many actions on cardiac tissues, the net result of which is to prolong the refractory period and reduce automaticity. Amiodarone also may depress contractility and may cause vasodilation. The drug produces noncompetitive beta-adrenergic blockade and blocks calcium channels. It is used for prophylaxis or therapy of life-threatening ventricular arrhythmias.

Absorption, distribution, and excretion. Oral absorption is variable, with most patients absorbing much less than half the administered dose. Amiodarone is highly lipid soluble and is sequestered in adipose tissue, as well as other sites. As a result the onset of action is measured in days or even months. The duration of action is also greatly prolonged. The drug may be detectable in plasma up to 9 months after it has been discontinued.

Side effects and toxicity. Sinus bradycardia is common, and arrest or heart block may occur. New arrhythmias may be generated in up to 5% of patients. Up to 15% of patients suffer significant pulmonary toxicity, which may be fatal. Neurotoxicity, signaled by weakness, numbness, or ataxia, may occur in up to 40% of patients. Sensitivity to sun, ocular toxicity, and hypothyroidism are also expected effects. Reversal of side effects may take months after cessation of therapy.

Bretylium

Bretylium has a mechanism of action different from that of other antiarrhythmic drugs. The drug increases the action potential duration and hence prolongs the refractory period. It does not directly suppress automaticity or conduction velocity. Bretylium accumulates in sympathetic neurons and causes an initial release of norepinephrine that may stimulate contractility, heart rate, and automaticity, but ultimately the drug produces an adrenergic blockade by preventing norepinephrine release. Bretylium is used primarily for life-threatening ventricular tachycardia, especially episodes refractory to lidocaine or cardioversion, and for ventricular fibrillation.

Absorption, distribution, and excretion. Bretylium is administered intravenously or intramuscularly. The duration of action is 6 to 8 hours and most of the drug is excreted by the kidneys.

Side effects and toxicity. The major reactions to this drug are precipitation of anginal attacks, bradycardia, and hypotension. Bretylium does not alter the electrocardiogram.

Class IV Antiarrhythmic Drugs (Table 19.1)

Antiarrhythmic drugs of this type primarily depress phase 4 depolarization and lengthen phase 1 and 2 repolarization. The heart rate may slow significantly.

Verapamil

Verapamil is a calcium channel blocking drug used not only as an antiarrhythmic agent but also as an antianginal agent (Chapter 14). The slow calcium ion current blocked by verapamil is more important for the activity of the AV node than for many other tissues in the heart. By interfering with this current, the calcium channel blockers achieve some selectivity of action. The major antiarrhythmic effect of verapamil is a delay in conduction through the AV node.

The drug is well absorbed by the oral route, but it is rapidly metabolized by the liver. This first-pass phenomenon significantly reduces its bioavailability (Chapter 2). Some of its metabolites may be active. Cirrhosis of the liver significantly diminishes drug elimination.

Verapamil may be administered intravenously when the oral route is inappropriate.

Miscellaneous Antiarrhythmic Drugs

Atropine

Atropine, a drug previously discussed as a blocker of muscarinic cholinergic receptors (Chapter 9), may also be used to treat certain arrhythmias. Its action as an antiarrhythmic drug depends on its ability to reduce the effects of vagal nerve stimulation, primarily on the SA node. Since stimulation of the vagus nerve slows heart rate, atropine is able to increase heart rate by blocking that effect. Because it also speeds conduction through the AV node, it may lessen heart block in certain cases.

Digitalis

Digitalis is primarily a cardiotonic agent (Chapter 18). However, in addition to its ability to strengthen contraction of the heart muscle, digitalis also increases vagal tone at the AV node. Through this action and the direct effects on nodal tissue, digitalis slows conduction through the AV node. This action is the primary one that is sought when digitalis is used as an antiarrhythmic agent.

As with all the other antiarrhythmic drugs, at higher concentrations digitalis may also *cause* arrhythmias of various types, most characteristically bradycardia and premature ventricular contractions. Bradycardia may be a sign of impending heart block (no impulse passes through the AV node to the ventricles). Premature ventricular contractions arise because digitalis increases the spontaneous rate of ventricular depolarization (phase 4 of the action potential). It increases the automaticity of Purkinje fibers in the ventricles.

Any digitalis preparation has the potential to be used as an antiarrhythmic agent. However, in practice digoxin is commonly used intravenously in an emergency and then continued orally for maintenance or prophylaxis (Table 19.3). *Deslanoside* (Cedilanid-D) may sometimes be used in emergencies.

Pharmacological Therapy of Arrhythmias

Atrial flutter and fibrillation are usually serious arrhythmias that demand treatment. Several useful drugs are available. The digitalis glycoside digoxin is frequently selected. The rationale for this therapy is that, by lowering the conduction of impulses through the AV node, digoxin protects the ventricles from overstimulation. The short-term therapeutic goal is not to slow the atrial rate, but to produce a partial heart block that allows fewer of the impulses from the atria to stimulate the ventricles to beat. The patient may therefore be maintained with rapid atrial rates but with ventricular rates from 60 to 80 beats per minute. Many patients spontaneously convert to normal sinus rhythm after a few days of treatment.

Beta-adrenergic blockers such as esmolol or propranolol can also slow ventricular rates in the face of atrial flutter, fibrillation, or tachycardia. These agents prolong AV conduction times and block beta adrenergic receptors, which may also reduce catecholamine stimulation of the heart. Both effects tend to slow heart rate.

Occasionally quinidine may be selected to control atrial flutter or fibrillation. Since its anticholinergic action may speed conduction through the AV node, the first result of this therapy may be a dramatic increase in the ventricular rate. Digoxin or a related drug should always be used before quinidine in this case to prevent a dangerous overstimulation of the ventricles during the initial phases of treatment. Once atrial rates have been sufficiently reduced, this action of quinidine on the AV node poses no particular problem to the patient.

Verapamil may also effectively slow AV conduction and protect the ventricles when atrial flutter or fibrillation is present.

Sinus tachycardia, a rapid atrial rate, may not be harmful unless the ventricular rate is also abnormally increased. Many physicians do not administer antiarrhythmic drugs to patients with rapid atrial rates and no other symptoms. Sinus tachycardia may be produced in normal persons by anxiety, by ingestion of coffee, tea, or alcoholic beverages, or by smoking. Drugs such as nitrites, sympathomimetics, anticholinergics, or phenothiazines may also induce transient sinus tachycardia.

Sinus bradycardia is usually of minor importance and is not treated. If bradycardia is associated with reduced cardiac output, atropine or isoproterenol may be prescribed. Atropine increases the heart rate by blocking the effects of vagal nerve stimulation, whereas isoproterenol directly stimulates the heart through the beta adrenergic receptors.

Ventricular premature contractions occur when the ventricles beat in response to both the SA node and an abnormal pacemaker. The ECG pattern shows a normal QRS complex following a P wave such as that shown in Figure 19.2, plus an abnormal QRS complex that is isolated from a P wave. These arrhythmias are found even among normal persons. If these premature contractions are rare, they are ordinarily not treated, unless the patient is recuperating from a myocardial infarction. If the patient complains of palpitations with the

PATIENT CARE IMPLICATIONS

General guidelines for patients receiving antiarrhythmic drugs

Drug administration

- Monitor the vital signs and blood pressure. Although a change in the heart rate is frequently a desired outcome of therapy, a heart rate less than 60 or greater than 120 beats per minute (in an adult) should usually be avoided. Establish specific guidelines for each patient in consultation with the physician.
- Monitor the electrocardiogram (ECG). In the acute care situation, monitor the continuous ECG tracing. Check the tracing on a regular basis on outpatients.
- Monitor other indicators of cardiovascular functioning as appropriate: blood pressure and pulse, intake and output, weight, heart and lung sounds. Assess for edema, especially in dependent areas, and jugular venous distention. Assess for activity tolerance with daily activities.
- Monitor the BUN, liver function studies, and serum drug levels if available.
- For intravenous administration, use microdrip tubing and an electronic infusion monitor. Usually, monitor the ECG during IV administration. Monitor the blood pressure and pulse. Keep patient supine after IV doses until vital signs are stable. Keep siderails up. Have emergency equipment and drugs available to treat toxicity or for resuscitation.

Patient and family education

- Teach patients about the desired effects and common side effects of prescribed drugs. Tell patients to report the development of any unexpected sign or symptom. Point out that drugs or doses may need to be changed or adjusted if unusual side effects are developing, so patients should not hesitate to contact the physician.
- Review with patients the importance of taking medications as ordered. Antiarrhythmic drugs are most effective when taken on a regular basis, as prescribed. If a dose is missed, patients should not double up for missed doses. Refer patients as appropriate to community-based nursing care agencies.
- Emphasize to patients not to discontinue antiarrhythmic medications without first consulting with the physician.
- Stress the importance of concomitant therapies, if ordered: diet therapy, weight reduc-

tion, sodium restriction, use of potassium replacements, diuretics, antihypertensives, limiting caffeine intake, stopping smoking.
- Assess the need for patients to monitor weight, pulse, blood pressure, or other parameters in the home setting. Consider the medical condition, prescribed medications, ability, and resources in making this decision.
- Suggest that the patient carry a medical identification tag or bracelet indicating that antiarrhythmics are being used.
- Avoid drinking alcoholic beverages unless approved by the physician.
- Keep all health care providers informed of all medications being used, including dentists.
- Keep all medications out of the reach of children.
- *Digoxin* is discussed in Chapter 18.
- *Beta-adrenergic receptor blockers* are discussed in Chapter 15.
- *Calcium channel blockers* are discussed in Chapter 14.
- *Phenytoin* is discussed in Chapter 47.

Amiodarone

Drug administration

- See the general guidelines for antiarrhythmic therapy.
- Assess breath sounds and respiratory rate for signs of pulmonary toxicity.
- Assess visual acuity at the start of therapy.

Patient and family education

- Review the general guidelines for antiarrhythmic therapy. Review the common side effects (see text). Instruct patient to report the development of respiratory difficulties, weakness, numbness, or ataxia.
- Review the hazards of photosensitivity (see Patient Problem: Photosensitivity on p. 647). Patients on this drug who develop photosensitivity may be sensitive even to sunlight coming through windows.
- Instruct the patient to report subjective visual or eye changes. Encourage patients who wear glasses to continue periodic ophthalmic examinations.
- Warn patients that the skin may turn a bluish-gray color, but the discoloration should fade when therapy is discontinued. Notify the physician if skin color begins to change.
- Review Patient Problems: Constipation on p. 187.

Continued.

PATIENT CARE IMPLICATIONS — cont'd

Atropine

Drug administration/patient and family education

- See the general guidelines for antiarrhythmic therapy, and review the patient care implications for anticholinergic drugs at the end of Chapter 13.
- See Patient Problem: Xerostomia on p. 169 and Patient Problems: Constipation on p. 187.
- Intravenous administration: May be given undiluted, or dilute dose in at least 10 ml of sterile water. Do not add to infusing fluids or drugs. Administer at a rate of 1.0 mg or less over 1 minute.

Bretylium

Drug administration

- See the general guidelines for antiarrhythmic therapy.
- Intramuscular administration: Administer in large muscle masses. Record and rotate injection sites. Do not dilute. Do not administer more than 5 ml into a single injection site; if a larger volume is ordered, divide the dose into two equal volumes for injection into two sites.
- IV push administration: May be given undiluted, one dose over 1 minute or less.
- Intermittent administration: Dilute drug in at least 50 ml of diluent, or use commercially prepared diluted solutions. Administer dose over 10 to 30 minutes. Too rapid infusion may contribute to nausea and vomiting.
- Continuous infusion: use microdrip tubing and an infusion control device.
- This drug is rarely used outside of the acute care setting. Keep patient and family informed of patient's condition.

Disopyramide

Drug administration

- See general guidelines for antiarrhythmic therapy.
- Assess for urinary retention: monitor intake and output, question patient about hesitancy or difficulty voiding, palpate bladder.
- Monitor blood sugar, as this drug can cause hypoglycemia.

Patient and family education

- See general guidelines for antiarrhythmic therapy.

- See Patient Problems: Xerostomia (p. 170), Orthostatic Hypotension (p. 237), and Constipation (p. 187). Tell patient to report any difficulty with urinating.
- Review the signs of hypoglycemia: fast heartbeat, cold sweats, headache, hunger, nausea, nervousness, shakiness, unsteady walk, anxious feeling. Tell patients to eat or drink a food containing sugar if this develops, and to notify the physician. Instruct diabetic patient to monitor blood glucose levels.
- Caution patients to avoid driving or operating hazardous equipment if dizziness or blurred vision develops; notify the physician.
- This drug may cause patients to sweat less. Tell patients to take frequent rest periods if engaging in strenuous activities, and to limit time in hot environments or in direct sunlight.
- Take disopyramide on an empty stomach, 1 hour before or 2 hours after meals. Tell patients taking the extended-release form to swallow the dose whole, without chewing or crushing.

Encainide and Flecainide

Drug administration/patient and family education

- See general guidelines for antiarrhythmic therapy.
- Tell patients to avoid driving or operating hazardous equipment if dizziness or visual changes develop. Notify the physician.
- Some patients experience a metallic taste. Monitor weight. If patient is unable to tolerate this side effect, consult physician. Remind patients not to discontinue medication without consulting physician.

Lidocaine

Drug administration/patient and family education

- See general guidelines for antiarrhythmic therapy.
- This drug is rarely used outside of the acute care setting. Keep patient and family informed of the patient's condition.
- Assess for the side effects noted in the text. Instruct the patient to report any subjective change.
- Intramuscular administration: Read labels carefully. Lidocaine with epinephrine is not given as an antiarrhythmic. Administer IM doses into the deltoid muscle. IM injection

PATIENT CARE IMPLICATIONS — cont'd

may cause elevations in the serum creatine phosphokinase (CPK or CK) levels.

- Intravenous administration: Read labels carefully. Lidocaine with epinephrine is not used as an antiarrhythmic. Bolus doses may be given undiluted at a rate of 50 mg/min; too rapid administration may cause seizures. For continuous infusion, dilute per agency protocol or consult manufacturer's literature. Use microdrip tubing and adjust dose to patient response.

Mexiletene

Drug administration

- See general guidelines for antiarrhythmic therapy.
- Monitor white blood cell count, white blood cell differential, and platelet count.
- Assess for ataxia, nystagmus, and development of CNS side effects.

Patient and family education

- See general guidelines for antiarrhythmic therapy.
- See Patient Problems: Bleeding Tendencies (p. 600) and Depressed White Blood Cell Production (p. 599). Instruct patients to report the development of these rare but serious side effects.
- Caution patients to avoid driving or operating hazardous equipment if dizziness, double vision, or confusion develops; notify the physician.
- Take doses with meals or snack to lessen GI irritation.

Procainamide

Drug administration

- See general guidelines for antiarrhythmic therapy.
- Monitor antinuclear antibody (ANA) tests.
- Intravenous administration: For direct IV injection, dilute each 100 mg with 10 ml of 5% dextrose in water or sterile water. Administer at a rate of 20 mg/min. For infusion, add 1 Gm to 500 ml 5% dextrose in water for a dilution of 2 mg/ml. Use microdrip tubing, and infuse at a rate of 2 to 6 mg/min.

Patient and family education

- See general guidelines for antiarrhythmic therapy.
- Take doses with a full glassful (8 oz. of water) to lessen GI symptoms. The drug is most effective when taken on an empty stomach,

1 hour before or 2 hours after meals or snack. If GI symptoms are intolerable, instruct the patient to take doses with meals, and to take doses consistently, either always on an empty stomach, or always with meals.

- Swallow sustained-release preparations whole, without chewing or breaking them.
- Instruct patients to report the development of arthritis, polyarthralgia, pleuritic pain, myalgia, skin lesions, or fever, or any other new sign or symptom.
- Caution patients to avoid driving or operating hazardous equipment if dizziness develops; notify the physician.

Quinidine

Drug administration

- See general guidelines for antiarrhythmic therapy.
- Read labels carefully; do not confuse quinidine with quinine.
- Monitor liver function tests, blood count, platelet count, and prothrombin time.
- A test dose may be ordered before the full dose to test for possible idiosyncrasy to quinidine.
- Assess for rash or skin changes.
- Intravenous administration: Dilute 800 mg (10 ml) in at least 40 ml of 5% dextrose in water. Do not add to IV solutions or mix with other drugs in a syringe. Administer at a rate of 1 ml (16 mg)/min.
- IM injections may be painful and may increase serum creatine phosphokinase (CPK or CK) levels.

Patient and family education

- See general guidelines for antiarrhythmic therapy.
- Review symptoms of cinchonism with patient: ringing in the ears, headache, nausea, and/or changes in vision. Tell the patient to notify the physician if these occur.
- Review Patient Problem: Photosensitivity (p. 647) with the patient.
- Warn patients to avoid driving or operating hazardous equipment if visual changes occur; notify physician.
- Doses are best taken on an empty stomach with a full glassful (8 oz) of water, 1 hour before or 2 hours after meals. If GI symptoms are severe, take doses with meals. Notify physician if diarrhea develops.
- Swallow sustained-release preparations whole, without swallowing or crushing them.

Continued.

PATIENT CARE IMPLICATIONS — cont'd

- Review Patient Problems: Bleeding Tendencies (p. 600), and Depressed White Blood Cell Production (p. 599) with patients. Tell patients to report the development of any unexpected sign or symptom.

Tocainide

Drug administration

- See general guidelines for antiarrhythmic therapy.
- Assess regularly for skin changes or rashes. Auscultate breath sounds and assess respiratory rate.

Patient and family education

- See general guidelines for antiarrhythmic therapy.
- Take doses with food or milk to lessen gastric irritation.
- Tell patients to notify physician immediately if rashes, skin changes, peeling or scaling of skin, blisters on skin or mouth, cough or shortness of breath develops.
- Warn patients to avoid driving or operating hazardous equipment if dizziness, lightheadedness, confusion, or visual changes develop; notify physician.

---

premature ventricular contractions, mild sedatives may be prescribed. Abstaining from coffee, tea, and cigarettes may also control the condition.

When ventricular premature contractions occur frequently or in rapid succession or when they occur with other signs of cardiac disease, treatment may be instituted with lidocaine, acebutolol, disopyramide, mexiletine, tocainide, quinidine, or procainamide. If these contractions are caused by a previous myocardial infarction, lidocaine is the drug of choice in the hospital.

Ventricular tachycardia is usually related to the presence of ectopic foci stimulating premature ventricular contractions. Lidocaine is again the drug of choice and may be used to control or to prevent this arrhythmia. Many other drugs can also be effective against ventricular tachycardia. Mexiletine, procainamide, propranolol, quinidine, and tocainide can be given for treatment or prophylaxis. Disopyramide can be used for therapy or prophylaxis of episodic arrhythmias of this type. Amiodarone, bretylium, encainide, and flecainide are reserved for life-threatening arrhythmias.

Digitalis-induced arrhythmias constitute a significant fraction of arrhythmias seen in most clinics, usually arising in patients receiving digitalis as a cardiotonic agent. Digitalis may induce any type of arrhythmia but the most common ones are bradycardia, ventricular premature contractions, and AV nodal tachycardia. The first step in therapy is to discontinue the digitalis. If the arrhythmia is not severe, no further therapy may be required. However, digitalis preparations routinely used as cardiotonics are relatively long-acting drugs, and it

may be necessary to treat the arrhythmia while the digitalis is being eliminated from the system. Potassium levels should be assessed in these patients since a low potassium level increases the sensitivity of the heart to digitalis and may predispose to arrhythmias. Potassium supplements may be given if required.

Phenytoin is the drug most often selected to treat digitalis-induced arrhythmias of all types. Empirically, phenytoin seems more effective in most patients than the other drugs, although a mechanistic explanation for this observation is lacking. If phenytoin does not control the arrhythmia satisfactorily, lidocaine or propranolol may be tried.

SUMMARY

Cardiac arrhythmias are any deviation from the normal rate or pattern of heart pacing: sympathetic overstimulation of the SA node produces tachycardia, whereas vagal nerve overstimulation produces bradycardia. Heart rates and ECG patterns may be altered when ectopic foci develop and begin to compete with the normal pacing of the heart by the SA node. Prolonged conduction times through the AV node can result in skipped beats and heart block.

Antiarrhythmic drugs are classified according to their effects on the action potential of heart cells. Class 1-A drugs (disopyramide, procainamide, quinidine) depress phase 0 and prolong action potential duration. These drugs share the properties of depressing automaticity, conduction velocity, and contractility of the heart. Quinidine and procainamide have virtually identical actions on the heart and share an atropine-like blockade of parasympathetic innervation in the heart. Quinidine may produce allergic reactions and cardiac toxicity. With prolonged use, procainamide can produce a syndrome resembling lupus erythematosus.

Class 1-B drugs (lidocaine, mexiletine, phenytoin, tocainide) depress phase 0 slightly and may shorten the action potential duration. These drugs are used primarily for ventricular arrhythmias. Phenytoin, a drug also used as an anticonvulsant, is especially useful in treating digitalis-induced arrhythmias. Lidocaine, a local anesthetic, is very rapidly destroyed by the liver and must be administered by continuous intravenous infusion. Mexiletine and tocainide have similar actions but can be used orally.

Class 1-C drugs (encainide, flecainide) markedly depress phase 0 and profoundly slow conduction in the heart. These drugs are reserved for life-threatening ventricular arrhythmias because both have been associated with fatal side effects.

Class II drugs (acebutolol, esmolol, propranolol) are beta-adrenergic receptor blockers and depress phase 4 depolarization in the heart. Blocking beta adrenergic effects in the heart may lower automaticity, but it may be dangerous in heart failure when sympathetic stimulation may be critical in maintaining cardiac output.

Class III drugs (amiodarone, bretylium) prolong phase 3 repolarization. These drugs are used for refractory or life-threatening ventricular arrhythmias.

Class IV drugs (verapamil) are calcium channel blockers that slow conduction through the AV node. Verapamil is the only drug of this class currently indicated for use as an antiarrhythmic agent.

Miscellaneous drugs used as antiarrhythmics include atropine and digoxin. Atropine blocks muscarinic cholinergic receptors and therefore blocks the action of the vagus nerve on the SA node. Atropine increases heart rates. Digoxin is a digitalis glycoside used primarily as a cardiotonic drug. As an antiarrhythmic, digoxin is used primarily to slow conduction through the AV node. Digoxin may induce arrhythmias, the most common of which is bradycardia.

STUDY QUESTIONS

1. What is an action potential?
2. What tissues in the heart are normally automatic?
3. Describe how the waves on an ECG are related to electrical activity of different portions of the heart.
4. What is the normal pacemaker of the heart?
5. What is the effect of vagus nerve stimulation on the heart?
6. What is the effect of sympathetic stimulation on the heart?
7. What is the refractory period?
8. What is reentry?
9. What are the classes of antiarrhythmic drugs? Upon what is the classification based?
10. What is the mechanism of action of quinidine and procainamide?
11. What secondary action do both quinidine and procainamide share?
12. How do the toxic effects of quinidine and procainamide differ?
13. What is the mechanism of action of disopyramide?
14. Lidocaine, mexiletine, and tocainide are most effective on which tissue in the heart?
15. How does the use of lidocaine differ from that of mexiletine and tocainide?
16. For what type of arrhythmia is phenytoin especially useful?
17. Encainide and flecainide are reserved for what special clinical indication? Why?
18. What is the mechanism of antiarrhythmic effect shared by acebutolol, esmolol, and propranolol?
19. What is the mechanism of action of amiodarone?
20. What are the uses of amiodarone?
21. What are the side effects of amiodarone?
22. What is the mechanism of action of bretylium used as an antiarrhythmic agent?
23. What is the mechanism of action of verapamil as an antiarrhythmic agent?

SUGGESTED READINGS

Andrews, L.K.: ECG rhythms made easier with algorithms, Am. J. Nurs. **89**(3):365, 1989.

Atchison, J.J.: Arrhythmia or artifact? Am. J. Nurs. **89**(2):210, 1989.

Benning, C.A., and Burke, P.A.: Tocainide in the cardiac ICU, Crit. Care Nurse **9**(2):45, 1989.

Breckenridge, A.M.: When should plasma levels of cardioactive drugs be monitored? Drug Therapy **14**(5):177, 1984.

Brodgen, R.N., and Todd, P.A.: Disopyramide: a reappraisal of pharmacodynamic and pharmacokinetic properties and therapeutic use in cardiac arrhythmias, Drugs **34**:151, 1987.

Brodgen, R.N., and Todd, P.A.: Encainide: a review of its pharmacological properties and therapeutic efficacy, Drugs **34**:519, 1987.

Crumpley, L.: An overview of antiarrhythmic drugs, Crit. Care Nurse **3**(4):57, 1983.

Drayer, D.: Basic clinical pharmacology of the antiarrhythmic drugs procainamide and quinidine, Cardiovasc. Rev. Rep. **2**(5):475, 1981.

Fenster, P.E., and Bressler, R.: Treating cardiovascular diseases in the elderly. I. Digitalis glycosides and beta-blockers, Drug Therapy **14**(2):125, 1984.

Fenster, P.E., and Bressler, R.: Treating cardiovascular diseases in the elderly. II. Antiarrhythmics, diuretics, and calcium channel blockers, Drug Therapy **14**(3):209, 1984.

Flaherty, K.K., and others: Hepatotoxicity associated with amiodarone therapy, Pharmacotherapy **9**(1):39, 1989.

Frye, and Lounsbury: Cardiac rhythm disorders: an introductory text using the nursing process. Baltimore, 1988, Williams & Wilkins.

Gever, L.N.: Giving procainamide safely, Nursing 84 **14**(5): 116, 1984.

Kupersmith, J.: Use of calcium channel blockers in cardiac arrhythmias, Prim. Cardiology **2**(suppl.):159, 1983.

Lazarus, M., Nolasco, V.M., and Luckett, C.: Cardiac arrhythmias: diagnosis and treatment, Crit. Care Nurse **8**(7):57, 1989.

Meola, D.R., and Walker, V.: Respond quickly to tachydysrhythmias, Nursing 87 **17**(1):34, 1987.

Nestico, P.F., Morganroh, J., and Horowitz, L.N.: New antiarrhythmic drugs, Drugs **35**:286, 1988.

Strathman, I., and others: Hypoglycemia in patients receiving disopyramide therapy, Drug Intell. Clin. Pharm. **17**(9):635, 1983.

Tordjman, T., and Estes, N.A.M. III: Encainide: its electrophysiologic and antiarrhythmic effects, pharmacokinetics and safety. Pharmacotherapy **7**(5):149, 1987.

Wilson, R.R., and Wallace, A.G.: Drug therapy: disopyramide, Cardiovasc. Rev. Rep. **3**(3):414, 1982.

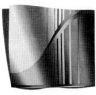

Agents Affecting Blood Coagulation

20

THE ROLE OF PLATELETS IN BLOOD COAGULATION

Platelets (thrombocytes) are the small cell fragments in blood that are derived from giant bone marrow cells called megakaryocytes. Ordinarily platelets do not stick to each other or to the endothelial lining of the blood vessels. When there is a break in the endothelial lining, however, platelets readily attach to the collagen in the exposed tissue. This attachment causes the platelets to aggregate, rapidly forming a plug that stops the bleeding and aids in the formation of a blood clot (thrombus). This aggregation of platelets in the presence of abnormal surfaces is the initial step in the normal repair system for the blood vessels. Drugs that interfere with this process have been termed either *antiplatelet* or *antithrombic* drugs.

In the late 1970s it was discovered that when the platelets adhere to a surface, they synthesize thromboxane A_2, a substance related to the prostaglandins. Thromboxane A_2 is a potent stimulus for the further aggregation of platelets and thereby accelerates the formation of the platelet plug. Therefore drugs blocking the synthesis of thromboxane A_2 inhibit the aggregation of platelets to form a plug. Aspirin and sulfinpyrazone (Anturane) are inhibitors of thromboxane A_2 synthesis. Dipyridamole (Persantine) and sulfinpyrazone prolong the survival of platelets in persons with thromboembolic diseases so that platelets do not initiate thrombus formation as readily. These drugs are listed in Table 20.1.

CLINICAL USE OF ANTIPLATELET DRUGS (Table 20.1)

The role of platelet aggregation as the initial step leading to blood coagulation is well established. In particular, the blood clots forming in the arterial system, as opposed to the venous system, are highly linked to conditions promoting platelet aggregation. Patients readily identified as at risk for developing arterial clots are those who have already suffered a myocardial infarction or a stroke. Among patients who have experienced a transient ischemic attack (TIA), or a ministroke, aspirin has been found effective in decreasing the incidence of further TIAs, strokes, or death. Sulfinpyrazone and dipyridamole were not found to be effective. Another established clinical use of antiplatelet drugs is for heart valve prostheses, disorders, and shunts.

The dose of aspirin may be important to its effectiveness in preventing thrombus formation. A low dose of aspirin (80 to 180 mg per day) inhibits the synthesis of thromboxane A_2 by the platelets as just discussed. A higher dose of aspirin (1000 mg per day) also inhibits the synthesis of prostacyclin (prostaglandin I_2) by the epithelial lining of the blood vessel. Prostacyclin inhibits the aggregation of platelets, an action directly opposite that of thromboxane A_2. Prostacyclin therefore prevents the formation of a platelet plug. For this reason a high dose of aspirin may be less effective than the low dose in preventing the formation of a thrombus. In fact, a recent study verified the effectiveness of taking one aspirin every other day as a method of reducing the risk of a heart attack. Over 22,000 doctors in the United States volunteered to take a buffered aspirin or a placebo every other day. At the end of 5 years, the aspirin takers had half the number of heart attacks and one third the deaths from heart attacks experienced by the placebo takers. However, these doctors were initially screened and found to be in normal health, so that the applicability of this study to the general population is not yet known.

Table 20.1 Antiplatelet Drugs

Generic name	Trade name	Administration/dosage	Comments
Aspirin		ORAL: *Adults*—After TIA: 325 mg with each meal and at bedtime or 650 mg twice a day. Prosthetic heart valve: 325 mg with each meal. AV shunt or fistula: 160 mg with each meal and at bedtime. Graft patency: 325 mg after each meal. Prevention of MI or sudden death in patient with unstable angina: 325 mg with each meal and at bedtime. Prevention of recurrent MI or coronary death post-MI: 325 to 1300 mg per day.	Taken with a coumarin for prosthetic heart valve. Taken with dipyridamole for graft patency.
Dipyridamole	Persantine* Apo-Dypridamole†	ORAL: *Adults*—75 mg 3 times a day. Aspirin, 325 mg, 3 times a day, is taken concurrently to prevent myocardial reinfarction (prophylactic). FDA Pregnancy Category B.	Taken to prevent thrombi formation with a prosthetic heart valve or to maintain graft patency. Taken with a coumarin for prosthetic heart valve. May also be taken with aspirin for a prosthetic heart valve or graft patency.
Sulfinpyrazone	Anturan† Anturane Antazone† Apo-sulfinpyrazone† Novopyrazone†	ORAL: *Adults*—200 mg 4 times a day.	Taken to prevent thrombi formation with a prosthetic heart valve, AV shunt or fistula, mitral stenosis, or to prevent sudden death after a myocardial infarction. Taken with a coumarin for prosthetic heart valve or mitral stenosis.

*Available in Canada and United States.
†Available in Canada only.

BLOOD COAGULATION AND THE MECHANISMS OF ANTICOAGULANTS

The schema of blood coagulation is diagrammed in Figure 20.1. The initial step can be an event in the intrinsic pathway, the activation of the blood component factor XII (the Hageman factor) by contact with exposed collagen, or an event in the extrinsic pathway, that is, the release of tissue factor by damaged tissue. Either pathway results in the activation of factor X. Factor Xa (activated factor X) forms a complex with platelet phospholipids, calcium, and factor V. This complex, which is sometimes called thromboplastin, catalyzes the conversion of prothrombin (factor II) to thrombin. Thrombin then catalyzes the conversion of fibrinogen to fibrin. After cross-linking of fibrin by factor XIIIa, fibrin becomes insoluble, forming a mesh that is the blood clot.

Blood clots in the arterial system are initially composed largely of platelets with a fibrin mesh (white thrombus). Blood clots in the venous system have only a few platelet aggregates and are composed largely of fibrin with trapped red blood cells (red thrombus). A thrombus in either the arterial or venous system may dislodge, becoming an embolus. Venous emboli often lodge in the small arteries of the pulmonary circulation, thereby markedly blocking the oxygenating capacity of the lungs and increasing the blood pressure in the pulmonary system, a life-threatening situation. Thrombi tend to form in veins when blood flow is low, favoring the accumulation of activated clotting factors. Patients at risk for experiencing venous thrombosis include those immobilized as a result of trauma or surgery and those with a history of thromboembolism.

Anticoagulant drugs are drugs that interfere with any of the steps depicted in Figure 20.1, leading to the formation of fibrin. Blood coagulation is often referred to as a *cascade phenomenon*, since

FIGURE 20.1   The stages of blood coagulation are diagrammed. Actions of drug classes discussed in this chapter include four stages.

Stage I:

  a. Antiplatelet drugs inhibit platelet aggregation in the intrinsic pathway.
  b. Citrate and EDTA, which chelate calcium, prevent the formation of factor Xa.
  c. Heparin, by activating antithrombin III, neutralizes factor Xa and stops coagulation at stage 1.
  d. Oral anticoagulants prevent the synthesis of factors VII, IX, and X, which are necessary for stage 1.
  e. Local hemostatic agents provide a contact to activate the intrinsic pathway.

Stage II: Oral anticoagulants prevent the synthesis of prothrombin.

Stage III: Heparin activates antithrombin III to prevent thrombin activity.

Stage IV:

  a. Aminocaproic acid inhibits the activation of profibrinolysin and so inhibits clot degradation.
  b. TPA, streptokinase, and urokinase activate profibrinolysin to aid clot digestion.

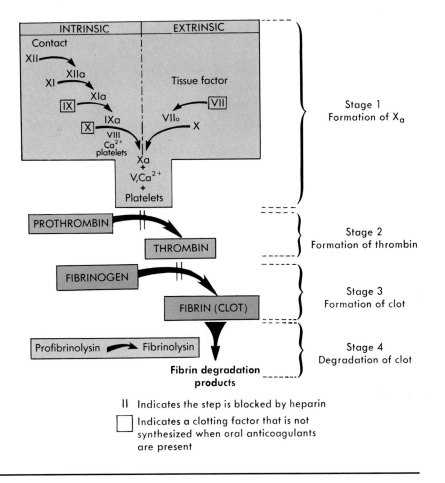

the process becomes magnified at every step. Each activated factor is a catalyst leading to the formation of many molecules of the next activated factor. The earlier in the process that a step can be blocked, the more efficient will be the inhibition of blood coagulation.

ANTICOAGULANTS

Anticoagulant drugs can be classified into three groups: (1) agents that remove calcium, (2) the drug heparin, and (3) oral anticoagulants.

Agents That Remove Calcium

Calcium is a cofactor for each of the steps through the activation of prothrombin. The removal of calcium will prevent the coagulation of blood. *Citrate* and *ethylenediaminetetraacetic acid (EDTA)* are compounds that complex calcium, making calcium unavailable for blood coagulation. When blood is drawn for testing or storage, citrate or EDTA may be present to keep the blood from clotting in the container. Since calcium is essential for many biochemical events, anticoagulants that complex calcium can be used only

in storage containers (in vitro), not in a patient (in vivo).

Heparin (Table 20.2)

Heparin is an anticoagulant that can either be administered to the patient or added to a storage container.

Mechanism. Heparin activates a plasma protein, antithrombin III. As the name indicates, antithrombin III will neutralize thrombin. However, antithrombin III also neutralizes factor Xa, the step before the activation of prothrombin to thrombin. This inhibition of factor Xa, rather than the inhibition of thrombin, appears to be primarily responsible for the effective anticoagulant action of heparin in low doses. Heparin may also serve as an antiplatelet drug. In vitro, heparin actually stimulates platelet aggregation. In vivo, however, heparin appears to coat the endothelial lining of the vessels. Since heparin is a highly negatively charged polymer, heparin adds a negative charge to the endothelium which keeps platelets from attaching and forming a thrombus.

Clinical uses of heparin. There are three clin-

Table 20.2   Anticoagulant Drugs

Generic name	Trade name	Administration/dosage	Comments
Heparin	Calciparine* Calcilean† Liquaemin Hepalean†	SUBCUTANEOUS: 10,000 to 20,000 units, then 8000 to 10,000 units every 8 hr or 15,000 to 20,000 units every 12 hr. INTRAVENOUS: *Intermittent*—10,000 units, then 5000 to 10,000 units every 4 to 6 hr. *Continuous*—20,000 to 40,000 units daily in 1000 ml. SUBCUTANEOUS: 5000 units 2 hr before surgery, then every 8 to 12 hr until ambulatory. FDA Pregnancy Category C.	High dose for therapeutic anticoagulation. Low dose for prophylaxis of postoperative thromboembolism.
ORAL ANTICOAGULANTS			
Anisindione	Miradon*	ORAL: 300 mg day 1, 200 mg day 2; 100 mg day 3, 25 to 250 mg daily for maintenance.	Half-life is 3 to 5 days. Peak effect in 2 to 3 days. Anticoagulant effect persists 1 to 3 days after discontinuance. Dermatitis is a side effect. Drug imparts an orange color to an alkaline urine.
Dicumarol (bishydroxycoumarin)		ORAL: 200 to 300 mg day 1; 25 to 200 mg daily for maintenance.	The prototype oral anticoagulant. Half-life is 1 to 2 days. Peak effect in 1 to 4 days. Anticoagulant effect persists 2 to 10 days after discontinuance. This coumarin is poorly and erratically absorbed.
Warfarin	Athrombin† Coumadin* Panwarfin Warfilone* Sofarin	ORAL, INTRAMUSCULAR, INTRAVENOUS: 10 to 15 mg daily until prothrombin time is in therapeutic range. 2 to 10 mg daily for maintenance. A loading dose of 40 to 60 mg (20 to 30 mg in the elderly) may be given initially.	Half-life is 2 days. Peak effect in 1 to 3 days. Anticoagulant effect persists 4 to 5 days after discontinuance.

*Available in Canada and United States.
†Available in Canada only.

ical uses of heparin that differ in dose and route of administration: (1) to achieve anticoagulation (in high doses), (2) to prevent postoperative thromboembolism (in low doses), and (3) to prevent coagulation of laboratory samples and stored blood in vitro.

High-dose administration. Heparin is used in the hospital to prevent the further growth of venous thrombi. Large doses (35 to 100 units/kg) must be administered intravenously to achieve this anticoagulation. Heparin cannot be taken orally, since it is not absorbed and it will cause a painful hematoma if administered intramuscularly. Heparin may be given as an intravenous injection, achieving immediate anticoagulation, with the same or lesser dose repeated every 4 to 6 hours. Blood levels of

heparin decrease by half every 1½ hours. Intermittent intravenous administration results in virtual incoagulability after administration and is associated with a higher risk of bleeding than continuous intravenous infusion. Thus an initial intravenous injection followed by continuous infusion at approximately 1000 units per hour is commonly given. An intravenous drip must be carefully monitored if used to deliver heparin, or overdosing may result, so an infusion monitor is usually used.

Low-dose administration. Heparin may also be given subcutaneously to achieve a slow, continual administration of heparin over an 8- to 12-hour period. Low-dose heparin is used for patients over 40 years of age undergoing thoracoabdominal surgery who are known to be at increased risk. It is not

THE NURSING PROCESS

ANTICOAGULANT DRUGS

Assessment

Anticoagulants are used in patients with a recent thrombus, who are immobilized after certain types of surgeries, have certain cardiac valve diseases, or require hemodialysis. Anticoagulation is done to prevent clot formation and does not dissolve existing clots. Baseline data to obtain would be related to the general physical condition of the patient, the history of problems with clots, bruising and/or easy bleeding, and blood coagulation studies that include prothrombin time (PT), partial thromboplastin time (PTT), platelet count, and clotting times. In addition, the presence of any bleeding should be documented.

Nursing diagnoses

Potential complication: hemorrhage

Potential altered health maintenance related to insufficient knowledge of the implications of anticoagulant therapy

Management

The blood coagulation studies should be monitored carefully, and the drug dosage calculated to maintain the desired range of anticoagulation. The patient should be monitored for bleeding from any site, and stools should be checked for occult blood. Any symptoms signaling possible embolus formation, such as chest pain or leg pain, or any symptom of internal bleeding, such as a headache, should be evaluated. An infusion monitoring device should be used for constant infusions of heparin, and dosages should be checked carefully. Discharge planning should be started by anticipating the level of anticoagulation desired, the drug to be used, and the length of time it will be taken. The antidotes for the drugs being used should be readily available during therapy.

Evaluation

The goals of anticoagulation therapy are to maintain the appropriate coagulation times within the desired range, to prevent thromboembolic problems, and to avoid side effects associated with bleeding. Before beginning self-management, the patient should be able to explain why the drug is needed, how to take the drug, the signs and symptoms of bleeding that should be reported, how to avoid injury and bruising, the side effects that may be related to the drug but that do not involve bleeding, and which additional side effects require notification of the physician. Finally, the patient should be able to state which other drugs, such as aspirin, should not be used while taking anticoagulants. For additional guidelines, see the patient care implications section at the end of this chapter.

---

used in brain, spinal cord, or eye surgery, in which even minor hemorrhage could be catastrophic. It is not effective in hip replacement surgery. Heparin is administered subcutaneously (5000 units) 2 hours before surgery, and then another 5000 units is administered every 8 to 12 hours until the patient is walking. This regimen can reduce the incidence of deep leg vein thrombosis by 50% in these patients without significantly affecting their bleeding or clotting times. The effectiveness of this therapy appears to result from heparin activating anti-thrombin III, which in turn rapidly inactivates newly formed factor Xa. After antithrombin III has inactivated factor Xa, the heparin can dissociate from this inactive complex and act again to cause further inactivation.

In vitro use. Heparin will prevent the coagulation of blood after it leaves the body. Tubing used to shunt blood can be pretreated with heparin to prevent clotting. The negative charge of the heparin coating on the wall of the tubing and preventing platelet adherence is probably the effective anti-

Table 20.3 Thrombolytic Drugs

Generic name	Trade name	Administration/dosage	Comments
TPA	Alteplase	INITIALLY: Intravenous bolus of 6-10 mg over 1-2 min, followed by intravenous infusion of 60 mg over the first hour and 20 mg over each of the second and third hours.	Monitor for dysrhythmias, reocclusion.
Streptokinase	Kabikinase Streptase*	Loading dose of 250,000 IU in 30 min, then intravenous infusion of 100,000 IU/hr. Dosage is continued for 24 to 72 hr for pulmonary embolism and for 72 hr for deep vein embolism. FDA Pregnancy Category C.	Thrombin times are monitored every 12 hr. Allergic reactions are common (15% of patients), usually of the milder variety: itching, flushing, nausea, headache. Treat with antihistamines.
Urokinase	Abbokinase Breokinase	Loading dose of 2000 IU/lb in 10 min by intravenous infusion, then 2000 IU/lb/hr for 12 hr. FDA Pregnancy Category B.	Isolated from human urine. Not as allergenic as streptokinase, but very expensive.

*Available in Canada and United States.

coagulant mechanism. Heparin is also added to containers to be used in the collection of blood. For transfusions, 4 to 6 units of heparin/ml of blood is used. For laboratory samples, 7 to 15 units of heparin/ml of blood is used.

Side effects. The major side effect of heparin is hemorrhage. Since the half-life of intravenously administered heparin is only 1½ hours, discontinuing heparin therapy is usually sufficient to reverse a hemorrhagic episode. If hemorrhaging must be stopped immediately, protamine sulfate may be given by slow intravenous infusion. Protamine is a highly positively charged molecule that complexes the negatively charged heparin. Protamine is itself an anticoagulant and has a longer half-life than does heparin. Protamine may persist and be the cause of bleeding after heparin is eliminated. One milligram of protamine sulfate neutralizes 100 units of heparin. No more than 50 mg of protamine sulfate should be administered in a 10-minute period.

Heparin is a natural compound, extracted from animal lungs or intestines for use in human beings. Some patients become allergic to heparin. The usual symptoms of heparin hypersensitivity are chills, fever, and urticaria, but other allergic reactions such as asthma, rhinitis, lacrimation, or even anaphylaxis have been reported. In some patients heparin has caused thrombocytopenia, so the platelet count should be measured daily after therapy.

Oral Anticoagulants (Table 20.2)

Four clotting factors—II (prothrombin), VII, IX, and X—are synthesized in the liver, with vitamin K as a necessary cofactor. If vitamin K is deficient, these clotting factors will be synthesized in a functionally inactive state, impairing blood coagulation.

Two classes of drugs, the *coumarins* and the *indandiones*, interfere with the regeneration of active vitamin K in the liver and thereby produce an effective vitamin K deficiency. Since it is the synthesis of functional clotting factors II, VII, IX, and X that is inhibited, the anticoagulant effect will not appear until preexisting factors II, VII, IX, and X are removed by normal degradation. This takes 1 day or longer. Factor II, prothrombin, is the longest lived of these clotting factors, and 24 hours is required to deplete half the existing prothrombin. A one-stage prothrombin test is frequently used to determine if the dose of oral anticoagulants is appropriate. Therapeutic doses of the oral anticoagulants increase the prothrombin time by 1½ to 2½ times the baseline values. Anticoagulant therapy must be individualized for each patient.

Anticoagulants that are vitamin K antagonists are ineffective in preventing coagulation of blood after it is drawn, since the clotting factors are already synthesized and present.

The major indication for the oral anticoagulants is the prophylaxis or treatment for a thrombus, either deep venous or pulmonary. However,

THE NURSING PROCESS

THROMBOLYTIC DRUGS

Assessment

The difference between anticoagulant therapy and thrombolytic therapy is that the goal of anticoagulant therapy is clot prevention and a clot already present will not be altered; in thrombolytic therapy, the clot is already present and the goal is clot dissolution. Both groups of drugs, however, alter the normal coagulation mechanism to cause anticoagulation. Baseline data needed for thrombolytic therapy are similar to those needed with heparin or coumarin therapy, with emphasis on assessment of the size and location of the clot and the signs and symptoms caused by the clot. A recent patient history of streptococcal infection would influence the choice of agents and should be documented.

Nursing diagnoses

Potential complication: hemorrhage

Potential complication: anaphylaxis or severe allergic reaction to streptokinase

Management

Thrombolytic drugs are used only in acute care settings and never on an outpatient basis. The use of an infusion monitoring device may be appropriate. Appropriate drugs to counteract bleeding, such as aminocaproic acid, should be available. The correct dose is calculated by patient size and should be done carefully in consultation with the pharmacist. The nurse should monitor the patient for signs of clot dissolution. As soon as possible, the patient will be switched to heparin therapy. In addition to monitoring the usual tests for blood coagulation, the nurse should also check the hematocrit daily because it may drop even when bleeding is not present. The nurse should check the patient frequently for signs of bleeding from any body orifice; hemorrhage is the major complication of therapy.

Evaluation

If effective, a thrombolytic drug will dissolve the existing clot without causing any hemorrhaging. The patient will not be discharged while still on thrombolytic therapy. For additional specific guidelines, see the patient care implications section at the end of this chapter.

---

low-dose heparin administered at surgery has significantly reduced the risk of thrombus formation. In the past, the oral coumarins were widely used as prophylaxis against myocardial reinfarction, a use never well substantiated by controlled studies. In recent years, the number of available oral anticoagulants has dropped dramatically to just three: two coumarins, warfarin and dicumarol; and one indandione, anisindione.

✳ Coumarins

Warfarin is the most widely used coumarin. It is the only coumarin that can also be administered intramuscularly or intravenously. Warfarin is well absorbed orally. Its peak effect occurs 36 to 72 hours

after administration, and the duration of action is 4 to 5 days.

Dicumarol is longer acting than warfarin. The peak action is 3 to 5 days after administration, and the duration of action is up to 10 days. Dicumarol is not well absorbed and causes flatulence and diarrhea.

Importance of protein binding to the pharmacokinetics of coumarins. The coumarins stay in the body a long time because they are bound tightly to plasma albumin. This tight binding has several consequences. First, only a small amount of the total drug in the body is free to diffuse to the site of action in the liver. Second, the liver also degrades the coumarin to inactive forms that are then ex-

Table 20.4 Hemostatic Agents

Generic name	Trade name	Administration/dosage	Comments
SYSTEMIC HEMOSTATIC AGENTS			
Aminocaproic acid	Amicar*	ORAL, INTRAVENOUS: *Adults*—5 to 6 Gm initially orally or by slow intravenous infusion, then 1 Gm hourly or 6 Gm every 6 hr. Maximum in 24 hr is 30 Gm. Reduced dosage is used with low renal output or renal disease. *Children*—100 mg/kg body weight every 6 hr for 6 days.	Prevents activation of plasminogen (fibrinolysis) so that blood clots are not broken down. Used in special surgical situations.
Phytonadione (vitamin K_1)	Aqua-MEPHYTON Konakion* Mephyton	ORAL, INTRAMUSCULAR, SUBCUTANEOUS: *Adults and children*—2.5 to 25 mg. INTRAMUSCULAR, SUBCUTANEOUS, INTRAVENOUS: *Newborns*—0.5 to 1 mg immediately after birth. Alternatively the mother is given 1 to 5 mg 12 to 24 hr before delivery.	Intravenous route can be dangerous. Use only in emergencies for oral anticoagulant overdose, and dilute so that no more than 1 mg is given per minute. Subcutaneous and intramuscular injection may be painful.
Menadiol sodium diphosphate (vitamin K_4)	Synkayvite*	ORAL, INTRAMUSCULAR, SUBCUTANEOUS, INTRAVENOUS: *Adults*—5 to 15 mg once or twice daily. *Children*—5 to 10 mg once or twice daily.	To correct secondary hypoprothrombinemia. Converted to menadione (vitamin K_3) in the body.
Tranexamic acid	Cykloapron*	ORAL: *Adults and children*—25 mg/kg 3 or 4 times the day before surgery and 2 to 8 days following surgery. INTRAVENOUS: *Adults and children*—10 mg/kg before surgery, administered with factor VIII or IX, and 10 mg/kg 3 or 4 times daily for 2 to 8 days after surgery. FDA Pregnancy Category B.	Indicated use is for hemophiliacs undergoing dental surgery.
LOCAL HEMOSTATIC AGENTS			
Absorbable gelatin sponge	Gelfoam	Blocks and cones of various sizes. Also a sterile (surgical) and nonsterile (dental) powder.	To control bleeding in a wound or at an operative site.
Absorbable gelatin film	Gelfilm	Thin film strips.	To repair membranes in neural, thoracic, and ocular surgery.
Oxidized cellulose	Oxycel*	Gauze-type pads or strips. Also as sponges 2 × 1 × 1 inch.	To control hemorrhage and absorb blood. May be left in wound. Not for packing around bone fractures or to be left on skin.
Oxidized regenerated cellulose	Surgicel	Knitted fabric strips.	Like oxidized cellulose, but may be left on skin.

*Available in Canada and United States.

Table 20.4 Hemostatic Agents—cont'd

Generic name	Trade name	Administration/dosage	Comments
LOCAL HEMOSTATIC AGENTS—cont'd			
Microfibrillar collagen hemostat	Avitene	Sterile powder. 1 Gm should cover 50 × 50 cm (20 × 20 inches) to control light bleeding	To control bleeding in a wound or at an operative site. May be used on skin. Discard unused material, since it cannot be resterilized.
Thrombin	Fibrindex Thrombin, topical	Sterile powder. Packaged by units. May be dissolved in sterile saline solution and applied in absorbable gelatin sponge.	To control bleeding in a wound or at an operative site. Discard unused material, since it cannot be resterilized and the solution is unstable.

THE NURSING PROCESS

HEMOSTATIC AGENTS

Assessment

Patients requiring hemostatic therapy are those in whom the retention or formation of a blood clot is desirable or who have been overmedicated by a drug causing anticoagulation. Baseline data would include assessment of the type, location, and amount of bleeding; the symptoms related to the bleeding such as pain, swelling, and level of consciousness; appropriate blood coagulation tests such as partial thromboplastin time, prothrombin time, clotting time, and platelet count; the hematocrit; and general physical condition of the patient. In most cases, these patients, by the nature of their presenting problems, will be in acute care units, and extensive monitoring will be ongoing.

Nursing diagnosis

Potential complication: deep vein thrombosis

Management

The route of administration depends on the drug being used. The nurse should monitor the appropriate coagulation studies and the hematocrit. The patient is observed for signs that bleeding is stopping and for side effects of the drugs. Overmedication with the systemic hemostatic agents is also possible, so care should be taken to ensure that the patient receives the correct dose.

Evaluation

The goal of therapy with hemostatic agents is to stop bleeding without causing excessive coagulation or side effects resulting from the drug therapy. These patients will rarely be sent home on hemostatic therapy but should be able to explain what to do if bleeding should recur. For more specific guidelines, see the patient care implications section at the end of this chapter.

creted in the urine, so only a small amount of the total coumarin is available for degradation. Third, several other drugs can displace coumarins from albumin. This displacement dramatically increases the effective concentration of coumarin. This can be appreciated by considering that if only 1% of the total coumarin is not bound and displacement causes another 1% to be free, the concentration of free coumarin drug has doubled. Fourth, the albumin-bound coumarin acts as a reservoir for the drug. Even after administration is discontinued, several days will be required for the drug to dissociate from the albumin and to be degraded by the liver.

Drug interactions. Drug interactions are especially numerous with the coumarins. Many drugs will alter the effectiveness of the coumarins. No drug should be added to or deleted from a therapeutic regimen that includes a coumarin without considering drug interactions and appropriately modifying dosages.

The anticoagulant action of both heparin and coumarins is *enhanced* by drugs that decrease platelet adhesion, that is, aspirin, clofibrate, dextran, dipyridamole, hydroxychloroquine, ibuprofen, indomethacin, and phenylbutazone. The anticoagulant action of coumarins is *enhanced* by drugs that inhibit coumarin degradation, such as clofibrate, disulfiram, metronidazole, oxyphenbutazone, phenylbutazone, and trimethoprim; drugs that displace bound anticoagulant, such as chloral hydrate, oxyphenbutazone, and phenylbutazone; and drugs that interact by unknown mechanisms, for example, anabolic steroids, cimetidine, D-thyroxine, glucagon, quinidine, and sulfinpyrazone. The anticoagulant action of coumarins is *diminished* by drugs that accelerate coumarin degradation, such as barbiturates, ethchlorvynol, glutethimide, griseofulvin, and rifampin; drugs that decrease gastrointestinal absorption of coumarins, for example, cholestyramine; and drugs that interact by unknown mechanisms, such as 6-mercaptopurine. Dicumarol is known to *enhance* the action of phenytoin. This list summarizes the major drug interactions but is by no means exhaustive.

Side effects. The principal side effect is hemorrhage. Signs of coumarin overdose can include blood in the urine or blood in the stools, causing them to turn red, orange, smoky, or black. The drug can be discontinued temporarily when minor hemorrhaging occurs. When hemorrhaging is severe, fresh or frozen plasma may be transfused to replace clotting factors immediately. Less severe hemorrhage may also be treated by administering 10 mg (up to 50 mg) of vitamin K_1, phytonadione. This adds excess vitamin K to overcome the block caused by the coumarins. Clotting factors are then again synthesized by the liver, returning the prothrombin time to normal about 24 hours later.

Side effects other than hemorrhaging are rare with the coumarins.

Indandiones

The indandiones more frequently cause side effects—including rashes, depression of the bone marrow, hepatitis, and renal damage—than do the coumarins and are not widely used in the United States. Drug interactions are not prominent with the indandiones.

Anisindione (Miradon) is the only indandione in clinical use in the United States and Canada. It is long acting, with the peak effect 48 to 72 hours after the initial dose. The prothrombin time returns to normal 24 to 72 hours after the last dose

THROMBOLYTIC DRUGS
Mechanisms and Use

Thrombolytic drugs have revolutionized the treatment of myocardial infarction (MI). Thrombolytics are drugs that promote the digestion of fibrin, thereby dissolving the clot. As shown in Figure 20.1, the plasma contains the enzyme fibrinolysin (also called plasmin), which degrade the fibrin into small, soluble fragments. Fibrinolysin normally exists in an inactive form, profibrinolysin (also called plasminogen). Profibrinolysin is activated to fibrinolysin by various factors in the plasma. Degradation products of fibrin act as anticoagulants, thereby limiting further clot formation.

Although the steps in coagulation occur very rapidly, the dissolution of a blood clot may take several days. Drugs to speed the clot dissolution process have become widely used. In recent years the treatment of choice for an acute MI has become the injection of a clot-dissolving drug as quickly as possible, which prevents the myocardial ischemia that leads to tissue death. Patients can leave the hospital after 3 days instead of 10 and may not require prolonged recovery at home. The drugs available are streptokinase, urokinase, and tissue plasminogen activator (TPA) (Table 20.3). Thrombolytic therapy is also used in acute pulmonary embolism, deep vein thrombosis, or peripheral arterial occlusion. This therapy is also helpful locally to clear arteriovenous shunts in patients receiving long-term renal dialysis; however, clotting often recurs.

The thrombolytic agents are proteins and must be infused. They are relatively short-acting—30 minutes or less. Tissue plasminogen activator (TPA, Alteplase) is a product of recombinant DNA technology; it activates fibrin-bound plasminogen. Streptokinase is isolated from group C beta-hemolytic streptococci; it acts by forming a complex with plasminogen to activate it. Urokinase is isolated from human urine; it is an enzyme that cleaves plasminogen to plasmin. Bleeding or its complications are potential side effects of all three agents. Streptokinase is antigenic and may cause allergic reactions.

HEMOSTATIC AGENTS
Systemic Hemostatic Drugs (Table 20.4)
Epsilon aminocaproic acid (Amicar)

Epsilon aminocaproic acid inhibits the activation of profibrinolysin (plasminogen) to the active enzyme fibrinolysin. The lack of fibrinolysin inhibits dissolution of blood clots. Aminocaproic acid is used primarily in selected instances in which it is desirable to protect blood clots, such as surgery on the prostate, following a ruptured cerebral aneurysm, or for patients with hemophilia, after a tooth extraction.

Aminocaproic acid can be given orally or intravenously. It is rapidly excreted in the urine. Most of the side effects are transient and minor: nausea, cramps, dizziness, headache, ringing in the ear, or stuffy nose. When intravenous therapy is used, aminocaproic acid can irritate the veins and give rise to thrombophlebitis. This effect may be minimized by diluting the drug before use and by carefully placing the needle.

Tranexamic acid (Cyklokapron)

Tranexamic acid, like epsilon aminocaproic acid, inhibits the activation of profibrinolysin (plasminogen) to the active enzyme fibrinolysin (plasmin). Tranexamic acid also directly inhibits fibrinolysin. As an antifibrinolytic agent, it is 5 to 10 times more potent than epsilon aminocaproic acid. The major indication for the drug is in hemophiliacs undergoing dental surgery.

Patients receiving tranexamic acid should be monitored to detect signs of thromboembolic complications. If they are to receive the drug for more than a few days, they should also receive an ophthalmologic examination; animal studies have indicated that high doses of the drug can cause focal areas of retinal degeneration. More frequent side effects are gastrointestinal upsets, including diarrhea, nausea, and vomiting. Tranexamic acid is eliminated largely unchanged in the urine.

Vitamin K

Vitamin K is a fat-soluble vitamin required for the synthesis of clotting factors II, VII, IX, and X in the liver.

Vitamin K is contained in many foods. Humans cannot synthesize vitamin K, but bacteria in the gastrointestinal tract can synthesize vitamin K for absorption by the host. Conditions that can produce vitamin K deficiency are the following:

1. Long-term intravenous feeding
2. Debilitation resulting from poor diet
3. Prolonged oral antibiotic therapy
4. Malabsorption syndrome
5. Acute diarrhea in infants
6. Biliary disease

In addition, the oral anticoagulant drugs—the coumarins and the indandiones—produce a relative vitamin K deficiency by inhibiting the reactivation of vitamin K.

Administration and side effects. Vitamin K is available as vitamin K_1, phytonadione, and vitamin K_3, menadione, for replacement therapy, but only vitamin K_1 is effective as an antidote for severe bleeding episodes caused by an overdose of one of the oral anticoagulants. Vitamin K_1 or K_3 is safest when taken orally. Intravenous injection must be made slowly with a dilute solution and even then may cause a severe reaction. Reactions to intravenous injection include flushing, a heavy feeling on the chest, sweating, vascular collapse, and an anaphylactic reaction. Intramuscular and subcutaneous administration may cause pain and bleeding at the injection site.

In infants and anyone with a deficiency of the enzyme glucose-6-phosphate dehydrogenase, menadione (K_3) can produce hemolysis but phytonadione (K_1) does not. Vitamin K_1 or K_3 will not promote clotting in a patient with liver disease or a hereditary deficiency of one of the vitamin K-dependent clotting factors.

Local Absorbable Hemostatics (Table 20.4)

Local absorbable hemostatics provide a surface that promotes platelet adhesion and thereby promotes blood clotting where the agent is applied.

Absorbable gelatin sponge (Gelfoam)

Gelfoam is a sterile material that is moistened with sterile saline solution and applied to bleeding capillary beds that cannot be readily sutured. It is absorbed in 4 to 6 weeks.

Absorbable gelatin film (Gelfilm)

Gelfilm is a thin sterile material used in neurological, thoracic, and ocular surgery to repair membrane surfaces. Reabsorption may take from 1 week to 6 months, depending on the size and site of the film.

Oxidized cellulose (Oxygel) and oxidized regenerated cellulose (Surgicel)

Oxidized cellulose material is used much like the absorbable gelatin sponge. Both celluloses interfere with bone regeneration and therefore cannot be packed around fractures.

Oxygel retards formation of new skin and cannot be used as a surface dressing. Small implants

Text continued on p. 340.

PATIENT CARE IMPLICATIONS

Aspirin

For a detailed discussion of aspirin, see Chapter 23.

Sulfinpyrazone

For a detailed discussion of sulfinpyrazone, see Chapter 23.

Dipyridamole

Patient and family education:

- Take doses with a full glassful (8 oz.) of water. It is best to take doses on an empty stomach, 1 hour before or 2 hours after meals. However, if gastric irritation is a problem, take doses with meals, milk, or a snack.
- Dipyridamole may be prescribed with aspirin or another anticoagulant. Review with the patient the importance of taking *both* drugs as prescribed.
- Remind patients to keep all health care providers informed of all drugs being taken. Tell patients not to take aspirin or any blood thinner unless it is prescribed by the same doctor who prescribed the dipyridamole.
- Tell patients to avoid over-the-counter medications, especially aspirin-containing products, unless approved by the physician.
- Instruct patients to space doses throughout the day. If a dose is missed, tell the patient to take the dose as soon as remembered, unless within 4 hours of the next dose, in which case the missed dose should be omitted and the usual schedule resumed with the next dose. Instruct patients not to double up for missed doses.
- Tell the patient to notify the physician if signs of bleeding occur: bruising, bleeding gums, nosebleeds, bleeding in the stool.

General guidelines for patients receiving anticoagulants

Drug administration

- Inspect the patient at least twice daily for the appearance of bruising and petechiae.
- Check stool for guaiac/blood at least twice a week.
- Monitor vital signs at regular intervals. Be alert to signs of hemorrhage: hypotension, rapid pulse, pale color, weakness. In pregnant women, hemorrhage occurs most often in the third trimester or immediate postpartum period.
- Avoid the use of restraints. If necessary to use them, pad the extremities well, and remove the restraints frequently to inspect the area.
- Handle patients carefully to avoid bruising.

Patient and family education

- Teach patients to notify the physician if bleeding occurs: nosebleeds, bleeding gums, blood in stool or urine, unexplained or severe bruising, severe headache, or stiff neck.
- Instruct patients to wear a medical identification tag or bracelet indicating that they are taking anticoagulants.
- Keep all health care providers informed of anticoagulant use, including dentists and oral surgeons.
- Avoid using razors with blades; use electric shavers instead.
- Do not take any medications except those prescribed without checking with the doctor. This applies especially to aspirin or over-the-counter drugs which might contain aspirin.
- Brush teeth with a soft-bristle brush if bleeding from gums is prolonged. Avoid flossing. Use water-spray oral care devices on low settings only.
- Do not go barefoot.
- Avoid rough contact activities or sports while on anticoagulants.

Heparin

Drug administration

- Review the general guidelines, above.
- Monitor blood work before administering doses, especially with high-dose heparin (>15,000 units/24 hours). Monitor activated PTT (aPTT): the goal of anticoagulation therapy is 1.5 to 2 times control in seconds. Other tests which may be monitored include the Lee-White whole blood clotting time and the activated clotting time (ACT). There will be little or no change when low-dose heparin is used. Blood specimens for these tests are usually obtained ½ hour before ordered doses for intermittent therapy. If the laboratory work indicates anticoagulation above the desired range, notify the physician before administering dose of heparin.
- Monitor platelet counts.
- If the patient is receiving heparin and an oral anticoagulant, monitor laboratory work appropriate to both drugs.
- For mild heparin overdose, the treatment is

PATIENT CARE IMPLICATIONS — cont'd

to discontinue heparin until the laboratory findings return to the therapeutic range. Keep protamine sulfate handy for treatment of severe overdose.

- Read labels carefully as there are several strengths available. Check calculations carefully; some institutions require that two nurses check doses of heparin before administration.
- Place a note above patient's bed (or as is customary in the institution) that the patient is receiving heparin therapy so that laboratory personnel will use care to avoid excessive bleeding after venipuncture.
- Avoid IM injections in patients on high dose heparin.
- Subcutaneous administration, intermittent doses:
  - Use any subcutaneous injection site (see Chapter 6), but the abdomen is preferred because it contains few muscles and bruising is less of a cosmetic problem. Avoid the arms.
  - Keep a record of sites used, and rotate sites, even if only the abdomen is being injected.
  - Avoid the area 2 inches around the umbilicus, and any abdominal scars.
  - Use careful technique to try to avoid bruising, but know that bruising may occur with even the best technique. Avoid areas that are already bruised. Do not rub the area after injecting drug.
  - After drawing up dose, change needles. Inject at 45 to 90 degree angle with ⅝ to ½ inch, 25 to 28 gauge needle, after careful assessment to avoid injection into a muscle. Do not aspirate before injecting drug.
  - There is disagreement about the desirability of pinching the skin, as would be done when administering insulin; pinching may contribute to more bruising.
- Continuous intravenous infusion of heparin:
  - Use microdrip tubing and an electronic infusion monitoring defice.
  - Many drugs are incompatible with heparin. If other IV drugs must be administered, establish a second IV infusion line for these medications, or flush the tubing containing heparin with normal saline before and after administering other medications. Note that heparin blood levels will be erratic if the heparin infusion is interrupted frequently or for long periods.
- Intermittent intravenous heparin via heparin well or other infusion access devices:
  - Insert heparin well (heparin lock) into vein using accepted venipuncture technique, and secure in place.
  - Prime the well with a small amount (1 to 2 ml) of heparin of the same strength as will be used for anticoagulation.
  - Inject each dose of heparin into the heparin well. The injected dose displaces the heparin remaining in the well each time a dose is given, so flushing the well after the dose is administered is not necessary. Follow agency procedures if different from those listed.
- Other intravenous medications via heparin well or heparin-primed infusion access devices:
  - Insert heparin well into vein using accepted venipuncture technique, and secure in place.
  - Prime the heparin well with 1 ml of a solution of normal saline containing 10 or 100 units of heparin/ml. Implanted ports may require up to 5 ml; consult manufacturer's literature. These solutions are available in prepackaged syringes, multiple dose vials, or can be prepared by the nurse or pharmacist. Some institutions use only normal saline for flushing.
  - Each time a dose of medications is given, flush the heparin well with 1 to 2 ml of saline (unless there is only saline in the heparin well); administer the prescribed medication via push or infusion; flush the well again with 1 to 2 ml of normal saline; finally, flush with 1 ml of the dilute heparin solution. Follow agency procedures if different from those listed.
- Check for patency and correct location of the heparin well before administering heparin or other medications. Assess for pain, tenderness, swelling, or redness. It should be possible to gently aspirate blood from the heparin well. It should be possible to smoothly but slowly inject drugs via the well with no patient discomfort and no resistance. If in doubt that the heparin well is patent and in the vein, it should be removed and another one inserted elsewhere.

Patient and family education

- See the general guidelines, above.
- If heparin is prescribed for home management, instruct the patient in the necessary

Continued.

PATIENT CARE IMPLICATIONS — cont'd

psychomotor tasks involved (subcutaneous injection or injection via implanted ports, heparin wells, or catheters). Provide positive reinforcement and encouragement. Supervise return demonstrations of the necessary techniques. Refer patients to a community-based nursing care agency.

- Tell patients that a variety of side effects may occur, including alopecia (hair loss), burning sensation of the feet, myalgia, and bone pain. Encourage the patient to notify the physician of any unusual sign or symptom.

Coumarins and indandiones

Drug administration

- See general guidelines for patients receiving anticoagulants.
- Monitor the prothrombin time (PT). The goal for anticoagulation is 1.2 to 2 times the control value in seconds. Check the daily laboratory work before administering dose, and if higher than the therapeutic range, notify physician before administering dose. If patient is receiving an oral anticoagulant as well as heparin, monitor laboratory studies of both drugs.
- Monitor white blood count, white blood cell differential, and platelet count.
- For mild overdose, the treatment is to withhold the anticoagulant until the blood chemistry returns to the therapeutic range. Keep vitamin K_1 or phytonadione available to treat severe overdose with the oral anticoagulants.
- Parenteral administration of warfarin: Reconstitute with diluent provided. May be given IM, although this route is used infrequently. For IV use, administer via IV push at a rate of 25 mg/min. May be mixed in a syringe with heparin. Do not mix with IV fluids.
- Pregnant women requiring anticoagulants are usually treated with heparin as the oral agents cross the placenta and cause birth defects. Anticoagulation will usually be discontinued at about the thirty-seventh week of pregnancy in anticipation of labor and delivery.

Patient and family education

- See general guidelines, above.
- Tell patients that anisindione may turn alkaline urine orange, which may be mistaken for blood. If in doubt, consult the physician.
- A variety of rare side effects may develop in patients taking oral anticoagulants. Emphasize the importance of notifying the physician if unexpected signs or symptoms develop.
- Instruct patients to avoid drinking alcoholic beverages while taking anticoagulants.
- Emphasize the importance of returning for follow-up visits to monitor laboratory studies.
- If a dose is missed, take it as soon as remembered if it is during the same day. If it is the next day, omit the forgotten dose and resume the original dosing schedule. Do not double up for missed doses.

Tissue plasminogen activator

Drug administration

- Monitor the vital signs. Be alert to signs of hemorrhage: hypotension, rapid pulse, or other signs of shock. Monitor pupil size and reactivity, and level of consciousness. Assess for any bleeding: nosebleeds, bleeding gums, blood in urine, stool, or vomitus; notify physician.
- Monitor laboratory work, including hemoglobin, hematocrit, thrombin time, aPTT, PT, and platelet count.
- Check stools daily for presence of blood/guaiac
- Use caution in handling and moving patients to avoid excessive bleeding or bruising. Do not restrain patients.
- If arterial puncture is necessary, apply presure to the puncture site for 30 minutes following the procedure. Check the site regularly for signs of bleeding.
- Monitor the electrocardiogram during therapy.
- For continuous infusion, use microdrip tubing and an electronic infusion monitoring device.
- Do not administer IM injections to patients receiving this drug.
- Avoid venipuncture unless absolutely necessary. Apply pressure to the site for at least 15 minutes following venipuncture. Label the bed (or as agency custom dictates) so personnel from the laboratory will use appropriate technique to minimize bleeding after venipuncture.
- This drug is used only in acute care settings. Keep patient and family informed of patient's condition.

PATIENT CARE IMPLICATIONS — cont'd

Streptokinase and urokinase

Drug administration

- Monitor the vital signs. Be alert to signs of hemorrhage: hypotension, rapid pulse, or other signs of shock. Monitor pupil size and reactivity, and level of consciousness. Assess for any bleeding: nosebleeds, bleeding gums, blood in urine, stool, or vomitus; notify physician.
- Temporary increases in blood pressure have been reported with streptokinase. If the systolic blood pressure increases more than 25 mm Hg, notify the physician.
- Monitor laboratory work, including hemoglobin, hematocrit, thrombin time (TT), aPTT, PT, and platelet count. If the patient has been receiving heparin therapy, streptokinase or urokinase is withheld until the TT is less than 2 times normal. If heparin is to be started after thrombolytic therapy, heparin is withheld until the TT is less than 2 times normal control.
- Check stools daily for the presence of blood/guaiac.
- Use caution in handling and moving patients to avoid excessive bleeding or bruising. Do not restrain patients.
- If arterial puncture is necessary, use the radial or brachial artery rather than the femoral. Apply pressure to the puncture site for 30 minutes following the procedure. Check the site regularly for signs of bleeding.
- Monitor the electrocardiogram during therapy.
- For continuous infusion, use microdrip tubing and an electronic infusion monitoring device.
- Do not administer IM injections to patients receiving these drugs.
- Avoid venipuncture unless absolutely necessary. Apply pressure to the site for at least 15 minutes following venipuncture. Label the bed (or as agency custom dictates) so personnel from the laboratory will use appropriate technique to minimize bleeding after venipuncture.
- Streptokinase is highly antigenic. Observe the patient for the signs and symptoms of allergic response: anaphylaxis, urticaria, itching, flushing, nausea, headache, and musculoskeletal pain. Have drugs, equipment, and personnel available to treat serious allergic response. Use antihistamines and corticosteroids to treat allergic response; do

not use aspirin to reduce fever.
- Before using these drugs to clear occluded cannulae, attempt to clear the occluded cannulae with heparinized saline. Follow institutional guidelines. Do not mix either of these drugs with any other drug in a syringe.
- These drugs are used only in acute care settings. Keep patient and family informed of patient's condition.

Aminocaproic acid

Drug administration

- This drug may be used to treat overdose with fibrinolytic drugs.
  INTRAVENOUS AMINOCAPROIC ACID
- Available in a concentration of 250 mg/ml or 1 Gm/4 ml. Further dilute with compatible solution, 50 ml of diluent for each 1 Gm of drug (4 ml). Administer at a rate of 5 Gm/hr for the first hour, then 1 Gm/hr after the first hour. Too rapid administration can cause cardiovascular side effects. Monitor the pulse, blood pressure, and if possible electrocardiogram during administration.
- Since the drug can cause clot formation, be alert to signs of possible thrombosis: pain in extremities, one extremity colder than another, loss of pulse in an extremity, shortness of breath, chest pain, Homan's sign.

Patient and family education

- Review the goals of therapy with the patient. Therapy is usually on a short-term basis, but side effects may develop. Encourage patients to notify the physician if any unexpected sign or symptom develops.
- Tell the patient to take any missed doses as soon as remembered, unless close to the time for the next dose, in which case the missed dose should be omitted. Do not double up for missed doses.

Tranexamic acid

Drug administration

- This drug may be used to treat overdose with fibrinolytic drugs.
  INTRAVENOUS TRANEXAMIC ACID
- May be given undiluted or further diluted in IV infusion solutions. Administer undiluted at a rate of 100 mg (1 ml)/min. Too rapid administration can cause cardiovascular side effects. Monitor the pulse, blood pressure, and if possible electrocardiogram during IV administration.

Continued.

PATIENT CARE IMPLICATIONS—cont'd

- Since the drug can cause clot formation, be alert to signs of possible thrombosis: pain in extremities, one extremity colder than another, loss of pulse in an extremity, shortness of breath, chest pain, Homan's sign.

Patient and family education

- Review the goals of therapy with the patient. Therapy with this drug is usually on a short-term basis, but side effects may develop. Encourage patients to notify the physician if any unexpected sign or symptom develops.
- Tell the patient to take any missed doses as soon as remembered, unless close to the time for the next dose, in which case the missed dose should be omitted. Do not double up for missed doses.
- The physician may recommend that patients on long-term tranexamic acid therapy receive an ophthalmic examination to detect side effects.

Phytonadione

Drug administration

- Assess for history of allergy before administering. Monitor vital signs and blood pressure. Remain with the patient for 5 to 10 minutes following administration. Have available drugs, equipment, and personnel to treat an acute allergic response.
- IM injection is painful, and the injection site may be tender. Use large muscle masses. Record and rotate injection sites.
- Monitor the prothrombin time.
- Read labels carefully. Konakion is for intramuscular injection only; AquaMEPHYTON may be given IM, IV, or subcutaneously.
  INTRAVENOUS PHYTONADIONE
- Dilute only with designated fluids (see manufacturer's instructions). Use only preserva-

tive-free diluents. Administer diluted solution at a rate of 1 mg/min. The drug is light sensitive. Administer immediately after preparing.
- Patients with bile deficiency who are receiving oral preparations need concomitant administration of bile salts.

Patient and family education

- Review with patients the expected benefits of therapy.
- Dietary deficiency of vitamin K is rare in adults. For dietary sources of vitamin K, see Dietary Consideration: Vitamins on p. 282.

Menadiol sodium diphosphate

Drug administration

- Assess for glucose-6-phosphate dehydrogenase deficiency before administering; if present, do not administer.
- IM injection is painful, and the injection site may be tender. Use large muscle masses. Record and rotate injection sites.
- Intravenous menadiol sodium diphosphate: May be given undiluted or added to most infusion solutions. Administer dose in undiluted form over at least 1 minute.
- Monitor the prothrombin time.
- Patients with bile deficiency who are receiving oral preparations need concomitant administration of bile salts.

Patient and family education

- Review with patients the expected benefits of therapy.
- Dietary deficiency of vitamin K is rare in adults. For dietary sources of vitamin K, see Dietary Consideration: Vitamins on p. 282.
- Take oral doses with meals to decrease gastric irritation.

---

are reabsorbed in 1 week, but large ones may require 6 weeks for reabsorption.

Microfibrillar collagen hemostat (Avitene)

Collagen hemostat is a water-insoluble powder that is applied to a bleeding surface to activate natural clotting. The collagen is absorbed in 7 weeks. Microfibrillar collagen is used in surgery to control bleeding in capillary beds, in the liver, and in skin graft sites. It does not interfere with the healing of skin or bone. Microfibrillar collagen must be kept

dry and cannot be resterilized after the container is opened.

Thrombin

Thrombin is an activated clotting factor (Figure 20.1). Thrombin is applied topically only as a sterile protein powder to bleeding surfaces. It must be kept cold and dry until use or it becomes inactive. Thrombin can be applied topically as a solution; however, it is important to note that it must not be injected.

SUMMARY

Blood coagulation is a complex process and is outlined in Figure 20.1.

Platelets are cell fragments capable of binding to an appropriate surface and aggregating to form a plug. This process appears to be a key step not only in the intrinsic pathway for blood coagulation, but also in initiating atherosclerotic plaques important in the etiology of strokes and myocardial infarctions. The recent elucidation of factors governing platelet aggregation has prompted clinical trials to determine whether drugs that inhibit platelet aggregation (antiplatelet or antithrombic drugs) will provide prophylaxis for patients with previous strokes or myocardial infarctions.

Anticoagulants in use include the following:

1. Drugs such as citrate and EDTA, which complex calcium and are used to prevent coagulation of stored blood
2. Heparin, which in low doses inhibits platelet adhesion in vivo and in high doses inhibits the activation of thrombin. Heparin is also an effective anticoagulant in vitro
3. Oral anticoagulants, the coumarins and indandiones, which inhibit the vitamin K-dependent synthesis of clotting factors by the liver

The prolonged onset of the oral anticoagulants (1 to 2 days) reflects the time for previously synthesized clotting factors to be destroyed. The coumarins are highly bound to plasma albumin and consequently have a long duration of action in the body. Coumarins interact with many other drugs because of protein binding, drug metabolism, and other factors, as described in the text.

Hemorrhaging is the most common toxicity of anticoagulants. Heparin has a short half-life (about 2 hours), and discontinuing administration is usually sufficient to control hemorrhaging. Protamine specifically complexes heparin and can be administered as an antidote. Vitamin K_1 is the specific antidote for an overdose with the oral anticoagulants, but in an acutely critical situation, transfusion of clotting factors is necessary.

T-PA, streptokinase and urokinase are enzymes used as thrombolytics to degrade blood clots in selected cases.

Hemostatic agents are systemic or local. Systemic hemostatics include aminocaproic acid and tranexamic acid, which inhibit the activation of profibrinolysin so that blood clots are not degraded, and vitamin K, the vitamin necessary for the synthesis of certain of the clotting factors by the liver. Local hemostatics include sponges and films of gelatin or cellulose, which can be sterilized and applied to areas to prompt blood clotting during surgical procedures. Thrombin and collagen can be applied as powders to promote blood clotting.

STUDY QUESTIONS

1. How do platelets initiate clot formation?
2. What drugs inhibit platelet aggregation?
3. What roles do thromboxane A_2 and prostacyclin play in platelet aggregation?
4. Describe the major steps in blood coagulation.
5. What are the three groups of anticoagulants and what is the mechanism of action of each group?
6. Describe the use of heparin in high-dose and low-dose therapy.
7. Which anticoagulants are effective when added to blood drawn for storage?
8. How do protamine and vitamin K each function as antidotes for hemorrhaging induced by drugs?
9. How does protein binding affect the pharmacodynamics of the coumarins?
10. What are the therapeutic limitations of the indandiones?
11. What is the action of thrombolytic drugs? Name the thrombolytic drugs.
12. What is the mechanism of action of aminocaproic acid? Of vitamin K?
13. List the agents used as local hemostatics. What is their mechanism of action?

SUGGESTED READINGS

Horwitz, C.A.: A practical approach to disorders of hemostasis, Postgrad. Med. **69**(3):79, 1981.

Marx, J.: Coagulation as a common thread in disease, Science **218**:145, 1982.

Myers, A.M.: Evaluation of the hemorrhage-prone patient, Postgrad. Med. **67**(4):161, 1980.

Antiplatelet therapy

Fields, W.S., Goldhaber, S.Z., and Lewis, H.D., Jr.: Who should have prophylactic aspirin? Patient Care **22**(8):28, 1988.

Mehta, J.: Platelets and prostaglandins in coronary artery disease, JAMA **249**:2818, 1983.

Pagano, T., Nair, C.K., and Sketch, M.H.: Use of common antiplatelet drugs for vascular diseases, Geriatrics **38**(11):75, 1983.

Relman, A.S.: Aspirin for the primary prevention of myocardial infarction, N. Engl. J. Med. **318**(4):245, 1988.

Rivera, V.M.: Stroke: a guide to differential diagnosis and prevention, Postgrad. Med. **77**(4):81, 1985.

Schwartz, L., and others: Aspirin and dipyridamole in the prevention of restenosis after percutaneous transluminal coronary angioplasty, N. Engl. J. Med. **318**:1714, 1988.

Steering Committee of the Physicians' Health Study Research Group: Preliminary report: findings from the aspirin component of the ongoing physicians' health study, N. Engl. J. Med. **318**:262, 1988.

Anticoagulant therapy

Bailey, R.E.: Clinically important interactions between warfarin and other drugs, Consultant **21**(1):281, 1981.

Errichetti, A.M., Holder, A., and Ansell, J.: Management of oral anticoagulant therapy, Arch. Intern. Med. **144**(10):1966, 1984.

McMahan, B.E.: Why deep vein thrombosis is so dangerous, RN **51**(1):20, 1987.

Painter, T.D.: Anticoagulation: current approach to heparin and warfarin therapy, Postgrad. Med. **74**(3):341, 1983.

Palmer, J.D.: Clinical uses of warfarin, Drug Therapy **6**(1):49, 1981.

Patrick, G.: Pros and cons of low dose heparin, Res. Staff Phys. **27**(5):81, 1981.

Paulsen, J.T., and Kersting, G.L.: A systematic approach to heparin administration for pediatric hemodialysis, ANNA J. **14**(4):265, 1987.

Swithers, C.M.: Tools for teaching about anticoagulants, RN **51**(1):57, 1988.

Todd, B.: Use heparin safely, Geriatr. Nurs. **8**(1):43, 1987.

VanBree, N.S., Hollerbach, A.D., and Brooks, G.P.: Clinical evaluation of three techniques for administering low-dose heparin, Nurs. Res. **23**(1):15, 1984.

Wallin, R., and Martin, L.F.: Vitamin K-dependent carboxylation and vitamin K metabolism in liver: effects of warfarin, J. Clin. Invest. **76**:1879, 1985.

Wilcox, C.M., and Truss, C.D.: Gastrointestinal bleeding in patients receiving long-term anticoagulant therapy, Am. J. Med. **84**:683, 1988.

Wilson, J.M.: Avoiding errors in intravenous heparin therapy, AD Nurse **3**:31, 1988.

Thrombolytic therapy

Dillon, J., and others: Rapid initiation of thrombolytic therapy for acute MI, Crit. Care Nurse **9**(2):55, 1989.

Guerci, A.D., and others: A randomized trial of intravenous tissue plasminogen activator for acute myocardial infarction with subsequent renadomization to elective coronary angioplasty, N. Eng. J. Med. **317**:1613, 1987.

Johnston, J.B.: T-PA: A panacea for heart attacks? Emerg. Nurs. Rep. **3**(1):1, 1988.

Joubert, D.W.: Drug update: T-PA or not T-PA? That is the question, J. Emerg. Nurs. **14**(4):240, 1988.

Korsmeyer, C., and others: The nurse's role in thrombolytic therapy for acute MI, Crit. Care Nurse **7**(6):22, 1987.

Loscalzo, J., and Braunwald, E.: Tissue plasminogen activator, N. Eng. J. Med. **319**(4):925, 1988.

Marder, V.J., and Sherry, S.: Thrombolytic therapy: current status, N. Eng. J. Med. **318**:1512, 1988.

McGrath, K.B., and Patterson, R.: Anaphylactic reactivity to streptokinase, JAMA **252**(10):1314, 1984.

Mich, R.J., and Bell, W.R.: Thrombolytic therapy of deep-vein thrombosis, Pract. Cardiol. **8**(9):43, 1982.

Olson, A.K.: What you should know about thrombolytic therapy, Nursing 87 **17**(12):52, 1987.

O'Neill, W., and others: A prospective randomized clinical trial of intracoronary streptokinase versus coronary angioplasty for acute myocardial infarction, N. Eng. J. Med. **314**:812, 1986.

Rafter, R.H.: Thrombolytic therapy orders and record sheets: nursing care made easier, J. Emerg. Nurs. **14**(4):237, 1988.

Rodman, M.J.: What to expect from the newest drugs, RN **51**(3):59, 1988.

Rodriguez, S.W., and Reed, R.L.: Thrombolytic therapy for MI, Am. J. Nurs. **87**(5):631, 1987.

Runge, M.S., Quertermous, T., and Haber, E.: Plasminogen activators: the old and the new, Circulation **79**(2):217, 1989.

Sherry, S.: Thrombolytic therapy of acute pulmonary embolism, Drug Therapy **8**(5):72, 1983.

Strauss, E., and Rudy, E.B.: Tissue-plasminogen activator: A new drug in reperfusion therapy, Crit. Care Nurse **6**(3):30, 1986.

Vitello-Cicciu, J.: Thrombolytic therapy . . . urokinase, J. Cardiovasc. Nurs. **1**(2):59, 1987.

White, H.D., and others: Effect of intravenous streptokinase on left ventricular function and early survival after acute myocardial infarction, N. Eng. J. Med. **317**:850, 1987.

Intravenous and intraarterial lines

Clarke, J., and Cox, E.: Heparinisation of Hickman catheters, Nurs Times **84**(15):51, 1988.

Cunliffe, M.T., and Polomano, R.C.: How to clear catheter clots with urokinase, Nursing 86 **16**(12):40, 1986.

Cyganski, J.M., Donahue, J.M., and Heaton, J.S.: The case for the heparin flush, Am. J. Nurs. **87**:796, 1987.

Dunn, D.L., and Lenihan, S.F.: The case for the saline flush, Am. J. Nurs. **87**:798, 1987.

Harper, J.: Use of heparinized intraarterial lines to obtain coagulation samples, Focus Crit. Care **15**(5):51, 1988.

Shearer, J.: Normal saline flush versus dilute heparin flush: a study of peripheral intermittent IV devices, NITA J. **10**(6):425, 1987.

21

Drugs to Lower Blood Lipid Levels

ORIGIN OF BLOOD LIPIDS AND THEIR ROLE IN ATHEROSCLEROSIS

There are two main types of lipids in the blood: triglyceride and cholesterol. These lipids are bound to special proteins to form soluble lipoproteins. There are four major classes of lipoproteins: chylomicrons, very low density lipoproteins (VLDL), low density lipoproteins (LDL), and high density lipoproteins (HDL). Chylomicrons and VLDL are composed largely of triglycerides and function to transport triglycerides to tissues for metabolic use or storage. LDL and HDL serve to transport cholesterol. The role and the composition of the lipoproteins are summarized in Figure 21.1.

Chylomicrons

Chylomicrons are very large lipoproteins that contain about 90% triglyceride by weight. After a meal the ingested fat is processed by the intestine into chylomicrons, which are transported through the lymphatic system to the plasma. Chylomicrons are normally found in the blood only during the 8 to 12 hours after a meal. Since chylomicrons represent dietary fat, patients being evaluated for triglyceride abnormalities should not eat for 12 to 16 hours before a blood sample is drawn.

Very Low Density Lipoproteins (VLDL)

The VLDL are 60% triglyceride by weight. This triglyceride pool is synthesized by the liver from carbohydrate sources for export as fuel to other tissues. Triglycerides cannot be transported directly into cells for use. Tissues that require triglycerides, particularly muscle and fat tissues, secrete an enzyme called *lipoprotein lipase,* which breaks down the triglycerides to fatty acids and glycerol, compounds that can be taken into the cells.

Low Density Lipoproteins (LDL)

The LDL are only 5% triglyceride but are 50% cholesterol by weight. The LDL are the remains of the VLDL after removal of triglycerides and some protein. When cells need cholesterol, they synthesize receptors for LDL. The LDL bind to these receptors and are taken into the cell by pinocytosis, and degraded. Most cells are also capable of synthesizing cholesterol, but this synthesis is turned off when the cholesterol from LDL is being utilized. When the cell has sufficient cholesterol, the cell stops making LDL receptors.

Role of LDL in atherosclerosis. Recent studies have examined the role of LDL in atherosclerosis because the concentration of LDL reflects the total cholesterol concentration. An increased total plasma cholesterol concentration is linked to an increased incidence of atherosclerosis. When there is an injury to the epithelial cells of arteries or when the amount of circulating LDL becomes very high, the receptor mechanism controlling LDL uptake no longer operates properly and the cell becomes overwhelmed with cholesterol. This is believed to be one origin of atherosclerotic plaques. Platelets may also play a role in initiating atherosclerosis. Aggregated platelets release factors that stimulate smooth muscle growth. This stimulation of growth heals the minute breaks in the normal blood vessel. When the epithelial cells are overloaded with cholesterol and aggregated platelets stimulate an overgrowth of smooth muscle cells, an atherosclerotic plaque is formed. The eventual outcome of atherosclerosis is the narrowing of an artery so that the blood flow is reduced and may not be sufficient to maintain tissue function. Reduced blood flow also favors the formation of a clot that may completely obstruct flow. A stroke may result when the cerebral arteries are involved, or a myocardial infarction may result when the coronary arteries are involved. When the legs are affected, limbs may be lost from gangrene. Renovascular hypertension is associated with atherosclerosis.

High Density Lipoproteins (HDL)

The last major category of lipoproteins is the high density lipoproteins (HDL). The HDL are 50%

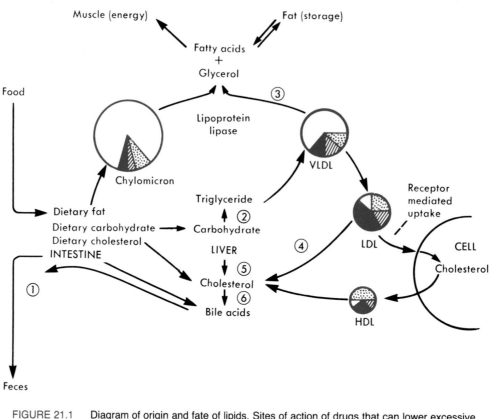

FIGURE 21.1   Diagram of origin and fate of lipids. Sites of action of drugs that can lower excessive plasma concentrations of lipids: (1) Drugs that lower cholesterol by increasing the excretion of bile acids-cholestyramine and cholestipol. (2) Drugs that lower triglycerides by inhibiting hepatic triglyceride synthesis-gemfibrozil and niacin. (3) Drug that lowers VLDL, inhibiting its release and activating lipoprotein lipase-clofibrate. (4) Drug that lowers cholesterol by stimulating LDL degradation-dextrothyroxine. (5) Drug that lowers cholesterol by inhibiting cholesterol synthesis-lovastatin, probucol. (6) Drug that lowers cholesterol by increasing cholesterol excretion into bile-clofibrate.

protein, 20% cholesterol, and 5% triglyceride by weight. Only about 20% of the total plasma cholesterol is found in HDL. Until recently the HDL were not widely studied. It now appears that the HDL play a very important role in removing excess cholesterol from peripheral tissues. HDL can remove cholesterol from cells and can inhibit the uptake of LDL by cells. Recent studies indicate that persons with high concentrations of HDL have a lower incidence of atherosclerosis and the related problems of heart disease and strokes.

The liver degrades cholesterol to bile acids, which are excreted into the small intestine. Bile acids emulsify lipids to aid in fat absorption. Some bile acids are absorbed into the portal vein for transport back to the liver. This circulation between the liver and small intestine is called *enterohepatic circulation*.

HYPERLIPIDEMIA
Origin and Types of Hyperlipidemia

Hyperlipidemia is associated with an abnormal concentration of one or more of the four lipoproteins. Five major types of hyperlipidemia have been described, depending on which lipoproteins are present in abnormally high concentrations. Since it is easier to measure cholesterol than LDL and easier to measure triglyceride than VLDL, hyperlipidemias are usually detected by measuring cholesterol and triglyceride. The characteristics of the five types of hyperlipidemia are given in Table 21.1. All hyperlipidemias can be genetically determined but may also be secondary to diabetes, obesity, alcoholism, hypothyroidism, and liver and kidney disease. Only two kinds of hyperlipidemias are commonly encountered: type II and type IV.

Type II hyperlipidemia is characterized by high concentrations of LDL but normal or modestly in-

Table 21.1   Types of Hyperlipidemias

	Type I	Type II	Type III	Type IV	Type V
Lipoprotein content of fasting plasma					
1. Chylomicrons	Markedly increased	Absent	May be present	Absent	Increased
2. VLDL	Normal or decreased	Normal or increased	Increased	Increased	Increased
3. LDL	Normal or decreased	Increased	Increased	Normal	Normal or decreased
Lipids					
Cholesterol	Increased	Increased	Increased	Normal or increased	Increased
Triglyceride	Increased	Normal or increased	Increased	Increased	Increased
Incidence	Rare	Common	Relatively uncommon	Common	Relatively uncommon
Usual age at detection	Early childhood	Early adulthood (can be detected in infancy or childhood)	Early adulthood	Adulthood (middle age)	Early adulthood
Risk of atherosclerosis	Normal	Greatly increased	Greatly increased	Probably increased	Unknown

creased amounts of VLDL. Persons with elevated LDL are those most at risk for atherosclerosis. In genetically determined type II hyperlipidemia, patients who are homozygous for the type II trait have evidence of severe heart disease by age 20. In addition, type II hyperlipidemia can occur in individuals who are obese, are hypothyroid, or suffer from liver or kidney disease.

Type IV hyperlipidemia is characterized by high concentrations of VLDL with relatively normal levels of LDL. It is the most common lipid abnormality and also carries a high risk of coronary artery disease. Type IV hyperlipidemia is common among patients who have diabetes, are obese, or are alcoholics. Oral contraceptives or estrogen can elicit type IV hyperlipidemia in some women.

The two common types of hyperlipidemia are associated with a high production of triglycerides (type IV) or cholesterol (type II) by the liver. Type IV hyperlipidemia (high VLDL) is often well controlled by calorie restriction with emphasis on losing weight and on reducing carbohydrates from which the liver synthesizes triglycerides. A decrease in foods high in cholesterol such as egg yolk, liver, and shellfish and a decrease in saturated fats are recommended dietary modifications for pa-

tients with type II hyperlipidemia. See Dietary Consideration: Cholesterol. When diet alone does not reduce blood lipid levels to acceptable ranges, a few drugs have been found effective for lowering the concentration of blood lipids. The type of hyperlipidemia determines which drug may be effective. These drugs have not been in use long enough to evaluate whether they are associated with long-term side effects.

Role of Drug Therapy in Treating Hyperlipidemia

The Lipid Research Study, conducted by the National Heart, Lung, and Blood Institute and completed in 1983, found that in a high-risk group whose cholesterol levels were lowered through diet and drug therapy there was as much as a 40% reduction in heart disease risk. The group had blood cholesterol levels above 265 mg/dl. They were treated with diet and up to 24 Gm daily of cholestyramine. The better the compliance of the test group, the greater the reduction in heart attacks and deaths from heart disease, the lower the need for bypass surgery, and the lower the incidence of heart disease symptoms. A 4.4% reduction in cholesterol concentration was associated with an 11% decrease in heart disease risk. A 19% reduction in

DIETARY CONSIDERATION: CHOLESTEROL

Dietary changes to lower serum cholesterol levels usually involve decreasing cholesterol intake, lowering the intake of saturated fat, and increasing the intake of polyunsaturated fat. As with all major dietary prescriptions, refer the patient to a dietitian for more extensive teaching and explanation if necessary.

Foods Allowed	Foods to Avoid or Limit

MEAT

Lean, well-trimmed meat. Prefer poultry, fish (not shrimp), veal, with occasional ham, pork, lamb, beef.	Fatty meat, regular ground beef, bacon, sausage, luncheon meat, fried meat; meat in gravy; shrimp, organ meats, fish roe.

EGGS AND OTHER MEAT ALTERNATIVES

Egg white only; no-cholesterol egg substitutes; legumes, soy protein, peanut butter, nuts (such as walnuts, pecans, almonds)	Egg yolk; canned pork and beans; cashews, macadamia nuts

MILK AND CHEESE

Skim milk and skim milk products; buttermilk; cheese, cottage cheese, and yogurt containing up to 1% milkfat; sherbet	Whole milk and milk; malted milk and milkshakes; cream (sweet and sour); ice cream and ice milk; nondairy substitutes for cream; whipped toppings containing coconut or palm oil; cheese made from cream or whole milk

VEGETABLES AND FRUITS

Fresh, canned, frozen, dried fruits or vegetables; juices; vegetables prepared without animal fat; vegetarian baked beans	Buttered, creamed, or fried vegetables; pork and beans; avocado (use sparingly)

FAT

Vegetable oils; soft margarine listing an allowed liquid oil as the first ingredient; mayonnaise and salad dressings not containing sour cream or cheese	Other margarines, including low-calorie; butter; hydrogenated vegetable shortening, bacon, lard, meat drippings, salt pork, suet, cream, coconut, palm and peanut oils; gravies unless made with allowed fat and skim milk

BREADS AND CEREALS

Cooked and dry cereal; rice; flour; pasta; breads made with a minimum of saturated fat; white, whole wheat, rye, pumpernickel, raisin, Italian, French, English muffins, hard rolls, matzo, pretzels, saltines; homemade breads made without whole milk, egg yolk, or saturated shortening	Egg noodles, egg bread; commercial biscuits, muffins, donuts, pancakes, waffles, butter rolls, mixes for above; corn chips, potato chips, and other deep-fried snacks; cheese crackers

SOUP

Bouillon; clear broths; fat-free vegetable soup and pot liquor; cream soups made with skim milk and allowed fat; packaged dehydrated soup	All other soups

DESSERTS AND SWEETS

Angel food cake; fruit ices; sherbet (1-2% fat); gelatin desserts; meringues, homemade pastries made with allowed fat, skim milk, and egg white; pure sugar candies; jam, jelly; honey, syrup made without fat; molasses, sugar	Commercial pies, cakes, mixes; desserts and candy containing nonallowed fat, egg yolk, and whole milk; chocolate; coconut

MISCELLANEOUS

Coffee, tea, caffeine-free coffee, carbonated beverages, relishes; fat-free barbecue sauce; catsup; chili sauce; spices, herbs, extracts, lemon juice, vinegar	

Table 21.2   Drugs That Reduce Blood Lipid Concentrations

Generic name	Trade name	Administration/dosage	Comments
Cholestyramine resin	Questran* Cholybar	ORAL: *Adults*—4 Gm 4 times daily (at meals and bedtime). May be increased to 6 Gm 4 times daily. Alternatively, the dosage may be divided into 2 or 3 doses. Material must be mixed with a liquid (1 oz for each gram). *Children*—over 6 yr, 8 Gm twice daily with meals. Total maximum dosage, 24 Gm daily.	Type II hyperlipidemia (high LDL). This resin stays in the intestine removing bile acids and thereby increasing cholesterol degradation by the liver. Available as a chewable bar, 4 Gm per bar.
Clofibrate	Atromid-S* Clariplex† Novofibrate	ORAL: *Adults*—500 mg 3 to 4 times daily.	Types III, IV, and V hyperlipidemia. Type II hyperlipidemia if VLDL is elevated. Inhibits triglyceride synthesis in the liver and inhibits the breakdown of triglycerides in fat tissue.
Colestipol hydrochloride	Colestid*	ORAL: *Adults*—15 to 30 Gm daily in 2 to 4 doses with meals. Mix 1 oz liquid with each 4 to 6 Gm. *Children*—not established.	Like cholestyramine.
Dextrothyroxine	Choloxin*	ORAL: *Adults*—with normal thyroid function, initially, 1 to 2 mg daily. May be increased monthly by 1 to 2 mg to a maximum of 8 mg daily (4 mg daily maximum in patients taking digitalis). *Children*—initially, 0.05 mg/kg body weight. May be increased monthly by 0.05 mg/kg to a maximum daily dose of 4 mg.	Type II hyperlipidemia. Lowers cholesterol by increasing LDL degradation.
Gemfibrozil	Lopid*	ORAL: *Adults*—600 mg twice daily 30 min before breakfast and dinner. FDA Pregnancy Category B.	Types IV and V hyperlipidemia. Lowers total triglyceride levels. Effects on cholesterol levels are mixed. LDL levels may fall and HDL levels increase.
Lovastatin	Mevacor*	ORAL: *Adults*—20 mg/day with the evening meal. May adjust at 4-week intervals. Maintenance dose: 20 to 80 mg daily. FDA Pregnancy Category X.	Type II hyperlipoproteinemia. Inhibits cholesterol synthesis in the liver.
Niacin (nicotinic acid)	Nicobid Niac Nicolar Tri-B3†	ORAL: *Adults*—initially 100 mg 3 times daily, increasing to a total of 2 to 6 Gm daily in divided doses with or after meals. FDA Pregnancy Category C.	Types II, III, IV, and V hyperlipidemia. Inhibits the synthesis of VLDL by the liver.
Probucol	Lorelco*	ORAL: *Adults*—500 mg twice daily (with breakfast and dinner). *Children*—not established.	Type II hyperlipidemia. Lowers cholesterol probably by inhibiting cholesterol biosynthesis in the liver.

*Available in Canada and United States.
†Available in Canada.

cholesterol concentration was associated with a 40% decrease in heart disease risk.

Earlier studies had not been as conclusive. The Coronary Drug Project trial studied men with coronary atherosclerosis who were treated with clofibrate, dextrothyroxine, or niacin to lower blood lipid concentration. None of the drugs reduced mortality, and dextrothyroxine increased mortality. It may be that in patients with established coronary atherosclerosis, reducing lipid levels may be less effective in preventing complications than in patients who have yet to develop clinical signs of heart disease and atherosclerosis.

THE NURSING PROCESS

BLOOD LIPID LEVELS

Assessment

The need for drugs to lower blood lipid levels is often diagnosed as an incidental finding in patients when blood is drawn for another purpose and elevated cholesterol and/or triglyceride levels are found. Occasionally a suspected family history of hyperlipidemia leads to the diagnosis. Finally, some physicians may elect to use these drugs in patients with a history of atherosclerosis, regardless of triglyceride or cholesterol levels. Baseline assessment would include a general assessment of the patient, including the following: weight, serum cholesterol and triglyceride levels, blood pressure, and dietary history.

Nursing diagnoses

Altered bowel elimination: diarrhea secondary to antilipemic therapy

Potential altered health maintenance related to scheduling of medication dosing times around dose of cholestyramine or colestipol

Management

These drugs have few associated side effects when used in usual doses. Any new sign or symptom should be evaluated. Discharge planning should include instruction by the dietitian, particularly if the type of hyperlipidemia can be better treated by dietary restriction and/or weight loss.

Evaluation

Ideally, effective use of these drugs would be validated by longer life span, but this cannot be easily proved. These drugs can be regarded as effective if the serum triglyceride or cholesterol levels approach normal. By the time of discharge, the patient should be able to explain why and how to take the prescribed drug, when it should be taken in relation to meals, anticipated side effects and what to do about them, which symptoms should be reported immediately to the physician, and how to plan meals within prescribed dietary restrictions. Finally, the patient should recognize that since the prescribed drug may interfere with other drugs, all health care providers should be kept informed about the drugs the patient is taking.

SPECIFIC DRUGS USED TO LOWER BLOOD LIPID LEVELS (Table 21.2)

Cholestyramine resin

Cholestyramine (Questran) is a resin with a sandlike texture that stays in the intestine and binds bile acids. Bile acids are the degradation products of cholesterol produced in the liver and excreted into the intestine through the biliary tract. The binding of bile acids by cholestyramine decreases the reabsorption of bile acid through the enterohepatic circulation and therefore increases the amount of fecal bile acid. Thus the effect of cholestyramine is to increase the excretion of cholesterol, but the drug must be taken several times a day to achieve this goal. Cholestyramine is effective in treating type II hyperlipidemia (high LDL) only.

The patient may experience bloating, nausea, and constipation at the beginning of therapy with cholestyramine. During therapy cholestyramine may interfere with the absorption of fat-soluble vitamins (A, D, K), digitalis, thyroxine, and coumarin anticoagulants.

Colestipol hydrochloride

Colestipol (Colestid) is similar to cholestyramine.

Clofibrate

Clofibrate (Atromid-S) reduces the plasma concentration of triglycerides by several mechanisms. One mechanism is the activation of the enzyme lipoprotein lipase. This accelerates the breakdown of VLDL. Another is to inhibit the release of VLDL by the liver. Clofibrate also decreases plasma cholesterol concentrations. This action appears to be the result of increased excretion of cholesterol into bile and subsequently into the feces. Clofibrate is used to treat type IV hyperlipidemia, type II if there is elevated VLDL, and the rare type III and V hyperlipidemias.

Clofibrate produces few side effects. About 10% of patients initially experience some gastrointestinal upset. Clofibrate may cause muscle cramps and impotence in men and should be used with caution in patients with liver or kidney disease. It is contraindicated during pregnancy or for nursing mothers. Clofibrate displaces several drugs from albumin, including coumarins, phenytoin, and tolbutamide. The higher concentration of displaced drug can cause toxic effects.

Long-term use of clofibrate increases the incidence of gallstones. In studies of men with ischemic heart disease or a history of a myocardial infarction, clofibrate was found to increase the incidence of gallstones and symptoms of ischemic heart disease while not decreasing, and perhaps increasing, the overall death rate.

Gemfibrozil

Gemfibrozil (Lopid) is chemically related to clofibrate. Like clofibrate, it lowers VLDL levels to lower total triglyceride levels. Gemfibrozil interferes with the transfer of fatty acids from adipose tissue to the liver and with the hepatic production of VLDL. Gemfibrozil has variable effects on total cholesterol levels. LDL levels appear to fall while HDL levels appear to rise. It is not known whether this is associated with a reversal of atherosclerotic risks.

Gemfibrozil is prescribed for the treatment of severe hypertriglyceridemia, Types IV and V. Side effects include gastrointestinal upset and rashes. Gemfibrozil increases the incidence of gallstones and therefore is contraindicated for patients with gallstones. Blood glucose levels may rise in diabetic patients.

Lovastatin

Lovastatin (Mevacor) is a new antilipemic drug that inhibits an early step in synthesis of cholesterol by the liver. This inhibition leads to an overall reduction in LDL production, making lovastatin effective in the treatment of type II hyperlipoproteinemia. LDL levels will start to decrease after 2 weeks of therapy; if therapy is discontinued, a therapeutic effect may remain for up to 6 weeks. Patients may complain of gastrointestinal discomfort, headaches, dizziness, or skin rash. Side effects may include muscle aches or cramps, fever, tiredness or weakness, and blurred vision. Liver function tests may change with therapy. Yearly ophthalmic examinations are recommended. Lovastatin is contraindicated during pregnancy because skeletal abnormalities have been noted in animal studies. Lovastatin is primarily excreted unchanged in the feces through the bile.

Niacin (nicotinic acid) and aluminum nicotinate

Niacin is a B vitamin for which the minimum daily requirement (MDR) is 20 mg. At doses 10 to 20 times higher than the MDR, niacin is a vasodilator (Chapter 15). At doses 100 to 200 times higher than the MDR, niacin depresses the synthesis of VLDL by the liver and thereby reduces LDL as well. Niacin is effective in treating types II, III, IV, and V hyperlipidemias. However, the high doses needed produce troublesome side effects in most patients, and only a few patients can tolerate continued use of niacin. Most patients experience marked flushing due to its vasodilator action. Itching and gastrointestinal upset are also frequent side effects. Tolerance may develop to all of these symptoms, so the dosage is usually low at first and increased gradually to avoid severe reactions. Niacin can cause or aggravate peptic ulcer, glucose intolerance (diabetes), and high plasma uric acid (gout).

Dextrothyroxine

Dextrothyroxine (Choloxin) is the inactive stereoisomer of the hormone thyroxine. It enhances the degradation of LDL and thereby lowers plasma cholesterol levels. Since the action is to lower LDL, dextrothyroxine is only useful for type II hyperlipidemia. When plasma cholesterol levels are high, it will produce a 20% to 30% decrease in 1 to 2 months. Side effects during this time include dizziness, diarrhea, and an altered sense of taste. Some patients show symptoms of hyperthyroidism: weight loss, nervousness, insomnia, sweating, and menstrual irregularities. Others may be hypersensitive to iodine with itching or a rash. Angina may be aggravated.

Dextrothyroxine can decrease glucose tolerance in diabetic patients. It enhances the action of coumarin anticoagulants. Contraindications to dextrothyroxine use include pregnancy and hypertension, as well as heart, renal, or liver disease. Since the latter conditions are common among patients with type II hyperlipidemia, the use of dextrothyroxine is limited.

Probucol

Probucol (Lorelco) inhibits cholesterol synthesis. It decreases plasma LDL and cholesterol and therefore is potentially useful in type II hyperlipidemia. Its main side effects are those of gastroin-

PATIENT CARE IMPLICATIONS

Patient and family education

- Most of these drugs cause GI side effects. Forewarn patients about this. Provide emotional support as needed. Reinforce to patients the importance of taking the drug as prescribed for best effect.
- Review Patient Problem: Constipation on p. 187.
- Tell patients to report persistent or severe diarrhea to the physician.
- Teach patients about necessary changes in diet to lower fat, carbohydrate, and cholesterol; see Dietary Consideration: Cholesterol on p. 346. Refer patients to the dietitian as appropriate.
- Teach patients that these drugs must be taken for weeks to months before full benefit can be seen. If the drugs prove to be beneficial, they may then be prescribed on a long-term basis.
- Remind patients not to discontinue taking the drugs without consulting the physician. Doses of other medications may be prescribed based on their effect when the patient is taking the prescribed antilipemic. Discontinuing the antilipemic therapy may result in incorrect or excessive doses of other drugs being taken.
- In familial hyperlipidemias, it may be appropriate to screen the children for its presence and if necessary to place them on therapeutic diets to lower lipid levels.

Cholestyramine and cholestipol

Drug administration

- Monitor intake and output and weight. Monitor urinalysis. Monitor vital signs. Assess for skin changes, rashes.
- Schedule drug administration times to allow as much time between cholestyramine or colestipol, and other drugs taken orally. At a minimum, take other drugs 1 hour before or 4 hours after cholestyramine or colestipol.

Patient and family education

- Review the general guidelines, above.
- The most common side effects are gastrointestinal. Instruct the patient to report the development of any unexpected sign or symptom.

- Review all of the drugs the patient is taking, and plan a dosing schedule to allow as much time as possible to elapse between the antilipemic and other medications.
- For the chewable bar, chew each bite well before swallowing.
- Do not take the powder in dry form. Always mix it with fluid or food or fruit having a high fluid content, such as applesauce, crushed pineapple, or thin soups, or with milk in hot or regular breakfast cereals. Fill a glass with 4 to 6 ounces of chosen fluid. Put the correct dose of medication on top of the fluid and let it stand, without stirring, for 1 to 2 minutes. This allows the medicine to absorb moisture and will help prevent formation of lumps. Stir and drink the mixture while the drug is still suspended. The drug will not dissolve in the fluid. Add a little more of the selected beverage to rinse the glass, and drink this also. If a carbonated beverage is chosen, use a large glass to prevent spillover, as the mixture will foam up. To prevent swallowing air, especially if a carbonated beverage is chosen, drink the mixture slowly. Take doses before meals and at bedtime, as ordered.
- Because these drugs interfere with absorption of fat-soluble vitamins, supplemental vitamins may be necessary; consult the physician.
- If these drugs are used to treat the pruritus of biliary stasis, the pruritus may reappear if the drug is discontinued.

Clofibrate

Patient and family education

- See the general guidelines, above.
- Nausea is the most common side effect, but others occasionally occur. Tell patients to report the development of any unexpected sign or symptom. Impotence and decreased libido have occurred; patients may be reluctant to mention these. Assess patient carefully for sexual side effects. Provide emotional support. It may be possible to change dose or drug; consult the physician.
- Take doses with meals to lessen gastric irritation. Nausea may diminish with continued use of the drug.

PATIENT CARE IMPLICATIONS — cont'd

Dextrothyroxine

Patient and family education

- Review general guidelines for antilipemic therapy.
- Refer to Chapter 52. The effects of treatment with dextrothyroxine mimic those of any thyroid replacement hormone. Overdose results in symptoms of hyperthyroidism.

Gemfibrozil

Patient and family education

- Review general guidelines for antilipemic therapy.
- Gastrointestinal upset is the most common side effect, but others occasionally occur. Tell patients to report the development of any unexpected sign or symptom.
- Caution diabetic patients to monitor blood glucose levels closely, as this drug may cause an increase in fasting glucose and a decrease in glucose tolerance. Changes in diet or insulin dose may be necessary.

Lovastatin

Patient and family education

- Review general guidelines for antilipemic therapy.
- Gastrointestinal discomfort may occur, and a variety of other side effects have been reported. Instruct patients to report the development of any unexpected sign or symptom.
- Warn patients to avoid driving or operating hazardous equipment if blurred vision or weakness develops; notify physician.
- Take doses with the evening meal.
- Encourage patients to have regular eye examinations.

Niacin

Patient and family education

- Review general guidelines for antilipemic therapy.
- As noted in the text, most patients experience flushing of the face and neck after taking the dose needed for its atilipemic effect. This usually diminishes with continued use of the drug. Starting with low doses and gradually increasing them may also help. Flushing may be ameliorated by taking 1 aspirin tablet 30 minutes before the niacin dose (check with physician).
- Gastrointestinal discomfort may occur, and a variety of other side effects have been reported. Instruct patients to report the development of any unexpected sign or symptom.
- Take doses with meals to lessen gastric irritation.
- For information about dietary sources of niacin, see Dietary Consideration: Vitamins, on p. 282.

Probucol

Patient and family education

- Review general guidelines for antilipemic therapy.
- Gastrointestinal discomfort may occur, and a variety of other side effects have been reported. Instruct patients to report the development of any unexpected sign or symptom. Impotence and decreased libido have occurred; patients may be reluctant to mention these. Assess patient carefully for development of such side effects. Provide emotional support. It may be possible to change dose or drug; consult the physician.
- Take doses with meals for best effect.

---

testinal upset: diarrhea, gas, abdominal pain, nausea, and vomiting. A clinical response to probucol occurs after 1 to 3 months of therapy. Cholesterol, but not triglyceride levels, is decreased. Patients with a history of cardiac arrhythmias should be monitored carefully.

Other Drugs Used as Lipid-Lowering Agents
Conjugated estrogens
Conjugated estrogens have been used as lipid-lowering agents because of the observation that premenopausal women have a low incidence of myocardial infarction. However, recent studies show that estrogen given to men not only causes feminization but also increases the incidence of heart attacks.

Progestins and androgens
Progestins may decrease hyperlipidemia in women with the rare type V hyperlipidemia. Progestins aggravate other types of hyperlipidemia and cannot be given to men. Anabolic androgens may reduce elevated plasma triglyceride concentrations in men only. Androgens can cause water retention

and therefore must be used with care in men with heart, kidney, or liver disease.

Neomycin

Neomycin is an antibiotic that is not well absorbed. Neomycin prevents cholesterol absorption in the intestine, thereby promoting bile acid secretion. These effects may lower elevated LDL levels in some patients with type II hyperlipidemia.

SUMMARY

Hyperlipidemia refers to greater than normal concentrations of plasma cholesterol or plasma triglycerides. High concentrations of plasma cholesterol are associated with an increased incidence of atherosclerosis, whereas high concentrations of plasma triglycerides are associated with an increased incidence of coronary heart disease. Genetics, diet, and metabolic disease each can be linked to hyperlipidemia.

Diet modification is the major therapeutic approach to treating the common types of hyperlipidemia. Drugs may be added if diet alone is not effective. Drugs acting to lower plasma cholesterol levels include cholestyramine, colestipol, dextrothyroxine, lovastatin, and probucol. Drugs acting to lower plasma triglyceride concentrations include clofibrate, gemfibrozil, and niacin.

STUDY QUESTIONS

1. List the four categories of lipoproteins and describe the role of each.
2. What is hyperlipidemia? What causes hyperlipidemia?
3. Name five drugs and their mechanism of action for lowering plasma cholesterol.
4. Name drugs and their mechanism of action for lowering triglycerides.

SUGGESTED READINGS

Antilipemics, Nursing 84 **14**(3):57, 1984.

Bissonnette, R.: Use of gemfibrozil in patients with dyslipidemia: a double-blind comparison with placebo, Intern. Med. **4**(9):132, 1983.

Borhani, N.O.: Coronary heart disease: an update on risk factors, Consultant **23**(5):77, 1983.

Brown, M.S., Kovanen, P.R., and Goldstein, J.L.: Regulation of plasma cholesterol by lipoprotein receptors, Science **212**:628, 1981.

Brown, W.V.: Treatment of hyperlipidemia, Prim. Cardiology **2**(suppl.):84, 1983.

Coronary Drug Project Research Group: Clofibrate and niacin in coronary heart disease, JAMA **231**:360, 1975.

Frick, M.H., and others: Helsinki heart study: primary prevention trial with gemfibrozil in middle-aged men with dyslipidemia, N. Engl. J. Med. **317**(20):1237, 1987.

Glueck, C.J.: Relationship of lipid disorders to coronary heart disease, Am. J. Med. **74**(5a):10, 1983.

Gotto, A.M., Jr.: Clinical diagnosis of hyperlipoproteinemia, Am. J. Med. **74**(5a):5, 1983.

Grundy, S.M.: Experience with individual lipid-lowering drugs: clofibrate, Cardiovasc. Rev. Rep. **3**(8):1179, 1982.

Grundy, S.M.: Cholesterol and coronary heart disease: a new era, JAMA **256**(20):2849, 1986.

Grundy, S.M.: HMG-CoA reductase inhibitors for treatment of hypercholesterolemia, N. Engl. J. Med. **319**(1):24, 1988.

Hartshorn, J.C., and Deans, K.: Treatment of hyperlipidemia with gemfibrozil, J. Cardiovasc. Nurs. **1**(4):76, 1987.

Havel, R.J.: Experience with individual lipid-lowering drugs: nicotinic acid, Cardiovasc. Rev. Rep. **3**(8):1982.

Hazzard, W.R.: Atherogenesis: why women live longer than men, Geriatrics **40**(1):42, 1985.

Herbert, P.N.: Experience with individual lipid-lowering drugs: probucol, Cardiovasc. Rev. Rep. **3**(8):1173, 1982.

Hoeg, J.M., Gregg, R.E., and Brewer, H.B., Jr.: An approach to the management of hyperlipoproteinemia, JAMA **255**(4):512, 1986.

Hunninghake, D.B.: Experience with individual lipid-lowering drugs: bile-acid sequestrants, Cardiovasc. Rev. Rep. **3**(8):1184, 1982.

Hunninghake, D.B.: Pharmacologic therapy for the hyperlipidemic patient, Am. J. Med. **74**(5a):19, 1983.

Kolata, G.: Cholesterol–heart disease link illuminated, Science **221**:1164, 1983.

Kolata, G.: Lowered cholesterol decreases heart disease, Science **223**:381, 1984.

Kuo, P.T.: Hyperlipoproteinemia and atherosclerosis: dietary intervention, Am. J. Med. **74**(5a):15, 1983.

Lovastatin Study Group II; Therapeutic response to lovastatin in nonfamilial hypercholesterolemia: a multicenter study, JAMA **256**(20):2829, 1986.

Lovastatin Study Group III; A multicenter comparison of lovastatin and cholestyramine therapy for severe primary hypercholesterolemia, JAMA **260**(3):359, 1988.

Luepker, R.V.: Hypercholesterolemia—contemporary recommendations for screening and treating, Consultant **22**(3):61, 1982.

Malinow, M.R.: Regression of atherosclerosis in humans, Postgrad. Med. **73**(5):232, 1983.

Nash, D.T.: Clinical investigation of gemfibrozil versus clofibrate, Cardiovasc. Rev. Rep. **3**(8):1207, 1982.

Nash, D.T.: Hyperlipidemia therapy—can it prevent coronary atherosclerosis? Postgrad. Med. **72**(2):207, 1982.

Nash, D.T.: Treatment that fights heart disease and checks atherosclerosis, Consultant **22**(12):165, 1982.

Nash, D.T.: Gemfibrozil in combination with other drugs for severe hyperlipidemia, Postgrad. Med. **73**(4):75, 1983.

Nash, D.T.: Hyperlipidemia: reducing the chances of cardiovascular disease, Geriatrics **39**(7):99, 1984.

Olsen, R.E.: Mass intervention vs. screening and selective intervention for the prevention of coronary heart disease, JAMA **255**(16):2204, 1986.

Peabody, H.D., Jr.: Clinical investigation of gemfibrozil: the treatment of primary hyperlipoproteinemia, Cardiovasc. Rev. Rep. **3**(8):1195, 1982.

Rifkind, B.M.: Gemfibrozil, lipids, and coronary risk, N. Engl. J. Med. **317**(20):79, 1987.

Ross, R.: The pathogenesis of atherosclerosis—an update, N. Engl. J. Med. **314**(8):488, 1986.

Samuel, P.: Effects of gemfibrozil on serum lipids. Am. J. Med. **74**(5a):23, 1983.

Schaefer, E.J., and Levy, R.I.: Pathogenesis and management of lipoprotein disorders, N. Engl. J. Med. **312**(20):1300, 1985.

Sloan, R.W.: Hyperlipidemia, Am. Fam. Physician **28**(3):171, 1983.

Todd, B.: Cholesterol reducers: worth the price? Geriatr. Nurs. **10**(1):39, 1989.

Vega, G.L., and Grundy, S.M.: Gemfibrozil therapy in primary hypertriglyceridemia associated with coronary heart disease, JAMA **253**(16):2398, 1985.

Williams, P.T., and others: Coffee intake and elevated cholesterol and apolipoprotein B levels in men, JAMA **252**(10):1407, 1985.

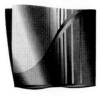

Drugs to Treat Nutritional Anemias

22

IRON
Functions of Iron

Iron is an essential component of several key proteins that function to carry oxygen or to utilize oxygen. Over 70% of body iron is part of hemoglobin, the protein of red blood cells that transports oxygen to tissues and carbon dioxide away from tissues. The red color of blood is due to the iron-oxygen complex in the heme portion of hemoglobin. Iron is also part of several of the electron transport enzymes of the mitochondria responsible for the oxidation-reduction reactions essential to every functioning cell.

Absorption, Storage, and Excretion of Iron

Given the importance of iron, it is not surprising that the body uses iron efficiently. The total iron content of a 70-kg man is about 4 Gm, yet iron is reused so efficiently that less than 1 mg of iron is lost daily. This small requirement is due to the extreme conservation of iron by the body. Not only is the iron of the red blood cell reused after cell degradation, but 10% to 35% of the iron is in a storage form for use when required. Iron is lost only as body cells are lost through shedding of cells from the gastrointestinal tract, skin, fingernails, and hair and in fluids such as bile, urine, and sweat are lost.

The absorption of iron from food is regulated. Iron is taken up by active transport into the mucosal cells of the duodenum and upper jejunum in the small intestine. These cells contain the protein ferritin, which binds the iron. When the ferritin is saturated with iron, further absorption of iron is limited. It remains in the mucosal cells unless transferred to the plasma protein transferrin. Iron not transferred within 5 days is lost in the feces as the mucosal cell is sloughed. Iron bound to transferrin is carried in the plasma and transferred to the proteins ferritin and hemosiderin, which act as storage forms of iron within the liver, spleen, and bone marrow.

Iron as a Therapeutic Agent

Iron deficiency anemia. When the intake of iron is inadequate to meet the demand, iron is first taken from the iron stores in hemosiderin and ferritin. Absorption of iron from the gastrointestinal tract can increase twofold when the ferritin within the mucosal cells is no longer saturated with iron. When iron stores are exhausted and the intake of iron is still inadequate, the newly made red blood cells are small (microcytic) and do not have much color (hypochromic) because there is not enough iron to make an adequate amount of hemoglobin to fill the cells. Iron deficiency anemia is therefore a microcytic, hypochromic anemia.

Requirements for iron. Iron deficiency anemia commonly results from one of two causes: blood loss or rapid growth. This is reflected in the varying requirements for dietary iron. The average American diet contains about 6 mg of iron per 1000 calories, and only 10% of dietary iron is actually absorbed, although up to 20% may be absorbed in an individual who is deficient in iron. Adult men and postmenopausal women have the lowest daily requirement for dietary iron (5 to 10 mg). Menstruating women have a higher daily requirement, depending on the amount of blood loss during menstruation (7 to 20 mg). Pregnant women have the highest daily requirement because of the added demand of the placenta and developing fetus (20 to 58 mg). Children and adolescents have a higher requirement per unit weight than adults because of their rapid growth (4 to 20 mg total). See Dietary Considerations: Iron.

Administration of replacement iron. Iron for replacement therapy is most commonly given orally as a ferrous salt. Iron preparations are listed in Table 22.1. Ferrous sulfate is the standard for these preparations. The usual daily dose in iron deficiency anemia is 50 to 100 mg of iron. The amount of iron per tablet depends on the ferrous salt used. A 300-mg tablet of ferrous sulfate con-

---

DIETARY CONSIDERATION: IRON

Iron deficiency contributes to iron deficiency anemia, the most common nutritional deficiency in the United States. Good dietary sources of iron include:

red meats   organ meats
legumes and nuts   green leafy vegetables
whole grains   enriched bread and
molasses   cereal
dried fruits   brewer's yeast

---

tains 60 mg of iron and 240 mg of sulfate; a 300-mg tablet of ferrous gluconate contains 37 mg of iron and 263 mg of gluconate; and a 300-mg tablet of ferrous fumarate contains 99 mg of iron and 201 mg of fumarate.

Iron is absorbed most readily in the ferrous form in the presence of acid. Therefore optimum absorption occurs when a tablet of ferrous sulfate or other soluble ferrous salt is taken before meals. However, iron is also highly irritating to the gastrointestinal tract; many patients cannot tolerate iron tablets taken on an empty stomach and have to take iron with meals. Enteric forms are not satisfactory, since they generally dissolve past the duodenum of the small intestine where there is little capacity for the absorption of iron. Infants and children given iron-supplemented formula or vitamins may develop an acute diarrhea from the gastrointestinal irritation.

Patients with iron deficiency anemia respond to iron therapy in the first 2 days with increased energy and appetite. Since this is too soon to correct the hemoglobin deficiency, the response may be due to restoration of the cellular enzymes containing iron. After 1 week there is an increase in the number of reticulocytes (immature red blood cells) and the rate of hemoglobin synthesis. Although the microcytic anemia of iron deficiency is eliminated after a few weeks of therapy, at least 6 months of therapy is necessary to restore iron storage sites.

Iron may also be given parenterally as iron dextran when oral administration is not possible. Slow intravenous injection is preferred. Deep intramuscular injection is painful and can discolor the injection site. An anaphylactic response is more common after intramuscular than after intravenous injection.

Food and drug interactions. Absorption of iron salts is increased with ingestion of large doses of ascorbic acid (vitamin C). Cereal and eggs decrease absorption, as do antacids, particularly magnesium trisilicate, and tetracyclines because all of these bind iron and prevent its uptake by the mucosal cells in the small intestine.

Iron Toxicity

Acute toxicity from excess iron. Acute toxicity from iron is uncommon in adults and is primarily seen in young children. The population most likely to be taking iron tablets are pregnant women who may also have small children. Many iron tablets are brightly colored and look like candy, leading young children to swallow many tablets at once. Most commonly the child experiences acute nausea and vomiting 30 to 60 minutes after ingesting the tablets. The primary treatment is gastric lavage with sodium phosphate or sodium bicarbonate to remove undissolved tablets, to create an alkaline environment that retards absorption, and to complex the ferrous iron into insoluble salts.

Within a few hours of ingestion, metabolic acidosis is common and cardiovascular collapse can occur. If supportive treatment carries the child through these stages, the next stage originates from tissue injury. The high concentration of iron overloads the uptake capacity of the mucosal cells so that a high concentration of free ferrous iron enters the portal circulation. Signs of extensive damage to the liver and kidney are evident in children who die of iron toxicity after 24 hours.

To avoid damage from high plasma concentrations of iron, a specific antidote, *deferoxamine mesylate (Desferal)*, is given as soon as possible and concurrently with lavage and supportive measures. Deferoxamine is given intramuscularly or intravenously, and in the plasma it combines with iron to form a water-soluble complex that is excreted in the urine (67%) and in the bile (33%). This complex gives a pink to red color to the urine and is evidence of elevated concentrations of iron in the plasma. The free deferoxamine imparts no color to the urine.

Chronic toxicity from iron overload. Since the body has no mechanisms to get rid of excess iron, excess intake can cause iron overload, called *hemosiderosis* (after the storage protein for iron). Chronic iron overload can occur in patients treated with parenteral iron or in patients who receive frequent blood transfusions, since each milliliter of blood contains 0.5 mg of iron. Some patients have a genetic tendency to store excess iron; this genetic disorder is called *hemochromatosis*. Iron overload traditionally causes a bronze color of the skin of the face, neck, upper chest, genitalia, hands, and forearms. The pancreas is especially sensitive to damage, and diabetes mellitus can result. Liver

Table 22.1 Drugs to Treat Nutritional Anemias

Generic name	Trade name	Administration/dosage	Comments
IRON SALTS FOR IRON DEFICIENCY ANEMIA			
Ferrous fumarate (33% elemental iron)	Femiron Fumerin* Feostat* Various others	Replacement therapy requires 90 to 300 mg of elemental iron daily in divided doses before meals if tolerated or with meals.	Timed-release or enteric coated forms considered less effective because of poor iron absorption beyond the duodenum.
Ferrous gluconate (11.6% elemental iron)	Fergon* Ferralet Various others	See above.	See above.
Ferrous sulfate (20% elemental iron)	Feosol* Fer-In-Sol Fero-Gradumet* Various others	See above.	See above.
Iron-dextran injection	Imferon* Dextraron* Various others	INTRAVENOUS: *Adults and children*— no more than 100 mg daily, no faster than 50 mg (1 ml) per minute of the undiluted solution, or dilute in 500 to 1000 ml normal saline solution and administer by drip over 10 hr. FDA Pregnancy Category C.	Reserved for use in severe iron deficiency anemia where oral iron is contraindicated (gastrointestinal disease) or unsuccessful. Serious toxic effects, including anaphylaxis, may accompany parenteral administration and are more common with intramuscular than with intravenous administration.
Iron-polysaccharide complex	Hytinic* Niferex*	See above.	Not well absorbed. May be milder to the stomach than other formulations.
ANTIDOTE FOR IRON TOXICITY			
Deferoxamine mesylate	Desferal*	INTRAMUSCULAR: preferred route; 1 Gm followed by 0.5 Gm at 4 hr and 8 hr. INTRAVENOUS: in face of cardiovascular collapse; as for intramuscular but infused at 15 mg kg/hr. Not to exceed 6 Gm in 24 hr.	A specific chelator for iron. To manage acute iron intoxication. Will turn urine pink to red. Can be administered long term to manage secondary hemochromatosis.
VITAMIN B$_{12}$ (CYANOCOBALAMIN) FOR PERNICIOUS ANEMIA			
Hydroxocobalamin	AlphaRedisol Acti-B$_{12}$*	As for cyanocobalamin.	Like cyanocobalamin. Somewhat longer acting.
Vitamin B$_{12}$ (cyanocobalamin)	Betalin 12* Redisol* Rubramin PC* Various others	INTRAMUSCULAR: 30 to 50 μg daily for 5 to 10 days, then 100 to 200 μg monthly.	For pernicious anemia, only intramuscular injection is effective. Oral forms may be taken for dietary deficiency.
FOLIC ACID FOR ANEMIA			
Folic acid	Apo-Folic† Folvite*	ANY ROUTE: *Adults or children*—1 mg daily.	Solutions of the sodium salt are used for parenteral administration.
Leucovorin calcium	Wellcovorin Generic	For megaloblastic anemia: 1 mg daily. To counter folic acid antagonists: give in amounts equal to the weight of antagonist.	The metabolically active form of folic acid. The expense does not justify its use for anemia, but protects normal tissue when given with methotrexate (antineoplastic drug) or pyrimethamine (antimalarial drug)

*Available in Canada and United States.
†Available in Canada.

THE NURSING PROCESS

IRON THERAPY

Assessment

Patients requiring iron therapy frequently are those with poor nutritional intake, blood loss, or excessive growth; they may be vegetarians, and they are often female. They may appear with fatigue, pallor, and lethargy. Folic acid deficiency and vitamin B_{12} deficiency are usually diagnosed from blood studies but may be seen in patients with iron deficiency anemia. Baseline data would include vital signs; weight; diet history; blood studies including hemoglobin, peripheral blood smear, and reticulocyte count; and the presence of any neurological symptoms such as tingling in the fingers or toes.

Nursing diagnoses

Altered bowel elimination: constipation secondary to iron therapy

Altered bowel elimination: diarrhea secondary to iron therapy

Management

In the usual prescribed dosages there are few side effects with these drugs. In planning for discharge, dietary instruction should be given when the source of the anemia is dietary. Since cyanocobalamin has occasionally produced anaphylaxis, appropriate drugs and equipment for resuscitation should be available when this drug is administered.

Evaluation

The goal of therapy is the return to and the maintenance of a normal blood count and blood profile. Before discharge the patient should be able to explain the kind or kinds of anemia present, the reasons for drug therapy, how to correctly take the prescribed medications, the anticipated side effects and what to do about them, and which symptoms related to the anemia can be expected to improve and which will not. (The neurological damage in pernicious anemia is occasionally permanent.) In addition, the patient should be able to identify dietary sources of needed iron or folic acid. For additional information, see the patient care implications section at the end of this chapter.

---

damage is seen on biopsy but is generally not serious unless superimposed on liver disease. Patients with iron overload generally die of heart failure. Treatment of iron overload is weekly bleeding (phlebotomy).

MEGALOBLASTIC MACROCYTIC ANEMIAS

Both vitamin B_{12} and folic acid are required for a key reaction in the synthesis of thymidylate, a component of deoxyribonucleic acid (DNA). Whereas folic acid is the immediate cofactor in this synthesis, vitamin B_{12} is necessary to regenerate the active form of folic acid. A deficiency of either folic acid or vitamin B_{12} results in the release of too few red blood cells. Those red blood cells that are released are large and immature because of the deficiency of DNA synthesis required for cell division and maturation. This is a *megaloblastic* (immature) *macrocytic* (large cell) anemia. Other tissue cells that turn over rapidly and require active DNA synthesis include some white cells and mucosal cells of the gastrointestinal tract. A deficiency in white cell counts may therefore appear, as can gastrointestinal upset in vitamin B_{12} or folic acid deficiency.

Vitamin B_{12} and Pernicious Anemia

Vitamin B_{12} is a unique vitamin because it requires a special binding protein for transport into the intestinal cells. This binding protein is called *intrinsic factor*, which is produced and released by the parietal cells of the stomach. (Parietal cells also release hydrochloric acid.) Pernicious anemia is the relative or complete lack of intrinsic factor so that vitamin B_{12} is no longer absorbed. The body has a large store of vitamin B_{12}, 4 to 5 mg, and a deficiency will not occur for 2 to 5 years after intrinsic factor is no longer released. Stomach atrophy is a normal part of the aging process, and pernicious anemia appears more frequently in patients over 50 years

General guidelines for patients receiving iron therapy

Drug administration

- Parenteral and oral iron preparations should not be given at the same time, as this will increase the incidence of toxic reactions.
- Parenteral doses of iron may cause anaphylactic reactions. Before the first dose of IM or IV iron dextran, a test dose of 25 mg should be given. Monitor the vital signs. Wait at least 1 hour before administering the remaining dose. Have available equipment, drugs, and personnel to treat anaphylactic reactions. Other reactions may include febrile reactions, arthralgias, myalgia, headache, transitory paresthesia, nausea, shivering, and rash.

INTRAMUSCULAR IRON DEXTRAN
- Use large muscle masses, preferably in the buttocks. The drug may stain the skin, which on the thigh is cosmetically unacceptable. Consult the physician when administering to small children and infants. Draw up the prescribed dose. Put a fresh needle on the syringe. Use the Z-track method of administration. For an illustration of the Z-track method, see Chapter 6.

INTRAVENOUS IRON DEXTRAN
- May be given undiluted or diluted in 50 to 250 ml normal saline. Administer a test dose over at least 5 minutes. Administer other doses at a rate of 50 mg/minute. Flush the IV line with normal saline before and after administering dose. Keep the patient in a supine position for 30 minutes following IV doses; monitor vital signs and blood pressure.

Patient and family education

- Review dietary sources of iron with patients (see Dietary Consideration: Iron on p. 355).
- Remind patients to keep all medications out of the reach of children. Tell patients to notify the physician immediately if overdose with iron is suspected.
- Take liquid iron preparations through a straw to avoid staining the teeth. Dilute the preparation well with water or fruit juice, and rinse the mouth well after taking the dose.
- Ideally, take iron preparations on an empty stomach, which may cause significant gastrointestinal upset. Take drug with meals or snack to reduce gastric irritation, but note that absorption is significantly reduced in the presence of milk, antacids, tetracycline, many cereals, and eggs. Ascorbic acid (vitamin C) increases the absorption of iron; some patients may wish to take the iron with orange or other citrus juice.

- Inform the patient that regular use of iron will cause the feces to turn dark green or black and to become more tarry in consistency. If there is doubt whether the cause of a change in color or consistency in stools is due to blood or ingestion of iron, the stool should be tested for presence of blood.
- Some patients experience constipation while taking iron preparations, while others experience diarrhea. See Patient Problem: Constipation on p. 187. If diarrhea is severe or persistent, notify the physician.
- To decrease gastric irritation, suggest that the patient take smaller but more frequent doses of iron.

Deferoxamine mesylate

Drug administration

- Deferoxamine may be administered via IM, IV, or subcutaneous injection, usually by subcutaneous pump. IM or subcutaneous injection may cause swelling, irritation, pain, and itching at the injection site.
- Deferoxamine has been associated with allergic reactions, including anaphylactic reactions. Monitor vital signs. Have equipment and drugs available to treat acute allergic reactions.

INTRAVENOUS DEFEROXAMINE
- Dilute as directed in the manufacturer's literature. Administer at a rate not exceeding 15 mg/kg/hr. Monitor the blood pressure and vital signs. Treatment of acute iron overdose should be done in the acute care setting.

Vitamin B_{12}

Drug administration

- Administer parenteral doses via the IM route only.
- Allergic reactions have been reported. Monitor vital signs and blood pressure. Have available drugs and equipment to treat acute allergic responses.

Patient and family education

- Teach patients with pernicious anemia about their disease. It may be difficult for patients to understand why the vitamin B_{12} cannot be taken orally, and why it must be continued for life.
- Review dietary sources of vitamin B_{12} (see Dietary Considerations: Vitamins on p. 282) with patients in whom vitamin B_{12} deficiency is due to dietary causes.
- Avoid the use of alcohol while taking vitamin B_{12}.

PATIENT CARE IMPLICATIONS—cont'd

Folic acid

Drug administration

- In addition to the more common oral administration, folic acid may be given IM, IV, or via the subcutaneous route.
- Intravenous administration:
  May be given undiluted or added to most IV solutions and given as an infusion. For direct IV administration, administer at a rate not to exceed 5 mg/min.
- Allergic reactions, though rare, have been reported. Monitor vital signs after parenteral administration. Have drugs and equipment available to treat acute allergic reactions.

Patient and family education

- Review dietary sources of folic acid (see Dietary Considerations: Vitamins on p. 282).
- Warn patients that self-treatment with large doses of vitamins is unwise, and may mask some health problems. Large doses of vitamins should be taken only under the direction of a physician.

Leucovorin

Drug administration/patient and family education

- Leucovorin is the calcium salt of folinic acid, a metabolite of folic acid. Read orders carefully. It may be given orally, IM, or IV. Parenteral administration is usually used when the drug is given to counteract some of the toxic effects of the folic acid antagonists, especially some cancer chemotherapy drugs (called leucovorin rescue). See Chapter 39.
- Parenteral administration:
  Reconstitute as directed on the vial. Further dilute in 100 to 500 ml of common IV fluid. Administer dilute volume over 15 minutes to 1 hour (depending on volume and patient condition). Monitor vital signs.
- Review with patients and families the reason leucovorin is being used. Instruct them to report the development of any unexpected sign or symptom.

---

of age than in younger patients. Any condition that damages the stomach can also cause pernicious anemia.

Origin, absorption, and distribution of vitamin B_{12}. A diet including animal protein, eggs, and dairy products contains adequate vitamin B_{12}. The usual American diet contains 5 to 15 μg of vitamin B_{12}, although the minimum daily requirement is only 1 to 2 μg of vitamin B_{12}. Only strict vegetarians may develop dietary vitamin B_{12} deficiency over a period of several years. Vitamin B_{12} bound to intrinsic factor is absorbed in the distal ileum, the part of the small intestine just ahead of the large intestine, and this absorption requires a slightly alkaline pH. Conditions in which the distal ileum is damaged or removed or in which the pancreas fails to secrete sufficient bicarbonate to keep the intestine at a slightly alkaline pH will slow absorption of vitamin B_{12}. After absorption, vitamin B_{12} is carried to storage sites. Some vitamin B_{12} is excreted in the bile but is later reabsorbed.

Neurological damage from vitamin B_{12} deficiency. A deficiency of vitamin B_{12} is especially serious because neurological damage may result. This damage arises because vitamin B_{12} is a cofactor for an enzymatic step necessary for producing the myelin sheath of nerves. A frequent initial neurological symptom of vitamin B_{12} deficiency is a tingling sensation of the extremities (paresthesia) from this neurological damage. Neurological damage becomes irreversible if vitamin B_{12} deficiency persists.

Administration of replacement vitamin B_{12} (Table 22.1). The intramuscular injection of vitamin B_{12} to bypass the intestine for systemic absorption is the treatment for pernicious anemia. Initial therapy is administered daily for about 1 week, then monthly throughout life. Oral vitamin B_{12} is indicated only for the rare dietary deficiency of vitamin B_{12} when there is an adequate amount of intrinsic factor released.

Vitamin B_{12} injections have been given indiscriminately to older patients as a general tonic, which it is not. Vitamin B_{12} injections are also not of therapeutic value for general neurological disorders, psychiatric disorders, general malnutrition, or loss of appetite. It is important also to realize that folic acid taken in large doses will overcome the block in DNA synthesis caused by the deficiency of vitamin B_{12}. Folic acid will thereby cure the anemia, but folic acid cannot affect the vitamin B_{12}–dependent reaction necessary for myelin synthesis. If folic acid is taken indiscriminately, the anemia of vitamin B_{12} deficiency will never appear, but neurological damage may proceed until it is irreversible.

Vitamin B_{12} injections are virtually free of side effects. Patients receiving vitamin B_{12} injections for pernicious anemia must understand that injections must be continued for the rest of their lives to avoid irreversible neurological damage.

Folic Acid and Anemia

Folic acid is found in most meats, fresh vegetables, and fresh fruits but is destroyed when these are cooked for longer than 15 minutes. Folic acid preparations are listed in Table 22.1. The minimum daily requirement is 50 μg, and the average American diet contains 200 μg to 300 μg. Unlike stores of vitamin B_{12}, stores of folic acid are not large and can be depleted in a few weeks when the diet is deficient in folic acid. Individuals with poor diets and chronic alcoholics may be deficient in folic acid. Pregnant women and nursing mothers have an increased requirement for folic acid, and it is commonly given as a routine supplement to these women. Folic acid, which is readily absorbed in the intestine, is administered orally.

Some drugs interfere with the utilization of folic acid: phenytoin, oral contraceptives, glucocorticoids, and aspirin. Methotrexate, antineoplastic drugs, and pyrimethamine, an antimalarial drug, are folic acid antagonists. When these drugs are used, *folinic acid (leucovorin)*, the metabolically active form of folic acid, can be given to protect normal tissues from folic acid deficiency. Folic acid itself is nontoxic. The greatest danger of indiscriminate ingestion of folic acid is that it may correct the anemia of pernicious anemia but leave the neurological damage untreated.

SUMMARY

The most common causes of nutritional anemias are deficiencies of iron, vitamin B_{12}, and folic acid.

Iron deficiency anemia is a microcytic, hypochromic anemia. Iron is a required part of hemoglobin, the red-colored protein that carries oxygen in the red blood cells. Normally the body stores 10% to 35% of its iron in reserve, but growth, pregnancy, and menstruation, in addition to a poor diet, can deplete these reserves.

The absorption of iron from the gastrointestinal tract is highly regulated. Because iron is so highly conserved, no route of excretion of any capacity exists for iron. Children ingesting an overdose of iron pills will suffer acute toxicity, which may cause death secondary to damage of the kidney and liver. Deferoxamine is a water-soluble iron chelator, which allows iron to be excreted into the urine and bile.

Pernicious anemia is a deficiency of vitamin B_{12} arising from a lack of intrinsic factor, a protein secreted by the parietal cells of the stomach and required to transport vitamin B_{12} throughout the body from the gastrointestinal tract. Pernicious anemia will give rise to a megaloblastic anemia because vitamin B_{12} is required to regenerate the folic acid needed for DNA synthesis. More serious is the damage to the myelin sheath of nerves, arising from the lack of vitamin B_{12}. This neurological damage can become irreversible if pernicious anemia is not treated. Replacement of vitamin B_{12} for pernicious anemia must be made by intramuscular injection.

A deficiency of folic acid gives rise to a megaloblastic anemia because folic acid is required for DNA synthesis and the maturation of red blood cells. Folic acid deficiency is most common during pregnancy and in alcoholics.

STUDY QUESTIONS

1. What is the role of iron?
2. Describe the factors governing the absorption of iron.
3. What are the symptoms of iron toxicity?
4. How does deferoxamine function as an antidote for iron toxicity?
5. What is pernicious anemia?
6. Why does vitamin B_{12} have to be injected intramuscularly to treat pernicious anemia?
7. What role do vitamin B_{12} and folic acid play in red blood cell maturation?
8. Why is folic acid contraindicated for treatment of pernicious anemia?

SUGGESTED READINGS

Beisel, W.R.: Iron nutrition: immunity and infection, Res. Staff Physician **27**(5):37, 1981.

Beutler, E.: The common anemias, JAMA **259**(16):2433, 1988.

Castle, W.B.: Megaloblastic anemia, Postgrad. Med. **64**(10):117, 1978.

Cohen, A.R.: Chelation therapy for iron overload, Drug Therapy **6**(9):47, 1981.

Emery, T.: Iron metabolism in humans and plants, Am. Scientist **70**:626, 1982.

Finch, C.A., and Huebers, H.: Perspectives in iron metabolism, N. Engl. J. Med. **306**:1520, 1982.

Fisher, D.S., Parkman, R., and Finch, S.C.: Acute iron poisoning in children, JAMA **218**:1179, 1971.

Froberg, J.H.: The anemias: causes and courses of action, RN, Part 1:**52**(1):24, 1989; Part 2:**52**(3):52, 1989.

Fuller, E.: Reviewing iron overload disorders, Patient Care **18**(19):102, 1982.

Hillman, R.S.: Blood-loss anemia, Postgrad. Med. **64**(10):88, 1978.

Hobbs, J., and Rodriguez, A.R.: Megaloblastic anemias, Am. Fam. Physician **22**(6):128, 1980.

How much workup for the anemic patient? Postgrad. Med. **64**(10):85, 1978.

Lanzkowsky, P.: Iron deficiency and resultant anemia in adolescents, Consultant **21**(8):164, 1981.

McArthur, J.R.: A clinical approach to anemia, Postgrad. Med. **64**(10):85, 1978.

O'Neil-Cutting, M.A., and Crosby, W.H.: The effect of antacids on the absorption of simultaneously ingested iron, JAMA **255**(11):1468, 1986.

Roach, E.S., and McLean, W.T.: Neurologic disorders of vitamin B$_{12}$ deficiency, Am. Fam. Physician **25**(1):111, 1982.

Stockman, J.A. III: Iron deficiency anemia: have we come far enough? JAMA **258**(12):1645, 1987.

Wallerstein, R.O.: Differentiating common anemias, Consultant **20**(8):65, 1980.

VI

DRUGS TO TREAT MILD PAIN AND FEVER, INFLAMMATION, ALLERGY, AND RESPIRATORY OBSTRUCTION

One area in classic pharmacology is that of the autacoids, those diverse "local mediators" whose functions are only now being understood. This section covers the pharmacological basis of mild pain and fever, inflammation, allergy, and respiratory obstruction in which autacoids play a major role.

The subject matter of Chapter 23, *Analgesic-Antipyretic, Nonsteroidal Antiinflammatory Drugs and Specific Agents to Treat Rheumatoid Arthritis and Gout,* may seem diverse but in fact relates the various uses of aspirin. Aspirin is recognized as an inhibitor of the synthesis of one class of autacoids, the prostaglandins. Certain prostaglandins play a role in inflammation. Another autacoid is histamine; hence Chapter 24, *Antihistamines.* Chapter 25, *Bronchodilators and Other Drugs to Treat Asthma,* deals with the therapeutics of a disease, asthma, in which autacoids play a major role but for which the therapeutic pharmacology principally involves adrenergic mechanisms. Chapter 26, *Drugs to Control Bronchial Secretions,* includes classes of drugs for treating respiratory problems, including nasal congestion, cough, and thickened mucus, to complete the coverage of respiratory pharmacology.

23

Analgesic-Antipyretic, Nonsteroidal Antiinflammatory Drugs and Specific Agents to Treat Rheumatoid Arthritis and Gout

This chapter is divided into four sections: analgesic-antipyretic drugs, nonsteroidal antiinflammatory drugs, drugs to treat rheumatoid arthritis, and drugs to treat gout. These are all classifications for the actions of aspirin, although aspirin is no longer used to treat gout. Aspirin is used for three basic pharmacological actions: antipyresis (reducing fever), analgesia for mild to moderate pain, and reducing inflammation. Although aspirin has been found to be an effective inhibitor of prostaglandin synthesis (Chapter 20), it is not clear that this explains more than the antiinflammatory action. In addition to aspirin, each of the four sections considers other drugs that are used clinically.

ANALGESIC-ANTIPYRETIC DRUGS
Analgesia

The analgesics discussed in this chapter, also called the *nonnarcotic analgesics*, all act by a peripheral mechanism through which they interfere with local mediators released in damaged tissue to stimulate nerve endings. In the presence of the nonnarcotic analgesics, the nerves are not stimulated. Objective pain, the component of pain that arises from stimulation of peripheral nerve endings, is therefore not felt. This mechanism is in contrast to that of the narcotic analgesics, which interfere with subjective pain at the level of the central nervous system (Chapter 44).

Antipyresis

An antipyretic drug is one that reduces a fever. Normally the balance between heat production and heat dissipation is regulated by the brain. An area of the preoptic anterior hypothalamus is considered the thermostat of the body. Fever results from an increase in the "set point" of this hypothalamic center. An endogenous fever-producing agent (pyrogen) is released by white cells engulfing foreign matter (phagocytic leukocytes). This endogenous pyrogen is the major, if not the only, final product that acts on the hypothalamic center to produce fever in response to infections, hypersensitivity, or inflammation. Even though it is clear that fever is produced by a protein synthesized by the body as part of an immunological reaction, it is not clear in what way fever is a beneficial response, although phagocytosis is enhanced by a higher body temperature. The nonnarcotic analgesics act as antipyretics by reversing the effect of the endogenous pyrogen on the hypothalamus so that the "thermostat" is returned to normal.

Analgesic-Antipyretic Drugs

Acetaminophen (Datril, Tylenol, Panadol, others) and several salicylates, including aspirin, are so widely used by the public that a patient may not think to mention them when asked, "What drugs have you taken recently?" Acetaminophen and the salicylates are similar in producing both analgesia and antipyresis and are safe enough to be available without a prescription. But, like all drugs, they do have side effects and can interact with other drugs. In addition to acetaminophen and the salicylates, the nonsteroidal antiinflammatory drugs discussed in the next section are also antipyretics and analgesics. Except for ibuprofen they are prescription drugs and are used primarily to treat inflammation and its pain.

Acetaminophen (Table 23.1)
Mechanism of action. Acetaminophen (Datril, Tylenol, Panadol, others) acts at the hypothalamus to reduce fever and at peripheral pain receptors to block activation. Although acetaminophen is identical to aspirin in its antipyretic and analgesic properties, there is no evidence that it inhibits prostaglandin synthesis. Acetaminophen is not effective

Table 23.1 Analgesic-Antipyretic Drugs

Generic name	Trade name	Administration/dosage	Comments
Acetaminophen	Tylenol* Datril Panadol* Liquiprin Various others	ORAL: *Adults*—325 to 650 mg every 6 to 8 hr. No more than 2.6 Gm in 24 hr. *Children*—7 to 12 yr, ½ adult dose; 3 to 6 yr, ⅙ adult dose. Available without prescription.	Analgesic and antipyretic only. Little antiinflammatory action. No inhibition of platelets. Contraindicated in patients with glucose 6-phosphate dehydrogenase deficiency. Nonprescription.
Aspirin (acetyl-salicylic acid)	A.S.A. Aspergum Bayer Aspirin Children's Aspirin Ecotrin* Measurin	*For analgesia or antipyresis:* ORAL, RECTAL: *Adults*—650 mg every 4 hr, or 1.3 Gm of timed-release every 8 hr. *Children*—65 mg/kg over 24 hr in divided doses, every 4 to 6 hours.	Oral doses should be taken with a large glass of water or milk to decrease stomach irritation. Some patients may need to take aspirin after a meal to avoid gastrointestinal distress. Nonprescription.
Aspirin, buffered	Aluprin Ascriptin Bufferin Alka-Seltzer Various others	Same as for aspirin. There are no smaller dose tablets for children.	Alka Seltzer contains 1.9 Gm sodium bicarbonate and 1 Gm citric acid per tablet. To avoid acid-base disturbances, limit ingestion to occasional use only. Remaining products contain magnesium and aluminum antacid salts. These salts are not absorbed systemically to any great extent. Nonprescription.
Salicylamide	Salicylamide	ORAL: *Adults and children over 12 yr*—650 mg every 6 hr.	Not as effective as aspirin. Nonprescription.
Sodium salicylate	Uracel Uromide	Same as for aspirin. An injectable form is available by prescription.	Less effective than an equal dose of aspirin. May be tolerated by patients who are allergic to aspirin. Does not affect platelet function, but does retain vitamin K antagonist effect, which can increase prothrombin time. Nonprescription.

*Available in Canada and United States.

in reducing the inflammation of rheumatoid arthritis but may be effective in reducing pain in mild osteoarthritis.

Administration and use. Acetaminophen is used for the same spectrum of analgesic-antipyretic actions as is aspirin and can be combined with aspirin or other analgesics, including codeine. Unlike aspirin, the drug can be formulated as a liquid for infants and young children. There are elixirs, solutions, suspensions, chewable tablets, wafers, tablets, caplets, and capsules available. Acetaminophen is preferred to aspirin in treating the fever and discomfort of "flu" and chickenpox in childhood and early adulthood. Aspirin is implicated in the development of Reye's syndrome in young people who experience those viral diseases. Acetaminophen has also become a popular alternative to aspirin for treating simple pain and fever because it does not cause gastric irritation or alter platelet funding and bleeding times, as does aspirin. Fur-

thermore, acetaminophen does not interact with the oral anticoagulants or other drugs.

Side effects. Acetaminophen can be the cause of allergic reactions, usually involving skin rashes. Persons with a known glucose 6-phosphate dehydrogenase deficiency can develop hemolytic anemia if they take the drug. In long-term use, acetaminophen can cause methemoglobinemia, which impairs the oxygen-carrying capacity of the blood. It is serious only in infants. There has been a report that chronic daily ingestion of acetaminophen is associated with an increased risk of renal disease.

Toxicity. In adults, overdose of acetaminophen causes liver damage. Alcoholics are especially prone to this occurrence. Children rarely suffer permanent liver damage from the drug, but adults who take more than 2.6 Gm in 24 hours may show mild symptoms of liver damage such as loss of appetite, nausea, vomiting, and slight jaundice. In deliberate overdoses of 10 Gm or more, adults are highly susceptible to severe liver damage; death has been reported following ingestion of 15 Gm. This toxicity arises because the liver normally conjugates toxic metabolites of acetaminophen with a sulfhydryl compound, glutathione, to produce an inactive, readily excreted compound. The amount of glutathione available for conjugation is exceeded when large amounts of acetaminophen are ingested. The unconjugated metabolites then bind to and destroy liver cells. Acetylcysteine is most effective if administered within 8 hours of an acetaminophen overdose. Cimetidine, which inhibits hepatic metabolism of acetaminophen, is being tested as an additional antidote for overdose.

Acetylcysteine (Mucomyst) is effective in preventing liver damage due to excessive acetaminophen. Acetylcysteine is used in respiratory therapy to degrade bronchial mucus (Chapter 26). When given to counteract acetaminophen, it provides the sulfhydryl groups needed to conjugate and inactivate the toxic metabolites of acetaminophen. Treatment should begin within 12 hours following overdose. The stomach is first emptied by lavage or induced vomiting. An initial dose of 140 mg/kg is given as a 5% solution; doses of 70 mg/kg are then administered every 4 hours for approximately 17 doses. Since acetylcysteine has the pervasive flavor of rotten eggs, it must be disguised in a flavored iced drink, and preferably drunk through a straw to minimize contact with the mouth.

Acetylsalicylic acid (aspirin) (Table 23.1)

Aspirin is effective in low doses (325 to 650 mg or 1 to 2 adult tablets) to reduce fever and relieve mild pain. Two aspirin tablets are considered the analgesic equivalent of 60 mg of codeine. Aspirin is an effective analgesic for most common mild to moderate headaches and to relieve generalized mild muscular aches. Aspirin or aspirin-codeine combinations are also useful in treating mild to moderate pain of tooth extractions, episiotomies, cancer, and bone fractures. A dose of 1.2 Gm per day of aspirin produces the maximum analgesic effect. At much higher doses (3 to 6 Gm per day) aspirin is the drug of choice in treating the inflammation of rheumatoid arthritis. At this concentration, aspirin is the prototype for the nonsteroidal antiinflammatory drugs, which will be discussed in the next section.

Absorption and distribution. Aspirin is a weak acid and is rapidly absorbed from the stomach and upper small intestine. Buffering agents are present in several aspirin brands to hasten dissolution of the tablet and to reduce gastric irritation from the tablet. These advantages of buffering agents are minimal, and if several doses are to be taken, the buffering agents may cause loose stools. The Alka-Seltzer brand contains so much sodium and bicarbonate that it should be used only on a short-term basis.

Once aspirin is absorbed, 50% to 90% binds loosely to plasma albumin. Aspirin can displace oral anticoagulants, oral hypoglycemic drugs, phenytoin, and methotrexate. Since the unbound drug is the effective concentration, the free drug may reach toxic levels when displaced by aspirin.

Metabolism and excretion. Aspirin is rapidly hydrolyzed in the blood. The acetyl group of aspirin is readily transferred to the enzyme cyclooxygenase of the blood platelets. Cyclooxygenase is the key enzyme for the formation of prostaglandins. The acetylation of cyclooxygenase is irreversible and therefore persists for the 3- to 7-day lifetime of the platelet. Acetylated cyclooxygenase is inactive, and synthesis of the prostaglandin thromboxane A_2 is therefore blocked. Thromboxane A_2, which is a potent agent promoting platelet aggregation, is normally synthesized by platelets as they begin to aggregate. Even one aspirin tablet inhibits blood clotting by inhibiting platelet aggregation. This observation has led to the examination of aspirin as a prophylactic agent to prevent myocardial infarctions and strokes, processes associated with an increased tendency toward platelet aggregation (Chapter 20).

Salicylic acid is the other product of the hydrolysis of aspirin. Salicylate (the basic salt to which salicylic acid dissociates at the pH of blood) is an analgesic-antipyretic and a reversible inhibitor of prostaglandin synthesis. Salicylate does not affect platelet aggregation, and therefore a salicylate salt is sometimes used in place of aspirin.

In an acidic urine, salicylic acid is uncharged and therefore diffuses back into the blood. Vitamin C (ascorbic acid) maintains an acidic urine when taken in large doses and can therefore delay the excretion of salicylic acid. This interaction can be dangerous if large doses of aspirin are being taken, as for arthritis. In an alkaline urine, salicylic acid dissociates to salicylate, which is charged, cannot diffuse back into the blood, and is therefore eliminated in the urine. Salicylate is metabolized to inactive salicyluric acid by the liver. However, a single 325-mg aspirin tablet will saturate this liver inactivation system; thus the liver cannot readily metabolize large doses of aspirin.

Side effects. Approximately 2% to 10% of those taking an occasional aspirin tablet will experience gastrointestinal upset. This may be felt as heartburn or nausea. Aluminum and calcium-urea salts of aspirin have been formulated to be less irritating to the stomach than aspirin. When aspirin is taken regularly in large doses, for arthritis, this incidence becomes 30% to 50% and may be the factor limiting the use of aspirin. Sometimes antacids are prescribed to minimize stomach irritation, but antacids also raise the pH of the urine and increase the rate of excretion of salicylic acid. Alternatively, therefore, enteric-coated or timed-release preparations may be tried to decrease gastric irritation.

Aspirin is directly irritating and damaging to gastric mucosal cells. Since alcohol also has these gastric effects, aspirin should not be taken when alcohol is in the stomach. The combination of alcohol and aspirin is greater than additive in producing gastric bleeding. Patients with active peptic ulcers should be advised not to use aspirin.

Long-term aspirin ingestion can cause the loss of 10 to 30 ml of blood daily from gastrointestinal irritation. This may lead to iron deficiency anemia in women with heavy menses. Rarely, massive gastrointestinal bleeding has been encountered in patients taking aspirin on a long-term basis.

Some people develop an allergy to aspirin. The most common form of aspirin intolerance is manifested as a rash. Patients with a skin rash caused by aspirin may tolerate other salicylates. A few people develop nasal polyps and sometime later develop an asthma that is triggered by aspirin.

Patients who are sensitive to aspirin may be sensitive to a variety of other compounds. Most commonly, individuals sensitive to aspirin may show *cross-sensitivity* to

1. Salicylin-containing foods, for example, apples, oranges, and bananas
2. Processed foods or drugs containing tartrazine dye or sodium benzoate
3. Iodide-containing substances
4. Various other nonsteroidal antiinflammatory agents
5. Tartrazine (see Patient Alert: Tartrazine)

As can be seen from this list, the origin of these cross-sensitivities is not always the classic cross-reactivity due to structural similarities of the agents.

Reye's syndrome. When treated with aspirin, children and teens who have an acute febrile illness, such as "flu" or chickenpox, seem to be at increased risk for contracting Reye's syndrome. Reye's syndrome is rare but serious. It is characterized by vomiting and rapidly progressive encephalopathy. Acetaminophen and other nonsteroidal antiinflammatory drugs have not been so implicated. Nonprescription aspirin products now contain a warning against administration to children and teenagers who manifest chickenpox or "flu" symptoms.

Salicylism. Mild intoxication with aspirin is called *salicylism* and is commonly experienced when the daily dosage is more than 4 Gm. Tinnitus (ringing in the ears) is the most frequent effect and may be accompanied by a degree of reversible hearing loss. Since salicylate stimulates the respiratory center, hyperventilation (rapid breathing) may be seen. Fever may even result because salicylate interferes with the metabolic pathways coupling oxygen consumption and heat production.

Toxicity. An acute overdose of aspirin causes serious disturbances in the body's acid-base balance. A child is more likely to die from a large overdose of aspirin than is an adult. Fatalities among children have been dramatically reduced since 1970 when the Poison Prevention Packaging Act required that orange-flavored "baby" aspirin (81 mg tablets) be limited to 36 tablets per bottle and that safety caps be used. If it has been determined that a child has ingested more than 150 mg/kg (36 baby tablets [one bottle] or 9 adult tablets for a 45-lb child), vomiting may be induced, or gastric lavage is used to get rid of undissolved tablets. Since charcoal absorbs about half its weight in aspirin, it is given orally to reduce absorption of aspirin.

Children, particularly those under 4 years of age, can rapidly develop metabolic acidosis. This is both because of the acidic nature of aspirin and its metabolites and because salicylate inhibits metabolism in a manner that favors the accumulation of organic acids, which would normally have been metabolized to carbon dioxide and water. The hyperthermia that is also produced with this metabolic block must be treated with sponge baths. The profuse sweating can produce dehydration. The supportive treatment of aspirin toxicity therefore consists of careful monitoring of the acid-base and electrolyte levels and appropriate fluid administration. Intravenous sodium bicarbonate can counter the tendency toward metabolic acidosis and produce an alkaline urine that hastens the excretion of salicylate. Osmotic diuretics or dialysis may be necessary in extreme cases to remove salicylate.

Salicylate is a weak vitamin K antagonist and in large doses will act like an oral anticoagulant. A day or two after massive aspirin ingestion, an increased bleeding tendency and signs of minor hemorrhaging may be noted. See the box on page 369 for a summary of the treatment of aspirin poisoning.

Drug interactions. The drug interactions characteristic of aspirin are especially important be-

PATIENT ALERT: TARTRAZINE

THE PROBLEM

Tartrazine (FD & C yellow dye #5) is used by many drug companies in manufacturing their drugs. Ingestion of this dye may cause an allergic reaction in susceptible individuals. This reaction, while rare, is seen more often in persons with aspirin hypersensitivity. A few of the drugs that contain tartrazine include Pronestyl brand procainamide; Choloxin brand 2 and 6 mg tablets dextrothyroxine; and Nicolar brand 500 mg niacin tablets.

SOLUTIONS

- Instruct patients with a known allergy to tartrazine to wear a medical identification tag or bracelet.
- Assess patients with an allergy to aspirin for associated allergy to tartrazine before giving medications that contain tartrazine.
- Instruct patients to warn the pharmacist of tartrazine allergy before prescriptions are filled, so that tartrazine-containing products can be avoided. Teach patients with this allergy not to switch brands of a drug without consulting the pharmacist, to avoid accidental exposure to tartrazine.

  Tartrazine is known to be associated with allergic reactions, but there are many other dyes, fillers, and preservatives used in the manufacture of drugs. Any patient experiencing an unusual reaction to a drug may be manifesting an allergic response to an ingredient used in its manufacture. Read ingredient labels carefully. Take a thorough drug history. Consult the pharmacist.

---

cause of its widespread and uncritical use. The mechanisms of these interactions have been described and are summarized here.

Drug interactions arise because aspirin

1. Enhances the potential for gastrointestinal bleeding and ulcers with glucocorticoids, alcohol, and phenylbutazone
2. Enhances anticoagulation with coumarins
3. Antagonizes the uricosuric effect of probenecid and sulfinpyrazone

Other Over-the-Counter Salicylates (Table 23.1)

Salicylamide

Salicylamide (Salrin) is a chemically modified form of salicylate. Salicylamide is not hydrolyzed to salicylic acid. It is less effective than aspirin or salicylic acid.

Sodium salicylate

Sodium salicylate does not alter platelet function as does aspirin. Salicylates bind to plasma albumin and displace other drugs, particularly the oral anticoagulants.

Methyl salicylate (oil of wintergreen)

Methyl salicylate is used topically only and is not listed in the drug table. It causes vasodilation in the applied areas and thereby creates a warmth that relieves muscle or joint stiffness.

NONSTEROIDAL ANTIINFLAMMATORY DRUGS

Aspirin is the prototype of the nonsteroidal antiinflammatory drugs. For many years aspirin has

TREATMENT OF ASPIRIN TOXICITY

Toxic salicylate plasma concentrations

Mild	45 to 65 mg/dl
Moderate	65 to 90 mg/dl
Severe	90+ mg/dl
Usually fatal	>120 mg/dl

Treatment steps

1. Undissolved tablets are removed through induced vomiting or absorption with charcoal.
2. Plasma salicylate, acid-base, glucose, sodium, and potassium concentrations are determined every 4 to 5 hours.
3. Hyperthermia is treated with sponge baths, and dehydration is treated with fluid replacement.
4. Fluids are administered as required to treat electrolyte imbalances and acidosis.
5. If the salicylate concentration is dangerously high or does not fall with supportive treatment, dialysis or exchange transfusions may be used.

been the first drug used to control the pain and inflammation of rheumatoid arthritis. During the recent years several new drugs have been developed, which like aspirin are analgesic, antipyretic, and antiinflammatory. These new drugs are all prescription drugs although ibuprofen is also available over-the-counter. They are prescribed as analgesic antiinflammatory drugs for patients with rheumatoid arthritis who cannot tolerate aspirin. In addition, they are prescribed for patients with painful

THE NURSING PROCESS

ANALGESIC-ANTIPYRETIC DRUGS

This section will cover only the use of these drugs for reducing fever. The nursing process for the use of these drugs as analgesics will be covered in the next section on nonsteroidal antiinflammatory drugs.

Assessment

The patient requiring a drug to reduce fever is one who has a temperature above 38.5° C (101° F) or above the locally accepted limit of normal. Fever is not a disease itself but is a symptom of an underlying process such as infection, some cancers, and drug reactions. Patient assessment relative to the fever includes determining the temperature and other vital signs; noting the presence of diaphoresis, chills, and/or seizures; and assessing the level of consciousness and the fluid intake and output. Since fever itself is a symptom, the nurse must evaluate the patient relative to the possible causes of fever. Thus the nurse should determine the respiratory status for possible pulmonary infections; wound status for possible wound infection; genitourinary system status for possible urinary tract infection; and so on.

Nursing diagnoses

Potential impaired home maintenance management related to knowledge deficit of safe use of anitpyretic agents

Management

The treatment of fever is twofold. Attempts are made (1) to reduce the fever and (2) to determine the cause of the fever and to treat or eliminate the cause. To reduce the fever, antipyretics are given either when the temperature exceeds the ordered upper limit or every 4 hours around the clock. The temperature should be monitored every 4 hours, adequate fluid intake maintained, fluid intake and output measured, blood counts monitored, and other vital signs checked. Maintaining patient comfort is important. If antipyretics are not successful, additional measures may be employed, including cool water or alcohol baths and use of cooling mattresses. If aspirin is being used, the patient should be monitored for the occurrence of bruising or bleeding.

Evaluation

Success with antipyretic therapy is a return of the patient's temperature to normal range. Hospitalized patients are rarely discharged with a fever. Antipyretics are used often as self-medication by the public for ailments such as colds and flu. Patients should be able to state the correct dose and frequency of administration, when medical assistance should be sought for fever, the possible side effects of antipyretics, and the other drugs and substances that should be avoided during antipyretic therapy. For more specific guidelines see the patient care implications at the end of this chapter.

---

joint disorders, with or without inflammation, such as osteoarthritis, ankylosing spondylitis, low back pain, and gout.

Mechanism of Action

The primary mechanism of action of the nonsteroidal antiinflammatory drugs (NSAIDs) is believed to be the inhibition of the enzyme cyclooxygenase so that prostaglandins are not formed. As discussed earlier, aspirin is an irreversible inhibitor of cyclooxygenase because cyclooxygenase is acetylated by aspirin. Other salicylates and nonsteroidal antiinflammatory drugs also inhibit cyclooxygenase but reversibly, for they do not acetylate cyclooxygenase.

How prostaglandins affect pain receptors is not known. The actions of one prostaglandin, prostaglandin E_2, include vasodilation and increased bone resorption. Large amounts of prostaglandin E_2 have been shown to be present in the synovial fluid of affected joints in patients with rheumatoid arthritis, synthesized by cells in the mesenchymal synovial lining. Presumably this production of prostaglandin E_2 contributes to the swelling and eventual bone erosion of rheumatoid arthritis. In addition, inflammation at other sites may involve the synthesis of prostaglandin E_2.

Dysmenorrhea (menstrual cramps) appears to be due to the overproduction of prostaglandins by the uterus at the time of menstruation. The prostaglandins can cause the uterus to contract to the point of cramping, producing dysmenorrhea. Aspirin is not a very effective drug for treating dysmenorrhea, but the nonsteroidal antiinflammatory drugs are proving very effective in averting menstrual cramps, particularly if therapy is begun a few days before the start of menses.

Recent studies have clarified other mechanisms of the NSAIDs that contribute to their action. These include inhibition of various enzymes, inhibition of transmembrane ion fluxes, and inhibition of the chemoattractant binding that plays an important role in the inflammatory process.

Side Effects

The major side effect of the NSAIDs is gastric irritation leading to an increase in peptic ulcers. Prostaglandins protect the gastric mucosa by inhibiting gastric acid secretion. The gastrointestinal irritation commonly caused by aspirin and other NSAIDs may arise because this protection is absent when these drugs, which inhibit prostaglandin synthesis, are present in the stomach. These effects can be minimized by taking the drugs with meals. All prescription NSAIDs now carry a warning label to reflect concern about the gastrointestinal side effects seen with their chronic use.

Misoprostol (Cytotec) is a new drug whose function is to control gastric irritation associated with aspirin and other NSAIDs. Misoprostol, an analog of prostaglandin E_1, is protective by inhibiting excessive gastric acid secretion. Thus it replaces the prostaglandin that is suppressed by the NSAIDs. (Misoprostol is discussed further in Chapter 13 and listed in Table 13.2.)

Inhibition of platelet aggregation is another common side effect of the NSAIDs. While this effect is irreversible in the case of aspirin, it is reversible as regards the other NSAIDs. The inhibition of prostaglandin synthesis is responsible also for the platelet phenomenon.

Patients who develop a rash or other allergic reaction to one of the NSAIDs may be intolerant of the others as well. This is especially true of patients who have experienced bronchospasm due to aspirin or who are sensitive to aspirin because they have asthma.

Elderly patients are more likely to develop gastrointestinal distress, liver toxicity, or renal damage while taking NSAIDs, and should be carefully monitored. In the main, use of NSAID in persons under 15 years of age has not been well studied.

Drug Interactions

In general, the NSAIDs are protein bound and displace other drugs, particularly hydantoins, sulfonamides, sulfonylureas, and calcium channel blockers, leading to exacerbation of side effects due to these drugs. NSAIDs may increase the risk of renal damage if acetaminophen is used concurrently over long periods. The risk of gastrointestinal complications, especially ulceration or hemorrhage, is increased if NSAIDs are taken concurrently with alcohol, anticoagulants, thrombolytics, or glucocorticoids. NSAIDs may diminish the effectiveness of diuretics and intensify the risk of renal failure. They potentiate drugs that inhibit platelet aggregation. NSAIDs should be discontinued when a gold compound or methotrexate is administered to treat rheumatoid arthritis, because of their potential for renal damage.

Salicylates (Table 23.2)

Aspirin

Aspirin is the drug given initially to control the symptoms of arthritis. Doses of 2.6 to 7.8 Gm/day are required to produce the plasma concentrations of 20 to 30 mg/dl needed for an effective antiinflammatory response. As previously discussed, these doses are associated with considerable gastric irritation with or without bleeding, salicylism, decreased platelet aggregation, and interactions with other drugs. Aspirin must be taken continuously for at least 2 weeks before an improvement may be noted. Timed-release or enteric-coated formulations may improve patient compliance by decreasing the number of times aspirin must be taken each day and by bypassing the stomach, thereby reducing gastric irritation.

Because aspirin is highly irritating to the stomach, a number of salicylate salts have been introduced that replace aspirin and cause less gastrointestinal upset. These salicylates do not affect plate-

Table 23.2   Nonsteroidal Antiinflammatory Drugs

Generic name	Trade name	Administration/dosage	Comments
ASPIRIN AND SALICYLATES			
Aspirin	Bayer Timed-Release Bufferin, Arthritis Strength Measurin Various others	ORAL: *Adults*—arthritis: 2.6 to 5.2 Gm daily in divided doses (every 8 hr for timed-release forms). For acute rheumatic fever, up to 7.8 Gm daily in divided doses. *Children*—65 mg/kg over 24 hr in divided doses every 6 hr. Available without prescription.	Dose needed to achieve blood levels for antiinflammatory activity (20 to 30 mg%) may vary from person to person. Doses given are average ones. Children who have a viral illness and are given aspirin have an increased risk of developing Reye's syndrome.
Choline salicylate	Arthropan	ORAL: *Adults and children over 12 yr*—870 mg (1 teaspoon) every 3 to 4 hr, up to 6 times daily. Available without prescription.	A mint-flavored liquid formulated for patients with arthritis.
Diflunisal	Dolobid*	ORAL: *Adults*—500 to 1000 mg daily, taken as 2 doses. Maximum dose is 1.5 Gm daily. Prescription drug.	A long-acting salicylic acid derivative. Has a lower incidence of the same side effects as aspirin.
Magnesium salicylate	Magan Mobidin	Same as aspirin. No pediatric forms. Prescription drug. FDA Pregnancy Category C.	Contains no sodium; low incidence of gastrointestinal upset. Contraindicated in renal failure.
Salsalate	Disalcid	ORAL: *Adults only*—1 Gm 3 times daily. Prescription drug. FDA Pregnancy Category C.	A dimer of salicylate. Absorption is from the intestine only after hydrolysis to salicylic acid. Delayed onset compared to free salicylic acid.
Sodium salicylate	Uromide	Same as aspirin. Available without prescription. An injectable form is available by prescription.	Less effective than an equal dose of aspirin. May be tolerated by patients with allergic reaction to aspirin. Does not affect platelet function but does retain vitamin K antagonist effect, which can increase prothrombin time.
Sodium thiosalicylate	Arthrolate Nalate Thiodyne Thiolate Th-Sal	INTRAMUSCULAR: *Adults*—prescription drug. For arthritis, 100 mg daily. For musculoskeletal disorders, 50 to 100 mg daily or every other day. For rheumatic fever, 100 to 150 mg every 4 to 6 hr for 3 days, then 100 mg twice daily.	An injectable, longer-acting form of salicylate that can be given in doses lower than for oral aspirin.
OTHER NONSTEROIDAL ANTIINFLAMMATORY DRUGS			
Carprofen	Rimadyl	ORAL: *Adults*—initially, 300 mg daily in divided doses. Reduce to lowest effective maintenance dose. FDA Pregnancy Category C.	Used to treat inflammation in rheumatoid arthritis and gout. Not available in Canada.
Diclofenac	Voltaren*	ORAL: *Adults*—150 to 200 mg daily divided into 2 to 4 doses. Also available in extended release form for once-daily administration. Available in Canada in suppository form. FDA Pregnancy Category B.	For rheumatoid arthritis, osteoarthritis, and ankylosing spondylitis.

*Available in Canada and United States.

Table 23.2   Nonsteroidal Antiinflammatory Drugs—cont'd

Generic name	Trade name	Administration/dosage	Comments
OTHER NONSTEROIDAL ANTIINFLAMMATORY DRUGS—cont'd			
Fenoprofen	Nalfon*	ORAL: *Adults*—300 to 600 mg 3 or 4 times daily for rheumatoid arthritis. For pain or dysmenorrhea, 200 mg every 4 to 6 hr.	For mild to moderate pain, dysmenorrhea, and rheumatoid arthritis.
Floctafenine	Idaract†	ORAL: *Adults*—200 to 400 mg every 6 to 8 hr.	For mild to moderate pain and inflammation. Not available in U.S.
Flurbiprofen	Ansaid* Froben*	ORAL: *Adults*—for arthritis, 100 to 200 mg daily in 3 or 4 divided doses. For dysmenorrhea, 50 mg 4 times daily. FDA Pregnancy Category B.	For arthritis or dysmenorrhea.
Ibuprofen	Advil Motrin* Nuprin Various others	ORAL: *Adults*—for mild pain, fever, or dysmenorrhea, 200 to 400 mg every 4 to 6 hr. For antiinflammatory response, 1.2 to 3.2 Gm daily in 3 or 4 divided doses.	Nonprescription for mild pain, fever, or dysmenorrhea. Higher doses available in prescription form for arthritis.
Indomethacin	Apo-Indomethacin† Indameth Indocid* Indocin Novomethacin	ORAL: *Adults*—25 mg 2 to 3 times daily. If necessary, total daily dose can be increased by 25 to 50 mg daily at weekly intervals, but the total daily dose should not exceed 200 mg. *Children*—1.5 to 2.5 mg/kg body weight per day, divided into 3 or 4 doses. Maximum dose is 4 mg/kg of body weight daily or 200 mg daily, whichever is less. *Premature infants*—0.3 to 0.6 mg/kg/24 hr to close the ductus arteriosus. Available in capsules, extended release capsules, oral suspension, and suppositories.	Administer with meals or with antacids to minimize gastric irritation. For acute inflammatory episodes. Also given to premature infants to close the ductus arteriosus.
Ketoprofen	Orudis*	ORAL: *Adults*—150 to 300 mg daily divided into 3 or 4 doses. Available in capsules, delayed-release capsules, and suppositories. FDA Pregnancy Category B.	For rheumatoid arthritis and dysmenorrhea.
Meclofenamate	Meclomen	ORAL: *Adults*—200 mg daily divided into 3 or 4 doses. May be increased up to 400 mg daily if necessary.	For rheumatoid arthritis. Not available in Canada.
Mefenamic Acid	Ponstel Ponstan*	ORAL: *Adults*—500 mg initially, then 250 mg every 6 hr as needed. FDA Pregnancy Category C.	For mild to moderate pain. Administer after meals to avoid gastric irritation.

*Available in Canada and United States.
†Available in Canada only

Continued.

Table 23.2   Nonsteroidal Antiinflammatory Drugs—cont'd

Generic name	Trade name	Administration/dosage	Comments
OTHER NONSTEROIDAL ANTIINFLAMMATORY DRUGS—cont'd			
Naproxen	Anaprox* Naprosyn*	ORAL: *Adults*—250 to 750 mg 2 times daily for rheumatoid arthritis; 500 mg initially, then 250 mg every 6 to 8 hr for mild to moderate pain, including dysmenorrhea; 750 mg initially, then 250 mg every 8 hr for acute gout. FDA Pregnancy Category B.	For dysmenorrhea, mild to moderate pain, acute gout, and rheumatoid arthritis.
Phenylbutazone	Azolid Butazolidin* Butazone	ORAL: *Adults*—initially, 300 to 600 mg daily divided into 3 or 4 doses. Maintenance dose is 100 mg 1 to 4 times daily. For acute gout, 400 mg initially, then 100 mg every 4 hr for 4 days or a maximum of 1 week. Available in capsules, tablets, delayed-release and buffered tablets. FDA Pregnancy Category C.	For rheumatoid arthritis and acute attacks of other arthritic conditions, including gout. Administer after meals to avoid gastric irritation.
Piroxicam	Feldene*	ORAL: *Adults*—20 mg once a day or 10 mg twice a day.	For rheumatoid arthritis and osteoarthritis. Administer after meals to avoid gastric irritation.
Sulindac	Clinoril*	ORAL: *Adults*—150 to 200 mg twice a day.	For rheumatoid arthritis, acute gout, and bursitis.
Tiaprofenic Acid	Surgam†	ORAL: *Adults*—600 mg daily divided into 2 or 3 doses.	For rheumatoid arthritis and osteoarthritis. Not available in U.S.
Tolmetin	Tolectin*	ORAL: *Adults*—initially, 400 mg every 8 hr, then 600 to 1800 mg daily, divided into 3 or 4 doses. FDA Pregnancy Category C.	For rheumatoid arthritis and osteoarthritis.

*Available in Canada and United States.
†Available in Canada only

let aggregation but do displace oral anticoagulants from albumin.

Diflunisal

Diflunisal (Dolobid) is a derivative of salicylic acid having a long duration of action. It is effective in relieving the symptoms of rheumatoid arthritis and osteoarthritis. Diflunisal has fewer side effects than does aspirin, but the side effects are the same: gastrointestinal reactions, dizziness, edema, and tinnitus.

Salicylate salts

Sodium salicylate, sodium thiosalicylate, magnesium salicylate, and *choline salicylate* are all salicylate salts that produce less gastrointestinal upset than aspirin.

Salsalate

Salsalate (Disalcid) is a dimer of salicylic acid. It is slowly hydrolyzed to two molecules of salicylic acid in the small intestine and absorbed into the bloodstream.

Thiosalicylate

Thiosalicylate (Arthrolate and others) is a chemically modified form of salicylate for intramuscular injection.

Nonsalicylate Nonsteroidal Antiinflammatory Drugs (NSAIDs) (Table 23.2)

Many NSAIDs have been introduced into clinical practice in recent years; three have been introduced and withdrawn because they were excessively toxic to kidneys in elderly patients. NSAIDs

THE NURSING PROCESS

NONSTEROIDAL ANTIINFLAMMATORY DRUGS

Assessment

Patients requiring analgesic and/or antiinflammatory drugs will have a wide variety of complaints, including headache, menstrual cramps, arthritis, musculoskeletal injury, and postoperative pain. Many of these patients will seek medical assistance for relief of their problem, whereas others will self-medicate with such drugs as aspirin or acetaminophen. Assessment should include a thorough collection of data related to the specific patient complaint. These data would include temperature, pulse, respiration, blood pressure, blood counts, a brief neurological examination, and other laboratory data relevant to the possible or probable diagnosis. Assessment of ability to perform activities of daily living may assist in planning for discharge.

Nursing diagnoses

Potential complication: gastrointestinal distress and/or bleeding

Potential complication: hematological disorders

Management

In general management is directed toward providing relief of the pain, improving the patient's condition, and determining a way to prevent and/or treat recurrences. Individualized planning requires that the health care team and the patient work together to develop a plan to reach the goal or goals of drug therapy, and therapy in addition to drugs is often required. Examples of additional therapy include application of heat or cold, immobilization, special exercises, and restricted activity. A plan may be proposed for the patient to begin a course of prophylactic drug therapy at a specific time in the future with the hope of preventing the problem; this is done for certain types of headache disorders and with menstrual cramps. By the time the patient is ready to begin self-management, goals and plan of therapy should be understood by the patient and the health care team. During the management phase, the nurse should monitor the vital signs and subjective and objective data related to the specific problem and the laboratory data appropriate to the problem and the drug therapy. For example, in the patient experiencing menstrual cramps associated with heavy bleeding who is being treated with ibuprofen (Motrin), the hematocrit and hemoglobin level might be monitored because of the heavy bleeding, whereas the uric acid level and liver function studies would be monitored because of the ibuprofen.

Evaluation

The question to ask in evaluating drug therapy with analgesics and antiinflammatory drugs is whether the short-term goal has been reached or will soon be reached while the patient remains free of side effects due to the medication. Before discharge the patient should be able to explain why and how to take the prescribed drugs and other therapies being used to treat the problem, which other drugs should be avoided while receiving therapy, whether alcohol should be avoided, what are reasonable expectations of the regimen (e.g., will joint pain disappear or only diminish), which are possible side effects and what to do if they occur, how to implement a plan for prophylactic treatment, and when to return for follow-up or assistance. For more specific guidelines see the patient care implications section at the end of this chapter.

are derived from several chemical classes and are discussed on the basis of their chemical group.

Ibuprofen and related NSAIDs

About half the NSAIDs are propionic acid derivatives. These include carprofen (Rimadyl), fenoprofen (Nalfon), floctafenine (Idarac), flurbiprofen (Ansaid), ibuprofen (Advil, Mediprin, Motrin, Nuprin, others), ketoprofen (Orudis), naproxen (Anaprox, Naprosyn) and tiaprofenic acid (Surgam). They provide good analgesic and antiinflammatory action. They are often effective in treating dysmenorrhea, rheumatoid arthritis, osteoarthritis, and gout. Specific indications are listed in Table 23.2.

Ibuprofen is available without a prescription. It is rapidly absorbed and has a plasma half-life of 2 hours. It appears to be well tolerated. Gastrointestinal irritation and bleeding occur less frequently than with aspirin and may be decreased by taking the drug with meals.

Diclofenac

Diclofenac (Voltaren) is new to the U.S. market. It is effective in treating rheumatoid arthritis, osteoarthritis and ankylosing spondylitis.

Indomethacin

Indomethacin (Indocin, Indocid, others) is prescribed for its analgesic and antiinflammatory actions. Gastrointestinal disturbances such as nausea, vomiting, loss of appetite, indigestion, or diarrhea are common, but they can be reduced by taking the drug after meals. Occasionally, indomethacin can cause ulceration along the gastrointestinal tract and this can become serious if bleeding or perforation results. Headaches and dizziness are the most common side effects. These can often be minimized if the dose is lowered and then increased gradually. Other central nervous system disturbances that can limit the use of indomethacin include confusion, light-headedness, fainting, or drowsiness.

Sulindac and tolmetin

Sulindac (Clinoril) and tolmetin (Tolectin) are chemically related to indomethacin. In general, their effects are similar to those of aspirin, although the incidence is less than with aspirin.

Sulindac has a plasma half-life of 8 hours and can be taken less frequently than indomethacin or tolmetin. It is a prodrug, activated following conversion by the liver. The active drug is excreted in the bile and reabsorbed from the intestine.

Tolmetin induces fewer side effects in the central nervous system than does indomethacin. Tolmetin is absorbed rapidly and has a plasma half-life of only 1 hour.

Meclofenamate and mefenamic acid

Meclofenamate (Meclomen) and mefenamic acid (Ponstel, Ponstan) are fenamate derivatives. Mefenamic acid is prescribed for mild to moderate pain. However, therapy with this drug is limited to 1 week because of the frequent occurrence of toxicity associated with the gastrointestinal, kidney, and blood-forming systems. Side effects may include gastrointestinal upset, diarrhea, and rash. Meclofenamate is prescribed for rheumatoid arthritis and osteoarthritis. However, side effects are similar to those of mefenamic acid.

Phenylbutazone

Phenylbutazone (Azolid, Butazolidin, Butazone) is a potent antiinflammatory drug with a long plasma half-life of 2 to 3 days. It binds strongly to plasma albumin and can displace other bound drugs, particularly oral anticoagulant and oral hypoglycemic drugs. Phenylbutazone causes fluid retention and gastric irritation, and prolongs platelet function, thereby inhibiting blood clotting. Occasionally, phenylbutazone causes liver damage or bone marrow suppression. Because of these problems, it is commonly prescribed for 1 to 2 weeks only to treat an acute inflammatory response.

Piroxicam

Piroxicam (Feldene) is well absorbed and has a long half-life of 45 hours, so that once-a-day dosing is adequate. Piroxicam is rapidly excreted in the urine as a glucuronide. Piroxicam is prescribed principally for rheumatoid arthritis and osteoarthritis.

DRUGS FOR RHEUMATOID ARTHRITIS
Rheumatoid Arthritis

Rheumatoid arthritis is a highly variable disease process. It frequently goes into remission for months or years. In early rheumatoid arthritis the synovial membranes only are inflamed, causing a painful swelling. In this situation aspirin and the other nonsteroidal antiinflammatory drugs may be effective. This effect added to the analgesic effect will ease the pain and help to increase the mobility of the affected joint. In mild cases NSAIDs may be sufficient to control symptoms. These drugs do not affect the progression of rheumatoid arthritis, how-

THE NURSING PROCESS

RHEUMATOID ARTHRITIS

Assessment

The patient with rheumatoid arthritis has a chronic illness. Assessment of an individual patient will vary in depth, depending on the frequency of contact with the health care team and whether the disease is in remission or exacerbation. A careful history of the presenting problem should be obtained in addition to vital signs, weight, and subjective and objective data related to the complaint and the overall condition of the patient. Laboratory work would include determining the hematocrit and hemoglobin level, blood counts; tests to confirm the diagnosis or to monitor the disease such as the rheumatoid factor, antinuclear antibody (ANA), complement, and erythrocyte sedimentation rate (ESR); and tests to monitor the activity or side effects of drugs the patient is taking. Finally, regular assessment of joint function and ability to perform activities of daily living should be done.

Nursing diagnoses

Potential complication: stomatitis (with gold compounds)

Potential complication: hematological disorders

Possible anxiety related to chronic disease, changing medical therapies, and use of drug(s) with a high potential for causing side effects

Management

There are no drugs that can cure rheumatoid arthritis. Goals of drug therapy are to provide analgesia, to reduce inflammation, which will in turn help to decrease pain, and to maintain or increase joint function. Management involves combining drugs with rest, application of heat, special exercises, and other therapies to improve or at least to maintain the current condition. The specific drugs will be determined by response to previous drugs or dosages and the severity of the disease. The nurse should monitor the response to the therapeutic regimen including such factors as pain, joint function, subjective and objective data related to the patient's complaints, new signs and symptoms possibly due to the therapy, and laboratory work specific for the drugs being used or the patient's problems. It is important for the nurse to engage in goal planning with the patient so that patient management is directed to a mutually satisfactory outcome. Maintaining ideal weight is less stressful to joints in cases of arthritis; dietary restriction and instruction may be necessary. Referral to occupational therapy, physical therapy, and visiting nurses may be helpful.

Evaluation

Because of the nature of the disease, evaluation of drug effectiveness will vary with the patient. That is, a specific drug used with a patient early in the disease process may decrease pain and inflammation and help increase joint mobility. In another patient the same drug may decrease pain and inflammation, but the bone changes may be too severe to allow for much if any improvement in joint function. Finally, most of these drugs have frequent and serious side effects. Before discharge and self-management, the patient should be able to explain the disease process and why specific drugs are being used, possible side effects of the drugs and what action to take if they should appear, how to take ordered drugs correctly, the need for frequent follow-up and data that will be obtained at these visits to monitor for effectiveness and side effects, and the need to avoid self-medication with over-the-counter drugs unless cleared by the physician. For additional specific information see the patient care implication section at the end of this chapter.

Table 23.3 Drugs Specific for Rheumatoid Arthritis

Generic name	Trade name	Administration/dosage	Comments
Auranofin	Ridaura	ORAL: *Adults*—6 mg daily. FDA Pregnancy Category C.	An investigational drug. Effective orally. Appears as effective as injected gold drugs in inducing remission of rheumatoid arthritis.
Aurothioglucose Gold sodium thiomalate	Solganal Myochrysine*	INTRAMUSCULAR (GLUTEAL): *Adults*—weekly injections of 10 mg wk 1, 25 mg wk 2, 25 to 50 mg wk 3, 50 mg each week thereafter until a total of 800 mg to 1 Gm has been administered. If the patient has improved and there are no toxic signs, 50 mg injections are continued every 2 wk (4 doses) then every 3 wk (4 doses), then every 3 to 4 week. *Children*—1 mg/kg (up to 25 mg) weekly for 20 wk, then every 2 to 4 wk if the therapy is beneficial. FDA Pregnancy Category C.	About 40% of patients develop serious side effects, most commonly an allergy marked by skin reactions or mouth ulcers. Blood counts and urinalysis are done routinely to monitor for suppression of blood cells and kidney damage. Therapy is discontinued if no improvement is seen in 5 mo.
Hydroxychloroquine sulfate	Plaquenil* Sulfate	ORAL: *Adults*—200 mg once or twice daily at meals, not more than 3.5 mg/lb.	Regular ocular examination to detect retinopathy if required.
Methotrexate	Rheumatrex	ORAL: *Adults*—2.5 to 5 mg every 12 hr for 3 doses weekly. FDA Pregnancy Category X.	Low dose weekly therapy.
Penicillamine	Cuprimine* Depen	ORAL: *Adults*—initially 125 to 250 mg daily as a single dose. May be raised every 2 to 3 mo by 250 mg daily to 500 to 750 mg daily.	Patient must be carefully monitored to detect suppression of blood cells and autoimmune responses.

*Available in Canada and United States.

ever, which is marked by erosion of the bone at the joint and eventual bone deformation. Drugs that may be effective in altering the progression of joint erosion include gold therapy, hydroxychloroquine, penicillamine, and the immunosuppressive drugs, tried in that order. Glucocorticoids have a restricted role in treating rheumatoid arthritis. All these antirheumatic drugs have potentially serious side effects which must be monitored carefully.

Specific Drugs (Table 23.3)

Aurothioglucose and gold sodium thiomalate

Aurothioglucose (Solganal) and gold sodium thiomalate (Myochrysine) are injectable gold salts. It is now known how gold affects the synovial tissues to suppress rheumatoid arthritis. Therapy is started with weekly injections into the gluteal muscle until 1 Gm has been given. Further therapy depends on the patient's response. Gold requires a long time to come to plateau levels in the tissues, and a response usually requires 2 to 6 months. Only 30% to 60% of patients treated with gold respond over a 2- to 3-year course of treatment. Patients in whom remission is induced usually continue receiving monthly injections.

The most common reason for discontinuing successful gold therapy is the appearance of serious side effects: skin reactions, mouth ulcers, fever, kidney damage, or abnormalities in the blood count. About 40% of patients develop an adverse reaction. Skin reactions and mouth ulcers are the most common side effects. If these are mild, the gold therapy may be halted temporarily and then tried again. Blood counts and a urinalysis to measure protein should be done before each dose early in gold therapy and continued periodically throughout therapy.

Auranofin

Auranofin (Ridaura) is a gold compound that can be taken orally. Clinical trials indicate that auranofin is as effective as the injectable gold drugs in inducing remission in rheumatoid arthritis. Auranofin is taken twice daily. Gastrointestinal re-

THE NURSING PROCESS

GOUT

Assessment

Patients may appear with the classic symptoms of pain in one or both large toes or other joints or be identified as individuals with high serum uric acid levels, even if asymptomatic. Assessment should include vital signs, weight, history of previous attacks and/or family history of gout, and assessment of subjective complaints and objective data. Blood work would include the serum uric acid level. X-ray films and joint aspiration may be required.

Nursing diagnoses

Possible impaired home maintenance management related to the need to increase daily fluid intake to 2500 ml

Potential complication: gastrointestinal distress

Management

The goals of drug therapy will be one or more of the following: symptomatic treatment of an existing attack, reducing the pool of urates and uric acid, and preventing recurrences. Drugs will be used to help achieve the goals in addition to rest for the affected joints, dietary restrictions to reduce purine intake on a short- or long-term basis, and a weight reduction diet if appropriate. To prevent the formation of kidney stones, a high urinary output should be maintained (2000 to 3000 ml per day), which requires a high fluid intake. A determination of fluid intake and output should be monitored in the hospitalized individual until it is certain that the high fluid output is being maintained. The nurse should monitor vital signs, blood pressure, the condition of affected joints, subjective complaints, objective signs, and appropriate laboratory work. Finally, drugs or dietary manipulation may be necessary to increase the alkalinity of the urine to help prevent urate crystal formation.

Evaluation

Therapy with these drugs is considered effective if the discomfort associated with an acute attack lessens, if further attacks are prevented, if the serum uric acid level drops toward normal and remains down, and kidney stones do not form as a result of therapy. It may be necessary to use two or more drugs to achieve these goals. Before discharge the patient should be symptomatically better or, if being treated as an outpatient, should be more comfortable in 2 to 3 days. The patient should be able to describe the disease, which medications have been prescribed and their actions, how to take the drugs to achieve maximum benefit, and the possible side effects and which ones should be reported immediately. In addition, the patient should be able to demonstrate how to plan meals within any prescribed dietary restrictions and be able to explain how to maintain a fluid intake that will ensure an adequate urinary output. For specific guidelines see the patient care implications section.

---

actions, including diarrhea, abdominal pain, nausea, and loss of appetite are common early in therapy but usually subside in the first month. The toxicity of auranofin is similar to that of the injectable gold compounds.

Hydroxychloroquine

Hydroxychloroquine (Plaquenil) is an antimalarial drug, which is also used as an alternative to gold therapy or when gold therapy has failed. A response may not be seen for 3 to 6 months after the start of therapy, and therapy is discontinued after 1 year if no response is seen. This drug is taken orally, and some remains in the body for months or years. Occasionally, patients develop retinopathy which can progress to blindness even when the drug is discontinued. Therefore regular ophthalmic examination is necessary. Skin rashes, peripheral neuropathy, and a depressed white cell count are other complications.

Penicillamine

Penicillamine (Cuprimine, Depen) is being evaluated for the treatment of rheumatoid arthritis. Side effects are frequent but are reversible when the dosage is reduced or the drug is discontinued. These include the loss of taste, nausea, depression of platelets and white cells, and proteinuria. Side effects are minimized by starting with a low dose and increasing the dose every 4 to 6 weeks until a response is obtained or a total of 1 Gm per day is given.

Methotrexate

Methotrexate (Rheumatrex) is a folic acid antagonist used to treat cancer and psoriasis. It has been approved for use in low doses to treat rheumatoid arthritis when other treatments have failed. Side effects include nausea, mucositis, gastrointestinal discomfort, rash, diarrhea, and headaches. Toxic reactions are possible, most of which are reversible if detected early; these include liver damage, lung disease, bone marrow depression, severe diarrhea, and ulcerative stomatitis. Baseline studies include blood chemistry, renal function, liver function, and chest x-ray films; these are repeated periodically throughout treatment. Contraindications to the use of methotrexate include pregnancy and nursing, alcoholism, blood dyscrasias, immunodeficiency syndromes, or hypersensitivity to the drug.

Glucocorticoids

Glucocorticoids relieve inflammation and the accompanying pain of arthritis in a dramatic fashion. One action of glucocorticoids is to indirectly inhibit prostaglandin E_2 synthesis. However, glucocorticoids do not alter the course of rheumatoid arthritis. Long-term administration suppresses the pituitary-adrenal axis with serious consequences (Chapter 51). Although oral administration is rarely given in rheumatoid arthritis, injection into the articular space of the joint may relieve acute inflammatory episodes without causing systemic reactions. Glucocorticoids may be used to treat certain nonarticular manifestations of rheumatoid arthritis, such as vasculitis and rheumatoid lung. Very small doses may sometimes be given to treat joint symptoms. *Hydrocortisone acetate, triamcinolone hexacetonide,* and depot *methylprednisone* are the preferred glucocorticoids because they have a longer duration of action than other injectable glucocorticoids. If a glucocorticoid is to be injected, the

DIETARY CONSIDERATION: PURINE

Uric acid is produced when purine is catabolized. Gout is a problem of elevated uric acid. Formerly, a mainstay of gout therapy was purine restriction in the diet. With better drug therapy, purine restriction is a less significant component of therapy. Patients should probably modify their diets to limit excessive purine intake, unless more severe restriction is indicated on an individual basis. High purine foods to avoid or limit include:

organ meats	roe
sardines	scallops
anchovies	broth and consomme
mincemeat	herring
shrimp	mackerel
gravies	yeast

patient should be warned to avoid strenuous use of the affected joint. This is because the drug masks the normal signals of stress at the joint, and therefore may damage the stressed joint.

DRUGS FOR GOUT
Gout

Gout is a metabolic disease in which total body pools of uric acid (a product of DNA and RNA degradation) are elevated. The uric acid crystallizes in joints or, less commonly, in tendons or bursae. The joint at the base of the big toe is most commonly affected. In an attack of acute gouty arthritis there is a marked inflammation of the joint accompanied by much pain. This acute attack is treated with the drug colchicine, which acts (in an unknown manner) to relieve the pain, with one of the nonsteroidal antiinflammatory drugs already discussed, or in special circumstances with ACTH (Chapter 51). Some patients develop a tophus in a joint—crystals of uric acid with fibrous tissue surrounding them. Patients with tophi or those with recurrent attacks of gouty arthritis need to receive long-term treatment, often for the rest of their lives, with drugs that will reduce the uric acid levels in the body.

Aspirin was once used to treat gout based on the action of salicylates, in doses over 5 Gm, to increase excretion of uric acid. (Lower doses have no effect, and doses of 1 to 2 Gm may decrease uric acid excretion.)

With the newer drug therapy, tophi, if present, will often regress with long-term therapy, thereby restoring the joint to a normal range of function. About 25% of such patients will be found to over-

Table 23.4   Drugs Used to Treat Gout

Generic name	Trade name	Administration/dosage	Comments
Allopurinol	Lopurin Zyloprim*	ORAL: *Adults*—200 to 300 mg daily as a single dose; maximum, 800 mg daily. Dose is reduced if there is renal insufficiency. FDA Pregnancy Category C.	Inhibits the formation of uric acid from hypoxanthine or xanthine; these are excreted instead.
Colchicine	Novocolchine†	ORAL: *Adults*—0.5 to 0.6 mg hourly or 1 to 1.2 mg initially and 0.5 to 0.6 mg every 2 hr. This is regimen for an acute gouty attack and is continued until the pain subsides or gastrointestinal symptoms appear. Maximum dose, 7 to 8 mg. For prophylaxis, 0.5 to 1 mg daily.	To terminate an acute gouty attack. Appearance of gastrointestinal distress usually limits the amount given.
		INTRAVENOUS: for an acute attack, 1 to 2 mg initially, then 0.5 mg every 3 to 6 hr or 1 dose of 3 mg; maximum dose, 4 mg. FDA Pregnancy Category D.	Dilute the drug 10-fold with sterile saline solution before injecting to minimize tissue damage.
Probenecid	Benemid* Benuryl†	ORAL: *Adults*—250 mg 2 or 3 times daily the first week, then 500 mg twice daily thereafter. May increase to 2.0 Gm daily if necessary.	Inhibits reabsorption of uric acid by the kidney. A prophylactic drug to reduce existing tophi and to prevent recurrence of a gouty attack.
Sulfinpyrazone	Anturan† Anturane	ORAL: *Adults*—100 to 200 mg 2 times daily with meals or with milk at bedtime. The dosage is raised as needed to control blood urate levels (400 to 800 mg daily). The dose is then reduced to the minimum effective level, usually 300 to 400 mg daily.	Acts like probenecid. May also prevent the recurrence of a myocardial infarction.

*Available in Canada and United States.
†Available in Canada only.

produce uric acid. These patients are treated with the drug allopurinol, which prevents the formation of uric acid from xanthine and hypoxanthine, the purine metabolites of DNA and RNA metabolism. The remainder of patients are treated with a uricosuric drug, probenecid or sulfinpyrazone. These drugs increase the renal excretion of uric acid by inhibiting its reabsorption from the proximal kidney tubule.

Specific Drugs (Table 23.4)

Colchicine

Colchicine provides relief from the pain of an acute attack of gouty arthritis, usually within 24 hours. The earlier in an episode colchicine is taken, the more effective it will be. (Antiinflammatory drugs are similarly more effective if taken early in an acute episode.) Colchicine taken orally at the doses required to treat an acute gouty attack may cause nausea and vomiting followed by diarrhea. These effects limit the amount of colchicine that can be taken. Alternatively, the drug may be given intravenously to minimize these side effects. Since it causes severe tissue inflammation, it is diluted before intravenous administration to minimize the effect of any drug leakage.

Colchicine may be continued at reduced dosages once the acute episode is over. Continuance of colchicine is most common if a drug to reduce uric acid is begun. A sudden change in body uric acid concentration will often precipitate a new acute attack of gouty arthritis. This can often be avoided with prophylactic colchicine.

Allopurinol

Allopurinol (Zyloprim) inhibits the formation of uric acid from xanthine or hypoxanthine so that xanthine or hypoxanthine is excreted instead. A patient who produces a morning urine with a ratio of uric acid to creatinine greater than 0.75 or whose 24-hour urine contains more than 600 mg of uric acid is classified as an overproducer of uric acid. These overproducers, and patients with renal uric acid crystals or with impaired renal function, are

Text continued on p. 387.

PATIENT CARE IMPLICATIONS

Acetaminophen

Patient and family education

- When used in usual doses, there are few side effects associated with this drug. Instruct patients to report the development of any new sign or symptom to the physician.
- Remind patients to keep these and all drugs out of the reach of children. Never encourage children to take medications by telling them that drugs are candy. Tell parents to seek medical help immediately if overdose is suspected.
- Tell patients to be alert to signs of acute toxicity: nausea, vomiting, abdominal pain. Severe poisoning may result in CNS stimulation, excitement, delirium, followed by CNS depression, stupor, hypothermia, rapid, shallow breathing, tachycardia, hypotension, and circulatory failure.
- Teach patients to read labels of all medications carefully. Many over-the-counter products for pain and for treatment of sinus problems or colds contain acetaminophen alone or in combination with other drugs. Tell patients to avoid taking several drugs simultaneously unless absolutely necessary.
- Review with parents the dosages appropriate for children of various sizes and ages. Assist parents in finding a drug form that is easy to administer. Note that absorption from a rectal suppository is variable, and there may be rectal irritation; this route may be the least desirable.
- Pain or fever that persists beyond 3 to 5 days may signal a more serious health problem. Instruct patients to seek medical help rather than to self-medicate indefinitely. Take only the recommended dose; too much may cause liver damage.
- Remind patients to keep all health care providers informed of all medications being taken.
- To take effervescent preparations, pour the granules into a glass. Fill the glass with 4 oz of cool water. Drink all of the contents of the glass, whether still fizzing or not.
- Avoid alcoholic beverages while taking acetaminophen.
- Instruct patients who are also taking tetracycline to take it at least 1 to 2 hours before or after acetaminophen.
- Acetylcysteine is discussed in Chapter 26.

Aspirin and related drugs

Drug administration

- Monitor the platelet count and hematocrit.
- Regularly check stools for presence of blood/guaiac.

Patient and family education

- Instruct patients about the signs of aspirin toxicity (see text). Instruct patients to report the development of tinnitus, unexplained bleeding or bruising, severe or persistent gastric irritation, blood in the stool. Note that salicylates do not affect platelet aggregation; see text.
- Warn parents that aspirin and other salicylates should not be used to treat the fever and discomfort of the "flu" or chickenpox in children, as aspirin has been associated with the development of Reye's syndrome. Acetaminophen is preferred over aspirin in treatment of childhood flu and chickenpox symptoms.
- Remind patients to keep these and all drugs out of the reach of children. Never encourage children to take medications by telling them that drugs are candy. Tell parents to seek medical help immediately if overdose is suspected.
- Teach patients to read labels of all medications carefully. Many over-the-counter products for pain and for treatment of sinus problems or colds contain salicylates alone or in combination with other drugs. Tell patients to avoid taking several drugs simultaneously unless absolutely necessary.
- To reduce gastric irritation, take oral doses with a full glassful of fluid, or take with meals or snack.
- Pain or fever that persists beyond 3 to 5 days may signal a more serious health problem. Instruct patients to seek medical help rather than to self-medicate indefinitely. Take only the recommended dose; too much may result in salicylism or other complications.
- Remind patients to keep all health care providers informed of all medications being taken, including aspirin; this includes dentists and oral surgeons. Note the drug interactions on p. 371.
- Do not take aspirin products which smell strongly of vinegar, as they may have begun to break down, and may no longer be effective.

PATIENT CARE IMPLICATIONS — cont'd

- To take effervescent preparations, pour the granules into a glass. Fill the glass with 4 oz. of cool water. Drink all of the contents of the glass, whether still fizzing or not.
- Swallow enteric-coated preparations whole, without chewing or crushing.
- Chewable aspirin tablets may be crushed, chewed, or swallowed whole.
- Chew aspirin chewing gum for several minutes (or as directed on the package label) for best effect.
- Extended-release preparations may be broken along scored lines. Some of these forms should not be chewed or crushed; consult the pharmacist about specific brands.
- Avoid alcoholic beverages while taking aspirin or salicylates.
- Buffered aspirin, choline and magnesium salicylates, or magnesium salicylates should not be taken at the same time as tetracyclines. Patients taking one of these drugs and tetracycline should allow 1 to 2 hours between doses.
- Patients on long-term therapy may find the extended-release preparations helpful, particularly at night, as blood levels of aspirin may not be so low in the morning.
- Teach patients taking aspirin for arthritis and other musculoskeletal conditions that the best effect is achieved through regular use of the drug, as prescribed.
- Warn diabetics that chronic or excessive use of aspirin-containing products may cause false urine sugar results. Monitor blood glucose levels. Consult physician or pharmacist as appropriate.
- Low-dose aspirin may be used for its antiplatelet effect. It may be prescribed for immobilized patients and for postoperative orthopedic patients, to decrease the incidence of thromboembolism. It is also used to prevent other vascular problems; see Chapter 20.
- Encourage patients who are allergic to aspirin to wear a medical identification tag or bracelet indicating their allergy.

Nonsteroidal antiinflammatory drugs

Drug administration

- Monitor vital signs, blood pressure, weight. Monitor the complete blood cell count, differential, platelet count, BUN, serum creatinine, liver functions tests.
- Check stools for presence of blood/guaiac.

- If diarrhea or vomiting is severe or persistent, monitor intake and output.
- Question patient about history of allergy to other drugs before administering. If in doubt that an allergy to a nonsteroidal antiinflammatory drug may exist, consult physician before administering the first dose.
- In patients with cardiovascular, renal, or hypertensive disease, assess for possible fluid retention. Auscultate lung sounds. Assess for jugular venous distention. Monitor daily weight.

Patient and family education

- Review the anticipated benefits and possible side effects of drug therapy. Instruct the patient to report the development of bruising, bleeding gums, nosebleeds, blood in stool, fever, rash, sore throat, mouth ulcers or irritation, jaundice, right upper quadrant abdominal pain, malaise. Encourage the patient to notify the physician if any unexpected sign or symptom develops.
- Tell patients with long-term musculoskeletal problems that several weeks of therapy may be necessary before full benefit is seen. Best effects are seen if the drugs are taken regularly, as ordered. Tell the patient not to discontinue or increase therapy without consulting the physician.
- Take doses with meals, snack, or full glassful of milk to reduce gastric irritation. Take with a full glassful (8 oz.) of fluid. Do not lie down for at least 15 to 30 minutes after an oral dose.
- Review the other medications and drug interactions noted in the text; counsel as appropriate. Remind patients to keep all health care providers informed of all drugs being taken, including dentists and oral surgeons. Tell the patient not to take over-the-counter products without consulting the physician. This applies especially to products containing aspirin or acetaminophen.
- Warn the patient to avoid driving or operating hazardous equipment if visual changes, dizziness, fatigue, or weakness occur; notify the physician.
- Avoid drinking alcoholic beverages while taking nonsteroidal antiinflammatory drugs.
- Some of these drugs may cause photosensitivity. Warn patients to limit time in the sun or under sun lamps until the effects of the drug can be evaluated. See Patient Problem: Photosensitivity on p. 647.

Continued.

PATIENT CARE IMPLICATIONS — cont'd

- Some of these drugs have been associated with visual changes with long-term therapy. If ophthalmic examinations are recommended, encourage the patient to follow through.
- Usually, enteric-coated forms should not be chewed or crushed, but swallowed whole. Capsules may be opened and the contents mixed with food. Some tablets may be crushed and mixed with food. Work with the patient to find a form the patient can take. Consult the pharmacist for information about crushing, breaking, or mixing an individual product.
- Instruct patients taking nonprescription nonsteroidal antiinflammatory drugs to review the manufacturer's literature supplied with the package. Emphasize the importance of continuing with other prescribed therapies, which might include a prescribed exercise program, weight reduction, application of heat and cold, physical therapy, and so forth.
- Some of these drugs cause fluid retention. Assess patient's ability, resources, and other health problems (e.g., hypertensive, cardiovascular, or renal disease). If appropriate, teach the patient to monitor and record weight on a daily basis. Report weight gain in excess of 2 pounds per day or 5 pounds per week to the physician.
- Remind pregnant or lactating women that no drugs should be used without consulting the physician.

Gold compounds

Drug administration

- Assess respiratory rate and auscultate lung sounds. Monitor intake, output, weight. Monitor complete blood count and differential, platelet count, BUN, serum creatinine, liver function tests. Monitor urinalysis to detect proteinuria, hematuria.
- Inspect skin and mouth for presence of rashes, ulcers, stomatitis, irritation.
- For IM injection, use large muscle masses. Record and rotate injection sites. Aspirate before administering dose to prevent inadvertent IV administration. Keep patient supine for at least 15 minutes after dose. Monitor vital signs and blood pressure. Have available drugs, equipment, and personnel to treat an acute allergic reaction in settings where parenteral gold compounds are administered
  INTRAMUSCULAR AUROTHIOGLUCOSE
- This drug form is an oil-based suspen-

sion. See Chapter 6 (box on p. 88) for instructions on administering oil-based drugs.

Patient and family education

- Review anticipated benefits and possible side effects of drug therapy with the patient. Instruct the patient to notify the physician if the following develop: severe or persistent vomiting or diarrhea; rashes, skin irritation, itching, mouth ulcers, oral irritation, stomatitis; metallic taste; unexplained bruising, bleeding of gums, bleeding in stool, nosebleeds; jaundice, right upper quadrant abdominal pain, malaise, fever, or sore throat; eye irritation or visual changes. Reinforce the importance of reporting any new sign or symptom to the physician.
- Take oral compounds with meals or snack to lessen gastric irritation.
- Review aspects of oral hygiene with the patient in the event stomatitis does develop. See Patient Problem: Stomatitis on p. 601.
- Review Patient Problem: Photosensitivity, on p. 647, with the patient.
- Point out that weeks to months of therapy may be necessary before full benefit of gold therapy can be seen. Emphasize the importance of continuing with other prescribed therapies, which might include a prescribed exercise program, weight reduction, application of heat and cold, physical therapy, and so forth.
- Women of childbearing age may wish to use some form of birth control while on gold therapy; discuss before initiating gold therapy.

Glucocorticoids

See Chapter 51 for a detailed discussion of these drugs.

Hydroxychloroquine

See Chapter 38 for a detailed discussion of this drug, which is also used to treat malaria.

Methotrexate

See Chapter 39 for a detailed discussion of this drug, which is used in higher doses to treat cancer.

Penicillamine

Drug administration

- Penicillamine is a copper chelating agent and is therefore used in the treatment of Wilson's disease, a disorder of copper metabolism. Patients with Wilson's disease should avoid

PATIENT CARE IMPLICATIONS — cont'd

foods higher in copper: chocolate, nuts, shellfish, mushrooms, liver, molasses, broccoli, and copper-enriched cereals.

- Monitor weight and blood pressure. Auscultate lung sounds. Inspect for presence of skin rashes and lesions. Monitor complete blood count and differential, platelet count, serum creatinine, BUN, liver function tests. Monitor urinalysis to detect proteinuria.
- Assess penicillin allergy before administering. Cross-sensitivity between the two drugs is possible, though rare.

Patient and family education

- Review anticipated benefits and possible side effects of drug therapy. Instruct patients to notify the physician if any of the following develop: severe or persistent vomiting or diarrhea; skin rashes, lesions, scaling, dermatitis, hair loss; fever; inflamed mouth, mouth lesions, stomatitis; swelling or edema; bruising, bleeding, nosebleeds, blood in stool, malaise, sore throat; jaundice, abdominal pain. Point out that side effects may develop any time during therapy. Report new signs and symptoms to the physician.
- Review Patient Problem: Stomatitis on p. 601.
- Emphasize the importance of taking the drug as ordered. Sporadic or intermitent use (unless prescribed by the physician) may contribute to further allergic reactions.
- Capsules may be opened and contents mixed with 15 to 30 ml of chilled applesauce, other pureed foods, or fruit juice for ease in administering.
- For treatment of arthritis, take doses 1 hour before meals or 2 hours after meals, and 1 hour apart from other medications, food, or milk.
- For treatment of Wilson's disease, take doses on an empty stomach, 30 to 60 minutes before meals or 2 hours after meals.
- For prevention of kidney stones (cystinuria), take the bedtime dose with at least two 8 oz glassfuls of water, and drink two more 8 oz glassfuls of water during the night. Take daytime doses with a full glassful of water.
- If oral iron preparations are also being administered, at least 2 hours should elapse between the two drugs.
- Avoid multivitamin preparations containing copper in patients with Wilson's disease.
- Penicillamine increases the body's require-

ment for pyridoxine. If pyridoxine is also prescribed, emphasize the importance of taking this supplement. See Dietary Considerations: Vitamins on p. 282 for dietary sources of pyridoxine.

- Women of childbearing age may wish to use some form of birth control while on penicillamine therapy; discuss before initiating therapy.
- Point out that weeks to months of therapy may be necessary before full benefit of penicillamine can be seen. Emphasize the importance of continuing with other prescribed therapies, which might include a prescribed exercise program, weight reduction, application of heat and cold, physical therapy, and so forth.

Colchicine

Drug administration

- Inspect the patient to detect hair loss and skin changes. Assess for gastrointestinal discomfort. Monitor serum creatinine, BUN, complete blood count, differential, platelet count, liver function tests, uric acid levels.

INTRAVENOUS COLCHICINE

- May be given undiluted or dilute with 0.9% sodium chloride without a bacteriostatic agent. Administer at a rate of 0.5 mg over 1 minute. Avoid extravasation or IM administration. Check that IV line is patent before administering.

Patient and family education

- Review anticipated benefits and possible side effects of drug therapy. Instruct patient to report the development of the following: change in the color of urine (hematuria); bruising, bleeding, nosebleeds, blood in stool; fever, sore throat, malaise; jaundice, abdominal pain. Gastrointestinal discomfort is very common. Encourage the patient to notify the physician of any GI discomfort.
- Tell the patient to maintain daily oral intake suficient to ensure a daily urinary output of at least 2 liters; this may require an intake of 2500 ml per day (about 10 8-oz glassfuls of water).
- Take oral doses with meals or snack to reduce gastric irritation.
- Caution patients to avoid the use of analgesics containing salicylates, without approval of the physician.

Continued.

PATIENT CARE IMPLICATIONS — cont'd

- Remind the patient to keep all health care providers informed of all drugs being taken. This drug may interfere with the desired effect of other drugs the patient is taking.
- Review Dietary Consideration: Purine.
- Limit the intake of alcoholic beverages.

Allopurinol

Drug administration

- Inspect to detect rash, skin changes. Assess vision. Monitor serum creatinine, BUN, uric acid levels, complete blood count, differential, platelet count, liver function tests.

- Review anticipated benefits and possible side effects of drug therapy. Instruct patient to report the development of the following: bruising, bleeding, nosebleeds, blood in stool; fever, sore throat, malaise; jaundice, abdominal pain. Gastrointestinal discomfort is common. Encourage the patient to notify the physician of GI discomfort.
- Tell the patient to maintain daily oral intake sufficient to ensure a daily urinary output of at least 2 liters; this may require an intake of 2500 ml per day (about 10 8-oz glassfuls of water).
- Caution patients to avoid the use of analgesics containing salicylates unless approved by the physician.
- Remind the patient to keep all health care providers informed of all drugs being taken. This drug may interfere with the desired effect of other drugs being taken.
- Take oral doses with meal or snack to reduce gastric irritation.
- Review Dietary Consideration: Purine.
- Limit the intake of alcoholic beverages.
- Do not take vitamin C while taking allopurinol as it may increase urine acidity and promote the formation of kidney stones.

Probenecid

Drug administration

- Inspect for development of skin changes. Monitor blood pressure. Monitor liver function tests, serum creatinine, BUN, uric acid levels.
- Probenecid is sometimes used concomitantly with some antibiotics, such as penicillins and cephalosporins; in this case, the probenecid helps increase the plasma and tissue antibiotic concentration.

Patient and family education

- Review anticipated benefits and possible side effects of drug therapy. Instruct patient to report the development of the following: malaise; jaundice, abdominal pain. Gastrointestinal discomfort is common. Encourage the patient to notify the physician of any GI discomfort.
- Tell the patient to maintain daily oral intake sufficient to ensure a daily urinary output of at least 2 liters; this may require an intake of 2500 ml per day (about 10 8-oz glassfuls of fluid).
- Warn patient to avoid driving or operating hazardous equipment if dizziness occurs; notify physician.
- Warn patients that flushing may occur following drug ingestion.
- Caution patients to avoid the use of analgesics containing salicylates without the physician's approval.
- Remind the patient to keep all health care providers informed of all drugs being taken. This drug may interfere with the desired effect of other drugs being taken.
- Alkalinization of the urine helps prevent crystallization of uric acid. For this reason, sodium bicarbonate, potassium citrate, or other alkalinizing agent may be prescribed concurrently.
- Review Dietary Consideration: Purine.
- Limit the intake of alcoholic beverages.
- There are combination products containing colchicine and probenecid. Review side effects of both drugs.

Sulfinpyrazone

Drug administration

- Assess for development of tinnitus and changes in hearing, gastrointestinal distress. Inspect for development of skin changes or rash.

Patient and family education

- Review anticipated benefits and possible side effects of drug therapy. Instruct patient to report the development of the following: bruising, bleeding, nosebleeds, blood in stool; fever, sore throat, malaise; ringing in the ears. Gastrointestinal discomfort is very common. Encourage the patient to notify the physician of any GI discomfort. Take oral doses with milk, meals, or snack to reduce gastric irritation.

PATIENT CARE IMPLICATIONS — cont'd

- Tell the patient to maintain daily oral intake sufficient to ensure a daily urinary output of at least 2 liters; this may require an intake of 2500 ml per day (about 10 8-oz glassfuls of fluid).
- Caution patients to avoid the use of analgesics containing salicylates without obtaining

the physician's approval.
- Remind the patient to keep all health care providers informed of all drugs being taken. This drug may interfere with the desired effect of other drugs being taken.
- Review Dietary Consideration: Purine.
- Limit the intake of alcoholic beverages.

---

the patients for whom allopurinol will be most effective. It is also effective for patients with gout resulting from drug therapy that increases uric acid production, particularly cancer therapy. Side effects are rare; they appear to be allergic reactions.

Probenecid and sulfinpyrazone

Probenecid (Benemid) and sulfinpyrazone (Anturane) inhibit the reabsorption of uric acid by the kidney tubules and thereby promote the excretion of uric acid in the urine. It is important that the patient drink at least eight glassfuls of water daily to keep the uric acid dilute so that it does not crystallize in kidney tubules or bladder. Since these drugs flood the kidney tubules with uric acid, they are contraindicated in patients with renal failure or with a history of renal stones.

Probenecid is generally well tolerated but occasionally causes gastrointestinal upset or an allergic reaction. It interferes with the renal excretion of many compounds.

Sulfinpyrazone is also well tolerated. The incidence of gastrointestinal upset is higher with sulfinpyrazone than with probenecid. Recent studies show that sulfinpyrazone decreases the incidence of sudden death in the first 8 months after an MI. This effect is believed due to decreased platelet aggregation. Since many patients with gout also have conditions such as diabetes, hypertension, or coronary artery disease (which are high-risk factors for MI), sulfinpyrazone may be more desirable than probenecid in spite of the higher incidence of gastrointestinal upset.

Drug Interactions in the Therapy of Gout

Factors that *diminish* the effectiveness of the uricosuric drugs probenecid and sulfinpyrazone include the following:
1. A diet high in purines produces too much uric acid. See Dietary Consideration: Purine.

2. Inhibition of uric acid secretion counteracts the block in reabsorption by the uricosuric drugs.
   a. Heavy alcohol consumption produces enough lactic acid to inhibit uric acid secretion.
   b. Aspirin and other salicylates at low doses (300 to 650 mg) inhibit uric acid secretion. Acetaminophen should be substituted for simple pain relief.
   c. Diuretics, particularly the thiazides, furosemide, ethacrynic acid, triamterene, and spironolactone inhibit uric acid secretion.

Drugs used to treat gout can *potentiate* other drugs.
1. Probenecid inhibits the renal secretion of these drugs, keeping their plasma levels high: penicillin, indomethacin, methotrexate, sulfonylureas (oral hypoglycemics), sulfinpyrazone, salicylates, and rifampin.
2. Sulfinpyrazone inhibits the degradation of these drugs: sulfonamides, particularly sulfadiazine and sulfisoxazole, sulfonylureas, and coumarins.
3. Allopurinol inhibits the degradation of these drugs: azathioprine, 6-mercaptopurine, antipyrine, coumarins, and cyclophosphamide.

SUMMARY

Aspirin is the prototype of analgesic-antipyretic and nonsteroidal antiinflammatory drugs (NSAIDs).

Aspirin and acetaminophen are over-the-counter drugs widely used for analgesia and for treating a fever. Analgesia results from the inhibition of peripheral pain receptors. Antipyresis results from an action on the hypothalamus to overcome the action of pyrogen, a fever-producing protein released by phagocytes. Acetaminophen does not cause gastrointestinal irritation and does not alter platelet function or bleeding times as does aspirin. Acetaminophen is also formulated as a liquid for infants and children.

Aspirin is well absorbed and is rapidly hydrolyzed to salicylic acid. It irreversibly inactivates the enzyme cyclooxygenase of platelets, a characteristic of aspirin only and not of other salicylates. This irreversible inactivation accounts for the inhibition of blood clotting characteristic of even low doses of aspirin. Gastrointestinal irritation is the other major side effect of aspirin. Salicylism is mild intoxication with aspirin. Symptoms of salicylism include tinnitus, hyperventilation, and, occasionally, fever. Drug interactions and cross-sensitivities for aspirin allergies are listed in the text.

Other analgesic-antipyretic drugs include the over-the-counter drugs salicylamide, sodium salicylate, and ibuprofen and the prescription drug mefenamic acid.

The major mechanism of action of the NSAIDs is the inhibition of prostaglandin synthesis. They are effective in treating the pain and inflammation of rheumatoid arthritis, osteoarthritis, other kinds of arthritis, muscle injury, gout, and dysmenorrhea. A common side effect is gastrointestinal upset. These drugs are variable in affecting platelet function and blood clotting.

Aspirin is an effective antiinflammatory drug but at much larger doses than are required for analgesia-antipyresis. Salicylates may be used if gastrointestinal upset becomes a problem. The other nonsteroidal antiinflammatory drugs are prescription drugs. Phenylbutazone is potent. Because it has potentially severe side effects and drug interactions, is used for only 2 weeks or less. Indomethacin and the related drugs sulindac and tolmetin are another group of NSAIDs. Limitations of indomethacin include gastrointestinal upset, headache, and dizziness. The propionic acids include ibuprofen, naproxen, fenoprofen, carprofen, floctafenine, flurbiprofen, ketoprofen, and tiaprofonic acid. These drugs have less severe side effects than the other antiinflammatory drugs and are proving suitable alternatives for patients with arthritis who cannot tolerate aspirin. Piroxicam is a new long-acting NSAID for arthritis. Meclofenamate and mefenamic acid are new NSAIDs. Their major side effect is gastrointestinal upset with diarrhea.

One role of selected NSAIDs is to reduce the pain and inflammation of rheumatoid arthritis until a remission occurs. If a remission does not occur and joint damage continues, a drug may be tried to induce a remission. Drugs include gold salts, hydrochloroquine, and penicillamine. Since each drug can cause serious side effects, careful monitoring of the patient is required during therapy. The immunosuppressive drugs azathioprine and cyclophosphamide and the glucocorticoids have restricted roles in the treatment of rheumatoid arthritis.

Gout is a metabolic disease characterized by elevated concentrations of uric acid. Gouty arthritis arises when uric acid crystallizes in one or more joints. Treatment is of two types: treatment of an acute attack marked by severe inflammation of the joint and long-term treatment designed to prevent recurrence. An acute attack may be treated with an NSAID, traditionally phenylbutazone, or indomethacin, or by the drug colchicine, whose mode of action is unknown. Long-term therapy is provided by allopurinol to inhibit the formation of uric acid, and/or probenecid or sulfinpyrazone to promote the excretion of uric acid. These drugs for long-term treatment have a number of drug interactions, which are listed in the text.

STUDY QUESTIONS

1. List the three pharmacological actions characteristic of aspirin.
2. How do the nonnarcotic analgesics produce analgesia?
3. What is the mechanism of antipyresis?
4. Which two paraaminophenols are found in over-the-counter analgesic-antipyretic drugs?
5. Why is acetaminophen considered safer than aspirin?
6. What are the side effects of acetaminophen?
7. What is the mechanism of acetaminophen toxicity?
8. What is the dosage difference between aspirin taken for analgesia-antipyresis and for an antiinflammatory response?
9. How does aspirin affect the stomach?
10. How does aspirin affect platelets?
11. What factors determine the metabolism and excretion of salicylate?
12. Describe salicylism.
13. Describe aspirin toxicity.
14. What pharmacological actions are characteristic of the NSAIDs?
15. Why is phenylbutazone used for 2 weeks or less?
16. What are the major side effects of indomethacin?
17. Which NSAIDS are chemically related to indomethacin?
18. Describe the uses of NSAIDs.
19. Which four drugs may be used to induce a remission in progressive rheumatoid arthritis?
20. Describe the role of colchicine in treating gout.

21. Describe the mechanisms of allopurinol, probenecid, and sulfinpyrazone for lowering the uric acid concentration of the body.

SUGGESTED READINGS

Analgesic-antipyretic drugs

Abramson, S., and others: Modes of action of aspirin-like drugs, Proc. Natl. Acad. Sci. **82:**7227, 1985.

Beaver, W.T.: Aspirin and acetaminophen as constituents of analgesic combinations, Arch. Intern. Med. **141**(3):293, 1981.

Brucker, M.C.: Management of common minor discomforts in pregnancy: managing minor pain in pregnancy, part 2, J. Nurse Midwife **33**(1):25, 1988.

Cooper, S.A.: Comparative pharmacokinetics of aspirin and acetophen, Arch. Intern. Med. **141**(3):282, 1981.

Eland, J.M.: Pharmacologic management of acute and chronic pediatric pain, Issues Compr. Pediatr. Nurse. **11**(2/3):93, 1988.

Fields, W.S.: Aspirin for prevention of stroke: a review, Am. J. Med. **74**(6A):61, 1983.

Hayes, A.H., Jr.: Therapeutic implications of drug interactions with acetaminophen and aspirin, Arch. Intern. Med. **141**(3):301, 1981.

Hurwitz, E.S., and others: Public Health Service study of Reye's syndrome and medications, JAMA **257**(14):1905, 1987.

Jick, H.: Effects of aspirin and acetaminophen in gastrointestinal hemorrhage, Arch. Intern. Med. **141**(3):316, 1981.

Kilmon, C.A.: Home management of children's fever, J. Pediatr. Nurs. **2**(6):400, 1987.

Langman, M.J.S., Coggon, D., and Spiegelhalter, D.: Analgesic intake and the risk of acute upper gastrointestinal bleeding, Am. J. Med. **74**(6A):79, 1983.

Mielke, C.H., Jr.: Comparative effects of aspirin and acetaminophen on hemostasis, Arch. Intern. Med. **141**(3):305, 1981.

Mielke, C.H., Jr.: Influence of aspirin on platelets and the bleeding time, Am. J. Med. **74**(6A):72, 1983.

Mustard, J.F., Kinlough-Rathbone, R.L., and Packham, M.A.: Aspirin in the treatment of cardiovascular disease: a review, Am. J. Med. **74**(6A):43, 1983.

Peters, B.H., Fraim, C.J., and Masel, B.E.: Comparison of 650 mg aspirin and 1000 mg acetaminophen with each other, and with placebo in moderately severe headache, Am. J. Med. **74**(6A):36, 1983.

Plotz, P.H., and Kimberly, R.P.: Acute effects of aspirin and acetaminophen on renal function, Arch. Intern. Med. **141**(3):343, 1981.

Prescott, L.F.: Treatment of severe acetaminophen poisoning with intravenous acetylcysteine, Arch. Intern. Med. **141**(3):386, 1981.

Rudolph, A.M.: Effects of aspirin and acetaminophen in pregnancy and in the newborn, Arch. Intern. Med. **141**(3):358, 1981.

Schachtel, B.P., and others: Rational scales for analgesics in sore throat, Clin. Pharmacol. Ther. **36**(2):151, 1984.

Settipane, G.A.: Adverse reactions to aspirin and related drugs, Arch. Intern. Med. **141**(3):328, 1981.

Spector, S.L.: Idiosyncratic reaction to aspirin in adult asthmatics and bronchitics, Intern. Med. **3**(10):69, 1982.

Stewart, R.B., Hale, W.E., and Marks, R.G.: Analgesic drug use in an ambulatory elderly population, Drug Intell. Clin. Pharm. **16**:833, 1982.

Temple, A.R.: Acute and chronic effects of aspirin toxicity and their treatment, Arch. Intern. Med. **141**(3):364, 1981.

Vale, J.A., Meredith, T.J., and Goulding, R.: Treatment of acetaminophen poisoning, Arch. Intern. Med. **141**(3):394, 1981.

Yaffe, S.J.: Comparative efficacy of aspirin and acetaminophen in the reduction of fever in children, Arch. Intern. Med. **141**(3):286, 1981.

Zimmerman, H.J.: Effects of aspirin and acetaminophen on the liver, Arch. Intern. Med. **141**(3):333, 1981.

Nonsteroidal antiinflammatory drugs

Abramson, S.B., and Weissmann, G.: The mechansism of action of nonsteroidal antiinflammatory drugs, Arthritis Rheumatism **32**(1):1, 1989.

Abruzzo, J.L.: The role of nonsteroidal antiinflammatory drugs in rheumatoid arthritis, Intern. Med. **3**(10):124, 1982.

Blackshear, J.L., and others: NSAID-induced nephrotoxicity—avoidance, detection, and treatment, Drug Therapy **8**(11):47, 1983.

Brater, D.C.: Drug-drug and drug-disease interactions with nonsteroidal anti-inflammatory drugs, Am. J. Med. **80**(Suppl 1A):62, 1986.

Butt, J.H., Barthel, J.S., and Moore, R.A.: Clinical spectrum of the upper gastrointestinal effects of nonsteroidal antiinflammatory drugs, Am. J. Med. **84**(Suppl 2A):5, 1988.

Calabro, J.J.: Analgesic and anti-inflammatory therapy in the elderly, Am. J. Med. **79**(Suppl 4B):33, 1985.

Chapman, J.D.: Dysmenorrhea: changing concepts and therapies, Mod. Med. **51**(3):164, 1983.

Coles, L.S., and others: From experiment to experience: side effects of nonsteroidal anti-inflammatory drugs, Am. J. Med. **74**:820, 1983.

Kantor, T.G., Kaplan, H., and Ward, J.R.: NSAID therapy made a little simpler, Patient Care **18**(12):89, 1984.

Khokhar, N.: Nephrotoxicity of nonsteroidal anti-inflammatory drugs, Am. Fam. Physician **30**(1):123, 1984.

Relieving pain: an analgesic guide, Am. J. Nurs. **88**(6):815, 1988.

Zawada, E.T.: Renal consequences of nonsteroidal antiinflammatory drugs, Postgrad. Med. **71**(5):223, 1982.

Zurier, R.B.: Prostaglandins—their potential in clinical medicine, Postgrad. Med. **68**(3):70, 1980.

Drugs to treat rheumatoid arthritis

Bartholomew, L.E., and Rynes, R.I.: Use of antimalarial drugs in rheumatoid arthritis: guidelines for ocular safety, Intern. Med. **3**(3):66, 1982.

Bombardier, C.: Auranofin therapy and quality of life in patients with rheumatoid arthritis, Am. J. Med. **81**(4):565, 1986.

Brassell, M.P.: Pharmacologic management of rheumatic disease, Orthop. Nurs. **7**(2):43, 1988.

Clegg, D.O., and Ward, J.R.: Slow-acting anti-rheumatic drug therapy for rheumatoid arthritis, Nurse Pract. **12**(3):44, 1987.

Christman, C.: Protocol for administration and management of chrysotherapy (gold therapy), Nurse Pract. **12**(10):30, 1987.

Conner, C.S.: Oral gold in arthritis, Drug Intell. Clin. Pharm. **18**(10):84, 1984.

Costello, P.B., and Green, F.A.: Serum salicylate measurement in the treatment of rheumatic disorders, Intern. Med. **4**(5):60, 1984.

Day, R.O., Dromgoole, S.H., and Paulus, H.E.: Getting the most out of aspirin and salicylates in rheumatoid arthritis, Mod. Med. **50**(8):125, 1982.

Fuller, E.: Aggressive drug therapy for RA, Patient Care **21**(5):22, 1987.

Harris, E.D.: Pathogenesis of rheumatoid arthritis, Am. J. Med. **80**(Suppl 4B):4, 1986.

Howell, D.S.: Pathogenesis of osteoarthritis, Am. J. Med. **80**(Suppl 4B):24, 1986.

Jaffe, I.A.: Penicillamine—an alternative to injectable gold, Consultant **22**(2):324, 1982.

Pisetsky, D.S.: Treating arthritis in the elderly, Drug Therapy **13**(3):47, 1983.

Robinson, D.R.: Management of gastrointestinal toxicity of nonsteroidal antiinflammatory drugs during the therapy of rheumatic diseases, Am. J. Med. **84**(Suppl 2A):1, 1988.

Roth, S.H.: The emerging new arthritis drugs—a clinician's opinion, Postgrad. Med. **73**(3):125, 1983.

Rynes, R.I.: Hydrochloroquine treatment of rheumatoid arthritis, Am. J. Med. **85**(Suppl 4A):18, 1988.

Schoen, R.T., and Vender, R.J.: Mechanism of nonsteroidal an-tiinflammatory drug induced gastric damage, Am. J. Med. **86**:449, 1989.

Strand, C.V., and Clark, S.R.: Adult arthritis: drugs and remedies, Am. J. Nurs. **83**(2):266, 1983.

Ziminski, C.M.: Treating joint inflammation in the elderly: an update, Geriatrics **40**(1):73, 1985.

Drugs to treat gout

Gordon, G.V., and Schumacher, H.R.: Management of gout, Am. Fam. Physician **19**(1):91, 1979.

Kweskin, S.: New and old options in gout therapy, Patient Care **13**:124, 1979.

Roberts, W.N., Liang, M.H., and Stern, S.H.: Colchicine in acute gout, JAMA **257**(14):1920, 1987.

Simkin, P.A.: Management of gout, Ann. Intern. Med. **90**:812, 1979.

Talbott, J.H.: Treating gout: successful methods of prevention and control, Postgrad. Med. **63**(5):175, 1978.

Antihistamines

24

EFFECTS OF HISTAMINE
Naturally Occurring Histamine

Histamine is a naturally occurring amine that is formed from the amino acid histidine. Histamine is found in three major sites. One is mast cells, which are numerous in the lung and skin, and basophils, the counterparts of mast cells in the blood. The histamine released from the mast cells causes many of the symptoms associated with allergic reactions. The second site is the gastrointestinal tract, where histamine is a potent stimulant for the secretion of acid in the stomach. The third site is certain parts of the brain, where histamine is believed to be a neurotransmitter. At present, the role of histamine in the brain is speculative but may involve regulating the level of arousal.

In this chapter the focus is on the role of histamine in allergic reactions and the drugs available to treat these reactions. The role of histamine in the stomach is discussed in Chapter 13.

Histamine Release

Histamine in mast cells and basophils is complexed with heparin and stored in granules. The typical allergic reaction such as hay fever or contact dermatitis involves the release of these granules in response to an antigen. Antibodies of the IgE class fix to the mast cells and basophils, and, when an antigen appears and binds to the fixed IgE, the cells degranulate, releasing histamine, heparin, and other compounds, which alter capillary permeability and attract phagocytes to degrade the bound antigen. This process is illustrated in Figure 24.1.

In addition to the antigen-induced degranulation, many drugs and venoms cause degranulation. These include drugs and dyes that carry a positive charge, large molecules as occur in animal sera and dextran solutions, and venoms and enzymes that damage tissue.

Allergic Responses Explained by the Action of Histamine

Local allergic responses involving histamine are as follows:

Angioedema: Swelling caused by plasma leakage and blood vessel dilation in the skin or mucous membranes. "Giant hives."

Anaphylaxis: Systemic. Onset is usually heralded by a generalized itching and tingling sensation and a feeling of apprehension. A profound hypotension leading to shock may follow, and the bronchioles are constricted, causing a choking sensation.

Asthma: Spasm of the bronchial smooth muscle.

Eczema: Inflamed areas of skin.

Purpura: Red spots on the skin caused by the leakage of blood from small vessels.

Rhinitis: Inflammation of the nasal mucous membranes that allows fluid to escape.

Urticaria: Hives, which are large wheals caused by leakage of plasma and are accompanied by severe itching.

Two actions of histamine are prominent in explaining allergic responses. First, histamine is a potent dilator of arterioles and renders the capillaries more permeable so that fluid and protein are lost into the extravascular space. This explains the bump that appears after an insect sting. Initially, there is a red spot reflecting the dilation of the small blood vessels, and as fluid leaks into the extravascular space, the bump, representing local edema, appears. Second, histamine stimulates the contraction of smooth muscle, particularly the bronchial smooth muscle. When mast cells are degranulated in the lung, as in asthma, the airway is narrowed and it becomes difficult to breathe.

Histamine released systemically causes anaphylaxis, which is characterized by a profound fall

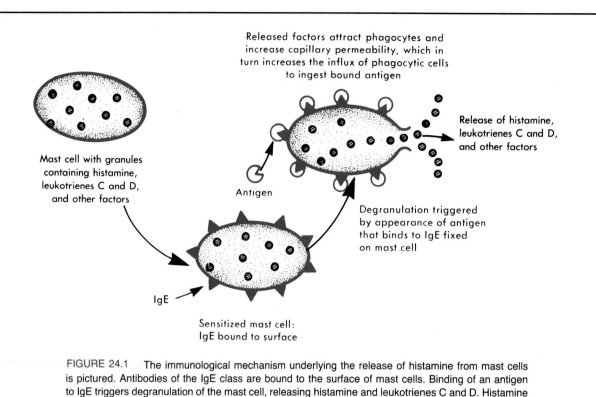

FIGURE 24.1   The immunological mechanism underlying the release of histamine from mast cells is pictured. Antibodies of the IgE class are bound to the surface of mast cells. Binding of an antigen to IgE triggers degranulation of the mast cell, releasing histamine and leukotrienes C and D. Histamine is responsible for many of the symptoms of allergies and asthma.

in blood pressure resulting from vasodilation and severe constriction of the bronchioles making breathing difficult. The loss of fluid from circulation resulting from the increased capillary permeability causes the shock that develops in an untreated anaphylactic response. Edema in the mucous tissue of the upper windpipe (laryngeal edema) can block the airway altogether. The drug of choice for anaphylactic shock is epinephrine. Epinephrine constricts blood vessels to raise the blood pressure and relieve laryngeal edema, and dilates the bronchioles, actions that reverse those of histamine (Chapter 14).

Histamine Metabolism

Once histamine is released, it is metabolized to inactive compounds in 5 to 15 minutes. One of the degradative pathways is inhibited by aspirin so that histamine may persist. This is the mechanism for one type of aspirin sensitivity.

ANTIHISTAMINES

Antihistamines have been available for over 50 years. Although these drugs are effective in blocking some actions of histamine, they are ineffective in blocking the histamine-mediated secretion of

acid in the stomach. The explanation is that there are two types of histamine receptors: the H-1 receptors, acting principally on blood vessels and the bronchioles, and the H-2 receptors, acting mainly on the gastrointestinal tract. The older antihistamines are specific antagonists for the H-1 receptors. Antagonists specific for the H-2 receptor are cimetidine (Tagamet), famotidine (Pepcid), nizatidine (Axid), and ranitidine (Zantac). These drugs, used primarily to decrease stomach acid, are discussed in Chapter 13. In this chapter, the term *antihistamine* refers to drugs that specifically block the H-1 receptors.

Absorption and Fate of Antihistamines

Antihistamines are given orally and are well absorbed. Their action is seen in 10 to 30 minutes and lasts for 4 to 6 hours. Timed-release forms are active for 8 to 12 hours. Antihistamines are metabolized to inactive compounds by the liver and kidneys.

Other Pharmacological Actions of Antihistamines

Although the antihistamines are so named because they specifically compete with histamine for

Table 24.1   Antihistamines Used to Control Allergic Reactions

Generic name	Trade name	Administration/dosage	Comments
Astemizole	Hismanol*	ORAL: *Adults*—10 mg once a day, taken on an empty stomach. *Children*—2 mg/10 mg body weight once a day, taken on an empty stomach.	New nonsedating antihistamine.
Azatadine maleate	Optimine*	ORAL: *Adults*—1 to 2 mg twice daily. *Children*—not established. FDA Pregnancy Category B.	Drowsiness is the most common side effect.
Brompheniramine maleate	Dimetane*‡ Various others	ORAL: *Adults*—4 to 8 mg 3 to 4 times daily or 8 to 12 mg of sustained-release form 2 to 3 times daily. *Children*—over 6 yr, ½ adult dose; under 6 yr, 0.5 mg/kg daily divided into 3 to 4 doses. FDA Pregnancy Category B.	Drowsiness is the most common side effect.
Carbinoxamine maleate	Clistin	ORAL: *Adults*—4 to 8 mg 3 to 4 times daily or 8 to 12 mg of sustained-release form 2 to 3 times daily. *Children*—over 6 yr, 4 mg 3 to 4 times daily; 3 to 6 yr, 2 to 4 mg 3 to 4 times daily; 1 to 3 yr, 2 mg 3 to 4 times daily. FDA Pregnancy Category B.	Low incidence of drowsiness. Anticholinergic effect is weak.
Chlorpheniramine maleate	Aller-Chlor‡ Chlortab Chlor-Trimeton† Teldrin‡ Various others	ORAL: *Adults*—4 mg 3 to 4 times daily or 8 to 12 mg of sustained-release form 2 to 3 times daily. *Children*—6 to 12 yr, 2 mg 3 to 4 times daily or 8 mg of sustained-release form once daily; 2 to 6 yr, 1 mg 3 to 4 times daily.	Low incidence of drowsiness. A common ingredient in cold remedies.
Clemastine	Tavist*	ORAL: *Adults*—2.68 mg 3 times daily. Not intended for children.	Low incidence of drowsiness. Very weak anticholinergic effects.
Cyproheptadine hydrochloride	Periactin	ORAL: *Adults*—4 to 20 mg daily, not more than 0.5 mg/kg. Dose is started at 4 mg 3 times daily. *Children*—7 to 14 yr, 4 mg 2 to 3 times daily to a maximum of 16 mg daily; 2 to 6 yr, 2 mg 2 to 3 times daily to a maximum of 12 mg daily. FDA Pregnancy Category B.	Used to relieve itching. Drowsiness is the most common side effect.
Dexchlorpheniramine maleate	Polaramine*	ORAL: *Adults*—1 to 2 mg 3 or 4 times daily or 4 to 6 mg 2 times daily or 6 mg of timed-release form 3 times daily. *Children*—under 12 yr, 0.15 mg/kg daily divided into 4 doses. FDA Pregnancy Category B.	Drowsiness is the most common side effect.

*Available in Canada and United States.
†Available in Canada only.
‡Available without a prescription.

Continued.

Table 24.1   Antihistamines Used to Control Allergic Reactions—cont'd

Generic name	Trade name	Administration/dosage	Comments
Diphenhydramine hydrochloride	Benadryl Hydrochloride‡ Bendylate Fenylhist Rohydra Valdrene Benyln Cough‡	ORAL: *Adults*—25 to 50 mg 3 to 4 times daily. *Children*—over 20 lb, 2.5 to 25 mg 3 to 4 times daily; under 12 yr, 5 mg/kg in 4 divided doses each day.	High incidence of drowsiness with little paradoxical stimulation in children. Also used to treat motion sickness and mild parkinsonism. Also used as an antitussive. May be used with epinephrine in treating an anaphylactic reaction.
Diphenylpyraline hydrochloride	Hispril	ORAL: *Adults*—2 mg every 4 hr or 5 mg of sustained-release form every 12 hr. *Children*—over 6 yr, 2 mg every 6 hr or 5 mg of sustained-release form once daily; 2 to 6 yr, 1 to 2 mg every 8 hr.	
Doxylamine succinate	Unisom†	ORAL: *Adults*—12.5 to 25 mg every 4 to 6 hr. *Children*—6 to 12 yr, 75 mg divided into 4 to 6 doses daily; under 6 yr, 2 mg/kg body weight divided into 4 to 6 doses daily. Decapryn available without prescription.	High incidence of drowsiness. Often included in nonprescription sleep aids.
Loratadine	Claritin†	ORAL: *Adults*—10 mg once a day.	New drug for seasonal rhinitis.
Methdilazine hydrochloride	Dilosyn† Tacaryl	ORAL: *Adults*—8 mg 2 to 4 times daily. *Children*—over 3 yr, 4 mg 2 to 4 times daily.	A phenothiazine derivative used primarily to relieve itching. Incidence of drowsiness is less than with other phenothiazines.
Phenindamine	Nolahist	ORAL: *Adults*—25 mg every 4 to 6 hr as needed. *Children* (6 to 12 yr)—12.5 mg every 4 to 6 hr.	For seasonal rhinitis.
Promethazine hydrochloride	Phenergan* Quadnite Remsed Zipan	ORAL: *Adults*—12.5 mg 4 times daily or 25 mg at bedtime. *Children*—½ adult dose.	A phenothiazine derivative with marked sedative action. Also used to treat motion sickness and to control nausea and vomiting.
Pyrilamine maleate	Dormarex	ORAL: *Adults*—25 to 50 mg 4 times daily. *Children*—6 to 12 yr, ½ adult dose. Available without prescription.	Low incidence of drowsiness.
Terfenadine	Seldane*	ORAL: *Adults*—60 mg every 8 to 10 hr as needed. FDA Pregnancy Category C.	New nonsedating antihistamine.

*Available in Canada and United States.
†Available in Canada only.
‡Available without a prescription.

Table 24.1   Antihistamines Used to Control Allergic Reactions—cont'd

Generic name	Trade name	Administration/dosage	Comments
Trimeprazine tartrate	Panectyl† Temaril	ORAL: *Adults*—2.5 mg 4 times daily or 5 mg of sustained-release form every 12 hr. *Children*—over 3 yr, 2.5 mg at bedtime or up to 3 times daily (over 6 yr can take 5 mg of sustained-release form once a day); 6 mo to 3 yr, 1.25 mg at bedtime or up to 3 times daily.	A phenothiazine derivative. Drowsiness is the most common reaction. Used primarily to relieve the itching of neurodermatitis, contact dermatitis, and chickenpox.
Tripelennamine citrate or hydrochloride	PBZ-SR Pyribenzamine* Hydrochloride† Ro-Hist	ORAL: *Adults*—25 to 50 mg every 4 to 6 hr or 100 mg of sustained-release form every 12 hr. *Children*—over 5 yr, 50 mg of sustained-release form every 12 hr; children and infants, 5 mg/kg daily divided into 4 to 6 doses.	Dizziness is a common side effect.
Triprolidine hydrochloride	Actidil*	ORAL: *Adults*—2.5 mg 3 to 4 times daily. *Children*—over 6 yr, ½ adult dose; under 6 yr, 0.3 to 0.6 mg 3 to 4 times daily. FDA Pregnancy Category B.	Low incidence of side effects, with drowsiness being the most common side effect.

*Available in Canada and United States.
†Available in Canada only.

the H-1 receptors, they have other pharmacological properties. The main secondary action is an anticholinergic or atropine-like action. This is the origin of side effects such as inhibition of secretions, blurred vision, urinary retention, fast heart rate (tachycardia), and constipation. In the central nervous system the anticholinergic effect can cause insomnia, tremors, nervousness, and irritability. These effects are particularly predominant in children. Sedation and drowsiness, the central antihistaminic effects, are more commonly seen in adults. The spectrum of antihistaminic and anticholinergic properties depends on the drug, the dose, and the individual.

Most antihistamines have a local anesthetic effect, which might relieve the itching of skin rashes. Antihistamines are rarely used for this purpose because they tend to be good antigens, thereby causing skin rashes themselves. There are other clinically important pharmacological actions limited to a few of the antihistamines. Some antihistamines are effective in preventing nausea and vomiting, particularly from motion sickness. A few antihistamines prevent vertigo (the feeling of movement, particularly rotational movement, when there is none). Antihistamines that are effective in suppressing the tremors of Parkinson's disease are discussed in Chapter 35.

Toxic Effects of Antihistamines

An overdose of an antihistamine can cause central nervous system depression or central nervous system stimulation, the latter being more common in children. The atropine-like symptoms (i.e., a flushed skin and fixed, dilated pupils) also become prominent. The treatment is to maintain an airway and to treat hypotension. In children a high temperature is common, which is reversed with ice packs and sponge baths. If the antihistamine is not a phenothiazine, vomiting is induced, gastric lavage is carried out, and cathartics are used to empty the gastrointestinal tract of remaining drug. Vomiting should not be induced because phenothiazines can cause uncoordinated movements of the head and neck, which would cause aspiration of vomitus. The antihistamines that are phenothiazine derivatives are identified in the drug tables.

Drug Interactions and Contraindications for Antihistamines

The main drug interaction associated with the antihistamines is the additive depression of the

THE NURSING PROCESS

ANTIHISTAMINES FOR ALLERGIC REACTIONS

Assessment

The patient requiring antihistamines for allergic reactions may be displaying nonacute symptoms such as red, watery eyes; nasal congestion; hives; or rash. Nausea, vomiting, and diarrhea may represent allergy to food or medications. An acute allergic response (anaphylaxis) manifests with rapidly developing edema of the face and hands, wheezing, bronchoconstriction, cyanosis, dyspnea, tachycardia, and hypotension, which can lead to death. Anaphylaxis is an emergency; the more delayed and chronic response may represent a source of annoyance to the patient but may never progress to an acute phase.

Vital signs, respiratory and cardiovascular status, relevant history of previous allergy and exposure to possible allergens, subjective symptoms, and objective data such as the extent and type of rash should be assessed.

Nursing diagnoses

Potential for injury: drowsiness related to antihistamine therapy

Potential altered bowel elimination: constipation related to antihistamine use

Management

The acute allergic reaction anaphylaxis requires immediate diagnosis and treatment, usually with 1:1000 epinephrine injected subcutaneously or intramuscularly, followed by parenteral antihistamines. Supportive care is symptomatic and based on rapid assessment of the cardiovascular and respiratory response. Management of the less acute allergic response is not an emergency. The nurse should monitor the vital signs, respiratory status, cardiovascular status, platelet count, and white blood cell count. The patient is observed for side effects of drug therapy, especially drowsiness; the fluid intake and output are monitored to determine urinary retention; and frequency of bowel movements is monitored to assess constipation. At the same time, the patient may be undergoing tests to identify the specific allergens responsible.

Evaluation

Before discharge, the patient should be able to explain why and how to take the prescribed medication, the side effects that may appear and which of these should be reported immediately, and what to do for specific side effects such as dry mouth, constipation, hypotension, and drowsiness. If specific allergens have been identified, the patient should be able to name them. The patient should be able to state the importance of wearing a medical identification tag or bracelet identifying specific allergens. The goal of therapy is primarily to reduce the histamine response and improve patient comfort. Treatment with antihistamines does not eliminate any allergies. Ideally, the patient would be symptomatically improved and free of drug side effects. In fact, most patients have some side effects resulting from antihistamine therapy. For additional information, see the patient care implications section at the end of this chapter.

---

central nervous system when taken with alcohol, hypnotics, sedatives, antipsychotics, antianxiety drugs, or narcotic analgesics. Because of their atropine-like effects, the antihistamines should be used with caution in patients with glaucoma, hyperthyroidism, cardiovascular disease, or hypertension.

Antihistamines are contraindicated for nursing mothers because the drugs are secreted in the milk.

Antihistamines taken by young children can cause paradoxical excitement, whereas the elderly are sensitive to the sedative actions.

CLINICAL USES OF ANTIHISTAMINES
Antihistamines for Allergic Reactions
(Table 24.1)

Antihistamines are effective primarily in decreasing the discomfort of acute allergic reactions

Table 24.2 Antihistamines Used to Control Nausea and Vomiting

Generic name	Trade name	Administration/dosage	Comments
Buclizine hydrochloride	Bucladin-S	ORAL: *Adults*—50 mg 30 min before travel, 50 mg 4 to 6 hr later for extended travel. 50 mg 2 to 3 times daily to control nausea. Not for children.	Most effective for preventing motion sickness. May alleviate nausea of disorders causing dizziness. Contraindicated in pregnancy. Drowsiness and anticholinergic effects are the most frequent side effects.
Cyclizine hydrochloride, cyclizine lactate	Marezine*	ORAL: *Adults*—50 mg 30 min before travel, 50 mg 4 to 6 hr later for extended travel, maximum dosage 200 mg daily. *Children*—6 to 10 yr, ½ adult dose. INTRAMUSCULAR: *Adults*—50 mg every 4 to 6 hr as needed.	Most effective for preventing motion sickness. Used for treating postoperative nausea and vomiting. Drowsiness and anticholinergic effects are the most frequent side effects.
Dimenhydrinate	Dramamine* Various others	ORAL: *Adults*—50 mg every 4 hr. *Children*—8 to 12 yr, 25 to 50 mg 3 times daily. INTRAMUSCULAR, INTRAVENOUS, RECTAL: same as oral, if required. Intravenous dose should take at least 2 min. FDA Pregnancy Category B.	Most effective for preventing motion sickness. Drowsiness is the most frequent side effect.
Diphenhydramine hydrochloride	Benadryl Hydrochloride‡ Various others	ORAL: *Adults*—50 mg 30 min before travel, 50 mg every 6 to 8 hr during travel. *Children*—over 20 lb, ¼ to ½ adult dose (5 mg/kg every 12 hr). INTRAMUSCULAR: *Adults*—10 to 50 mg every 2 to 3 hr up to 400 mg/day. *Children*—5 mg/kg in 4 doses up to 300 mg/day.	Most effective for preventing motion sickness. Drowsiness is a frequent side effect.
Hydroxyzine hydrochloride, hydroxyzine pamoate	Atarax‡ Vistaril Various others	ORAL: *Adults*—25 to 100 mg 3 to 4 times daily. *Children*—over 6 yr, 50 to 100 mg daily in divided doses; under 6 yr, 50 mg daily in divided doses. INTRAMUSCULAR: *Adults*—25 to 50 mg. *Children*—0.5 mg/lb.	A sedative that controls nausea and vomiting.
Meclizine hydrochloride	Antivert‡ Bonine†	ORAL: *Adults*—25 to 50 mg 1 hr before travel, repeated every 24 hr during the journey. Not recommended for children.	Most effective for preventing motion sickness and vertigo. Contraindicated in pregnancy. Drowsiness and anticholinergic effects are the most common side effects.

*Available in Canada and United States without prescription.
†Available without prescription.
‡Available in Canada and United States.

Continued.

Table 24.2   Antihistamines Used to Control Nausea and Vomiting—cont'd

Generic name	Trade name	Administration/dosage	Comments
Promethazine hydro-chloride	Phenergan‡ Prorex Remsed V-Gan Various others	ORAL, RECTAL: *Adults*—25 mg 30 to 60 min before travel, repeat in 8 to 12 hr. During journey, 25 mg on arising and at dinner. *Children*—½ adult dose. *Postoperatively:* 25 mg every 4 to 6 hr; children's dose ½ adult dose. INTRAMUSCULAR: ½ oral dose.	A phenothiazine derivative. Used to treat motion sickness and postoperative nausea and vomiting.

‡Available in Canada and United States.

THE NURSING PROCESS

ANTIHISTAMINES AS ANTIEMETICS

Assessment

There are a variety of conditions and situations that may produce nausea and vomiting in susceptible individuals, including the flu, motion sickness, general anesthesia, certain medications, pain, or odors. The nurse should assess the patient's overall condition, checking skin turgor, fluid intake and output, weight and weight changes, and vital signs. The history should include the causes, amount, frequency, and characteristics of vomitus and subjective complaints.

Nursing diagnoses

Potential for injury: drowsiness related to antiemetic therapy

Potential altered bowel elimination: constipation related to antiemetic use

Management

Nausea and vomiting from many causes are self-limiting. Antiemetic therapy is symptomatic until time cures the problem or a specific cause can be found. The nurse should monitor the vital signs, the fluid intake and output, the skin turgor, and the level of consciousness and should check for constipation.

The patient should be provided with a clear liquid diet. Comfort measures may be helpful, including decreasing or eliminating environmental odors, keeping food out of the patient's sight, applying a cool washcloth to the head, and providing regular mouth care. These measures should be individualized, based on the patient's response. Appropriate laboratory tests include the white blood cell count, and the serum electrolyte levels.

Evaluation

Ideally, antiemetics will decrease nausea and vomiting, permit the patient to eat without difficulty and to be more comfortable, without causing side effects. In fact, many patients have side effects with antihistamine therapy, although some patients may welcome drowsiness that promotes sleep if the nausea and vomiting have been severe. In most cases, antiemetics are needed on a short-term basis, usually only 1 week to 10 days, but this time period varies with the cause of the nausea. Before beginning self-medication, the patient should be able to explain what the prescribed dose is, and how to take the prescribed medication, what the side effects are and how to treat them, which side effects require immediate contact with a physician, what to do if the nausea and vomiting do not improve within a specified period of time, and what to do to prevent dehydration and fluid and electrolyte imbalance with continued vomiting.

PATIENT CARE IMPLICATIONS

Drug administration

- Monitor blood pressure, pulse, intake and output. Auscultate breath sounds. Inspect for development of rash. Monitor complete blood count, white blood cell count and differential, platelets.
- Supervise ambulation, especially of the elderly. Keep side rails up and a nightlight on. Supervise smoking.
- Assess for urinary retention: difficulty initiating voiding, feelings of incomplete bladder emptying. Palpate the bladder.
  INTRAMUSCULAR ADMINISTRATION
- Use large muscle masses (see Chapter 6). Record and rotate injection sites. Aspirate before injecting medication to prevent accidental intravenous administration. Warn patients that IM injection of antihistamine may burn as the medication is injected.
- Read labels carefully. Some forms are for IM use only and should not be used for intravenous administration.
- Antihistamines may be prescribed with narcotic analgesics for pain relief. They may decrease nausea, and may potentiate CNS depression, but they do not enhance the analgesic effect of the narcotic. It may be necessary to lower the dose of one or the other of the two drugs because of the hypotension, sedation, and other side effects which may occur when both drugs are used.
  INTRAVENOUS BROMPHENIRAMINE
- May be given undiluted, but further dilution is preferred. Check with the pharmacist regarding compatibility with other drugs. Administer a single bolus injection over at least 1 minute.
  INTRAVENOUS CHLORPHENIRAMINE
- May be given undiluted. Administer at a rate of 10 mg over 1 minute, or longer if possible.
  INTRAVENOUS DIMENHYDRINATE
- Dilute 50 mg of drug in 10 ml of sodium chloride injection. Administer at a rate of 25 mg/min.
  INTRAVENOUS DIPHENHYDRAMINE
- May be given undiluted. Administer at a in, or longer if possible.
  INTRAVENOUS PROMETHAZINE
- Dilute to at least 25 mg/ml, preferably to 2.5 to 5 mg/ml. Administer at a rate of 25 mg/min. Slightly yellow solutions may be safely used; discard highly discolored solutions.

Patient and family education

- Warn patients to avoid driving or operating hazardous equipment if drowsiness, blurred vision, or dizziness occurs. Notify physician if blurred vision develops.
- Review Patient Problems: Constipation (p. 187); Dry Mouth (p. 170); Orthostatic hypotension (p. 237); and Photosensitivity (p. 647) with the patient.
- Instruct patients to report the development of fever, sore throat, rash, unexplained bleeding or bruising, as these may be signs of rare but serious hematologic side effects.
- Take oral doses with meals or light snack to decrease gastric irritation.
- Swallow sustained release forms whole, without crushing or chewing. Scored tablets may be broken before swallowing. Capsules may be opened and content poured into soft food for ease in taking. Chew gum forms for 15 minutes or longer (see manufacturer's literature).
- For motion sickness, take doses 30 to 60 minutes before beginning travel.
- When traveling by car, have the affected person face forward, in the center of the front seat, if possible.
- Avoid the use of alcohol, as well as other central nervous system depressants (see text).
- Remind patients to keep all health providers informed of all medications being used, even over-the-counter preparations. Regular use of antihistamines may mask side effects developing from other drugs in use, especially ototoxic effects.
- Teach patients to read labels of over-the-counter preparations carefully. Patients using remedies for colds, hay fever, insomnia, and other problems may be taking unnecessary drugs, or taking the same drug in two or more combination products. Consult the pharmacist for assistance.
- Remind patients that antihistamines may also cause allergies. Encourage patients to report the development of any unexpected sign or symptom to the physician.
- Encourage patients with allergies to wear a medical identification tag or bracelet indicating the nature of the allergies.
- Pregnant women should not take any medication without the approval of the physician.
- Remind patients to keep these and all drugs out of the reach of children.

that involve the upper respiratory system, such as hay fever, or the skin, such as hives.

Hay fever is most successfully treated when the antihistamine therapy is begun while the pollen count is still low. The symptoms of sneezing, runny nose, and swollen eyes are reduced in more than 70% of patients. The swelling and itching (pruritus) of hives (urticaria) and related conditions are reduced.

Antihistamines do not prevent or treat colds effectively, although they are present in many over-the-counter cold remedies. Because most antihistamines have anticholinergic actions, they can "dry up" a runny nose and relieve the symptoms of a cold. Antihistamines are ineffective in treating asthma, probably because substances other than histamine are responsible for the prolonged bronchiole constriction characteristic of asthma. Since the drugs have a drying effect because they inhibit bronchial secretions, they can aggravate asthma.

Antihistamines exert no effect of their own on histamine receptors. Because of this, some allergic responses are not effectively treated with antihistamines. Anaphylaxis, the response to the systemic release of histamine, represents a true emergency for which an antihistamine is inadequate because it neither acts fast enough nor reverses the histamine reactions. Epinephrine acts rapidly, and its pharmacological actions reverse those of histamine.

Antihistamines to Control Vomiting (Antiemesis) (Table 24.2)

Antihistamines are principally effective in preventing the nausea of motion sickness, but the drug must be taken before the motion starts. *Cyclizine (Marzine), meclizine (Antivert, Bonine),* and *dimenhydrinate (Dramamine)* are the antihistamines most effective in preventing motion sickness. Dimenhydrinate causes considerable sedation.

Nausea and vomiting caused by factors acting on the chemoreceptor trigger zone are best treated with the antipsychotic drugs, the phenothiazines. These drugs are chemically related to the antihistamines but also block the dopamine receptor in the chemoreceptor trigger zone. *Promethazine (Phenergan, Remsed)* is the antihistamine considered most effective as an antiemetic. It is chemically related to the phenothiazines.

Antihistamines as Sedatives
(Tables 24.1 and 24.2)

Sedation is a common side effect of antihistamines, and some are used principally for this purpose. Many over-the-counter sleeping aids use an antihistamine as the active agent. The three antihistamines approved as sleep-aid ingredients are pyrilamine, doxylamine succinate, and diphenhydramine.

Hydroxyzine (Vistaril, Atarax)

Hydroxyzine is a prescription drug sometimes used as an antianxiety agent when it is desirable to have the antiemetic and antihistaminic properties, such as in treating motion sickness, in an allergic skin reaction, or in a preanesthetic medication. For the nursing process with drugs used for sedation, see Chapter 27.

SUMMARY

Histamine, a naturally occurring amine in the body, plays a role in allergic reactions, in stomach acid secretion, and probably as a neurotransmitter in the central nervous system.

Two classes of histamine receptors, the H-1 and H-2 receptors, have been identified. In humans, activation of the H-1 receptors by histamine results in vasodilation (blood vessels) and in constriction of bronchial smooth muscle, whereas activation of H-2 receptors (stomach) results in gastric acid secretion.

The term *antihistamine* refers to drugs that block the H-1 receptor. Antihistamines are effective for treatment of hay fever and hives. Selected antihistamines also produce anticholinergic, antiemetic, and sedative effects.

STUDY QUESTIONS

1. Describe the origin, location, and role of histamine.
2. What factors mediate histamine release?
3. What are five pharmacological actions of antihistamines?
4. What are the drug interactions and contraindications for the antihistamines?
5. Describe three clinical uses of the H-1 receptor antihistamines.
6. How does cimetidine differ from the H-1 receptor antihistamines?

SUGGESTED READINGS

Ballow, M.: Allergic rhinitis and conjunctivitis: help for the weeping nose and eyes, Postgrad. Med. **76**(1):197, 1984.

Brodoff, A.: Keeping current on allergy treatment, Patient Care **18**(3):137, 1984.

Brucker, M.C.: Management of common minor discomforts in pregnancy: managing upper respiratory infections in pregnancy, part 1, J. Nurse Midwife **32**(6):349, 1987.

Clark, M.: Allergy: new insights, Newsweek, p. 40, Aug. 23, 1982.

Council on Scientific Affairs: In vitro testing for allergy: Report II of the allergy panel, JAMA **258**(12):1639, 1987.

Dolan, B.: Rapid desensitization, Am. J. Nurs. **82**(10):1532, 1982.

Druce, H.M., and Kaliner, M.A.: Allergic rhinitis, JAMA **259**(2):260, 1988.

Levinson, A.I.: Urticaria and angioedema: current approach to common problems, Postgrad. Med. **76**(1):183, 1984.

Norman, P.S.: New developments in treating allergic rhinitis, Drug Therapy **14**(8):117, 1984.

Pepper, G.A.: OTCs vs. Rx for allergic rhinitis, Nurse Pract. **12**(6):58, 1987.

Schuller, D.E.: Acute urticaria in children, Postgrad. Med. **72**(2):179, 1982.

Serafin, W.E., and Austen, K.F.: Mediators of immediate hypersensitivity reactions, N. Engl. J. Med. **317**(1):30, 1987.

Sheffer, A.L.: Angioedema: better treatment is in sight, Consultant **21**(9):173, 1981.

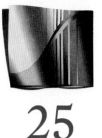

Bronchodilators and Other Drugs to Treat Asthma

25

Drugs that dilate the bronchioles (bronchodilators) and other drugs that are used to treat asthma are discussed in this chapter.

ASTHMA

Asthma is a disease of reversible obstruction of the bronchioles. An attack of asthma involves not only constriction of the bronchioles but also edema of the bronchial mucosa and excess secretion of mucus, all of which combine to restrict the caliber of the airway, as diagrammed in Figure 25.1. Asthma is classified as *extrinsic* if an allergic response is the primary stimulus for bronchial constriction. When no such response can be identified, asthma is classified as *intrinsic*.

Mechanisms in Extrinsic Asthma

Extrinsic asthma involves an immunological mechanism. The mast cells play a major role in precipitating the attack. In the lung, mast cells are primarily located in the epithelial layer and exposed to the surface. IgE antibodies bind to mast cells, and when an antigen appears it becomes bound to the IgE. The formation of the antigen-antibody complex causes the mast cells to degranulate, releasing several substances, including histamine and leukotrienes C and D.

The leukotrienes are potent bronchoconstrictors, chemically related to the prostaglandins. Histamine, also a bronchoconstrictor, additionally induces vasodilation and increased capillary permeability, which results in the mucosal edema that is characteristic of asthma.

Drug therapy for extrinsic asthma includes one or more bronchodilator drugs in addition to cromolyn sodium, which prevents the mast cells from degranulating so that an asthma attack does not start. In severe cases, glucocorticoids may be used to reverse the severe inflammation of the bronchioles. Antihistamines are sometimes administered to prevent mild episodes. Because antihistamines have a drying effect that turns the excess mucus into hard plugs, they are contraindicated for patients with severe asthma.

Adrenergic Mechanisms in Asthma

In recent years much has been learned about the molecular pharmacology of the bronchial smooth muscle and the mast cell. This knowledge has led to an understanding of some of the mechanisms involved in reversible airway obstruction. As diagrammed in Figure 25.2, the beta adrenergic system plays a major role in effecting relaxation of bronchial smooth muscle and inhibiting degranulation of the mast cells. Activation of the beta-2 receptor stimulates an enzyme, adenylate cyclase, to synthesize more cyclic adenosine 3′,5′-monophosphate (cyclic AMP), which is a second messenger for the beta-2 receptor (Chapter 10). Cyclic AMP activates intracellular pathways that result in (1) relaxation of smooth muscle, (2) inhibition of mast cell degranulation, and (3) stimulation of the ciliary apparatus to remove secretions more effectively. This means that drugs that increase cyclic AMP are bronchodilators as well as inhibitors of mast cell degranulation and promoters of secretion flow in the bronchioles. Drugs that increase cyclic AMP include the beta adrenergic agonists, which stimulate the beta-2 receptor, and the phosphodiesterase inhibitors, which inhibit the breakdown of cyclic AMP. The xanthine compounds are used clinically as bronchodilators because they inhibit phosphodiesterase. Prostaglandins E_1 and E_2 also stimulate adenylate cyclase, but at present there are no drugs available clinically that mimic these prostaglandins.

Cholinergic Mechanisms Controlling Bronchioles

The bronchioles have little, if any, direct innervation by the sympathetic nervous system. However, there is indirect involvement, since sympathetic nerve terminals in pulmonary blood vessels release norepinephrine, which can act on the beta-2 receptors in the bronchioles. Norepinephrine is not a potent stimulant of beta-2 receptors, however. The beta-2 receptors are activated by epinephrine released from the adrenal medulla in response to stress. Acetylcholine, the neurotransmitter of the parasympathetic nervous system, acts on the muscarinic receptors to cause bronchoconstriction through the intracellular second messenger, cyclic 3',5'-guanyl monophosphate (cyclic GMP). Mast cell degranulation is also promoted by agents that stimulate the formation of cyclic GMP. Intrinsic asthma is believed to arise from direct stimulation of the enzyme guanyl cyclase, which synthesizes cyclic GMP. Irritants such as noxious gases can stimulate guanyl cyclase. Asthmatic individuals respond to low doses of inhaled methacholine, a cholinomimetic drug, with bronchospasm, whereas high doses are needed to induce bronchospasm in the nonasthmatic individual. Intrinsic asthma may therefore primarily involve a parasympathetic response, mediated by cyclic GMP, to inhaled bronchial irritants. Blocking the muscarinic receptor with atropine or scopolamine causes bronchodilation, but muscarinic antagonists do not at present play a major role in the treatment of asthma.

Prostaglandin F_{2a} is another potent bronchoconstrictor that acts by stimulating the synthesis of cyclic GMP. However, the factors causing the release of prostaglandin F_{2a} are not well understood, and it is not clear whether prostaglandin F_{2a} plays a major role in asthma.

Other Pulmonary Diseases with Airflow Obstruction

Obstruction of airflow is a component of many pulmonary diseases. Chronic obstructive pulmonary disease (COPD) describes conditions in which the common feature is limitation of the airflow. In long-standing pulmonary disease, irreversible changes take place so that the elastic smooth muscle tissue is replaced with inelastic scar tissue. This can occur in the bronchioles in chronic bronchitis or in the alveoli in emphysema. These irreversible changes cannot be modified with drugs. However, since the early stages of chronic bronchitis and emphysema often involve reversible bronchospasm, bronchodilators can provide some relief.

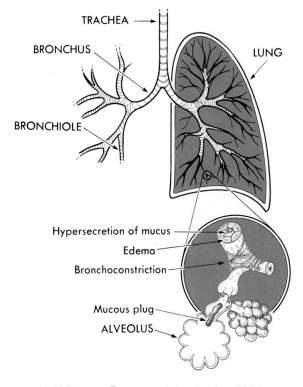

FIGURE 25.1   Factors restricting the airway. Major factors include hypersecretion of mucus, mucosal edema, and bronchoconstriction. Mucous plugs may form in the alveoli.

BRONCHODILATORS

Beta Adrenergic Agonists

Mechanism of action. The mechanism by which the beta adrenergic agonists increase cyclic AMP to cause dilation of the bronchioles has been discussed. The beta receptors of the bronchial smooth muscle are beta-2 receptors, whereas cardiac beta receptors are beta-1 receptors. The goal has been to develop drugs that stimulate only beta-2 receptors because stimulation of the heart is not desirable and can limit the use of the drug. In theory, stimulation of the alpha receptors causes vasoconstriction of the blood vessels around the bronchioles, limiting the edema, a desirable action. However, systemic constriction of alpha receptors can cause an undesirable increase in blood pressure. Also, there is some evidence that alpha receptors constrict bronchiolar smooth muscle, at least in disease states. Table 25.1 summarizes the alpha, beta-1, and beta-2 activities of the adrenergic drugs used as bronchodilators.

Administration and fate. Also important to the

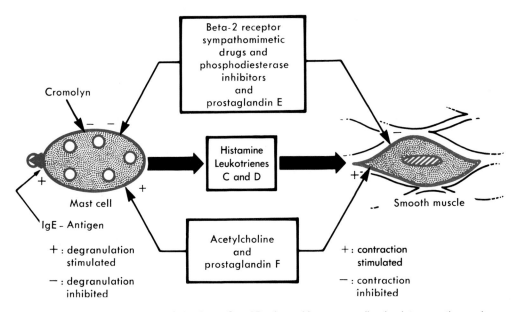

FIGURE 25.2   Histamine and leukotrienes C and D released from mast cells stimulate smooth muscle contraction to produce bronchoconstriction. Mast cell degranulation and smooth muscle contraction are both stimulated by acetylcholine and prostaglandin F. Smooth muscle relaxation and inhibition of mast cell degranulation are both promoted by beta-2 receptor agonists, phosphodiesterase inhibitors, and prostaglandin E.

selection of a bronchodilator is the route of administration and the onset and duration of action. Table 25.2 summarizes these points. Inhalation is a particularly effective route of administration for the bronchodilators. Not only are epinephrine, isoproterenol, and isoetharine degraded if swallowed, but inhalation places the drug near the site of action. When inhalation is the route, alpha agonist activity is desirable because it both reduces congestion and limits systemic absorption of the drug. In fact, cyclopentamine or phenylephrine, which stimulate alpha but not beta receptors, are included in some inhalation preparations of isoproterenol to relieve congestion and to slow systemic absorption, thereby limiting cardiac effects while increasing the duration of action of the beta agonist.

Many of the bronchodilators are administered by inhalation. This requires that the drug be in a solution that is contained in a nebulizer or pressurized cartridge (aerosol), which will disperse the drug solution in tiny drops to be taken into the lungs by deep inhalation. The metered aerosols are particularly easy to use, and deliver a measured dose with each push of the cartridge. The disadvantage is that the inert carrier substances may irritate the bronchioles and cause bronchospasm. Also, the patient must be well instructed in inha-

lation therapy to ensure that the drug is inhaled, and that there is no gagging and swallowing of the drug.

In a severe attack, the patient may not be able to inhale the drug. A subcutaneous injection of epinephrine or terbutaline would then be appropriate. An orally or subcutaneously administered bronchodilator would also be preferred if there is a great deal of mucosal edema and bronchoconstriction, which would limit the access of the inhaled drug.

Nonselective Beta Adrenergic Bronchodilators (Table 25.3)

The older beta adrenergic bronchodilators—ephedrine, epinephrine, and isoproterenol—are not selective for the beta-2 adrenergic receptor. They have a range of side effects resulting from their nonselective action.

Epinephrine (Asmolin, Medihaler-Epi, Adrenalin and others)

Epinephrine can be administered subcutaneously for the relief of an acute asthmatic attack. The drug will cause not only bronchodilation but also vasoconstriction to relieve bronchial edema. Given subcutaneously, an aqueous suspension of epinephrine (Sus-Phrine) lasts 8 hours; the hydro-

Table 25.1 Sympathomimetic Bronchodilators' Adrenergic Receptor Specificity*

Drug	Alpha effects	Beta-1 effects	Beta-2 effects
Albuterol	0	0	+
Bitolterol	0	0	+
Cyclopentamine	+	0	0
Ephedrine	+	+	+
Epinephrine	+	+	+
Ethylnorepinephrine	0	0	+
Fenoterol	0	0	+
Isoetherine	0	0	+
Isoproterenol	0	+	+
Metaproterenol	0	(±)	+
Phenylephrine	+	0	0
Pirbuterol	0	0	+
Terbutaline	0	0	+

ALPHA EFFECTS
Vasoconstriction
1. Systemic: increased blood pressure.
2. Inhaled: decreased bronchial congestion, increased duration of action for co-administered beta-2 drug.

BETA-1 EFFECTS
1. Stimulation of heart, increasing rate, force of contraction, and rate of repolarization. Overstimulation causes palpitations, arrhythmias.
2. Increased lipolysis (breakdown of fat).
3. Relaxation of gastrointestinal tract.

BETA-2 EFFECTS
1. Bronchiole dilation.
2. Stimulation of skeletal muscle to cause a tremulous or shaky feeling.
3. Vasodilation (mainly in blood vessels supplying muscle).
4. Glycogenolysis (breakdown of stored glucose).

CENTRAL NERVOUS SYSTEM EFFECTS
Stimulation, causing nervousness, anxiety, insomnia, irritability, dizziness, sweating.

*0, No stimulation; +, stimulation; (±), modest stimulation.

chloride salt lasts only 3 hours. Epinephrine is also available in metered-dose inhalers as an aerosol or in solution for use in a nebulizer.

The most common side effects of epinephrine are an increased heart rate, muscle tremors, and stimulation of the central nervous system to produce anxiety, nervousness, or excitability. Large doses can produce an acute hypertensive episode and cardiac arrhythmias.

Ephedrine (Ephed II)

Ephedrine has a spectrum of action similar to that of epinephrine, but is effective orally. Ephedrine is a weaker bronchodilator than epinephrine and of no use for an acute asthma attack. Its major use is a prophylactic one for patients with mild to moderate asthma. Several formulations combine ephedrine with theophylline and a sedative in a single pill.

The major action of ephedrine is the release of stored norepinephrine from sympathetic neurons, an indirect sympathomimetic effect that explains the weak bronchodilator action. The major metabolite is phenylpropanolamine, an active alpha adrenergic drug by itself that is frequently used as a decongestant.

The most common side effect of ephedrine is stimulation of the central nervous system manifested as nervousness, excitability, and insomnia. The development of orally active, beta-2 selective bronchodilators is making its use obsolete.

Ethylnorepinephrine (Bronkephrine)

Ethylnorepinephrine acts on both beta-1 and beta-2 adrenergic receptors. It also exerts some vasoconstrictive activity that helps to reduce bronchial congestion. Ethylnorepinephrine is available only for subcutaneous or intramuscular administration.

Isoproterenol (Isuprel Hydrochloride, Vapo-Iso, Medihaler-Iso, Norisodrine Sulfate)

Isoproterenol was the first widely used adrenergic drug with selectivity for beta rather than receptors. It is not selective for beta-2 receptors and therefore stimulates the heart. Isoproterenol is primarily given by inhalation and is effective for up to 2 hours in relieving bronchoconstriction. If swallowed, it is degraded in the gut wall. The drug is available as a sublingual tablet, but absorption is so erratic that this route is not often used.

Some side effects are related to stimulation of the heart: palpitation, fast heart rate, and arrhyth-

Table 25.2   Adrenergic Bronchodilators: Onset and Duration of Action

Generic name	Trade name	Administration	Onset (min)	Duration (hr)
Albuterol	Proventil	Inhalation Oral	30	4 to 6
Bitolterol	Tornalate	Inhalation	3	5 to 8
Ephedrine	Ventolin	Oral	15	2 to 4
Epinephrine hydrochloride		Subcutaneous Inhalation	5 2	1 to 3 2 to 3
Epinephrine suspension	Sus-Phrine	Subcutaneous	15	Up to 8
Ethylnorepinephrine	Bronkephrine	Subcutaneous	10	1 to 2
Isoetharine	Bronkometer Bronkosol Dilabron	Inhalation	2	1
Isoetharine and phenylephrine	Bronkosol-2	Inhalation	2	2
Isoproterenol	Isuprel Vapo-Iso	Inhalation	2	½ to 2
Isoproterenol and cyclopentamine	Aerolone Compound Aludrine	Inhalation	2	3½
Isoproterenol and phenylephrine	Nebu-Prel	Inhalation	2	3½
Metaproterenol	Alupent Metaprel	Inhalation Oral	2 15	2 to 4 3 to 4
Pirbuterol	Maxair	Inhalation	5	5
Terbutaline	Bricanyl Brethine	Oral Subcutaneous	10 15	4 to 7 2 to 4

mias. Isoproterenol can also cause tremors, headache, nervousness, and hypotension. Excessive inhalation can cause bronchial constriction for which the drug no longer has a bronchodilator effect. Drug effectiveness returns when the drug is discontinued for a few days.

Selective Beta Adrenergic Bronchodilators
(Table 25.3)

The newer beta adrenergic bronchodilators are relatively selective for the beta-2 receptor, the adrenergic receptor mediating bronchodilation. Because of this selective action, these drugs are less likely to cause unwanted cardiac effects or to cause a breakdown of liver glycogen to glucose. Patients with hypertension, cardiac disease, or diabetes can better tolerate the selective beta adrenergic bronchodilators. Occasionally, nervousness or restlessness are experienced as side effects.

Many of the new bronchodilators are available in metered aerosol form so that one inhalation delivers a given amount of a drug. These include bitolterol, fenoterol, isoetharine, metaproterenol, pirbuterol, and terbutaline. If more than one inhalation is administered, it is usually preferable to wait a minute or so between inhalations. The metered-dose inhaler has emerged as the standard for aerosol therapy. One advantage is that since only about 10% of the delivered drug is actually deposited in the lung, the likelihood of overdosing is small. Albuterol, fenoterol, metaproterenol, and terbutaline are available in oral forms. While oral administra-

Table 25.3 Bronchodilators and Other Drugs to Treat Asthma—cont'd

Generic name	Trade name	Administration/dosage	Comments
BETA RECEPTOR AGONISTS—cont'd			
Metaproterenol ulfate	Alupent* Metaprel*	ORAL: *Adults*—10 mg 3 or 4 times daily initially, increased to 20 mg 3 or 4 times daily over 2 to 4 wk. FDA Pregnancy Category C. *Children*—6 to 9 yr, 10 mg 3 or 4 times daily; over 9 yr or over 60 lb, 20 mg 3 or 4 times daily.	Relatively selective for beta-2 (bronchial) receptors. More effective orally than ephedrine. Shakiness (a stimulation of skeletal muscle) is the most frequent side effect.
		INHALATION (metered aerosol): *Adults and children over 12 yr only:* 2 to 3 inhalations every 3 to 4 hr not to exceed 12 inhalations daily.	Longer acting than isoproterenol. Patients are less likely to develop tolerance to metaproterenol than to isoproterenol.
Pirbuterol	Maxair*	INHALATION: *Adults*—1 or 2 inhalations every 6 hr as needed. FDA Pregnancy Category C.	A new beta-2 selective bronchodilator.
Terbutaline sulfate	Brethine* Bricanyl*	SUBCUTANEOUS: *Adults*—0.25 mg repeated in 15 to 30 min if necessary, with no more than 0.5 mg administered in any 4 hr period. FDA Pregnancy Category B. *Children*—0.01 mg/kg body weight to a maximum of 0.25 mg.	Subcutaneous route used for relief of an acute asthma attack.
		ORAL: *Adults*—initially 2.5 mg every 8 hr, increased to 5 mg every 8 hr 3 times daily over 2 to 4 wk. Dose may be lowered to 2.5 mg if side effects are too disturbing. *Children 12 yr and younger*—1.25 to 2.5 mg 3 times daily during waking hours.	Shakiness (a stimulation of skeletal muscle) is the most frequent side effect.
	Brethaire*	INHALATION (metered aerosol): *Adults and children over 12 yr*—2 inhalations 1 min apart, every 4 to 6 hr.	Side effects are mild. Headache, nausea, and GI upset are the most common.
XANTHINES			
Aminophylline (theophylline ethylenediamine)	Sold mainly under generic name	For acute asthma attack: INTRAVENOUS: Solutions should be diluted to 25 mg/ml and injected no more rapidly than 25 mg/min to avoid circulatory collapse. Loading dose, 5.6 mg/kg over 30 min. Maintenance dose, no more than 0.9 mg/kg/hr by continuous infusion. Dose is determined by age, cardiac and liver status, and smoking history. RECTAL: *Adults*—250 to 500 mg 1 to 3 times daily. FDA Pregnancy Category C. *Children*—5 mg/kg not more often than every 6 hr. ORAL: *Adults*—500 mg for an acute attack. Maintenance dose, 200 to 250 mg every 6 to 8 hr. *Children*—7.5 mg/kg for an acute attack. Maintenance dose, 5 mg/kg every 6 hr.	85% theophylline, so 116 mg of aminophylline is equivalent to 100 mg theophylline. Watch for nausea, wakefulness, restlessness, and irritability as early symptoms of toxicity. Serious toxic effects of intravenous administration include delirium, convulsions, hyperthermia, and circulatory collapse.

*Available in Canada and United States.

Continued.

Table 25.3   Bronchodilators and Other Drugs to Treat Asthma—cont'd

Generic name	Trade name	Administration/dosage	Comments
XANTHINES—cont'd			
Dyphylline	Dilor* Dyflex* Lufyllin* Neothylline*	ORAL: *Adults*—200 to 800 mg every 6 hr. FDA Pregnancy Category C. *Children*—2 to 3 mg/lb/24 hr given in divided doses every 6 hr. Maximum dose, 15 mg/kg every 6 hr. INTRAMUSCULAR: *Adults*—250 to 500 mg.	Not a theophylline salt. Has a short half-life (2½ hr) and is not excreted in the urine without being metabolized.
Oxtriphylline (choline theophyllinate)	Protophylline† Choldeyl* Novotriphyl†	ORAL: *Adults*—200 mg every 6 hr. FDA Pregnancy Category C. *Children 2 to 12 yr*—100 mg/60 lb every 6 hr.	64% theophylline, so 156 mg is equivalent to 100 mg theophylline.
Theophylline	Many names, elixirs, syrups, tablets, capsules, timed-release preparation, suppositories	ORAL: *Adults, children*—Initial dose, 3 to 5 mg/kg every 6 hr. For maintenance: *Adults*—100 to 200 mg every 6 hr. FDA Pregnancy Category C. *Children*—50 to 100 mg every 6 hr. RECTAL: *Adults*—250 to 500 mg every 8 to 12 hr. *Children*—10 to 12 mg/kg/24 hr. Administered no more frequently than every 6 hr.	Headache, dizziness, nervousness, nausea, vomiting, and epigastric pain are the most common side effects of oral administration. Therapeutic levels are 10 to 20 mg/ml serum.
Theophylline sodium glycinate	Synophylate*	ORAL: *Adults*—330 to 660 mg every 6 to 8 hr after meals. *Children*—over 12 yr, 220 to 300 mg; 6 to 12 yr, 165 to 220 mg; 3 to 6 yr, 110 to 165 mg; 1 to 3 yr, 55 to 110 mg every 6 to 8 hr after meals.	49% theophylline, so 200 mg is equivalent to 100 mg theophylline.

*Available in Canada and United States.
†Available in Canada only.

tion is convenient, especially for children, the patient is exposed to more side effects with oral administration than with aerosol administration.

Albuterol (Proventil, Ventolin)

Albuterol is available in forms for oral and inhalation administration for treatment of acute asthma or for prophylaxis in chronic asthma. The inhalation forms include a metered aerosol and a solution. The solution is administered by nebulizer or intermittent positive pressure breathing (IPPB). The onset of action is 5 to 15 minutes and the duration of action 3 to 6 hours. For oral administration, albuterol is available as a syrup, tablets, or extended-release tablets. The onset of action is 15 to 30 minutes and the duration of action is 8 hours.

In Canada, an injectable form is also available with a duration of action of 12 hours. Albuterol is metabolized by the liver to an inactive form and excreted in the urine.

Bitolterol (Tornalate)

Bitolterol is available in metered aerosol form for treatment of acute asthma or for prophylaxis in chronic asthma. The onset of action is 3 to 4 minutes and the duration of action is 5 to 8 hours. Bitolterol is conjugated and excreted in the urine.

Fenoterol (Berotec)

Fenoterol is available in metered aerosol form, solution, and as tablets for the treatment of acute asthma or for prophylaxis in chronic asthma. While

THE NURSING PROCESS

BRONCHODILATORS

Assessment

Patients requiring bronchodilator therapy are those with asthma or other respiratory diseases that have bronchospasm as a component, such as some cases of bronchitis and emphysema. Although a general assessment of the patient should be done, the focus is often on the respiratory system. The nurse should check the vital signs, the amount and characteristics of secretions, and the level of fatigue; auscultate breathing sounds; determine the arterial blood gas levels, the vital capacity, subjective complaints, and the ability to perform activities of daily living and tolerance for activity; and obtain relevant history such as smoking, exposure to irritants, infection, and stress. In addition, the nurse should monitor the level of consciousness and send the sputum to the laboratory for culture and drug sensitivity if ordered.

Nursing diagnoses

Anxiety related to difficulty breathing, air hunger, tachycardia, and drug side effects

Potential complication: hypertension

Management

The initial use of these drugs is to provide symptomatic relief of dyspnea (shortness of breath) and inadequate oxygenation. Coupled with drug therapy are efforts to stabilize the patient for discharge. The vital signs are monitored, and an acute care unit may be appropriate for the patient in acute respiratory distress. The nurse should monitor the fluid intake and output, the level of consciousness, the blood gas levels, vital capacity, and the treatment of any infectious process. An infusion control device should be used for intravenous drugs. Serum xanthine levels are monitored and the blood glucose concentration is measured when patients receive xanthine therapy. In addition to drug therapy, the plan of care should be individualized to include instruction in additional aspects of maintenance such as breathing exercises, irritants and inhalants to be avoided, and how to use supplies at home, including oxygen, nebulizers, and intermittent positive pressure breathing machines. The patient may be referred to appropriate agencies for respiratory therapy, social services, or the local visiting nurse association. Finally, the nurse should work with the physician and the patient to determine the best combination of drugs for management of the respiratory problem in the home setting.

Evaluation

These drugs are successful if the patient is both subjectively and objectively improved. The vital capacity should be increased, arterial blood gas levels should be closer to normal values, the respiratory rate should be decreased, and the patient should appear to be in less respiratory distress. Subjectively, the patient should be able to report easier breathing, less shortness of breath, less fatigue, and better tolerance for activities of daily living. Before discharge for home management, the patient should be able to explain which drugs are to be taken and how to take them correctly, to explain what situations would require notification of the physician either because of exacerbation of the disease process or because of effects resulting from drug therapy, and to demonstrate how to perform any other measures such as exercises for respiratory management and the correct use of oxygen. The patient should be able to demonstrate correct use of any equipment such as intermittent positive pressure breathing machines or drug administration devices such as an inhaler or nebulizer. The patient should be able to explain which specific respiratory irritants should be avoided.

Table 25.4   Other Drugs to Treat Asthma

Generic name	Trade name	Administration/dosage	Comments
Beclomethasone dipropionate	Beclovent* Becotide† Vanceril*	INHALATION (metered dose inhaler): each dose is 50 μg. *Adults*—2 inhalations 3 to 4 times daily. *Children 6 to 12 yr*—1 to 2 inhalations 3 to 4 times daily.	An inhaled glucocorticoid. Patients transferring from oral glucocorticoids to beclomethasone must be carefully monitored because adrenal function is impaired and may require months to begin functioning adequately.
Cromolyn sodium	Intal* Fivent†	INHALATION: *Adults and children over 5 yr*—20 mg capsule inhaled 4 times daily. (Spinhaler); 2 inhalations 4 times daily (inhalation aerosol). FDA Pregnancy Category B.	Prophylactic drug to inhibit mast cell degranulation. Cough or bronchospasm is occasionally experienced after inhaling the dry powder.
Dexamethasone sodium	Decadron Respihaler*	INHALATION (metered dose inhaler): each dose is 84 μg. *Adults*—3 inhalations 3 or 4 times per day. *Children*—2 inhalations 3 or 4 times per day.	An inhaled glucocorticoid. See warnings for beclomethasone
Flunisolide	AeroBid*	INHALATION (metered dose inhaler): each dose is 250 μg. *Adults and children over 6 yr*—2 inhalations 2 times per day initially. Patients over 15 years may increase dose to 4 inhalations twice daily if necessary.	An inhaled glucocorticoid. See warnings for beclomethasone
Ipratropium	Atrovent*	INHALATION (metered dose inhaler): each dose is 18 μg. *Adults*—1 or 2 inhalations 3 or 4 times daily. FDA Pregnancy Category B.	A new anticholinergic bronchodilator.
Triamcinolone	Azmacort*	INHALATION (metered dose inhaler): each dose is 100 μg. *Adults*—2 sprays 3 or 4 times daily, up to 12 to 16 sprays daily. *Children 6 to 12 yr*—1 or 2 sprays 3 or 4 times daily, up to 12 sprays daily for severe cases.	An inhaled glucocorticoid. See warnings for beclomethasone

*Available in Canada and United States.
†Available in Canada only.

available in Canada, fenoterol is not currently available in the United States.

Isoetharine (Bronkometer, Bronkosol, others)

Isoetharine is available in metered aerosol form and as a solution for the treatment of acute asthma or for prophylaxis in chronic asthma. The onset of action is 1 to 6 minutes and the duration of action is 1 to 4 hours. Isoetharine is metabolized by the liver and excreted in the urine.

Metaproterenol (Alupent, Metaprel)

Metaproterenol is available as a metered aerosol and as a solution for inhalation administration, and as a syrup and tablet for oral administration. Metaproterenol is used to treat acute asthma or as prophylaxis in chronic asthma. The aerosol form has an onset of action of 1 minute and a duration of action of 1 to 5 hours. The solution, administered by hand-bulb nebulizer or intermittent positive pressure breathing (IPPB), has a slower onset of action, 5 to 30 minutes, and a duration of action of 2 to 6 hours. The oral forms are effective in 15 to 30 minutes, for up to 4 hours. Metaproterenol is metabolized by the liver and excreted in the urine.

Pirbuterol (Maxair)

Pirbuterol is available as a metered aerosol for the treatment of acute asthma or for prophylaxis in chronic asthma. The onset of action is 5 minutes and the duration of action is 5 hours. Pirbuterol is conjugated and excreted in the urine.

Terbutaline (Bricanyl, Brethine)

Terbutaline is available in metered aerosol form, in tablets, and as an injection for the treatment of acute asthma or for prophylaxis in chronic asthma. With inhalation, terbutaline is effective in 5 to 30 minutes and has a duration of action of 3 to 6 hours. With oral administration, the onset of action is 1 to 2 hours and the duration of action 4 to 8 hours. With an injection, the onset of action is within 15 minutes and the duration of action 1.5 to 4 hours. Terbutaline is metabolized by the liver and excreted in the urine.

Xanthines
Theophylline
Mechanisms of action. Theophylline is the prototype of the xanthines used to treat asthma. Like the beta adrenergic agonists, theophylline is thought to act by increasing cellular cyclic AMP concentrations, an action that relaxes bronchial smooth muscle and inhibits mast cell degranulation. Theophylline and the other xanthines accomplish this by inhibiting the degradation of cyclic AMP by the enzyme phosphodiesterase. This action complements that of the beta agonists, and the two kinds of agents may both be included in therapy when the effect of either drug alone is insufficient to control bronchospasm.

Administration and fate. Theophylline is an effective bronchodilator that can be given intravenously (as aminophylline) for the control of acute bronchospasm in status asthmaticus; or it can be given orally to control the bronchospasm of mild, moderate, or severe asthma. Theophylline is not highly water soluble, and there are many formulations to improve the solubility. Studies have shown that theophylline tablets are well absorbed, with more than 96% of the drug appearing in the plasma within 2 hours. Aminophylline, the most common soluble form of theophylline, is the only form that can be administered intravenously.

Several soluble salts of theophylline are available, and dosage is determined by the theophylline content. In addition, the drug is available in slow-release preparations, a fast-release preparation, alcoholic or aqueous solutions, and suppositories. Only the suppository preparation is so erratically absorbed as to be unreliable, however; rectal solutions are well absorbed. Theophylline is combined with ephedrine and a sedative in several combination products for treating asthma. Most clinicians prefer to individualize doses of each ingredient to minimize side effects while maximizing therapeutic effects and therefore do not favor combination drugs. Theophylline is not effective when administered by inhalation. Intramuscular injections of theophylline are not used because they are painful.

Variability of plasma levels. Theophylline is metabolized by the liver into inactive compounds that are excreted in the urine. There is a wide variability among individuals as to the plasma half-life of theophylline. In normal, nonsmoking adults, the plasma half-life is about 6 hours, but this can vary from 3 to 12 hours. In smokers and children, the plasma half-life is shorter, whereas in the elderly, premature infants, and patients with liver disease or congestive heart failure with pulmonary edema, the plasma half-life is prolonged.

Side and toxic effects. The most common side effects of theophylline after oral administration are nausea and epigastric pain. Headache, dizziness, and nervousness are also common. The effectiveness of theophylline is determined by its plasma concentrations, with the therapeutic range being 10 to 20 µg/ml. Agitation, exaggerated reflexes, and mild muscle tremors (fasciculations) are often seen when plasma levels are 20 to 30 µg/ml. Seizures and cardiac arrhythmias may be seen when plasma levels exceed 30 µg/ml but have been occasionally reported with plasma concentrations between 20 and 30 µg/ml.

Other actions of theophylline seen in the therapeutic dose range are dilation of blood vessels and a mild diuresis due to the increased renal blood flow and glomerular filtration. Stomach acid secretion is increased, and this may be a problem for a patient with an ulcer. Another effect is stimulation of the medullary centers of respiration, which is beneficial if the asthmatic patient is hypoxic. Theophylline is useful for treating Cheyne-Stokes respiration, a condition in which the medullary sensitivity to hypoxia is decreased. Theophylline is administered to stimulate respiration in newborns who are not breathing well.

Dyphylline

Dyphylline (Airet, Dilor, Lufyllin, Neothylline) is related to theophylline but is less potent and shorter acting. Dyphylline has a half-life of 2½ hours and is eliminated largely unchanged in the urine.

Other Drugs

Cromolyn sodium (Table 25.4)

Cromolyn sodium (Intal) is a prophylactic drug that acts by inhibiting mast cell degranulation and the release of bronchospastic agents caused by immunological (antigen IgE) or nonimmunological (exercise, hyperventilation) stimulation. Cromolyn is of no value in treating an ongoing asthma attack or in preventing asthma attacks brought on by vagal reflexes rather than by mast cell degranulation. By itself, cromolyn does not have bronchodilator or antiinflammatory activity.

Cromolyn can be administered by inhalation using a "Spinhaler," a hand-held and hand-operated device that when activated punctures a capsule, releasing a dry powder. This powder is dispersed by the air current from a small rotor blade and enters the lungs during deep inhalation.

Cromolyn is now available as a metered inhalation aerosol, which will probably replace the "Spinhaler." In addition, cromolyn is now formulated for nasal administration (Nasalcrom, Rynacrom) as prophylaxis for allergic rhinitis, and for ophthalmic administration (Opticrom, Vistacrom) for allergic conjunctivitis.

Given orally or parenterally, cromolyn is so rapidly excreted in the urine that effective drug levels cannot be maintained. Because of this rapid clearance, cromolyn is practically nontoxic. The major side effect that can limit use is bronchospasm caused by the dry powder in sensitive individuals. Some individuals become allergic to cromolyn.

Cromolyn is usually added to bronchodilator therapy to avoid the use of glucocorticoids or to allow the gradual reduction in dose of glucocorticoids. No tolerance develops to the drug. Cromolyn is reported to be more effective in treating children than in treating adults for asthma.

Glucocorticoids (corticosteroids)

Glucocorticoids are used to treat the asthmatic patient who has severe symptoms that are not controlled by bronchodilator therapy. Initially, very high doses (up to 1 Gm of methylprednisolone) of

a glucocorticoid may be administered for as long as 5 days to bring a severe asthma attack under control when intravenous aminophylline and sympathomimetics have proved inadequate. As discussed in Chapter 51, high doses of glucocorticoids can be tolerated for a short period of time, but on a long-term basis they cause many severe side effects. Few patients with asthma will require glucocorticoids even after an acute attack. The mechanisms by which these drugs specifically act to alleviate asthma are not known, but they do potentiate the action of the bronchodilators. To minimize the long-term toxic effects of glucocorticoids, they are administered in small doses (20 mg) every other day. This schedule minimizes suppression of adrenal function and also avoids excessive use, which could cause Cushing's syndrome (characteristic of excessive glucocorticoid administration; Chapter 51).

Aerosol glucocorticoids

Aerosol glucocorticoids have been developed that can be inhaled daily without producing adrenal suppression or Cushing's syndrome. As with other aerosol medications, the patient must be carefully instructed in the administration of the drug. The aerosol cannot be used during an episode of acute bronchospasm because the powder will cause further irritation and the bronchospasm will prevent adequate inhalation. An oral glucocorticoid is indicated instead. Patients using these aerosols should gargle after use to prevent the drug trapped in the throat from being swallowed and absorbed systemically; gargling should also be done to avoid a candidal infection (a type of fungal infection) in the mouth or throat.

Glucocorticoids available as aerosols include beclomethasone, dexamethasone, flunisolide, and triamcinolone.

Ipratropium (Atrovent)

Ipratropium bromide is the first anticholinergic drug available for the treatment of asthma and conditions such as chronic bronchitis and emphysema in which bronchoconstriction is present. It opens narrowed breathing passages by blocking vagal nerve impulses that tighten the muscles in the walls of the bronchial tubes. Mucus secretion is also reduced. Ipratropium is not appropriate for treating acute asthma. The onset of action is 5 to 15 minutes and the duration of action is 3 to 6 hours. The drug is primarily excreted unchanged in the feces. It has negligible cardiovascular effects. Atropine-like side effects are rare with inhalation administration.

PATIENT CARE IMPLICATIONS

General guidelines for bronchodilator therapy

Drug administration

- Review the side effects discussed in the text and the information on tables 25.1 to 25.3.
- Monitor the pulse, blood pressure, and respiratory rate. Auscultate lung sounds. The frequency of monitoring will vary with the drug, dose, and route of administration, as well as patient condition. During intravenous administration, monitor vital signs every 5 to 15 minutes until stable. With subcutaneous administration, monitor every 15 minutes. With inhalation administration, monitor every 5 to 15 minutes.
- Monitor all patients requiring bronchodilators carefully, but especially the elderly, and patients with cardiovascular or hypertensive disease, or diabetes mellitus.
- Monitor acutely ill patients in the intensive care setting. Monitor electrocardiogram.
- Anxiety, insomnia, fear, and other emotional responses may aggravate bronchospasm and air hunger. Maintain a calm but efficient attitude in caring for patients. Do not leave the patient unattended for long periods. Keep the call bell within easy reach.
- With subcutaneous or IM injection, aspirate before administering dose to avoid inadvertent intravenous administration.
- For continuous IV infusion, use an infusion control device, and usually, microdrip tubing. Monitor intake and output, as well as vital signs.
- Monitor the blood glucose level of diabetic patients carefully, as these drugs may produce hyperglycemia.

Patient and family education

- Review the common side effects of the prescribed drug(s). Wait until the patient is out of acute respiratory distress.
- If tachycardia is a problem, suggest that the patient limit caffeine intake.
- Tell the patient with respiratory problems to stop smoking.
- Before discharge, check that the patient can describe or demonstrate the correct way to take ordered medications: frequency, route of administration, use of devices, and under what circumstances to return to the physician or emergency room if the drugs are not effective. Caution patients to use these drugs only as prescribed, and not to increase dose size or frequency unless directed to do so by the physician. It is not unusual for patients who find relief with metered dose inhalers to begin using them more often than prescribed, or to conclude that if one puff is good, two are better, then three or more. These drugs soon become ineffective, or the patient may suffer significant side effects.
- Warn diabetic patients to monitor blood glucose levels carefully, especially when changing doses of bronchodilator.
- Let sublingual tablets dissolve under the tongue. Do not swallow saliva until the tablet is completely dissolved.
- Take oral doses with meals or snack to lessen gastric irritation.
- Make certain the patient can use the metered dose inhaler correctly when using it for the first time. Review manufacturer's instruction sheet with the patient. Have the patient assemble the inhaler and shake the canister. Exhale deeply, then put the mouthpiece into the mouth with the opening directed to the back of the throat. Grasp the mouthpiece with the teeth and lips. Inhale deeply while depressing the aerosol container or activating the spray mechanism. Hold the breath as long as possible before exhaling. Wait several minutes before taking a second dose (if prescribed). For children, it may be necessary to hold the nose shut. When finished, wash off and dry the mouthpiece.
- There are special devices made to help children use inhalation medications if they are having difficulty using the metered-dose inhaler; examples include the InspirEase and Inhal-Aid devices. Counsult the pharmacist.
- When two drugs are ordered via inhalation, use the bronchodilator first, then the second drug, such as beclomethasone.
- Teach patients to check the supply of drug on hand to avoid running out at inopportune times. To check the amount in a canister, drop the canister into water (without mouthpiece). The full container sinks to the botom, the half-full container floats with the bottom slightly out of the water. The empty container floats on its side, half submerged. Consult the manufacturer's literature for additional information.
- Remind patients to keep all health care providers informed of all drugs being taken. Remind patients to avoid over-the-counter drugs unless first approved by the physician. Many decongestants and cold remedies contain products which will duplicate the effects

Continued.

PATIENT CARE IMPLICATIONS — cont'd

of the bronchodilators, causing increased side effects.

- Keep these and all drugs out of the reach of children.
- No drugs should be used during pregnancy or lactation unless first approved by the physician.

Nonselective beta adrenergic bronchodilators

Drug administration

- Epinephrine hydrochloride (Adrenalin Chloride) is used via subcutaneous injection or intramuscular injection to treat anaphylactic allergic reactions. The dose is 0.1 to 0.5 mg (0.1 to 0.5 ml) of 1:1000 injection.
- See general guidelines above. Monitor the pulse and blood pressure carefully.
- Sus-Phrine is a suspension. Rotate the vial between the hands to mix the suspension before preparing the dose, and administer immediately so the drug does not settle out of suspension.
- See Chapter 14 for a discussion of use of these drugs in shock.

Patient and family education

- Review the general guidelines.
- Review Patient Problem: Dry Mouth on p. 170.
- Review Patient Problem: Orthostatic Hypotension on p. 237.

Selective beta adrenergic bronchodilators

Patient and family education

- Review the general guidelines.
- Review Patient Problems: Dry Mouth on p. 170 and Orthostatic Hypotension on p. 237.
- Generally, sustained-release formulations should be swallowed whole, without chewing or crushing. If there is a question about a specific product, consult the pharmacist.

Xanthines

Drug administration

- Review the general guidelines for bronchodilator therapy.
- Monitor the vital signs, blood pressure, and auscultate lung sounds. Hypotension may be pronounced. Supervise ambulation. Keep side rails up.
- Monitor serum theophylline levels.
  INTRAVENOUS AMINOPHYLLINE
- Only the concentration of 25 mg/ml may be given undiluted, by direct IV push, at a rate of 20 mg/min. Usually, aminophylline is diluted in at least 100 to 200 ml of 5% dextrose in water and given as an infusion, based on serum levels, patient response, or both. Available prediluted. Incompatible with many drugs, so should not usually be administered "piggyback"; rather, a separate IV should be started and maintained for replacement fluids and other drugs.

Patient and family education

- Review the general guidelines for bronchodilator therapy.
- Review Patient Problem: Orthostatic Hypotension, p. 237.
- Warn the patient to avoid driving or operating hazardous equipment if dizziness, lightheadedness, or vertigo develops; notify physician.
- Teach patients to read drug prescriptions and labels carefully. Many of these drugs are available in regular formulations and sustained-release formulations; the two cannot be interchanged on the same dosing schedule. See Chapter 6 for a discussion of sustained release products.
- Limit or avoid the use of coffee, tea, chocolate, and other methylxanthines, as they may affect xanthine metabolism.
- Avoid smoking cigarettes or marijuana, as they may alter serum levels.

Inhaled glucocorticoids

Drug administration

- See Chapter 51 or a detailed discussion of glucocorticoid therapy. Systemic side effects with inhaled forms are uncommon, but may occur. See the general guidelines for bronchodilator therapy for a discussion of the use of metered dose inhalers. As noted in the text, teach patients to gargle and rinse the mouth after each use of the inhaler to help prevent fungal infections.

Cromolyn

Patient and family education

- See the general guidelines for a discussion of metered dose inhalers. The "Spinhaler" is packaged with detailed instructions, which should be reviewed with the patient.
- Teach patients the importance of taking this drug as ordered, on a regular basis. This drug

PATIENT CARE IMPLICATIONS—cont'd

is useful for prophylactic treatment of asthma, but will not help control an acute attack of asthma.
- See Patient Problem: Dry Mouth on p. 170.
- Side effects are rare, but encourage the patient to report the development of any unexpected sign or symptom.

Ipratropium

Patient and family education

- See the general guidelines for a discussion of metered dose inhalers.
- Review Patient Problems: Dry Mouth on p. 170, and Constipation on p. 187. See Chapter

13 for a more detailed discussion of anticholinergics.

Alpha-1-proteinase inhibitor

Drug administration

- Consult the manufacturer's literature for current guidelines.
- Store the drug in the refrigerator before reconstitution.
- The patient may also be immunized against hepatitis B since the drug is prepared from pooled human plasma.
- Monitor vital signs.
- Administer IV at a rate of 0.08 ml/kg/min.

Alpha-1 proteinase inhibitor in chronic obstructive lung disease (COPD)

Chronic bronchitis and emphysema are together referred to as chronic obstructive lung disease or COPD. Patients with COPD commonly have some degree of reversible airflow obstruction. As with asthma, bronchodilators and corticosteroids play a major role in supportive therapy.

Research has shown that lung damage in COPD results from the destruction of elastin, a major structural protein of the lung. Elastin is destroyed when there is an imbalance between the lung proteinase, elastase, which breaks down elastin, and alpha-1-proteinase inhibitor (also called alpha-1-antitrypsin), a protein that inhibits elastase. Smoking seems to depress alpha-1-proteinase inhibitor, which can account for the high association between smoking and COPD. Some people have a genetic defect that results in low levels of alpha-1-proteinase inhibitor. Alpha-1-proteinase inhibitor (Prolastin) is now available for replacement therapy in those patients with a congenital deficiency of alpha-1-proteinase inhibitor. This drug is currently purified from human plasma and administered intravenously. The recommended dosage is 60 mg/kg body weight administered once weekly.

SUMMARY

Asthma is a disease in which there is reversible obstruction of the bronchioles involving constriction of the bronchial smooth muscle, edema of the bronchial mucosa, and excessive secretion of mucus (Figure 25.1). Extrinsic asthma is the best characterized form of asthma and involves an immunological mechanism that releases histamine and

other active compounds from mast cells. Drugs acting to increase intracellular cyclic AMP have proven especially efficacious in treating extrinsic asthma. These drugs include the beta adrenergic receptor agonists and the xanthines. Beneficial actions mediated through cyclic AMP include (1) bronchial dilation, (2) inhibition of mast cell degranulation, and (3) stimulation of the ciliary apparatus to remove secretions.

Cholinergic mechanisms may be important in the etiology of intrinsic asthma and may involve the intracellular second messenger cyclic GMP. The pharmacological factors affecting cyclic GMP are not completely understood.

Bronchodilators include beta adrenergic receptor agonists and the xanthines. Beta adrenergic receptor agonists vary in their effective route of administration and include inhalation, oral, sublingual, and subcutaneous routes. Uses vary from prophylaxis to treatment of an acute attack. The most common side effects include cardiovascular, muscular, and central nervous system stimulation. The beta receptor agonists are relatively specific for the beta-2 adrenergic receptors and have a lesser incidence of cardiac stimulation. Xanthines, chiefly forms of theophylline, are used both prophylactically and to control an acute attack.

Other drugs include cromolyn and the aerosol glucocorticoids. Cromolyn prevents mast cell degranulation and is a prophylactic drug only. Aerosol glucocorticoids help to control severe asthma.

New drugs for chronic obstructive lung disease (COPD) include ipratropium, an anticholinergic bronchodilator, and alpha-1-proteinase inhibitor.

STUDY QUESTIONS

1. What are the three components that restrict the airway in extrinsic asthma?
2. Contrast the mechanisms responsible for extrinsic and intrinsic asthma.
3. What is the mechanism of action of the bronchodilators (beta adrenergic receptor agonists and theophylline)? List three beneficial responses attributed to this mechanism.
4. Which of the beta adrenergic agonists used as bronchodilators are relatively specific for the beta-2 receptor?
5. What are the side effects associated with the bronchodilators?
6. What role does cromolyn play in the treatment of extrinsic asthma? What is the mechanism of action?
7. What role does beclomethasone play in the treatment of extrinsic asthma? What is the mechanism of action?

SUGGESTED READINGS

Austen, K.F.: The heterogeneity of mast cell population and products, Hosp. Pract. 19(9):135, 1984.

Brim, S.: A quick guide for home use of inhalant medications, Pediatr. Nurs. 15(1):87, 1987.

Dickerson, M.: Anaphylaxis and anaphylactic shock, Crit. Care Nurse Q. 11(1):68, 1988.

DiPalma, J.R.: Beta-2 agonists for acute asthma, Am. Fam. Phys. 31(5):184, 1985.

Easton, P.A., and others: A comparison of the bronchodilating effects of a beta-2 adrenergic agent (albuterol) and an anticholinergic agent (ipratropium bromide), given by aerosol alone or in sequence, N. Engl. J. Med. 315:735, 1986.

Fanta, C.H., Rossing, T.H., and McFadden, E.R. Jr.: Treatment of acute asthma: is combination therapy with sympathomimetics and methylxanthines indicated? Am. J. Med. 80:5, 1986.

Greenberg, S.D.: The lungs and their response to disease, Res. Staff Physician 29(11):28, 1983.

Gross, N.J.: The clinical recognition of asthma, Pract. Cardiol. 7(4):75, 1981.

Gross, N.J., and Skorodin, M.S.: Role of the parasympathetic system in airway obstruction due to emphysema, N. Engl. J. Med. 311(7):421, 1984.

Gross, N.J.: Ipratropium bromide, N. Engl. J. Med. 319(8):486, 1988.

Kaliner, M., Eggleson, P.A., and Mathews, K.P.: Rhinitis and asthma, JAMA 258(20):2851, 1987.

Marx, J.L.: The leukotrienes in allergy and inflammation, Science 215:1380, 1982.

McFadden, E.R. Jr: Methylxanthine therapy and reversible airway obstruction, Am. J. Med. 79(6A):1, 1985.

Melethil, S., Carlson, J.D., and Haug, M.T.: Predictability of theophylline levels, Drug Intell. Clin. Pharm. 16:695, 1982.

Miller, M., and others: Theophylline metabolism: variation and genetics, Clin. Pharmacol. Ther. 35(2):170, 1984.

Nemec, M.A.: Inhalation medications for chronic asthma, J. Pediatr. Health Care 1(4):223, 1987.

Newhouse, M.T., and Dolovich, M.B.: Control of asthma by aerosols, N. Engl. J. Med. 315(14):879, 1986.

Newman, S.P., and Clarke, S.W.: Inhalation technique with aerosol bronchodilators: does it matter? Pract. Cardiol. 9(9):157, 1983.

Petty, T.L.: Future trends in the management of asthma and chronic obstructive pulmonary disease, Am. J. Med. 79(Suppl 6A):38, 1985.

Samuelsson, B.: Leukotrienes: mediators of immediate hypersensitivity reactions and inflammation, Science 220:568, 1983.

Skorodin, M.S.: Pharmacologic management of obstructive lung disease: current perspectives, Am. J. Med. 81(5a):8, 1986.

Summers, R., and Smith, L.: Asthma management: new perspectives, improved options, Postgrad. Med. 76(1):209, 1984.

Drugs to Control Bronchial Secretions

26

Drugs to Treat Nasal Congestion

ALPHA ADRENERGIC AGONISTS AS NASAL DECONGESTANTS

Mechanism of action. Nasal congestion results when the blood vessels in the nasal passage become dilated as a result of infection, inflammation, allergy, or emotional upset. This dilation increases capillary permeability and allows fluid to escape into the nasal passage. Drugs that stimulate alpha receptors cause blood vessels to constrict, thereby relieving the congestion. These drugs are alpha adrenergic agonists because they mimic the action of the neurotransmitter norepinephrine (Chapter 10).

Topical Nasal Decongestants

Several alpha adrenergic agonists are applied topically as drops or sprays. Because these nasal decongestants have an immediate and direct contact with the nasal mucosa, they have a rapid action and provide temporary symptomatic relief by opening up the nasal passages. However, when the effect of the drug wears off, the congestion reappears (rebound congestion). If the nasal decongestant is used with increasing frequency, it has less and less effect. The drug ultimately irritates the nasal passages and causes the congestion to become worse rather than better. For this reason decongestants are most effective when used only occasionally and for no longer than 3 to 5 days. Nasal decongestants are available without a prescription.

Administration of nose drops. When a nasal decongestant is applied as drops into the nostril, the patient should be lying on a bed with the head hanging over the edge and turned to one side. The drops are then instilled into the upper nostril. After a few seconds the head is turned to allow administration to the other nostril. Use of this lateral, head-low position allows the drops to coat the nasal mucosa

without being immediately swallowed. The drops may cause a stinging or burning sensation or induce sneezing.

With repeated use of a nasal congestant, more of the drug is absorbed and systemic effects become possible. The symptoms of an overdose are those expected from a sympathomimetic drug (Chapter 10): nervousness, dizziness, palpitation, and transient high blood pressure readings. Children are especially vulnerable to overdoses of nasal decongestants, and they may have reactions that include sweating, drowsiness, shock, or coma.

Orally Active Decongestants

Those alpha adrenergic agonists most commonly found in cold remedies include *phenylpropanolamine, phenylephrine,* and *pseudoephedrine.* Cold remedies are syrups, tablets, or capsules that may also include an antihistamine, an analgesic, or other miscellaneous ingredients. Cold remedies are discussed in Chapter 4.

Drug interactions with nasal decongestants. Patients with hyperthyroidism, diabetes mellitus, hypertension, or heart disease are vulnerable to the sympathomimetic side effects of nasal decongestants and should avoid these drugs. A hypertensive reaction to a nasal decongestant may occur in a patient taking a monoamine oxidase inhibitor. Patients receiving tricyclic antidepressants are vulnerable to the cardiac effects of sympathomimetic agents.

Specific Sympathomimetic Drugs Used as Nasal Decongestants (Table 26.1)

Phenylephrine

Phenylephrine (Coricidin, Neo-Synephrine, and others) is a potent alpha adrenergic agonist that is administered orally or topically. It is available both alone and in many combination cold preparations.

Table 26.1 Nasal Decongestants (Nonprescription Drugs)

Generic name	Trade name	Administration/dosage	Comments
Epinephrine hydrochloride	Adrenalin Chloride*	TOPICAL: 0.1% aqueous solution as a spray or 1 to 2 drops every 4 to 6 hr. Not recommended for children under 6 yr.	Short acting. Frequently causes rebound congestion. Can cause central nervous system stimulation, headaches, and palpitations.
Ephedrine sulfate	Ectasaale Epedsol	ORAL: *Adults*—25 to 50 mg every 3 to 4 hr. *Children*—3 mg/kg body weight daily in 4 to 6 divided doses. TOPICAL: *Adults and children*—3 to 4 drops of a 1% or 3% solution in each nostril every 3 to 4 hr, no more than 4 times daily. Also may apply as a pack or tampon.	Can cause central nervous system stimulation, transient hypertension, and palpitations, so contraindicated for patients with heart disease, diabetes, hypertension, and hyperthyroidism. Rebound congestion is common.
Naphazoline hydrochloride	Privine Hydrochloride*	TOPICAL: 0.05% and 0.1% solutions. Two drops in each nostril no more than every 3 hr or 2 sprays every 4 to 6 hr.	An imidazoline. Can cause rebound congestion. Systemic effects from overuse include arrhythmias, transient hypertension, slowing of the heart rate, and drowsiness. Do not use in an atomizer with aluminum parts.
Oxymetazoline hydrochloride	Afrin* Nafrine†	TOPICAL: *Adults*—2 to 4 drops or 2 to 3 sprays of 0.05% solution in each nostril at morning and at bedtime. *Children*—over 6 yr, as for adults; 2 to 5 yr, 0.025% solution is used as above.	An imidazoline. Long acting. Side effects are mild, generally safe.
Phenylephrine hydrochloride	Coricidin Decongestant Nasal Mist Neo-Synephrine hydrochloride* Super Anahist nasal spray	TOPICAL: *Adults*—drops of 0.25% to 1% solution in each nostril (head in lateral, head-low position) every 3 to 4 hr. Nasal spray or nasal jelly may be used. *Children over 6 yr*—as for adults. *Infants and young children*—0.125% solution is used as above.	Less potent and longer acting than epinephrine. No central nervous system stimulation, but can cause transient hypertension, headaches, and palpitations.
Phenylpropanolamine hydrochloride	Various combination drugs	ORAL: *Adults*—25 mg every 3 to 4 hr or 50 mg every 6 to 8 hr. *Children 8 to 12 yr*—20 to 25 mg 3 times daily. Not recommended for children under 8 yr.	Similar to ephedrine but with less central nervous system stimulation.
Propylhexidrine	Benzedrex	TOPICAL (inhalation): 2 inhalations in each nostril as needed.	A volatile drug safe for adult use; children should be supervised. Inhaler should be warmed by the hands if cold.
Pseudoephedrine hydrochloride	Novafed Sudafed* Robidrine†	ORAL: *Adults*—60 mg every 6 to 8 hr. *Children*—4 mg/kg body weight in 4 divided doses.	The stereoisomer of ephedrine with a lesser incidence of central nervous system stimulation and hypertension than ephedrine. Useful for relief of a runny nose or congestion leading to an earache.

*Available in Canada and United States.
†Available in Canada only.

Table 26.1   Nasal Decongestants (Nonprescription Drugs)—cont'd

Generic name	Trade name	Administration/dosage	Comments
Pseudoephedrine sulfate	Afrinol Repetabs	As for pseudoephedrine hydrochloride.	
Tetrahydrozoline hydrochloride	Tyzine	TOPICAL: *Adults*—2 to 4 drops of a 0.1% solution in each nostril. Do not repeat more frequently than every 3 hr. *Children*—6 yr and over, as for adults; 2 to 6 yr, 2 to 3 drops of a 0.05% solution in each nostril every 4 to 6 hr.	An imidazoline. Adverse reactions can be severe: hypertension, drowsiness, sweating, rebound hypotension, bradycardia, and cardiac arrhythmias. May cause a high fever and coma in young children. Rebound congestion may persist a week after discontinuing.
Xylometazoline hydrochloride	Neo-Synephrine II, Long-acting Otrivin-Spray* Sinutab Long-Lasting Sinus Spray	TOPICAL: *Adults*—2 to 3 drops of 0.1% solution or 1 to 2 inhalations of 0.1% spray in each nostril every 8 to 10 hr. *Children*—6 mo to 12 yr, 2 to 3 drops of 0.05% solution in each nostril every 4 to 6 hr. *Infants*—1 drop of 0.05% solution in each nostril every 6 hr.	An imidazoline. A relatively safe, long-acting decongestant but should not be used excessively or for more than a few days. Do not use in atomizers with aluminum parts.

*Available in Canada and United States.
†Available in Canada only.

Phenylpropanolamine

Phenylpropanolamine (Propadrine) is used mainly in oral combination cold remedies. It is an alpha adrenergic agonist and also acts indirectly, releasing norepinephrine from nerve terminals.

Pseudoephedrine

Pseudoephedrine (Novafed, Sudafed, and others) is included in many oral combination cold remedies. It is a beta agonist as well as an alpha agonist.

Propylhexedrine

Propylhexedrine (Benzedrex) is a volatile drug that stimulates alpha receptors. It causes little stimulation of the central nervous system and is therefore generally safer than some of the other nasal decongestants.

Imidazolines (Table 26.1)

There is a subgroup of four nasal decongestants that are chemically related, the imidazolines. These all stimulate the alpha adrenergic receptors to produce vasoconstriction. They are potent, and only xylometazoline is considered safe for young children. All are used topically. Naphazoline and xylometazoline will react with aluminum and should not be used in atomizers with aluminum parts.

Naphazoline

Naphazoline (Privine) is a very effective nasal decongestant but can produce a severe rebound congestion resulting from irritation and swelling of the nasal mucosa. Overdosage of naphazoline has been reported to produce coma in children and systemic effects such as hypertension, sweating, cardiac arrhythmias, and drowsiness in adults.

Oxymetazoline

Oxymetazoline (Afrin) is a relatively long-lasting nasal decongestant that has not been implicated in as many severe systemic effects as naphazoline. However, rebound congestion does occur with repeated use.

Tetrahydrozoline

Tetrahydrozoline (Tyzine) is an effective nasal decongestant similar to naphazoline in its adverse effects.

Xylometazoline

Xylometazoline (Neo-Synephrine II, Sinutab Long-Lasting Spray, and others) is similar to oxymetazoline in its effects.

Other Drugs Used to Relieve Nasal Congestion

Nasal congestion is common in allergies such as hay fever. As discussed in Chapter 24, antihis-

Table 26.2 Expectorants*

Generic name	Trade name	Administration/dosage	Comments
Guaifenesin (glycerol guaiacolate)	Anti-tuss Glycotuss Nortussin Robitussin† Various others	ORAL: *Adults*—200 to 400 mg every 3 to 4 hr. *Children*—6 to 12 yr, 100 mg every 3 to 4 hr; 2 to 6 yr, 50 mg every 3 to 4 hr.	Use for symptomatic relief of a dry, unproductive cough. Occasionally causes nausea or drowsiness. Available without prescription.
Iodinated glycerol	Organidin†	ORAL: *Adults*—20 drops of solution (50 mg) or a 60 mg tablet or 5 ml elixir (60 mg) 4 times daily. *Children*—no more than ½ adult dose daily.	See potassium iodide.
Potassium iodide	Potassium Iodide SSKI Pima Iodo-Niacin	ORAL: *Adults*—300 mg every 4 to 6 hr. *Children*—60 to 500 mg daily, divided in 2 to 4 doses.	Contraindicated for patients with hyperkalemia, hyperthyroidism, or hypersensitivity to iodide. Symptoms of hypersensitivity include a skin rash. Iodism (overdose of iodide) causes a metallic taste, fever, skin eruptions, nausea, vomiting, mucous membrane ulcerations, and salivary gland swelling.

*Only those expectorants available alone have been listed. Other drugs included in cough or cold mixtures as an expectorant include potassium guaiacolsulfonate, ammonium chloride, terpin hydrate, ipecac, calcium iodide, and citric acid.
†Available in Canada and United States.

tamines are useful in treating hay fever because they block the receptors for histamine on the blood vessels and thereby prevent the dilation that causes nasal congestion. Antihistamines are also frequently included in cold remedy preparations. The anticholinergic action characteristic of antihistamines aids in reversing the vasodilation of the nasal blood vessels.

Drugs to Treat a Cough

EXPECTORANTS, ANTITUSSIVES, AND MUCOLYTIC DRUGS

Origin of Secretions

Respiratory secretions in the trachea, bronchi, and bronchioles originate from the goblet cells and from the bronchial glands (Figure 26.1). The goblet cells lie on the surface, making up part of the epithelial layer. The tracheal epithelium consists of about 20% goblet cells, whereas the bronchiolar epithelium consists of only 2% goblet cells. These cells produce a gelatinous mucus that they peri-

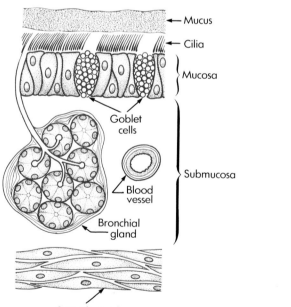

FIGURE 26.1   Mucous layer at top is the lumen of the airway. Relative position of goblet cells and bronchial glands, secretions of which make up the mucus, are shown. Mucous layer is normally swept up toward the throat by the cilia to cleanse the airway.

Table 26.3   Antitussives

Generic name	Trade name	Administration/dosage	Comments
Chlophedianol	Ulo Ulonet†	ORAL: *Adults*—25 mg 3 or 4 times daily. *Children 6 to 12 yr*—12.5 to 25 mg 3 or 4 times daily. *Children 2 to 6 yr*—12.5 mg 3 or 4 times daily.	Prescription drug. Side effects include drowsiness and nausea.
Codeine, codeine phosphate, codeine sulfate		ORAL: *Adults*—10 to 20 mg every 4 to 6 hr, no more than 120 mg in 24 hr. *Children 6 to 12 yr*—5 to 10 mg every 4 to 6 hr, no more than 60 mg in 24 hr; *2 to 6 yr*—2.5 to 5 mg every 4 to 6 hr, no more than 30 mg in 24 hr.	A Schedule II drug. Codeine is included in some Schedule III and Schedule V combination formulations, usually including a decongestant, an antihistamine, and an expectorant. For adverse effects, see Chapter 31.
Dextromethorphan hydrobromide	Coughettes Sucrets cough control lozenge Romilar CF Various others	ORAL: *Adults*—10 to 20 mg every 4 hr or 30 mg every 6 to 8 hr. *Children 6 to 12 yr*—½ adult dose; *2 to 6 yr*—¼ adult dose.	Nonnarcotic, available without prescription. No tolerance develops. Has no analgesic or hypnotic effect, does not depress respiration. Does not cause constipation as readily as codeine.
Diphenhydramine hydrochloride	Benylin Cough Syrup† Benadryl*	ORAL: *Adults*—25 mg every 4 hr, no more than 100 mg in 24 hr. *Children 6 to 12 yr*—½ adult dose. *2 to 5 yr*—¼ adult dose.	An antihistamine. Side effects include drowsiness and a drying effect.
Hydrocodone bitartrate	Codone Dicodid Robidone†	ORAL: *Adults*—5 to 10 mg every 6 to 8 hr. *Children*—0.6 mg/kg body weight daily in divided doses.	A Schedule II drug. Hydrocodone is included in some Schedule III and Schedule V combination formulations, usually including a decongestant, an antihistamine, and an expectorant. For adverse effects, see Chapter 31.
Noscapine	Tussacapine Noscatuss†	ORAL: *Adults*—15 to 30 mg every 4 to 6 hr; maximum 120 mg in 24 hr. *Children 6 to 12 yr*—15 mg, 3 or 4 time daily, maximum 60 mg in 24 hrs. *2 to 6 yr*—7.5 to 15 mg, 3 or 4 times daily, maximum 4 doses.	Available without prescription as tablets or syrup. May cause drowsiness in large doses.

*Available in Canada and United States.
†Available in Canada only.

odically secrete. What factors normally control the goblet cells is not known, but chronic exposure to irritants increases their size, number, and activity. An example is the phlegm coughed up by smokers. The bronchial glands lie several layers beneath the epithelium. The grapelike (acinar) cells are controlled by the cholinergic nervous system, and when stimulated these cells secrete a plentiful watery fluid into a duct that empties onto the surface.

The secretions of the goblet cells and bronchial glands combine to form a mucus called the *respi-ratory tract fluid*. Much of the water in the respiratory secretions evaporates to humidify the air taken into the lungs. If too much water is lost to humidification, the mucus forms thick plugs that cannot be readily eliminated. Normally, the respiratory tract fluid forms a lining that is swept upward by the action of the ciliary hairs into the throat (pharynx), where it is swallowed. This activity, the *mucociliary escalator*, provides a cleansing mechanism for the lungs, since any foreign particles or bacteria are trapped in this viscous layer

THE NURSING PROCESS

DRUGS MODIFYING RESPIRATORY SECRETIONS

Assessment

Patients who require drugs to modify bronchial secretions are those who are self-medicating for symptomatic treatment of colds and upper respiratory infections, those with serious upper respiratory problems, and those few with chronic pulmonary diseases characterized by problems with coughing or secretions. The nurse should assess the patient as a whole in addition to focusing on the subjective complaints. An appropriate history would include questions related to the onset of symptoms, possible irritants for the symptoms that are present, the times of the day when symptoms are worse (such as a cough which is more troublesome at night), therapies used by the patient that have successfully relieved the symptoms, and the history of irritants or environmental conditions that may be aggravating the symptoms. Objective data might include the respiratory rate, the vital signs, the character and quantity of any secretions, an examination of the nose, throat, and ears, and an assessment of the lungs.

Nursing diagnoses

Ineffective airway clearance related to suppressed ability to cough

Potential altered health maintenance related to misuse/overuse of nasal decongestants

Management

Since the patient is usually being treated for relief of symptoms, the nurse needs to monitor these symptoms during the course of therapy. The nurse should monitor the vital signs, and in some patients it may be necessary to monitor the fluid intake and output. The nurse should work with the patient to identify nonmedical solutions for troublesome symptoms. For patients receiving mucolytic agents, a suction machine should be at the bedside if there is doubt that the patient can adequately handle secretions.

Evaluation

These drugs are successful if the patient's symptoms are relieved or if the underlying condition requiring the drugs has improved because of therapy. Before discharge for self-management, the patient should be able to explain how to take the drugs correctly, to demonstrate how to administer the drugs correctly, to explain what side effects might occur that would require notification of the physician, to explain the need to discontinue the drugs after symptoms have improved, and to explain what actions to take if the symptoms return or do not improve.

---

and eliminated. If the ciliary hairs are paralyzed by tobacco smoke or by alcohol, the secretions cannot be cleared naturally, and give rise to the "smoker's cough."

Cough

A cough is a protective reflex initiated by irritation in the airway. As long as material is being brought up by the cough, it is beneficial. Several common situations cause an unproductive cough. The air of heated rooms can dry the airway enough to cause irritation. A sore throat can produce an unproductive cough and can be self-perpetuating when the cough itself further irritates the throat. A cough can result from irritants responsible for asthma or pulmonary edema, which also stimulate the cough receptors. Congestion of the nasal mucosa results in a postnasal drip, which irritates the throat and produces the cough associated with a cold or the flu.

When a cough is not productive and disrupts sleep and rest, relief is sought. Therapy for a cough depends on the cause. If the air is dry, a vaporizer or steamer may be sufficient to liquefy the secre-

Table 26.4 Mucolytic Drug

Generic name	Trade name	Administration/dosage	Comments
Acetylcysteine	Mucomyst* Airbron†	NEBULIZATION USING FACE MASK, MOUTHPIECE, OR TRACHEOSTOMY: 1 to 10 mg of a 20% solution or 2 to 20 ml of a 10% solution every 2 to 6 hr. DIRECT INSTILLATION: 1 to 2 ml of a 10% or 20% solution as often as every hour.	Has the odor of rotten eggs, which may cause gastrointestinal upset. Solutions can be diluted with sterile water for nebulization. Reacts with iron, copper, and rubber, so nebulization equipment should not contain these materials.

*Available in Canada and United States.
†Available in Canada only.

tions so that they do not become irritating. A dehydrated state limits respiratory secretions, so having the patient drink plenty of fluids prevents or overcomes the dehydration that accompanies common illnesses. Patients with sore throats can suck hard candies to increase flow of saliva to coat the throat. If these simple measures do not eliminate the cough, expectorants may be used. An *expectorant* is a drug that increases the output of respiratory tract fluid to coat the trachea and bronchi. In addition, a cough suppressant or *antitussive* drug may be taken. Expectorants and antitussive drugs are widely available as over-the-counter drugs.

Expectorants (Table 26.2)

Although many drugs are used as expectorants, no expectorant has proved effective. Iodide, usually given as potassium iodide, is one widely used expectorant. After entering the bloodstream, potassium iodide is believed to stimulate the bronchial glands to secrete more fluid. Use of iodides is associated with a high incidence of adverse effects. Some people develop a skin rash. A few patients become hypothyroid. One symptom of iodide excess is a mumpslike swelling of the parotid glands, presumably a result of stimulation of the glands. Iodides are seldom used today.

Another mechanism that stimulates the secretion of respiratory tract fluid is the reflex activity carried by the vagal nerve characteristic of nausea. Some drugs used as expectorants are believed to initiate this reflex by irritating the stomach when swallowed. One such drug is *guaifenesin (glycerol guaiacolate)*, a widely used expectorant for which there is some evidence of efficacy. Other drugs acting by this mechanism include *syrup of ipecac* and *ammonium chloride*. Potassium iodide is believed to act in part by this latter mechanism as well as by the secretory mechanism just described. Syrup

of ipecac is more commonly used to induce vomiting (emesis) than as an expectorant.

Other agents added as expectorants to cough suppressant mixtures include *terpin hydrate, citric acid, sodium citrate, iodinated glycerol,* and *cal-*

Antitussives (Table 26.3)

Tussis is the Latin word meaning cough, and cough suppressants are called antitussives.

Codeine and hydrocodone

Codeine and hydrocodone are good antitussives, but they are opiates and therefore capable of producing drug dependence. Hydrocodone has a greater potential for producing drug dependence than codeine. Most preparations containing codeine or hydrocodone are prescription drugs. Some preparations are available as Schedule V drugs and may be obtained by signing for them with a registered pharmacist. The opiates suppress a cough by directly inhibiting the medullary center for the cough reflex. The doses required to suppress a cough are less than those to produce analgesia or respiratory depression. Side effects at antitussive doses are uncommon, but they include nausea, dizziness, and constipation.

Nonopiate antitussives include *dextromethorphan, diphenhydramine,* and *benzonatate*.

Dextromethorphan hydrobromide

Dextromethorphan hydrobromide is the most widely used antitussive in over-the-counter cough mixtures. It is related to the opiates but has no analgesic effect and causes no drug dependence. Dextromethorphan is an effective cough suppressant that inhibits the medullary center for the cough reflex. It is very well tolerated and only occasionally causes drowsiness or dizziness.

PATIENT CARE IMPLICATIONS

Nasal decongestants

Drug administration

- Monitor blood pressure and pulse. Monitor blood glucose levels in diabetic patients.
- Assess for GI symptoms. Persistent or severe GI symptoms indicate a need to change drug or dose.

Patient and family education

- Review the side effects (discussed in the text) with the patient.
- Teach patients to choose over-the-counter remedies appropriate for their symptoms, and to read product labels. Use products only as directed. Consult the pharmacist to assist in choosing an appropriate remedy for a specific problem.
- Remind patients to keep all health care providers informed of all drugs being used, even over-the-counter preparations. In particular, patients with thyroid disease, diabetes mellitus, hypertension, or heart disease should use nasal decongestants only with physician approval (see text).
- Remind patients to keep all drugs out of the reach of children, even nasal sprays and drops. Only pediatric preparations and pediatric doses should be used for children.
- Review Chapter 6 for information about using nose drops and nose sprays correctly. To prevent contamination of equipment, family members should not share droppers or spray applicators. Rinse and dry applicators after each use.
- To prevent insomnia, take the last dose of the day around the time of the evening meal.
- If photophobia occurs, instruct the patient to avoid brightly lit areas and to wear sunglasses.
- To use nasal jelly (phenylephrine, others): First, blow the nose. Wash hands. Place a pea-sized amount of jelly in each nostril. Sniff well to move jelly back into nose. Wipe off the tip of the tube with a tissue and replace the cap.

Expectorants and antitussives

Patient and family education

- Teach patients about the difference between an antitussive and an expectorant.
- Remind patients to read labels carefully on over-the-counter preparations to avoid taking unnecessary medications. Consult the pharmacist for assistance as needed.
- Remind patients to keep these and all drugs out of the reach of children. Only products for pediatric use and in pediatric doses should be administered to children.
- Remind patients to avoid driving or operating hazardous equipment if drowsiness is a problem.
- Tell patients with cough to stay well hydrated (daily fluid intake of at least 2500 ml for an adult); avoid smoking; and to keep the room air moist through use of a vaporizer or humidifier.
- For preparations containing iodide: question about history of allergy to iodine or shellfish before administering. Swallow enteric-coated tablets whole, without swallowing or crushing, and take with a full glass of liquid. Dilute liquid preparations with water, milk, or juice. Take doses with meals or snack to reduce gastric irritation. Discuss signs of chronic iodine poisoning: headache, swelling of eyelids, metallic taste, nausea, vomiting, diarrhea, skin changes, mouth ulcers. Remind patients to report any unexpected sign or symptom to the physician.
- As noted in the text, codeine and hydrocodone have the same potential for side effects as all narcotics; see Chapter 44.

Mucolytic agents

Drug administration

- Supervise patients receiving acetylcysteine during and after treatment to see that the airway is still patent in the presence of increased pulmonary secretions. Have a suction machine at the bedside of patients who are elderly, immobilized, or intubated, or anyone who may not be able to handle secretions.
- Before using a mucolytic agent with a patient for the first time, review the purpose and desired effects of the drug. Tell the patient to cough up and expectorate loosened secretions.
- Supervise patients with asthma who are receiving acetylcysteine, as it may cause bronchospasm. If bronchospasm develops, discontinue nebulization; if severe, notify the physician.
- Assess for other common side effects: stomatitis, rhinorrhea, nausea.

PATIENT CARE IMPLICATIONS—cont'd

■ Acetylcysteine is administered orally for treatment of acetaminophen overdose. The dose is based on the time since acetaminophen ingestion and serum level of acetaminophen. The regimen involves a loading dose, followed by 17 doses at 4-hour intervals. Dilute doses in juice or cola beverages before administering. If the patient vomits within 1 hour after receiving a dose, the dose should be repeated; consult the physician.

Noscapine

Noscapine (Tusscapine) is chemically related to the opiates. Its antitussive potency is equivalent to that of codeine, but noscapine does not have the side effects characteristic of codeine.

Chlophedianol

Chlophedianol (Ulo) is a centrally acting antitussive with some local anesthetic and anticholinergic action. Use of this drug may cause some patients to become excited and hyperirritable. Large doses cause sedation.

Diphenhydramine

Diphenhydramine (Benylin) is an antihistamine with antitussive action. Adverse effects include the drowsiness common to the antihistamines and the anticholinergic drying effect that hinders a productive cough.

Mucolytic Drugs

The value of water, taken as liquid or inhaled as vapor, has already been mentioned as a useful method for keeping the mucus from becoming too viscous. The use of expectorants to stimulate the watery secretion of the bronchial glands has also been covered.

Mucolytics are agents that break up a viscous mucus so that it can be coughed up or otherwise drained. A viscous mucus is most likely to occur in the patient with a pulmonary infection or with chronic obstructive lung disease where the normal mechanisms for clearing the lungs are compromised.

Table 26.4 lists dosages and administration of the mucolytic drugs currently available.

Acetylcysteine

Acetylcysteine (Mucomyst) is a sulfhydryl compound that can break disulfide bonds. A viscous mucus has long molecules linked by disulfide bonds; when these disulfide bonds are broken, the molecules separate, reducing the viscosity.

Acetylcysteine is administered by nebulizer through a face mask, mouthpiece, or tracheostomy. Acetylcysteine has a rotten egg odor and may irritate the nasal passages.

SUMMARY

A runny nose and a cough are two of the most common cold symptoms for which people seek relief.

Nasal congestion and a runny nose result from dilation of the blood vessels in the nasal mucosa and leakage of fluid from these vessels. Drugs that stimulate alpha adrenergic receptors cause vasoconstriction and thereby relieve nasal congestion. Commonly these drugs are applied as drops or sprays. Abuse results in the blood vessels becoming unresponsive, and rebound congestion occurs. A few sympathomimetic drugs are effective orally. The imidazolines are selective alpha receptor agonists for topical use.

Secretions arise from goblet cells and bronchial glands in the respiratory tract to form mucus. This mucus normally traps particulate matter in the lungs and is swept up to the throat by ciliary hairs. Expectorants are drugs such as iodides and guaifenesin that stimulate the production of these secretions.

Irritation of the throat causes a cough, which is a protective reflex mediated through the medullary cough center. Suppression of a cough may be desired to provide rest or when the cough is unproductive. Codeine, hydrocodone, dextromethorphan, diphenhydramine, chlophedianol, and noscapine act at the medullary cough center to suppress a cough.

Mucolytic drugs break up a viscous mucus that cannot be coughed up or drained. Acetylcysteine breaks the disulfide bonds holding together the long molecules that compose mucus.

STUDY QUESTIONS

1. Explain how alpha adrenergic agonists act to relieve nasal congestion.
2. Describe the technique for administering topical nasal decongestants.
3. What are the side effects, drug interactions, and contraindications for the use of nasal decongestants?
4. What is rebound congestion?
5. Categorize the drugs used as nasal decongestants as topical sympathomimetics, oral sympathomimetics, and imidazolines.
6. Describe the origin and function of mucus.
7. List the expectorants and their mechanisms of action.
8. Describe the mucolytic drug and its mechanism of action.
9. List the antitussives and their mechanisms of action.
10. What are the nonmedicinal approaches for treating a cough?

SUGGESTED READINGS

Barbieri, E.J.: Mucolytics, Am. Fam. Physician **28**(2):175, 1983.

Brown, L.H.: The effective cough, Crit. Care Nurse **8**(2):77, 1988.

Ellenbogen, C.: The common cold, Am. Fam. Physician **24**(3):181, 1981.

Janoff, A.: New insights into the pathogenesis of emphysema: clinical significance, Intern. Med. **3**(3):56, 1982.

Thurkauf, G.E.: Acetaminophen overdose, Crit. Care Nurse **7**(1):20, 1987.

VII

DRUGS AFFECTING THE IMMUNE SYSTEM

This section presents the pharmacology of the immune system. Chapter 27, *Basic Function of the Immune System*, relates the basic functions of the immune system so that the rationale for pharmacological intervention can be understood. Chapter 28, *Immunomodulators*, discusses drugs intended to either enhance or block immune responses. The situations in which these drugs are indicated are also discussed.

Basic Function of the Immune System

27

The immune system is a complex and diffuse system that is present throughout the body. Its main function is to protect the body from damage caused by any environmental agent that is foreign to it. Foreign agents include invading microorganisms such as bacteria, fungi, parasites, and viruses, as well as foreign tissue such as transplanted kidneys, hearts, and livers. Any foreign agent capable of inducing an immune response is termed an *antigen*. The immune system also serves to protect the self, ridding the body of malignant cells as they arise and preventing the body from taking action against its own tissues. Like all other body systems, the immune system can exhibit pathology and abnormal responses.

INNATE AND ACQUIRED IMMUNITY

Two basic forms of immunity exist: innate and acquired. *Innate immunity* is derived from all elements with which a person is born and which are always present and available on short notice to protect the body from challenges by foreign materials. Innate immunity is conferred by physical, cellular, and chemical barriers. Physical barriers include skin, mucous membranes, and the cough reflex. Phagocytic cells make up the cellular barrier. *Phagocytosis* is ingestion and destruction of foreign particles such as bacteria by individual cells of the immune system. Biologically active substances that include degradative enzymes, toxic free radicals, lipids, and low pH serve as chemical barriers to invasion by foreign agents.

Acquired immunity, as the name implies, is not present at birth but develops as the individual grows and matures. Although a person has the capacity at birth for developing acquired immunity, this form of immunity is not exhibited until the person has had two sequential exposures to the same foreign agent. Acquired immunity has two main arms—the humoral immune response and the cellular immune response. *Humoral immunity* consists of the production of antibodies, which are soluble proteins present in normal serum. *Cellular immunity* consists of responses such as the delayed-type of hypersensitivity, which are mediated by cells rather than by soluble substances. Lymphocytes are the main providers of acquired immunity.

ORGANS AND CELLS OF THE IMMUNE SYSTEM

The immune system is comprised of five white blood cell types: lymphocytes, monocytes/macrophages, polymorphonuclear leukocytes (PMNs), basophils, and eosinophils. All of these, as well as the red blood cells and the platelets, are derived from a common precursor cell type found in the bone marrow. This precursor cell type is the *stem cell.*

Monocytes and macrophages represent different states of cell maturation. Monocytes circulate freely within the body; with differentiation, they become macrophages. Macrophages may be fixed within the tissues, where they may persist for years; some, however, recirculate through secondary lymphoid organs. Either fixed or recirculating macrophages can assist lymphocytes in generating immune responses, and can phagocytize foreign particles. Macrophages can become activated to kill tumor cells.

Lymphocytes are subdivided into two major groups: the thymus-derived or T cells, and the bone marrow-derived or B cells. The B lymphocytes produce antibodies. T lymphocytes are further subdivided into helper T cells and cytotoxic T cells. Helper T cells assist B cells to respond to an antigen, and are the cells which mediate the delayed-type of hypersensitivity. Cytotoxic T cells are responsible for the rejection of grafts, and for destroying virus-infected cells. The ratio of helper cells to cytotoxic cells normally ranges from 1.2 : 1 to 2:1. In the acquired immunodeficiency syndrome (AIDS) this ratio is usually reversed and can be as low as 0.2 (1:5).

Polymorphonuclear leukocytes (PMNs) are the predominant phagocytes within the circulation. They are usually the first cells to arrive at the site of an infection. Besides phagocytosis, the PMN has two other means of killing foreign invaders. The first is the oxidative burst of the PMN, which leads to release of superoxide dismutase and hydrogen peroxide. Second, contained within azurophil granules are antimicrobial substances including lysozyme, lactoferrin, cathepsin G, and defensins, which are released upon activation of the PMN.

Basophils participate in allergic and inflammatory responses. These cells contain densely staining granules in their cytoplasm. Within these granules are mediators of allergic and inflammatory responses such as histamine, complement components, and leukotrienes C and D. Degranulation occurs when antigen interacts with IgE molecules bound to the cell surface of the basophil.

Eosinophils also participate in allergic reactions but perform another major role in host defense—the killing of parasites. Contained within the cytoplasmic granules of the eosinophil are some of the same mediators as found in basophil granules, such as leukotrienes C and D, as well as a number of proteins that are toxic to parasites. Eosinophils can also cause histamine to be released from mast cells and basophils. Eosinophils are also phagocytic, but their role as phagocytes is not as important as is that of the PMNs.

Organs of the immune system are classified as primary or secondary. The *primary lymphoid organs* are the thymus and the bone marrow. Maturation of lymphocytes occurs in these structures. The spleen, lymph nodes, and Peyer's patches are the *secondary lymphoid organs.* Peyer's patches are clusters of lymphocytes spread throughout the lining of the intestinal wall, tonsils, and appendix. Secondary lymphoid tissues are highly effective in trapping and concentrating foreign substances and are the main sites of antibody production and generation of antigen-specific T lymphocytes.

GENERATION OF IMMUNE RESPONSES

Generation of either humoral or cellular immunity requires three steps: (1) activation, (2) proliferation, and (3) differentiation. Activation of T lymphocytes requires that antigen be processed and presented by specialized cells called *antigen-presenting cells.* The antigen-presenting cells also secrete soluble factors necessary for the proliferation of T cells. The major antigen-presenting cells are monocytes and macrophages. Other cells that can also present antigen include dermal Langerhans' cells, dendritic cells in various locations, and hepatic Küpffer cells. The antigen-presenting cells take up antigen, process it, and then express it on the cell surface together with histocompatibility antigens. T lymphocytes are activated by interaction with this complex of processed antigen and histocompatibility antigen on the surface of the antigen-presenting cells. B lymphocytes are activated by interacting directly with unprocessed antigen via antibody molecules on their surface.

Once activated, both T and B lymphocytes express receptors for growth factors synthesized and released primarily by activated helper T cells. In response to these growth factors, the T and B cells proliferate. Having undergone proliferation, B and T cells can then respond to other soluble mediators secreted by activated helper T cells, and will differentiate into functional effector cells. B lymphocytes differentiate into antibody-secreting plasma cells. T lymphocytes differentiate into cells capable of mediating a delayed-type of hypersensitivity or killing virus-infected cells. Generation of humoral and cellular immune responses is summarized in Figure 27.1.

SOLUBLE MEDIATORS INVOLVED IN IMMUNE RESPONSES

Communication within the immune system occurs mainly through release of soluble factors by the cells that respond to the foreign agent. In addition, certain immune functions are also mediated by soluble factors. Most of these soluble factors are named *interleukins,* because they allow one type of leukocyte to influence the function of other leukocytes. Some of these mediators can in fact act on or be produced by cells outside of the immune system. The genes for most of these factors have been cloned so that they can be produced outside the body in large amounts. These recombinant DNA techniques have made it possible to use those factors in clinical trials in humans. The names and major actions of the soluble factors are summarized in Table 27.1. It should be noted that overproduction of some of these agents can lead to pathologic states, as in the production of tumor necrosis factor in shock.

Immunoglobulins, the soluble mediators of humoral immunity, are divided into five classes: IgM, IgG, IgA, IgE, and IgD (Table 27.2). The immunoglobulin molecule itself is comprised of two light chains and two heavy chains. Figure 27.2 is a schematic diagram of an antibody molecule. The light

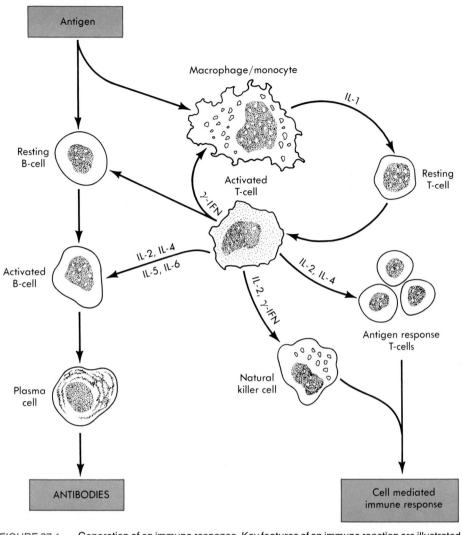

FIGURE 27.1   Generation of an immune response. Key features of an immune reaction are illustrated, with factors responsible for humoral immunity shown on the left and factors responsible for delayed, cell-mediated immunity shown on the right.

chain is made up of a variable region (V) and a constant region (C). Heavy chains contain three or four constant regions and the variable region. Each variable portion of the immunoglobulin molecule includes three hypervariable regions, which, as their name implies, vary widely in amino acid composition. The combination of these hypervariable regions makes up the antibody-combining site of the immunoglobulin molecule. This portion of the molecule actually binds the antigen against which the antibody was generated. Each antibody molecule has two combining sites.

Five different constant regions define the major immunoglobulin classes. IgG is the major immunoglobulin in serum and has four subclasses. Two subclasses of IgA molecules exist. IgG, IgE, and IgD

are monomeric, each composed of one antibody molecule. IgM is composed of five antibody molecules and IgA is composed of two. A protein, the J chain, joins the five basic molecules that make up the IgM molecule. Secretory component, synthesized by epithelial cells, connects the two IgA molecules that compose the dimer. Table 27.2 summarizes the immunoglobulin classes and their functions.

COMPLEMENT SYSTEM

Complement is a system of enzymes found in serum. The major functions of the complement system include opsonization, or coating, of antigenic particles (including microorganisms), causing damage to the membrane of pathogens which often re-

Table 27.1 Properties of Human Lymphokines

Lymphokine	Biologic properties
Interleukin-1 (IL-1)	Activates resting T cells; is a cofactor for hemopoietic growth factors; stimulates synthesis of lymphokines; increases natural killer cell activity; chemotaxin for neutrophils, lymphocytes, and macrophages.
Interleukin-2 (IL-2)	Growth factor for activated T cells; induces lymphokine production by T cells; activates cytotoxic T cells; increases natural killer cell activity; induces lymphokine-activated killer cells.
Interleukin-3 (IL-3)	Supports the growth of pluripotent bone marrow stem cells; growth factor for mast cells.
Interleukin-4 (IL-4)	Growth factor for activated B cells; induces class II histocompatibility antigens on B cells; growth factor for T cells; growth factor for mast cells; induces IgE synthesis.
Interleukin-5 (IL-5)	Induces differentiation of eosinophils; increases IgM and IgG secretion by activated B cells.
Interleukin-6 (IL-6)	Induces differentiation of activated B cells into plasma cells; growth factor for T cells.
Interleukin-7 (IL-7)	Growth factor for T cells.
Interferon-gamma (gamma-IFN)	Exerts antiviral activity; induces expression of class II histocompatibility antigens on macrophages; decreases IgE synthesis by B cells; increases natural killer cell activity.
Tumor Necrosis Factor (TNF)	Directly cytotoxic to some tumor cells; stimulates synthesis of lymphokines; activates macrophages; mediates inflammation and septic shock.

cell walls of some bacteria, cell walls of yeast, endotoxin derived from cell walls of gram-negative bacteria, aggregated IgA, and by a factor present in cobra venom.

Several steps in the complement cascade result in the release of a fragment of some of the proteins of the complement system. These small molecules are very potent mediators of a number of reactions. C3a and C5a are *chemotaxins* and *anaphylatoxins*. Chemotaxins are substances that cause phagocytic cells to migrate from an area where there is less chemotaxin to an area of higher concentration. Anaphylatoxins are molecules that cause mast cell degranulation, smooth muscle contraction, and increased capillary permeability. C3b opsonizes anything to which it binds. C3b and C5b activate the lytic pathway, leading to the formation of the membrane attack complex, a series of proteins with detergent properties that produce "holes" in the target cell membrane, resulting in lysis of the target cell.

sults in lysis of the pathogen, and mediating inflammatory responses. Nineteen distinct proteins make up the complement system. An enzyme cascade, proteins of the complement system interact such that the products of one reaction form the enzyme needed for the next step in the enzyme cascade. In this manner, a small stimulus can be amplified to activate large amounts of complement.

Complement can be activated by two pathways, the *classical* pathway and the *alternate* pathway. Both pathways share many components but differ in the ways in which they become activated. The classical pathway is activated by antigen-antibody complexes. The alternate pathway is activated by suitable surfaces or molecules including

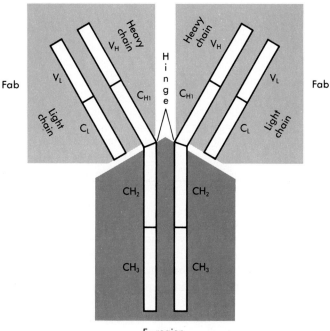

FIGURE 27.2 Schematic diagram of an antibody molecule. Heavy and light chains composed of variable (V_H, V_L) regions and constant (C_H, C_L) regions. The Fab portions of the molecule are responsible for antigen binding and the Fc portion mediates biological activity.

Table 27.2 Major Classes of Immunoglobulins

Class	Distribution	Biologic properties
IgG	Intra- and extravascular	Majority of secondary response to most antigens; activation of complement; opsonin; sensitize target cells for destruction by killer cells; neutralization of toxins and viruses; can pass placenta; immobilization of bacteria.
IgM	Mostly intravascular	First class produced during primary immune response; activates complement well; efficient agglutinating antibodies; natural isohemagglutinins.
IgA	Intravascular and secretions	Most common antibody in secretions where it protects mucous membranes; bactericidal in presence of lysozyme; efficient antiviral antibody.
IgE	On basophils and mast cells; in saliva and nasal secretions	Mediates hypersensitivity and allergic reactions; protection against parasite infections.
IgD	Surface of B lymphocytes; trace in serum	Serves as antigen-specific receptor on B cells; may be involved in differentiation of B lymphocytes.

IMMUNE SYSTEM DISORDERS AND PATHOLOGY

The immune system is very tightly regulated to ensure optimal function. Disorders in the development of immune cells, during the generation of immune responses, and/or in the synthesis of the products of the immune system may cause immunologic disorders ranging in severity from mild to fatal. The disorders can be classified into two broad categories: deficiencies of immune cells or their soluble products, and overproduction of immune cells or their products.

Immune deficiencies are divided into two groups—primary and secondary. *Primary immune deficiencies* are diseases in which the immune deficiency is the cause of the disease; they may be hereditary or acquired. *Secondary immune deficiencies* occur as a result of other disease(s). These patients invariably suffer from recurrent infections, and many times it is this development that leads to the diagnosis of an immune deficiency.

PRIMARY IMMUNE DEFICIENCIES

B cell deficiencies can result in the absence of one class of immunoglobulin or of all immunoglobulin classes. Persons with B cell deficiencies suffer mainly from recurrent bacterial infections. Although immunoglobulin replacement therapy may maintain them for as long as 20 to 30 years, the prognosis is poor, and many succumb to chronic lung disease.

T cell deficiencies affect not only cell-mediated immune responses, but also synthesis of antibody, as T cells are necessary for most antibody responses. Patients with T cell disorders are extremely susceptible to fungal, viral, and protozoal infections.

Severe combined immunodeficiencies are a result of defects in both T and B cells. As the name implies, these disorders are very serious. Untreated infants will rarely survive beyond 1 year of age. These patients are susceptible to every type of infection. Treatment with drugs alone is ineffective. Infants can be cured by bone marrow transplantation provided the transplantation is done before there are irreversible complications of the disease.

Phagocytic cell dysfunctions also give rise to severe disorders. Phagocytes play an important role in both innate and acquired immunity. Defects may be a consequence of deficiencies of antibody, lymphokines, or complement deficiencies, and can also result from defects within the cells themselves.

Abnormalities in the complement system can lead to immunodeficiencies. Not only is the complement system important in fighting infections, but it is thought that an intact complement system helps prevent diseases characterized by inappropriate response to the self. These diseases are termed *autoimmune* diseases. Genetic defects are associated with nearly all of the individual components of the complement system.

SECONDARY IMMUNE DEFICIENCIES

Secondary immunodeficiencies occur as complications of other diseases. Easily the most common cause of these disorders is the deliberate immune suppression associated with the use of chemotherapeutic agents in cancer treatment or the immunosuppressive drugs used to prevent rejection of transplanted organs. The best known secondary immune deficiency is the acquired immunodeficiency syndrome, or AIDS. This disease is caused by infection with human lymphotropic virus III, now called human immunodeficiency virus (HIV). A significant reason for the immune deficiency associated with AIDS is the loss of helper T cells. These cells are not the only immune cells affected by the virus, as the profound immune suppression associated with AIDS cannot be explained only on the basis of loss of helper T cells. Patients with secondary immunodeficiencies suffer severe recurrent infections by opportunistic organisms normally not pathogenic.

GAMMOPATHIES

Several neoplastic diseases arise as a result of abnormal proliferation of B cells and plasma cells. These diseases are termed *gammopathies*. The three principal gammopathies are multiple myeloma, macroglobulinemia, and heavy chain disease.

Multiple myeloma is the most common of the gammopathies, resulting from the malignant proliferation of plasma cells. The disease is characterized by synthesis of large amounts of a given isotype of immunoglobulin and may be accompanied by the production of free light chains (called Bence Jones proteins). Multiple myeloma involves multiple organ systems due to infiltration of them by malignant plasma cells. Patients are susceptible to recurrent bacterial and viral infections due to suppression of the synthesis of normal antibodies.

Macroglobulinemia occurs due to synthesis of large amounts of IgM. The excess immunoglobulin leads to increased viscosity of serum, and this in turn leads to decreased blood flow, thrombosis, disorders of the central nervous system, and bleeding. Decreased synthesis of the other immunoglobulin classes is observed, leading ultimately to hypogammaglobulinemia.

Heavy chain disease is characterized by the appearance of large amounts of protein in the serum and urine resembling the Fc portion of the immunoglobulin molecule. This disorder is uncommon. Patients have recurrent bacterial infections, anemias, and enlarged lymphoid organs.

SUMMARY

Two forms of immunity exist: innate and acquired. Innate immunity is constant and immediate, being conferred by physical, cellular, and chemical barriers. Acquired immunity arises in response to repeated exposure to antigen, and consists of humoral factors such as antibodies and cellular components that mediate delayed reactions. The cells of the immune system are white blood cells: lymphocytes, monocytes/macrophages, polymorphonuclear leukocytes (PMNs), basophils, and eosinophils. Macrophages and PMNs are the primary phagocytes. Lymphocytes of the B cell type produce antibody. T cell lymphocytes mediate delayed hypersensitivity and assist B cells. Bone marrow and thymus gland are classified as primary lymphoid organs because maturation of B cells occurs in the bone marrow and maturation of T cells occurs in the thymus. Secondary lymphoid organs (spleen, lymph nodes, Peyer's patches) are sites of antibody production and generation of antigen-specific T lymphocytes. Generation of an immune response requires activation, proliferation, and differentiation of specific cells. Soluble mediators called interleukins modulate these steps. The final products of B cells are also soluble factors called antibodies. The five classes of antibodies (IgG, IgM, IgA, IgE, IgD) serve different functions in the body. The complement system is an enzyme cascade that leads to production of soluble mediators which attract cells of the immune system to sites of infection and inflammation and can lead to lysis of foreign cells. Disorders of the immune system can result from deficiencies in T cells, B cells, macrophages, and components of the complement system, or overproduction of cells or soluble mediators of the immune system.

STUDY QUESTIONS

1. What is innate immunity?
2. Define acquired immunity.
3. What are the two forms of acquired immunity?
4. What white blood cell types are responsible for phagocytosis?
5. What are T cells? Where are they formed?
6. What are B cells? Where are they formed?
7. What cell type forms antibodies?
8. What cell type produces the delayed-type of hypersensitivity?
9. What are interleukins?
10. What are the five classes of antibodies?
11. What are the primary functions of each class of antibody?
12. What is the complement system?
13. What are the two major functions of the complement system?
14. Define primary and secondary immunodeficiency.
15. Define gammopathy.

SUGGESTED READINGS

Benjamini, E., and Leskowitz, S.: Immunology: a short course, New York, 1988, Alan R. Liss, Inc.

Delafuente, J.C.: Immunodeficiency diseases, in Pharmacotherapy: a pathophysiologic approach, edited by DiPiro, J.T. and others, New York, 1989, Elsevier, pp. 845–855.

Dinarello, C.A., and Mier, J.W.: Current concepts: lymphokines, N. Engl. J. Med. 317(15):940, 1987.

Fonger, P.A., and others: Nursing care of the child with severe combined immune deficiency . . . SCIDS, J. Pediatr. Nurs. 2(6):373, 1987.

Male, D.: Immunology: an illustrated outline, London, 1986, Gower.

O'Garra, A.: Peptide regulatory factors: interleukins and the immune system 1, Lancet 1:943, 1989.

O'Garra, A.: Peptide regulatory factors: interleukins and the immune system 2, Lancet 1:1003, 1989.

O'Garra, A., Umland, S., De France, T., and Christiansen, J.: B-cell factors are pleiotropic, Immunol. Today 9(2):45, 1988.

Pohl, L.R., and others: The immunologic and metabolic basis of drug hypersensitivities, Am. Rev. Pharmacol. 28:367, 1988.

Reckling, J.B., and Neuberger, G.B.: Understanding immune system dysfunction, Nursing87 17(9):34, 1987.

Tartaglione, T.A., and Collier, A.C.: Principles and management of the acquired immunodeficiency syndrome in Pharmacotherapy: a pathophysiologic approach, edited by DiPiro, J.T. and others, New York, 1989, Elsevier, pp. 1306–1334.

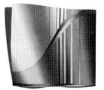

Immunomodulators

28

Drugs That Stimulate or Enhance the Immune System

Enhancement of the immune system can be accomplished by two methods, both falling in the category of acquired immunity. *Active acquired immunity* refers to the administration of substances, such as vaccines, that stimulate the immune system to produce a response against a foreign material. Vaccines usually contain killed or attenuated bacteria or viruses, but protection can also be conferred with immunogenic proteins or toxoids from the pathogen in question (Tables 28.1 and 28.2). Once the immune response has occurred, "memory" of the response is retained by specific cells in the immune system, and a secondary immune response will occur rapidly upon a subsequent encounter with the antigen. This principle is illustrated in Figure 28.1. Active immunity usually persists for years.

Passive acquired immunity refers to the administration of preformed substances, such as immune serum or antibodies, that can immediately combat the foreign agent to which they are directed. The passive immunity conferred by immune sera, antibodies, or globulins lasts only a matter of weeks.

FETAL AND NEONATAL IMMUNITY AND IMMUNIZATION

The fetus is protected from bacterial and viral infections and from microbial toxins by maternal IgG antibodies, which pass to the fetus through the placenta to confer passive immunity. Immunoglobulin G is the only antibody that is able to cross the placenta. Newborn infants do not have a fully functional immune system; human milk, however, contains factors that aid the newborn response against infectious agents. Some of these factors enhance the growth of beneficial intestinal flora, while others nonspecifically inhibit the growth of harmful microorganisms. The inhibitory factors include lysozyme, lactoferrin, interferon, and leukocytes. Antibodies are also found in breast milk and are especially abundant in colostrum (first milk). Immunizations can begin when the infant is 2 months of age and is able to mount an effective immune response on its own. Table 28.3 indicates the recommended schedule for active immunizations.

ABSORPTION AND FATE OF IMMUNOSTIMULANTS

Intramuscular (IM) injection is the usual route of administration of the immune serums and globulins (Table 28.4). Oral administration is not usually possible with these agents as the degradative processes in the digestive tract would render them inactive before they could be absorbed. Distribution is fairly rapid after IM injection, but if very rapid therapy is required, these agents can be given intravenously, resulting in immediate distribution. The immunity provided by immune globulins and serums lasts from 1 to 6 weeks. Once injected, the antibodies interact with the entire organism against which they were generated, thus facilitating phagocytosis of the organism by monocytes/macrophages and PMNs. Antibodies made against toxins of pathogenic microorganisms form complexes with the toxin, and these immune complexes are also cleared by phagocytes. Immunity is lost as the injected antibodies are cleared from the system.

Vaccines are administered by either IM or subcutaneous (SC) injection (Table 28.4). Two exceptions to these routes are smallpox vaccine, which is given intradermally (ID), and oral poliovaccine.

Table 28.1   Vaccines Useful in Preventing Bacterial and Rickettsial Diseases

Disease	Vaccine characteristics	Vaccine administration
Bubonic plague	Inactivated *Yersinia pestis* confers immunity.	Administered during outbreaks or to persons heavily exposed.
Cholera	Killed strains of *Vibrio cholerae* confer resistance.	Used in persons entering a country where cholera is known to exist.
Diphtheria, tetanus, and pertussis (whooping cough)	This combination, known as DTP, contains absorbed toxoids and a vaccine to protect against all three diseases.	Given routinely to children between the ages of 2 months and 7 years. In event of injury additional protection against tetanus may be needed.
Haemophilus influenzae type B	Based upon polysaccharide from the organism.	Recommended for all children 2 years of age or older.
Meningitis	Meningococcal polysaccharide mixtures give protection against group A, group C, or both.	Used only in outbreaks or in exposed persons who also receive antibiotics to protect against infections by serogroup B.
Pneumococcal pneumonia	Mixed capsular material from cultured pneumococci confers resistance to lobar pneumonia and bacteremia caused by one of the strains used as a source of capsular material.	Given only to high-risk patients, weak convalescents, or patients over 50 years of age.
Tetanus and diphtheria	Mixed absorbed toxoids are used in patients over 6 years.	Used for routine prophylaxis in patients who have not received DTP.
Tetanus toxoid	Absorbed tetanus toxoid confers immunity	May be used for routine immunization but DTP is preferred. Most commonly given following an injury that poses risk of tetanus infection.
Tuberculosis	Attenuated strain of *Mycobacterium bovis* confers variable temporary immunity.	Given to exposed but uninfected patients who cannot receive drug therapy.
Typhoid	Killed *Salmonella typhosa* gives prolonged protection.	Used in persons known to have been exposed or persons traveling where typhoid is endemic.
Typhus	Killed *Rickettsia prowazekii* confers resistance.	Given to persons entering areas where exposure to the louse-born disease is likely.

Duration of protection is usually from 1 to 10 years. Since vaccines stimulate the recipient's immune system to respond actively rather than providing passive protection, as discussed above, protection persists even after the injected agent has disappeared. The fate of vaccines is similar to that of immune globulins. As vaccines are antigens and not antibodies, they are taken up and processed by antigen-presenting cells as described in Chapter 27 for the generation of immune responses. Some, but not necessarily all, of the injected agent will be metabolized in this manner. Once antibodies have been produced, any remaining injected material can become complexed with the antibodies and cleared by phagocytes.

SIDE EFFECTS AND TOXICITY OF IMMUNOSTIMULANTS

Many of the known side effects of immune serum or globulin injections are dose-related. Patients may have pain at the injection site, mild chest pain, and chills. Less common side effects include malaise, headache, nausea and vomiting, dyspnea, faintness, and back pain. Hepatitis B immune glob-

**Table 28.2   Vaccines Useful in
Preventing Viral Diseases**

Disease	Characteristics of vaccine
Poliomyelitis	Oral vaccine containing attenuated live poliovirus mimics natural form of the disease without risk of central nervous system involvement.
Rubella (German measles)	Attenuated live rubella vaccine confers long-term resistance.
Measles (rubeola)	Attenuated live virus vaccine stimulates protective antibodies in 95% of children receiving vaccine.
Mumps	Attenuated live virus vaccine stimulates protective antibodies in 95% of those receiving vaccine.
Influenza	Inactivated viruses of types causing recent outbreaks. Differs from year to year.
Smallpox	Success of vaccination is judged by response at vaccination site.
Yellow fever	Live attenuated virus confers resistance to most persons receiving vaccine.
Rabies	Killed, fixed virus confers resistance to most patients exposed to infection.
Hepatitis	Developed from surface antigens from hepatitis B virus.

ulin can also cause urticaria and angioedema. Varicella zoster immune globulin injections can result in a mild rash, usually observed 10 to 14 days after immunization.

Immune serums, especially those employing nonhuman proteins, can cause anaphylaxis in patients with a history of hypersensitivity reactions to immune globulin injections. This serum sickness is due to an immune response directed against proteins in the injected serum. Massive immune complex formation occurs, followed by deposition of these complexes in the kidney and circulatory system leading to nephritis and arteritis. The deposited immune complexes also initiate mediator release from platelets, basophils, and PMNs. This massive mediator release can be life-threatening. A local deposition of insoluble immune complexes at the site of injection produces the Arthus reaction, in which redness and edema occur near blood ves-

sels. Caution must always be taken when injections of foreign serum are repeated. Other signs of serum sickness include arthralgia, lymphadenopathy, and pruritus. In serious cases abdominal pain, fever, headache, and malaise may be present. Use of immune serums may be contraindicated in patients with thrombocytopenia, as excessive bleeding may occur at the site of injection. Live virus vaccines should not be used in patients receiving immunosuppressive therapy, as these vaccines have the potential to cause progressive disease in immunocompromised patients. Live virus vaccines are also contraindicated in pregnant women, as they have the potential to damage the fetus.

DRUG INTERACTIONS

There are no known drug interactions associated with the use of the passive immunostimulants, immune serum, and globulins. All immunosuppressive agents have the potential of interfering with the generation of active immunity induced by vaccines and toxoids. Corticosteroids, azathioprine, cyclosporine, and a variety of agents used in cancer chemotherapy are immunosuppressives that fall in this category.

INTERFERONS AND INTERLEUKINS

The interferons and interleukins, especially interleukin-2 (IL-2), are new forms of therapy whose use is growing rapidly. Both interferons and interleukins are employed mainly in the treatment of cancer. Interferons exhibit direct antiproliferative effects, while the anticancer effects of interleukin-2 are indirect. Interleukin-2 stimulates a population of lymphocytes to become killer cells capable of destroying tumor cells. Since therapy with these agents can be life-threatening, they warrant special consideration.

These agents were initially thought to be devoid of significant toxicity since they are natural human substances. However, in early trials, four cancer patients treated with alpha-interferon died. This event led to a careful examination of the effects of the interferons and interleukins administered to human subjects. Though these substances occur in the body naturally at very low concentrations, therapy with them usually involves administration of high doses, which leads to a wide range of adverse reactions. Their toxic effects are summarized in Table 28.5. It should be noted that these reactions refer to intravenous administration. No toxic effects have been reported following local injection into tissue. In the trials, the major dose-limiting effect of the interferons was severe fatigue.

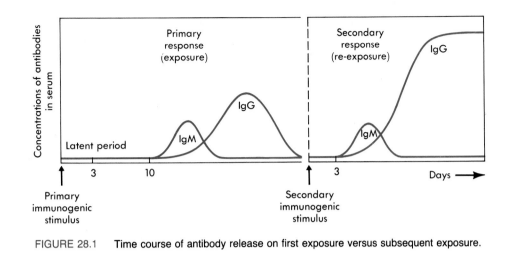

FIGURE 28.1   Time course of antibody release on first exposure versus subsequent exposure.

Marked fluid retention due to a generalized increase in vascular permeability is the most serious adverse reaction of IL-2 therapy.

Drugs That Suppress the Immune System

Immunosuppressive drugs are used in two important clinical areas—organ transplantation and autoimmune diseases. Patients who have received kidney, heart, liver, bone marrow, or skin allografts require immunosuppressive agents to prevent rejection of the foreign graft by their immune system. Combinations of these agents are sometimes necessary during a rejection episode. Certain immunosuppressive drugs are used only immediately following transplantation. The major immunosuppressive drugs are listed in Table 28.6.

Corticosteroids are immunosuppressive agents commonly given to treat autoimmune disorders such as rheumatoid arthritis. Prednisone was the drug of choice for maintenance immunosuppression in organ transplantation before the advent of cyclosporine. Methylprednisolone and another immunosuppressive agent, azathioprine, were routinely used during a rejection episode. Steroid immunosuppressive drugs are thought to bind to cytoplasmic receptors and to be carried into the cell's nucleus, where they alter cellular metabolism. These drugs markedly reduce certain populations of lymphocytes. The corticosteroids are discussed in more detail in Chapter 51.

Certain *anticancer agents* are also used as

Table 28.3   Active Immunization Schedule

Age	Vaccine
2 months	Diphtheria, tetanus, pertussis (DTP-1), trivalent oral polio (TOP-1)
4 months	DTP-2, TOP-2
6 months	DTP-3, TOP-3
15 months	Measles, mumps, rubella
18 months	DTP-4, TOP-4, *Haemophilus influenzae* Type B
4-6 years	DTP-5, TOP-5
14-16 years (and each 10 years thereafter)	Tetanus toxoid and reduced adult dose of diphtheria toxoid
18-24 years	Measles, mumps (especially for susceptible males), rubella
25-64 years	Measles (for persons born after 1956), mumps (especially for susceptible males), rubella (for females up to 45 years)
>65 years	Influenza, pneumococcus

Data from Benjamini, E., and Leskowitz, S.: Immunology—a short course, 1988, New York, Alan R. Liss, p. 334.

Table 28.4 Clinical Use of Major Immunostimulants

Generic name	Route	Duration of effect	Contraindications
Antirabies serum	IM	3 wk	Allergy to equine serum
Cholera vaccine	IM, SC	6 mo	Previous allergic reaction to vaccine
Crotaline antivenin, polyvalent	IV	3 wk	Allergy to equine serum
Digoxin immune Fab	IV; ID: for allergy testing	1 wk	Allergy to sheep products or serum products
Diphtheria antitoxin	IV, IM	3 wk	Allergy to equine serum; pregnancy
Diphtheria toxoid, adsorbed	IM: children 6 wk to 6 yr; second dose 6 to 8 wk after first; third dose 1 yr after second dose	10 yr	CNS disease; not used in adults
Diphtheria and tetanus toxoids	IM: adults only	10 yr; boosters required	History of neurologic reaction to diphtheria-tetanus toxoids
Diphtheria and tetanus toxoids and adsorbed pertussis vaccine	IM: children: 6 wk to 6 yr—four doses at 2, 4, 6, 18 mo; booster at 4 to 6 yr	10 yr; boosters required for tetanus toxoid	Encephalopathy, seizures, or other signs of CNS damage; not used in adults
H. influenzae type B vaccine	SC: children: 1.5 to 4 yr	Not clearly known	Children younger than 1.5 yr or older than 5 yr; not used in adults
Hepatitis B vaccine	IM, SC: 3 doses; second dose 1 mo after first; third 6 mo after first dose	At least 5 yr	Severe cardiovascular disease with pulmonary dysfunction; pregnancy
Immune globulin	IV, IM	4 wk, more often if needed	Selective IgA deficiency; thrombocytopenia; pregnancy
Influenza virus vaccine	IM: adults and children over 12 yr—single dose; children 3 to 12 yr—2 doses 4 or more wk apart	1 yr	Allergy to eggs or chicken; history of Guillain-Barre syndrome; pregnancy
Measles virus vaccine live	SC	8 yr or longer	Immune deficiencies; febrile seizures or cerebral trauma; pregnancy; women should not become pregnant within 3 months after vaccination
Mumps virus vaccine live	SC	Permanent immunity (develops in only 75-90% of patients receiving vaccine)	Immune deficiencies; pregnancy; women should not become pregnant within 3 months after vaccination
Pertussis immune globulin	IM	3 weeks	Hypersensitivity to IgG; not used in adults
Pneumococcal vaccine polyvalent	IM, SC	Months to years, exact duration not known	Recent pneumococcal pneumonia; children under 2 yr; pregnancy

Table 28.4   Clinical Use of Major Immunostimulants—cont'd

Generic name	Route	Duration of effect	Contraindications
Poliovirus vaccine in-activated	SC: 4 doses; adults—first 2 doses at least 4 wk apart; third and fourth doses a few mo apart; children—first 3 doses at 4 to 8 wk intervals; final dose 6 to 12 mo after third dose	Years, exact duration not known	Acute febrile illness; pregnancy
Poliovirus vaccine live oral	ORAL: adults—single dose but adults should receive inactivated vaccine; children—3 doses; two schedules—6 to 12 wk, 8 wk later, 8 to 12 mo after second dose or at 2, 4, 18 mo	Years, exact duration not known	Elderly; pregnancy except single doses may be given when rapid immunization is needed
Rabies immune globulin	IM	3 wk	Thrombocytopenia
Rabies vaccine	IM	Years; boosters may be required	None
Rh_o (D) immune globulin	IM	3 wk; treatment required after each subsequent pregnancy	RH_o (D) positive blood type; elderly
Rubella virus vaccine live	SC	Years; boosters not recommended although exact duration not known	Immune deficiencies; recent treatment with blood products or immune globulins; pregnancy; women should not become pregnant within 3 months after vaccination
Smallpox vaccine	ID	Complete protection for 1 to 3 yr; significant protection for 20 yr	Viral diseases other than smallpox; pregnancy
Tetanus antitoxin	IM, SC	3 wk	Allergy to equine serum; pregnancy
Tetanus immune globulin	IM	32 days	Allergic reactions to immune globulins; pregnancy
Tetanus toxoid	IM, SC: tetanus toxoid only if SC	10 years; boosters required	Prior reactions to tetanus toxoid preparations; children under 6 wk of age; pregnancy
Typhoid vaccine	SC, ID: 2 doses 4 wk apart	3 years; boosters can be given when needed	Severe febrile illness; pregnancy
Varicella-zoster immune globulin	IM	3 to 4 wk	Allergy to immunoglobulin; pregnancy
Yellow fever vaccine	SC	10 years; boosters may be given when needed	Allergy to eggs or chicken; immune deficiencies; pregnancy

Table 28.5   Toxic Effects of Interleukin-2 and Interferons

Immunomodulator	Common effects
Alpha-interferon	Neurotoxicity (fatigue, lethargy) Hematological (leukopenia, neutropenia, thrombocytopenia) Allergic (skin reaction, fever, chills) Gastrointestinal (anorexia, diarrhea, nausea) Other (tachycardia, headache, myalgia, arthralgia)
Beta-interferon	As for alpha-interferon, but fever and gastrointestinal side effects, and less thrombocytopenia
Gamma-interferon	Similar to beta-interferon
Interleukin-2	Cardiovascular/renal (fluid retention, elevated serum creatinine) Neurotoxicity (fatigue, lethargy) Hematological (anemia) Hepatic (hyperbilirubinemia) Pulmonary (interstitial edema, dyspnea)

immunosuppressants. Cyclophosphamide, methotrexate, and mercaptopurine are employed when the goal is to severely suppress immune function or to aid in complete destruction of the immune system before bone marrow transplantation. Drugs of this type function by blocking proliferation of cells of the immune system. When used in this manner, they are usually combined with whole body irradiation or total lymphoid irradiation. These agents are discussed in more detail in Chapter 39.

Anti-thymocyte globulin (ATG), or serum and *antilymphocyte globulin (ALG)* or *serum* are employed in organ transplantation, usually during the first 14 to 28 days after surgery or during an acute rejection episode. Antibodies in these preparations bind to lymphocytes, leading either to their destruction or to inhibition of their actions. These agents are usually produced in horses, though goats and rabbits may be used for this purpose if allergic reactions to the equine material occur.

Muromonab-CD3 is a monoclonal antibody directed against the CD-3 molecule present on the surface of all T lymphocytes. Monoclonal antibodies are much more specific than antibodies prepared against whole lymphocytes, since the antibody can bind only to cells that express the CD-3 molecule. Other cells of the immune system are thus spared

the effects of the antibody preparation. Muromonab-CD3 is utilized to prepare bone marrow before infusion, to rid the marrow of immunocompetent cells and increase the likelihood that only stem cells will be injected. This process aids in preventing graft-versus-host disease, which is a common and possibly fatal outcome of bone marrow transplantation. Muromonab-CD3 is also used during graft rejection when other therapy has proved ineffective.

Azathioprine functions in a manner similar to that of the antiproliferative drugs discussed above. While this drug does exert effects in its native form, it can be converted in the body to mercaptopurine, which may account for its immunosuppressive action.

Cyclosporine is rapidly becoming the drug of choice for immunosuppression in organ transplantation. Originally isolated from fungi found in soil, it is currently being made synthetically. Cyclosporine, unlike most of the other immunosuppressive agents, is relatively selective for cells of the immune system, especially the helper subset of T lymphocytes. Myelosuppression, a common problem with many immunosuppressive drugs, is not seen with cyclosporine. Cyclosporine may produce its effects by preventing synthesis of IL-2 by activated helper T lymphocytes. It can be used in maintenance immunosuppression in kidney transplantation without the need for any other agents, and is combined with low doses of corticosteroids in liver and heart transplantation.

ABSORPTION AND FATE OF IMMUNOSUPPRESSANTS

Absorption and fate of the corticosteroids are discussed in detail in Chapter 51, and the anticancer agents are discussed in Chapter 39.

The usual route of administration of antilymphocyte globulin and antithymocyte globulin is by intravenous infusion. Distribution is therefore immediate. The half-life of equine IgG is 6 days. Small amounts of these preparations can be given intradermally to test for allergic responses to the material. A wheal with localized erythema and edema observed within 60 minutes of injection indicates a positive test and may prohibit safe administration of the globulin.

Muromonab-CD3 is given by rapid IV injection. Immediately upon administration, the antibody binds to CD-3 positive T lymphocytes. Its effects persist for about 1 week after therapy is discontinued.

Azathioprine is usually given orally but can be given IV immediately following surgery until the patient is able to tolerate oral dosing. The drug is

Table 28.6   Major Immunosuppressants in Clinical Use

Generic name	Route	Half-life	Contraindications
Antithymocyte globulin	INTRAVENOUS: daily for 14 days then alternate days for 14 days; ID: for allergy testing	6 days	Previous allergy to equine materials or serum products; pregnancy
Antihuman lymphocyte globulin	INTRAMUSCULAR, INTRAVENOUS: single dose prior to transplantation with prednisone, daily after transplantation for 4 weeks, alternate days for weeks 5 and 6, every third day until patient leaves hospital	6 days	Known allergy to equine materials or serum products; pregnancy
Azathioprine sodium	ORAL: daily for transplantation until patient leaves hospital; IV: until patient can tolerate oral dose	In plasma-1 hr	Renal impairment; pregnancy
Cyclosporine	ORAL: single daily dose, first dose preceding transplantation; IV: single dose by infusion until patient can tolerate oral dose	19 to 27 hr	Allergy; pregnancy
Muromonab-CD3	INTRAVENOUS: daily by rapid injection for 10 to 14 days	Effect lasts for 1 wk	Recent exposure to chickenpox or herpes zoster; fluid overload or pulmonary edema; fever above 37.8° C; pregnancy; dose in children not established

readily absorbed orally, is distributed rapidly throughout the tissues, and is metabolized extensively. Metabolites of azathiprone, including the antiproliferative compound mercaptopurine, are excreted by the kidney.

Cyclosporine is available as both an oral and an IV solution. As with azathioprine, IV injections can be given until the patient can take oral doses. Bioavailability after oral doses of cyclosporine is variable. Maximum absorption is about 30%. Peak plasma levels are observed 3.5 hours after an oral dose. Because of its relatively high lipid solubility, cyclosporine is distributed to most tissues and fluids including the fetus and breast milk. The drug is extensively metabolized by the liver, and a first-pass effect is observed following oral administration. The elimination half-time for cyclosporine is variable, ranging from 19 to 27 hours. Metabolized drug appears in the bile but little is seen in urine.

SIDE EFFECTS AND TOXICITY OF IMMUNOSUPPRESSANTS

Two important complications are shared by virtually all immunosuppressant drugs—increased incidence of infections and of certain cancers, predominantly lymphomas. The increased incidence of infection is especially noteworthy as many of these infections are unusual and difficult to treat. The risk of developing cancer is confirmed when patients are carefully monitored over months and years, and their incidence of cancer is compared to that of age-matched controls.

Antithymocyte globulin and antilymphocyte globulin share certain side effects. Lymphocytopenia is the desired action of these drugs but a more general leukocytopenia may develop. Thrombocytopenia may also occur. The incidence of leukocytopenia and thrombocytopenia can be as high as 20%. Fever and malaise are common and should be expected during the early phases of therapy. Allergic reactions ranging from local skin reactions to serum sickness and anaphylaxis may be observed in 15% of patients. Gastrointestinal upset, marked by diarrhea, nausea, vomiting, and abdominal distention, can result from treatment with antithymocyte globulin. Cardiovascular problems, including hypotension, hypertension, tachycardia, generalized and pulmonary edema, and chest pain, have occurred with antithymocyte globulin therapy. Hypoglycemia is possible, and diabetic patients should be monitored closely. CNS involvement is less common but can include seizures.

Azathioprine therapy is limited by a number of side effects. Bone marrow suppression is the most common toxic effect limiting use of the drug. In-

THE NURSING PROCESS

IMMUNOMODULATORS

Assessment

Patients receiving immunomodulators may present with no health problems—such as those receiving routine immunizations—to those critically ill with cancers, tissue rejection, or AIDS. Assessment is based on the age of the patient, severity of the presenting problems, acuity level, and planned drug intervention.

Nursing diagnoses

Potential complication: immunosuppression and risk of infection

Potential complication: serum sickness

Management

The nurse should monitor the vital signs and temperature, and appropriate laboratory work, including the complete blood count, white blood cell differential, and platelet count. Seriously ill patients will require more extensive and frequent monitoring. Because the field of immunotherapy is changing rapidly, new guidelines may be available, and new side effects recognized. Study the manufacturer's current literature for update information.

Evaluation

Immunizations are successful if the disease is prevented, with a minimum of side effects. In organ transplant, success is measured by a slowing of the rejection process. In cancers, immunomodulators may slow disease progression, and perhaps eventually lead to cure. In AIDS, ongoing research with immunomodulators may lead to significant extension of life, or eventually to cure or prevention. Before discharge, review with patients any side effects of drug therapy, and make certain they feel free to call the physician or nurse with questions or concerns.

---

dications of bone marrow suppression include leukocytopenia, macrocytic anemia, pancytopenia, and thrombocytopenia which can lead to unexplained bleeding and bruising. Anorexia, nausea, vomiting, and diarrhea occur, especially with large doses. Toxic hepatitis with biliary stasis, leading to jaundice, may be observed in renal transplantation patients. Allergic reactions can accompany azathioprine therapy. Rashes, fever, and serum sickness may arise.

Complications associated with cyclosporine therapy involve nearly every physiological system. Nephrotoxicity is the dose-limiting toxic effect of cyclosporine. This toxicity is dose related, with up to 38% of patients showing an elevated BUN and serum creatinine. Tremor develops in up to 50% of treated patients. Less common are confusion, headaches, flushing, and seizures. Hypertension also is seen in up to 50% of patients, and may require treatment with antihypertensives. Anemia, leukopenia, and thrombocytopenia are rare. Gastrointestinal symptoms include diarrhea, nausea, and vomiting, with reports of gastrointestinal bleeding. Hirsutism develops in one quarter to nearly one half of patients, and acne may also appear. Hepatotoxicity is seen in a small percentage of patients; it is usually reversed when doses are lowered. Cyclosporine may induce lymphomas, especially when given in conjunction with other immunosuppressive agents. Lastly, gingival hyperplasia develops in 30% of treated patients.

Muromonab-CD3 has several toxic effects associated with the first dose, which seldom recur upon subsequent doses. Trembling and shaking of hands, chest pain, diarrhea, nausea, and vomiting fall in this category. Allergic symptoms are also common after the first dose, but persistence of these symptoms should be investigated. Causes include infection, severe pulmonary edema, and fluid overload.

DRUG INTERACTIONS

Treatment with immunosuppressive drugs in general will lead to decreased effectiveness of any

PATIENT CARE IMPLICATIONS

Vaccines

- Any serum product containing proteins such as immunoglobulins can cause acute allergic reactions and an allergic reaction called serum sickness (see text). Review with patients the signs and symptoms of serum sickness, and instruct patients to notify the physician if it develops. Note that serum sickness may not develop for up to 6 to 12 days after immunization.
- Have available epinephrine 1:1000 solution in settings where protein-containing products are administered. Have drugs, equipment, and personnel available to treat acute allergic reactions.
- Question women about the possibility of pregnancy before administering. Live virus vaccines are contraindicated in pregnant women.
- For IM administration, use anatomical landmarks in selecting injection sites. Use the deltoid muscle for administration of most vaccines and similar medications of older children and adults. Usually, avoid the injection sites in the gluteal area unless large-volume doses must be divided into two or more injections or the patient is receiving two or more drugs that cannot be administered in the same site. Use the vastus lateralis in infants and small children. Aspirate before injecting drug to avoid inadvertent IV administration; if blood is aspirated, withdraw needle, discard syringe and needle, and prepare a fresh dose.
- Review manufacturer's instructions when preparing unfamiliar medications.
- Sensitivity tests may be ordered on patients prior to administering the full dose for the following immunostimulants: antirabies serum, crotaline antivenin (snakebite antivenin), diphtheria antitoxin, tetanus antitoxin. Consult physician, and read manufacturer's literature.

Patient and family education

- Review with patients the anticipated benefits and possible side effects of drug therapy. With small children, if regular immunizations usually cause a fever, suggest that the mother use acetaminophen to treat this side effect (consult physician).
- Warn patient to avoid scratching injection sites. Brief application of an ice pack may lessen irritation.

- When appropriate, review with patients the schedule for additional doses of immunizations.
- Refer patients to the local health department if appropriate.
- Instruct patients who manifest an allergic response to wear a medication identification tag or bracelet listing the allergic response, and to be cautious in taking vaccines or immunomodulators without consulting the physician.

Interferons

Drug administration

- Review the side effects listed in Table 28.5.
- Assess for development of side effects. Be alert to signs of depression: insomnia, weight loss, withdrawal, anorexia, lack of interest in personal appearance.
- Monitor pulse and blood pressure. Auscultate lung sounds and heart sounds. Monitor intake, output, and weight.

Patient and family education

- Review anticipated benefits and possible side effects of drug therapy.
- Review the dosing schedule, and discuss with patients what to do if a dose is missed, in the event that they are self-administering these drugs in the home setting. Make certain they can inject dose correctly.
- Warn patients to avoid driving or operating hazardous equipment if fatigue or dizziness develops.
- These drugs often cause a flu-like reaction, with fever, chills, and headache. Consult with physician about appropriate instructions for the patient related to notifying the doctor and self-medicating with antipyretics.
- Do not change to other brands of interferon without consulting the physician.
- Avoid other drugs which may also cause drowsiness or fatigue, unless specifically approved by the physician.
- Review Patient Problem: Depressed White Blood Cell Count on p. 599.
- Take doses at night to lessen daytime fatigue.

Interleukins

Drug administration

- Review the information given in Table 28.5 for interferons, above.
- Monitor weight, and assess for edema. Monitor blood pressure.

Continued.

PATIENT CARE IMPLICATIONS — cont'd

- Consult manufacturer's literature for current guidelines.

Glucocorticoids
- These drugs are discussed in Chapter 51.

Antithymocyte globulin

Drug administration
- Monitor blood pressure and pulse. Auscultate breath sounds. Assess for jugular venous distention. Monitor intake, output, and weight, and inspect for skin changes.
- Monitor complete blood count and differential, platelet count, blood glucose levels, serum electrolytes.
- Thrombophlebitis is common. Assess the IV line for patency before administering. Instruct the patient to report pain or redness at the IV site.
- Fistulas or shunts may clot in some patients. Assess fistulas or shunts per agency procedure (through palpation or auscultation) at least every 2 hours while the patient is receiving this drug. If the patient knows how to assess shunts or fistulas, engage the patient in monitoring also.

Patient and family education
- Review anticipated benefits and possible side effects of drug therapy. Note that serum sickness may develop (see text). Teach patients that serum sickness may not develop for up to 10 to 14 days following drug therapy.
- Instruct diabetic patients to monitor blood glucose levels carefully, as antithymocyte globulin may cause changes in blood glucose levels.
- See Patient Problem: Depressed White Blood Cell Count (p. 599) and Patient Problem: Bleeding Tendencies (p. 600).

Antihuman lymphocyte globulin

Drug administration
- Assess blood pressure, temperature, and pulse. Inspect for skin changes.
- Monitor complete blood count and differential.
- See manufacturer's literature for current guidelines.

Patient and family education
- Review anticipated benefits and possible side effects of drug therapy. Note that serum sickness may develop (see text). Teach patients

that serum sickness may not develop for up to 10 to 14 days following drug therapy.
- See Patient Problem: Depressed White Blood Cell Count (p. 599) and Patient Problem: Bleeding Tendencies (p. 600).

Muromonab-CD3

Drug administration/patient and family education
- Monitor blood pressure and pulse. Remain with the patient for 15 to 30 minutes after the first dose. Chest pain may follow the first dose, but is rare thereafter.
- Forewarn patients that trembling and shaking of the hands following the first dose is common.
- Monitor intake, output, and weight. Auscultate breath sounds.
- See manufacturer's literature for current guidelines.

Azathioprine

Drug administration
- Monitor intake, output, and weight. Assess for skin changes.
- Monitor complete blood count and differential, platelet count, liver function tests.
  INTRAVENOUS ADMINISTRATION
- Reconstitute as directed on the vial. A solution of 10 mg/ml may be given by direct IV injection or further diluted in 0.9% sodium chloride or 5% dextrose. Administer ordered dose over 30 to 60 minutes.

Patient and family education
- Review the benefits and possible side effects of drug therapy.
- Tell patients that weeks to months of therapy with this drug may be necessary for full benefit to be seen.
- Warn patients that serum sickness may occur, but may not develop for 10 to 14 days after taking a dose.
- Review Patient Problem: Depressed White Blood Cell Count (p. 599) and Patient Problem: Bleeding Tendencies (p. 600).
- Take oral doses after meals to lessen gastric irritation.
- Do not have any immunizations while taking this drug without first consulting with the physician.
- Oral ulcers may develop. See Patient Problem: Stomatitis on p. 601.

PATIENT CARE IMPLICATIONS—cont'd

Cyclosporine

Drug administration

- See information on the side effects, listed in the text.
- Monitor blood pressure and pulse. Monitor intake, output, and weight. Inspect teeth and gums regularly.
- Monitor complete blood count and differential, liver function tests, BUN, and serum creatinine.
- Review manufacturer's instructions when preparing oral doses, as doses must be measured with a dropper, then diluted.
  INTRAVENOUS ADMINISTRATION
- Dilute each 50 mg in 20 to 100 ml of 0.9% sodium chloride or 5% dextrose in water. Infuse over 2 to 6 hours. Monitor vital signs.

Patient and family education

- Review the anticipated benefits and possible side effects of drug therapy.
- Warn patients that tremor may develop.
- Warn patients to avoid driving or operating hazardous equipment if confusion develops; notify physician.
- Instruct patients not to stop therapy without consulting the physician.
- Reinforce the importance of regular dental hygiene including flossing, brushing, and visits to the dentist.
- Do not have any immunizations while taking cyclosporine without physician approval.

---

therapy whose purpose is to enhance immunity. Live vaccines are contraindicated with most immunosuppressants, as their use can lead to serious, even fatal, disease—instead of immunity. Combination therapy with two or more immunosuppressive agents can profoundly impair normal host defense mechanisms, in turn progressing to increased risk of infection or development of malignancies, especially lymphomas.

Antithymocyte globulin or antilymphocyte globulin administration can enhance the effectiveness of other immunosuppressive agents given at the same time, which further impairs host defenses. This may be life-threatening, or may lead to blood dyscrasias.

Allopurinol interferes with the metabolism of azathioprine, leading to accumulation of azathioprine and thus increasing the risk of bone marrow suppression.

Cyclosporine-induced nephrotoxicity precludes the use of aminoglycoside antibiotics. Amphotericin B should similarly be avoided. Administration of corticosteroids and ketoconazole may provoke an increase in the serum level of cyclosporine by diminishing the normal hepatic metabolism of the latter.

IMMUNOTOXINS

With recombinant DNA technology a new class of agents has been developed that may allow for more selective therapy in organ transplantation,

treatment of cancer, and treatment of AIDS. *Immunotoxins* are drugs that contain a highly toxic agent coupled to a protein that selectively binds to the cells rejecting transplanted organs, cancer cells, or cells infected with the human immunodeficiency virus (HIV).

Early immunotoxins were monoclonal antibodies to tumor antigens, coupled chemically to ricin, an agent that inactivates ribosomes, thereby preventing protein synthesis and leading to cell death. One molecule of ricin was sufficient to kill a cell. Animal studies showed limited success with the immunotoxins. A critical problem with monoclonal antibodies directed against tumor antigens is that they frequently cross-react with normal tissue. New immunotoxins were developed to overcome this problem. *Pseudomonas* exotoxin is composed of three domains: one for binding to the cell and one for translocation into the cell; the third inactivates elongation factor 2 and prevents protein synthesis. By joining the DNA sequences for the translocation and toxic domains of the exotoxin with DNA sequences that code for proteins targeting the immunotoxin, agents have been produced that are highly and selectively toxic against human cells. Similarly, diphtheria toxin has been used in animal studies. This toxin cannot be administered in humans once they are immunized against diphtheria. In mice, toxin coupled to interleukin-2 (IL-2) has been shown to prolong survival of transplanted hearts. The cells that reject the graft express receptors for IL-2, which can bind the immunotoxin, and can be killed by the toxin. In mice, this toxin has also been shown to prevent the delayed-type of hypersensitivity. Coupling the toxin to transforming growth factor-alpha generates a toxin capable of killing cells that express a high number of epidermal growth factor receptors, as seen in certain types of cancer. Lastly, the exotoxin has been coupled to CD4, a cell surface molecule expressed on T cells, which is recognized by the HIV virus. A cell infected with the HIV virus expresses on its surface a protein which binds CD4. The CD4-exotoxin protein is very effective in eliminating HIV-infected cells in vitro but does not kill noninfected cells. At this writing, clinical trials with this agent are under way.

SUMMARY

Enhancing the immune system can be accomplished in two ways. Active acquired immunity can be produced by administration of vaccines that stimulate the immune system in basically the same way that natural infection would, producing immunity that typically persists for years. Passive acquired immunity is accomplished by supplying immune serum or antibodies directed toward a particular antigen. This form of immunity persists only so long as the proteins remain in the body, which is usually less than 6 weeks. Drugs that suppress immune responses are useful in organ transplantation and in treating autoimmune diseases. Glucocorticoids and certain anticancer drugs are potent immunosuppressants, blocking proliferation of cells of the immune system. Azathioprine has a similar mechanism of action. More specific suppression can be achieved with antithymocyte globulin, antilymphocyte globulin, or muromonab-CD3 because these agents interfere with more selective populations of cells. Cyclosporine is the current drug of choice for organ transplantation, selectively inhibiting the helper T cells. Immunotoxins may provide highly selective therapy in the future by delivering potent toxins directly to cancer cells, cells rejecting transplanted organs, or cells infected with the HIV virus.

STUDY QUESTIONS

1. Explain active acquired immunity and how it is achieved. How long does it last?
2. Explain passive acquired immunity and how it is achieved. How long does it last?
3. What immune protection does the fetus have?
4. What is a common side effect of immune serums?
5. Name a pharmacological role for interferons and for interleukin-2.
6. What are the clinical indications for immune suppressants?
7. How do corticosteroids cause immune suppression?
8. How do anticancer drugs such as cyclophosphamide or mercaptopurine produce immune suppression?
9. How do antithymocyte globulin and antilymphocyte globulin act?
10. What is the mechanism of action of muromonab-CD3?
11. What is the mechanism of action of azathioprine?
12. What is the mechanism of action of cyclosporine?
13. Name two important side effects of immunosuppressant drugs.
14. Why must live vaccines not be given to patients receiving immunosuppressant drugs?
15. What are immunotoxins? How do they act?

SUGGESTED READINGS

Barrett, L.V., and others: Treatment with a diphtheria toxin-related interleukin 2 fusion protein prolongs cardiac allograft survival in mice, Transplant. Proc. **21**(1):1130, 1989.

Benjamini, E., and Leskowitz, S.: Immunology: a short course. 1988, New York, Alan R. Liss.

Bertino, J.S., and Chiarello, L.A.: Vaccines, toxoids, and other immunobiologics, in Pharmacotherapy: a pathophysiologic approach, edited by DiPiro, J.T. and others, 1989, New York, Elsevier, pp. 1288-1305.

Burlingame, M.B., and Delafuente, J.C.: Systemic lupus erythematosus in Pharmacotherapy: a pathophysiologic approach, edited by DiPiro, J.T. and others, 1989, New York, Elsevier, pp. 856-864.

Chaudhary, V.K., and others: Activity of a recombinant fusion protein between transforming growth factor type alpha and *Pseudomonas* toxin, Proc. Natl. Acad. Sci. **84**(13):4538, 1987.

Chaudhary, V.K., and others: Selective killing of HIV-infected cells by recombinant human CD4-*Pseudomonas* exotoxin hybrid protein, Nature **335**(6188):369, 1988.

DiJulio, J.E.: Treatment of B-cell and T-cell lymphomas with monoclonal antibodies, Sem. Oncol. Nurs. **4**(2):102, 1988.

Dillman, J.B.: Toxicity of monoclonal antibodies in the treatment of cancer, Sem. Oncol. Nurs. **4**(2):107, 1988.

Fent, K., and Zbinden, G.: Toxicity of interferon and interleukin, Immunol. Today **8**(3):100, 1987.

Foon, K.A.: Advances in immunotherapy of cancer: monoclonal antibodies and interferon, Semin. Oncol. Nurs. **4**(2):112, 1988.

Hahn, M.B., and Jassak, P.F.: Nursing management of patients receiving interferon, Sem. Oncol. Nurs. **4**(2):95, 1988.

Karb, V.B., Queener, S.F., and Freeman, J.B.: Enhancing agents: vaccines, toxoids, and sera. In Handbook of drugs for nursing practice, St. Louis, 1989, C.V. Mosby Co., pp. 444-468.

Karb, V.B., Queener, S.F., and Freeman, J.B.: Immune suppressants. In Handbook of drugs for nursing practice, St. Louis, 1989, C.V. Mosby Co., pp. 469-476.

Kelley, V.E. and others: Interleukin 2-diphtheria toxin fusion protein can abolish cell-mediated immunity in vivo, Proc. Natl. Acad. Sci. **85**(11):3980, 1988.

Kreis, H., and others: Prolonged administration of a monoclonal anti-T3 cell antibody (Orthoclone OKT3) to kidney allograft recipients. Transplant. Proc. **18**(4):954, 1986.

Mackie, J.D., and others: Immunotherapy using interleukin-2 diphtheria toxin chimer prolongs murine allografts. Transplant. Proc. **21**(1):2718, 1989.

Matas, A.J., and others: ALG treatment of steroid-resistant rejection in patients receiving cyclosporine, Transplantation **41**(5):579, 1986.

Minnefor, A.B., and Oleske, J.M.: IV immune globulin: efficacy and safety, Hosp. Pract. **22**(10):171, 1987.

Ortho Multicenter Transplant Study Group: A randomized clinical trial of OKT3 monoclonal antibody for acute rejection of cadaveric renal transplants. N. Engl. J. Med., **313**(6):337, 1985.

Pastan, I., Willingham, M.C., and FitzGerald, D.J.P.: Immunotoxins, Cell **47**(5):641, 1986.

Ponticelli, C., and others: Clinical experience with Orthoclone OKT3 in renal transplantation, Transplant. Proc. **18**(4):942, 1986.

Ptachcinski, R.J., Venkataramanan, R., and Burckart, G.J.: Drug therapy in transplantation in Pharmacotherapy: pathophysiologic approach, edited by DiPiro, J.T. and others, 1989, New York, Elsevier, pp. 75-86.

Rieger, P.T.: Immunology: monoclonal antibodies, Am. J. Nurs. **87**(4):469, 1987.

Starzl, T.E., and Fung, J.J.: Orthoclone OKT3 in treatment of allografts rejected under cyclosporine-steroid therapy, Transplant. Proc. **18**(4):937, 1986.

ANTIINFECTIVE AND CHEMOTHERAPEUTIC AGENTS

This section discusses drugs that are effective by acting as selective poisons against certain organisms or types of cells. Chapter 29, *Introduction to the Use of Antiinfective Agents*, introduces the principle of selective toxicity that underlies all the information in the remaining chapters and focuses on the use of selective poisons to treat disease caused by bacteria or closely related microorganisms. Chapters 30 through 35 discuss specific antiinfective agents, grouping drugs into chapters on the basis of similar mechanisms of action (Chapters 30 to 32), similar toxic reactions and side effects (Chapter 33), and similar uses (Chapters 34 and 35).

Chapters 36 to 38 consider several types of drugs. Each chapter not only discusses specific drugs but also delineates the differences between therapy of diseases produced by viruses, fungi, or eucaryotic parasites from the therapy of bacterial disease.

Chapter 39, *Drugs to Treat Neoplastic Diseases*, presents the individual antineoplastic agents and the necessary information on the nature of neoplastic disease to make obvious the rationale behind the use of these agents. The mechanism of drug action is emphasized so that toxicity may be more readily understood. Understanding the mechanism of action allows the clinical properties of these drugs to be more easily appreciated and puts the nursing procedures into proper perspective.

CHAPTER

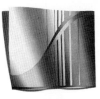

Introduction to the Use of Antiinfective Agents

29

The preceding chapters presented the use of drugs intended to alter processes occurring naturally in the body. For example, cardiotonic drugs alter existing patterns of ion flow in heart cells; the therapeutic goal of increasing contractility of the heart is achieved by this direct action of the drug. Similarly, a direct action on normal physiological functions can be cited for each drug discussed previously. In contrast, the drugs considered in this section ideally do not directly affect any physiological process in the patient. The antiinfective agents may rightfully be considered to be selective poisons, since the goal of therapy with these drugs is to poison invading, pathogenic microorganisms without poisoning the patient.

This introductory chapter presents concepts important in understanding antibiotic therapy. The microbiological principles that make antibiotic therapy effective are reviewed, the general mechanisms by which these drugs act are discussed, and the major problems associated with antimicrobial therapy are presented. Specific drugs are discussed in subsequent chapters.

THE PRINCIPLE OF SELECTIVE TOXICITY

Although the microbial world was discovered by Anton Van Leeuwenhoek in 1676, the impact of these tiny organisms on human destiny was not appreciated until the last third of the nineteenth century. During this period, Louis Pasteur and Robert Koch, working in separate laboratories and on different microorganisms, clearly showed that bacteria could cause human disease. Once this fundamental fact was appreciated, two subsequent developments became almost inevitable. The first was that microbiologists and physicians began to classify human diseases in terms of the organism that produced the disease. By the early part of the

twentieth century, the microorganisms that cause cholera, typhoid, bubonic plague, gonorrhea, leprosy, malaria, syphilis, and a host of other diseases were isolated and identified.

The second inevitable consequence of this new knowledge was that therapy of microbially induced diseases was put on a more rational basis. The first attempts at controlling diseases caused by microorganisms involved immunization. This form of therapy allowed certain diseases to be prevented. However, immunization was neither effective for all diseases nor effective once the disease was established. Thus, chemists began to explore the possibility of finding agents that could eradicate invading pathogens in a living patient. A leader in this area was Paul Ehrlich, who in 1912 introduced Salvarsan, a drug specific for syphilis. Salvarsan and a related drug, Neosalvarsan, established the validity of the principle of selective toxicity. In 1935 a synthetic agent was discovered that could cure streptococcal infections, and in 1939 development was begun on an extract of culture fluid from the mold *Penicillium*. These discoveries marked the beginnings of the sulfonamides and penicillin. From that day to now, the search for more effective antimicrobial agents has not ceased. As subsequent chapters illustrate, that search has been extraordinarily fruitful.

THE MICROBIOLOGICAL BASIS FOR SELECTIVE TOXICITY

Many similarities exist in the chemical processes of all life forms on this planet. Deoxyribonucleic and ribonucleic acids (DNA and RNA) carry the genetic information for all living things, and all use the same code to translate DNA and RNA into proteins. Proteins, or enzymes, carry out all the metabolic transformations required for life.

Some important differences in chemical or molecular organization do exist among living things. Based on these differences, life forms may be divided into two major categories: procaryotes and eucaryotes. Procaryotic cells are those in which the genetic material exists free within the cell protoplasm, whereas eucaryotic cells have membrane-bounded nuclei that contain the genetic material. Other distinguishing characteristics exist. For example, procaryotes possess cell walls composed in part of peptidoglycan, a complex molecule containing amino acids and sugars. Eucaryotic cells from multi-celled organisms usually contain no cell wall at all but only a cell membrane. Single-celled eucaryotic organisms such as algae and fungi may possess complex, rigid cell walls, but these walls do not contain peptidoglycan.

Procaryotes and eucaryotes also differ in certain internal functions. For example, the ribosomes in eucaryotes are larger than those in procaryotes, and the two forms differ in their response to certain chemicals (see Chapters 31 to 33). Likewise, folic acid metabolism may differ in the two types of organisms. Many procaryotes cannot utilize folic acid from the environment but must synthesize the vitamin from simpler starting materials. In contrast, eucaryotes cannot synthesize folic acid but must absorb it from the diet.

The structural and metabolic differences just cited between procaryotes and eucaryotes form the basis for selective toxicity. Selective toxicity is defined as the selective poisoning of an invading, disease-causing organism by means of an agent that has no effect on the person in whom the disease exists.

An ideal antimicrobial agent would have no effect at all on the patient's tissue but would destroy the pathogens causing disease. However, no drug yet approaches that ideal, and every antiinfective agent discussed causes some direct effect on the host. We therefore must consider some way to evaluate the degree of selective toxicity that may be achieved with a drug. One way to do this is by means of the therapeutic index (see Chapter 2). The therapeutic index (TI) is defined as the ratio of the dose of a certain drug that kills 50% of the test animals to the dose of that drug that is effective in 50% of the animals (TI = LD_{50}/ED_{50}). A drug that is relatively nontoxic may be given in very large doses before the animals are killed. If the drug is also potent, it may require small doses to achieve the desired clinical effect, which in this case would be cure of the infection. Such a drug would have a large TI and would be considered to display good selective toxicity, that is, it attacked the pathogen at doses well below those that were dangerous to the host. In contrast, a drug with low TI would not have good selective toxicity. A drug with a TI of 1 would be equally toxic to the bacteria and to the patient.

The TI is obviously derived from studies performed on laboratory animals. Since correlating animal studies with the clinical effectiveness of a drug is sometimes difficult, other indices of selective toxicity have been used to indicate clinical experience with a drug. For example, the *safety margin* of a drug is defined as the percentage increase above the standard therapeutic dose that may be required to produce serious toxic reactions in a certain percentage of patients. This evaluation is based entirely on clinical experience. A drug with a large TI and a wide safety margin may be given to patients in larger than normal doses without causing significant toxicity in most patients. To illustrate this principle, consider the antibiotics gentamicin and penicillin G. Gentamicin must be given in carefully controlled doses because it can damage the kidneys if the concentration in the bloodstream becomes too high. Gentamicin has a low TI and a narrow safety margin. Increasing the dose by 50% may cause significant toxicity (see Chapter 33). In contrast, penicillin G, which was the first clinically useful penicillin, has a very wide safety margin and a high TI. Direct toxicity with this drug is very low, and doses three or four times the standard dose may be administered with very little risk of toxic reactions in most patients (see Chapter 30).

MECHANISMS BY WHICH ANTIBIOTICS ACHIEVE SELECTIVE TOXICITY

Most antibiotics act on microorganisms in one of the following five ways: they (1) inhibit cell wall formation, (2) block protein synthesis, (3) disrupt cell membranes, (4) interfere with nucleic acid synthesis, or (5) prevent synthesis of folic acid. Each mechanism of action exploits a biochemical difference between eucaryotic and procaryotic cells.

In addition to categorizing antibiotics in terms of specific mechanisms, they may be broadly categorized as bacteriostatic or bactericidal drugs. The term *bactericidal* refers to drugs that directly kill the bacterial cell. For example, several antibiotics, by interfering with cell wall synthesis, may cause the bacterial cell literally to explode as the osmotic forces generated within the cytoplasm can no longer be contained by the defective cell wall. Likewise, antibiotics that disrupt the bacterial cell membrane allow the cytoplasmic contents of the cell to leak out, and the cell dies.

Bacteriostatic drugs, on the other hand, may

THE NURSING PROCESS

ANTIINFECTIVE THERAPY

Assessment

Patients requiring drugs for antiinfective therapy usually have some sign of infection. These signs usually include fever, purulent drainage, elevation of the white blood cell count, and signs of inflammation such as redness, swelling, or tenderness. Occasionally, infections are diagnosed because of a positive culture even though the patient is asymptomatic, as occurs with some urinary tract infections. Infections can occur in patients of any age, both inpatients and outpatients. Some infections would be self-limiting if left untreated. Some cause few symptoms, whereas others can cause debilitating symptoms and eventually death. The data base for a patient with a known or suspected infection should include a thorough total assessment. In addition, the nurse should emphasize the temperature and vital signs; subjective and objective evaluation of any area thought to be infected; results of culture and sensitivity testing, other appropriate laboratory work, such as complete blood counts that might indicate elevated white blood cell counts; history of exposure to infecting organisms; and assessment of preexisting medical conditions.

Nursing diagnoses

Altered bowel elimination: diarrhea and cramping secondary to antiinfective use

Potential complication: ototoxicity due to antiinfective therapy

Potential complication: vaginal superinfection with *Candida*

Management

Once the decision is made to treat with one or more antiinfective agents, the nurse should then obtain additional data about particular organs or areas that might be affected by the prescribed antibiotics. For example, an assessment of the patient's hearing should be done before starting antibiotics that may cause ototoxicity; assessment of renal function should be done before starting antibiotics that are known to cause nephrotoxicity. In addition, the health care team members should remember that, when used together, certain antibiotics are more prone to cause toxicity to certain organs.

During the management phase the nurse should monitor the temperature and vital signs. Appropriate laboratory work, such as blood counts, liver function tests, and renal function tests, should be done to monitor for the desired effects and possible side effects of the drugs. The nurse also should monitor the patient's subjective and objective signs of infections regularly. Other therapies may be needed to help control the infectious process, such as application of warm moist soaks, debridement of infected areas, and special wound-cleaning procedures. Adequate nutritional and fluid intakes should be maintained, and it may be appropriate to measure intake and output. Other drugs may be prescribed to assist in providing patient comfort, such as antipyretics for fever and bladder analgesics for severe urinary tract infections.

The nurse should check for known side effects of antibiotic therapy, such as candidal overgrowth of the oral cavity or the vagina. The nurse should evaluate carefully the appearance of new symptoms that may or may not indicate a potentially serious reaction to the antibiotic. For example, diarrhea that occurs in the patient being treated with ampicillin may be a troublesome but not too serious side effect; diarrhea that appears in the patient being treated with clindamycin, however, may indicate a serious side effect and may warrant discontinuing the medication. Because some antiinfective agents are known to cause allergic responses more often than others, appropriate drugs and equipment for resuscitation should always be available for a possible acute allergic response.

Continued.

THE NURSING PROCESS—cont'd

Evaluation

The goal of therapy with antiinfective agents is to help the body eliminate the infection without causing side effects. Frequently this is exactly what happens, and many patients take antibiotics with no reported side effects. Occasionally, side effects persist after therapy is discontinued or occur days to weeks after therapy has stopped. In preparation for discharge, the patient should be able to explain why and how to take the drug ordered, the necessity of continuing the course of therapy for as long as prescribed, side effects that may occur, side effects that warrant notifying the physician immediately, symptoms that would indicate that the medication is not effective (e.g., continuing fever or discomfort persisting 3 to 4 days after the start of therapy), recommended guidelines about diet and fluids that have been prescribed, and the importance of not sharing antiinfective agents with other individuals. For additional information about specific kinds and locations of infections, refer to appropriate textbooks. For specific information about individual antiinfective agents, see the remaining chapters in this text and the patient care implications section at the end of this chapter.

not directly kill the bacterial cell but rather halt the cell's growth and reproduction. With bacteriostic drugs it may be possible to remove the bacteria from exposure to the drug and have them resume growth. If bacterial death is not caused directly, then how may these drugs achieve a cure? The key to this question is that the host's immune system must attack, immobilize, and eliminate the pathogens in order for therapy with bacteriostatic drugs to achieve a long-term cure. In theory, cures can be effected with bactericidal drugs independent of the immune system. In fact, such cures are not easily achieved; any cure of bacterial disease in normal persons depends strongly on immunological factors. In immunosuppressed patients, cures of bacterial infections are much more difficult to achieve, even with appropriately prescribed bactericidal drugs.

To classify a drug as exclusively bactericidal or bacteriostatic is, in a sense, misleading. Many antibiotics may be either bacteriostatic or bactericidal depending on dose, site of infection, and the causative organism. For example, consider sulfonamides, which prevent folic acid synthesis in sensitive bacteria. These drugs might be considered bacteriostatic for a systemic infection but, because of the high drug concentration in urine, may be bactericidal in urine. Other examples would be cases in which two types of microorganisms differed greatly in sensitivity to a certain antibiotic. For the more sensitive organism, the serum and tissue levels achievable with normal dosage may

be sufficient for bactericidal action, whereas the more resistant organism may simply suffer growth inhibition, that is, a bacteriostatic effect, at that same antibiotic concentration.

Based on this discussion, the term *antimicrobial spectrum* may be defined as the type of microorganisms against which a particular drug is effective. Table 29.1 lists common pathogenic microorganisms according to criteria established by microbiologists. A drug effective against only a few of these organisms would be considered *narrow spectrum*, such as penicillin G, which is primarily effective against gram-positive bacteria. In contrast, a drug that could be used against several groups of organisms would be classified as *broad spectrum*, such as tetracycline, which is effective against gram-positive and gram-negative bacteria, as well as against *Rickettsia* and *Chlamydia*.

The terms *minimum inhibitory concentration (MIC)* and *minimum bactericidal concentration (MBC)* are intimately related to the concept of the antimicrobial spectrum. For each antibiotic and microorganism, it is possible to determine in the laboratory the amount of that drug required to halt the growth of the organism and the amount required to kill the organism. The concentrations are the lowest ones at which growth inhibition or cell death can be observed. A consideration of these figures as well as determination of safe blood levels for an antibiotic are involved in determining an effective therapeutic regimen. For example, a blood concentration above the MBC is desirable, but

Table 29.1 Microbial Pathogens of Human Beings

Organisms	Common diseases produced
VIRUSES	
Influenza	"Flu"; upper respiratory tract infections
Herpes simplex	Skin, eye, brain infections
CHLAMYDIA	Psittacosis; eye, genital infections
RICKETTSIA	Typhus; Q fever; Rocky Mountain spotted fever
SPIROCHETES	Syphilis; yaws
EUBACTERIA, GRAM NEGATIVE	
Haemophilus	Meningitis
Escherichia	Urinary tract infections
Proteus	Urinary tract infections
Klebsiella	Urinary tract infections; pneumonia
Pseudomonas	Urinary tract infections; meningitis
Neisseria	Meningitis; gonorrhea
Salmonella	Typhoid; gastroenteritis
Shigella	Dysentery
EUBACTERIA, GRAM POSITIVE	
Staphylococcus	Soft tissue infections
Streptococcus	Upper respiratory tract infections
MYCOBACTERIA	Tuberculosis; leprosy
ACTINOMYCETES	Organ lesions and abscesses
FUNGI	
Candida	Minor skin, mild respiratory; severe systemic infections
Cryptococcus	
Histoplasma	
Blastomyces	

whether that concentration can be obtained will depend on the pharmacological properties governing drug absorption and elimination, as well as the threshold for toxicity produced by the drug in the host.

MICROBIAL RESISTANCE TO ANTIBIOTICS

As already discussed, not all microorganisms are sensitive to all antibiotics. Resistance to antibiotics may be classified as *inherent* or *acquired*. Inherent resistance to an antibiotic is unrelated to prior exposure of the microbe to the drug. For example, the first time a culture of *Pseudomonas aeruginosa* was ever exposed to penicillin G, it was found to be resistant; that is, penicillin resistance was an inherent quality of the microorganism.

In contrast, acquired resistance refers to resistance that depends on prior exposure of the microbe to the drug. For example, when penicillin G was first tested against *Staphylococcus aureus*, the organism was exquisitely sensitive. If the organism was exposed to sublethal doses of the drug for long periods, however, more and more penicillin-resistant microbes began to appear. This tells us that the entire population of a strain of *S. aureus* can be converted from penicillin sensitivity to penicillin resistance by continuous low-level exposure to the drug, which allows genetic variants displaying penicillin resistance to proliferate. This phenomenon is called *acquired resistance.* Not only can acquired resistance be demonstrated in the laboratory; it also occurs clinically. *S. aureus* is again a good example, since strains isolated from clinical infections during the 1940s were almost always penicillin sensitive, whereas today clinically isolated *S. aureus* strains are mainly penicillin resistant.

Plasmids are small, circular pieces of DNA found separate from the chromosome in bacteria. Many genes for antibiotic resistance reside on plasmids. Since plasmids may be rapidly passed between bacterial cells, antibiotic resistance can spread rapidly through an entire bacterial population. This mechanism for acquired resistance usually results in serious therapeutic difficulty, since resistance to several antibiotics may occur simultaneously.

The precise mechanisms by which microorganisms achieve resistance to an antibiotic may be divided into three categories. The first of these mechanisms is actual destruction of the antibiotic by the microorganism. This process usually involves enzymes that chemically alter and thereby inactivate the antibiotic. Examples of this process include penicillinase, which destroys penicillin, and the acetylase, phosphorylase, and adenylating enzymes that inactivate the aminoglycoside antibiotics.

A second mechanism by which bacteria may achieve antibiotic resistance is by reducing the uptake of the drug into the bacterial cell. Many antibiotics freely enter and in some cases are concentrated within bacterial cells. By blocking this uptake, resistance may be achieved. An example of this type of resistance is seen with tetracyclines, which can be shown to freely enter sensitive bacteria but not resistant strains.

The third mechanism for resistance involves a mutation or an alteration in the target of the antibiotic in the microorganism. For example, erythromycin inhibits protein synthesis by binding to certain sites on the bacterial ribosome. Certain resistant microorganisms form altered ribosomes that do not bind erythromycin and are therefore resistant to the inhibitory action of that drug. Some types of streptomycin resistance may occur through similar means. A clinically important example of this type of resistance is methicillin-resistant *Staphylococcus aureus.*

FACTORS THAT AFFECT THE OUTCOME OF ANTIBIOTIC THERAPY

In antibiotic therapy the first step is the proper identification of the microorganism causing the disease. In some infections the symptoms are sufficiently clear-cut to allow accurate diagnosis with a physical examination only. In other cases, culturing must be done to identify the organism. In some institutions nursing personnel are trained to take specimens for culture, whereas in others laboratory personnel or physicians perform this function.

The second step in treatment is the selection of the proper antibiotic, a process that obviously depends on knowledge of the pathogen involved. This decision may be based entirely on clinical experience or may be aided by antibiotic sensitivity testing carried out in the microbiology laboratory on the pathogen isolated from the patient.

Even when the proper drug has been selected, several factors may influence the effectiveness of therapy. One is the site of infection. For example, meningitis is difficult to treat partly because many antibiotics do not penetrate the blood-brain barrier very well, making an effective drug concentration at the infection site difficult to obtain. Similarly, many abscesses or soft tissue infections are not easily treated, since the areas of infections are poorly perfused, and many drugs do not penetrate well into these areas. Healing is frequently hastened by surgical drainage.

Other drugs the patient is receiving may influence the outcome of antibiotic therapy. Immunosuppressant drugs are good examples of agents that limit antibiotic effectiveness by depressing immune mechanisms. Large doses of glucocorticoids cause significant immunosuppression. Other specific interactions may occur and are mentioned with individual drug classes in subsequent chapters.

Finally, the clinical status of the patient can alter the outcome of antibiotic therapy. In particular, renal function is very important to consider, since many available antibiotics are excreted by the kidney. If renal function is impaired, drugs eliminated through the kidney may accumulate. Likewise, hepatic disease may cause accumulation of drugs that are eliminated primarily by liver mechanisms. Patients with insufficiencies in either of these organ systems must be watched closely for signs of drug toxicity, and these signs may occur at lower doses than would be expected in normal persons.

PROBLEMS IN ANTIBIOTIC THERAPY

Direct drug toxicity is observed with many classes of antibiotics. Each antibiotic should be considered for its potential toxicity to the patient when it is administered. These direct toxic effects are frequently highly characteristic. For example, any aminoglycoside antibiotic can cause kidney damage and loss of hearing or loss of equilibrium. When these drugs are given, therefore, the patient should be observed closely for these characteristic toxic signs. Even very safe drugs occasionally may cause direct toxic reactions, such as penicillin effects on the central nervous system. Nursing personnel should be alert to these signs. Many direct toxic reactions to antibiotics are dose dependent and would be expected to be more frequent and serious when high doses of drugs are given or when drug accumulation occurs in patients with renal or hepatic impairment.

Allergies occur frequently with several antibiotics. The best examples are the penicillins, which can produce allergic reactions ranging from simple rashes to anaphylactic shock. Allergies occur in patients who have previously been exposed to the antibiotic, either in the medical setting or in the environment. Although in theory animals intended for immediate slaughter may not be treated with antibiotics also used in human beings, meat occasionally has contained sufficient quantities of antibiotics to sensitize some people who consumed the meat.

Superinfections are infections that arise during antibiotic therapy. By definition, they involve microorganisms that are resistant to the antibiotic originally used; thus superinfections are often serious and difficult to treat. Such infections are more common with broad spectrum than narrow-spectrum antibiotics. This observation is apparently based on the fact that broad spectrum antibiotics eliminate much more of the natural bacterial flora and upset the ecological controls that normally keep the resistant pathogens in check. With tetracyclines, for example, yeasts such as *Candida* are often involved in superinfections.

Misuses of Antibiotics

Antibiotics are often misunderstood and misused. One of the most common misconceptions is that antibiotics will cure any type of infectious dis-

PATIENT CARE IMPLICATIONS

Drug administration

- Question patients about history of allergy to antibiotics or antiinfectives prior to administering dose. Phrase questions appropriately. For example, "Are there any medicines you should not take, and why?" may elicit a better response than "Are you allergic to any antibiotics?" Have the patient describe previous problems. A gastric upset is probably a side effect; the development of hives is probably an allergic reaction. If there is a question whether or not the patient is allergic to the medication, consult the physician before administering the dose.
- Label the patient's health record, chart, medication kardex, armband, and so on (per agency procedure) if the patient is allergic to any medications. In some hospitals patients with allergies wear a second specially marked or colored identification bracelet indicating allergies.
- Observe all patients receiving antiinfective agents for possible allergic reactions. Monitor vital signs. Have available equipment and personnel to treat acute allergic reactions. Have available drugs to treat allergic reactions: epinephrine, antihistamines, steroids.
- Nurses who are allergic to any antiinfective agent should wear gloves when preparing or administering doses of that drug.
- Read orders and labels carefully. Within a class of antiinfectives, there may be several drugs with similar names.
- Reconstitute parenteral forms as directed by the label or in the manufacturer's literature. Date and initial the vial if some of the drug will be saved for later use. Do not use undated reconstituted medications. Observe expiration dates.
- For intramuscular administration, use large muscle masses (see Chapter 6). Aspirate before administering to prevent inadvertent IV administration. Record and rotate injection sites. If the ordered dose is a large volume of medication, divide the dose and administer in two injections.

Patient and family education

- When antiinfective agents are prescribed, review the anticipated benefits and possible side effects of drug therapy with the patient. Instruct the patient to report the development of any unexpected sign or symptom.
- Encourage patients with a known severe allergy to any medication to wear a medical identification tag or bracelet indicating the allergies.
- Tell patients to take antiinfective agents for as long as prescribed (usually 1 week to 10 days), even if they begin to feel better. Do not share antiinfectives with other family members. Do not save remaining doses to treat later infections.
- Antiinfectives work best when taken at evenly spaced intervals throughout the day. Discuss with patients an appropriate dosing schedule based on the prescribed drug frequency.
- Tell pregnant or lactating women not to take any antiinfective agents without prior consultation with the physician.
- Shake suspensions thoroughly before pouring dose. Use the same spoon or medicine cup to ensure the same dose each time.
- Some oral liquids are dispensed in bottles with droppers, though the medicine is to be taken orally.
- Chewable tablets should be chewed and swallowed for best effect. Enteric coated preparations should be swallowed whole, without crushing or chewing. If in doubt about a specific preparation, consult the pharmacist.
- Review with patients any restrictions about taking the drug with meals, milk, or snack, and special storage considerations, such as refrigeration. The pharmacist will usually label drugs which must be refrigerated.
- If a dose is missed, tell patients to take it as soon as remembered, unless close to time for the next dose, in which case the forgotten dose should be omitted. The exact guidelines will vary depending on the frequency doses are to be taken. Do not double up for missed doses.
- Remind parents to keep drugs out of the reach of children. Pediatric dosage forms are often disguised in pleasant-tasting syrups and diluents, and children may wish to take more than ordered doses. Tell parents to give children only the drugs and doses prescribed for children.
- Keep all health care providers informed of all drugs being taken. Review all drugs a patient is taking. If there are questions about drug incompatibilities, consult the physician or pharmacist.

ease, including those caused by viruses. In fact, no effective drugs exist to treat minor viral infections such as colds. As discussed in Chapter 37, very few drugs are available for use in *any* viral infections, and certainly none of the commonly employed antibiotics are effective in viral diseases.

Many infectious diseases resolve quickly once appropriate antibiotics are administered. Thus it is tempting for patients to discontinue medication much earlier than the physician planned, namely as soon as they feel better. This practice is dangerous for several reasons. Antibiotics with bacteriostatic action inhibit growth of bacteria, but the cells remain viable, at least until the immune system can eliminate them. Therefore, if therapy is discontinued too early, these organisms may again proliferate and relapse may occur. Not only does this event prolong recovery, but it may also make the disease more difficult to treat. If we consider that the organisms most resistant to the drugs being used are the ones that will probably survive longest, we can appreciate that these resistant organisms may cause the relapse. Therapy may therefore be difficult, since some degree of drug resistance has occurred.

One of the excuses frequently given when patients discontinue antibiotic therapy early is that they wish to have the medication on hand in case they ever need it again. This practice is dangerous not only for the reasons just discussed but also because it assumes the patient will be able to diagnose future illnesses accurately. Self-medication with old, unused antibiotic prescriptions may delay proper medical attention and prolong or worsen the patient's disease. Once medication has been started, culture results become relatively unreliable and proper diagnosis may be impossible. Thus patients should be discouraged from saving previously prescribed antibiotics to take them "just until I can get to the doctor."

Finally, many drugs require special storage conditions and do not remain active for very long when exposed to the warm, humid environment of most bathroom medicine cabinets. Drugs stored for weeks or months under such conditions may be inactive or may convert to forms that are more toxic. Penicillin in solution, for example, tends to form polymers that have been implicated in an increased incidence of anaphylactic episodes. Tetracyclines tend to be light-sensitive and break down to toxic compounds.

Any drug that remains in the household may be a hazard to children. Proper use and disposal of drugs is important to protect children from accidental poisoning. In addition, as seen in subsequent chapters, very young children may be much more sensitive to certain antibiotics than adults. Antibiotics should never be given to children without first consulting a physician.

SUMMARY

Successful therapy of diseases caused by pathogenic microorganisms depends on the use of selectively toxic agents, that is, agents that are nontoxic to the patient yet destroy the pathogenic microorganisms causing the disease. Selective toxicity is measured by the therapeutic index or the safety margin. Drugs that are highly toxic to pathogenic microorganisms but relatively nontoxic to the host have a high therapeutic index and a wide safety margin. Good selective toxicity is achieved by using drugs that antagonize a process in the microorganism that is absent or insensitive in human beings.

Resistance to various antibiotics is an inherent property of certain microorganisms. The antimicrobial spectrum of an antibiotic describes the array of microorganisms that are sensitive to the drug. Microorganisms may also acquire resistance to antibiotics. Acquired resistance results from a genetic change in the organism that causes the formation of enzymes to inactivate the antibiotic, blocks the uptake of the antibiotic, or alters the biochemical target of the antibiotic in the microbial cell.

The success of antibiotic therapy depends on using the proper antibiotic for the particular pathogen causing the disease. In addition, the site of the infection, other drugs the patient may be receiving, as well as the patient's clinical status may influence the outcome of antibiotic therapy. Poor patient compliance may also compromise therapy. Discontinuing antibiotics before the prescribed time increases the risk of relapse and superinfection. Use of antibiotic prescriptions from previous illnesses risks creating additional toxicity from outdated or degraded drugs and may interfere with proper diagnosis if medical attention is sought after the drugs are taken.

STUDY QUESTIONS

1. What is the principle of selective toxicity?
2. Why is selective toxicity possible to achieve?
3. How is selective toxicity achieved?
4. How is selective toxicity measured?
5. What is the difference between a bacteriostatic and a bactericidal drug?
6. What is the antimicrobial spectrum of a drug?
7. Define the terms *minimum inhibitory concentration (MIC)* and *minimum bactericidal concentration (MBC)*.

8. What is the difference between inherent and acquired resistance?
9. What are the three types of mechanisms by which microorganisms become resistant to antibiotics?
10. Name five factors that influence the outcome of antibiotic therapy.
11. What are the three general types of problems that may arise during antibiotic therapy?
12. What are some of the common misuses of antibiotics?
13. What are the dangers associated with premature cessation of antibiotic therapy?
14. What are two of the dangers associated with saving leftover antibiotics in the home?

SUGGESTED READINGS

Bint, A.J., and Burtt, I.: Adverse antibiotic drug interaction, Drugs **20**:57, 1980

Brown, J.M.: Innovative antibiotic therapy at home, J. Intravenous Nurs. **11**(6):397, 1988.

Gahart, B.L.: Intravenous medications: a handbook for nurses and other allied health personnel, ed. 5, St. Louis, 1989, C.V. Mosby Co.

Ma, M.: Brush up on antibacterial agents, Nursing89 **19**(1):76, 1989.

Novick, R.P.: Plasmids, Sci. Am. **243**(6):102, 1980.

Rhodes, K.H., and Johnson, C.M.: Antibiotic therapy for severe infections in infants and children, Mayo Clin. Proc. **62**(11):1018, 1987.

Rosenblatt, J.E.: Laboratory tests used to guide antimicrobial therapy, Mayo Clin. Proc. **62**(9):799, 1987.

Smith, I.M.: Infections in elderly patients: practical guidelines for treatment, Drug Therapy **23**(4):93, 1983.

Strenz, M.H., and Barfoot, K.S.: Total parenteral nutrition: compatibility of antibiotic admixtures, J. Intravenous Nurs. **11**(1):43, 1988.

Todd, B.: Antibiotics: interactions with maintenance medication, Geriatr. Nurs. **9**(6):364, 1988.

Van Scoy, R.E., and Wilkowske, C.J.: Prophylactic use of antimicrobial agents, Mayo Clin. Proc. **62**(12):1137, 1987.

Van Scoy, R.E., and Wilson, W.R.: Antimicrobial agents in patients with renal insufficiency, Mayo Clin. Proc. **62**(12):1142, 1987.

Welch, H.G.: Antibiotic resistance: a new kind of epidemic, Postgrad. Med. **76**(6):63, 1984.

Wilkowske, C.J., and Hermans, P.E.: General principles of antimicrobial therapy, Mayo Clin. Proc. **62**(9):789, 1987.

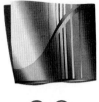

Antibiotics: Penicillins, Cephalosporins, and Related Drugs

30

This chapter is intended as an introduction to the most widely used family of antibiotics in medical practice today: the beta-lactam antibiotics, of which penicillins and cephalosporins are the most important representatives. The chapter first discusses the properties common to all members of this family of antibiotics and then considers the special features of individual agents.

PROPERTIES COMMON TO ALL PENICILLINS AND CEPHALOSPORINS
Mechanism of Action and Bacterial Resistance

Penicillins and cephalosporins are irreversible inhibitors of a bacterial enzyme called *transpeptidase*. The function of this enzyme is to cross-link parallel strands of cell wall material called *peptidoglycan*. When cross-linking occurs, peptidoglycan becomes very rigid and is an effective cell wall. When cross-linking is blocked by penicillin or cephalosporin, cell wall synthesis continues without cross-linking. Ultimately, the unreinforced strands that are formed are unable to resist the osmotic forces within the bacterial cell. The bacterium may literally explode. Since exposed bacteria may be directly killed, the beta-lactam antibiotics are classified as bactericidal drugs. However, even at doses below those required to kill bacteria, penicillins and cephalosporins may be effective in some circumstances. Minimum disruption of the bacterial cell wall by these drugs may make the bacterium more liable to elimination by the immune system of the host.

Penicillins and cephalosporins do not destroy existing bacterial cell wall; these drugs instead prevent formation of new, intact cell wall. Thus penicillins and cephalosporins are most effective against actively multiplying bacteria.

Resistance to penicillins and cephalosporins develops in microorganisms. The most common mechanism for resistance involves enzymes called *beta-lactamases*. These enzymes usually are referred to as penicillinases or cephalosporinases, depending on which type of drug the enzyme is most effective against. These enzymes destroy the penicillin or cephalosporin nucleus (Figure 30.1), rendering the drug inactive. Some organisms possess these enzymes as part of their normal metabolic makeup and therefore are intrinsically resistant to beta-lactam antibiotics. Other organisms may acquire the enzyme and thus be converted from antibiotic sensitivity to resistance. Clinically important examples of acquired penicillin resistance are *Staphylococcus aureus* and *Neisseria gonorrhoeae*. Although 25 years ago both organisms could routinely be considered to be sensitive to penicillin G, today significant resistance to penicillin G exists for both organisms. In some hospitals more than 90% of *S. aureus* strains are resistant.

Though resistance to penicillins is most commonly acquired by developing beta-lactamase, other important forms of resistance are known. The most clinically relevant example may be methicillin–resistant *Staphylococcus aureus* (MRSA). In this organism resistance is conferred by altered penicillin targets.

Excretion

Penicillins and cephalosporins are excreted by the kidney, primarily by active secretion. For all the penicillins except nafcillin and for most of the cephalosporins, the kidney is the main route of excretion. Exceptions are cefotaxime and ceftriaxone,

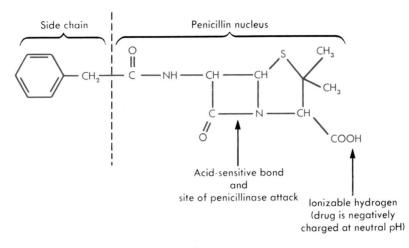

FIGURE 30.1   Structure of penicillin G. All the penicillin antibiotics contain the penicillin nucleus shown. Any chemical disruption of the nucleus, such as that produced by acid or penicillinase, results in loss of antibiotic activity. The ionizable hydrogen may be replaced with sodium or potassium ion without effect on drug activity. Alterations of the side chain of penicillin affect the acid stability, penicillinase resistance, and antimicrobial spectrum of the drug. The penicillins used clinically differ from one another in their side chain structures. Cephalosporins contain a slightly different nucleus and side chains than penicillins.

which are metabolized by the liver and cefoperazone, which is excreted in bile.

Toxicity of Penicillins and Cephalosporins

Allergies are the most common adverse reaction to the penicillins. Many patients experience skin rashes or urticaria, but anaphylaxis is a much more dangerous allergic response. Whereas allergic rashes and drug fevers usually appear after several days of therapy, the onset of anaphylaxis is nearly always within 10 minutes. Injections of penicillin are responsible for most anaphylactic episodes, but any form of exposure to penicillin may produce anaphylaxis in sensitive individuals.

A patient beginning penicillin therapy should be asked to remain in the clinic for about 30 minutes after a penicillin injection so that if anaphylaxis develops, medical help will be immediately available. If anaphylaxis occurs, medical personnel first should administer subcutaneous epinephrine. Anaphylaxis involves profound vasomotor collapse, and laryngeal edema may further complicate resuscitation efforts. Steroids may be required, as well as a tracheostomy and oxygen under positive pressure. All these emergency supplies should be at hand in any clinical setting where antibiotics are administered.

Some physicians perform a skin test before administering penicillins to try to identify allergic patients. An estimated 3% to 5% of the population is allergic to penicillin; about 10% of those who have previously received penicillin in a medical setting may be allergic. Patients about to receive penicillin must be asked if they have ever been given penicillin before and if they have ever had a rash or other allergic symptom during penicillin therapy. This information, although necessary, is somewhat unreliable in that many patients who report allergy to penicillin in the past do not experience allergic reactions when reexposed to the drug. In part this may be because the original reaction was not a true penicillin allergy. Ampicillin, for example, may cause a benign macular eruption rather than a urticarial reaction. This toxic rash is not a sign of allergy but may be reported as an allergy by the patient. Another explanation for apparent changes in sensitivity to penicillins is that some patients are allergic to contaminants present in early penicillin preparations but absent from the more purified modern preparations.

Some patients who report no previous allergies to penicillin and some who claim never to have received penicillin still may experience an allergic response when they receive the drug. In some cases the patient might be unaware of what drug was prescribed and thus not be a reliable source. Although rare, some persons have become sensitized

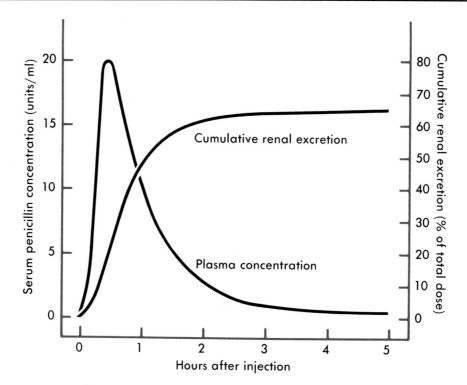

FIGURE 30.2   Serum concentration and urinary excretion of an intramuscular dose of penicillin G. Penicillin G is efficiently and rapidly absorbed following intramuscular injections. Peak plasma concentrations of the drug appear 20 to 30 minutes after injection. Penicillin G is actively secreted in the renal tubule, accounting for the very rapid elimination half-time of about 20 to 30 minutes. Most of the drug dose ends up in the urine as unaltered penicillin.

by being exposed to penicillin in the environment or in the food chain. For example, animals destined for human food use can be treated with penicillins by the feed lot owner, although sufficient time should be allowed before slaughter so that the drug can be removed from the animal's system.

Cephalosporins are good allergens much like penicillins, and many patients suffer allergic reactions to the drugs. Rashes are most common, but anaphylaxis is possible. Many patients who are allergic to penicillins are also allergic to cephalosporins, and vice versa.

Direct drug toxicity with penicillin is very low; massive doses have been given with no ill effect. The tissue most sensitive to direct effects is the central nervous system. Intrathecal injection (into the subarachnoid space or cerebrospinal fluid) may produce convulsions. Convulsions also occur occasionally in patients given high doses intramuscularly or intravenously, especially if there is some renal impairment and the drug accumulates. A relatively high concentration in the cerebrospinal fluid must be achieved before convulsions occur.

This complication could occur in an elderly patient being treated for a serious infection such as streptococcal endocarditis. This patient may receive 25 to 40 million units of penicillin daily to maintain continuous bactericidal drug concentrations. Whereas normal persons can readily eliminate these large amounts through their kidneys, elderly persons may have diminished renal function. Therefore drug accumulation may occur, and penicillin may begin to enter the central nervous system. The first sign may be loss of consciousness or myoclonic movements. Generalized seizures may follow.

Another group of patients with reduced ability to excrete penicillin are newborn infants. Because of this, neonates receive carefully adjusted penicillin doses based on their body weight and reduced clearance of penicillin.

Cephalosporins also are excreted primarily by the kidney and, as with the penicillins, may accumulate in patients with impaired renal function. Hence cephalosporin dosage may be reduced when renal function is lower than normal.

Table 30.1   Antimicrobial Spectrum of Penicillin G

Organism	Typical infections
GRAM-POSITIVE BACTERIA	
Streptococcus, selected strains	Upper respiratory infections, endocarditis, bacteremia
Streptococcus pneumoniae	Abscesses, bronchitis, meningitis, pneumonia, bacteremia
Staphylococcus aureus, non-penicillinase	Skin and soft tissue infections, bronchitis, endocarditis, otitis, pneumonia, meningitis, bacteremia
Bacillus anthracis	Anthrax
Corynebacterium diphtherium	Diphtheria
Clostridium tetani	Tetanus
Clostridium perfringens	Gas gangrene
GRAM-NEGATIVE BACTERIA	
Neisseria gonorrhoeae	Gonorrhea
Neisseria meningitidis	Meningitis
SPIROCHETE	
Treponema pallidum	Syphilis

Oral penicillin preparations cause gastrointestinal distress in some patients. Reactions include irritation and inflammation of the upper gastrointestinal tract, nausea, vomiting, and diarrhea. Orally administered cephalosporins may also cause gastric irritation, nausea, and vomiting.

Several penicillin and cephalosporin preparations contain sufficient sodium or potassium to alter electrolyte balance in some patients. For example, 1 million units of penicillin G and penicillin V may contain 1.5 mEq of potassium. Given in high enough doses for long enough periods, potassium intoxication and cardiac arrhythmias may occur. Carbenicillin and some preparations of penicillin G contain high concentrations of sodium, which may cause difficulties in patients with preexisting cardiac or renal dysfunction.

Penicillins and cephalosporins require some care in handling and diluting for intramuscular or intravenous therapy. Many penicillins require properly buffered solutions for best stability, and thus not all are compatible with common intravenous fluids. Medical personnel should check the package insert or refer to the pharmacist before adding penicillins or cephalosporins to any intravenous fluid.

Probenecid is a drug sometimes used with penicillins to increase their effective duration of action by slowing excretion in the kidney. Probenecid itself may cause toxic reactions difficult to distinguish from a penicillin reaction. For example, probenecid may produce chills, fever, and rash as well as gastrointestinal irritation and anemia. Probenecid also blocks renal excretion of some cephalosporins.

PROPERTIES OF INDIVIDUAL PENICILLINS

Penicillin G

Absorption. Penicillin G was the first penicillin adopted for widespread clinical use. This drug is one of several so-called natural penicillins, being formed spontaneously by the *Penicillium* mold and released into the culture fluid. Of these naturally occurring compounds, penicillin G has the most potent antibacterial action. The structure of penicillin G is shown in Figure 30.1; it differs from the other penicillins only in the side chain. The penicillin nucleus is found in all clinically useful penicillins.

The penicillin nucleus must remain intact to retain antibacterial activity. As pointed out in Figure 30.1, at least one bond in the nucleus is sensitive to acid, a fact that explains the lability of penicillin G in the stomach. Approximately 30% of an orally administered dose is absorbed, the rest being destroyed in the stomach or retained in the intestine and destroyed by bacteria in the large bowel. Because of the incomplete and somewhat variable absorption of penicillin G by this route, oral doses of penicillin G are not recommended.

Penicillin G is rapidly and completely absorbed following intramuscular injection (Figure 30.2). Serum concentrations reach a peak within 20 to 30 minutes of the injection. Unfortunately this peak concentration persists for only a very short time, primarily because the kidney so efficiently removes penicillin from the bloodstream. Within 2 to 3 hours after intramuscular injection about 60% of the penicillin dose has appeared in the urine. The drug in urine is unchanged and still possesses antibacterial activity. Penicillin enters the urine by a process called *active secretion* in the renal tubule. This process involves a specific transport system for which several drugs may compete. Physicians may take advantage of this trait by using a drug

---

⬟ **DRUG ALERT: PATIENTS WITH IMPAIRED RENAL FUNCTION**

THE PROBLEM

Most beta-lactam antibiotics are excreted primarily through the kidneys, with biliary excretion as an alternative route. If renal function is impaired, excretion may be slowed and the drug can accumulate. Healthy geriatric patients may have significantly lower renal function than younger adults and may need to be considered as renally impaired.

SOLUTIONS

- Monitor renal function
- Adjust doses for renal function, as prescribed or as described in package insert

---

such as probenecid to block penicillin excretion, thereby increasing the peak penicillin concentration in the serum and increasing its effective duration.

Distribution. Penicillin G is generally well distributed throughout many body tissues, with high concentrations found in blood, liver, kidney, and bile. Virtually none is found in brain or cerebrospinal fluid in normal persons. If the meninges are inflamed, as in meningitis, penicillin can penetrate the central nervous system in significant amounts.

Uses. Penicillin G is a narrow-spectrum antibiotic; the organisms against which it is effective are summarized in Table 30.1. Most of the sensitive organisms are gram-positive bacteria. These bacteria are characterized by thick, peptidoglycan-rich cell walls, which react with the Gram stain. Some of these gram-positive organisms, such as *S. aureus*, *Streptococcus* species, and *Streptococcus pneumoniae*, cause common infections of the upper respiratory tract and soft tissues, as well as more serious infections. Other rare gram-positive organisms, such as the ones which cause anthrax, gas gangrene, tetanus, and diphtheria, are also sensitive to penicillin. Among gram-negative organisms, clinically significant sensitivity to penicillin G is seen only with *N. meningitidis* (meningococcus) and *N. gonorrhoeae* (gonococcus). Other common gram-negative organisms normally found in the bowel and those frequently responsible for urinary tract infections are clinically resistant to penicillin G. In the laboratory, some of these gram-negative bacteria can be affected by very high doses of penicillin G, but these high drug levels cannot routinely be achieved in patients. Although penicillin G is not effective against common pathogens in routine urinary tract infections, it is very effective against syphilis and gonorrhea. Syphilis, caused by a spirochete, and gonorrhea, caused by *N. gonorrhoeae*, frequently may be treated effectively by single-dose penicillin therapy.

Repository penicillins: procaine penicillin G and benzathine penicillin G

Absorption. One disadvantage of penicillin G is its very short duration of action. The repository penicillins were designed to slow absorption from intramuscular injection sites and thereby prolong the duration of action. Along with slower absorption comes a lower peak serum concentration (see Chapter 2). Once the drug is absorbed from the depot sites, it is hydrolyzed to release penicillin G, which is the active form of the drug.

The repository penicillins are procaine penicillin G and benzathine penicillin G. Procaine penicillin G reaches its peak serum concentration 3 to 4 hours after injection, and significant serum concentrations may persist for up to 48 hours. With a single dose of 300,000 units of aqueous penicillin G, peak serum levels for penicillin may reach 6 to 8 units/ml, whereas for procaine penicillin G at that same dose, the peak concentration will be only 1 to 2 units/ml. Benzathine penicillin G is absorbed even more slowly and reaches maximum concentration by 8 hours after injection. This concentration decreases very slowly, and significant serum levels are observed for 2 weeks or longer. A common adult dose of 1.2 million units produces peak serum levels of only 0.1 to 0.3 units/ml (Table 30.2).

Toxicity. The repository penicillins are intended only for deep muscular injections. Both preparations are stabilized suspensions of relatively insoluble forms of penicillin and contain up to about 2% weight/volume of emulsifying agents in addition to buffers. Such preparations should never be given intravenously. Care must be taken on intramuscular injection to prevent the accidental entry of these preparations into blood vessels, since occlusion of the blood vessel may result.

Uses. The repository penicillins are not appropriate for very serious infections when high serum concentrations of drug are required. Rather, these drugs are appropriate to maintain modest serum levels for relatively long periods. These conditions would occur when very sensitive organisms were involved in mild to moderately serious infections or when prophylaxis was required.

Procaine penicillin G is associated with central nervous system toxicity due to the procaine. After

THE NURSING PROCESS

THERAPY WITH PENICILLINS, CEPHALOSPORINS AND RELATED DRUGS

Refer to the nursing process section in Chapter 29 for general guidelines on the nursing process with antibiotic therapy. The material below relates specifically to the penicillins, cephalosporins and related drugs.

Assessment

Penicillins and cephalosporins are prescribed for patients with many types of infections. Assessment should be carried out with emphasis on the organ in which the infection is thought to be present, if the infection is localized. Other clinical signs of infection should be monitored. The nurse should pay special attention to subjective data that suggest the patient has a history of allergy either to penicillins or to other agents. Since penicillins and cephalosporins are excreted mainly by the kidney, the nurse should assess renal function.

Nursing diagnoses

Potential complication: allergic reactions

Potential complication: gastrointestinal distress

Management

Once the decision is made to administer penicillins or cephalosporins, the nurse should determine that emergency supplies are at hand to treat a possible anaphylactic reaction. The patient should be observed closely for at least 20 to 30 minutes after the medication is administered. If the patient will continue to receive these antibiotics on an outpatient basis, the nurse should instruct the patient in the proper timing of doses and the need to continue therapy for the prescribed time. The nurse also should inform the patient about side effects such as rashes or gastrointestinal distress and teach the patient that these reactions may necessitate contacting the physician.

Evaluation

Penicillins and cephalosporins seldom cause long-term side effects and are usually very effective in treating common infections. Patients should show rapid objective and subjective improvement for most infections treated with these agents. The patient should demonstrate the ability to judge improvement in the infection and should be able to tell the nurse what reactions might be expected to the medications and when it would be appropriate to call the physician.

---

injection, procaine may be released in significant amounts into the bloodstream and may produce anxiety, lowered blood pressure, respiratory depression, and convulsions. These central nervous system reactions to procaine are usually transient, lasting less than 1 hour.

✗ Phenoxy penicillins: penicillin V

Absorption. Attempts to improve the oral absorption of penicillin G have led to the development of phenoxy derivatives of penicillin. The most useful member of this class is penicillin V.

Penicillin V is more acid stable and thus more efficiently absorbed from the gastrointestinal tract than penicillin G, but is less potent as an antibacterial agent.

Uses. The uses of penicillin V are restricted to those circumstances in which oral antibiotic therapy is appropriate. Mild to moderately serious infections caused by penicillin-sensitive organisms may be treated with penicillin V. Penicillin V also may be used in prophylaxis, especially in patients who have had rheumatic fever. In these patients penicillin V prophylaxis may prevent recurrent

Table 30.2 Common Dosages of Representative Penicillins

Generic name	Trade name	Administration/dosage
BIOSYNTHESIZED PENICILLINS		
Penicillin G	Crystapen Megacillin P-50† Pentids Pfizerpen	ORAL: *Adults*—200,000 to 500,000 units every 6 to 8 hr administered ½ hr before or 2 hr after meals. *Children*—25,000 to 90,000 units/kg body weight daily in 3 to 6 doses. INTRAMUSCULAR: *Adults*—1 million to 5 million units daily in divided doses. *Children*—50,000 to 250,000 units/kg body weight daily divided among 6 doses. INTRAVENOUS: *Adults and children*—same as for intramuscular. Higher doses have been used for severe infections.
Penicillin V	Pen-Vee-K V-Cillin K* Veetids	ORAL: *Adults*—125 to 500 mg every 4 to 6 hr. *Children*—25 to 50 mg/kg body weight daily in divided doses.
REPOSITORY PENICILLINS		
Benzathine penicillin G	Bicillin* Permapen	ORAL: *Adults*—400,000 to 600,000 units (base) every 4 to 6 hr. *Children*—25,000 to 90,000 units/kg daily, divided into 3, 4, or 6 doses. INTRAMUSCULAR: *Adults*—600,000 to 1.2 million units every 2 to 4 weeks. *Children*—50,000 units/kg body weight once.
Procaine penicillin G	Crysticillin Duracillin A.S. Wycillin*	INTRAMUSCULAR: *Adults and children*—600,000 to 1.2 million units every 12 to 24 hr. For uncomplicated gonorrhea, 4.8 million units in 1 dose divided between two sites. *Infants*—50,000 units/kg body weight once daily.
PENICILLINASE-RESISTANT PENICILLINS		
Cloxacillin	Orbenin† Tegopen	ORAL: *Adults*—0.25 to 1 Gm every 4 to 6 hr. *Infants*—50 to 100 mg/kg body weight daily divided into 4 doses. Administer 1 hr before or 2 hr after meals.
Dicloxacillin	Dycill Dynapen* Pathocil	ORAL: *Adults*—0.125 to 1 Gm every 4 to 6 hr. *Children*—12.5 to 25 mg/kg body weight daily divided into 4 doses. Administer 1 hr before or 2 hr after meals.
Methicillin	Staphcillin	INTRAMUSCULAR: *Adults*—1 Gm every 4 to 6 hr. *Children*—100 to 200 mg/kg body weight daily divided into 4 to 6 doses. INTRAVENOUS: *Adults*—1 to 2 Gm diluted into 50 ml Sodium Chloride Injection USP injected at a rate of 10 ml/min every 4 to 6 hr. *Children*—same as for intramuscular.
Nafcillin	Nafcil Nallpen Unipen*	ORAL: *Adults*—0.25 to 1 Gm every 4 to 6 hr. *Children*—50 to 100 mg/kg body weight daily divided into 4 doses. *Neonates*—30 to 40 mg/kg body weight daily divided into 3 or 4 doses. INTRAMUSCULAR: *Adults*—500 mg every 4 to 6 hr. *Children*—40 to 100 mg/kg body weight daily divided into 4 doses. INTRAVENOUS: *Adults*—0.5 to 1 Gm every 4 hr. *Children*—150 mg/kg body weight daily divided into 4 doses.
Oxacillin	Bactocill Prostaphlin	ORAL: *Adults*—0.5 to 1 Gm every 4 to 6 hr. *Children*—50 to 100 mg/kg body weight daily divided into 4 doses. Administer 1 hr before or 2 hr after meals. INTRAMUSCULAR: *Adults*—0.25 to 2 Gm every 4 to 6 hr. *Children*—50 to 100 mg/kg body weight daily divided into 4 to 6 doses. INTRAVENOUS: *Adults*—same as for intramuscular. The drug should be diluted to 20 mg/ml or less before injection.
EXTENDED SPECTRUM PENICILLINS		
Amdinocillin	Coactin	INTRAMUSCULAR OR INTRAVENOUS: *Adults*—10 mg/kg body weight every 4 hr. FDA Pregnancy Category B.

*Available in Canada and United States.
†Available in Canada.

Table 30.2   Common Dosages of Representative Penicillins—cont'd

Generic name	Trade name	Administration/dosage
EXTENDED SPECTRUM PENICILLINS—cont'd		
Amoxicillin	Amoxil* Axicillin† Polymox* Trimox	ORAL: *Adults*—250 to 500 mg every 8 hr. *Infants and children 8 to 20 kg*—20 to 40 mg/kg body weight daily divided into 3 doses.
Amoxicillin + K clavulanate	Augmentin Clavulin†	ORAL: *Adults*—250 or 500 mg amoxicillin + 125 mg K clavulanate every 8 hr. FDA Pregnancy Category B. *Infants*—amoxicillin 20 to 40 mg/kg body weight + 5 to 10 mg K clavulanate daily divided into 3 doses
Ampicillin	Amcill* Omnipen Penbritin† Polycillin Principen Totacillin	ORAL: *Adults*—250 to 500 mg every 6 hr. *Infants*—50 to 100 mg/kg body weight daily divided into 4 doses. INTRAMUSCULAR: *Adults*—same as for oral. *Infants*—100 to 200 mg/kg body weight daily divided into 4 doses. INTRAVENOUS: *Adults*—same as for oral. *Infants*—same as for intramuscular. Higher doses have been administered for serious infections.
Ampicillin + sulbactam	Unasyn	INTRAMUSCULAR OR INTRAVENOUS: *Adults*—1 to 2 Gm ampicillin and 0.5 to 1 Gm sulbactam every 6 hr. FDA Pregnancy Category B.
Bacampacillin	Penglobe† Spectrobid	ORAL: *Adults*—280 to 560 mg ampicillin every 12 hr (400 mg bacampacillin = 280 mg ampicillin). FDA Pregnancy Category B. *Children*—17.5 mg ampicillin every 12 hr.
Cyclacillin	Cyclapen-W	ORAL: *Adults*—250 to 500 mg every 6 hr. *Children*—125 to 250 mg every 8 hr.
ANTI-*PSEUDOMONAS* PENICILLINS		
Azlocillin	Azlin	INTRAVENOUS: *Adults*—3 Gm every 4 hr or 4 Gm every 6 hr by slow injection. Up to 24 Gm may be given daily for life-threatening infections. FDA Pregnancy Catebory B.
Carbenicillin	Geocillin Geopen* Pyopen*	INTRAMUSCULAR: *Adults*—1 to 2 Gm every 6 hr. Doses increased for life-threatening infections but should not exceed 40 Gm daily. *Children*—50 to 200 mg/kg body weight daily divided into 4 to 6 doses. INTRAVENOUS: *Adults and children*—same as for intramuscular.
Carbenicillin indanyl ester	Geocillin	ORAL: *Adults*—382 to 764 mg (1 or 2 tablets) every 6 hr.
Mezlocillin	Mezlin	INTRAMUSCULAR, INTRAVENOUS: *Adults*—3 to 4 Gm every 4 to 6 hr. Severe infections may be treated with up to 24 Gm daily in equally divided doses. FDA Pregnancy Category B. *Children*—50 mg/kg body weight every 4 hr.
Piperacillin	Pipracil*	INTRAMUSCULAR, INTRAVENOUS: *Adults*—3 to 4 Gm every 4 to 6 hr. Intravenous doses by slow injection. Up to 24 Gm may be given daily for life-threatening infections. FDA Pregnancy Category B.
Ticarcillin	Ticar*	INTRAMUSCULAR: *Adults*—1 Gm every 4 to 6 hr. *Children*—50 to 100 mg/kg body weight daily divided into 3 or 4 doses. INTRAVENOUS: *Adults and children*—200 to 300 mg/kg body weight daily in 4 to 6 doses. Drug should be infused over 10 to 20 min.
Ticarcillin + clavulanate	Timentin	INTRAVENOUS: *Adults*—as for ticarcillin, based on ticarcillin content of preparation. FDA Pregnancy Category B.

*Available in Canada and United States.
†Available in Canada.

Table 30.3 Common Dosages of Representative Cephalosporins

Generic name	Trade name	Administration/dosage
FIRST GENERATION		
Cefadroxil	Duricef* Ultracef	ORAL: *Adults*—1 to 2 Gm daily in divided doses. FDA Pregnancy Category B. *Children*—30 mg/kg body weight daily divided into 2 equal doses.
Cefazolin	Ancef* Kefzol*	INTRAMUSCULAR, INTRAVENOUS: *Adults*—250 mg every 8 hr, up to 1.5 Gm every 6 hr. FDA Pregnancy Category B. *Children*—25 to 50 mg/kg body weight total daily dose in 3 or 4 divided doses.
Cephalexin	Ceporex* Keflex* Novolexin*	ORAL: *Adults*—1 to 4 Gm daily. FDA Pregnancy Category B. *Children*—25 to 100 mg/kg body weight total daily dose divided into 4 doses.
Cephalothin	Ceporacin* Keflin* Seffin	INTRAMUSCULAR, INTRAVENOUS: *Adults*—1 to 2 Gm every 4 to 6 hr. FDA Pregnancy Category B. *Children*—80 to 160 mg/kg body weight total daily dose.
Cephapirin	Cefadyl*	INTRAMUSCULAR, INTRAVENOUS: *Adults*—500 mg to 1 Gm every 4 to 6 hr. FDA Pregnancy Category B. *Children*—40 to 80 mg/kg body weight total daily dose.
Cephradine	Anspor Velosef*	ORAL, INTRAMUSCULAR, INTRAVENOUS: *Adults*—1 to 6 Gm total daily dose. FDA Pregnancy Category B. *Children*—25 to 100 mg/kg body weight divided into 4 daily doses.
SECOND GENERATION		
Cefaclor	Ceclor*	ORAL: *Adults*—1 to 4 Gm daily. FDA Pregnancy Category B. *Children*—20 to 40 mg/kg body weight, not to exceed 1 Gm daily.
Cefamandole	Mandol*	INTRAMUSCULAR, INTRAVENOUS: *Adults*—500 mg to 2 Gm every 4 to 6 hr. FDA Pregnancy Category B. *Children*—50 to 100 mg/kg body weight daily divided into 3 to 6 doses.
Cefonicid	Monocid	INTRAMUSCULAR, INTRAVENOUS: *Adults*—1 to 2 Gm once daily. No more than 1 Gm should be given at a single intramuscular site. FDA Pregnancy Category B. *Children*—safety and effectiveness have not been established.
Ceforanide	Precef	INTRAMUSCULAR, INTRAVENOUS: *Adults*—0.5 to 1 Gm twice daily. FDA Pregnancy Category B. *Children*—20 to 40 mg/kg body weight daily in 2 equally divided doses.
Cefotetan	Cefotan	INTRAMUSCULAR, INTRAVENOUS: *Adults*—1 to 2 Gm every 12 hr. Do not exceed 6 Gm daily. FDA Pregnancy Category B. *Children*—Safe dosage not established.
Cefoxitin	Mefoxin*	INTRAMUSCULAR, INTRAVENOUS: *Adults*—3 to 12 Gm daily in 3 or 4 equal doses. FDA Pregnancy Category B. *Children*—50 to 150 mg/kg body weight daily divided into 4 to 6 doses.
Cefsulodin	Cefomonil†	INTRAVENOUS: *Adults*—2 to 12 Gm total daily dose, divided into 4 equal doses.
Cefuroxime axetil	Ceftin Zinnat	ORAL: *Adults*—250 to 500 mg every 12 hr. FDA Pregnancy Category B. *Children*—125 mg every 12 hr.
Cefuroxime	Kefurox Zinacef*	INTRAMUSCULAR, INTRAVENOUS: *Adults*—0.75 to 1.5 Gm every 6 to 8 hr. FDA Pregnancy Category B. *Infants to 3 mo*—30 to 100 mg/kg divided into 2 or 3 daily doses. *Children over 3 mo*—75 to 120 mg/kg body weight daily divided into 3 equal doses.
THIRD GENERATION		
Cefoperazone	Cefobid* Cefobine	INTRAMUSCULAR, INTRAVENOUS: *Adults*—2 to 4 Gm daily divided into 2 equal doses. More severe infections may require up to 12 Gm daily divided into 2 to 4 doses. FDA Pregnancy Category B. *Children*—safe use has not been established.

*Available in Canada and United States.
†Available in Canada only.

Table 30.3   Common Dosages of Representative Cephalosporins—cont'd

Generic name	Trade name	Administration/dosage
THIRD GENERATION—cont'd		
Cefotaxime	Claforan*	INTRAMUSCULAR, INTRAVENOUS: *Adults*—3 to 4 Gm daily divided into 3 or 4 equal doses. More severe infections may require up to 12 Gm daily. FDA Pregnancy Category B. *Children*—50 to 180 mg/kg body weight doses have been used.
Ceftazidime	Fortaz* Magnacef* Tazicef	INTRAMUSCULAR, INTRAVENOUS: *Adults*—0.5 to 2 Gm every 8 to 12 hr. FDA Pregnancy Category B. *Children*—30 to 50 mg/kg body weight every 8 to 12 hr.
Ceftizoxime	Cefizox	INTRAMUSCULAR, INTRAVENOUS: *Adults*—3 Gm daily divided into 2 equal doses. Severe infections may require up to 12 Gm daily, divided into 3 doses. FDA Pregnancy Category B. *Children*—safety and effectiveness have not been established.
Ceftriaxone	Rocephin	INTRAMUSCULAR, INTRAVENOUS: *Adult*—1 to 2 Gm as a single dose or divided into 2 doses daily. FDA Pregnancy Category B. *Children*—50 to 75 mg/kg body weight daily, divided into 2 doses.
Moxalactam	Moxam* Oxalactam	INTRAMUSCULAR, INTRAVENOUS: *Adults*—2 to 4 Gm daily divided into 3 equal doses. FDA Pregnancy Category C. *Children*—50 mg/kg body weight every 6 to 8 hr.

*Available in Canada and United States.

streptococcal infections, which could lead to heart or kidney damage.

Other than being better absorbed orally, penicillin V resembles penicillin G. Penicillin V has the same antimicrobial spectrum, same pattern of distribution and excretion, and same toxicity as penicillin G. Penicillin V should be given 1 hour before or 2 hours after meals, since food can interfere with absorption.

Penicillinase-resistant penicillins: methicillin

Absorption. Methicillin is not acid stable and therefore must be administered parenterally.

Toxicity. Methicillin can cause significant blood dyscrasias as well as interstitial nephritis. These reactions are uncommon with other penicillins. Methicillin is also unusual in that resistance to the drug involves cell tolerance rather than the development of penicillinase. When methicillin resistance does occur, the organism also becomes resistant to penicillin G, cephalosporins, other penicillinase-resistant penicillins, and other antibiotics as well.

Uses. Methicillin was the first penicillin developed to be resistant to attack by penicillinase. This important breakthrough in pharmaceutical development allowed penicillin therapy of penicillinase-producing staphylococcal infections. Methicillin is best used only in treatment of infections caused by this pathogenic organism; in all other penicillin-sensitive infections penicillin G is preferred, because it is more potent than methicillin.

Acid-stable, penicillinase-resistant penicillins: nafcillin, oxacillin, cloxacillin, and dicloxacillin

Absorption and excretion. This group combines two of the most useful features of penicillin derivatives: acid stability, which allows oral dosage; and resistance to staphylococcal penicillinase, which allows the drugs to be used against many penicillin G–resistant organisms. One member of this group, nafcillin, is unique among all the penicillins in that it is excreted primarily in the bile. All other penicillins are excreted primarily by the kidney. Although nafcillin is occasionally used orally, it is not as well absorbed as the other members of this class—oxacillin, cloxacillin, and dicloxacillin. With these latter drugs oral absorption can be approximately doubled by fasting. These drugs are all more potent than methicillin but less potent than penicillin G.

Uses. The primary use of this group of drugs is in initial therapy when a penicillinase-producing organism is suspected. If the infection is later demonstrated by culture results to be caused by a non-penicillinase-producing organism, the patient may

Table 30.4   Clinical Summary of Aztreonam and Imipenem

Generic name	Trade name	Administration/dosage
Aztreonam	Azactam	INTRAMUSCULAR, INTRAVENOUS: *Adults*—1 to 8 Gm daily, divided into 2 to 4 equal doses. FDA Pregnancy Category B.
Imipenem-cilastatin	Primaxin	INTRAVENOUS: *Adults*—1 to 4 Gm daily, divided into 3 or 4 equal doses. FDA Pregnancy Category C.

frequently be switched to penicillin V or penicillin G. One of the dangers in too common use of these drugs is that the unusual drug tolerance type of resistance may develop in more and more bacterial populations. As discussed for methicillin, this type of resistance then affects all beta-lactam antibiotics and makes the resistant organism quite dangerous and difficult to eradicate.

Extended spectrum penicillins: amdinocillin, ampicillin, amoxicillin, bacampacillin, and cyclacillin

Absorption. Ampicillin may be administered orally, but only 35 to 50% of an oral dose is absorbed. Bacampacillin and cyclacillin are prodrug forms that were designed to be more rapidly and completely absorbed than ampicillin but on breakdown in the body to release ampicillin. Amoxicillin is chemically related to ampicillin, but is more acid stable and therefore better absorbed orally. Amdinocillin is not absorbed orally and must be administered parenterally.

Uses. All the penicillins discussed earlier have relatively narrow antimicrobial spectra, being primarily useful against gram-positive bacteria. The development of ampicillin and related drugs significantly broadened the penicillin spectrum to include several common gram-negative pathogens. These drugs penetrate gram-negative cell walls better than does penicillin G and are therefore more effective against these organisms than penicillin G. The extended spectrum penicillins are not resistant to penicillinase and so may not be effective against *S. aureus* strains resistant to penicillin G.

Ampicillin is available in a fixed combination with sulbactam, and amoxicillin is available in a fixed combination with clavulanic acid. Sulbactam and clavulanic acid are inhibitors of penicillinases. Inclusion of these inhibitors in the fixed combinations is designed to protect the active drugs from

destruction, allowing their use against some organisms that would otherwise be resistant.

Anti-*Pseudomonas* penicillins: azlocillin, carbenicillin, mezlocillin, piperacillin, and ticarcillin

Absorption. These drugs must be administered parenterally. For carbenicillin, an indanyl ester is available, which allows the drug to be used orally. However, indanyl carbenicillin does not produce high enough serum levels of carbenicillin to make the drug effective for most infections. Therefore it is reserved for use in urinary tract infections, since the drug does accumulate to high concentrations in the urine following oral dosage.

Uses. One pathogenic organism that is not sensitive to ampicillin or amoxicillin is *Pseudomonas aeruginosa*. This gram-negative bacterium is responsible for certain urinary tract infections, bacteremias, and infections in burn patients, and is unusually resistant to many antibiotics. Thus the anti-*Pseudomonas* drugs were developed specifically for use against this organism.

Anti-*Pseudomonas* penicillins may be used with gentamicin (see Chapter 33) for the treatment of severe *Pseudomonas* infections. Gentamicin must never be directly mixed in the syringe or intravenous bottle with these agents, since these penicillins inactivate gentamicin.

CEPHALOSPORINS

The cephalosporins are conveniently divided into three subgroups, referred to as *generations*. Among the first-generation cephalosporins, cephalothin and cefazolin are the most widely used parenteral agents and cephalexin is the most widely used oral agent, although other members of this class differ little from these three. Second-generation cephalosporins differ from the first-generation drugs in having slightly extended activity against gram-negative bacteria. For example, the second-generation drug cefamandole has better activity than first-generation cephalosporins against *Enterobacter*. Other second-generation cephalosporins are especially active against *Haemophilus*. Third-generation cephalosporins are characterized by lower activity against gram-positive organisms than first-generation drugs, but the third-generation cephalosporins have significant activity against the important gram-negative pathogen *Pseudomonas aeruginosa*. They are the only cephalosporins to possess such activity. In addition, several third-generation cephalosporins are distributed reliably into the central nervous system.

Absorption. Several cephalosporins are currently available for oral use (Table 30.3). These preparations are well absorbed and produce effective serum concentrations of antibiotic. Absorption of cephalosporins from the gastrointestinal tract is slowed by food in the stomach, but about the same amount of drug is ultimately absorbed as in a fasting patient.

Most cephalosporins are given parenterally (Table 30.3), being well absorbed from intramuscular sites. The elimination half-times of all these drugs are about twice as long as that of penicillin G and are roughly equivalent to those of ampicillin or the penicillinase-resistant penicillins.

Distribution. Cephalosporins are distributed in the body in a manner similar to that of penicillins, except that first- and second-generation cephalosporins do not penetrate the central nervous system well enough to be used in meningitis. Cephalosporins, with the exception of cefoperazone and ceftriaxone, are excreted primarily by the kidney and are highly concentrated in the urine, making them useful in treating several common types of urinary tract infections.

Toxicity. Many cephalosporins cause pain at the injection site. When given intravenously, the drugs cause phlebitis or thrombophlebitis and pain along the affected vein. Orally administered cephalosporins may cause gastric irritation, nausea, and vomiting.

Interstitial nephritis occasionally has been observed with these drugs. The danger of synergistic nephrotoxicity should be considered when any cephalosporin is given with other nephrotoxic agents, such as the antibiotics gentamicin, kanamycin, and polymyxin or the diuretics furosemide and ethacrynic acid.

Uses. The primary usefulness of cephalosporins is based on the differences in the antimicrobial spectra of penicillins and cephalosporins. First-generation cephalosporins resemble ampicillin in their effectiveness against gram-negative bacteria. Unlike ampicillin, however, cephalosporins resist the action of staphylococcal penicillinase and can be used when the organism is resistant to penicillin G. Second- and third-generation cephalosporins are used for specific, serious infections caused by gram-negative bacteria.

Related Beta-Lactam Antibiotics

Beta-lactam antibiotics related to penicillins and cephalosporins have become available for clinical use. These include imipenem (a carbapenem) and aztreonam (a monobactam).

Aztreonam (Table 30-4)

Aztreonam has a mechanism of action similar to that of other beta-lactam antibiotics, interfering with bacterial cell wall synthesis. Unlike most penicillins and cephalosporins, aztreonam inhibits or destroys primarily gram-negative aerobic bacteria and has little effect on gram-positive or anaerobic bacteria.

Aztreonam must be administered parenterally in order to obtain useful concentrations in plasma. The drug is distributed well to many body tissues and fluids, but is relatively low in cerebrospinal fluid. Excretion is primarily via the kidneys, with only minor amounts of drug being eliminated by hepatic mechanisms.

The principal adverse reactions to aztreonam include pain and/or phlebitis at the injection site in up to 2.4% of patients. Gastrointestinal symptoms including nausea, diarrhea, and/or vomiting occur in up to 1.3% of patients. Rash and other symptoms of allergic reactions can occur, as with all beta-lactam antibiotics.

Aztreonam is given to treat urinary tract infections, septicemia, infections of the lower respiratory tract, intraabdominal or gynecologic infections, and soft-tissue infections. These infections are typically cuased by gram-negative bacteria, including *Pseudomonas*.

Imipenem

Imipenem is an extremely potent inhibitor of bacterial cell wall synthesis. The mechanism of action resembles that of other beta-lactam antibiotics. Imipenem has a very broad antimicrobial spectrum that includes gram-positive, gram-negative, and anaerobic bacteria. Imipenem is effective against penicillinase-producing *Staphylococcus aureus*.

Imipenem is well distributed to many tissues, but is low in cerebrospinal fluid. Excretion is

Text continued on p. 478.

Table 30.5   Guide for Rate of Direct Infusion for Penicillins, Cephalosporins and Related Drugs

Drug	Recommended dilution*	Rate of administration†
Ampicillin	500 mg in at least 5 ml diluent	1 dose/10-15 min
Ampicillin + sulbactam	1.5 Gm in 4 ml diluent	1 dose/15-30 min
Azlocillin	1 Gm/10 ml diluent	3-5 min
Carbenicillin	Dilute as directed on vial, then further dilute each gram in at least 10 ml diluent	1 Gm/5 min
Methicillin	500 mg reconstituted drug in at least 25 ml diluent	10 ml/min
Mezlocillin	1 Gm in at least 10 ml diluent	1 dose/3-5 min
Nafcillin	Desired amount of drug in 15 to 30 ml diluent	500 mg/5-10 min
Oxacillin	1 Gm/10 ml diluent	1 ml/min
Piperacillin	1 Gm/5 ml diluent	1 dose/3-5 min
Ticarcillin	1 Gm in at least 4 ml diluent, then further diluted to 1 Gm/10 ml	1 Gm/5 min
Ticarcillin + clavulanate	3.1 Gm/13 ml diluent; further dilute in 50 to 100 ml of fluid	1 dose/30 min
Cefamandole	1 Gm/10 ml diluent	1 Gm/3-5 min
Cefazolin	1 Gm/10 ml diluent	1 Gm/5 min
Cefonicid	0.5 Gm/2 ml diluent	1 dose/3-5 min
Cefoperazone	1 Gm/5 ml diluent	1 dose/3-5 min
Ceforanide	0.5 Gm/5 ml diluent	1 dose/3-5 min
Cefotaxime	1 dose/10 ml diluent	1 dose/3-5 min
Cefotetan	1 Gm/10 ml diluent	1 dose/3-5 min
Cefoxitin	1 Gm/10 ml diluent	1 Gm/3-5 min
Ceftazidime	0.5 Gm/5 ml	1 dose/3-5 min
Ceftizoxime	1 Gm/10 ml diluent	1 dose/3-5 min
Ceftriaxone	250 mg/2.4 ml; further dilute in 50 to 100 ml of fluid	1 dose/30 min
Cefuroxime	750 mg with 9 ml diluent	1 dose/3-5 min
Cephalothin	1 Gm/10 ml diluent	1 Gm/3-5 min
Cephapirin	1 Gm/10 ml diluent	1 Gm/5 min
Cephradine	500 mg/5 ml diluent	1 Gm/3-5 min
Moxalactam	1 Gm/10 ml diluent	1 dose/3-5 min

*For information about appropriate diluents, preparations for constant infusion, compatibilities with infusion fluids, storage conditions, and other questions, consult the pharmacist and the manufacturer's information. Because the cephalosporins are so irritating to the vein, diluting these drugs more than is indicated in the table is preferable, when possible.
†These rates are for direct IV unless otherwise noted. When diluted in 50 to 100 ml or more, the rate is determined in part by the total volume.

Table 30.5   Guide for Rate of Direct Infusion for Penicillins, Cephalosporins and Related Drugs—cont'd

Drug	Recommended dilution*	Rate of administration†
Aztreonam	1 dose/6 to 10 ml diluent	1 dose/3-5 min
Imipenem and cilastatin	1 dose/10 ml diluent; further dilute in 100 ml fluid	1 dose/20-30 min

*For information about appropriate diluents, preparations for constant infusion, compatibilities with infusion fluids, storage conditions, and other questions, consult the pharmacist and the manufacturer's information. Because the cephalosporins are so irritating to the vein, diluting these drugs more than is indicated in the table is preferable, when possible.
†These rates are for direct IV unless otherwise noted. When diluted in 50 to 100 ml or more, the rate is determined in part by the total volume.

PATIENT CARE IMPLICATIONS

Drug administration

- Review the Patient Care Implications presented in Chapter 29.
- Assess for history of allergy before administering these drugs.
- Monitor vital signs, temperature. Inspect for development of rash.
- Monitor serum creatinine and BUN, liver function tests, complete blood count, and differential count. Monitor serum electrolytes of patients with hypertensive, renal, or cardiovascular disease, and in patients receiving drugs high in potassium or sodium (see text).
- For intravenous administration, consult the manufacturer's literature or Table 30.5 for the approximate rate of IV push administration. Too rapid administration of penicillins has resulted in the occurrence of seizures. Too rapid administration of the cephalosporins contributes to venous irritation and patient discomfort.
- Warn patients that IM injection may be painful. Use large muscle masses. Record and rotate injection sites. See Chapter 6 for a description of IM injection sites.
- Read labels and orders carefully. Products containing procaine, benzathine, or a combination of these are never given intravenously. Occasional patients are sensitive to procaine; symptoms include anxiety, confusion, agitation, fear of impending doom, and convulsions.

Patient and family education

- Review the Patient Care Implications given in Chapter 29.
- The following drugs should be taken on an empty stomach, 1 hour before or 2 hours after meals, with a full glassful (8 oz) of water: ampicillin, liquid bacampicillin, carbenicillin, cloxacillin, dicloxacillin, methicillin, nafcillin, oxacillin, penicillin G.
- The following drugs can be taken without regard to meals or snack: amoxicillin, amoxicillin and clavulanate, the tablet form of bacampicillin, penicillin V, and oral cephalosporins.
- Cefuroxime axetil tablets may be crushed and mixed with food for ease in taking and to help disguise the taste.
- The penicillins, cephalosporins, and related drugs may cause false-positive reactions with copper sulfate urine glucose tests. Check with the physician before changing insulin or diet. Instruct patients to monitor blood glucose levels, if possible.
- Warn the patient that amoxicillin, amoxicillin and clavulanate, ampicillin, bacampicillin, penicillin G, and penicillin V may cause the tongue to discolor or darken during therapy, but this is not significant.
- If chewable tablets are prescribed, tell patients to chew or crush the tablets before swallowing them.
- These drugs may cause diarrhea. If severe or persistent, notify the physician. For mild diarrhea, only medicines containing kaolin or attapulgite should be used.
- Warn patients taking cefamandole, cefoperazone, cefotetan, or moxalactam to avoid the use of alcohol while taking these drugs and for several days after completing the course of therapy. Ingestion of alcohol may cause a disulfiram-type of reaction; see Patient problem: Disulfiram reaction on p. 637.

through the kidney. When given alone, imipenem is hydrolyzed in the kidneys and excreted as inactive products. The clinical preparation includes cilastatin, an agent chemically related to imipenem but with no antibacterial activity. Cilastatin inhibits destruction of imipenem in the kidneys and allows active imipenem to accumulate in renal tissue and urine.

Imipenem can cause mild to serious allergic reactions, as can other beta-lactam antibiotics. Imipenem can also cause rare CNS reactions, which may include seizures. Pseudomembranous colitis can also occur.

Because imipenem has such a broad antimicrobial spectrum, it is used to treat a variety of infections at many sites. *Pseudomonas aeruginosa* is usually sensitive, but resistant strains may occur.

SUMMARY

Penicillins and cephalosporins are beta-lactam antibiotics that share many common properties. Both inhibit cell wall biosynthesis in actively growing bacteria, are inactivated by bacterial enzymes, and are excreted primarily by the kidney. Direct drug toxicity from these antibiotics is relatively low, with allergic reactions being the most common side effect. Oral forms of penicillins and cephalosporins may cause various forms of gastrointestinal distress. Many penicillin and cephalosporin preparations contain sufficient sodium or potassium to alter electrolyte balance in some patients. Many are unstable in solution and must be diluted with care for intramuscular or intravenous use.

Penicillin G is the most potent penicillin against many gram-positive bacteria. The disadvantages of this drug are rapid excretion, narrow antimicrobial spectrum, variable oral absorption, and sensitivity to *Staphylococcus aureus* penicillinase. Procaine penicillin G and benzathine penicillin G are long-acting repository forms of penicillin G and are suitable only for intramuscular administration. These preparations differ from penicillin G only in having a long duration of action as a result of slowed absorption from injection sites. Penicillin V differs from penicillin G in being more acid stable and therefore more reliably absorbed orally. The penicillins developed for resistance to *S. aureus* penicillinase include methicillin, an agent used only parenterally, and nafcillin, an agent unique among the penicillins in being excreted primarily in bile. Penicillinase-resistant penicillins that are well absorbed orally include oxacillin, cloxacillin, and dicloxacillin. Bacterial resistance does develop against these penicillinase-resistant drugs, but the mechanism involves cell tolerance to the

antibiotic rather than destruction of it. Penicillins with an extended spectrum toward gram-negative bacteria include ampicillin and amoxicillin. Both agents are used orally, although amoxicillin is the better absorbed of the two. Bacampacillin and cyclacillin are also well-absorbed oral agents; these drugs are converted to ampicillin in the body. Amdinocillin is an extended spectrum penicillin but is not used orally. Azlocillin, carbenicillin, mezlocillin, piperacillin, and ticarcillin are currently listed as anti-*Pseudomonas* penicillins and are used only parenterally.

Cephalosporins differ from penicillins in having an extended spectrum against gram-negative microorganisms and in being resistant to *S. aureus* penicillinase.

Related beta-lactam antibiotics include aztreonam and imipenem. Aztreonam is a parenteral agent with activity mainly against gram-negative aerobic bacteria. Imipenem is a very potent, broad spectrum antimicrobial agent. It is administered in fixed combination with cilastatin to prevent destruction of imipenem in the kidney.

STUDY QUESTIONS

1. What is the mechanism of action of penicillins and cephalosporins?
2. What is the effect of beta-lactam antibiotics on existing bacterial cell wall?
3. How do most bacteria gain resistance toward beta-lactam antibiotics?
4. What is the mechanism of excretion for most penicillins and cephalosporins?
5. What is the most common toxic reaction to penicillins and cephalosporins?
6. What is the purpose of skin tests for penicillin allergies?
7. What is the effect of penicillin on the central nervous system?
8. Name two groups of patients most at risk of accumulating penicillins given at normal doses.
9. What type of patient would be most at risk from the potassium and sodium contained in many penicillin and cephalosporin preparations?
10. Why is probenecid sometimes administered with penicillin G?
11. What is the effect of destroying the penicillin nucleus?
12. What is the effect of altering the penicillin side chain structure?
13. Why is penicillin G absorbed erratically from the gastrointestinal tract?
14. When does the peak concentration of penicillin

G appear in the bloodstream following an intramuscular dose of the drug?

15. What is the elimination half-time for penicillin G in normal patients?

16. How does the penetration of penicillin G into the cerebrospinal fluid differ in normal patients and in those with meningitis?

17. Name three groups of microorganisms that are sensitive to penicillin G.

18. Why do procaine penicillin G and benzathine penicillin G have longer durations of action than penicillin G?

19. By what route must the repository penicillins be administered?

20. Which would produce a higher serum concentration of antibiotic, 1 million units of penicillin G or 1 million units of procaine penicillin G?

21. What advantage does penicillin V have over penicillin G?

22. Why would methicillin be useful in treating infections caused by penicillinase-producing *Staphylococcus aureus?*

23. How do bacteria become resistant to methicillin?

24. What is the route of excretion of nafcillin?

25. What advantages do oxacillin, cloxacillin, and dicloxacillin possess over methicillin?

26. How does the antimicrobial spectrum of ampicillin and amoxicillin differ from that of penicillin G?

27. What advantage does amoxicillin possess over ampicillin?

28. How do bacampacillin and cyclacillin differ from ampicillin?

29. Why is clavulanic acid or sulbactam included in fixed combination with ampicillin, amoxicillin, or ticarcillin?

30. Infections caused by what pathogen are appropriately treated with carbenicillin or ticarcillin?

31. How does indanyl carbenicillin differ from carbenicillin?

32. Why are first-generation cephalosporins not useful in treating meningitis?

33. What is the most common reaction expected from most cephalosporins when the drugs are administered intravenously?

34. How does the antimicrobial spectrum of the cephalosporins differ from that of penicillin G?

35. What is the antimicrobial spectrum of aztreonam?

36. What is the antimicrobial spectrum of imipenem?

37. Why is imipenem given with cilastatin?

SUGGESTED READINGS

Childs, S.J., and Bodey, G.P.: Aztreonam: a review of its pharmacologic, microbiologic, and clinical properties, Pharmacotherapy 6(4):138, 1986.

Choice of cephalosporins, Med. Lett. Drugs Ther. **25**:57, June 10, 1983.

Eichenwald, H.F.: Using cephalosporins in children, Drug Therapy **13**(1):221, 1983.

Gever, L.N.: Primaxin: an antibiotic for (nearly) all bacterial infections, Nursing87 **17**(3):102, 1987.

Jaresko, G.S., and Barriere, S.L.: Imipenem monotherapy versus combination therapy in the management of mixed bacterial infection, Pharmacotherapy 8(6):324, 1988.

Link, D.L.: Antibiotic therapy in the cancer patient: focus on third generation cephalosporins, Oncol. Nurs. Forum **14**(5):35, 1987.

Selwyn, S.: The evolution of the broad-spectrum penicillins, J. Antimicrob. Chemother. 9(suppl. B):1, 1982.

Smith, B.R., and LeFrock, J.L.: Azlocillin, mezlocillin, and piperacillin: a review of the newer penicillins, Intern. Med. **4**(2):47, 1983.

Smith, C.R.: Cefotaxime and cephalosporins: adverse reactions in perspective, Rev. Infect. Dis. 4(suppl.):S481, Sept.-Oct. 1982.

Thompson, R.L., and Wright, A.J.: Cephalosporins, carbapenem, and monobactam, Mayo Clin. Proc. **62**(9):821, 1987.

Wright, A.J., and Wilkowske, C.J.: The penicillins, Mayo Clin. Proc. **62**(9):806, 1987.

CHAPTER

Antibiotics: Erythromycin, Clindamycin, and Miscellaneous Penicillin Substitutes

31

This chapter introduces several antibiotics with antimicrobial spectra similar to those of narrow spectrum penicillins. Because of this property, these drugs are sometimes grouped together as penicillin substitutes. The mechanisms of action, modes of bacterial resistance, absorption properties, drug distribution and excretion, as well as the unique toxic reactions these drugs may induce are discussed.

ERYTHROMYCIN

Mechanism of Action and Bacterial Resistance

Erythromycin binds to bacterial ribosomes and thus prevents bacterial protein synthesis. At low concentrations, this effect is bacteriostatic, but at high concentrations the drug may be bactericidal.

Bacteria become resistant to erythromycin by one of two mechanisms. Gram-negative organisms seem to be relatively impermeable to erythromycin and are therefore intrinsically resistant. Cell wall–deficient forms of these bacteria (L-forms) are permeable to erythromycin and are highly sensitive to the drug. Gram-positive organisms acquire resistance by chemically altering their ribosomes so that the ribosomes no longer bind erythromycin; thus protein synthesis is not inhibited. This ribosomal alteration is catalyzed by an enzyme that is synthesized from genes carried on a bacterial plasmid. Plasmids are discrete circular molecules of deoxyribonucleic acid (DNA) that exist separate from the bacterial chromosome (see Chapter 43). These plasmids can be transferred directly from one bacterial cell to another. Therefore resistance to erythromycin may spread rapidly throughout a bacterial population.

Absorption

Erythromycin is sensitive to acid and therefore may be extensively degraded in the stomach. Thus erythromycin base is formulated with acid-resis-

tant coatings so that the drug will pass intact through the stomach and be dissolved and absorbed in the small intestine. This tactic is based on the knowledge that the pH of the duodenum is near neutrality (see Chapter 2).

Certain chemical forms of erythromycin are used clinically primarily because of their increased resistance to acid and better oral absorption. These compounds are the stearate, ethylsuccinate, and estolate esters of erythromycin (Table 31.1). Erythromycin stearate and erythromycin ethylsuccinate are absorbed more rapidly and more completely from the gastrointestinal tract than erythromycin base. Free erythromycin apparently is absorbed from the duodenum with these agents following hydrolysis of the esters. With erythromycin estolate, much better oral absorption of drug is achieved, and serum levels may be four times higher than with other forms of erythromycin. However, with erythromycin estolate most of the drug in the serum is actually the ester, and controversy exists as to whether this form of the drug has biological activity. Many physicians prefer the erythromycin estolate because of the high tissue and blood levels and note that many tissues and many bacteria can hydrolyze the ester form of the drug to release free erythromycin at the infection site.

Food may interfere with the oral absorption of most erythromycin preparations. Erythromycin estolate and erythromycin ethylsuccinate are the exceptions, being well absorbed even when food is present.

Erythromycin is available as the lactobionate or the gluceptate for intravenous injection (Table 31.1). These water-soluble products may be diluted with sterile water for injection but should not be diluted in sterile water containing preservatives. Erythromycin lactobionate or erythromycin gluceptate may be rapidly inactivated if added to fluids below pH 5.5. This sensitivity to extremes of pH

480

Table 31.1   Clinical Summary of Erythromycins

Generic name	Trade name	Drug form	Administration/dosage
Erythromycin base	E-Mycin* Erythromid Ilotycin Robimycin	Enteric or film-coated tablets	ORAL: *Adults*—250 mg 4 times per day (15 to 20 mg/kg body weight per day). *Children*—30 to 100 mg/kg per day in 3 or 4 doses. *Patients with very severe infections*—up to 4 Gm per day.
Erythromycin stearate	Erypar Erythrocin Stearate Ethril Wyamycin-S	Film-coated tablets	ORAL: *Adults and children*—same as for erythromycin base.
Erythromycin estolate	Ilosone* Novorythro	Tablets, capsules, suspension, chewable tablets	ORAL: *Adults and children*—same as for erythromycin base.
Erythromycin ethylsuccinate	E.E.S.* E-Mycin E Pediamycin	Drops, suspension, chewable tablets, film-coated tablets	ORAL: *Adults*—400 mg 4 times per day. *Children*—same as for erythromycin base.
Erythromycin lactobionate	Erythrocin Lacto-bionate-IV	Powder stabilized with benzyl alcohol; to be reconstituted with diluent suggested by manufacturer	INTRAVENOUS: *Adults and children*—15 to 20 mg/kg body weight per day, preferably by continuous infusion; intervals between doses for intermittent therapy should be 6 hr or less. Doses of up to 4 Gm per day may be used for very severe infections.
Erthromycin gluceptate	Ilotycin Glucep-tate-IV*		

*Available in Canada and United States.

makes erythromycin incompatible in solution with a number of other drugs. Before adding erythromycin to any other drug solution, compatibility of the agents should be verified with the pharmacist. Erythromycin lactobionate and erythromycin gluceptate should be infused slowly into the vein to avoid pain.

Intramuscular administration of erythromycin is avoided because injections are extremely painful.

Distribution and Excretion

Erythromycin readily enters body tissues, and tissue concentrations of the drug may persist well beyond the time when drug can be detected in the serum. Erythromycin is especially concentrated in the liver and spleen. It enters fluids of the middle ear and pleural fluids but not cerebrospinal fluid, unless the meninges are inflamed. The drug does cross the placenta, but fetal blood levels are less than 20% of maternal blood levels. Erythromycin also enters breast milk, where the concentrations may equal that of maternal serum.

The liver is the major excretory organ for erythromycin. A large percentage of orally administered drug is concentrated in bile and excreted in the feces. Some reabsorption from the intestine occurs in a process called *enterohepatic circulation* (see Chapter 2). Another significant proportion of erythromycin is apparently inactivated in the liver. Less than 10% of orally administered erythromycin appears as active drug in the urine. With intravenous dosage, about 15% of the dose appears in the urine. Because of the relative importance of the liver and the kidney in drug excretion, patients with mild renal insufficiency might be expected to receive normal doses of erythromycin, whereas a patient with hepatic insufficiency might require reduced drug doses.

Toxicity

The most common patient complaint with oral erythromycin is some form of gastrointestinal difficulty. Abdominal discomfort and cramping are dose-related reactions to these drugs. At normal doses, nausea, vomiting, and diarrhea are apparently less frequent than with oral penicillins or tetracyclines.

Allergic reactions to erythromycin have occurred, although these are rare. Reactions ranging from urticaria to anaphylaxis have been noted.

Rarely patients who receive more than 4 Gm of erythromycin lactobionate per day have experienced hearing loss.

The most significant toxicity occurs with erythromycin estolate. This drug damages the liver, either by direct drug toxicity or by an immune reaction. This reaction, called *cholestatic hepatitis,* usually appears 10 to 12 days after therapy is begun but may appear earlier in patients previously exposed to the drug. These patients may experience severe abdominal pain, liver enlargement, fever, and jaundice. When the drug is discontinued, these symptoms rapidly disappear in most patients.

Drug Interactions

Erythromycin is metabolized in the liver and may therefore compete with other drugs for the limited metabolic capacity of the liver. For example, alfentanil, carbamazepine, warfarin, and theophylline are drugs that also must be eliminated by hepatic mechanisms. When erythromycin is given concurrently, the result is that the aforementioned drugs are eliminated more slowly, serum levels rise, and the drugs may accumulate. Because all of these drugs have dose-related toxicity, the effect of erythromycin is not only to increase serum levels but also to increase the risk of serious toxicity.

Erythromycin may rarely cause hepatotoxicity, especially when used at high doses or for long periods of time. The risk of liver damage is increased if erythromycin is given concurrently with other hepatoxic agents, such as acetaminophen (high dose), anabolic steroids, androgens, estrogens, isoniazid, ketoconazole, phenothiazines, rifampin, azlocillin, mezlocillin, piperacillin, sulfonamides, or valproic acid.

Erythromycin can antagonize the antibacterial effects of lincomycin or clindamycin because these drugs share the same target in bacteria and may displace each other from the target. Erythromycin should not be used concurrently with clindamycin or lincomycin.

Uses

Erythromycin has a similar antimicrobial spectrum to penicillin G but is chemically unrelated to penicillins and is not cross-allergenic with them. Therefore it is a very useful penicillin substitute in patients allergic to penicillins. In addition, since penicillins and erythromycin act by entirely different mechanisms, bacteria that become resistant to one of these drugs are still sensitive to the other.

Erythromycin is the drug of choice for some conditions, including atypical pneumonias, such as *Mycoplasma* pneumonia and Legionnaires' disease. Erythromycin also may be preferred over penicillin G for diphtheria, since it effectively eradicates the diphtheria carrier state. Erythromycin also may be exceedingly useful in relapsing urinary tract infections; the relapse is frequently caused by L-forms of gram-negative organisms such as *Escherichia coli* and *Proteus mirabilis*. These L-forms lack cell walls and are therefore resistant to penicillins. The L-form bacteria remain latent during penicillin therapy, revert to normal, and again produce disease when penicillin therapy is stopped. Since erythromycin penetrates these L-forms and blocks protein synthesis, the infection may be eradicated.

Clinical studies suggest that pregnant women have variable absorption of oral erythromycin, and many do not achieve effective serum concentrations of the drug. Because of this lack of effect and because erythromycin can accumulate over long periods in fetal livers, the drug may not be recommended during pregnancy.

CLINDAMYCIN AND LINCOMYCIN
Mechanism of Action and Bacterial Resistance

Clindamycin and lincomycin inhibit the action of bacterial ribosomes in a manner analogous to that of erythromycin. These drugs halt bacterial protein synthesis and may be bacteriostatic or bactericidal, depending on drug concentrations. Bacterial resistance to lincomycin and clindamycin apparently develops in several ways. Some organisms may become impermeable to the drugs. Others alter the ribosome so that it does not bind lincomycin or clindamycin. With this latter mechanism, organisms may become resistant to both lincomycin and erythromycin. In practice, most clinically observed resistance to clindamycin and lincomycin develops slowly and in a gradual, stepwise manner.

Absorption

Lincomycin may be administered by oral, intramuscular, or intravenous route (Table 31.2). When given orally, peak serum concentrations occur about 4 hours after the dose is administered. Food significantly hinders lincomycin absorption and results in serum levels much lower than those observed in the fasting state. Thus the drug should be administered between meals so that no food is taken for 1 to 2 hours before and 1 to 2 hours after the drug.

In contrast to lincomycin, clindamycin absorption is not significantly impaired by the presence of food. Clindamycin is more rapidly absorbed orally than is lincomycin and produces higher

Table 31.2   Clinical Summary of Lincomycin and Clindamycin

Generic name	Trade name	Drug form	Administration/dosage
Clindamycin	Cleocin HCl Dalacin C*	Capsules (hydrochloride hydrate)	ORAL: *Adults*—150 to 450 mg 4 times daily.
Clindamycin palmitate	Cleocin Pediatric Dalacin C*	Granules in suspension	ORAL: *Children*—8 to 25 mg/kg body weight per day in 3 or 4 doses for children over 10 kg. Smaller children should receive no more than 37.5 mg 3 times daily.
Clindamycin phosphate	Cleocin Phosphate Dalacin C*	Solution with benzyl alcohol, disodium edetate, and/or hydrochloric acid or sodium hydroxide	INTRAMUSCULAR, INTRAVENOUS: *Adults*—300 to 600 mg every 6 to 8 hrs to an upper limit of 2.4 Gm per day (no more than 0.6 Gm per injection site intramuscularly). *Children over 1 mo*—15 to 40 mg/kg body weight daily in 3 or 4 doses.
Clindamycin phosphate	Cleocin T	1% topical gel or solution	TOPICAL: *Adults and children*—For acne vulgaris apply thin film to affected area twice daily.
Lincomycin	Lincocin	Capsules, syrup	ORAL: *Adults*—500 mg 3 or 4 times daily. *Children over 1 mo*—30 to 60 mg/kg body weight per day in 3 or 4 divided doses.
		Solution with 0.9% benzyl alcohol	INTRAMUSCULAR: *Adults*—600 mg once or twice daily. *Children over 1 mo*—10 mg/kg body weight once or twice daily.
		Solution with 0.9% benzyl alcohol	INTRAVENOUS: *Adults*—600 mg to 1 Gm 2 or 3 times daily; 8.4 Gm is the upper limit for daily doses. *Children over 1 mo*—10 mg/kg body weight once or twice daily.

*Available in Canada.

blood concentrations, at least during the first few hours of therapy. Clindamycin palmitate is also available as flavored granules to be used in suspension for oral administration. The palmitate is apparently rapidly removed to release active clindamycin.

Lincomycin or clindamycin-2-phosphate may be injected intramuscularly (Table 31.2). Clinical reports suggest that local pain following injection may be a problem with clindamycin-2-phosphate, but this has rarely been reported for lincomycin. Absorption of drug by this route is good, with serum peaks being achieved 30 to 60 minutes after injection. These two drugs are also suitable for intravenous use. By this route clindamycin-2-phosphate causes pain and phlebitis, whereas this reaction has not been observed with lincomycin. Clindamycin-2-phosphate is inactive as an antibiotic but is rapidly converted to clindamycin in the body.

Distribution and Excretion

Clindamycin and lincomycin are well distributed to most body tissues, with the exception of the central nervous system. Lincomycin does not appear in the cerebrospinal fluid of normal patients but may enter the central nervous system when the meninges are inflamed by infection. Clindamycin does not appear in the cerebrospinal fluid even when meningitis is present. Both lincomycin and clindamycin appear in the milk of lactating females treated with these drugs.

Both clindamycin and lincomycin are extensively biodegraded in the body; the liver is the primary site of biotransformation. Since less than 20% of the total drug administered shows up as active antibiotic in the urine or feces, these drugs are used at normal dosages in patients with renal insufficiency or renal failure. Neither lincomycin nor clindamycin is removed by hemodialysis.

Toxicity

The most serious reaction to lincomycin or clindamycin is colitis. Symptoms range from mild diarrhea to a severe, life-threatening condition called *pseudomembranous colitis*. Any increase in frequency of bowel movements or softness of the stools may be reason to discontinue the drug, especially in elderly patients. Significant diarrhea should prompt discontinuation of the drug and may be relieved by that measure alone. The appearance of blood or mucus in the stool may be a sign of severe colitis.

Pseudomembranous colitis is caused by a toxin produced by *Clostridium difficile.* Overgrowth of this organism in the bowel can occur as a result of antibiotic perturbation of the bacterial flora in the bowel. This superinfection and its associated colitis may be specifically treated with vancomycin. Fluid and electrolyte replacement and other supportive therapy also may be required. Agents that slow peristaltic action may worsen the condition or prolong it; thus opiates or diphenoxylate with atropine are not appropriate for use in these patients.

In addition to colitis, clindamycin and lincomycin may produce gastrointestinal irritation ranging from nausea and vomiting to glossitis and stomatitis.

Allergies to clindamycin and lincomycin range from mild rashes to drug fever and anaphylactic shock. These reactions may occur in any patient but are more common in those with other allergies. The appearance of any allergic response is cause for discontinuing the drug.

Some reports suggest that blood dyscrasias and liver dysfunction occur during lincomycin or clindamycin therapy. A direct cause-and-effect relationship between the drugs and these reactions has not been demonstrated.

Lincomycin administered intravenously has caused hypotension in a few patients. Cardiopulmonary arrest has occurred. These reactions are apparently related to a too-rapid intravenous injection. Lincomycin should be administered in an intravenous solution no more concentrated than 1 Gm/dl at a rate no more rapid than 100 ml per hour. Clindamycin should be administered in an intravenous solution no more concentrated than 0.6 Gm/dl at a rate no more rapid than 100 ml in 20 minutes.

Drug Interactions

Lincomycin is incompatible in solution with the antibiotics novobiocin and kanamycin. Clindamycin is incompatible with aminophylline, ampicillin, barbiturates, calcium gluconate, magnesium sulfate, and phenytoin.

Since both clindamycin and lincomycin have neuromuscular blocking properties, they may enhance the action of various neuromuscular blocking agents and inhalation anesthetics.

The absorption of oral doses of lincomycin may be decreased by food and other agents. The use of kaolin-pectin antidiarrheal agents given at the time oral lincomycin is ingested markedly lowers the serum concentrations of lincomycin.

Uses

Clindamycin and lincomycin have antimicrobial spectra similar to those of penicillin G or erythromycin, being primarily effective against gram-positive organisms. Lincomycin and clindamycin are not as effective as penicillin against *Neisseria gonorrhoeae* or other gram-negative cocci. Clindamycin is effective against several anaerobic organisms, particularly *Bacteroides fragilis.* Infections caused by these organisms are a major indication for clindamycin use.

The dangers of severe colitis have largely restricted the use of clindamycin and lincomycin to cases in which patients are allergic to safer drugs or the pathogenic organism is demonstrated by the microbiology laboratory to be sensitive to these agents. Clindamycin is more effective and less toxic than lincomycin and is much more commonly used.

VANCOMYCIN
Mechanism of Action and Bacterial Resistance

Vancomycin prevents synthesis of bacterial cell walls by blocking peptidoglycan strand formation. This site of action is different from the sites sensitive to penicillin and other antibiotics interfering with cell wall synthesis.

Resistance to vancomycin is relatively uncommon and tends to develop slowly. As the drug is used clinically, it is a rapidly bactericidal agent, which may partly explain the low incidence of bacterial resistance to vancomycin.

Absorption

Vancomycin is a complex glycopeptide that may be positively or negatively charged, depending on the pH. Therefore vancomycin does not easily cross biological membranes and is not absorbed significantly following oral administration (Table 31.3). Vancomycin is most often administered intravenously by intermittent infusion; 500 mg may be dissolved in 10 ml of sterile water and then added to 100 to 200 ml of 0.9% sodium chloride injection or 5% dextrose in water for infusion over 20 to 30 minutes. This regimen may be repeated every 6 hours.

Vancomycin may rarely be given by mouth for intestinal infections. Bactericidal concentrations of

PATIENT CARE IMPLICATIONS

Erythromycin

Drug administration

- See Patient Care Implications in Chapter 29.
- Assess for history of allergy before administering.
- Assess baseline hearing acuity. Assess for gastrointestinal symptoms and signs of liver dysfunction. Monitor intake, output, and weight.
- Monitor liver function tests.

INTRAVENOUS ERYTHROMYCIN LACTOBIONATE OR GLUCEPTATE

- Dilute each 500 mg with 10 ml of sterile water for injection, and further dilute as instructed in drug insert. Administer at a rate of 1 Gm diluted in 100 ml over 20 to 60 minutes. Monitor vital signs.

Patient and family education

- See Patient Care Implications in Chapter 29.
- Instruct the patient to report the development of ringing in ears or hearing loss, malaise, fever, jaundice, right upper quadrant abdominal pain, change in the color or consistency of stools.
- Take oral doses with meals or snack to reduce gastric irritation.

Clindamycin and lincomycin

Drug administration

- See Patient Care Implications in Chapter 29.
- Assess for history of allergy before administering.
- Assess for signs of diarrhea or gastrointestinal distress. Monitor intake, output, and weight.
- Monitor complete blood count and differential, platelet count, liver function tests, serum electrolytes.

INTRAVENOUS CLINDAMYCIN

- Dilute each 300 mg with at least 50 ml suitable diluent; see drug insert. Administer at a rate of 300 mg or less over at least 10 minutes. Do not administer too rapidly. Monitor vital signs. Supervise ambulation.

INTRAVENOUS LINCOMYCIN

- Dilute 1 Gm with at least 100 ml of suitable diluent; see drug insert. Administer at a rate of 1 Gm or less/hr. Monitor vital signs. Do not administer too rapidly. Supervise ambulation.

Patient and family education

- See Patient Care Implications in Chapter 29.
- Instruct patients to report the development of diarrhea.
- Take oral doses of clindamycin with a full glassful (8 oz) of fluid, whether with or without meals.
- Take oral lincomycin with a full glassful (8 oz) of fluid on an empty stomach, 1 hour before or 2 hours after meals or snack.

Vancomycin

Drug administration

- See Patient Care Implications in Chapter 29.
- Assess for history of allergy before administering.
- Assess baseline hearing acuity.
- Monitor serum creatinine, BUN, complete blood count, and differential count. Monitor urinalysis.

INTRAVENOUS VANCOMYCIN

- Dilute each 500 mg with 10 ml of sterile water for injection. Further dilute with compatible fluid; see drug insert. Administer each diluted dose over 60 minutes. Monitor vital signs. Too rapid IV administration may be associated with hypotension, cardiac arrest, or "red man's syndrome" or "red-neck syndrome": maculopapular or erythematous rash of the face, head, chest, and arms; fever, chills, fainting, nausea, vomiting, tachycardia, or itching.

Patient and family education

- See Patient Care Implications in Chapter 29.
- Instruct patient to report ringing in ears or hearing loss.
- Do not take oral doses within 4 hours of doses of cholestyramine or colestipol.

Bacitracin

Drug administration/patient and family education

- See Patient Care Implications in Chapter 29.
- Topical use of this drug is rarely associated with side effects.

Spectinomycin

Drug administration/patient and family education

- See Patient Care Implications in Chapter 29.
- Warn patients that IM injections may cause burning at the site. Use diluent supplied by the manufacturer. Dilute as directed on the vial label.

the drug is chemically unrelated to penicillins and has a different mechanism of action, it is effective against organisms that are resistant to penicillins, including methicillin-resistant staphylococci. Since vancomycin and penicillin are not cross-allergenic, vancomycin is very useful in patients allergic to penicillins. Vancomycin also has special utility in treating antibiotic-induced colitis, which arises from a superinfection with *Clostridium difficile* in the bowel.

BACITRACIN
Mechanism of Action and Bacterial Resistance

Bacitracin blocks the regeneration of a lipid carrier that transports cell wall material through the bacterial cell membrane. This site of action is different from that of penicillins or other antibiotics that inhibit cell wall formation. In addition to this action, the drug interferes with bacterial cell membrane function.

Inherent resistance to bacitracin exists in gram-negative organisms, but acquired resistance among the gram-positive organisms is uncommon. Organisms resistant to bacitracin are not necessarily resistant to other antibiotics.

Absorption, Distribution, and Excretion

Bacitracin is well absorbed from intramuscular injection sites and penetrates all body organs. The kidney eliminates the drug, primarily by glomerular filtration.

The most common route of administration is topical, either on the skin or in the eye (Table 31.3). When applied to the body surface or when used to lavage the peritoneal cavity, the drug seems not to be absorbed to any significant degree.

Toxicity

Bacitracin is extremely nephrotoxic. Glomerular and tubular necrosis have occurred. Protein may appear in the urine and azotemia (excess urea and other nitrogen-containing compounds in the blood) may develop. Because of the great risk of permanent kidney damage, bacitracin is not used systemically. Other less toxic drugs can usually be substituted. When used topically, the drug is practically nontoxic.

Uses

Bacitracin is effective against gram-positive bacteria, especially staphylococci.

The most common use of bacitracin is as a topical ointment for superficial skin infections. The drug may be obtained alone or in combination with various other antibiotics in several nonprescription preparations. Special formulations of bacitracin exist for use in the eye.

SPECTINOMYCIN
Mechanism of Action, Bacterial Resistance, and Clinical Use

Spectinomycin inhibits bacterial protein synthesis. Both gram-positive and gram-negative bacteria may be affected, but the ability of spectinomycin to inhibit *N. gonorrhoeae* is the basis for its clinical usefulness. On this basis it is classified as a penicillin substitute. Resistance to spectinomycin may occur.

Absorption, Distribution, and Excretion

Spectinomycin is administered by intramuscular injection in the treatment of gonorrhea (Table 31.3). Absorption is adequate to produce high serum concentrations of drug and to maintain those concentrations long enough after a single injection to eradicate *N. gonorrhoeae* from the infection site. Within 2 days, nearly all of the injected drug appears in active form in the urine.

Toxicity

Single doses of spectinomycin have caused nausea, chills, and dizziness. Some patients report pain at the injection site, urticaria, or fever. Urine output may be diminished, but renal damage has not been verified.

SUMMARY

Penicillin substitutes are antibiotics that have an antimicrobial spectrum similar to that of penicillin G and are frequently used in patients allergic to the penicillins or against organisms that have acquired resistance to penicillins.

Erythromycin is primarily used orally, with the esters of erythromycin being less acid sensitive and better absorbed than erythromycin base. Erythromycin lactobionate or gluceptate may be given intravenously but may cause pain. Erythromycin is excreted primarily by the liver. Erythromycin estolate may rarely produce cholestatic hepatitis. Allergies and hearing loss are rare reactions to erythromycins. The most common limiting toxicity with these drugs is gastrointestinal distress. Erythromycin has special utility in treating atypical pneumonias, infections resulting from bacterial L-forms, and diphtheria.

Clindamycin may be used orally or, when used as the phosphate, may be injected parenterally. Clindamycin does not enter the cerebrospinal fluid but is otherwise well distributed to body tissues.

The liver degrades the drug extensively and is the main route of drug elimination. Clindamycin use can lead to a superinfection of the bowel with *Clostridium difficile*. This organism produces a toxin that induces severe colitis. Diarrhea and the danger of this severe reaction limit the use of clindamycin.

Vancomycin is a parenteral agent well distributed to most body tissues and fluids. The drug is excreted primarily by the kidney and may accumulate when kidney function is reduced. Vancomycin can produce deafness, nephrotoxicity, and an acute reaction on injection. Bacterial resistance to vancomycin is rare. One unique use of the drug is in treating antibiotic-induced colitis caused by *C. difficile*.

Bacitracin is used primarily as a topical agent because it is too toxic to the kidney for routine systemic use. Spectinomycin is used primarily in the treatment of gonorrhea when penicillin is inappropriate.

STUDY QUESTIONS

1. Why are erythromycin, clindamycin, vancomycin, bacitracin, and spectinomycin called *penicillin substitutes*?
2. What are two mechanisms that account for bacterial resistance to erythromycin?
3. What advantages do the esters of erythromycin possess over erythromycin base?
4. Which of the erythromycin esters is best absorbed orally and may be taken with meals?
5. Which forms of erythromycin can be used parenterally?
6. What property limits the parenteral use of erythromycin?
7. What is the major route of excretion of erythromycin?
8. What is the most common reaction to erythromycin?
9. What toxic reaction is unique to erythromycin estolate?
10. Name four clinical uses of erythromycin.
11. Bacterial resistance to clindamycin is associated with resistance to which other antibiotic?
12. How do clindamycin and lincomycin differ in oral absorption?
13. What form of clindamycin is appropriate for parenteral use?
14. How do clindamycin and lincomycin differ in their distribution to the central nervous system?
15. How is clindamycin eliminated from the body?
16. What is the limiting toxicity to clindamycin?
17. How is clindamycin-induced colitis best treated?
18. Why is bacterial resistance to vancomycin relatively rare?
19. By what route is vancomycin usually administered?
20. What is the major route of excretion of vancomycin?
21. What toxic reactions are most common with vancomycin?
22. Name three clinical uses for vancomycin.
23. By what route is bacitracin usually administered?
24. What toxicity is associated with the systemic use of bacitracin?
25. What is the primary clinical indication for spectinomycin?
26. What pharmacological property of spectinomycin makes this drug a useful replacement of penicillin in the treatment of gonorrhea?

SUGGESTED READINGS

Dipiro, J.T., and others: Oral neomycin sulfate and erythromycin base before colon surgery, Pharmacotherapy 5(2):91, 1985.

Hermans, P.E., and Wilhelm, M.P.: Vancomycin, Mayo Clin. Proc. **62**(10):901, 1987.

Keighley, M.R.B.: Antibiotic-associated pseudomembranous colitis: pathogenesis and management, Drugs **20**:49, 1980.

Wilson, W.R., and Cockerill, F.R. III: Tetracyclines, chloramphenicol, erythromycin, and clindamycin, Mayo Clin. Proc. **62**(10):906, 1987.

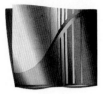

CHAPTER

Antibiotics: Tetracyclines and Chloramphenicol

32

In this chapter antibiotics with very broad antimicrobial spectra, tetracyclines and chloramphenicol, are introduced. The tetracyclines are a large family of chemically related compounds, many of which are clinically useful. Chloramphenicol is the only member of its chemical class that is approved for use in the United States.

TETRACYCLINES
Mechanism of Action and Bacterial Resistance

The tetracyclines block bacterial growth by preventing ribosomes from binding messenger RNA, thereby preventing the initiation of protein synthesis. Members of this drug family are, therefore, bacteriostatic rather than bactericidal.

For tetracyclines to be effective, they must first be transported into the bacterial cell. Antibiotic uptake is accomplished by an energy-dependent transport system. Resistant bacteria lose the ability to transport tetracyclines into the bacterial cell, and the antibiotic does not come in contact with its intracellular target. Much of the observed tetracycline resistance involves a plasmid (Chapter 29), which is transmitted from bacterium to bacterium and may therefore spread rapidly throughout bacterial populations. For example, families of patients treated on a long-term basis with low doses of tetracyclines may show a conversion of the normal tetracycline-sensitive bacterial flora to tetracycline-resistant forms. Cross-resistance between the older tetracyclines is complete. The newer tetracyclines minocycline and doxycycline, however, are more lipid soluble than the older drugs and are transported into the bacterial cell by different mechanisms than the older drugs. These drugs may therefore penetrate bacterial cells that do not concentrate the older tetracyclines. For example, strains of *Staphylococcus aureus* resistant

to tetracycline do not accumulate tetracycline but may accumulate minocycline and may be sensitive to it.

Absorption

Tetracyclines are administered primarily by the oral route (Table 32.1). They are frequently administered as the hydrochloride or the phosphate salt to increase solubility and thereby increase absorption.

Tetracyclines are variably absorbed from the gastrointestinal tract. Absorption is influenced by three factors: acid lability, water solubility, and lipid solubility. All the tetracyclines with the exception of doxycycline and minocycline are acid labile and are partly destroyed by stomach acid. Tetracyclines are not highly water soluble and this solubility may be further reduced by complex formation with metal ions or with solid material in the intestine. In these insoluble forms the drugs are not absorbed but remain in the intestine and are excreted in the feces. Doxycycline and minocycline are the exceptions, being highly lipid soluble; both drugs tend to pass freely through the gastrointestinal membranes and are much more completely and rapidly absorbed than most of the other tetracyclines.

Absorption of tetracyclines from intramuscular sites is generally poor and frequently causes local tissue irritation and pain at the injection site. Intramuscular use of tetracyclines is therefore limited.

Tetracyclines may be used intravenously in serious infections. Tetracycline, oxytetracycline, doxycycline, and minocycline all can be obtained in a form suitable for intravenous use. These drugs have a relatively low water solubility, however, and must be diluted extensively before use by this route. When used intravenously, tetra-

Table 32.1   **Clinical Summary of Tetracyclines**

Generic name	Trade name	Administration/dosage
Tetracycline HCl	Achromycin* Bristacycline Cyclopar Panmycin Sumycin Tetracyn*	ORAL: *Adults*—1 to 2 Gm per day in 2 to 4 doses. *Children over 8 yr*—25 to 50 mg/kg per day in 2 to 4 doses.
	Achromycin IM Tetracyn IM	INTRAMUSCULAR: *Adults*—300 mg to 800 mg per day in divided doses. *Children over 8 yr*—15 to 25 mg/kg not to exceed 250 mg per dose.
	Achromycin IV Tetracyn IV	INTRAVENOUS: *Adults*—250 to 500 mg every 12 hrs. *Children over 8 yr*—15 to 25 mg/kg per day in 2 doses.
Oxytetracycline HCl	Oxlopar Terramycin*	ORAL: As for tetracycline.
	Terramycin IM	INTRAMUSCULAR: As for tetracycline.
	Terramycin IV	INTRAVENOUS: As for tetracycline.
Methacycline HCl	Rondomycin	ORAL: *Adults*—600 mg per day in 2 or 4 doses. *Children over 8 yr*—10 mg/kg per day in 4 doses.
Demeclocycline HCl	Declomycin*	ORAL: *Adults*—600 mg to 1 Gm per day in 4 doses. *Children over 8 yr*—6 to 12 mg/kg per day in 2 to 4 doses.
Doxycycline	Doxycycline hyclate Vibramycin*	ORAL: *Adults*—100 to 200 mg per day in 2 doses. *Children over 8 yr*—2 to 4 mg/kg per day in 2 doses.
	Vibramycin IV	INTRAVENOUS: As for oral route.
Minocycline HCl	Minocin*	ORAL: 200 mg initially, then 100 mg every 12 hr.
	Minocin IV	INTRAVENOUS: As for oral route.

*Available in Canada and United States.

cyclines may cause thrombophlebitis. Improper dilution of the drug or repeated infusion into the same vein increases the likelihood of thrombophlebitis.

Distribution and Excretion

Tetracyclines are well distributed in most body tissues and fluids, appearing in liver, spleen, bone marrow, bile, and cerebrospinal fluid even in the absence of inflammation. The drugs pass the placental barrier and enter fetal circulation in appreciable amounts. Tetracyclines also appear in the milk of nursing mothers.

Differences in lipid solubility among the tetracyclines affect their elimination. The more polar or water-soluble drugs are eliminated through the kidney in greater amounts than are the lipid-soluble tetracyclines. All the tetracyclines enter the urine by passive glomerular filtration. However, the lipid-soluble drugs are more completely reabsorbed from the kidney tubule than drugs that are charged at the acid pH of the tubular fluid. This high degree of reabsorption is reflected in the longer elimination half-life for doxycycline and minocycline (about 12 to 15 hours) than that of less lipid-soluble tetracyclines such as oxytetracycline, tetracycline, or chlortetracycline (about 6 to 9 hours).

The second major route of elimination is by biliary excretion. Tetracyclines are concentrated in the liver and bile and carried into the intestine, where they may be reabsorbed by the process called *enterohepatic circulation*. The liver is also the site for biotransformation of several of the tetracyclines. In general, the more lipid-soluble drugs penetrate the liver cells and are more extensively biotransformed. Minocycline is in particular extensively biotransformed. The high lipid solubility of doxycycline and its tendency to form insoluble complexes with intestinal solids account for an unusual mode of elimination for this drug. It seems to diffuse directly into the intestine, where the drug is sequestered by complex formation with fecal material. Because of this unusual mechanism for excretion, doxycycline does not accumulate in renal failure.

Toxicity

Tetracyclines cause a wide variety of adverse reactions. Perhaps the most common complaint with these drugs is gastrointestinal irritation. Many patients suffer nausea, vomiting, or pain with oral tetracyclines. Diarrhea may occur as a result of irritation by unabsorbed tetracycline remaining in the bowel. Diarrhea may also result from changes in the intestinal flora. Occasionally the effects of these broad-spectrum drugs on intestinal flora are so extensive that overgrowth of drug-resistant bacteria occurs. Staphylococcal enterocolitis may result and may be life-threatening, producing bloody diarrhea and extensive damage to the intestinal epithelium. *Candida* superinfections of the throat, vagina, and bowel also occur occasionally.

Allergies to tetracyclines are uncommon. Urticaria, morbilliform rashes, and dermatitis have occurred, as well as more serious reactions such as asthma, angioedema, and anaphylaxis.

Tetracyclines are not entirely specific for bacterial ribosomes and may inhibit mammalian protein synthesis to a small degree. This fact may explain their toxic effect on various tissues. For example, kidney function may be impaired by tetracyclines, and the effects may be worse in a kidney already damaged by disease or trauma. Renal function should therefore be carefully watched in patients receiving these drugs. Likewise the liver is sensitive to tetracyclines. Hepatotoxicity may progress to jaundice, fatty liver, and death unless the drug is discontinued at the first sign of difficulty. Pregnant women are most sensitive to this complication and should rarely, if ever, be given tetracyclines. Elderly patients who are extremely debilitated or patients recovering from extensive surgery or traumatic injuries may suffer metabolic derangement when given tetracyclines. These patients commonly show negative nitrogen balance. This reaction is thought to result from tetracycline inhibition of mammalian protein synthesis.

Tetracyclines also delay blood coagulation. The exact mechanism for this reaction is not known but it may involve binding the calcium that is required in coagulation.

The ability of tetracyclines to bind calcium also leads to their deposition in bones and teeth. In adults this binding produces little visible effect, but in children under 8 years of age the newly formed permanent teeth may be stained by the drug. This staining is irreversible. Binding of tetracyclines to bones may slow bone growth visibly in fetuses or very young children. Infants may also display an increase in intracranial pressure with bulging fontanelles when given tetracyclines.

Specific tetracyclines may cause unique adverse reactions. For example, minocycline can cause damage to vestibular function, thereby impairing balance. No other tetracyclines produce this effect, although other antibiotics do. Another specific reaction to a single tetracycline is the phototoxic effect of demeclocycline. All tetracyclines can be degraded to toxic products by exposure to light, but demeclocycline seems to be most effective in producing these reactions. The drug appears to be broken down by the action of ultraviolet light on the skin, and the toxic products released cause an intense sunburn reaction. Since tetracyclines other than demeclocycline have the potential of causing this reaction, it is prudent to suggest that patients receiving these drugs limit their exposure to direct sunlight, especially in subtropical or tropical climates.

Outdated tetracycline preparations have been implicated in occasional severe adverse reactions, apparently caused by toxic breakdown products of the drugs. A reaction called the *Fanconi syndrome* has been observed, in which the patient loses amino acids, proteins, and sugar in the urine and suffers polyuria and polydipsia, acidosis, nausea, and vomiting. These reactions slowly disappear after the drug is discontinued. In other cases patients show symptoms reminiscent of systemic lupus erythematosus.

Drug Interactions

Several tetracycline interactions with other drugs are the result of the ability of tetracyclines to form insoluble complexes with metal ions. For example, oral tetracyclines frequently cause gastric irritation, and for this reason patients may wish to take antacids along with the antibiotic. This practice should be discouraged, since common antacids include magnesium and aluminum salts, which complex with tetracyclines and prevent their absorption from the gastrointestinal tract. The antacids, therefore, reduce the antibacterial effect of the antibiotic. Likewise, iron-containing preparations such as vitamin or mineral supplements may prevent tetracycline absorption. Milk and other dairy products are high in calcium and also impair absorption. Sodium bicarbonate taken with a tetracycline tablet may impede tablet dissolution in the stomach and thereby reduce absorption of the drug.

Food in the stomach impairs absorption of oral tetracyclines, with the exception of doxycycline and minocycline. These lipid-soluble tetracyclines are absorbed well even in the presence of food or milk products in the stomach.

Several tetracyclines, but especially doxycycline and minocycline, are metabolized to some degree by the liver. Drugs such as barbiturates, which increase hepatic drug-metabolizing enzymes, shorten the duration of action of doxycycline and minocycline. This action may decrease the antibacterial effectiveness of these agents.

The bacteriostatic mechanism of action of tetracyclines leads to interactions with two different types of drugs: immunosuppressants and penicillins. Immunosuppressant drugs such as glucocorticoids depress the host defense mechanisms against bacterial infections. Since tetracyclines are bacteriostatic drugs, they depend on the patient's immune system to eliminate the pathogen. If this elimination cannot occur, the bacteria may overcome the inhibitory effects of the tetracycline and the effect of the drug is lost. Penicillins given with tetracyclines may be less effective than penicillin given alone. Penicillins are bactericidal drugs that are effective against actively multiplying bacteria. Tetracyclines inhibit bacterial growth, thereby making them resistant to the action of penicillins.

Tetracycline nephrotoxicity may become significant and dangerous when these antibiotics are given with other nephrotoxic agents. One example involves the anesthetic methoxyflurane (Penthrane). This anesthetic gas is itself nephrotoxic; when given to patients receiving tetracyclines, it may exacerbate kidney damage.

Uses (Table 32.1)

Tetracyclines are clinically important by virtue of their very wide antibacterial spectrum. Most gram-positive organisms are sensitive to tetracyclines; however, most infections due to these organisms are best treated by other agents because penicillins, cephalosporins, erythromycin, and clindamycin are equally or more effective against these organisms and are less toxic. Nevertheless, when laboratory results confirm the organism to be sensitive to tetracyclines, these drugs can be used in some gram-positive infections.

Gram-negative bacteria found in the bowel are usually sensitive to tetracyclines, but resistance does develop. *Serratia, Proteus,* and *Pseudomonas* strains are usually resistant.

Neisseria gonorrhoeae is sensitive to tetracyclines. Clinically, however, tetracyclines are used to treat gonorrhea only when penicillin is contraindicated.

Tetracyclines are clinically effective for a number of bacterial infections that are relatively rare in the United States: chancroid *(Haemophilus ducreyi)*, rabbit fever or tularemia *(Francisella tularensis)*, black plague *(Yersinia pestis)*, brucellosis *(Brucella* species*)*, and cholera *(Vibrio cholerae)*.

Tetracyclines are highly effective for diseases caused by rickettsiae (tick fever, Rocky Mountain spotted fever, typhus, and Q fever), chlamydia (parrot fever or psittacosis, trachoma, lymphogranuloma venereum), and *Mycoplasma pneumoniae* (atypical or "walking" pneumonia).

Tetracyclines are useful in treating Lyme disease *(Borrelia burgdorferi)*, relapsing fever *(Borrelia recurrentis)*, syphilis *(Treponema pallidum)*, and yaws *(Treponema pertenue)*, which are all diseases caused by spirochetes.

Tetracyclines may have a useful role in treating amebic dysentery. Minocycline in particular may be useful in nocardial infections.

Tetracyclines have been widely used in for the treatment of acne. Relatively low doses may be prescribed over long periods of time. Although this treatment is effective for many patients, questions arise as to long-term adverse effects of the drugs and to the contribution this practice makes to the development of tetracycline-resistant bacterial populations.

Pharmaceutical formulations of tetracyclines are quite varied. These antibiotics are available in 100 to 500 mg tablets or capsules, syrups for pediatric use, ophthalmic ointments or drops, and various forms for topical use.

CHLORAMPHENICOL
Mechanism of Action and Bacterial Resistance

Chloramphenicol inhibits bacterial protein synthesis. The mechanism of action is different from that of tetracyclines in that chloramphenicol inhibits late rather than early steps in ribosomal function. Like tetracyclines, chloramphenicol is bacteriostatic rather than bactericidal.

Bacterial resistance to chloramphenicol nearly always involves destruction of the antibiotic by bacterial enzymes. These enzymes are not always present but may be induced by exposure of potentially resistant bacteria to sublethal doses of chloramphenicol. The genes required for synthesizing this enzyme are usually carried on small DNA molecules called *plasmids*, which may exist separately from the bulk of genetic material in the cell. Plasmids may be transmitted from bacterium to bac-

Table 32.2   Clinical Summary of Chloramphenicol

Generic name	Trade name	Administration/dosage	Comments
Chloramphenicol	Chloromycetin Novochloro-cap* Pentamycetin*	ORAL: *Adults*—50 to 100 mg/kg per day in 4 doses. *Children*—25 mg/kg per day or less, depending on liver function.	Blood levels should ordinarily not exceed 20 µg/ml.
Chloramphenicol palmitate	Chloromycetin	ORAL: *Children*—as for other oral forms.	This tasteless suspension is intended for pediatric use.
Chloramphenicol succinate	Chloromycetin Pentamycetin*	INTRAVENOUS: As for oral.	Should be administered as a 10% solution and injected slowly into the vein.

*Available in Canada.

terium, and resistance to chloramphenicol may thereby be transmitted widely throughout bacterial populations.

Absorption, Distribution, and Excretion

Chloramphenicol is nearly completely absorbed from the gastrointestinal tract following oral administration. The peak serum concentration achieved by an oral dose is about the same as that produced by an equivalent dose given intravenously, although the attainment of the peak serum concentration is somewhat delayed with oral administration (Table 32.2). Intramuscular injection produces lower blood levels than oral administration and for this reason is not recommended. Seriously ill patients should receive chloramphenicol intravenously, since oral absorption may be impaired in these patients. The succinate form of chloramphenicol is used for intravenous administration only, whereas the parent drug, chloramphenicol, is used orally.

Chloramphenicol is very well distributed throughout body tissues and fluids. Significant and effective concentrations of the drug enter the eye, joint fluid (synovial), and pleural fluids. Unlike many other antibiotics, chloramphenicol enters the cerebrospinal fluid relatively easily, even when the meninges are not inflamed. Chloramphenicol also easily crosses the placenta and appears in human milk.

Most of a dose of chloramphenicol is inactivated in the liver. The drug is conjugated with glucuronic acid to form chloramphenicol glucuronide. This inactive drug form may be excreted in the kidney by tubular secretion, whereas unaltered chloramphenicol is excreted solely by glomerular filtration. The actual concentration of active chloramphenicol in the urine is high enough to be an-

tibacterial, but the active chloramphenicol in the urine is only a small fraction of the total drug excreted via this route.

Toxicity

Chloramphenicol is a very effective antibiotic, but its clinical usefulness has been limited by its potential for bone marrow toxicity. A reversible form of bone marrow depression causes a reduction of reticulocytes and leukopenia. These symptoms usually resolve quickly when chloramphenicol is discontinued. Patients receiving chloramphenicol should have routine blood tests performed during therapy to detect early signs of this toxic reaction.

Chloramphenicol may also induce an irreversible bone marrow depression, which leads to aplastic anemia, a condition with a high mortality. This condition is usually characterized by pancytopenia (loss of all forms of blood cells), but in some cases one or more of the major blood cells will continue to be formed. Aplastic anemia, although rare, may appear weeks or months after chloramphenicol therapy. This time lag between drug administration and appearance of aplastic anemia complicates the accurate calculation of drug-associated risk, especially considering that most patients will have received more than one other drug during the interim between chloramphenicol therapy and development of aplastic anemia. Best estimates of the actual incidence suggest that roughly one in 30,000 chloramphenicol-treated patients will develop aplastic anemia. Although this incidence is low, the frequently fatal outcome is sufficient cause to restrict the use of chloramphenicol to the treatment of very serious infections.

Less severe problems may also occur with

THE NURSING PROCESS

TETRACYCLINES AND CHLORAMPHENICOL

Refer to the nursing process section in Chapter 29 for general guidelines on the nursing process with antibiotic therapy. The additional material below relates specifically to the broad spectrum antibiotics: tetracyclines and chloramphenicol.

Assessment

Tetracyclines may be prescribed for a very wide variety of infections, including bacterial and rickettsial diseases. Tetracyclines are not usually prescribed for pregnant patients or for children under the age of 8 years. Chloramphenicol is usually reserved for seriously ill patients, primarily those with typhoid fever or with bacteremia or meningitis caused by a chloramphenicol-sensitive organism. A thorough assessment should be carried out with emphasis on the organ in which the infection is thought to be present (if the infection is a localized one) and on liver and kidney function. Other clinical signs of infection should be monitored.

Nursing diagnoses

Potential complication: gastrointestinal distress

Possible altered home maintenance management related to insufficient knowledge of how to take tetracycline preparations

Potential complication: bone marrow depression

Management

Once the decision is made to treat the patient with tetracyclines, the nurse should obtain additional data for the data base about kidney and liver function. Patients receiving chloramphenicol should be carefully checked for adequate liver function. The nurse should also question the patient about having received chloramphenicol in the past, since a history of treatment with the drug may predispose the patient to the development of toxicity. The nurse should give special care to the proper timing of tetracycline doses, since the absorption of this drug from the gastrointestinal tract is so strongly influenced by the presence of food and other drugs. Most tetracyclines are best absorbed on an empty stomach. These drugs do cause gastrointestinal irritation, and the patient will need instruction on how to deal with this problem, since common remedies such as milk or nonprescription antacids greatly impair drug absorption. Patients receiving chloramphenicol should receive routine blood testing during and after therapy. The nurse should explain to the patient the need for this type of follow-up and encourage compliance.

Evaluation

Tetracyclines and chloramphenicol may cause reactions during and after therapy. Patients receiving tetracyclines not only should be evaluated for clearing of the infection being treated, but also should be observed for renal damage and signs of superinfection. *Candida* superinfections of the mouth, vagina, and bowel are relatively common with the use of tetracyclines. One of the tetracyclines, minocycline, can cause symptoms of vestibular damage. Chloramphenicol can cause blood dyscrasias, which appear long after the end of drug therapy. Patients should be watched for development of signs of blood abnormalities. Outpatients should demonstrate the ability to judge improvement in the infection being treated and should be able to tell the nurse what reactions might be expected with the medications and when it would be appropriate to call the physician.

PATIENT CARE IMPLICATIONS

Tetracyclines

Drug administration

- See Patient Care Implications in Chapter 29.
- Assess for allergy prior to administering.
- Assess for dizziness, vertigo in patient receiving minocycline. Inspect for bruising, bleeding, blood in stool.
- Monitor BUN, serum creatinine, liver function tests, complete blood count and differential, platelet count.
- Palpate the fontanelles of infants every 4 hours; report bulging to the physician.
- Do not administer to children under 8 years of age unless absolutely necessary.
- Administer IV doses slowly, and well diluted to lessen the chance of venous irritation and phlebitis. Make certain IV is patent before administering to avoid extravasation.
  INTRAVENOUS OXYTETRACYCLINE AND TETRACYCLINE
- Dilute as directed in drug insert. Administer at a rate of 100 mg or less over at least 5 minutes.
  INTRAVENOUS DOXYCYCLINE
- Dilute each 100 mg with 10 ml sterile water for injection or normal saline. Further dilute as directed in drug insert with 100 to 1000 ml of compatible fluid. Administer at a rate of 100 mg over 1 to 4 hours.
  INTRAVENOUS MINOCYCLINE
- Dilute as directed in drug insert. Final dilution will be in a volume of 500 to 1000 ml. Administer at an appropriate rate for the fluid volume.
- Warn patients that IM injections will be painful.

Patient and family education

- See Patient Care Implications for Chapter 29.
- Take oral doses with a full glassful (8 oz) of water
- Usually, take oral tetracyclines on an empty stomach, 1 hour before or 2 hours after meals. However, if the drug causes stomach upset, the physician may permit it to be taken with meals or snack. Doxycycline and minocycline may be taken on a full or an empty stomach.
- Do not take tetracyclines within 1 to 2 hours of drinking milk, milk products, or formula, or any of the following medications: antacids, calcium supplements, choline and magnesium salicylate combinations, magnesium salicylate, magnesium-containing laxatives, or sodium bicarbonate. Review the patient's other medications with the patient to clarify these instructions.
- Do not take iron preparations or vitamin preparations containing iron within 2 to 3 hours of taking a tetracycline preparation.
- Warn patients that tetracyclines may cause the tongue to become darkened or discolored. This effect is not significant, and will clear when the drug is stopped.
- Contraceptive pills containing estrogen may not be effective while the patient is taking tetracyclines; other forms of birth control should be used. Discuss this effect with the physician or pharmacist.
- This drug may cause patients to develop photosensitivity. See Patient Problem: Photosensitivity, p. 647.
- Demeclocycline may be used to treat the syndrome of inappropriate antidiuretic hormone (SIADH), and when used for this, functions as a diuretic. This diuretic action is effective in patients with SIADH, but is not satisfactory in other patients who may require diuretics.
- When tetracyclines are used in children under the age of 8, there may be discoloration of the teeth. Notify the physician if this occurs.
- Teach patients to observe expiration dates on all medications, but especially tetracyclines. As noted in the text, use of outdated preparations, or those that look as if they have deteriorated or changed color, may cause severe adverse reactions.
- Warn patients taking minocycline to avoid driving or operating hazardous equipment if vertigo or dizziness occurs; notify the physician.
- Tell diabetics that tetracyclines may contribute to false results in urine glucose tests. Consult physician before changing diet or insulin. Monitor blood glucose if possible.

Chloramphenicol

Drug administration

- See Patient Care Implications in Chapter 29.
- Assess for history of allergy before administering.
- Assess visual acuity before beginning therapy and at regular intervals. Assess for gastrointestinal side effects, skin changes, and signs of hematologic side effects.

PATIENT CARE IMPLICATIONS—cont'd

- Monitor infants for appearance of gray syndrome. Assess for failure to feed, abdominal distention, progressive pallid cyanosis, and irregular respiration. Note that gray syndrome can develop in infants of women who received chloramphenicol during labor or the last few days of pregnancy.
- Monitor serum drug levels, complete blood count and differential, platelet count, BUN, serum creatinine, and liver function tests.
INTRAVENOUS CHLORAMPHENICOL
- Dilute 1 gm with 10 ml of sterile water or 5% dextrose in water. May be further diluted with 50 to 100 ml of compatible solution; see drug insert. Administer IV push at a rate of 1 Gm over at least 1 minute. For infusion, administer volume of 50 to 100 ml over 30 to 60 minutes. Warn patients that they may experience a bitter taste after IV administration; this should resolve after a few minutes.

Patient and family education

- See Patient Care Implications in Chapter 29.
- Instruct patients to report the development of unexplained bruising or bleeding, nosebleed, bleeding from gums, or blood in stools; fever, sore throat, malaise, fatigue, or symptoms of infection. Tell the patient to report these symptoms even if they develop after the drug has been stopped.
- Take oral doses with a full glassful (8 oz) of water on an empty stomach, 1 hour before or 2 hours after meals, for best effect.
- Caution patients to avoid driving or operating hazardous equipment if confusion or visual changes occur.
- Warn diabetic patients that chloramphenicol may cause false results with urine glucose tests. Consult the physician before changing diet or diabetes medications. Monitor blood sugar levels if possible.

chloramphenicol therapy. Allergies of various types may occur, as well as gastrointestinal irritation. Long-term therapy has been associated with neuritis, which may involve the optic nerve. Blindness has occurred in a few patients. Central nervous system symptoms are also seen in some patients: headache, mental confusion, depression, or delirium.

Patients with reduced liver function are at risk of severe toxic reactions due to drug accumulation. The liver normally converts over 90% of administered chloramphenicol, which is toxic, to the glucuronide, which is nontoxic. Therefore any reduction in the liver's ability to detoxify the drug may result in accumulation of the toxic drug in the body, unless dosages are appropriately reduced. One group of patients especially at risk for this complication is newborn infants. Neonates have an immature liver that lacks the enzyme to form the glucuronide. When these infants are given a weight-adjusted dosage based on adult doses, many develop a condition that has been called the *gray syndrome*. Drug accumulation proceeds without symptoms for 3 to 4 days, after which time the infant may develop abdominal distention, emesis, progressive pallid cyanosis, and irregular respiration. In a high percentage of cases vasomotor collapse and death may re-

sult. Infants receiving smaller doses are less likely to develop these symptoms. If early signs of the condition are noted by alert health care personnel and the drug is discontinued, most infants will recover.

Chloramphenicol crosses the placenta and may concentrate in fetal liver. For this reason the drug is not given to pregnant women near term.

Drug Interactions

Chloramphenicol can inhibit drug-metabolizing enzymes of the liver. This property may lead to dangerous interactions with drugs that have two characteristic properties: (1) a relatively low therapeutic index and (2) a major route of elimination by microsomal enzymes of the liver. The three drugs that fall into this category are phenytoin, tolbutamide, and coumarin anticoagulants. When a patient who is receiving one of these drugs on a long-term basis is given chloramphenicol, these liver-metabolized drugs tend to accumulate. As a result well-controlled diabetics may become hypoglycemic, successfully anticoagulated patients may develop spontaneous bleeding, and controlled epileptics may develop phenytoin toxicity.

Since chloramphenicol is rarely used, these interactions are also rather rare. In the unusual case in which these drugs must be combined in the same patient, the early signs of drug interactions should be anticipated.

Uses (Table 32.2)

Because of dangerous toxic reactions, chloramphenicol is reserved for use only in serious infections. Chloramphenicol is the drug of choice for typhoid fever. In addition, life-threatening infections such as bacteremias or meningitis may be treated with chloramphenicol when the pathogen has been tested and proved sensitive to the drug. The antibacterial spectrum of chloramphenicol is quite similar to that of tetracyclines, being especially effective against gram-negative bacteria (except *Pseudomonas aeruginosa*), rickettsiae, and chlamydia.

Chloramphenicol is especially effective against the important anaerobic pathogen *Bacteroides fragilis*.

SUMMARY

Tetracyclines are bacteriostatic drugs that inhibit bacterial protein synthesis. They are primarily used as oral agents, but only doxycycline and minocycline are efficiently absorbed from the gastrointestinal tract. All other tetracyclines are sensitive to acid and tend to form insoluble complexes in the intestine, and are therefore incompletely absorbed. Tetracycline, oxytetracycline, doxycycline, and minocycline may be used intravenously but must be extensively diluted, since the drugs tend to cause thrombophlebitis. Intramuscular use of tetracycline is limited by poor absorption and local tissue irritation. The tetracyclines are well distributed in body fluids and tissues. The more polar tetracyclines are largely eliminated by the kidney, whereas the newer lipid-soluble tetracyclines (doxycycline and minocycline) are eliminated primarily in the bile or by direct intestinal adsorption. These drugs frequently irritate the gastrointestinal tract following oral use and may extensively alter the bacterial flora. Superinfections in the mouth, vagina, and bowel may result from tetracycline therapy. These drugs may also damage the liver and kidneys as well as interfere with blood coagulation. Tetracyclines bind to calcium in bones and teeth and may discolor the teeth if administered to children during the years when teeth are forming. Tetracyclines in general, and especially demeclocycline, may cause phototoxic reactions. Minocycline may cause vestibular damage. Outdated tetracycline preparations may be more toxic than newly prepared drugs, since the breakdown products are highly toxic. Tetracyclines are most useful in practice because of their very wide antimicrobial spectrum.

Chloramphenicol has a similar mechanism of action and antimicrobial spectrum to the tetracyclines. Chloramphenicol is well absorbed orally and may be used intravenously in the succinate form. The drug penetrates the central nervous system efficiently. Most of the chloramphenicol administered is converted to inactive products by the liver and then eliminated by the kidney. It may accumulate in patients with impaired liver function. Chloramphenicol may also produce various blood dyscrasias, the most serious being aplastic anemia. Aplastic anemia is a rare complication and occurs weeks to months after therapy, but it is a fatal drug reaction. The danger of this severe toxic reaction limits the clinical use of this otherwise very effective drug.

STUDY QUESTIONS

1. What is the mechanism of action of tetracycline antibiotics?
2. What is the mechanism by which bacteria become resistant to tetracyclines?
3. What factors influence the oral absorption of tetracycline antibiotics?
4. How does the absorption of minocycline and doxycycline differ from that of other tetracyclines?
5. What factors limit the intramuscular use of tetracyclines?
6. What precautions are necessary for using tetracyclines intravenously?
7. What are the three main routes of excretion for the tetracyclines?
8. Are minocycline and doxycycline eliminated in the same way as the other tetracyclines?
9. What are the main toxic reactions common to all tetracycline antibiotics?
10. What toxic reaction is especially associated with demeclocycline?
11. What toxic reaction is especially associated with minocycline?
12. What toxicity is associated with the use of outdated tetracycline preparations?
13. What is the effect of administering tetracyclines with antacids?
14. Why do immunosuppressant drugs interfere with the clinical effect of tetracyclines?
15. Why do tetracyclines interfere with the antimicrobial action of penicillins?

16. Name three groups of organisms against which the tetracyclines are effective.
17. What is the mechanism of action of chloramphenicol?
18. What is the mechanism by which bacteria become resistant to chloramphenicol?
19. Which routes of administration give the most rapid and complete absorption of chloramphenicol?
20. Does chloramphenicol efficiently enter the cerebrospinal fluid?
21. What is the primary route of elimination of chloramphenicol from the body?

22. What is the most dangerous toxic reaction associated with chloramphenicol?
23. What is the gray syndrome?
24. Name one clinical indication for chloramphenicol.

SUGGESTED READINGS

Bryant, S.G., Fisher, S., and Kluge, R.M.: Increased frequency of doxycycline side effects, Pharmacotherapy 7(4):125, 1987.

Nursing Update: Tetracyclines, Nursing84 14(1):46, 1984.

Wilson, W.R., and Cockerill, F.R. III: Tetracyclines, chloramphenicol, erythromycin, and clindamycin, Mayo Clin. Proc. 62(10):906, 1987.

Antibiotics: Aminoglycosides and Polymyxins

33

In this chapter two groups of antibiotics with primary usefulness against gram-negative bacteria are introduced. The aminoglycosides are antibiotics composed of three or four amino sugars held together in glycosidic linkage. Great variability in structure is possible in these component sugars, and as a result several antibiotics of this type exist. Polymyxins are peptide antibiotics created by a spore-forming bacillus found in the soil. These two groups of drugs are considered together, since they have similar antimicrobial spectra and share certain toxic properties.

AMINOGLYCOSIDES
Mechanism of Action and Bacterial Resistance

The aminoglycosides inhibit early steps in bacterial protein synthesis by binding to bacterial ribosomes. Under certain conditions bacterial protein synthesis may continue in the presence of aminoglycosides but with a greatly increased error rate. Defective proteins formed may damage the bacterial cell. Aminoglycosides also have a somewhat delayed effect on the bacterial cell membrane. Aminoglycosides are usually considered to be more bactericidal than many other antibiotics that inhibit bacterial protein synthesis.

Resistance to aminoglycosides occurs by one of three mechanisms: decreased antibiotic uptake, changes in antibiotic binding to the ribosome, and enzymatic destruction of the aminoglycosides. By far the most common mechanism for resistance involves antibiotic destruction. To understand this mechanism of bacterial resistance to aminoglycosides, two facts must be appreciated. First, many sites for enzymatic attack exist on the amino sugar components of aminoglycosides. Second, several different enzymes exist that modify the aminogly-

cosides by different mechanisms. The primary sites of attack are amino groups and hydroxyl groups on the sugars. Amino groups may be acetylated and hydroxyl groups may have a phosphate or an adenylate group added. Any of these substitutions may render the aminoglycoside inactive. At least 13 separate enzymes catalyzing these reactions have been identified. Table 33.1 lists the clinically useful aminoglycosides and indicates how many of these degrading enzymes can attack an individual drug. As would be predicted, those drugs sensitive to fewer enzyme forms have a broader antimicrobial spectrum.

Rarely, bacterial resistance may result from reduced drug uptake. This mechanism has been observed especially with amikacin. An equally rare mechanism of resistance involves lowering drug binding to the ribosome. Occasional streptomycin-resistant strains arise by this mechanism.

Absorption

Aminoglycosides are polycationic molecules at physiological pH. As a result of being charged, these drugs do not penetrate mammalian membranes readily and are not absorbed orally. Therapy with aminoglycosides is therefore by intramuscular or intravenous routes and usually involves a hospitalized patient suffering from a moderate to severe infection. Absorption of aminoglycosides from intramuscular injections sites is rapid, and peak serum concentrations occur between 1 and 1.5 hours after injection.

Distribution and Excretion

Aminoglycosides do not enter the central nervous system to any significant extent in normal persons. Some drug does appear in cerebrospinal fluid when meningitis is present. Aminoglycosides enter most other body fluids and tissues with the

Table 33.1 Sensitivity of Clinically Useful Aminoglycoside Antibiotics to Antibiotic-Degrading Enzymes in Bacteria

Drug	Number of aminoglycoside degrading enzymes that inactivate drug
Amikacin	2
Gentamicin	4
Kanamycin	6
Neomycin	3
Netilmicin	4
Streptomycin	4
Tobramycin	5

exception of bile. These drugs cross the placenta and achieve significant concentrations in the fetus.

Aminoglycosides are excreted by glomerular filtration in the kidney. Active drug is concentrated in the urine. Since the kidney is the primary site for elimination of these drugs, any reduction in renal function may lower the excretion sufficiently to cause aminoglycoside accumulation. The approximate half-time for elimination of these drugs is normally about 2 to 4 hours but in renal failure may be greatly prolonged. Excretion is also lower in neonates, who have immature kidneys and in elderly patients, whose renal function is diminished simply as a function of age.

Toxicity (Table 33.2)

The aminoglycosides exert significant toxicity of three major types: ototoxicity, renal toxicity, and neuromuscular blockade. Ototoxicity may be manifested by progressive hearing loss, loss of equilibrium control, or both. Hearing loss in some patients continues even after the drug is discontinued. Loss of equilibrium may be less obvious than hearing loss but can usually be revealed by appropriate tests. Nausea or dizziness may be a patient complaint that signals disturbance of equilibrium. Ototoxicity is usually more severe when serum concentrations of aminoglycosides exceed 8 to 10 μg/ml. Total dose administered may also be a factor, since some patients treated over long periods may display these symptoms in spite of never having excessively high serum levels of the drug. Amino-

glycosides may damage both tubules and glomeruli in the kidney, especially when high doses are given. This toxic potential can cause a rapid clinical deterioration, since renal damage can cause drug accumulation, which in turn causes further damage to the kidney. This cycle of accumulation and increasing renal damage can destroy kidney function. Patients who accumulate the drug due to renal dysfunction are also more prone to ototoxicity.

The third characteristic toxic reaction to aminoglycosides is neuromuscular blockade. This reaction is usually observed in surgical patients when an aminoglycoside is used in peritoneal lavage. Neuromuscular blockade in this case usually is manifested by respiratory paralysis, since the muscles of the chest involved in breathing are prevented from functioning. Some of the aminoglycosides produce a competitive neuromuscular blockade, which may be reversed by neostigmine. Others, such as kanamycin, produce an irreversible blockade, which neostigmine does not affect, although calcium may relieve the blockade in some cases. Patients who have recently received muscle relaxants are more prone to suffer neuromuscular blockade with aminoglycosides. Patients with myasthenia gravis are also more sensitive to this effect.

Less common adverse reactions include effects on a variety of organ systems. Blood dyscrasias, while rare, may occur with any aminoglycoside. Likewise, rare neurotoxicity may be manifested by headaches, paresthesias, tremor, confusion, and disorientation. The aminoglycosides are also somewhat irritating, and may cause pain at the injection site.

Drug Interactions

The ototoxicity and nephrotoxicity of aminoglycoside antibiotics may be enhanced by a variety of agents. For example, if a patient who is receiving an aminoglycoside is also given a nephrotoxic drug such as a cephalosporin or methoxyflurane (Penthrane), the risk of kidney damage is increased. Likewise, ototoxic drugs such as ethacrynic acid may enhance ototoxicity in a patient receiving an aminoglycoside antibiotic.

All aminoglycosides possess neuromuscular blocking activity. This action has led to enhancement of agents used for neuromuscular blocking action during surgery.

Gentamicin is frequently combined with an anti-*Pseudomonas* penicillin to treat *Pseudomonas aeruginosa* infections. Although these drugs may be used in the same patient, they should never be physically mixed, since penicillins chemically inactivate gentamicin in solution.

Table 33.2   Summary of Toxicity Observed with Clinically Useful Aminoglycosides

Drug	Ototoxicity Vestibular	Hearing	Renal toxicity	Neuromuscular blockade
Amikacin	Lower incidence than hearing impairment.	From 3% to 11% of treated patients may show measurable hearing impairment.	More patients show rise in serum creatinine than with gentamicin. Up to 20% of patients may be affected.	Expected from animal studies.
Gentamicin	About 2% of treated patients suffer permanent mild to severe vestibular damage.	Less frequent than vestibular damage and usually involves high-tone hearing loss.	Acute renal failure has occurred. Blood urea and creatinine may rise; proteinuria may occur. Damage is usually but not always reversible.	May occur, but is less common than with kanamycin, neomycin, and streptomycin.
Kanamycin	Vertigo or other symptoms of vestibular damage affect about 7% of patients receiving high doses.	Up to 30% of patients receiving high doses suffer detectable hearing loss; fewer patients develop complete deafness.	Blood urea and creatinine may rise; hematuria and other signs of renal irritation may occur. Most signs of damage disappear when drug is discontinued.	Occurs following peritoneal lavage; usually not reversed by neostigmine and occasionally not reversed by calcium.
Neomycin	Not common.	Irreversible hearing loss progressing to complete deafness is common.	Reversible, progressive kidney toxicity causing an increase in blood urea.	Occurs following peritoneal lavage; usually reversed by neostigmine.
Netilmicin	Possible but less likely than hearing loss.	About 1% to 2% of treated patients show hearing impairment.	From 3% to 8% of treated patients show some sign of changes in renal function.	May be twice as potent as gentamicin in producing blockade.
Streptomycin	May affect 75% of patients receiving 2 Gm daily for 2 to 4 mo and 25% of patients receiving 1 Gm daily.	Loss usually partial but may be complete; affects 4% to 15% of patients receiving drug longer than 1 wk.	Not common unless high drug doses are used and the urine is acid.	May occur following peritoneal lavage; reversed by neostigmine and/or calcium.
Tobramycin	From 1% to 11% of treated patients show measurable impairment.	Incidence is the same as for vestibular damage.	Serum creatinine may be elevated, but the incidence may be less than with gentamicin or amikacin.	Expected from animal studies.

Aminoglycosides are many times more effective at the slightly alkaline pH of normal serum (pH 7.4) than at the acidic pH of normal urine (pH 5). Therefore, in the treatment of urinary tract infections with these drugs, a therapeutic advantage may be gained by alkalinizing the urine.

Oral neomycin causes mucosal alterations in the bowel, which may in extreme cases lead to malabsorption syndrome. Oral neomycin may also impair absorption of orally administered drugs. This potential interaction has been documented with penicillin V, digoxin, and vitamin B_{12}. If these drugs must be given to a patient receiving oral neomycin, extra care may need to be taken to ensure that adequate amounts of the other orally administered medications are being absorbed.

Uses

The clinical use of these drugs is limited by their toxic potential. As a general rule the aminoglycosides are reserved for serious infections caused by aerobic gram-negative bacteria or by mycobacteria (Chapter 35). Individual drugs in this family differ in specific uses as a result of differences in relative toxicity and antibacterial activity. Table 33.3 lists the most important clinical uses of individual aminoglycosides. Streptomycin is most useful today in combination with other agents to

Table 33.3 Clinical Uses of Aminoglycoside Antibiotics

Drug	Indications
Amikacin	Serious infections due to aerobic gram-negative bacteria including *Pseudomonas aeruginosa*
Gentamicin	Serious infections due to aerobic gram-negative bacteria including *P. aeruginosa*.
Kanamycin	Serious infections due to aerobic gram-negative bacteria other than *Pseudomonas*. Oral use to reduce bacterial population of the bowel.
Neomycin	Oral use for reducing bacterial population of the bowel.
Netilmicin	Serious infections due to aerobic gram-negative bacteria including *P. aeruginosa*.
Streptomycin	Used alone to treat tularemia (rabbit fever) and plague (bubonic or black plague). Used in combination with other antibiotics to treat bacterial endocarditis (with penicillin G), tuberculosis (with isoniazid or other antituberculosis agents), brucellosis (with tetracyclines), *Listeria* infections (with ampicillin or penicillin G).
Tobramycin	Primarily for *P. aeruginosa* infections; may also substitute for gentamicin in other infections.

treat infections in which strict bactericidal action is required for most effective therapy. Examples of these infections are bacterial endocarditis and tuberculosis (Chapter 35). Neomycin is too toxic for parenteral use but may be administered orally with the intent that the drug will remain in the bowel and lower the bacterial population. This effect may be useful before bowel surgery or in hepatic coma. Certain specific infections of the bowel may also respond to this therapy. Kanamycin may occasionally be used orally in a manner similar to neomycin; however, kanamycin is most useful for serious systemic infections.

One difference among aminoglycosides is their different degree of activity against *P. aeruginosa*. Amikacin, gentamicin, and tobramycin are most effective against this pathogen. Kanamycin usually is not effective. Amikacin differs from other aminoglycosides in being less sensitive to common aminoglycoside-degrading enzymes. Amikacin is therefore active against some bacterial strains that are resistant to other aminoglycosides.

Table 33.4 lists the common dosages for aminoglycosides employed in patients with normal renal function. When renal function is significantly impaired or is in question, it may be necessary to monitor serum levels of these drugs in order to prevent intoxication.

POLYMYXINS
Mechanism of Action and Bacterial Resistance

Polymyxins alter the permeability of bacterial cell membranes, causing the loss of required small molecules and ions from the cell. This action is made possible by the combination of highly ionic groups along with lipid-soluble hydrocarbon chains all within the same molecule. The positively charged portion of the polymyxin molecule is attracted to the negatively charged surface of the bacterial membrane. Membrane disruption occurs when the hydrocarbon chain portion of the polymyxin is inserted into the lipid-rich bacterial membrane. Bacterial cell death is an inevitable consequence of the loss of cell nutrients and cofactors required for energy production. Polymyxins are effective in either actively growing or static bacterial cells.

Polymyxins are of clinical interest because of their bactericidal action on gram-negative bacteria. With the exception of *Proteus, Neisseria,* and *Bacteroides,* most gram-negative organisms including *P. aeruginosa* are sensitive to the polymyxins. Gram-positive organisms are usually considered resistant to the polymyxins.

Clinical resistance to polymyxins has not increased since the drugs were first introduced into clinical practice in 1947. Organisms that are nat-

Table 33.4   Administration and Dosage of Aminoglycoside Antibiotics

Generic name	Trade name	Administration/dosage
Amikacin	Amikin*	INTRAMUSCULAR, INTRAVENOUS: *Adults, children, infants*—15 mg/kg body weight daily in 2 or 3 doses. Do not exceed 1.5 Gm daily. Intravenous doses are given by slow infusion. FDA Pregnancy Category D.
Gentamicin	Cidomycin† Garamycin* Gentafair	INTRAMUSCULAR, INTRAVENOUS: *Adults*—3 to 5 mg/kg daily in 3 doses. FDA Pregnancy Category C. *Children*—6 to 7.5 mg/kg daily in 3 doses. *Neonates*—5 mg/kg daily in 2 or 3 doses.
Kanamycin	Kantrex* Klebcil	ORAL: *Adults*—up to 12 Gm daily in 4 to 6 doses. FDA Pregnancy Category D. *Children and infants*—50 mg/kg daily in 4 to 6 doses. INTRAMUSCULAR, INTRAVENOUS, INTRAPERITONEAL: *Adults and children*—not to exceed 15 mg/kg daily, divided into 2 or 3 doses.
Neomycin	Mycifradin† Myciguent*	ORAL: *Adults*—4 to 8.4 Gm daily in up to 6 doses. *Children*—Up to 4.8 Gm/M² daily divided into 4 doses. TOPICAL: *Adults and children*—commonly used as 0.35% creams and ointments. Also used in numerous combinations with other antibiotics.
Netilmicin	Netromycin*	INTRAMUSCULAR, INTRAVENOUS: *Adults*—4 to 6.5 mg/kg daily divided into 3 equal doses. FDA Pregnancy Category D. *Children*—5.5 to 8 mg/kg daily divided into 2 or 3 doses. *Neonates to 6 wk*—adult dose.
Streptomycin	Streptomycin	INTRAMUSCULAR, INTRAVENOUS: *Adults*—1 to 4 Gm daily in 2 or 3 doses (15 to 25 mg/kg daily). Elderly patients may require less drug. Lower doses are used for long-term treatment of mild tuberculosis. Intravenous route rarely used. *Children*—20 to 40 mg/kg daily in 2 doses.
Tobramycin	Nebcin*	INTRAMUSCULAR, INTRAVENOUS: *Adults, infants*—3 to 5 mg/kg daily divided into 3 doses. FDA Pregnancy Category D. *Children*—6 to 7.5 mg/kg daily divided into 2 or 3 doses.

*Available in Canada and United States.
†Available in Canada.

Table 33.5   Clinical Summary of Polymyxins

Generic name	Trade name	Administration/dosage	Clinical use
Colistimethate sodium (colistin methane sulfonate)	Coly-Mycin M*	INTRAMUSCULAR, INTRAVENOUS: *Adults and children*—2.5 to 5 mg/kg body weight daily in 2 to 4 doses up to 300 mg daily. Dosage must be reduced if renal impairment exists.	Reserve drug for treatment of *Pseudomonas aeruginosa.*
Polymyxin B sulfate	Aerosporin*	INTRAMUSCULAR: *Adults and children*—25,000 to 30,000 units/kg daily in 4 to 6 doses. INTRAVENOUS: *Adults and children*—15,000 to 25,000 units/kg daily by infusion in 300 to 500 ml 5% dextrose. INTRATHECAL: *Adults*—50,000 units daily in single dose. *Children under 2 yr*—20,000 units in single daily dose.	Not recommended due to extreme pain at injection site. Reserve drug for treatment of *Pseudomonas aeruginosa.* Reserve drug for *Pseudomonas aeruginosa* meningitis.

*Available in Canada and United States.

urally resistant to these drugs apparently possess barriers that prevent polymyxin from contacting the cell membrane.

Absorption, Distribution, and Excretion

Polymyxins are not absorbed from the gastrointestinal tract, but effective systemic concentrations of the drugs can be achieved by parenteral administration (Table 33.5). Peak blood levels are ordinarily reached about 2 hours after intramuscular injection, but severe pain may result with this route of administration.

Intravenous administration of the polymyxins is by relatively slow infusion. These drugs should

THE NURSING PROCESS

AMINOGLYCOSIDES AND POLYMYXINS

Refer to Chapter 29 for general guidelines on the nursing process with antibiotic therapy. The additional material below relates specifically to the aminoglycosides and polymyxins.

Assessment

Aminoglycoside antibiotics are prescribed for a relatively limited number of indications, primarily in moderate to severe infections (Table 33.3). Since the drugs are administered parenterally, the patient population is primarily in hospital. Polymyxins are not widely used to treat systemic infections; they are used in seriously ill patients with very specific diseases (Table 33.5). A full assessment of the patient should be carried out with emphasis on the organ in which the infection is thought to be present, if the infection is a localized one. Other clinical signs of infection should be monitored. Renal function, hearing acuity, and vestibular function should be assessed carefully. Other medications the patient may be receiving should be noted.

Nursing diagnoses

Potential complication: ototoxicity

Potential complication: renal damage/renal failure

Management

Once the decision is made to administer aminoglycosides or polymyxins, the nurse should gather the proper supplies for proper administration by the parenteral route chosen. The nurse should note whether the patient has received any other neuromuscular blocking agents or whether the patient has any other condition (such as myasthenia gravis) that would predispose the patient to respiratory paralysis. Equipment should be on hand to deal with respiratory paralysis if it occurs. The nurse should see that the medications are administered exactly at the times prescribed. If samples are being taken for the measurement of blood levels of these drugs, these samples must be taken exactly as ordered, since the timing is critical for proper interpretation of the information.

Evaluation

In the short term, the vital signs of the patient should be closely monitored, and evidence of objective and subjective recovery from serious illness should be noted. Hearing loss caused by aminoglycosides and polymyxins may progress during and after therapy. The nurse should continuously evaluate the patient for this symptom and for any loss of control of equilibrium as evidenced by difficulty in walking, staggering, or dizziness.

---

never be given rapidly by vein, since the resulting high blood levels can produce respiratory paralysis in some patients.

Polymyxins are bound to various tissues and persist at those sites for up to 3 days after therapy is stopped. Significant concentrations of polymyxins do appear in fetuses when these drugs are administered to the mother.

Excretion of polymyxins is primarily by the kidney. The serum half-life for polymyxins in the body is on the order of 2 to 3 hours in a patient with normal renal function.

Toxicity

Since the detergent-like action of polymyxins on cell membranes is nonspecific, this family of drugs has a low therapeutic index. Significant neurotoxicity, nephrotoxicity, and neuromuscular blockade can be produced.

Neuromuscular blockade is due to a curare-like action of polymyxin at the neuromuscular junction. This effect is most often observed clinically as respiratory paralysis. Calcium chloride may relieve the blockade in some patients, but neostigmine does not.

PATIENT CARE IMPLICATIONS

Aminoglycosides

Drug administration

- See Patient Care Implications in Chapter 29.
- Assess for history of allergy before administering.
- Review Table 33.2 for a summary of toxicity observed with these drugs. Assess for changes in hearing, balance, development of tinnitus. Monitor intake and output, and weight. Monitor vital signs, auscultate lung sounds.
- Monitor serum creatinine, BUN, urinalysis, liver function tests, serum electrolytes, complete blood count and differential, and platelet count.
- Monitor serum drug levels. Peak and trough levels may be available. Peak levels indicate serum levels after a dose is given, and reflect the highest serum level for that patient at that dose. Trough levels are drawn shortly before a dose is given and reflect the lowest serum level for that patient at that dose. If peak and trough levels are ordered, notify the laboratory of the time a dose will be given so blood levels can be obtained at the necessary times for drug level calculations.
- Have neostigmine and calcium chloride available in settings where aminoglycosides are used with high-risk patients, such as in the operating room, recovery room, and intensive care units. Monitor respiratory status. Have a suction machine available at the bedside.
- A separate form of gentamicin without preservatives is available for intrathecal administration.
- Do not mix aminoglycosides in a syringe with other medications.
  INTRAMUSCULAR STREPTOMYCIN
- Dilute as directed on the label of the vial. Use a large muscle mass. This drug is not administered IV.
  INTRAVENOUS AMIKACIN
- Dilute 500 mg in 200 ml of normal saline or 5% dextrose in water and administer over 30 to 60 minutes.
  INTRAVENOUS GENTAMICIN
- Dilute a single dose in 50 to 200 ml of normal saline or 5% dextrose in water. The concentration should not exceed 0.1% (1 mg/ml). Administer each dose over 30 to 60 minutes. Prepared dilutions are available.

INTRAVENOUS KANAMYCIN
- Dilute the prescribed dose in normal saline, 5% dextrose in normal saline, or 5% dextrose in water to a concentration of 500 mg in 100 to 200 ml. Administer over 30 to 60 minutes.
  INTRAVENOUS NETILMICIN
- Dilute a single dose in 50 to 200 ml of diluent; see drug insert. Administer over 30 minutes to 2 hours.
  INTRAVENOUS TOBRAMYCIN
- Dilute dose in 50 to 100 ml of 5% dextrose in water or normal saline and administer over 20 to 60 minutes.
- For pediatric doses and dilutions, consult the manufacturer's literature.
- Because of the possibility of hypotension or vertigo, keep side rails up. Supervise ambulation.
- Neomycin may be ordered orally or via enema to inhibit ammonia-forming bacteria in the GI tract of patients with hepatic encephalopathy.

Patient and family education

- See Patient Care Implications in Chapter 29.
- Instruct the patient to report the development of hearing loss, nausea, dizziness or vertigo, or decreased urinary output.
- Streptomycin is often given in long-term therapy for tuberculosis, in combination with other drugs. Streptomycin may cause false results in urine glucose tests. Warn diabetic patients about this. Monitor blood glucose if possible.
- With topical preparations, systemic side effects are rare, but can occur. Factors which influence the likelihood of toxicity would include the frequency of application, the size of the area to which the preparation is being applied, whether the skin surface was intact, and the amount and kind of other ototoxic or nephrotoxic drugs the patient might be receiving concomitantly.
- Photosensitivity has been reported with topical preparations. See Patient Problem: Photosensitivity on p. 647.

Polymyxins

Drug administration

- See Patient Care Implications in Chapter 29.
- Assess for history of allergy before administering.

PATIENT CARE IMPLICATIONS — cont'd

- Review the text for a summary of toxicity observed with use of these drugs. Assess for confusion, slurred speech, ataxia. Monitor intake and output, and weight. Monitor vital signs, auscultate lung sounds.
- Monitor serum creatinine, BUN, urinalysis, liver function tests, serum electrolytes, complete blood count and differential, and platelet count.
- Have calcium chloride available in settings where polymyxins are used with high-risk patients, such as in the operating room, recovery room, and intensive care units. Monitor respiratory status. Have a suction machine available at the bedside.
- Warn patients that IM injections may cause pain at the injection site.
  INTRAVENOUS COLISTIMETHATE
- Dilute the 150 mg vial with 2 ml sterile water for injection. Further dilute each dose with 20 ml sterile water for injection. Administer at a rate of 75 mg or less over 5 minutes. May also be further diluted and administered as an infusion; see drug insert.
  INTRAVENOUS POLYMYXIN B
- Dilute 500,000 units of powder with 5 ml sterile water or normal saline for injection. Further dilute dose in 300 to 500 ml compatible fluid. Administer diluted dose over 60 to 90 minutes. For intrathecal use, dilution is different; consult literature. Monitor vital signs, especially respirations.

Patient and family education
- See Patient Care Implications in Chapter 29.
- Caution patients to avoid driving or operating hazardous equipment if dizziness, vertigo, confusion, ataxia, or blurred vision develops; notify the physician.

Nephrotoxicity, manifested by decreased glomerular filtration rates and increased serum creatinine and BUN, occurs when polymyxin concentrations in the blood exceed recommended levels. Nephrotoxicity is usually reversible. However, patients in whom renal toxicity is not recognized may suffer a rapid deterioration in clinical status due to the cycle of drug accumulation, increasing renal deterioration, further drug accumulation, and additional drug toxicity.

Neurotoxicity of polymyxins is manifested by symptoms of numbness, tingling of the extremities, generalized pruritus, and dizziness. Paresthesias are observed fairly commonly. At higher doses or in patients suffering drug accumulation, more severe symptoms may be observed. These symptoms include giddiness or mental confusion, slurring of speech, ataxia, convulsions, or coma. The signs of neurotoxicity usually disappear when polymyxins are discontinued.

Drug Interactions

The most important clinical interaction of polymyxins occurs with muscle relaxing agents. In some patients unexpected neuromuscular blockade and respiratory paralysis have occurred when the patient received both polymyxin and another antibiotic with curare-like action. Potential for this interaction exists with kanamycin, streptomycin, neomycin, and probably other aminoglycoside antibiotics as well.

The muscle-relaxing agents used in conjunction with surgery are the drugs most commonly involved in drug interactions with polymyxins. These curariform muscle relaxants include ether, tubocurarine, succinylcholine, gallamine, decamethonium, and sodium citrate. Patients who are receiving or have recently received these drugs should be most carefully observed for development of respiratory paralysis if polymyxins must be administered.

Uses

Because of their relatively narrow antimicrobial spectrum and relatively high toxicity, the uses for these drugs are limited. Specific indications for the individual members of this drug class are listed in Table 33.5.

Polymyxins are also used in various ointments and creams intended for topical application. For this purpose they are frequently combined with neomycin and bacitracin.

SUMMARY

Aminoglycoside antibiotics inhibit bacterial protein synthesis, producing bactericidal as well as bacteriostatic effects. Bacterial resistance to aminoglycosides arises by decreased antibiotic uptake, decreased antibiotic binding to the ribosome, or enzymatic destruction of the antibiotic. The most common mode of resistance involves aminoglycoside destruction, which may be carried out by as many as 13 different enzymes. Aminoglycosides are not absorbed orally but are rapidly and efficiently absorbed from intramuscular sites. They do not enter the central nervous system very efficiently but are well distributed to most other tissues. The drugs are excreted almost exclusively by the kidney. Aminoglycosides may cause hearing loss, vestibular damage, nephrotoxicity, and neuromuscular blockade. Ototoxicity and nephrotoxicity are more extreme when the drugs accumulate in the body or are used at too high a dose. Neuromuscular blockade is more likely in patients with preexisting impairment at the neuromuscular junction, that is, a patient with myasthenia gravis or one who has recently received a neuromuscular blocking agent in conjunction with surgery. Streptomycin is used in combination with penicillins to treat certain serious infections caused by gram-positive bacteria and in combination with other agents for the treatment of tuberculosis. Neomycin is too toxic for systemic use. Kanamycin may be used for serious infections due to gram-negative bacteria, but gentamicin, tobramycin, netilmicin, or amikacin must be used if the pathogen is *Pseudomonas aeruginosa*.

Polymyxins disrupt cell membranes of gram-negative bacteria, causing bacterial cell death. Resistance to polymyxins has not been observed. These drugs are not absorbed from the gastrointestinal tract. Intramuscular administration causes pain at the injection site. Intravenous infusion can produce respiratory paralysis if the rate of infusion is too rapid. These drugs do not enter the cerebrospinal fluid from the bloodstream. Polymyxins are excreted by the kidney and are inactivated by body tissues. Polymyxins may produce neuromuscular blockade and nephrotoxicity. In addition, these drugs may produce neurotoxicity, including numbness, paresthesias, and tingling of the extremities. More serious central nervous system reactions may result with higher drug doses.

STUDY QUESTIONS

1. What is the mechanism of action of aminoglycoside antibiotics?
2. What are the three mechanisms by which bacteria gain resistance to aminoglycoside antibiotics?
3. What is the most common mechanism for bacterial resistance to aminoglycosides?
4. Which routes of administration are appropriate for aminoglycosides?
5. What is the primary route of excretion of aminoglycosides?
6. What effect may aminoglycoside antibiotics have on the function of the ear?
7. What effects do the aminoglycoside antibiotics have on the kidney?
8. What groups of patients might be more prone to aminoglycoside ototoxicity and nephrotoxicity?
9. What is the effect of aminoglycosides on the neuromuscular junction?
10. What groups of patients are most likely to develop respiratory paralysis following therapeutic use of aminoglycoside antibiotics?
11. What special precautions must be taken when gentamicin and carbenicillin are used in the same patient?
12. What drugs may be poorly absorbed when neomycin is used orally?
13. Name three clinical uses of streptomycin.
14. Name two clinical indications for neomycin.
15. How does the clinical indication for the use of kanamycin differ from the indications for gentamicin, tobramycin, netilmicin, and amikacin?
16. What is the mechanism of action of polymyxins?
17. By what routes are polymyxins best administered?
18. How is polymyxin eliminated?
19. What are the three most common toxic reactions to polymyxins?
20. What patients are most at risk of neuromuscular blockade with polymyxins?

SUGGESTED READINGS

Brummett, R.E.: Drug-induced ototoxicity, Drugs **19**:412, 1980.

Burkle, W.: Comparative evaluation of the aminoglycoside antibiotics for systemic use, Drug Intell. Clin. Pharm. **15**:847, 1981.

Edson, R.S., and Terrell, C.L.: The aminoglycosides, Mayo Clin. Proc. **62**(10):916, 1987.

Guay, C.R.P.: Netilmicin, Drug Intell. Clin. Pharm. **17**(2):83, 1983.

Matthews, A. and others: Clinical pharmacokinetics, toxicity and cost effectiveness analysis of aminoglycosides and aminoglycoside dosing services, J. Clin. Pharm. Ther. **12**:(5):273, 1987.

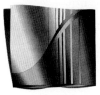

CHAPTER

Antibiotics: Sulfonamides, Trimethoprim, Quinolones, and Furantoins

34

This chapter focuses on drugs used mainly in urinary tract infections. Four separate chemical families are represented: (1) sulfonamides, (2) trimethoprim, (3) quinolones, and (4) nitrofurantoins. The special antimicrobial mechansims and pharmacokinetic properties that make these drugs useful in a variety of infections are considered.

SULFONAMIDES AND TRIMETHOPRIM
Mechanism of Action and Bacterial Resistance

Sulfonamides are metabolic inhibitors that block bacterial synthesis of folic acid, a vitamin required for the synthesis of amino acids and nucleic acids (Figure 34.1). The metabolically active form of folic acid, tetrahydrofolic acid (THFA), is synthesized in bacteria by two enzymes working in sequence. The first enzyme, dihydropteroate synthetase, converts paraaminobenzoic acid (PABA) and other small molecules to dihydropteroate which becomes dihydrofolic acid. The second enzyme, dihydrofolic acid reductase, forms THFA. The sulfonamides competitively inhibit the first enzyme in this sequence, dihydrofolic acid synthetase.

Sulfonamides are selectively toxic to organisms that must form folic acid from paraaminobenzoic acid and the other precursors. Fortunately, humans are not sensitive to this action, since we cannot synthesize folic acid but must absorb it preformed in our diet. Sulfonamides are primarily bacteriostatic against those organisms they affect.

Trimethoprim inhibits the second step in THFA synthesis, the enzyme dihydrofolic acid reductase. Trimethoprim therefore also prevents THFA formation in bacteria. Dihydrofolic acid reductase functions both in humans and in bacteria, since much of the vitamin in the mammalian diet is converted to dihydrofolic acid. Therefore trimethoprim might be expected to be toxic to humans as well as to bacteria. This is not the case, however, since dihydrofolic acid reductase in humans is relatively resistant to the action of trimethoprim, and the drug may be given at doses that inhibit this enzyme in bacteria but not in humans.

Sulfonamides are potentially active against a wide range of gram-positive and gram-negative organisms as well as *Nocardia*, *Chlamydia*, and *Actinomyces*. Bacterial resistance to the sulfonamides has become widespread, however, and has reduced the clinical usefulness of these drugs. Some bacteria such as pneumococci acquire an altered dihydrofolic acid synthetase, which is less sensitive to sulfonamides. Overproduction of paraaminobenzoic acid is a common mechanism of resistance for several pathogens, including staphylococci, pneumococci, and gonococci. Since sulfonamides are only competitive inhibitors of paraaminobenzoic acid incorporation into folic acid, excess paraaminobenzoic acid will overcome the sulfonamide inhibition.

Trimethoprim has a spectrum of antimicrobial activity similar to that of the sulfonamides with the following exceptions: (1) trimethoprim is more active against the gram-negative bacteria *Proteus*, *Klebsiella*, and *Serratia*; (2) trimethoprim is not useful alone against *Chlamydia* or *Nocardia*; and (3) trimethoprim resistance has not yet become widespread. Trimethoprim is used in the United States most commonly in combination with a sulfonamide. A preparation of trimethoprim alone is available for use in urinary tract infections.

Absorption, Distribution, and Excretion

Sulfonamide antibacterial agents with a wide variety of pharmacokinetic properties are available (Tables 34.1 to 34.3). Some of these drugs are not

509

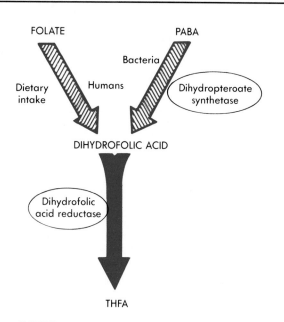

FOLATE   PABA

Bacteria

Dietary intake   Humans   Dihydropteroate synthetase

DIHYDROFOLIC ACID

Dihydrofolic acid reductase

THFA

FIGURE 34.1   Synthesis of tetrahydrofolic acid (THFA) in bacteria and humans. THFA is a vitamin required for nucleic acid and amino acid synthesis. Many bacteria form this vitamin from paraaminobenzoic acid (PABA) and other small molecules. Two enzymes are involved in this synthesis: dihydrofolic acid synthetase and dihydrofolic acid reductase. Sulfonamides inhibit the first of these enzymes, thereby blocking THFA synthesis in bacteria. Mankind is immune from this action, since preformed folate and dihydrofolic acid are taken in the diet.

GERIATRIC DRUG ALERT: SULFONAMIDES

THE PROBLEM

The elderly are more likely to suffer severe blood and skin reactions to sulfonamides than are younger adults. Diuretics, commonly taken by the elderly for high blood pressure, compound the risk.

SOLUTIONS

- Monitor blood tests for signs of bone marrow depression
- Watch for bleeding or reduced platelet counts
- Inspect carefully for rash or purpura
- Ascertain if patient is taking thiazide diuretic, either alone or as component of other preparations

absorbed from the gastrointestinal tract and are intended to remain within the bowel and reduce the bacterial population there. Some systemic absorption of these agents can occur through ulcerated regions of the bowel. Systemic absorption can likewise occur when sulfonamides are used on extensive areas of burned skin.

The sulfonamides used for treatment of systemic infections are all well absorbed from the gastrointestinal tract. Distribution of these drugs to body tissues, and to the brain, is good. Concentrations of sulfonamides in cerebrospinal and other body fluids may approach that of serum. Sulfonamides also pass the placental barrier and enter the fetus.

Elimination of sulfonamides from the body involves both the liver and kidneys. The liver converts a portion of the sulfonamide in the bloodstream to an acetylated derivative, which is usually bacteriologically inactive. Both the acetylated and the free drug are eliminated by the kidney primarily by glomerular filtration. Tubular reabsorption is significant for some sulfonamides. Since absorbed sulfonamides are excreted by the kidney in part in

the free, unacetylated form, the urine contains antibacterial activity. Excretion of the sulfonamides is favored by alkalinizing the urine. This procedure increases the solubility of these drugs in urine and also converts the drugs to a charged form that does not undergo renal tubular reabsorption.

The use of trimethoprim in fixed combination with sulfamethoxazole (Table 34.2) represents a clever exploitation of drug properties for good therapeutic effect. These drugs are administered in tablets containing the agents in the ratio of 1:5, trimethoprim:sulfamethoxazole. Both drugs are well absorbed from the gastrointestinal tract. Serum concentrations of the free drug not bound to serum proteins are usually in the ratio 1:20, trimethoprim:sulfamethoxazole. At this concentration ratio, the drugs have maximum antibacterial activity. The combination is actually synergistic, that is, more effective in combination than would be expected from the action of either drug alone. Synergy may result, since both drugs ultimately starve sensitive bacteria for THFA, but the drugs work on two different enzymes in the sequence of reactions leading to THFA. The sequential blockade of this metabolic pathway is much more effective than blockade of a single step by one drug at high concentrations.

Trimethoprim has synergistic effects with any of the systemically effective sulfonamides. Sulfamethoxazole was chosen for use in the fixed combination with trimethoprim because the kinetics of elimination of the two drugs are quite similar. Therefore use of this fixed combination does not lead to accumulation of one or the other of the drugs.

Trimethoprim penetrates body tissues better than sulfamethoxazole. Trimethoprim concentra-

Table 34.1   Clinical Summary of Sulfonamides: Single Component Formulations

Generic name	Trade name	Administration/dosage	Clinical use
Sulfacytine	Renoquid	ORAL: *Adults*—500 mg loading dose, then 250 mg 4 times daily. Not for children under 14 yr.	Urinary tract infections.
Sulfadiazine	Microsulfon Sulfadi-azine*	ORAL: *Adults*—single loading dose of 2 to 4 Gm, then 2 to 4 Gm daily in 3 to 6 doses. *Children over 2 months*—75 mg/kg body weight to load, then 150 mg/kg daily in 4 to 6 doses.	Nocardiosis, rheumatic fever prophylaxis.
Sulfamethizole	Thiosulfil*	ORAL: *Adults*—0.5 to 1 Gm, 3 or 4 times daily. *Children over 2 mo*—30 to 45 mg/kg daily in 4 doses.	Urinary tract infections only.
Sulfamethoxazole	Gantanol*	ORAL: *Adults*—single 2 Gm loading dose, then 1 Gm 2 or 3 times daily. *Children over 2 mo*—50 to 60 mg/kg loading dose, then 25 to 30 mg/kg twice daily, not to exceed 75 mg/kg daily.	Conjunctivitis, nocardiosis, otitis media, trachoma, and urinary tract infections.
Sulfapyridine	Dagenan†	ORAL: *Adults*—500 mg 4 times daily. Reduce by 500 mg increments as improvement allows.	Dermatitis herpetiformis
Sulfasalazine	Azulfidine Salazopyrin* SAS-500*	ORAL: *Adults*—3 to 4 Gm daily in divided doses. *Children*—40 to 60 mg/kg daily in 3 to 6 doses.	Two thirds of oral dose remains in bowel for treatment of ulcerative colitis.
Sulfisoxazole	Gantrisin* SK-Soxazole Sulfafura-zole*	ORAL: *Adults*—2 to 4 Gm loading dose, then 4 to 8 Gm daily in 3 to 6 doses. *Children over 2 mo*—75 mg/kg loading dose, then 150 mg/kg daily in 4 to 6 doses.	Urinary tract infections and systemic infections due to sensitive organisms, nocardiosis.

*Available in Canada and United States.
†Available in Canada only.

tions in breast milk, bile, prostatic fluid, vaginal fluids, liver, spleen, skin, and kidney actually may exceed plasma concentrations of the drug. Penetration into other tissues is adequate, including the central nervous system.

Trimethoprim appears in the urine at a concentration approximately 100 times the plasma concentration, most of the drug being in the active form. Sulfamethoxazole in the urine is mostly in the acetylated form, and the urinary concentration is about five times the plasma concentration.

Sulfonamides are available in a number of fixed combinations (Table 34.2). Those combinations that contain only sulfonamides are formulated so that the amount of any one agent is well below the recommended dosage; dosage is calculated on total sulfonamide content. These formulations are designed to avoid sulfonamide insolubility in the urine. Each drug in the combination dissolves independently of the others so that total sulfonamide concentration in the urine exceeds that possible with a single agent.

Sulfonamides may be combined with phenazopyridine for the treatment of urinary tract infections (Table 34.2). The sulfonamide component supplies antibacterial activity while the phenazopyridine, which is excreted in the urine, exerts an analgesic effect on the mucosa of the urinary tract. The added phenazopyridine therefore relieves the symptoms of pain, burning, and itching associated with the urinary tract infection.

Sulfonamide preparations are available for vaginal application, but no evidence of effectiveness exists. Moreover, sensitization may be produced.

Toxicity

Sulfonamides induce allergic reactions in a significant proportion of patients receiving the drugs. The most common reactions are skin rashes and pruritus, but drug fever and other more serious reactions may occur. Anaphylaxis has been reported. Since sulfonamides are chemically related to the thiazide diuretics, acetazolamide, and oral hypoglycemic agents, a patient who becomes allergic to

Table 34.2   Clinical Summary of Sulfonamides: Fixed Combinations for Oral Use

Components of combination		Drug form	Trade name	Dosage	Clinical use
Sulfamethoxazole Trimethoprim	400 mg 80 mg	Tablet	Bactrim* Cotrim Protrim Roubac Septra*	*Adults*—2 tablets every 12 hr. For pneumocystis pneumonia, 25 mg/kg sulfamethoxazole and 5 mg/kg trimethoprim every 6 hr. *Children*—8 mg/kg trimethoprim and 40 mg/kg sulfamethoxazole daily in 2 doses.	Urinary tract infections, otitis media, enteritis due to sensitive *Shigella*, pneumocystis pneumonia
Sulfadiazine Trimethoprim	410 mg 90 mg	Tablet	Coptin†	*Adults*—1 tablet every 12 hr. *Children 3 mo to 5 yr*—¼ to ½ tablet every 12 hr. *Children 5 to 12 yr*—½ to 1 tablet every 12 hr.	Urinary tract infections
Sulfadoxine Pyrimethamine	500 mg 25 mg	Tablet	Fansidar	*Adults*—for treatment, 2 to 3 tablets as single dose; or 1 tablet for chemoprophylaxis. *Children 1 mo to 4 yr*—½ tablet once for therapy or every 7 days for chemoprophylaxis. *Children 5 to 8 yr*—1 tablet once for therapy or every 7 days for chemoprophylaxis. *Children 9 to 12 yr*—2 tablets once for therapy or every 7 days for chemoprophylaxis.	Malaria
Sulfamerazine Sulfadiazine Sulfamethazine	167 mg 167 mg 167 mg	Tablet or per 5 ml suspension	Lantrisul Terfonyl Triple Sulfa	*Adults*—2 to 4 Gm total sulfonamide loading dose, then 2 to 4 Gm daily in 3 to 6 doses. *Children*—75 mg/kg to load, then 150 mg/kg daily in 4 to 6 doses.	Urinary tract infections
Sulfamethoxazole Phenazopyridine	500 mg 100 mg	Tablet	Azo-Gantanol UroGantanol	*Adults*—4 tablets to load, then 2 tablets every 12 hr for 3 days.	Urinary tract infections only.
Sulfamethizole Phenazopyridine	250 or 500 mg 50 mg	Tablet	Thiosulfil-A	*Adults*—2 to 4 tablets 2 or 3 times daily. *Children*—30 to 45 mg sulfamethizole/kg daily in 4 doses.	Urinary tract infections only.
Sulfisoxazole Phenazopyridine	500 mg 50 mg	Tablet	Azo-Gantrisin Suldiazo	*Adults*—4 to 6 tablets to load, then 2 tablets every 6 hr for 3 days. *Children*—dose as for sulfisoxazole alone.	Urinary tract infections only.

*Available in Canada and United States.
†Available in Canada only.

a sulfonamide may also become allergic to one or more of these agents.

Gastrointestinal disturbances also occur with the sulfonamides. In addition to nausea, vomiting, and diarrhea, pancreatitis, hepatitis, and stomatitis may occur.

Central nervous system alterations have been observed, including headache, ataxia, hallucinations, and convulsions.

Deaths from aplastic anemia and other blood dyscrasias, although rare, have been reported in connection with sulfonamide therapy. Sore throat, fever, or pallor may signal a serious blood dyscrasia.

Renal toxicity was of great concern with the

Table 34.3   Clinical Summary of Sulfonamides: Topical Agents

Generic name	Trade name	Application form	Clinical use	Comments
Mafenide acetate	Sulfamylon*	Cream: 85 mg mafenide acetate/Gm.	Treatment of second- and third-degree burns.	Drug is effective against a broad spectrum of pathogens, including *Pseudomonas aeruginosa*. Drug may be absorbed through burned tissues.
Silver sulfadiazine	Silvadene Flamazine† Thermazene	Cream: 10 mg/Gm	Treatment of second- and third-degree burns.	Drug is effective against a broad spectrum of pathogens, including *P. aeruginosa* and certain yeasts. Drug may be absorbed through burned tissues.
Sulfacetamide	Bleph Liquifilm* Cetamid* Ocu-Sul Sulamyd*	Solution: 10%, 15%, or 30% Ointment: 10%	Ophthalmic only. For conjunctivitis, corneal ulcer, trachoma.	Drug allergy may develop in sensitive patients.
Sulfisoxazole diolamine	Gantrisin Ophthalmic*	Solution: 4% Ointment: 4%	Ophthalmic only. For conjunctivitis, corneal ulcer, trachoma.	Drug allergy may develop in sensitive patients.

*Available in Canada and United States.
†Available in Canada only.

PEDIATRIC DRUG ALERT: SULFONAMIDES

THE PROBLEM
Sulfonamides displace bilirubin from serum proteins. In neonates, who typically have elevated bilirubin, this displacement may be sufficient to produce kernicterus.

SOLUTIONS
- Avoid sulfonamides in pregnancy near term
- Avoid sulfonamides in infants younger than 1 month

sulfonamides in use before about 1960. Most of the renal damage associated with these older agents was produced by drug precipitation or crystallization in the urine. These drugs precipitated because of their low solubility in normal acidic urine. The newer sulfonamides are much more soluble under these conditions, and drug precipitation is seldom a problem. However, patients should receive sufficient fluids to produce at least 1 liter of urine daily while receiving sulfonamides. Solubility of the sulfonamides in urine may be increased by alkalinizing the urine. Sulfamethizole and sulfasalazine produce a yellow-orange coloration in alkaline urine.

This coloration, also observable in skin, is not harmful.

Patients with preexisting renal or hepatic disease may be more prone to develop toxic reactions, since these organs are the primary means of removal of sulfonamides from the body. Patients with a known genetic deficiency of glucose 6-phosphate dehydrogenase are also at greater risk of hemolytic anemia induced by sulfonamides. The highest frequency of glucose 6-phosphate dehydrogenase deficiency is observed among blacks and Mediterranean racial groups; patients from these groups should be watched with special care for signs of anemia.

Trimethoprim appears to be less toxic than the sulfonamides, although it may affect the bone marrow. When trimethoprim is used in combination with sulfamethoxazole, patients should be observed for all signs of sulfonamide toxicity.

Drug Interactions

Certain sulfonamides are highly bound to serum proteins and may therefore displace other drugs from protein binding sites. This displacement can occur with oral anticoagulants, sulfonylureas (oral hypoglycemic agents), and with the antineoplastic agent methotrexate.

Paraaminobenzoic acid may interfere with the action of sulfonamides. Procaine, a local anesthetic

Table 34.4 Clinical Summary of Quinolone and Related Antibiotics

Generic name	Trade name	Administration/dosage	Comments
Cinoxacin	Cinobac Cinobactin†	ORAL: *Adult*—250 mg every 6 hr or 500 mg every 12 hr. FDA Pregnancy Category B.	Primarily for urinary tract infections
Ciprofloxacin	Cipro	ORAL: *Adult*—500 to 700 mg every 12 hr. FDA Pregnancy Category C.	Bone and soft tissue infections, pneumonia, and bacterial diarrhea may respond
Nalidixic acid	NegGram*	ORAL: *Adult*—1 Gm 4 times daily for 1 to 2 wk	Urinary tract infections only; emergence of resistant bacterial strains is a common cause of treatment failure
Norfloxacin	Noroxin*	ORAL: *Adult*—400 mg every 12 hr for 3 to 21 days. FDA Pregnancy Category C.	Currently indicated primarily for urinary tract infections

*Available in United States and Canada.
†Available in Canada.

that is derived from paraaminobenzoic acid, may also block the action of sulfonamides on dihydrofolic acid synthetase (Figure 34.1).

QUINOLONES
Mechanism of Action and Bacterial Resistance

Quinolone and related antibiotics interfere with DNA replication in bacteria by inhibiting the proper functioning of DNA gyrase. DNA gyrase is the enzyme that allows bacterial DNA to unwind ("relax") so that replication may proceed. The quinolones block this action and ultimately lead to breaks in the double-stranded DNA. At achievable clinical concentrations, these agents are bactericidal. Ciprofloxacin and norfloxacin have broad antibacterial spectra, with activity toward aerobic gram-positive bacteria and aerobic gram-negative bacteria, including *Pseudomonas aeruginosa*. Cinoxacin and nalidixic acid have more restricted spectra, covering many common gram-negative pathogens but not *Ps. aeruginosa*.

Resistance to these drugs can occur, but plasmid-mediated resistance is not significant. One mechanism of resistance may involve blockage of antibiotic transport into the bacterial cell.

Absorption, Distribution, and Excretion

Quinolone and related antibiotics are generally well absorbed when given orally. Portal circulation carries absorbed drug directly to the liver, where metabolism occurs. Nalidixic acid is the most extensively metabolized drug of this group, with glucuronide and hydroxylated derivatives being formed.

PEDIATRIC DRUG ALERT: QUINOLONES

THE PROBLEM
Quinolones, including nalidixic acid and cinoxacin, have damaged cartilage in tests in young animals, leading to permanent joint impairment.

SOLUTION
■ Avoid quinolones in children

The hydroxylated form of nalidixic acid is biologically active and comprises a significant proportion of the active drug in the bloodstream and in urine. Over 90% of nalidixic acid in the bloodstream is bound to serum proteins. Little enters most body tissues. The only organ in which the drug concentration exceeds the plasma concentration is the kidney. Nalidixic acid has the lowest plasma concentration of any drug in this group.

Ciprofloxacin, norfloxacin, and cinoxacin are less extensively metabolized than nalidixic acid. From 30% to 60% of an oral dose of these drugs appears in the urine unchanged. Tissue penetration is greater with ciprofloxacin and norfloxacin than with cinoxacin or nalidixic acid. Ciprofloxacin and norfloxacin also persist longer in plasma than the other quinolones.

Doses of the quinolones may need to be adjusted in patients with renal impairment because the kidneys are the primary organ of excretion of either active drug or metabolites. Ciprofloxacin is

---

PATIENT PROBLEM: URINARY TRACT INFECTIONS

THE PROBLEM

Urinary tract infections are more common in women than in men, because the urethra is shorter in women. They are also more common in patients wearing urinary retention catheters (Foley catheters), and in patients requiring intermittent catheterization or urinary tract manipulation. Drugs may be prescribed when an infection develops, or prophylactically when genitourinary examination or manipulation is planned, or when there is a history of chronic urinary tract infection.

SIGNS AND SYMPTOMS

Burning on urination, frequent urination, irritation, burning, or itching in the area of the urinary meatus, fever, malaise.

PATIENT AND FAMILY EDUCATION

- Drink sufficient fluids to ensure a daily urine output of 1500 to 2000 ml. Usually, this means drinking at least 6 to 8 glassfuls (8 oz) for an adult.
- In women, always wipe after voiding or defecating from front to back, to avoid accidental contamination of the urinary meatus with bacteria from the anal region.
- Avoid bubble baths. Some patients, especially women, may have to limit all baths, taking showers instead.
- Wash soap off the perineal region well, to avoid irritation from the soap. Some patients may have to wash with water only, avoiding soaps.
- Void immediately after sexual intercourse.
- Some drugs for urinary tract infections are most effective if the pH of the urine is changed. This is difficult to do through diet alone, so other drugs may be prescribed by the physician. If sodium bicarbonate or other drugs are prescribed, take as ordered for best treatment of the urinary tract infection.
- Take drugs for the full prescribed dose (often 7 to 10 days); do not stop when symptoms begin to subside.

FOR PATIENTS WITH URINARY CATHETERS

- Secure the catheter well, so there is minimal pulling on the meatal area.
- Wash the catheter insertion area with soap and water, but avoid rough scrubbing. Rinse well.
- Avoid opening the drainage system unless necessary.
- Clean the tubing and bag as directed (unless replacing them with new device), usually with a dilute bleach solution or as instructed by the discharge nurse.
- In the hospital, use sterile technique to insert catheters. In the home, use clean technique as instructed.
- Maintain a good fluid intake, as noted above.

---

also eliminated by transintestinal transport, with about 15% of each dose appearing in feces.

Toxicity

Quinolones have two major side effecs. The first involves the central nervous system. Symptoms range from headache, dizziness, tinnitus, insomnia, shakiness, and changes in vision to seizures. These drugs should not be given to patients with preexisting CNS disease, because they can exacerbate the problem. The second side effect shared by the quinolones is a tendency to damage cartilage, especially in the young. This reaction has been observed in the young of several animal species and has led to permanent damage and lameness. For this reason, quinolones are not given to children.

Drug Interactions

Antacids containing aluminum or magnesium compounds can block absorption of ciprofloxacin and norfloxacin. The result is lower plasma and urinary concentrations of antibiotic and loss of antibacterial effectiveness.

Sodium bicarbonate, citrates, carbonic anhydrase inhibitors, and antacids containing calcium may alkalinize the urine, which renders ciprofloxacin less soluble. The drug may crystallize in the urinary tract, causing pain and obstruction. Avoiding these agents and maintaining an adequate fluid intake lessen the risk of crystalluria developing.

Ciprofloxacin use lowers hepatic clearance of theophylline, which can cause theophylline to accumulate. As serum theophylline levels increase, so does the risk of CNS toxicity; there may be nausea, vomiting, tremors, restlessness, agitation, and palpitations.

NITROFURANTOINS
Mechanism of Action and Bacterial Resistance

Nitrofurantoin apparently functions as an inhibitor of certain bacterial enzymes required for metabolism of sugar and perhaps other compounds. The drug is effective against a variety of gram-positive and gram-negative organisms, including most common pathogens of the urinary tract. *Pseudomonas* and *Proteus* species are, however, usually intrinsically resistant. Development of resistance to nitrofurantoin therapy is not a significant problem.

Absorption, Distribution, and Excretion

Many compounds that are effective antibacterial agents in the laboratory are ineffective when

THE NURSING PROCESS

SULFONAMIDES, QUINOLONES, AND NITROFURANTOINS

The student should refer to Chapter 29 for general guidelines on the nursing process with antibiotic therapy. The additional material below relates specifically to the sulfonamides, quinolones, and other drugs discussed in this chapter.

Assessment

The drugs described in this chapter are used mainly for the treatment of urinary tract infections. Assessment should be carried out with emphasis on renal function. Other clinical signs of infection should be monitored as well. Objective data such as blood tests, history of allergies, and mental function should also be obtained.

Nursing diagnoses

Possible altered home maintenance management related to the need to increase fluid intake to 1500 ml or more per day

Potential complication: blood dyscrasias

Management

Progress of treatment for urinary tract infections may be monitored by clinical signs alone, such as relief of pain and itching, or by culturing the urine. The nurse should be certain that urine samples are appropriately collected to prevent trivial contamination, which renders the culture results meaningless. Blood tests may be required for patients receiving sulfonamides. All patients being treated for urinary tract infections should receive adequate fluids to maintain good urine flow. Patient teaching should include instruction in the signs of blood dyscrasias for those receiving sulfonamides, signs of pulmonary distress and peripheral neuropathy for those receiving nitrofurantoins, and signs of central nervous system distress in those receiving nalidixic acid or cinoxacin. These side effects are usually sufficient cause for the physician to discontinue medication.

Evaluation

These drugs are all capable of curing urinary tract infections. However, relapses or failure of therapy are not uncommon, for several reasons. First, bacterial resistance may develop. This form of therapeutic failure is relatively common with nalidixic acid. Second, reinfections may occur frequently in some people. In some cases the reinfection may reflect inadequate hygiene, whereas in others it may reflect a defect within the urinary tract that impedes urine flow and promotes infections.

The nurse should make certain that the patient can explain how to take the prescribed medication and can point out which side effects are sufficient reasons to call the physician. The patient should also be capable of properly collecting urine for testing.

---

used to treat systemic infections because of the unfavorable pharmacokinetics of the drugs. One example of such a compound is nitrofurantoin. This drug, in spite of being well absorbed from the small intestine, never achieves satisfactory blood levels. Low blood levels result from a rapid excretion of the drug in the kidney. Removal of the drug from the system occurs so quickly that it fails to accumulate in the bloodstream. Therefore, despite its broad antibacterial spectrum, it is ineffective against systemic infections. However, nitrofuran-

toin is concentrated in the kidney and achieves antibacterial concentrations in the urine. In the renal tubule, it diffuses into kidney tissues so that the final concentration in the kidney is much greater than would be expected from the very low blood concentrations of the drug. These properties make the drug effective against urinary tract infections.

Toxicity

One of the more common reactions to nitrofurantoin is gastric irritation, with anorexia, nau-

PATIENT CARE IMPLICATIONS

Sulfonamides and trimethoprim

Drug administration

- Review Patient Care Implications listed at the end of Chapter 29.
- Question the patient about history of allergy to other sulfonamides, thiazide diuretics, acetazolamide, or oral hypoglycemic agents before administering the sulfonamides.
- Inspect for development of rashes or skin changes and gastrointestinal distress. Monitor temperature.
- Monitor complete blood count and differential, platelet count, BUN, serum creatinine, liver function tests, urinalysis.
- Topical sulfonamide preparations are used in the treatment of burns (Table 34.3). Wear sterile gloves when applying medication. The drugs are most effective when the area is cleaned of debris and pus. Dressings are not necessary but may be used. Medicate for pain before redressing wounds. Monitor serum drug levels and serum electrolytes, in addition to blood work noted above.

  INTRAVENOUS TRIMETHOPRIM-
  SULFAMETHOXAZOLE

- Dilute each 5 ml ampule in 125 ml 5% dextrose in water. Administer diluted dose over 60 to 90 minutes. Flush tubing well after administration. For patients on fluid restriction, see package insert.

Patient and family education

- Review Patient Care Implications given at the end of Chapter 29.
- Review the benefits and possible side effects of drug therapy. Instruct the patient to report the development of fever, sore throat, unexplained bleeding or bruising, malaise, jaundice, rashes, skin changes.
- Review Patient Problem: Urinary Tract Infections on p. 515.
- Tell patients receiving sulfamethizole or sulfasalazine that these drugs may turn urine or skin a yellow-orange color.
- Tell patients taking combination products that contain phenazopyridine that this compound will turn urine reddish-orange in color. In addition, this dye may produce false results with urine glucose tests. Tell diabetic patients about this effect. Instruct such patients not to change insulin or diet without discussing with the physician. Monitor blood glucose if possible.

- Take doses with a full glassful (8 oz) of water or other liquid.
- Do not give sulfonamide drugs to children under 12 years unless specifically prescribed by a physician.
- Review Patient Problem: Photosensitivity (p. 647) with patients.
- Caution patients to avoid driving or operating hazardous equipment until the effects of this medication are known. Report dizziness to the physician.
- Sulfonamides are available for ophthalmic use. See Chapter 6 for a discussion of application of drops and ointment.
- Sulfonamides are available for intravaginal use. Make certain the patient can apply the ordered dose correctly. See Patient Problem: Treatment of Vaginal Infections on p. 540.
- Remind patients to keep all health care providers informed of all drugs being used.

Quinolones

Drug administration

- See Patient Care Implications listed at the end of Chapter 29.
- Assess for history of allergy before administering.
- Assess for CNS side effects: headache, dizziness, tinnitus, insomnia, shakiness, and changes in vision.
- Monitor complete blood count and differential, and platelet count, BUN, serum creatinine and liver function tests.

Patient and family education

- See Patient Care Implications given at the end of Chapter 29.
- Review anticipated benefits and possible side effects of drug therapy. Instruct the patient to report the development of any new sign or symptom.
- Reinforce the importance of not giving quinolones to children.
- Take oral doses with a full glassful (8 oz) of water or fluid.
- See Patient Problems: Urinary Tract Infections (p. 515); Photosensitivity (p. 647); and Dry Mouth (p. 170).
- Note the drug interactions. Take ciprofloxacin or norfloxacin 1 hour before or 2 hours after antacids containing aluminum or magnesium. Review the patient's other medications, and counsel as necessary. Remind pa-

Continued.

PATIENT CARE IMPLICATIONS—cont'd

tients to keep all health care providers informed of all drugs being used.

- Caution patients to avoid driving or operating hazardous equipment if CNS symptoms develop. Report dizziness, tinnitus, visual changes to the physician.
- If photophobia develops (eyes have increased sensitivity to light), instruct the patient to wear sunglasses and avoid bright lights or sunlight.
- Tell diabetic patients taking nalidixic acid that the drug may interfere with urine glucose results. Do not change diet or insulin without consulting the physician. Monitor blood glucose levels.

Nitrofurantoins

Drug administration

- See Patient Care Implications described at the end of Chapter 29.

- Assess for GI disturbance, skin changes, peripheral neuropathy. Assess lung sounds and respiratory rate. Monitor weight.
- Monitor complete blood count and differential, liver function tests.

Patient and family education

- See Patient Care Implications listed at the end of Chapter 29.
- Review anticipated benefits and possible side effects of drug therapy. Instruct the patient to report the development of any new sign or symptom.
- Review Patient Problem: Urinary Tract Infections on p. 515.
- Take oral doses with meals or snack to reduce gastric irritation. Warn patients that oral suspensions may stain teeth. Dilute doses of suspension with milk or juice before taking.

Table 34.5   Clinical Summary of Nitrofurantoin and Trimethoprim

Generic name	Trade name	Administration/dosage	Comments
Nitrofurantoin	Furadantin Furalan Nitrex	ORAL: *Adults*—50 to 100 mg 4 times daily. *Children*— 5 to 7 mg/kg daily in 4 divided doses. The drug should not be given to children under 3 mo.	Gastric irritation may be minimized by administering the drug with food or milk.
Nitrofurantoin macrocrystals	Macrodantin*	As for nitrofurantoin.	Large crystal size minimizes gastric irritation.
Trimethoprim	Proloprim* Trimpex	ORAL: *Adults*—100 mg every 12 hr. *Children*—the drug has not been extensively tested in children and is not recommended.	Blood changes can occur with this drug.

*Available in Canada and United States.

---

sea, and emesis. This reaction is apparently lessened if the drug is administered as large crystals (Macrodantin, Table 34.5) rather than in the original microcrystalline form. The large crystals are more slowly absorbed, but this does not interfere with clinical effectiveness.

Rashes, allergies, and reversible blood dyscrasias have been observed with nitrofurantoin. Hemolytic anemia similar to that seen with sulfonamides may also be seen. Infants under 3

months of age have undeveloped enzyme systems that make them especially susceptible to hemolytic anemia induced by nitrofurantoin. It should be used with care in pregnant patients.

Oral suspensions may stain the teeth. Nitrofurantoin also causes the urine to turn brown, but this is a harmless effect. An occasional patient may suffer hair loss while receiving the drug.

Peripheral neuropathy is one of the most serious toxic effects of nitrofurantoin. If detected early, the condition disappears following discontinuation of the drug. Damage may be permanent if the drug is continued after signs of peripheral neuropathy have developed. As with any drug that is excreted primarily by the kidney, nitrofurantoin may accumulate in patients with a degree of renal failure. These patients are more likely to suffer from significant side effects of nitrofurantoin therapy. Vitamin B deficiency, a common finding in alcoholics, may also predispose a patient to peripheral neuropathy. Diabetes mellitus, a disease that may itself cause peripheral neuropathies, may produce added risk of neural complications.

Patients receiving nitrofuranotin for long periods should be observed for the occurrence of pneumonitis or pulmonary fibrosis, which may develop gradually or appear as an acute illness.

Nitrofurantoin is used clinically to treat certain types of urinary tract infections, especially when the causative organism is a sensitive strain of *Escherichia coli*.

SUMMARY

Sulfonamides are metabolic inhibitors that block bacterial synthesis of tetrahydrofolic acid (THFA), a vitamin required for the synthesis of amino acids and nucleic acids. Sulfonamides are effective against a wide range of gram-positive and gram-negative bacteria. They are available for topical use and for use as nonabsorbable oral agents. However, most are well absorbed orally and penetrate most body tissues, including the brain. Sulfonamides are acetylated by the liver and excreted by the kidneys. Since the drugs are present in a high concentration in an active form in the urine, they are very useful in urinary tract infections. Sulfonamides cause allergies, gastrointestinal distress, and blood dyscrasias. Patients should receive 2 to 2.5 L of fluid daily to prevent urinary precipitation of the drug.

Trimethoprim blocks the conversion of dihydrofolic acid to THFA in bacteria. Trimethoprim is synergistic when used with sulfonamides and for that reason is most frequently used in fixed combination with sulfamethaxazole. Trimethoprim is well distributed to tissues and is excreted by the kidney, with most of the drug remaining in the active form. It appears to be relatively nontoxic, but may affect the bone marrow.

Quinolones inhibit bacterial DNAgyrase and may be rapidly bactericidal in both gram-positive and gram-negative bacteria, including *Pseudomonas aeruginosa*. Resistance to quinolones is not mediated by plasmids and hence is not transmitted between bacterial strains. Quinolones are well absorbed orally and excreted mostly in urine as both active drug and metabolites. Nalidixic acid, cinoxacin, and norfloxacin are administered primarily in urinary tract infections. Ciprofloxacin is given in bone infections, pneumonia, diarrhea, and soft tissue infections as well. All quinolones can cause CNS symptoms or exacerbate seizures. These drugs may also damage cartilage and should be avoided in children.

Nitrofurantoins are orally administered antibacterial agents that achieve effective concentrations only in the urine. They may irritate the gastrointestinal tract, especially when administered in the microcrystalline form. Rashes, allergies, and blood dyscrasias may also develop. Peripheral neuropathy and pneumonitis are associated with long-term use of nitrofurantoin.

STUDY QUESTIONS

1. What is the mechanism for the antibacterial effect of sulfonamides?
2. Why are sulfonamides not equally toxic to humans and bacteria?
3. What is the effect of paraaminobenzoic acid on sulfonamide action in bacterial cells?
4. By what routes may sulfonamides be administered?
5. Do sulfonamides enter the cerebrospinal fluid from the bloodstream?
6. What is the route of elimination of sulfonamides?
7. What is the purpose of combining sulfonamides with phenazopyridine in the treatment of urinary tract infections?
8. What are the major toxic reactions to sulfonamides?
9. How has the renal toxicity of the sulfonamide preparations used clinically changed since the early 1940s?
10. What is the mechanism for the antibacterial effect of trimethoprim?
11. Why is trimethoprim not equally toxic to humans and bacteria?
12. Why are trimethoprim and sulfamethoxazole combined for the treatment of urinary tract infections and infections at other sites?
13. What is the mechanism of the antibacterial effect of quinolones?
14. By what route are quinolones given?
15. What is the major clinical use of nalidixic acid, cinoxacin, and norfloxacin?
16. What is the major route of excretion of the quinolones?

17. What type of toxicity is associated with quinolones?
18. Why are quinolones not used in children?
19. Why is nitrofurantoin not effective for systemic infections?
20. By what route is nitrofurantoin administered?
21. What reactions to nitrofurantoin are commonly encountered with short-term therapy?
22. What reactions to nitrofurantoin are associated with long-term therapy?

SUGGESTED READINGS

Cockerill, F.R. III, and Edson, R.S.: Trimethoprim-sulfamethoxazole, Mayo Clin. Proc. **62**(10):921, 1983.

Conti, M.T., and Eutropius, L.: Preventing UTIs: what works? Am. J. Nurs. **87**(3):307, 1987.

Fiorelli, R.L.: Recurrent urinary tract infections in women: pathogenesis and treatment, J. Urol. Nurs. **7**(4):510, 1988.

Glatt, A.E.: Treating *P. carinii* pneumonia in patients with AIDS, Drug Therapy **19**(4):69, 1989.

Karb, V.B.: Two new fluoroquinolones: ciprofloxacin and norfloxacin, J. Neurosci. Nurs. **20**(5):327, 1988.

Manzo, M.: Ciprofloxacin and norfloxacin—potent oral antiinfectives, Nursing **19**(2):30, 1989.

Millette-Petit, J.M.: Urinary tract infections in older adults, Nurse Pract. **13**(12):21, 1988.

Osborne, S.: Ciprofloxacin—a new fluoroquinolone antimicrobial agent, J. Urol. Nurs. **7**(4):505, 1988.

Walker, R.C., and Wright, A.J.: The quinolones, Mayo Clin. Proc. **62**(11):1007, 1987.

Wilhelm, M.P., and Edson, R.S.: Antimicrobial agents in urinary tract infections, Mayo Clin. Proc. **62**(11):1025, 1987.

Drugs to Treat Tuberculosis and Leprosy

35

Tuberculosis and leprosy are diseases produced by *Mycobacterium* infections. Both diseases have been known since ancient times and are among the earliest examples of diseases that were recognized as infectious. Tuberculosis, or the white plague, was a major cause of death in Europe and the Orient throughout the Middle Ages and until recent times. Leprosy, although less common, was greatly feared because of the disfigurement it caused. This grim picture changed in the early 1940s when the first effective antituberculosis agent, streptomycin, was discovered. Around the same time a sulfone was discovered to be effective in controlling leprosy. With these and other more recently discovered agents, both diseases may now be treated effectively in most patients. *Mycobacterium avium* complex in AIDS patients has a poor prognosis. In this chapter the clinical features of *Mycobacterium* infections, which make their treatment more difficult than that of most other bacterial diseases, are considered. Second, the properties of the drugs used to treat these diseases and the ways in which they are employed are covered.

TREATMENT OF TUBERCULOSIS
Clinical Features of Tuberculosis

Tuberculosis is produced by *Mycobacterium tuberculosis*, or less commonly by other mycobacteria harbored by cattle or birds. Three features of *M. tuberculosis* are especially important to recall in considering how disease is produced in humans by these organisms. First, mycobacteria are strict aerobic organisms. This property decrees that the organism must live in an oxygen-rich environment and may explain the fact that the first site of infection in humans is usually along the alveoli of the lung. Second, mycobacteria induce activity of macrophages, causing these cellular immunity factors to phagocytize *M. tuberculosis*. Rather than

helping prevent infection, this action actually may enhance survival and spread of the disease-causing organisms, since *M. tuberculosis* is resistant to the acids and enzymes that usually destroy bacteria within macrophages. *M. tuberculosis* reproduces within macrophages at a near-normal rate and may be carried by them throughout the body. Third, mycobacteria are slow-growing organisms relative to other bacteria. The time required for the tubercle bacilli to reproduce is 10 to 12 hours, as compared to 20 to 30 minutes for other bacteria such as *Escherichia coli* or *Pseudomonas aeruginosa*. This slow growth contributes to the difficulty encountered in treating the disease, since it is during active growth that the organism is most susceptible to metabolic interference.

The disease may pass through several phases. The initial or primary infection usually occurs in the lung as a result of inhaling droplets containing live *M. tuberculosis*. These infective aerosols are generated when a patient with an established active case of tuberculosis coughs or sneezes. Once in the alveoli, the *M. tuberculosis* is phagocytized and begins to multiply. Infected macrophages may remain in the lung, but a significant number enter the lymphatic system and a few enter the bloodstream and are carried throughout the body. In response to the increasing number of tubercle bacilli in the lung, a pneumonia-like condition may develop within a few weeks. This inflammatory response to the infection may continue for a few weeks, but in most people this process is ultimately halted by the delayed immune reaction provoked by the infection. This acquired cellular immunity results in increased effectiveness of macrophages in destroying the *M. tuberculosis*. Lesions within the lung resolve as infective loci become calcified. Living tubercule bacilli no longer appear in sputum at this stage, and the disease is said to be inactive. Living

THE NURSING PROCESS

TREATMENT OF TUBERCULOSIS

Assessment

Antituberculosis therapy is used in patients who are diagnosed as having active tuberculosis or those whose tuberculosis skin tests convert from negative to positive. In some instances patients receiving high doses of adrenocortical steroids may require antituberculosis therapy. In the latter group of patients, the concern is that the high doses of steroids will alter the patient's ability to resist infection from tuberculosis or will cause reactivation of earlier tubercular infections. Initially, patients may show a picture of chronic illness, may be seriously ill, or may be well in appearance and have been diagnosed only through conversion of the tuberculin skin test. The initial assessment needs to be based in part on the patient's obvious condition. Certainly a thorough total assessment should be done, with an emphasis on subjective complaints, possible history of tuberculosis in the patient and family, and recent activities such as travel or moving that might have influenced exposure to the disease. Not all patients have the characteristic cough historically associated with tuberculosis. If a cough with sputum production exists, the sputum should be sent for culture and drug sensitivity testing. Tuberculosis can appear in other organs besides the lung (e.g., tuberculosis meningitis). Obviously the focus of the assessment would be different if the patient had a nontraditional form of tuberculosis.

Nursing diagnoses

Anxiety related to diagnosis and long-term drug therapy

Potential altered home maintenance management related to lack of knowledge about how to incorporate drug therapy into daily activities

Management

The diagnosis of tuberculosis still causes many health care professionals and patients to develop unnecessary anxiety and fear about this disease. As soon as the diagnosis is made, it is important to begin patient education so that unreasonable fears can be calmed. If health care personnel are unsure of the local standards regarding care of tuberculosis patients, the local health department or hospital infection control department should be contacted. The hospitalized patient will be placed in isolation. It is beyond the scope of this book to go into detail about such procedures as isolation for the various forms of tuberculosis; refer to appropriate nursing textbooks for these procedures. It is important to remember that many tuberculosis patients are diagnosed and treated entirely on an outpatient basis. Because drug therapy for tuberculosis is lengthy, usually lasting 2 years or longer, the management phase can be thought of as a long-term process. New cases of tuberculosis should be reported to the local health department so that they can follow up possible family and social contacts of the patient who has been diagnosed with this disease.

Evaluation

Success with antituberculosis therapy is manifested by a resolution of the disease. Many factors influence the success of therapy, such as patient motivation to continue the long-term course of therapy, actual patient compliance, and the incidence of side effects that occur with the drugs. In fact, noncompliance is a major cause of treatment failures. Before beginning self-management, the patient should be able to explain why and how to take the drugs ordered, possible side effects, ways to treat minor side effects such as nausea associated with taking the medication, and side effects that require notification of the physician. The patient should also be able to explain when and why return visits for evaluation of laboratory work and other patient data are scheduled and should be able to explain and demonstrate the measures to take to decrease the possibility of spreading the disease to others. With a markedly positive skin test, the individual

THE NURSING PROCESS—cont'd

should be able to explain that skin tests in the future should be refused, and that follow-up should be made via x-ray film. If side effects have occurred with the drugs, such as peripheral neuropathy with isoniazid therapy, patients will receive appropriate additional pharmacological management. Although these measures are not related directly to actions with the patient, it is important the health care personnel accept responsibility for having TB skin tests or chest x-ray films on a regular basis to diagnose possible exposure to tuberculosis. For further specific information, see the patient care implications section at the end of this chapter.

M. tuberculosis remains within the body, however, for relapses may occur months or years after the initial infection. When relapse occurs, localized areas again become sites of active multiplication of tubercle bacilli. Local necrosis develops as the cellular immunity factors attempt to isolate the infection. Necrosis may spread as a result of this inflammatory response and may cause large cavities within the lungs or other tissues.

M. tuberculosis, like most other bacteria, has the ability to acquire resistance to drugs. Development of resistance is common when patients are treated with a single drug. To minimize this therapeutic complication, multiple drug therapy is used. The rationale for this therapy is that since mutations are required for the development of resistance to a drug, if two drugs that have different mechanisms of action are administered, then the organism must acquire two independent mutations to become resistant to both drugs. Since mutations are rare events, the likelihood of simultaneously acquiring two specific mutations is very small. The probability of developing resistance is further reduced by using three drugs with independent mechanisms of action.

The traditional method of chemotherapy for established tuberculosis has been to administer a combination of drugs for 2 years and perhaps longer. Patients so treated rapidly cease to be infectious, but chemotherapy must be continued for long periods to eliminate most of the dormant tubercle bacilli. Frequency of relapse seems inversely proportional to the duration of therapy. Recent clinical studies in Great Britain and the United States have suggested that shorter treatment periods may be employed if three drugs are used continuously for the first 2 months of therapy, followed by an additional 6 to 9 months with two of the drugs. Clin-

ical trials are also being conducted with intermittent therapy in which drugs are administered twice weekly. Intermittent therapy at present seems best suited to patients who do not reliably take their medication without direct medical supervision. For these patients the drugs may be administered by a visiting nurse.

Many drugs are now available for antituberculosis therapy. These agents may be divided into two categories, depending in part on their potency and spectrum of activity and in part on their toxicity. The so-called first-line drugs are isoniazid, rifampin, streptomycin, and ethambutol. The second-line, or reserve, drugs are aminosalicylate (PAS), pyrazinamide, cycloserine, ethionamide, and capreomycin. The properties and proper uses of these drugs are considered in the following sections.

Properties of Individual Agents

Isoniazid

Clinical use. Isoniazid is considered to be the best antituberculosis drug available. Isoniazid, also referred to as *INH*, is the most commonly used first-line drug and the only antituberculosis agent used routinely for prophylaxis.

Mechanism of action. Although isoniazid is known to alter several metabolic processes in mycobacteria, it is not yet known which of these actions is critical for destruction of the microorganism in vivo. Isoniazid is a potent inhibitor of an enzyme involved in cell wall synthesis and also blocks pyridoxine (vitamin B_6) utilization in a number of intracellular enzymes. Isoniazid is bactericidal and affects both intracellular (within macrophages) and extracellular mycobacteria.

Whatever the precise mechanism of action of isoniazid, mycobacteria possess the ability to rap-

Table 35.1   Summary of First-Line Antituberculosis Drugs

Generic name	Trade name	Administration/dosage	Clinical use	Patient populations with increased risk of toxicity
Isoniazid or isonicotinic acid hydrazide (INH)	Isotamine† Laniazid* Nydrazid Rimifon*	ORAL: *Adults*—300 mg daily maximum. *Children*—10 to 20 mg/kg daily.	In multidrug therapy for active tuberculosis. Alone for prophylaxis.	Patients also receiving rifampin have an increased risk of drug-induced hepatitis. Older patients have a higher risk of drug-induced hepatitis. Malnourished patients, alcoholics, and diabetics may suffer vitamin B_6 depletion and are therefore more at risk of peripheral neuropathies. Patients with impaired liver or renal function may be at greater risk of isoniazid toxicity. Fetuses and neonates may be at risk during therapy of the mother. Patients receiving phenytoin for convulsive disorders may require dosage adjustment because isoniazid decreases the metabolism of phenytoin.
	Nydrazid	INTRAMUSCULAR, INTRAVENOUS: As for oral.	As for oral in treatment of acute active tuberculosis.	
Ethambutol	Etibi* Myambutol†	ORAL: *Adults*—15 mg/kg in a single daily dose. *Children under 13 yr should not receive the drug.* ORAL: *Adults*—25 mg/kg in a single daily dose for 2 mo, after which dose may be reduced to 15 mg/kg daily. ORAL: *Adults*—45 to 50 mg/kg twice weekly or 90 mg/kg once weekly.	In multidrug initial therapy of tuberculosis. In multidrug treatment of tuberculosis. In multidrug intermittent therapy of tuberculosis.	Patients with reduced renal function require reduced drug doses. Patients with preexisting visual defects may be difficult to evaluate for drug-induced visual changes. Pregnant women or nursing mothers should be observed to see if ethambutol is harming the fetus or nursing infant.
Rifampin	Rifadin† Rimactane† Rofact*	ORAL: *Adults*—600 mg daily in 1 dose. *Children*—10 to 20 mg/kg up to 600 mg daily.	In multidrug initial therapy or retreatment for pulmonary tuberculosis.	Patients with prior liver disease are more likely to suffer drug-induced hepatotoxicity. Pregnant women or nursing mothers should be observed to see if rifampin is harming the fetus or nursing infant. Patients receiving coumarin anticoagulants, oral hypoglycemic agents, methadone, or digitalis may require adjustment of the dosage of these agents because rifampin induces the liver microsomal enzymes that degrade these drugs. Patients receiving oral contraceptives or replacement doses of cortisol may lose the effectiveness of these agents because rifampin accelerates breakdown of the steroids.

*Available in Canada and United States.
†Available in Canada only.

Table 35.1   Summary of First-Line Antituberculosis Drugs—cont'd

Generic name	Trade name	Administration/dosage	Clinical use	Patient populations with increased risk of toxicity
Streptomycin		INTRAMUSCULAR: *Adults*—1 Gm daily for 2 to 4 mo or longer. After initial therapy dosage may be reduced to 1 Gm 2 or 3 times weekly. *Children and elderly patients*—may require smaller doses.	In multidrug therapy for all forms of tuberculosis.	Patients with renal insufficiency are more prone to accumulate streptomycin and develop ototoxicity. Elderly patients are more sensitive to ototoxic effects of streptomycin. Patients receiving muscle relaxants may suffer excessive action of these drugs because streptomycin is a weak neuromuscular blocking agent.

idly acquire resistance to it. In very early clinical trials when isoniazid was used alone to treat active pulmonary tuberculosis, 11% of the patients carried isoniazid-resistant strains at the end of 1 month of therapy. At the end of the 3 months, 71% of these patients harbored resistant *Mycobacterium*. Observations such as these have led to the clinical practice of combining isoniazid therapy with one or two other drugs. Combined drug therapy successfully suppresses the appearance of resistant organisms in most patients.

Isoniazid is used alone for prophylaxis. The drug is prescribed for persons exposed to tuberculosis or patients who have recently converted from negative to positive reactions in the skin test for tuberculosis. The latter patients usually have smaller numbers of *Mycobacterium* than would be found in an active, symptomatic case of tuberculosis, and for them the use of isoniazid alone is usually successful.

Isoniazid is most effective against *M. tuberculosis*, inhibiting the growth of over 90% of tested strains at a concentration of 0.2 mg/ml. Some evidence suggests that resistant strains of *M. tuberculosis* are less pathogenic than sensitive strains. For this reason isoniazid therapy may be continued even after isoniazid-resistant strains are cultured.

Mycobacterium kansasii, which rarely causes disease in humans, is less sensitive to isoniazid than is *M. tuberculosis*. Other mycobacteria are resistant to the drug.

Absorption, distribution, and excretion. Isoniazid is well absorbed following oral administration, achieving peak serum levels in 1 to 2 hours. The drug enters body tissues relatively efficiently, and bactericidal concentrations are found in most tissues, including pleural fluids and caseous exudates

surrounding active loci of tuberculosis infections in the lung.

Isoniazid undergoes a number of metabolic conversions in the liver, most resulting in inactive drug, which is excreted primarily in the kidney. The major metabolite is an acetylated form of isoniazid. The rate of drug acetylation differs markedly among populations, and two genetically determined types may be distinguished. The so-called *rapid acetylators* inactivate isoniazid two to three times as rapidly as the *slow acetylators*. As would be expected, rapid acetylators have lower blood concentrations of active drug than slow acetylators. Nevertheless, both types of patients respond well to standard therapeutic doses administered once daily. Increasing the drug dose or the frequency of administration in slow acetylators is not wise, since these patients tend to accumulate the acetylated metabolite, which is hepatotoxic.

Slow acetylators comprise 45% to 65% of the Northern European and American white or black populations. Oriental and Eskimo populations contain predominantly rapid acetylators.

Toxicity. Isoniazid is a relatively nontoxic drug. Nevertheless, as with any drug, untoward reactions can occur in a small percentage of treated patients. The most commonly encountered toxic reaction is peripheral neuropathy. Diabetics, alcoholics, and malnourished persons are more prone to this complication than the general population. At least some of these reactions are related to low pyridoxine (vitamin B_6) levels and may be prevented by administration of 5 mg of the vitamin daily. Peripheral neuropathies are more likely to occur in slow acetylators.

Hepatotoxicity is the most serious side effect associated with isoniazid. Fatalities resulting from liver failure have been noted, even among persons receiving the drug prophylactically. Hepatitis caused by isoniazid is rare among patients under 20 years of age, and occurs in patients aged 20 to 34 years at a rate of approximately 3 cases per 1000 patients. After age 50, the incidence increases to 23 cases per 1000 patients. Patients also have an increased risk of hepatitis if they are rapid acetylators of isoniazid, if they ingest ethanol daily, or if they also receive the drug rifampin. Liver function should be monitored in all patients receiving isoniazid and most carefully watched in those patients at high risk. Various other reactions have occasionally been reported with isoniazid, including allergies, blood dyscrasias, gastric distress, and metabolic acidosis.

Ethambutol

Clinical use. Ethambutol is an effective antituberculosis drug that is chemically unrelated to other antituberculosis drugs or antibiotics. It is apparently effective only against mycobacteria and no other bacteria, viruses, or fungi tested. Ethambutol, a first-line drug in conventional antituberculosis therapy, is frequently used as one of the drugs in intermittent therapeutic programs.

Mechanism of action. The precise antibacterial action of ethambutol is unknown. The drug interferes with the formation of several cellular metabolites and cell walls of *Mycobacterium*; death follows in about 24 hours. Nearly all strains of *M. tuberculosis* are sensitive to the drug. Nearly all strains of *M. avium* are resistant. Other mycobacteria have intermediate sensitivity to ethambutol.

Resistance to ethambutol will develop in vivo if the drug is used alone in therapy. Since ethambutol is chemically unrelated to other antituberculosis drugs and presumably has a different mechanism of action, it does not induce cross-resistance to other antituberculosis agents.

Absorption, distribution, and excretion. Ethambutol is administered orally and is well absorbed from the gastrointestinal tract in either the presence or the absence of food. Peak serum concentrations are observed 2 to 4 hours after an oral dose. Ethambutol is less extensively metabolized than isoniazid and up to 50% of the drug excreted in the urine is in the unaltered active form. Up to 15% of the drug in the urine is in the form of a metabolite. Fecal concentrations of the drug represent unabsorbed material.

Ethambutol has been detected in cerebrospinal fluid following oral therapy, although the levels are below those found in plasma. The drug is also known to concentrate in erythrocytes.

Toxicity. Ethambutol has become a first-line antituberculosis drug because of its relatively wide spectrum of activity against *Mycobacterium* species and its relatively low toxicity. These advantages have outweighed the disadvantage that the drug is somewhat less potent than several other antituberculosis agents.

The most commonly reported toxic reaction to normal therapeutic doses of ethambutol is a visual disturbance. Some patients report changes in color vision, whereas others suffer a more prominent loss of visual acuity. These signs are cause to terminate ethambutol use. If the drug is discontinued when these visual signs appear, the changes are reversible, although full recovery may take months.

Other reactions to ethambutol appear rare. Allergic reactions have occasionally been reported. Peripheral neuritis is a rare complication, occurring with higher doses. Some reactions attributed to ethambutol may actually have been caused by other drugs administered concomitantly. Elevated uric acid levels have been reported in patients receiving ethambutol, although evidence linking this action directly to ethambutol is scanty.

Rifampin

Clinical use. Rifampin, originally developed as an antibacterial drug, was observed to be effective against *Chlamydia*, some viruses, and mycobacteria. Rifampin is as potent as isoniazid against mycobacteria and has the broadest spectrum of activity of any antituberculosis agent against species of mycobacteria. These advantages have placed rifampin in the group of first-line antituberculosis agents. The disadvantages of the drug include its expense and its tendency to cause increased toxicity when administered intermittently.

Mechanism of action. Rifampin inhibits DNA-dependent RNA polymerase in sensitive organisms. As a result, gene transcription halts and protein synthesis is prevented. Metabolic activity in the *Mycobacterium* stops, and the cell ultimately dies or is eliminated by host defenses.

Resistance to rifampin can occur when the drug is used alone against *Mycobacterium*. Resistant strains have an altered DNA-dependent RNA polymerase that is no longer inhibited by the drug. Cross-resistance to other antituberculosis drugs does not occur.

Absorption, distribution, and excretion. Rifampin is absorbed orally in adequate amounts in the presence or absence of food. The slightly slower absorption observed in the presence of food is apparently not clinically important.

Rifampin is a relatively lipid-soluble agent.

This property explains why it is found in higher concentrations in body tissues than in serum. Its lipid solubility also explains the ability of this drug to penetrate white blood cells and attack *Mycobacterium* living there.

Roughly 40% of a dose of rifampin is excreted in the bile and a little less in the urine. The drug is also deacetylated by the liver, and the deacetylated metabolite is excreted via the bile into the feces.

Toxicity. Rifampin can cause a variety of mild reactions such as gastrointestinal upset and central nervous system disturbances. The drug also turns body fluids such as tears, sweat, saliva, and urine an orange-red color, which might be mistaken for blood. This coloration is harmless.

Liver abnormalities seem to be the most common reaction observed with rifampin. Mild abnormalities in liver function may return to normal without discontinuing the drug, but increases in alkaline phosphatase or the appearance of jaundice signals that the drug should be discontinued.

High doses given intermittently may cause an immune reaction that is associated with a variety of symptoms. This flulike syndrome may progress from chills, fever, vomiting, diarrhea, and myalgia to acute renal failure. Deaths have occurred. Since these symptoms occur when therapy is resumed, patients should be advised not to miss doses of rifampin, especially if they are receiving relatively high doses. Some treatment centers have significantly lowered rifampin dosage for intermittent therapeutic programs and have reduced these immune reactions (Table 35.1) (see also Appendix A).

Rifampin induces liver enzymes involved in drug and hormone metabolism in humans. This action leads to the drug interactions listed in Table 35.1.

Rifampin also seems to be an immunosuppressant in humans, producing delayed effects on the immune system. The implication of this action on the clinical effectiveness of rifampin is unknown.

Streptomycin

Clinical use. The first of the antituberculosis drugs to be discovered, streptomycin is still a reliable first-line agent. Streptomycin is frequently used as part of a three-drug regimen for initial therapy (Table 35.1). It is usually discontinued after the number of infective organisms has been greatly reduced, usually 2 to 4 months. The patient may continue to receive the remaining two drugs throughout the treatment period. Streptomycin has also been used as part of intermittent treatment programs where the drug is given two or three times a week for the first 2 months of therapy.

Mechanism of action. Streptomycin inhibits protein synthesis in sensitive bacteria (Chapter 33) and mycobacteria. The drug is highly effective against most types of pathogenic mycobacteria with the exception of *M. avium.*

Resistance to streptomycin may develop when the drug is used alone. When streptomycin is used in combination with isoniazid or another first-line agent, development of resistance is minimized.

Absorption, distribution, and excretion. Streptomycin is not absorbed orally and must be administered by intramuscular injection for routine clinical use (Chapter 33). This property restricts its use to the hospital setting or to a well-supervised outpatient program. Because of the difficulties of daily injections, patients are frequently taken off streptomycin after 2 to 4 months of therapy, so long as bacteriological improvement is obvious. Therapy is continued in these cases with other antituberculosis drugs.

Streptomycin is well distributed in the body and may be used to treat tuberculosis meningitis and other forms of nonpulmonary tuberculosis.

The excretion of streptomycin has been discussed in Chapter 33.

Toxicity. Streptomycin has the potential to produce any toxic reaction seen with other aminoglycoside antibiotics (Chapter 33), but ototoxicity is the most commonly encountered reaction in tuberculosis patients. Careful attention to maintaining dosage within safe limits (Table 35.1) will prevent the reaction in most patients. Patients with renal insufficiency, elderly patients, and patients receiving long-term streptomycin therapy are more prone to develop toxic reactions.

Reserve Drugs Used in Tuberculosis Therapy

Aminosalicylate (PAS)

Clinical use. Aminosalicylate (PAS) use has declined with the introduction of ethambutol and rifampin. PAS was in the past included in the standard three-drug regimen for tuberculosis in which streptomycin, isoniazid, and PAS were administered for 3 to 4 months. After active mycobacteria had disappeared from sputum and other fluids, PAS and isoniazid were continued for another 2 years. Currently, treatment protocols are more likely to include ethambutol or rifampin than PAS. PAS is not effective in short-course regimens. PAS is now a second-line or reserve drug.

Mechanism of action. PAS inhibits mycobacterial growth by interfering with folic acid metabolism. The mechanism is probably similar to

Table 35.2   Summary of Second-Line Antituberculosis Drugs

Generic name	Trade name	Administration/dosage	Clinical use	Toxic reactions
Amikacin	Amikin*	INTRAMUSCULAR, INTRAVENOUS: *Adults*—15 mg/kg daily, not to exceed 1.5 Gm daily for 10 days.	Atypical mycobacterial infections.	See Chapter 33.
Aminosalicylate sodium	Nemasol* P.A.S. Teebacin	ORAL: *Adults*—10 to 12 Gm daily in 3 or 4 doses. *Children*—200 to 300 mg/kg daily in 3 or 4 doses.	Drug-resistant tuberculosis.	Patients with active hypertension or other diseases in which sodium overload is undesirable may be unable to tolerate the sodium load with this drug; outside the U.S. calcium salts and the free acid are available.
Capreomycin	Capastat	INTRAMUSCULAR: *Adults*—1 Gm daily in single dose. Not recommended for children.	Retreatment of tuberculosis.	Nephrotoxicity; low blood potassium level; eighth cranial nerve toxicity.
Cycloserine	Seromycin	ORAL: *Adults*—15 mg/kg daily in 2 doses up to maximum daily dose of 1 Gm. Dosage not established for children.	Retreatment of tuberculosis; urinary tract tuberculosis.	Central nervous system toxicity, including psychotic reactions.
Ethionamide	Trecator SC	ORAL: *Adults*—0.5 to 1 Gm daily in 1 to 3 doses. Dosage not established for children.	Any form of tuberculosis when primary drugs are inappropriate; retreatment.	Nausea and vomiting induced by central nervous system effects; liver toxicity.
Pyrazinamide	Pyrazinamide* Tebrazid†	ORAL: *Adults*—20 to 35 mg/kg daily up to 3 Gm. Dosage not established for children.	Retreatment of tuberculosis.	Hepatotoxicity; increased blood concentrations of uric acid (hyperuricemia).

*Available in Canada and United States.
†Available in Canada.

sulfonamide inhibition of bacterial growth. Mycobacteria can develop resistance to PAS, and the drug is never used alone in therapy. *M. tuberculosis* is usually sensitive to PAS, but other types of mycobacteria are generally resistant.

Absorption, distribution, and excretion. PAS is efficiently absorbed by the oral route and is well distributed to most body tissues. It does not enter the cerebrospinal fluid in the absence of inflamed meninges. Excretion is primarily via the kidney, but PAS is also acetylated in the liver and inactivated.

Toxicity. PAS is not well tolerated by most patients. Nearly all patients receiving the drug report gastrointestinal irritation of one form or another. Taking the drug with food or antacids prevents some but not all of the irritation produced by the large amount of drug contained in a normal dose (Table 35.1).

Various allergic symptoms have also been reported with PAS, including exfoliative dermatitis and severe organ damage.

The low patient acceptance of PAS and the availability of better tolerated and more effective agents have combined to restrict the use of PAS.

The major properties of other second-line, or reserve, drugs used to treat tuberculosis are summarized in Table 35.2. The wide use of these drugs is limited by various factors. As a group, the reserve drugs are more toxic than the first-line drugs. Moreover, many of the reserve drugs are not as potent as the more commonly used drugs. Nevertheless, these reserve agents are quite useful when strains of mycobacteria resistant to first-line drugs appear

THE NURSING PROCESS

TREATMENT OF LEPROSY

Assessment

In the United States the diagnosis of leprosy is very unusual. Baseline assessment data should include a thorough total assessment, with special emphasis on subjective and objective deviations from normal.

Nursing diagnoses

Anxiety related to diagnosis and long-term drug therapy

Potential complication: depression related to change in skin color secondary to drug side effect.

Management

Perhaps more than tuberculosis, the diagnosis of leprosy causes a great deal of fear and anxiety in patients. As soon as the diagnosis is made, referral to appropriate agencies for education and support should be offered, and patient and family education should be begun. Appropriate agencies would include the local health department and the Centers for Disease Control in Atlanta, Georgia. The ongoing management of the patient would include regular total patient assessment, with a focus on identifying possible toxic and side effects of the drugs being prescribed. Early in the management phase, instruction should be started about the drugs that will be used and their possible side effects.

Evaluation

Therapy for leprosy, as indicated in the text, is often continued for 5 years or longer. Before discharging the patient for self-management, the nurse should be certain that the patient is able to explain why and how to take the drugs prescribed, side effects that may occur, side effects that require notification of the physician, possible ways to treat more commonly seen side effects, and any additional measures that may be prescribed related to the stage of the disease as it was diagnosed. This disease needs to be reported to the local health department for family follow-up.

DIETARY CONSIDERATION: GLUTEN-FREE DIET

Gluten, which is found in many grains, is restricted in the management of several health problems, including celiac disease (nontropical sprue) and dermatitis herpetiformis. Food items to *avoid* on a gluten-free diet include the following: cereal grains including wheat, barley, oats, rye, bran, graham, millet, wheat germ, bulgur, and malt, and products containing these grains. Products made with gluten-containing grains include prepared meats, thickened stews, breaded vegetables, root beers, pastas, macaroni products, gluten stabilizer, brewer's yeast, flour (when the source is not indicated), pizza.

The following foods are *permitted*: rice, corn, and flours made from soybeans, buckwheat, lima beans, gluten-free wheat starch; cornmeal, hominy.

Encourage patients to read labels carefully.

Refer patients as needed to the dietitian.

or when a patient develops intolerable toxic reactions to these first-line drugs.

TREATMENT OF LEPROSY

Leprosy, like tuberculosis, is currently found primarily in developing countries and rarely encountered in the United States or Canada. Also like tuberculosis, leprosy is a disease that is curable with appropriate drug therapy. Patients are usually treated for at least 4 years and some must be treated for life. Long-term treatment is required because *Mycobacterium leprae,* the causative agent of leprosy, is a very slow-growing organism and may remain dormant for long periods in the human body.

The primary drug used to treat leprosy is a sulfone called *dapsone,* but alternatives are now available. *Clofazimine* seems as effective as dapsone. Moreover, strains of *M. leprae* that acquire resistance to dapsone remain sensitive to clofazimine.

PATIENT CARE IMPLICATIONS

General guidelines for patients with tuberculosis or leprosy

- Provide emotional support for patients and their families when a diagnosis of tuberculosis or leprosy is made. Both diseases may be associated with patient fears and misunderstandings. Teach patients and families about the diseases, their spread, and control, as well as about drug therapy.
- Review anticipated benefits and possible side effects associated with drug therapy.
- Emphasize the importance of long-term therapy for best effect.
- Encourage patients to return as scheduled for follow-up appointments. Blood work must be monitored to rule out side effects.
- Refer patients to the local health department for teaching and follow-up.
- Health care personnel should obtain a routine tuberculosis screening test regularly (annually).
- Keep all health care providers informed of all drugs being taken.

Isoniazid

Drug administration

- Review Patient Care Implications at the end of Chapter 29.
- Assess for peripheral neuropathy: numbness, tingling, paresthesia, and feelings of heaviness of the fingers, arms, and legs.
- Monitor complete blood count and differential, platelet count, liver function tests, blood glucose.
- Intramuscular injection may produce pain at the injection site; warn patients about this.

Patient and family education

- Review the general guidelines, above.
- Instruct patients to report the development of any new sign or symptom.
- Emphasize to patients the importance of taking pyridoxine if prescribed. Review Dietary Consideration: Vitamins (p. 282) for information about dietary sources of pyridoxine.
- Avoid the use of alcohol while taking isoniazid.
- Take oral doses with meals to avoid gastric irritation.
- See Patient Problem: Dry Mouth (p. 170).
- Caution patients to avoid driving or operating hazardous equipment if dizziness, ataxia, tinnitus, or vision changes occur; notify physician.

- Ingestion of food or cheese by patients taking isoniazid may cause a reaction. Symptoms include headache, flushing, nausea, vomiting, and tachycardia, itching skin, or lightheadedness. Tell patients to limit or avoid cheese or fish. Notify physician if these symptoms develop.
- Tell diabetic patients that isoniazid may cause false results in urine glucose tests. Do not change diet or insulin without contacting the physician. Monitor blood glucose levels if possible.
- Do not take aluminum-containing antacids within 1 hour of taking isoniazid.

Ethambutol

Drug administration

- See general guidelines for patients with tuberculosis, and the Patient Care Implications at the end of Chapter 29.
- Assess for visual changes and peripheral neuropathy.
- Monitor complete blood count and differential, uric acid levels.

Patient and family education

- Review general guidelines, above.
- Take oral doses with meals or snack to lessen gastric irritation.
- Report changes in vision to the physician.
- Avoid driving or operating hazardous equipment until the effects of this medication are known; it may cause drowsiness or dizziness.

Rifampin

Drug administration

- See general guidelines for patients with tuberculosis, and the Patient Care Implications at the end of Chapter 29.
- Assess complete blood count and differential, platelet count, liver function tests.

Patient and family education

- Review general guidelines, above.
- If tolerated, take rifampin on an empty stomach, 1 hour before or 2 hours after meals. Take with meals if gastric irritation is severe when taken on an empty stomach.
- Warn patients that body fluids (tears, sweat, feces, and urine) may turn orange-red while on rifampin therapy. Soft contact lenses may become permanently stained.

PATIENT CARE IMPLICATIONS — cont'd

- It is especially important not to miss rifampin doses. Take regularly, as prescribed, for best results.
- Do not take doses of rifampin within 6 hours of doses of aminosalicylates (PAS).
- Avoid driving or operating hazardous equipment if drowsiness, dizziness, or visual changes occur; notify the physician.
- Avoid alcoholic beverages while taking rifampin.
- Contraceptive pills may not be effective in patients who are also taking rifampin. Use another means of birth control while taking rifampin; consult the physician.
- Capsules may be opened and the contents mixed with applesauce or jelly for ease in taking.
- A suspension can also be made; consult the pharmacist.

Streptomycin

Streptomycin was discussed in Chapter 33.

Aminosalicylate

Nursing care, drug administration/patient and family education

- See general guidelines for patients with tuberculosis, above.
- Take oral doses with meals or snack to lessen gastric irritation. Provide positive reinforcement. This drug is difficult to take: a 10 Gm/day dose requires 20 500-mg tablets, divided into 3 or 4 doses.
- Discard discolored tablets and obtain a fresh supply.
- To prevent crystalluria, maintain a fluid intake of 2000 to 2500 ml per day.
- For the powder form of the drug, dissolve contents of the package in a glassful of water and stir well. Drink all of the fluid to obtain the full dose.
- Do not take aminosalicylates within 6 hours of doses of rifampin.
- Do not take aminosalicylate calcium within 1 to 3 hours of the time tetracycline doses are taken.
- If photophobia develops, wear sunglasses and avoid areas of bright lights or sunlight.

- Warn diabetic patients that aminosalicylates may cause false urine glucose results. Do not change diet or insulin without consulting the physician. Monitor blood glucose levels if possible.

Dapsone

Nursing care, drug administration/patient and family education

- See general guidelines for patients with tuberculosis and leprosy.
- Assess for skin changes and peripheral neuropathy.
- Monitor complete blood count and differential, platelet count, BUN, serum creatinine. Monitor urinalysis.
- Take ordered doses with meals or snack to lessen gastric irritation.
- If insomnia occurs, take once-daily doses in the morning.
- Avoid driving or operating hazardous equipment if dizziness or lightheadedness occurs; notify physician.
- Patients with dermatitis herpetiformis may be placed on a gluten-free diet. See Dietary Consideration: Gluten-free Diet.

Clofazimine

Nursing care, drug administration/patient and family education

- Take oral doses with meals or snack to lessen gastric irritation.
- Warn patients that this drug may cause red to brown pigmentation of the skin and eyes. Assess for discoloration. If the skin changes produce depression or extreme sadness, notify physician.
- See Patient Problem: Photosensitivity on p. 647.
- Clofazimine may discolor feces, sputum, sweat, tears, and urine. It may also produce black, tarry or bloody stools; notify physician if this occurs.
- Use a lotion or skin cream to treat dry, scaly skin.
- Avoid driving or operating hazardous equipment if drowsiness or dizziness occurs; notify physician.

Table 35.3   Summary of Drugs Used to Treat Leprosy

Generic name	Trade name	Administration/dosage	Toxicity	Comments
Dapsone	Avlosulfon Dapsone*	ORAL: *Adults*—100 mg daily for 4 yr to life, with rifampin for first 6 to 36 months. *Children*—1.4 mg/kg daily.	Mild, rare gastrointestinal disturbance. Serum sickness reactions are possible.	Patients with glucose 6-phosphate dehydrogenase deficiency are more prone to hemolytic reactions and must receive reduced doses.
Clofazimine	Lamprene	ORAL: *Adults*—50 to 100 mg daily for 4 yr to life, with rifampin for first 6 to 36 months.	Gastrointestinal distress. FDA Pregnancy Category C.	Primary use is for dapsone-resistant leprosy. Red drug imparts a dark red color to skin and other body tissues. This coloration is harmless.
Rifampin	Rifadin* Rimactane* Rofact†	ORAL: *Adults*—600 mg daily for 6 to 36 months, with dapsone or clofazimine.	Liver toxicity; abdominal distress.	Not yet approved for this use in the United States.

*Available in Canada and United States.
†Available in Canada.

The antituberculosis drugs rifampin and more rarely ethionamide have also been used to treat leprosy.

Resistance to dapsone is appearing more frequently today than in years past. Therefore, combination therapy has become the accepted policy in the United States because combining of drugs lessens the likelihood that resistance will occur and increases the likelihood that all mycobacteria will be eradicated and a permanent cure will be achieved. Rifampin is combined with either dapsone or clofazimine for the first 6 months to 3 years, after which dapsone or clofazimine alone may be continued for as long as is necessary (Table 35.3).

The properties of drugs used to treat leprosy are summarized in Table 35.3.

SUMMARY

Tuberculosis is caused by four strains of *Mycobacterium*. Mycobacteria are slow-growing strict aerobes that resist the digestive action of macrophages. These properties of the organism make tuberculosis more difficult to treat than many other bacterial infections. The disease is contagious only during active phases. Long dormant periods are common. Mycobacteria can develop resistance to antituberculosis drugs, causing therapeutic failures. To minimize this complication, multiple drug therapy is the rule.

Isoniazid may be used in combination with other drugs to treat tuberculosis or alone for prophylaxis in patients who have been exposed to the disease. The drug inhibits cell wall biosynthesis and utilization of pyridoxine in mycobacteria. Isoniazid is well absorbed orally and is actively metabolized by the liver. Rapid acetylators and slow acetylators exist in most normal populations. Isoniazid is associated most prominently with hepatotoxicity, especially in older patients.

Ethambutol is an effective first-line drug; it is as well absorbed as isoniazid but less extensively metabolized. Ethambutol may cause visual disturbances, which are reversible if therapy is stopped when this reaction appears.

Rifampin inhibits DNA-dependent RNA polymerase in several stains of mycobacteria. This oral agent is relatively lipid soluble and may concentrate in body tissues. The drug is eliminated via the bile. Rifampin may produce a flulike syndrome leading to life-threatening complications, especially if the drug is used intermittently.

Streptomycin inhibits protein synthesis in mycobacteria as well as in other types of bacteria. The drug is administered only by the intramuscular route and is therefore most frequently used in initial therapy as part of a two- or three-drug treatment program.

Aminosalicylate (PAS) inhibits folic acid metabolism in *Mycobacterium*. It is absorbed by the oral route and excreted by the kidney. PAS produces significant gastrointestinal toxicity in most patients. Other toxicity is related to allergic reactions to the drug and electrolyte imbalances produced by the high ion content of the PAS preparations.

Capreomycin, cycloserine, ethionamide, and pyrizinamide are considered second-line drugs for tuberculosis primarily because of lower activity and higher toxicity of these agents.

Leprosy, a disease that develops very slowly and is produced by a strain of *Mycobacterium leprae*, is effectively treated with dapsone or clofazimine in combination with rifampin. Therapy usually continues for several years to ensure that the disease will be cured.

STUDY QUESTIONS

1. What organisms cause tuberculosis?
2. What properties of mycobacteria make control of tuberculosis more difficult than that of many other bacterial diseases?
3. Where is the initial site of tuberculosis infection?
4. During what phase of tuberculosis is the disease contagious?
5. Why is tuberculosis usually treated by multiple drug therapy?
6. What is the duration of therapy for tuberculosis?
7. What is the mechanism of action of isoniazid?
8. What is the outcome of using isoniazid alone to treat active tuberculosis?
9. When may isoniazid be used alone in therapy of tuberculosis?
10. How is isoniazid administered in tuberculosis therapy?
11. What is the fate of isoniazid in the body?
12. What toxicity is associated with isoniazid?
13. What is the mechanism of action of ethambutol?
14. How is ethambutol administered in tuberculosis therapy?
15. What toxicity is associated with ethambutol?
16. What is the mechanism of action of rifampin?
17. How is rifampin administered in tuberculosis therapy?
18. How may the timing of rifampin therapy influence the toxicity the drug produces?
19. What is the mechanism of action of streptomycin?
20. How is streptomycin administered?
21. What toxicity is associated with the use of streptomycin?
22. What is the mechanism of action of PAS?
23. How is PAS administered in tuberculosis therapy?
24. What toxicity is associated with the use of PAS?
25. Why are certain drugs classed as second-line drugs in tuberculosis therapy?
26. What drugs are most useful in treating leprosy?
27. How long must therapy continue for control of leprosy?

SUGGESTED READINGS

Cornell, C.: TB in hospital employees, Am. J. Nurs. **88**(4):484, 1988.

Gangadharam, P.R.J.: Antimycobacterial drugs, Antimicrobial Agents Annual **3**:15, 1989.

Hastings, R.C., and Franzblau, S.G.: Chemotherapy of leprosy, Ann. Rev. Pharm. Tox. **28**:231, 1988.

Jacobson, R.R.: Antibiotic therapy for leprosy, Antimicrobial Agents Annual **3**:41, 1989.

Lancaster, E.: TB on the rise, Am. J. Nurs. **88**(4):484, 1988.

Todd, B.: Treating tuberculosis, Geriatr. Nurs. **9**(4):250, 1988.

Van Scoy, R.E., and Wilkowske, C.J.: Antituberculous agents, Mayo Clin. Proc. **62**(12):1129, 1987.

Antifungal Agents

36

Fungal diseases range from mild infections in localized areas of the skin to grave systemic infections. Diseases of various types may be produced by a wide range of fungi, and to a great extent the seriousness of the infection is determined by the nature of the infective organism and the immune status of the host. In this chapter some of the more common and the more serious fungal diseases are examined and the drugs that are used to control these specific infections are considered.

SELECTIVE TOXICITY IN THE TREATMENT OF FUNGAL DISEASES

Although the fungi that cause disease in humans are single-celled organisms, they are eucaryotes (Chapter 29) and therefore resemble humans more than bacteria in their biochemical properties. These biochemical similarities to humans present therapeutic problems. For instance, none of the antibiotics that inhibit bacterial protein synthesis affect that process in fungi. The ribosomes that form protein in fungi are very much like those in humans and are sensitive to the same drugs. Therefore selective toxicity cannot be achieved by this mechanism. Likewise, fungi resist the action of sulfonamides as do mammalian cells. Moreover fungal cells do not contain a peptidoglycan cell wall, which renders them resistant to all antibiotics that block peptidoglycan synthesis (e.g., penicillins). For these reasons the antimicrobial agents considered in previous chapters are useless in treating fungal disease.

Design of new antifungal agents is limited by the number of known biochemical differences between fungal and mammalian cells. A few individual enzymes seem to possess different drug sensitivities in humans and fungi. However, the only systematically exploited difference between humans and fungi lies in the outer membranes of the two cell types. The cells of humans contain cholesterol in their membranes, whereas those of fungi contain ergosterol. This feature of membrane structure is the basis of action of the polyene antifungal drugs. Polyene antifungal agents have a greater affinity for ergosterol than for cholesterol and therefore somewhat selectively react with ergosterol from fungal cell membranes. This action destroys the integrity of the cell membrane, cytoplasmic components are lost, and the cell dies. However, the selectivity of these drugs is not so great as that of most drugs used for treating bacterial infections. Imidazole antifungal agents inhibit the synthesis of ergosterol. This action also impairs the function of the fungal cell membrane.

Fungal cells do possess many cell surface antigens, which ultimately provoke host immune responses. Most fungal infections resolve in this way, many times without the host ever being aware of an active disease. This pattern is especially common with the fungal diseases spread by breathing in spores from contaminated soil. Examples of diseases of this type are histoplasmosis, blastomycosis, coccidioidomycosis, cryptococcosis, and aspergillosis. Several of these diseases are concentrated in specific geographic areas. For example, coccidioidomycosis is most common, or endemic, in the southernmost portions of California, Nevada, Utah, Arizona, New Mexico, and Texas, whereas histoplasmosis is most common in the states bordering the Mississippi and Ohio rivers. Blastomycosis is common in isolated areas along the Mississippi and Ohio Rivers, around the Great Lakes, the St. Lawrence River, and in the Carolinas.

Some fungal diseases are spread by contact with soil contaminated with bird droppings. Birds are not necessarily affected by these diseases, but they do frequently carry the organisms. Cryptococcosis frequently follows exposure to high concentrations

Table 36.1   Summary of Drugs Used to Treat Systemic Fungal Infections

Generic name	Trade name	Administration/dosage	Clinical use	Principal toxic reactions
Amphotericin B	Fungizone*	INTRAVENOUS: *Adults and children*—0.25 to 1 mg/kg per day infused at 0.1 mg/ml in 5% dextrose over 6 hr. Total drug course usually less than 4 Gm.	Disseminated, symptomatic fungal disease due to *Histoplasma, Blastomyces, Coccidioides, Cryptococcus, Aspergillus, Candida,* and others.	Initial headache, nausea, vomiting, and fever. Progressive nephrotoxicity, anemia, and renal electrolyte imbalance.
Flucytosine	Ancobon Ancotil†	ORAL: *Adults and children*—50 to 150 mg/kg daily in 4 doses. Lower drug doses are required when renal function is impaired.	Disseminated fungal infections due to sensitive *Candida* strains; cryptococcal meningitis and other infections; usually combined with amphotericin B.	Nausea and diarrhea are relatively common. Blood dyscrasias are also possible. Rare instances of fatal bowel perforation.
Itraconazole	—	ORAL: *Adult*—200 mg daily. Investigational agent.	Dermatophytoses, vaginal candida, histoplasmosis, coccidioidomycosis, and cryptococcosis.	Minor alterations in liver enzymes.
Ketoconazole	Nizoral*	ORAL: *Adults*—200 to 400 mg daily in a single dose. Higher doses have been suggested to improve response. *Children under 20 kg*—50 mg once daily. *Children 20 to 40 kg*—100 mg once daily. *Children over 40 kg*—200 mg once daily.	Disseminated infections caused by *Histoplasma, Paracoccidioides,* and *Candida.*	Nausea, pruritus, headache, and gastrointestinal disturbances. Gynecomastia occurs in about 10% of treated males. Rare fatal hepatic necrosis. FDA Pregnancy Category C.
Miconazole nitrate	Monistat-IV*	INTRAVENOUS: *Adults*—highly variable, depending upon the causative organism. Daily doses as low as 200 mg or as high as 3.6 Gm, divided into 3 equal doses, may be indicated. *Children*—total daily dose 20 to 40 mg/kg with no single infusion exceeding 15 mg/kg.	Systemic infections caused by *Candida, Cryptococcus,* and *Aspergillus.* Also used topically (see Table 36.2).	Thrombophlebitis, gastrointestinal distress, blood dyscrasias, and allergic reactions have been reported with intravenous use.

*Available in Canada and United States.
†Available in Canada only.

of pigeon droppings. Histoplasmosis is associated with avian excreta such as chicken or starling droppings or bat guano.

Although pulmonary forms of the aforementioned diseases are usually mild and limited by effective development of immunity in the victim, in rare cases the fungus may become disseminated and invade other body tissues. A notorious example is the yeast *Cryptococcus neoformans*, which can cause meningitis as well as pulmonary disease and infections at many other sites. The disseminated, or systemic, fungal diseases are most likely to develop in patients whose immune system is de-

pressed by disease or drug therapy, especially with glucocorticoids or immunosuppressant antineoplastic agents.

The yeast *Candida* may cause a range of infections from serious systemic disease to annoying mucous membrane infections. Since *Candida* is normally found on the skin and mucous membranes of healthy persons, the growth of *Candida* to cause disease usually represents an opportunistic infection. *Candida* infections are therefore most common in persons receiving broad-spectrum antibacterial drugs such as tetracyclines (superinfections, Chapter 29) or in persons with suppressed

Text continued on p. 540.

THE NURSING PROCESS

FUNGAL INFECTIONS

Assessment

Fungal infections are relatively common and can occur in patients of any age. Examples include thrush in the infant, athlete's foot, and vaginal monilial infections in the female. Serious systemic infections are possible with a variety of fungi and, although relatively uncommon, are life-threatening. Initially the patient should receive a thorough total assessment, with a focus on the specific subjective complaints or objective signs that indicate possible fungal infection. Parts of the history that may be important include recent exposure to possible new sources of infection, previous recent use of drugs that may alter the patient's immune response, and measures the patient has tried to this point for eradication of the problem. Obviously the depth of assessment will vary according to the nature of the problem as the patient presents it; the patient with a systemic infection could be obviously seriously ill and would need a different kind of assessment than an infant with the relatively common problem of oral thrush. Early diagnosis is enhanced through a high degree of awareness. Patients most likely to have fungal infections include those receiving cancer chemotherapy, immunotherapy, antibiotic therapy, or drugs that alter the normal pH of such areas as the vagina; those receiving nutritional support via peripheral or central venous catheters; and those taking high doses of adrenocortical steroids.

Nursing diagnoses

Potential altered comfort: nausea and vomiting as a side effect of drug therapy

Potential complication: renal damage and failure

Management

The management phase is often two-pronged. One aspect of the management phase is treatment with an appropriate drug for the fungal infection itself. The second aspect of care is removal of possible causative agents, including discontinuing drugs that may predispose the patient to fungal infections. For example, the adolescent female taking tetracycline for control of acne may need to have this drug discontinued at least temporarily to successfully treat vaginal monilial infections. During the management phase the nurse needs to teach the patient about the drugs prescribed, about the infection itself, and about possible ways to limit the spread of the infection and to prevent its recurrence. Treatment of systemic fungal infections is more serious. Patients with such infections often require long-term hospitalization with regular intravenous antifungal drug therapy. The nurse should monitor the vital signs and appropriate laboratory work to evaluate possible side effects. It may be appropriate, depending on the patient's response, to measure the fluid intake and output; to use additional drugs to control side effects such as headache, nausea, and vomiting; and to adjust meals and other patient activities to times in the day when the patient is better able to tolerate them. The use of an infusion monitoring device may be appropriate.

Evaluation

Therapy with antifungal agents should eradicate the infection. With the exception of the systemically used drugs, side effects are relatively uncommon. Before a patient is discharged for self-management with an antifungal agent, that patient should be able to explain why the drug is being used, exactly how it should be used and under what circumstances, what to do if side effects should occur, and which side effects require notification of the physician. The patient should be able to explain any other measures suggested to provide relief of symptoms or treatment of the infection and what to do if symptoms do not begin to clear within 3 to 7 days. For further information, see the patient care implications section at the end of this chapter.

Table 36.2   Summary of Drugs Used to Treat Topical Fungal Infections

Generic name	Trade name	Administration/dosage	Clinical use	Principal side effects	Comments
Amphotericin B	Fungizone	TOPICAL: *Adults and children*—3% cream, lotion, or ointment applied two to four times daily.	Rx—*Candida* infections of skin or mucous membranes.	Local tissue irritation.	Ciclopirox, clotrimazole, econazole or miconazole are preferred.
Benzoic and salicylic acids	Whitfield's ointment	TOPICAL: *Adults and children*—6% benzoic and 3% salicylic acids, or double strength, applied two or three times daily.	OTC—Ringworm.	Local tissue irritation.	Ointment is also keratolytic.
Butoconazole	Femstat	INTRAVAGINAL: *Adults*—2% cream applied once daily for 3 days. FDA Pregnancy Category C.	Rx—Vaginal infections caused by *Candida*.	Vaginal burning is possible.	Has been used by pregnant women.
Calcium undecylenate	Caldesene Cruex	TOPICAL: *Adults and children*—10% powder applied as needed.	OTC—Tinea cruris (jock itch); also used for diaper rash or other skin irritations of groin area.	Powder should not be inhaled or allowed to contact eyes or mucous membranes.	Diabetics and others with impaired circulation should use only with physician's advice.
Carbol-fuchsin (Castellani paint)	Castel Plus	TOPICAL: *Adults and children*—Solution swabbed over affected area one or two times daily.	Rx—Tinea pedis (athlete's foot) and ringworm.	Contact sensitivity may cause reactions.	Carbol-fuchsin is poisonous if ingested.
Ciclopirox olamine	Loprox	TOPICAL: *Adults*—1% cream applied twice daily. FDA Pregnancy Category B.	Rx—Tinea infections including tinea versicolor; cutaneous candidiasis.	Redness, itching, burning, and stinging of skin.	Avoid contact with eyes; do not use occlusive dressing.
Clioquinol (iodochlorhydroxyquin)	Iodo Torofor Vioform	TOPICAL: *Adults and children*—3% cream, ointment or powder applied several times daily.	Rx—Localized dermatophytoses.	Irritation of skin usually mild, but eyes must be avoided.	Can cause a false-positive result in the ferric chloride test for phenylketonuria (PKU).
Clotrimazole	Canesten† Lotrimin Mycelex	TOPICAL: *Adults and children*—1% cream, lotion, or solution applied twice daily. FDA Pregnancy Category B.	Rx—Tinea and cutaneous *Candida*.	Skin irritation, pruritus, urticaria; general irritation may be severe enough to cause drug to be discontinued.	Do not use around eyes.
	Canesten† Gyne-Lotrimin Myclo†	INTRAVAGINAL: *Adults*—tablets or creams containing 100 mg inserted once daily. FDA Pregnancy Category B.	Rx—Vulvovaginal candidiasis.		

†Available in Canada.

Continued.

Table 36.2   Summary of Drugs Used to Treat Topical Fungal Infections—cont'd

Generic name	Trade name	Administration/dosage	Clinical use	Principal side effects	Comments
Clotrimazole—cont'd	Mycelox	ORAL: *Adults and children over 4*—10 mg lozenge dissolved in mouth five times daily. FDA Pregnancy Category C.	Rx—Candidiasis, oropharyngeal.		
Econazole	Ecostatin† Prevaryl† Spectazole	TOPICAL: *Adults and children*—1% cream applied to skin 1 or 2 times daily. FDA Pregnancy Category C.	Rx—*Candida*, mucocutaneous; tinea.	Skin irritation.	Do not use around eyes.
	Ecostatin*	VAGINAL: *Adults*—single 150 mg suppository once daily for 3 days.	Rx—*Candida*, vulvovaginal.	Vaginal irritation.	
Gentian violet	—	TOPICAL: *Adults and children*—0.5%, 1% or 2% solution two or three times daily for 3 days.	Rx—*Candida* infections of skin or vagina.	Irritation of vagina can be damaging.	This dye will stain skin and clothing.
	Genapax	INTRAVAGINAL: *Adults*—One tampon (Genapax) inserted once or twice daily for 12 days. FDA Pregnancy Category C.			
Griseofulvin	Fulvicin* Grifulvin Grisactin Gris-PEG	ORAL: *Adults*—500 mg microcrystalline form in single or divided dose. *Children*—5 to 10 mg/kg daily.	Rx—Tinea infections with exception of tinea versicolor. Not for *Candida*.	Blood dyscrasias occur rarely. Headache occurs early in treatment. Gastrointestinal disturbances, neuritis, allergies, and hepatotoxicity may occur.	Warfarin anticoagulant activity blocked. Barbiturates decrease griseofulvin activity. Avoid during pregnancy.
Haloprogin	Halotex	TOPICAL: *Adults and children*—1% cream or solution applied twice daily. FDA Pregnancy Category B.	Rx—Tinea and other superficial fungal infections.	Local tissue irritation or maceration.	Do not use around eyes.
Ketoconazole	Nizoral	TOPICAL: *Adults and children*—2% cream applied once daily. FDA Pregnancy Category C.	Rx—Tinea and other superficial fungal infections.	Irritation is rare.	See drug listing.
Miconazole nitrate	Micatin Monistat-Derm	TOPICAL: *Adults and children*—2% cream, lotion, or aerosol applied twice daily.	Rx—Dermatophytoses or *Candida* infections.	Local tissue irritation or maceration.	Do not use around eyes.
	Monistat	INTRAVAGINAL: *Adults*—2% cream, tampon, or suppositories once daily.			

*Available in United States and Canada.
†Available in Canada.

Table 36.2   **Summary of Drugs Used to Treat Topical Fungal Infections—cont'd**

Generic name	Trade name	Administration/dosage	Clinical use	Principal side effects	Comments
Naftifine	Naftin	TOPICAL: *Adults and children*—1% cream, applied to skin twice daily.	Rx—Tinea.	Local irritation.	New drug.
Natamycin	Natacyn	OPHTHALMIC: *Adults and children*—5% ophthalmic suspension 1 drop every 2 to 6 hours.	Rx—Fungal blepharitis, conjunctivitis, or keratitis.	Eye irritation.	New drug chemically related to amphotericin.
Nystatin	Mycostatin Nadostine† Nilstat Nystex	ORAL: *Adults and children*—0.5 to 1 million units three times daily. *Infants*—0.1 to 0.2 million units four times daily.	Rx—oropharyngeal *Candida* infections.	Nausea, vomiting, or diarrhea.	Drug is not absorbed from intestinal tract.
		TOPICAL: *Adults and children*—ointments, creams, lotions (0.1 million units/g) applied twice daily.	Rx—*Candida* infections of skin.	Irritation of skin.	—
		INTRAVAGINAL: *Adults*—tablets, 0.1 to 0.2 million units daily.	Rx—*Candida* infections of vagina.	Irritation is rare.	Relief of symptoms is rapid, but dosage should be continued for 2 weeks or longer if necessary.
Sodium thiosulfate	—	TOPICAL: *Adults and children*—25% lotion or solution applied twice daily for weeks.	OTC—Tinea versicolor.	Irritation is possible.	Avoid the eyes.
Terconazole	Terazol	VAGINAL: *Adults*—5 Gm 0.4% cream or 80 mg suppository once daily. FDA Pregnancy Category C.	Rx—Candida vulvovaginal.	Vaginal burning.	New drug.
Tolnaftate	Aftate Tinactin	TOPICAL: *Adults and children*—1% cream, gel, solution, powder, or aerosol applied twice daily.	OTC—Tinea infections only; not effective against *Candida*.	Rarely causes irritation or sensitization.	Avoid eyes; 2 to 3 weeks of therapy is usually sufficient.
Undecylenic acid	Desenex Ting Undecylenic compound Unde-Jen	TOPICAL: *Adults and children*—ointment (5%, with 20% zinc undecylenate), powder (2%, with 20% zinc undecylenate), 10% solution, 2% soap applied twice daily.	OTC—Tinea pedis and ringworm in areas other than around nails or hairy areas.	Should not be allowed to contact eyes or mucous membranes.	Diabetics and others with impaired circulation should use only with physician's advice.

†Available in Canada.

PATIENT PROBLEM: VAGINAL INFECTION

THE PROBLEM

The dark, moist environment of the vagina is prone to infection by a variety of organisms. Some chronic health problems, such as diabetes mellitus, increase susceptibility to vaginal infection. Treatment with some groups of drugs, such as antibiotics, may increase susceptibility to fungal superinfection. Finally, some invading organisms are passed as venereal diseases. Treatment of vaginal infection may be messy and difficult. It is difficult to reach all mucosal surfaces, and, since the woman is upright during most of the day, medications drain out due to gravity.

THE SOLUTION

- Use prescribed agents for the full course of therapy; do not stop just when symptoms disappear.
- Do not wear tampons during therapy. Wear sanitary napkins to prevent staining of clothing.
- Continue therapy through the menstrual period.
- Wash hands carefully before and after using prescribed medications.
- Use once-daily doses of vaginal medication in the evening, before retiring. Insert vaginal suppository, ointment, or cream just before going to sleep, to allow the medication to remain in the vaginal area as long as possible.
- If douching is prescribed, wash douche equipment carefully after each use, and dry it.
- Depending on the infecting agent, it may be necessary to treat the sexual partner also; consult physician.
- Usually, avoid sexual intercourse during the course of therapy. If not possible, the sexual partner should wear a condom.

TO HELP PREVENT VAGINAL INFECTION

- Wear clean underwear daily, preferably of cotton material. Synthetic fabrics do not allow air to circulate as well, so keep the vaginal area more moist than normal. Avoid pantyhose for the same reason.
- Wipe from front to back following voiding or defecation.
- Do not douche unless prescribed by the physician. Do not douche between doses of vaginal medications.
- Avoid bubble baths and soaps that may irritate vaginal mucosa. Wash the vaginal area gently, and rinse soap off well. Some women may need to wash with water only, if soap is irritating to the vaginal area.
- Use water-soluble lubricants, if needed, in the vagina. Do not use oil-based products such as petroleum jelly.

---

immune systems. *Candida* infections are very common in AIDS patients.

Fungi whose growth is almost always restricted to the skin of humans are termed *dermatophytes.* These fungi cause the annoying infections commonly known as *ringworm* and *athlete's foot,* as well as several others. This group of infections is frequently referred to as *tinea.* Drugs used for these superficial infections are not the same as those employed for systemic fungal infections. Many of the drugs used topically are not absorbed extensively through the skin. Therefore much more toxic agents may be employed and selective toxicity is achieved against many dermatophytes.

DRUGS TO TREAT SYSTEMIC FUNGAL INFECTIONS

Amphotericin B

Mechanism of action. Amphotericin B is a polyene antifungal drug whose action depends on selectively damaging membranes containing ergosterol, that is, fungal membranes. Unfortunately, this membrane-disruptive effect is not entirely selective, and some of the cholesterol-containing membranes of mammalian cells are also damaged. Nevertheless, amphotericin B can be clinically useful in treating a broad spectrum of fungal diseases, including those caused by *Histoplasma, Blastomyces, Cryptococcus, Aspergillus,* and others. Amphotericin B may also be used to treat systemic *Candida* and *Coccidioides* infections.

Absorption, distribution, and excretion. Amphotericin B is not absorbed orally and must be administered intravenously, although the drug is irritating to vascular tissue and frequently causes phlebitis. The drug, which is lipid soluble, is administered as a colloidal suspension stabilized with small amounts of the detergent desoxycholate. Amphotericin B must be infused at a concentration of less than 0.1 mg/ml in a 5% dextrose solution. Higher drug concentrations will cause the precipitation of the drug in the intravenous solution and will endanger the patient.

Since amphotericin B has a high affinity for lipid, the drug tends to bind to tissues rather than remain in the bloodstream. The elimination half-life of the drug is about 12 hours following a single intravenous dose. During long-term therapy only a fraction of the daily dose can be recovered in the urine or feces. The unrecovered drug is apparently held in tissues, since amphotericin B continues to appear in the urine for long periods after therapy is halted. The tissue-binding properties and the relative water insolubility of amphotericin B prevent the drug from entering body fluids efficiently. For this reason concentrations of the drug in the cerebrospinal fluid or in ocular fluid are rather low and may not be high enough to effectively eliminate infections at those sites. To overcome this problem, amphotericin B may be injected intrathecally (into the cerebrospinal fluid) in meningitis.

Toxicity. Most patients are begun on low doses of the drug, and the dosage is increased as tolerance to the ensuing toxic reactions develops. Headache, fever, nausea, and vomiting may occur after the first few injections, but these side effects usually subside as therapy continues. Renal damage progresses with length of therapy and may become irreversible when total doses of amphotericin B approach 4 Gm. Anemia also develops with time, as do a number of electrolyte disturbances including acidosis and hypokalemia (low blood potassium).

Amphotericin B therapy must be continued for long periods to create the possibility of a cure for disseminated fungal disease. No firm guidelines for therapy exist, although as a general rule physicians try to limit the total drug dose to under 4 Gm. Even with doses approaching this limit, cures are not always obtained. For many patients therapy must be discontinued early because of toxic effects of the drug.

Amphotericin B has been experimentally administered encapsulated in liposomes (lipid vesicles). Patients whose therapy was ineffective with the standard preparation responded to the liposomal form of the drug. This experimental method of administration may also reduce the drug's toxicity. Development of this interesting technique is continuing.

Flucytosine

Mechanism of action. Flucytosine is a pyrimidine analog that is apparently converted to the cytotoxic agent 5-fluorouracil in sensitive fungi. Since this metabolite is not freely formed in humans, a degree of selective toxicity is achieved. Unfortunately, a relatively narrow range of fungi are sensitive to the drug, including *Cryptococcus, Candida,* and a few other very rarely encountered pathogenic fungi. Intrinsic resistance to flucytosine may exist in a significant number of clinically encountered *Candida* strains, and resistance to the drug may be acquired by *Cryptococcus* during ther-

apy. This pattern of resistance has limited the drug's usefulness.

Absorption, distribution, and excretion. Flucytosine is a water-soluble drug that is well absorbed from the gastrointestinal tract and well distributed into body fluids. Drug concentration in cerebrospinal fluid may be 50% to 70% of serum levels, in contrast to amphotericin B for which cerebrospinal fluid levels are less than 5% of serum levels. The primary organ of excretion for flucytosine is the kidney; more than 90% of an oral dose can be recovered intact in the urine. Urine concentrations of the drug tend to be high. The elimination half-time is about 6 hours.

Toxicity. Flucytosine therapy is usually continued for several weeks to several months. Unlike the situation with amphotericin B, few patients are forced to discontinue medication because of toxic reactions. Nausea and diarrhea appear in roughly one fourth of the patients. Blood dyscrasias and transient liver abnormalities have been reported. Since flucytosine is now frequently administered with amphotericin B, it may be difficult to distinguish which toxic reactions are caused by flucytosine.

The rationale for combining flucytosine and amphotericin B therapy for serious infections caused by fungi is twofold. First, the combination allows the dose of amphotericin B to be lowered somewhat, thereby reducing toxicity. Second, the development of resistance to flucytosine is minimized by combination chemotherapy.

Imidazole antifungals: Itraconazole, Ketoconazole, and Miconazole

Mechanism of action. Imidazole antifungals inhibit synthesis of ergosterol. As a result, the function of the fungal cell membrane is impaired. Development of invasive hyphae by fungal cells may be retarded, enhancing the ability of the host immune system to eliminate the fungi.

Imidazole antifungal agents are used to treat superficial fungal infections such as dermatophytoses, keratomycosis, and vaginal *Candida.* Ketoconazole is used against *Histoplasma* and *Paracoccidioides.* The drug may also be effective in certain patients with disseminated candidiasis, blastomycosis, coccidioidomycosis, and cryptococcosis. Itraconazole has been tested against many of these same infections and others. Miconazole may be used against systemic coccidioidomycosis, cryptococcosis, and candidiasis, but is primarily used as a topical agent (Table 36.1).

Absorption, distribution, and excretion. Ketoconazole is adequately absorbed orally, but bio-

PATIENT CARE IMPLICATIONS

Amphotericin B

Drug administration

- Side effects with topical preparations are uncommon. The cream form may stain skin. Fabric discoloration from lotion or cream can be removed with soap and water. Discoloration from ointment can be removed with cleaning fluid. The remaining comments about amphotericin B focus primarily on parenteral administration.
- Assess for side effects: nausea, vomiting, chills, phlebitis, headache, anemia, electrolyte imbalances.
- Monitor temperature, vital signs, intake, output, weight.
- Monitor complete blood count and differential, platelet count, serum creatinine, BUN, serum electrolytes.
- Use an infusion monitoring device to assist in regulating the rate. Too rapid infusion may be associated with cardiac toxicity.
- To prevent side effects, corticosteroids may be administered prior to or during therapy, or may be added to the infusion. Monitor blood glucose levels.
- Antiemetics may be prescribed 30 minutes before starting the infusion to help prevent nausea and vomiting.
- Acetaminophen may be administered before or during infusion to treat fever and/or headache. Codeine or other analgesics may also be used to treat headache.
- Other drugs may be administered to prevent or treat side effects. Heparin may be added to infusions to help prevent thrombophlebitis; IV meperidine may be used to treat rigors (shaking chill); diphenhydramine may be administered to prevent chills.
- There is disagreement about the need to cover the tubing and fluid reservoir containing amphotericin B. Follow agency custom; most agencies still cover the bag with a plastic or paper bag.
- Keep side rails up and call bell within easy reach. Do not leave patient unattended for long periods.
- Use of IV filters is controversial. If an IV filter is used, it must be at least 1.0 micron in diameter.
- Prepare IV doses as directed in the package insert. Dissolve doses in sterile water with no bacteriostatic agent. Further dilute to desired volume in 5% dextrose in water; no other diluent may be used. Do not administer other IV medications via the amphotericin B line without flushing well before and after the dose with 5% dextrose in water. If other IV medications are to be administered during amphotericin B infusion, start and maintain a separate IV access line.
- The diluted drug is a suspension. Gently agitate the bag or bottle regularly during the infusion to promote uniform dilution.

Patient and family education

- Review anticipated benefits and possible side effects of drug therapy. Patients may need not only teaching, but continued emotional support, as IV therapy is continued for weeks to months. Some patients are suitable candidates for home therapy. Assess patient and consult physician.
- Instruct the patient to report the development of any new sign or symptom.
- Refer home therapy patients to a community-based nursing care agency.
- Monitor serum electrolytes and hematocrit and hemoglobin. Provide instruction on dietary sources of sodium, potassium, and iron as indicated.
- Warn patients to avoid driving or operating hazardous equipment if visual changes occur; notify physician.
- Remind patients to keep all health care providers informed of all drugs being used.

Flucytosine

Drug administration

- Inspect patient for bruising, bleeding, or other signs and symptoms of blood dyscrasias. Assess for development of gastrointestinal side effects. Monitor weight.
- Monitor BUN, serum creatinine, complete blood count and differential, platelet count, and liver function tests.
- Check stools for blood/guaiac regularly.

Patient and family education

- Review anticipated benefits and possible side effects of drug therapy. Tell the patient to report the appearance of any new sign or symptom.
- Provide emotional support as needed; weeks to months of therapy may be needed for adequate treatment.
- Take oral doses with meals or snack to lessen gastric irritation. Take doses over 15 minutes or longer to lessen gastric irritation.

PATIENT CARE IMPLICATIONS—cont'd

- Warn patients to avoid driving or operating hazardous equipment if vertigo or sleepiness occurs; notify physician.

Ketoconazole

Drug administration

- Monitor for evidence of side effects: CNS effects and gastrointestinal distress.
- Monitor liver function tests.

Patient and family education

- Review anticipated benefits and possible side effects of drug therapy. Tell patients to report the development of any new sign or symptom.
- Warn patients to avoid driving or operating hazardous equipment if dizziness or lethargy develops; notify physician.
- Do not take H_2 receptor blocking drugs (e.g., cimetidine, ranitidine) or antacids within 2 hours of doses of ketoconazole.
- Avoid alcoholic beverages while taking ketoconazole.
- If photophobia develops (sensitivity of the eyes to light), wear sunglasses and avoid bright lights and sunlight.
- Absorption of this drug requires an acid pH in the stomach. For patients with achlorhydria, dissolve each 200 mg of ketoconazole in 4 ml of 0.2N HCl solution. Administer the solution through a straw to avoid contact with the teeth. Follow the dose with a full glassful of water. Consult pharmacist and physician as needed.

Miconazole

Drug administration

- Perform neurologic assessment regularly. Monitor vital signs, weight. Inspect injection site for development of phlebitis and pruritus.
- Monitor complete blood count and serum electrolytes.
  INTRAVENOUS MICONAZOLE
- Dilute dose in 200 ml of normal saline or 5% dextrose in water. Administer dose over 30 to 60 minutes. Monitor vital signs with IV doses, and do not administer too rapidly.

Patient and family education

- Review anticipated benefits and possible side effects of drug therapy. Instruct patients to report the development of any new sign or symptom. Provide emotional support as needed as therapy may be needed for weeks to months.

Itraconazole

Nursing care, drug administration/patient and family education

- Consult drug insert for current information.
- Monitor liver function tests.
- Instruct the patient to report the development of any new sign or symptom.

Topical antifungal agents

Patient and family education

- For best effect, these agents must be used regularly, as prescribed.
- With ointments and creams, apply dose as directed, and gently rub into the area. Do not cover with a dressing unless instructed to do so.
- With aerosol powders or solutions, shake well before using. Hold spray opening 6 to 10 inches away from area to be treated, and spray well. Do not inhale powder or solution, or get it into the eyes.
- With powder forms, sprinkle liberally on the affected area (such as the toes and feet).
- When treating toes and feet, make certain drug reaches area between toes and on bottom of feet. Sprinkle or spray onto socks or in shoes, if directed to do so.
- See Patient Problem: Vaginal Infections on p. 540.
- Remind women that no medications, even topical ones, should be used during pregnancy or lactation without prior consultation with the physician.

Griseofulvin

Nursing care, drug administration/patient and family education

- Assess for development of any side effects.
- Monitor complete blood count and differential, urinalysis.
- Take oral doses with meals or snack to lessen gastric irritation.
- Review Patient Problem: Photosensitivity on p. 647.
- Avoid drinking alcoholic beverages while taking griseofulvin.
- Warn patients to avoid driving or operating hazardous equipment if dizziness or sleepiness occurs; notify physician.

Continued.

- Oral contraceptives may be ineffective if taken concurrently with griseofulvin. Other forms of birth control should be used. Consult the physician.

Nystatin

Nursing care, drug administration/patient and family education

- Side effects are uncommon. Tell patients to report the development of any new sign or symptom.
- With nystatin suspension, the drug may be dispensed with a dropper; use this to measure the dose. Place half the dose in one side of the mouth, and the other half in the other side. Hold, swish, and gargle, for as long as possible, then swallow.
- With nystatin powder, add dose (about ⅛ tsp) to 4 to 5 ounces of water, and stir well. Take a mouthful of the suspension, hold it, swish and gargle for as long as possible before swallowing. Repeat with another mouthful until the entire dose has been taken.
- With lozenge form, allow the lozenge to dissolve slowly in the mouth, which may take 15 to 30 minutes. Swallow the saliva as needed. Do not chew or break the lozenge. Do not let young children under 5 years have lozenges, as they may choke on them.

availability is dependent upon sufficient stomach acidity. Ketoconazole is best absorbed on an empty stomach and should not be administered within 2 hours of administration of antacids or H_2-histamine receptor blocking drugs such as cimetidine. Ketoconazole is not well distributed to all tissues and is especially low in cerebrospinal fluid. Elimination is primarily by the liver, which forms inactive metabolites and excretes the drug into bile.

Itraconazole is relatively lipid soluble and is absorbed following oral administration, but miconazole must be administered intravenously in systemic infections. Miconazole metabolites are formed in the liver and excreted in urine.

Toxicity. Ketoconazole is relatively nontoxic for many patients. Nausea and pruritus occur in less than 5% of treated patients. Dizziness, nervousness, and headache have been reported less frequently. Ketoconazole may inhibit testosterone and cortisol synthesis. Gynecomastia (excessive development of mammary glands) has been noted in about 10% of males receiving ketoconazole. Liver changes have also been noted, which in rare cases progress to hepatitis or fatal hepatic necrosis.

Miconazole may produce rashes, itching, redness at the injection site, or phlebitis. Reversible platelet dysfunction, thrombocytopenia, and anemia may also occur with systemic administration.

Itraconazole appears to cause less hepatic toxicity than ketoconazole and alters platelet function less than miconazole. Further clinical experience is required to fully assess the side effects.

DRUGS TO TREAT LOCALIZED OR TOPICAL FUNGAL INFECTIONS

In this section the drugs that are useful to treat fungal infections restricted to skin, mucous membranes, or gastrointestinal tract are considered. The properties of specific drugs are listed in Table 36.2. Most of these agents are used strictly locally, being applied at the site of infection. For example, *tolnaftate* is an effective agent for simple cases of tinea, but the effectiveness is limited by the accessibility of locally applied drug to the infective fungi. For this reason tinea infections around nails and heavily keratinized skin are hard to eradicate.

Griseofulvin is an effective drug for the treatment of several types of dermatophytic infections. It is administered orally rather than used topically. For this reason griseofulvin is especially useful for treating fungal infections of the scalp. The usefulness of this drug as an oral agent depends on its ability to localize in the skin following oral absorption. Those skin cells containing high concentrations of griseofulvin are resistant to infection by dermatophytes. Ultimately, all infected cells will be lost through the natural sloughing off of skin cells and the disease will be cured. This process takes a considerable period of time and, accordingly, griseofulvin therapy may need to be continued for several weeks or several months, depending on the site and severity of the infection.

Nystatin is sometimes administered orally to treat intestinal fungal infections. This treatment may be considered topical, since nystatin is not absorbed orally and is retained in the intestinal tract. Nystatin is also used for treating vaginal infections, such as those caused by *Candida*. This treatment is also local, since the drug is administered intravaginally and is not significantly absorbed from that site. Nystatin is too toxic to be used for systemic infections.

Numerous over-the-counter preparations are available for treating fungal infections of the skin. Some of these preparations contain useful antifungal agents, whereas others are practically useless. The most effective preparations are identified in Table 36.2.

Antifungal agents are also available in combination with various antibacterial drugs. The rationale for these combinations is that many infections diagnosed as fungal are, in fact, mixed bacterial and fungal infections. Full resolution of symptoms may therefore require treatment with an antibacterial and an antifungal agent. However, this therapy is best accomplished by using two separate preparations so that the most effective drugs for the specific infection may be chosen. Moreover, dosage adjustment is easier with separate preparations.

SUMMARY

Fungi are eucaryotic organisms and therefore offer few targets for selectively toxic agents. The polyene antifungal agents achieve some selective toxicity by interacting with fungal cell membranes more readily than with mammalian cell membranes. Imidazole derivatives (clotrimazole, econazole, ketoconazole, and miconazole) affect fungal cell membranes by inhibiting synthesis of ergosterol.

Fungal diseases range from mild, self-limited pulmonary disease to serious systemic disease. Very few drugs are available for the treatment of systemic fungal infections. Amphotericin B is used to treat various systemic mycoses, but the drug is very toxic and successful therapy is difficult to achieve. The drug tends to bind to body tissues; nephrotoxicity, anemia, and electrolyte imbalances often occur during therapy.

Flucytosine is less toxic than amphotericin B but is frequently ineffective, since resistance can develop easily. Amphotericin B and flucytosine are sometimes used in combination. Combining the two drugs allows the dose of amphotericin B to be lowered, thereby lowering toxicity, and minimizes the development of resistance to flucytosine.

Ketoconazole is an effective oral antifungal agent that may be used for systemic fungal infections. Miconazole is rarely used for systemic infections, but it may be used, like econazole and clotrimazole, for treating fungal infections of the skin.

Fungal infections localized to the skin are called dermatophytes. Since drugs can be applied topically in many cases, these infections may be treated with much more toxic agents than can systemic infections. An exception is the drug griseofulvin, which concentrates in the skin after oral administration and helps eliminate fungal infections of the skin.

STUDY QUESTIONS

1. Why are fungi resistant to drugs like penicillins and tetracyclines?
2. What animal species commonly spread fungal diseases to humans?
3. What types of infections are commonly caused by *Candida*?
4. What are dermatophytes?
5. What is the mechanism of action for the polyene antifungal agent amphotericin B?
6. By what route is amphotericin B administered?
7. What types of fungal infections are properly treated with amphotericin B?
8. How does the lipid solubility of amphotericin B influence its tissue distribution?
9. What are the characteristic toxic reactions associated with systemic use of amphotericin B?
10. What is the mechanism of action of flucytosine?
11. May flucytosine be employed as an oral agent?
12. What is the main route of excretion of flucytosine?
13. What toxic reactions occur with the use of flucytosine?
14. Why are flucytosine and amphotericin B sometimes combined for antifungal therapy?
15. What is the mechanism of action of ketoconazole?
16. By what route is ketoconazole administered?
17. What type of fungal infections respond to ketoconazole?
18. How may econazole be used clinically? Itraconazole?
19. May miconazole be employed for systemic fungal infections?
20. What is the mechanism of action of griseofulvin?
21. How is griseofulvin administered?
22. Is therapy with griseofulvin long or short term?
23. What types of fungal disease may be treated with the polyene nystatin?

SUGGESTED READINGS

Angeles, A.M., and Sugar, A.M.: The polyene macrolide antifungal drugs, Antimicrobial Agents Annual 3:257, 1989.

Antifungal agents: In AMA drug evaluations, ed. 6, Philadelphia, 1986, W.B. Saunders Co.

Kauffman, C.A.: Flucytosine, Antimicrobial Agents Annual **3**:246, 1989.

Lesher, J.L. Jr., and Smith, J.G.: Athlete's foot: a logical approach to treatment, Drug Therapy **14**(9):113, 1984.

Maddux, M.S., and Barriere, S.L.: A review of complications of amphotericin-B therapy: recommendations for prevention and management, Drug Intell. Clin. Pharm. **14**:177, 1980.

Mahon, S.M.: Taking the terror out of amphotericin B, Am. J. Nurs. **88**(7):960, 1988.

Sipes, C.: Giving amphotericin B in the home, Am. J. Nurs. **88**(7):965, 1988.

Terrell, C.L., and Hermans, P.E.: Antifungal agents used for deep-seated mycotic infections, Mayo Clin. Proc. **62**(12):1116, 1987.

Wack, E.E., and Galgiani, J.N.: The azoles: miconazole, ketoconazole, itraconazole, Antimicrobial Agents Annual **3**:251, 1989.

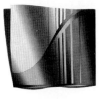

37

Treatment of Viral Diseases

Viral diseases are among the most common infections in humans, yet the prevention and treatment of these diseases has lagged far behind the ability to control bacterial infections. This chapter discusses the properties of viral diseases that make them difficult to prevent or treat and the mechanisms of action of antiviral drugs that have been developed.

NATURE OF VIRAL DISEASES

Viruses cause a wide variety of clinical disease, including some conditions that have only recently been recognized as viral in origin. Viral diseases may be classified as acute, chronic, or slow. Acute illnesses include the common cold, influenza, and various other respiratory tract infections. These illnesses frequently resolve very quickly and leave no latent infections or sequelae. Chronic infections are those in which the disease runs a protracted course with long periods of remission interspersed with reappearance of the disease. An example of this type of viral disease is herpes infection of the conjunctiva, skin, or genitalia in which active disease alternates with latent periods during which the virus remains dormant in nervous tissue. Slow virus infections are diseases that progress over a number of months or years, causing cumulative damage to body tissues and ultimately ending in death of the host. Diseases that involve infection with slow-acting viruses include multiple sclerosis, amyotrophic lateral sclerosis, Alzheimer-Pick disease, and various other degenerative diseases of the central nervous system.

Viral diseases may also be classified as local or generalized. Examples of local viral diseases include those that affect only the tissues of the respiratory tract. For these diseases, symptoms develop as the infection spreads from the original site to immediately adjacent cells. The severity of symptoms depends in part on how many host cells are affected.

Some viruses have the potential for more generalized invasion of tissues throughout the body. This spread may come about in several ways. Viruses such as rabies travel along the nervous tissue and eventually invade the brain, causing the characteristic symptoms of rabies. Other viruses spread via the bloodstream; this mechanism is called *viremic spread*. The details of viremic spread are given in Table 37.1. The most important feature to recognize in this process is that clinical symptoms do not appear in most diseases spread in this manner until very late in the disease, when the secondary viremia occurs. At this stage most viral infections are self-limiting and will resolve even without medical attention. However, certain viruses can attack the brain following the secondary viremia. An example is the poliovirus, which causes relatively mild disease during the respiratory phase and secondary viremic stage but becomes life-threatening when it invades the central nervous system. Even with polioviruses, invasion of the central nervous system is a rare event and most infections end with the secondary viremia.

The fact that symptoms appear late in most viral diseases has implications for chemotherapy; since symptoms occur after most of the virus particles have reproduced, therapy instituted at this stage of the disease can be expected to have limited effectiveness. This pattern is different from that of bacterial diseases, in which active bacterial reproduction accompanies the worst clinical symptoms. This relative delay in appearance of clinical symptoms in viral diseases is one of the most important reasons that drug therapy of viral diseases is difficult once the disease is established.

Table 37.1 Viremic Spread in Mammalian Body

Site	Symptoms
PRIMARY SITE OF INFECTION (e.g., lung in pox, measles, mumps; gastrointestinal tract in polio)	First wave of replication produces no symptoms.
BLOODSTREAM (viruses free or bound to blood cells)	Primary viremia produces no symptoms.
SECONDARY SITES OF INFECTION (e.g., liver, spleen, bone marrow, or lymphoid tissue)	Second wave of replication may produce mild symptoms for some viral diseases.
BLOODSTREAM (viruses free or bound to blood cells)	Secondary viremia may produce fever, rashes, and other symptoms whose severity depends on the number of viruses released.
CENTRAL NERVOUS SYSTEM (rarely involved)	Serious illness; specific care determined by the area of brain attacked.

VACCINES TO PREVENT VIRAL DISEASES

The external surface of viruses contains antigenic substances that promote the production of antibodies. These humoral factors limit the spread of many types of viral disease and ultimately allow the body to eliminate the virus. Infected cells are also changed sufficiently in many viral diseases so that these cells are also eliminated.

Many viral diseases are best controlled by inducing antibodies in healthy individuals prior to exposure to the viral disease. This prophylaxis is successful for many diseases (Table 28.2, Chapter 28). Vaccines cannot be produced efficiently for many viral diseases, however. One example is rhinoviruses, which cause respiratory disease. Among these viruses there are approximately 100 strains, each of which induces a specific antibody in humans; however, no antibody attacks more than one of the serotypes. Therefore successful immunization would require that an antibody be developed against each of the 100 pathogenic strains. Such a program is not feasible.

Influenza viruses illustrate another difficulty in immunizing against viral diseases. With influenza the antigenic properties shift every few years so that those persons who were immunized either naturally or artificially against the prevalent strain of

GERIATRIC DRUG ALERT: AMANTADINE

THE PROBLEM
The elderly are more sensitive to the antimuscarinic side effects of amantadine than are younger adults.

SOLUTIONS
- Normal adult dose is cut by one-half for the elderly
- Watch carefully for antimuscarinic signs such as confusion or difficulty in urination

the virus are unprotected when the new viral type arises. Therefore influenza immunizations are effective only for a specific viral strain and should not be expected to carry over when new strains appear. Rapid antigenic shift is also a characteristic of human immunodeficiency virus (HIV), the virus that causes AIDS.

The most successful immunization programs are for those viral diseases in which few pathogenic strains exist and with which antigenic properties do not change. The vaccine for poliovirus fits these criteria. The oral vaccine is directed against the three major viral strains; these strains have not shifted in antigenic properties.

In addition to the traditional immune responses to viral infection, the body has another mechanism by which it limits the spread of viral diseases. This mechanism is the production of glycoproteins called *interferons* (Chapter 27). Interferons, released from virus-infected cells, alter the metabolism of uninfected cells to prevent the virus from attacking these new cells. This mechanism prevents the spread of the viral disease to new cells and allows the immune system to eliminate the viruses and infected cells.

Interferons have several properties that make them difficult to use as antiviral drugs. First, interferons are host specific and not virus specific. This property means that interferons induce resistance to several types of viruses at once. Host specificity of interferons determines that only human interferon is effective in preventing viral disease in humans.

In the past, this host specificity limited development of interferons for clinical use because no ready source of the material was available. Today, human proteins of many kinds are made by recombinant DNA technology, which allows human interferons to be produced in large quantities by recombinant organisms.

The second property of interferons that makes them less than ideal for use as drugs is that the resistance they confer is transient. Long-term protection does not develop as with antibody production. To overcome some of these problems, inducers of interferons have been tested. Although compounds have been developed that successfully induce interferons, the protection produced is again transient. Moreover, cells exposed to the inducers become refractory to further induction for a period of time, making it impossible to continuously maintain high interferon levels. For these reasons interferons remain an interesting class of substances whose clinical usefulness as routine antiviral agents has not yet been proven. These drugs limit cell proliferation and are used as anticancer agents (Chapter 39).

SELECTIVE TOXICITY IN THE TREATMENT OF VIRAL DISEASES

Since viral reproduction is carried out mostly by host cell enzymes and ribosomes, targets for selective toxicity are difficult to identify. Virus reproduction can be divided into four steps (Table 37.2). Study of the details of each of these processes has revealed more potential for selective toxicity than was originally thought. It is now known that a few viral enzymes are involved in forming viral nucleic acid, for example. Viral enzymes or processes that occur only in virus-infected cells are likely points for attack with selectively toxic agents. Many agents have been tested as antiviral drugs, but only a few meet the test of effective action against virus-infected cells with low toxicity to uninfected host cells.

SPECIFIC ANTIVIRAL DRUGS (Table 37.3)

Acyclovir

Acyclovir is the most highly selective of the antiviral agents in use in the United States. The drug is activated by *viral* thymidine kinase, an enzyme found only in virus-infected cells. The activated form of the drug preferentially and irreversibly inhibits the viral DNA polymerase present in infected cells, effectively halting virus production. Much higher concentrations of acyclovir are required to halt normal human cell metabolism. Therefore effective doses for antiviral activity are relatively nontoxic to normal cells of the host.

Acyclovir has been tested clinically for a number of conditions. Initial lesions of genital herpes respond well to intravenous acyclovir and to a topically applied ointment. Oral administration is also effective. Acyclovir controls mucocutaneous herpes simplex infections in immunocompromised pa-

tients and is under study for the control of herpes zoster infections in the same patient population.

Acyclovir is used intravenously to treat mucocutaneous herpes simplex in immunocompromised patients and in severe genital herpes. Oral administration of acyclovir leads to incomplete absorption, but this route is effective when used for mild to moderate genital herpes. Once absorbed, acyclovir is widely distributed to tissues. The drug does not seem to penetrate to all tissue sites where latent herpes viruses reside, however. Recurrence of herpes infections can occur following treatment with acyclovir.

Acyclovir appears to be relatively nontoxic. Nephrotoxicity, including crystallization of drug in the renal tubule, can be minimized by giving the drug as a slow infusion rather than as a rapid bolus. Increasing water intake also helps. Phlebitis at the injection site may also occur with acyclovir administration intravenously.

Amantadine

Amantadine has a narrow antiviral spectrum, being effective only against influenza type A. Moreover, clinical information suggests the drug is most effective at preventing the disease and has very limited ability to alter the course of the disease once symptoms have appeared. There is limited clinical evidence that if the drug is administered by a nebulizer so that it is breathed into the lungs, it may help reduce the severity of the symptoms and the duration of influenza type A infections. At present, however, the drug is limited to prophylaxis in patients at great risk in influenza epidemics, that is, in elderly patients or others in whom influenza is likely to lead to life-threatening complications.

Rimantadine, a chemical relative of amantadine, may be more concentrated in the lung than amantadine. Rimantadine may also have less CNS toxicity. This new drug has been extensively used in the Soviet Union and is under investigation in the United States.

Routine administration of amantadine is by the oral route, with most of the drug being excreted unchanged in the urine. The concentration of amantadine that reaches the epithelial surfaces of lung tissues is the determining factor in protecting against influenza A infections.

Toxicity with amantadine prophylaxis for viral diseases is ordinarily low, unless kidney failure is present and the drug accumulates in the bloodstream. Amantadine can cause amphetamine-like stimulation of the central nervous system, as well as lethargy, ataxia, slurred speech, and other symptoms. Because of these central nervous system ef-

Table 37.2   Sequence of Events in Virus Reproduction in Mammalian Cells

Step in reproduction	Biochemical events	Drugs that block process
1. Adsorption	Initial ionic, dissociable association become irreversible adsorption of virus to cell surface.	No clinically useful drugs block this process
2. Penetration and uncoating	Virus particles enter the cell and the outer coats dissolve, releasing the viral genetic material (either DNA or RNA).	Amantadine
3. Replication and transcription	All viruses synthesize new messenger RNA and, using host ribosomes, synthesize viral proteins.	Acyclovir Idoxyuridine (IUdR) Trifluridine Vidarabine (ara-A) Zidovudine
4. Assembly and release	Viral nucleic acids and proteins are assembled to form mature viruses, which are then released either by budding off from infected cell or by lysis of infected cell.	Methisazone

fects, the drug should be used cautiously, if at all, in elderly patients with cerebral arteriosclerosis or in patients with a history of epilepsy.

Amantadine has been used to treat Parkinson's disease (Chapter 48). Since doses used for this purpose are about twice those for influenza prophylaxis, toxic reactions are more common.

Idoxuridine

Idoxuridine, also referred to as 5-iodo-2'-deoxyuridine or IUdR, is an analog of the thymidine normally found in DNA. Idoxuridine is incorporated into DNA in place of the normal thymidine, thereby preventing normal DNA replication and halting virus formation. Unfortunately, idoxuridine does not have a good therapeutic index and will harm rapidly growing normal host cells as well as virus-infected cells. For this reason its use is restricted to topical treatment of herpes simplex infections of the cornea, conjunctiva, and eyelids. These infections tend to recur, and idoxuridine does not prevent reappearance of the infection, nor does it prevent scarring and resultant loss of sight in serious cases.

When used topically in the eye, little idoxuridine enters the systemic circulation. The drug can produce local reactions in the eye, the most serious being corneal defects. It may also interfere with corneal epithelial regeneration and healing. Systemic toxic reactions to idoxuridine include anorexia, nausea, stomatitis, vomiting, hair loss (alopecia), blood dyscrasias, and cholestatic jaundice. These toxic reactions preclude the safe use of this

drug systemically. Idoxuridine is potentially mutagenic and carcinogenic.

Ribavirin

Ribavirin is a synthetic purine nucleoside that interferes with multiple steps leading to synthesis of viral nucleic acids. In the United States, ribavirin is indicated only for therapy of severe respiratory syncytial virus (RSV) in children, but in other parts of the world the drug has been used to treat various viral-induced hemorrhagic fevers.

Ribavirin is administered as an aerosol to treat respiratory viruses. In this way, drug levels in the lung are maximized, but systemic absorption is low, which minimizes side effects. High oral doses of ribavirin may produce blood dyscrasias such as anemia.

Trifluridine

Trifluridine, like idoxuridine, is activated by viral and host cell thymidine kinase to a form of drug that inhibits DNA polymerase. Trifluridine is not selective in its action, but it inhibits DNA polymerase in normal as well as virus-infected cells. Therefore trifluridine is not tolerated systemically.

Trifluridine is effective for topical therapy of herpes infections of the eye. This agent may be less damaging to the cornea than idoxuridine or vidarabine; nevertheless, burning of the conjunctiva and cornea can occur when the drug is placed into the eye. Swelling of the eyelids (palpebral edema) has also been noted.

Like idoxuridine and vidarabine, trifluridine is

Table 37.3   Summary of Drugs Used to Treat Viral Diseases

Generic name	Trade name	Administration/dosage	Clinical use	Principal toxic reactions
Acyclovir	Zovirax*	ORAL: *Adults*—200 mg 5 times daily. FDA Pregnancy Category C. INTRAVENOUS: *Adults*—5 mg/kg infused at a constant rate over 1 hr, repeated every 8 hr. *Children under 12*—250 mg/M² infused at a constant rate over 1 hr, repeated every 8 hr. TOPICAL: 5% ointment applied directly to initial lesions of genital herpes.	Mucosal and cutaneous herpes simplex infections in immuno-compromised patients; severe initial episodes of genital herpes; varicella–zoster infections.	Renal toxicity usually mild; phlebitis.
Amantadine	Symadine Symmetrel*	ORAL: *Adults*—100 mg twice daily. *Geriatrics*—100 mg once daily. FDA Pregnancy Category C. *Children*—4.4 to 8.8 mg/kg, up to 150 mg daily.	Prophylaxis of influenza type A infections in high-risk patients.	Central nervous system stimulation, ataxia, slurred speech, lethargy.
Idoxuridine	Herplex* Stoxil	OPHTHALMIC: *Adults and children*—0.1% solution, 0.5% ointment used 5 times daily.	Topical use in the eye for herpes keratitis.	Local irritation and pitting defects in the cornea. Systemic toxicity is possible but rare by this route.
Ribavirin	Vilona* Viramid* Virazid* Virazole	INHALATION: *Children*—20 mg/ml in a Viratek Small Particle Aerosol Generator Model SPAG-2 12 to 18 hr/day.	Severe viral pneumonia in children only.	Few side effects when used by aerosol; FDA Pregnancy Category X.
Trifluridine	Viroptic*	OPHTHALMIC: *Adults and children*—1% solution applied up to 9 times daily.	Topical use in the eye for herpes keratitis.	Local irritation.
Vidarabine	Vira-A*	OPHTHALMIC: *Adults and children*—3% ointment used 5 times daily. FDA Pregnancy Category C.	Topical use in the eye for herpes keratitis.	Local irritation, superficial punctate keratitis, allergy.
Zidovudine	Retrovir	ORAL: *Adults*—200 mg every 4 hr around the clock. FDA Pregnancy Category C.	HIV infection (AIDS, ARC).	Bone marrow depression may cause fever, chills, bleeding, tiredness, or weakness.

*Available in Canada and United States.

potentially mutagenic and carcinogenic. Since these drugs are not well absorbed from the eye into systemic circulation, it is not clear how important this potential may be when these agents are used topically.

Vidarabine

Vidarabine, also referred to as *adenine arabinoside,* inhibits viral DNA synthesis in a variety of DNA viruses. Vidarabine is activated by host cell enzymes to ara-ATP, a potent and selective inhibitor of viral DNA polymerase. Clinically important selectivity of action is achieved against herpes virus–infected cells. Therefore this agent is employed to treat various herpes infections.

Vidarabine is used topically in eye infections caused by herpes in much the same way as idoxuridine. Vidarabine administered parenterally may also be effective in other serious herpes infections, especially in immunosuppressed patients, but acy-

THE NURSING PROCESS

VIRAL DISEASES

Assessment

Most patients who are diagnosed as having viral illnesses are treated symptomatically and not with an antiviral agent. Examples include patients who have the "flu," the common cold, influenza, and other kinds of viremias. Use of antiviral agents is limited to patients in whom supportive therapy has not been helpful or who have viruses known to be particularly virulent or frequently fatal. A total thorough assessment should be done. Emphasis should be placed on the subjective and objective complaints related to the virus, and data to be obtained would include appropriate laboratory work, cultures, and other studies that would be helpful in monitoring the progress of the disease.

Nursing diagnoses

Potential complication: blood dyscrasias

Potential for injury related to ataxia as a drug side effect

Management

Even when antiviral agents are used, much of the care is supportive and symptomatic in nature. The nurse should monitor appropriate laboratory work, vital signs, and other objective data that will help chart the progress of the disease. If antiviral agents are being used, the nurse should monitor for the side effects known to occur with that drug. If it is anticipated that the patient will be receiving antiviral drug therapy after discharge, patient and family instruction should be given. If the virus is known to be a particularly virulent one, patient isolation may be necessary during the hospitalization phase. For information about specific viruses, consult the infection control department, the local health department, or the Centers for Disease Control in Atlanta, Georgia. Many of the serious viral illnesses should be reported to the local health department, since this information is used for epidemiological charting of viral spread; examples include polio and rabies. Finally, immunization of family members and health care team members should be done if appropriate for the specific virus being treated.

Evaluation

Success with antiviral agents is manifested by recovery from the virus being treated. Side effects with the most commonly used antiviral agents in the United States are relatively uncommon. Because new drugs and new dosage regimens are being used with the antiviral agents, it is important that health care personnel monitor these patients carefully for the appearance of signs and symptoms that may indicate possible side or toxic effects to the drugs. If patients are being discharged while taking these agents, before discharge they should be able to explain how to take the drug correctly, should know side effects that may occur, and should be able to describe situations that require notification of the physician.

clovir is better. The drug is not effective in treating genital herpes.

Vidarabine is rapidly metabolized when administered parenterally, and the metabolites formed are less active than vidarabine itself. The drug is poorly absorbed orally or from intramuscular sites and is suitable only for intravenous use when systemic absorption of the drug is desired. Large infusion volumes are required because the drug is not highly soluble in water solution.

Vidarabine may produce transient gastrointestinal distress when administered intravenously. Central nervous system disturbances, including tremors, ataxia, confusion, and psychoses, may rarely occur. High doses are cytotoxic and produce blood dyscrasias. Vidarabine is teratogenic and po-

PATIENT CARE IMPLICATIONS

Acyclovir

Drug administration

- Assess for GI symptoms and CNS side effects. Inspect for development of skin rashes.
- Monitor intake, output, and weight.
- Monitor complete blood count and differential, platelet count.
  INTRAVENOUS ADMINISTRATION
- Dilute as directed in the drug insert. Administer dose over 1 hour. Use an infusion control device and/or microdrip tubing to help regulate rate of infusion. Inspect IV site frequently, and question patient regarding symptoms of phlebitis or irritation.

Patient and family education

- Review anticipated benefits and possible side effects of drug therapy.
- Warn patients to avoid driving or operating hazardous equipment if dizziness, fatigue, or vertigo develops; notify physician.
- Teach patients taking oral or IV doses to increase fluid intake to 2500 to 3000 ml per day.
- For topical application, use a glove or finger cot to apply ointment, to avoid contamination of the finger. Use the drug on a regular basis, as prescribed, for best effect.
- Teach the patient with genital herpes how to lessen the chance of spreading the virus: avoid sexual activity when open lesions or scabs are present. Male partners should wear condoms. Acyclovir will not prevent the spread of herpes.
- Keep areas of infection clean and dry. Wear loose-fitting garments. Do not use other creams or ointments on viral lesions unless prescribed by the physician.
- Encourage women with genital herpes to have regular "Pap" smears to check for development of cervical cancer.

Amantadine

See Patient Care Implications in Chapter 48.

Rimantidine

See drug package insert for current information.

Ribavirin

Nursing care, drug administration/patient and family education

- Review anticipated benefits and possible side effects of drug therapy with patient and family. Encourage the patient or family to report the development of new signs or symptoms.
- Auscultate lung sounds and assess respiratory status. Monitor temperature and vital signs.
- Check drug package insert for current information. Do not administer with other aerosolized medications simultaneously. Use only the aerosol generator specified by the manufacturer.

Vidarabine

Drug administration

- Assess for CNS and GI side effects.
- Monitor intake and output, weight.
- Monitor complete blood count and differential, platelet count.
  INTRAVENOUS ADMINISTRATION
- Review drug package insert for dilution guidelines. Administer diluted dose over 12 to 24 hours, at a constant rate. Use an infusion monitoring device and/or microdrip tubing to ensure correct rate. Use an in-line filter of 0.45 micron. Inspect infusion site and assess patient for signs of phlebitis.

Patient and family education

- Review anticipated benefits and possible side effects of drug therapy with patients and family. Encourage the patient to report the development of new signs or symptoms.
- Make certain patient can apply eye drops correctly if that route is ordered. See Chapter 6 for a discussion of administration of eye drops.

Zidovudine

Drug administration

- Assess for headaches, anxiety, and confusion. Inspect for rashes. Monitor temperature and pulse.
- Monitor complete blood count and differential, platelet count.

Patient and family education

- Review anticipated benefits and possible side effects of drug therapy with patient and family. Encourage the patient to report the development of new signs or symptoms.
- Review drug package insert for current information.

tentially carcinogenic. Ophthalmic use is not usually associated with serious side effects.

Zidovudine

Zidovudine is used in AIDS (acquired immune deficiency syndrome) and in ARC (AIDS-related complex), conditions caused by infection with HIV (human immunodeficiency virus). HIV is a retrovirus that has borne several names, including LAV (lymphadenopathy-associated virus) and HTLV-III (human T-cell lymphotropic virus type III). Retroviruses use RNA as their genetic material and must therefore convert RNA into DNA within the host cell, in order for viral replication to take place. This unusual reaction, which does not normally occur in the host cell, is catalyzed by an enzyme called *reverse transcriptase*. Zidovudine inhibits reverse transcriptase. In addition, some of the drug may be incorporated into viral DNA, where it causes premature chain termination. Both actions will block viral replication.

Zidovudine does not cure AIDS or ARC, but may lower the incidence of opportunistic infections and prolong useful life in these patients. In order to be effective, the drug must be administered continuously throughout life. The short half-life and toxicity of the drug make this ideal difficult to achieve. Zidovudine has a half-life of only 1 hour, and is quickly metabolized to an inactive glucuronide on first pass through the liver. For this reason, the drug is taken every 4 hours around the clock to attempt to maintain virustatic concentrations.

Nearly all patients suffer toxicity from zidovudine. The most common reactions are granulocytopenia and anemia. Routine blood monitoring is extremely important. Withdrawal from zidovudine may be necessary to allow recovery from drug-induced blood dyscrasias.

Development of anti-HIV drugs is proceeding very rapidly in major laboratories around the world. Reverse transcriptase inhibitors such as *suramin*, *HPA-23*, and *phosphonoformate* are virustatic but produce no clinical or immunological improvement in patients. *Ribavirin* has slowed progression of ARC to AIDS in at least one trial group of patients. *Rifabutin, D-penicillamine*, and *2',3'-dideoxynucleoside* derivatives are all in trials.

Agents with the ability to improve immune function in AIDS patients are also being treated. *Imuthiol* (sodium diethyldithiocarbamate), *isoprinosine* (inosine prabonex), and *ampligen* (poly rIn.r[C12,U]n) not only influence the immune system but also may have direct inhibitory effects on the virus.

The status of these investigational agents changes very quickly. Current information can be obtained by consultation with the AIDS section at the National Institutes of Health or by consulting current publications devoted to AIDS research.

SUMMARY

Viral diseases are of three types: acute diseases that resolve quickly and leave no latent infections or sequelae; chronic infections in which the disease runs a protracted course with long periods of remission interspersed with reappearance of disease; and slow viral infections in which the disease progresses over a number of months or years, causing cumulative damage to body tissues and ultimately killing the host. Viral diseases may remain localized in certain tissues or may spread by viremia. For most viral diseases the appearance of symptoms occurs late in the disease. This fact makes pharmacological treatment of viral diseases difficult.

The body produces antibodies against viruses. Immunization is therefore possible against some viral diseases. However, some viruses have too many virulent strains or change antigenic properties too often to allow efficient immunizations to be developed.

Interferons are part of the body's natural defense against viral disease, blocking the spread of viruses to uninfected cells. Only the human form of interferon is effective in humans. Unlimited supplies of these agents are available through recombinant DNA techniques. Disease resistance produced by interferons appears to be transient.

Selective toxicity against viral diseases is possible by attacking those viral enzymes that are involved in producing the viral genome in infected human cells. Idoxuridine, trifluridine, and vidarabine are used only as topical agents for herpetic infections of the eye.

Acyclovir is a highly selective antiviral agent that may be given intravenously for treating serious cases of genital herpes; the drug may also be effective in controlling herpes infections in immunosuppressed patients. Amantadine blocks the penetration and uncoating of the influenza A_2 virus and is used in prophylaxis. Ribavirin is administered as an aerosol to treat respiratory syncytial virus infections in children.

Zidovudine is used in ARC and AIDS patients to lower the incidence of opportunistic infections and to prolong useful life. The drug inhibits the HIV virus but does not cure AIDS or ARC. Anemia and granulocytopenia are common reactions to zidovudine. Patients must take the medication every 4 hours around the clock because the drug is rapidly metabolized and excreted.

STUDY QUESTIONS

1. What are the differences between acute, chronic, and slow viral diseases?
2. What is viremic spread of viral disease?
3. What factors limit our ability to develop pharmacological agents to treat viral diseases?
4. Why is immunization not possible against all viral diseases?
5. What is interferon?
6. What are the drawbacks of interferon that make it less than ideal as an antiviral agent?
7. What is the mechanism of action of acyclovir?
8. How is acyclovir used in the therapy of viral diseases?
9. What side effects are associated with acyclovir?
10. What is the mechanism of action of amantadine?
11. How is amantadine used in the therapy of viral diseases?
12. What side effects are associated with amantadine therapy?
13. What is the mechanism of action of idoxuridine?
14. How are idoxuridine, trifluridine, and vidarabine used in the therapy of viral disease?
15. What side effects are associated with the use of idoxuridine, trifluridine, and vidarabine?
16. What is the mechanism of action of ribavirin?
17. How is ribavirin used in therapy of viral disease?
18. What is the mechanism of action of zidovudine?
19. How is zidovudine used in therapy of viral disease?
20. What side effects are associated with the use of zidovudine?
21. Why is zidovudine given every 4 hours around the clock?

SUGGESTED READINGS

Armstrong-Esther, C., and Hewitt, W.E.: AIDS: the knowledge and attitudes of nurses, Canadian Nurse **85**(6):29, 1989.

Balfour, H.H. Jr.: Acyclovir, Antimicrobial Agents Ann. **3**:345, 1989.

Barnard, J.: AIDS and the nurse, Canadian Nurse **83**(6):15, 1987.

Beaufoy, A., Goldstone, I., and Riddell, R.: AIDS: what nurses need to know, Canadian Nurse **84**(7):16, 1988.

Bettoli, E.J.: Herpes: facts and fallacies, Am. J. Nurs. **82**(6):924, 1982.

Dolin, R.: Amantadine and rimantadine, Antimicrobial Agents Ann. **3**:361, 1989.

Galasso, G.J.: Vidarabine, Antimicrobial Agents Ann. **3**:400, 1989.

Hall, C.B.: Ribavirin, Antimicrobial Agents Ann. **3**:384, 1989.

Hendricksen, C.: The AIDS clinical trials unit experience: clinical research and antiviral treatment, Nurs. Clin. N. Am. **23**(4):697, 1988.

Hermans, P.E., and Cockerill, F.R. III: Antiviral agents, Mayo Clin. Proc. **62**(12):1108, 1987.

Langtry, H.D., and Camppoli-Richards, D.M.: Zidovudine, Drugs **37**(4):408, 1989.

Rudd, C.C.: Acyclovir: profile of a unique antiviral agent, Drug Therapy Hosp. **8**(9):41, 1983.

Taelman, H., van der Groen, G., and Piot, P.: Human immunodeficiency virus: prospects for antiviral therapy, Antimicrobial Agents Ann. **3**:432, 1989.

Whiteman, K.F.: Why bother about flu shots? Am. J. Nurs. **87**(11):1412, 1987.

CHAPTER

Drugs to Treat Protozoal and Helminthic Infestations

38

On a worldwide scale, chronic diseases caused by protozoal or helminthic infestations are the most common afflictions of mankind. Although these diseases flourish primarily in tropical regions of the world, several are also encountered in North America. In this chapter the discussion centers on the treatment of diseases that occur in the continental United States. The first sections of this chapter relate individual drugs to specific diseases and explain the rationale for their use. The last section covers the pharmacological properties of the drugs.

THE TREATMENT OF DISEASES CAUSED BY PROTOZOANS

Amebic Diseases

Entamoeba histolytica is a frequent pathogen of humans, commonly being passed from host to host by oral ingestion of fecally contaminated food or water. The organism is ingested as the cysts form. Cysts have thick walls and are resistant to desiccation or to the action of stomach acids. Once in the intestine, the nonmotile cysts change to a motile, sexually active form called a *trophozoite*. Trophozoites produce the active disease as they reproduce and invade various tissues. Homosexual males have a high incidence of infection with *Entamoeba*.

Amebic disease may be restricted to the intestinal lumen. However, trophozoites invade the intestinal lining in the course of the disease and may penetrate the intestinal wall and create abscesses in other tissues and organs. The liver and lung are most commonly affected in this way.

The choice of drug for treating amebic disease depends on the stage of the disease. For the acute colitis that occurs while the disease is limited to the intestinal tract, several drugs are available

(Table 38.1). Antibiotics such as tetracycline may be used as adjuncts to therapy of this form of the disease. For more extensive intestinal disease or for abscesses in other organs, metronidazole is the safest and most effective agent. Metronidazole therapy is usually followed by iodoquinol or diloxanide, drugs that more effectively destroy free amebae within the intestinal lumen. Alternative therapy is dehydroemetine followed by iodoquinol alone or iodoquinol and chloroquine.

Malaria

Malaria is caused when an infected mosquito injects a species of *Plasmodium* into the bloodstream of a person. Four species of *Plasmodium* produce human disease: *P. falciparum*, *P. vivax*, *P. ovale*, and *P. malariae*.

Plasmodia have complex life cycles. The form that enters the human bloodstream (sporozoites) travels immediately to the liver and may persist in the tissue for prolonged periods. Clinical malaria is produced when merozoites, the plasmodial form produced in liver cells, are released into the bloodstream. The merozoites attack red blood cells and ultimately cause them to rupture, thus producing the fever, chills, and sweating characteristic of the disease. A few gametocytes are also formed, which means that the patient at this stage of the disease can transmit the parasites to mosquitoes and thence to other human hosts. Only gametocytes cause a mosquito to become infectious and capable of transmitting the disease.

Therapy of malaria depends upon the stage of the disease and which plasmodial species is involved. *P. falciparum* and *P. malariae* appear not to produce persistent tissue forms of the parasite. Therefore therapy that destroys blood forms of the protozoan will be curative. With *P. vivax* and

Table 38.1 Drugs Used to Treat Amebic Infestations (Amebiasis)

Disease form	Drug used	Administration/dosage
Asymptomatic	Iodoquinol	ORAL: *Adults*—650 mg 3 times daily for 3 wk. *Children*—30 to 40 mg/kg divided in 3 doses daily for 3 wk. Maximum daily dose 2 Gm.
	Diloxanide furoate	ORAL: *Adults*—500 mg 3 times daily for 10 days. *Children over 2 yr*—20 mg/kg daily in 3 divided doses for 10 days.
Intestinal symptoms only	Metronidazole + iodoquinol	ORAL: *Adults*—750 mg 3 times daily for 10 days. *Children*—35 to 50 mg/kg divided into 3 doses daily for 10 days. As above.
	Dehydroemetine + iodoquinol	INTRAMUSCULAR (deep), SUBCUTANEOUS: *Adults*—1 mg/kg up to 60 mg daily in a single dose for 5 days. As above
Abscesses in liver or other organs	Metronidazole + iodoquinol	As above. As above.
	Dehydroemetine + iodoquinol and chloroquine phosphate	As above. As above. As above. ORAL: *Adults*—250 mg four times daily for 2 days, then 250 mg twice daily for 2 or 3 wk. *Children*—10 mg/kg up to 500 mg daily for 3 wk.

P. ovale, however, therapy must include a drug that destroys the persistent tissue forms of *Plasmodium*. A drug such as chloroquine is quite effective against blood forms (Table 38.2). Using chloroquine phosphate plus primaquine phosphate allows control of all four species of *Plasmodium*.

Chloroquine has been a mainstay in treating malaria for a number of years. Unfortunately, chloroquine-resistant malaria has now developed in several regions of the world. This type of disease should be treated with the combination of quinine, pyrimethamine, and sulfadoxine. Pyrimethamine and sulfadoxine are synergistic in activity and are given together for maximum benefit.

Several of the drugs used to treat malaria may also be used for prophylaxis. Chloroquine, hydroxychloroquine, primaquine, and pyrimethamine/sulfadoxine are give in once weekly doses. Clindamycin, doxycycline, and tetracycline have been included in treatment or prophylaxis regimens in other countries, but are not officially recognized for this use in the United States.

Trichomoniasis

Vaginal infections caused by *Trichomonas vaginalis* occur commonly. The disease is marked by watery discharge from the vagina and signs of tissue irritation. *Trichomonas* may be unnoticed in the urinary tract and in the rectum, but these sites can serve as sources of infection.

PEDIATRIC DRUG ALERT: CHLOROQUINE AND HYDROXYCHLOROQUINE

THE PROBLEM

Infants and children are more sensitive to 4-aminoquinolines than are adults. Children have died after swallowing as little as 750 mg of chloroquine. Severe reactions and sudden death have been reported with parenteral use.

SOLUTIONS

- Use minimal effective doses in children
- Do not give these drugs long-term to children
- Carefully observe children receiving these drugs

Vaginal trichomoniasis may be treated with local agents applied as gels or douches (Table 38.3). Complete cure of the sites outside the vagina and of infections in the male urinary tract may require a systemic agent. Metronidazole is the drug of choice.

Giardiasis

Giardiasis is an intestinal infection caused by the protozoan *Giardia lamblia*. This disease, which is passed between human hosts by ingestion of fecally contaminated food, may be asymptomatic in

Table 38.2 Drugs Used to Treat Malaria

Disease form	Drug used	Administration/dosage
Blood forms causing clinical symptoms	Chloroquine phosphate	ORAL: *Adults*—600 mg initially; 300 mg at 6, 24, and 48 hr. *Children*—10 mg/kg initially; 5 mg/kg at 6, 24, and 48 hr.
	Chloroquine hydrochloride	INTRAMUSCULAR, INTRAVENOUS: *Adults*—3 mg/kg every 6 hr (maximum 900 mg/24 hr). *Children*—2 to 3 mg/kg repeated in 6 hr. Not for intravenous use in children under 7 yr.
	Hydroxychloroquine sulfate	ORAL: *Adults*—620 mg initially (four 200 mg tablets as the sulfate equals 620 mg base); 310 mg at 6, 24, and 48 hr. *Children*—10 mg/kg initially; 5 mg/kg at 6, 24, and 48 hr.
	Quinine sulfate	ORAL: *Adults*—650 mg 3 times daily for 3 days. *Children*—25 mg/kg per day in three doses for 3 days.
	Quinine dihydrochloride	INTRAVENOUS: *Adults*—600 mg in 300 ml saline every 8 hr. *Children*—25 mg/kg divided into two 1 hr infusions daily.
Persistent tissue forms of *Plasmodia* (*P. ovale, P. vivax*) or gametocytes	Primaquine phosphate	ORAL: *Adults*—15 mg for 14 days following therapy with one of the drugs listed above. *Children*—0.3 mg/kg for 14 days following therapy with one of the drugs listed above.
Chloroquine-resistant *P. falciparum*	Quinine sulfate or hydrochloride + pyrimethamine/sulfadoxine	As above. ORAL: *Adults and children over 4 yr*—tablets contain 25 mg pyrimethamine and 500 mg sulfadoxine. One to 3 tablets as a single dose may be followed with quinine or primaquine.

many patients. For others, the disease may be much more severe, producing diarrhea, gastrointestinal distress, and malabsorption.

Quinacrine is the most commonly recommended drug for giardiasis in adults. Children should receive metronidazole. Many adults now also receive metronidazole (Table 38.3).

Toxoplasmosis

In the United States toxoplasmosis is primarily acquired from ingestion of the oocyte of *Toxoplasma gondii*. The most common source of infection is cat feces. In adult humans the disease is usually mild and transitory, with symptoms resembling those of mild mononucleosis. Occasionally, the disease may involve the eyes or nervous system in adults.

One dangerous form of toxoplasmosis is congenital, resulting from infection in a pregnant woman. Congenital toxoplasmosis is usually fatal, causing severe damage to eyes, brain, and other organs of the fetus. Because of the dangers this disease poses to fetuses, many obstetricians suggest that pregnant women not handle used cat litter and avoid close contact with cats.

Pyrimethamine and sulfadoxine or sulfadiazine are employed in combination to treat this disease (Table 38.3).

Toxoplasmosis is a common cause of death in AIDS patients, with death coming from encephalitis. Aggressive therapy with pyrimethamine and sulfonamides is usually attempted, but for patients who cannot tolerate sulfonamides other drugs such as clindamycin may be combined with pyrimethamine.

Pneumocystosis

The parasite *Pneumocystis carinii* seldom causes disease in healthy humans, but it can produce severe pulmonary disease in patients receiving immunosuppressive drugs or in patients suffering from AIDS. Young, malnourished children are also susceptible. As many as half the patients who acquire this disease may die unless treated. Patients receiving immunosuppressive cancer chemotherapy or those receiving immunosuppressive drugs to prevent rejection of a transplanted organ usually respond well to the fixed combination of sulfamethoxazole/trimethoprim (Chapter 34). Many of these patients may receive sulfamethoxazole/trimethoprim to prevent development of *P. carinii* pneumonia.

Table 38.3   Drugs Used to Treat Trichomoniasis, Giardiasis, Toxoplasmosis, and Pneumocystosis

Disease form	Drug used	Administration/dosage
Trichomoniasis	Povidone-iodine	VAGINAL: *Adults*—10% gel applied nightly; 10% douche applied every morning. Therapy continues for 2 wk or longer.
	Metronidazole	ORAL: *Adults*—250 mg 3 times daily for 7 to 10 days.
Giardiasis	Quinacrine	ORAL: *Adults*—100 mg 3 times daily for 5 to 7 days. *Children*—6 mg/kg daily in 3 divided doses for 5 days. Daily dose should not exceed 300 mg in children.
	Metronidazole	ORAL: *Adults*—250 to 500 mg 3 times daily for 5 to 7 days.
Toxoplasmosis	Pyrimethamine	ORAL: *Adults*—50 to 100 mg daily for 1 or 2 wk, then 25 mg daily for up to 5 wk. *Children*—1 mg/kg daily in 2 doses for 2 to 4 days. Continue 0.5 mg/kg for 30 days.
	+ sulfadiazine	ORAL: *Adults*—75 mg/kg up to 4 Gm for 1 or 2 wk, then 100 mg/kg daily divided into 2 or 3 doses. *Children*—150 mg/kg total divided in 4 to 6 daily doses after an initial dose equivalent to one half the daily total.
Pneumocystosis	Trimethoprim with sulfamethoxazole	ORAL, INTRAVENOUS: *Adults and children*—20 mg/kg trimethoprim and 100 mg/kg sulfamethoxazole daily divided into 4 doses.
	Pentamidine isethionate	INTRAVENOUS, INTRAMUSCULAR: *Adults and children*—4 mg/kg daily as a single dose for 12 to 14 days or longer. AEROSOL: *Adults*—approved for prophylaxis.

Sulfamethoxazole/trimethoprim may also be given to treat *P. carinii* pneumonia in AIDS, but these patients suffer an unusually high incidence of serious reactions to these drugs. Pentamidine isethionate is also effective against *P. carinii* pneumonia, but this drug can often cause serious toxicity, as well. Experimental regimens in *P. carinii* pneumonia in AIDS patients include clindamycin with primaquine, dapsone with trimethoprim, and trimetrexate with leucovorin. Intermittent administration of aerosolized pentamidine is currently a popular method of prophylaxis. Because this area of medicine is changing so rapidly, nursing personnel should consult a current publication from the Centers for Disease Control, or another official source for up-to-date information.

TREATMENT OF DISEASES CAUSED BY HELMINTHS

Ascariasis

Ascariasis, also called *roundworm infestation,* is produced by ingesting the eggs of *Ascaris lumbricoides.* This common disease is spread by fecally contaminated food and water. Larvae and adult worms migrate through lungs, liver, gallbladder, and other organs and may cause severe damage.

Ascaris infestations may be treated effectively with several agents, including mebendazole, pyrantel pamoate, and piperazine (Table 38.4).

Enterobiasis (Pinworm Infestation)

Pinworms are freely passed between individuals living in close proximity. Constant reinfection is the rule, since the eggs of these parasites are passed in great numbers and adhere to clothing, towels, and hands. The disease is usually mild and may be asymptomatic. However, patients may suffer pruritus ani and pruritus vulvae or more serious symptoms.

Since pinworms tend to stay within the intestinal tract, treatment of the disease is relatively simple. Mebendazole, pyrantel pamoate, and pyrvinium pamoate are all nearly 100% effective after a single dose. Piperazine is also effective, but therapy continues over a period of several days (Table 38.4).

Whipworm Infestation

This intestinal infestation is usually asymptomatic, although large numbers of worms in small children may produce diarrhea, anemia, and cachexia. Whipworm infestations are easily and effectively treated with mebendazole (Table 38.4).

Threadworm Infestation

This disease, also called *strongyloidiasis,* is more serious than many infestations because the worms may reproduce in the human body. Larvae migrate from the wall of the intestine into systemic

Table 38.4 Drugs Used to Treat Infestations by Helminths

Disease form	Drug used	Administration/dosage
Roundworms (ascariasis)	Pyrantel pamoate Mebendazole Piperazine	ORAL: *Adults and children*—single dose of 11 mg/kg up to 1 Gm. ORAL: *Adults and children*—100 mg twice daily for 3 days. ORAL: *Adults*—2 Gm 3 times in 12 hr. Repeat in 2 weeks. *Children*—75 mg/kg up to 3.5 Gm once or twice in 12 hr; repeat in 2 weeks.
Pinworms (enterobiasis)	Mebendazole Pyrantel pamoate Pyrvinium pamoate Piperazine	ORAL: *Adults and children*—100 mg single dose. ORAL: *Adults and children*—single dose of 11 mg/kg up to 1 Gm. ORAL: *Adults and children*—single dose of 5 mg/kg. ORAL: *Adults and children*—65 mg/kg up to 2.5 Gm once daily for 1 wk.
Whipworms (trichuriasis)	Mebendazole	ORAL: *Adults and children*—100 mg daily for 3 days.
Threadworms (strongyloidiasis)	Thiabendazole	ORAL: *Adults and children*—25 mg/kg up to 3 Gm twice daily for 1 or 2 days.
Hookworms (necatoriasis)	Mebendazole Pyrantel pamoate	ORAL: *Adults and children*—100 mg twice daily for 3 days. ORAL: *Adults and children*—11 mg/kg up to 1 Gm as single dose for 3 days.
Cutaneous larva migrans	Thiabendazole	ORAL: *Adults and children over 13.6 kg*—25 mg/kg twice daily for 2 to 5 days plus topical application of suspension (500 mg/5 ml) 4 times daily for 5 days.
Pork roundworms (trichinosis)	Thiabendazole	ORAL: *Adults and children*—25 mg/kg up to 3 Gm twice daily for 2 to 7 days.
Tapeworms (cestodiasis)	Niclosamide	ORAL: *Adults*—2 Gm as a single dose. *Children weighing more than 34 kg*—1.5 Gm as a single dose. *Children 11 to 34 kg*—1 Gm as a single dose. For all patients, tablets should be thoroughly chewed and taken on an empty stomach. For treatment of dwarf tapeworm infestations, doses must be continued for 5 days and repeated 1 to 2 weeks after initial therapy.
	Praziquantel	ORAL: *Adults and children over 4 yr*—10 to 25 mg/kg as a single dose.

circulation and thence return to the intestine to mature and further increase the numbers of worms in the host. Malabsorption syndrome, diarrhea, and duodenal irritation may occur.

Most drugs used against worm infestations are ineffective against threadworms, since these worms live within the intestinal tissue. Thiabendazole is well distributed to the tissues where this parasite lives and is effective in eliminating the infestation (Table 38.4).

Hookworm Infestation

This disease, also called *necatoriasis*, is found in the southern United States. Although two species of hookworms are known, most infestations encountered in the United States are caused by *Necator*. Therefore most patients may be treated with mebendazole or pyrantel pamoate.

Another type of hookworm from dogs and cats produces a cutaneous lesion called *creeping eruption*, or *cutaneous larva migrans*. Thiabendazole, either topically or orally, may be effective to kill the parasites and limit the allergic responses, which cause itching, burning, and skin damage (Table 38.4).

Trichinosis

This condition, also known as *pork roundworm infestation*, is much less common today than it once was. Ingested cysts from raw or improperly cooked meat develop into adult worms in the human intestine. Larvae are ultimately released into the circulation and enter muscle to form cysts. Patients suffer gastrointestinal upset, fever, muscle aches, and eosinophilia (accumulation of certain white cells in the blood).

Table 38.5   Common Reactions to Antiparasitic Drugs

Generic name	Trade name	Toxicity	References for uses and dosages
Chloroquine	Aralen*	Gastrointestinal distress is most common. Vision changes, central nervous system irritability, hemolysis can occur.	Malaria: treatment of clinical attacks or prophylaxis (Table 38.2).
Dehydroemetine		Gastrointestinal irritation and cardiac toxicity are common.	Amebiasis: severe colitis with or without tissue abscesses (Table 38.1).
Diloxanide furoate	Furamide	Flatulence is common. Other gastrointestinal symptoms are rare.	Amebiasis: eliminates cysts; eradicates carrier state (Table 38.1).
Hydroxychloroquine	Plaquenil sulfate*	As for chloroquine.	Malaria: treatment of clinical attacks or prophylaxis (Table 38.2).
Iodoquinol (Diiodohydroxyquin)	Diodoquin† Diquinol Yodoxin	Gastrointestinal upset and skin eruptions are most common. Blood levels of iodine may rise; optic neuritis may occur rarely.	Amebiasis: intestinal forms of disease (Table 38.1).
Mebendazole	Vermox*	Abdominal discomfort may occur. Mebendazole is teratogenic in rats. FDA Pregnancy Category C.	Roundworms, pinworms, whipworms, hookworms (Table 38.4).
Metronidazole	Flagyl* Metryl Protostat	Gastrointestinal distress and pelvic discomfort may occur. Bone marrow suppression is possible. FDA Pregnancy Category B.	Amebiasis: intestinal or tissue abscesses (Table 38.1). Trichomoniasis, giardiasis (Table 38.3).
Niclosamide	Niclocide Yomesan†	Mild gastrointestinal upset on day of therapy. FDA Pregnancy Category B.	Tapeworms (Table 38.4).
Pentamidine	Lomidine† Pentam	Hypoglycemia and hypotension may occur quickly. Blood dyscrasias, hyperglycemia, and diabetes mellitus are later reactions.	Pneumocystis pneumonia (Table 38.3)
Piperazine	Antepar Vermizine	Gastrointestinal upset may occur. Skin rashes and transient neurological signs may be seen.	Roundworms, pinworms (Table 38.4).
Povidone-iodine	Betadine*	Tissue irritation may occur with topically applied drug.	Trichomoniasis (Table 38.3).
Praziquantel	Biltricide Cysticide†	Gastrointestinal distress, dizziness, or drowsiness may occur. Drug is well tolerated by most patients.	Alternative drug for tapeworms (Table 38.4) but a primary drug for schistosomiasis (snail fever).
Primaquine		Gastrointestinal distress can occur. Hemolysis may occur, especially when G-6-PD deficiency exists. Avoid during pregnancy.	Malaria: persistent tissue forms (Table 38.2).
Pyrantel pamoate	Antiminth	Mild gastrointestinal upset and transient changes in liver function occur. Headaches and dizziness are more rare.	Roundworms, pinworms, and hookworms (Table 38.4).

*Available in Canada and United States.
†Available in Canada.

Continued.

Table 38.5 Common Reactions to Antiparasitic Drugs—cont'd

Generic name	Trade name	Toxicity	References for uses and dosages
Pyrimethamine	Daraprim*	Nausea and vomiting as well as blood dyscrasias occur, especially with higher doses.	Malaria: with quinine and sulfadoxine (Table 38.2). Toxoplasmosis: with sulfadiazine (Table 38.3).
Pyrvinium pamoate	Vanquin†	Intestinal distress occurs in some patients. Bright red drug stains teeth, intestinal contents.	Pinworms (Table 38.4).
Quinacrine	Atabrine*	Gastrointestinal distress, dizziness, or headache may occur. Yellow discoloration of skin is harmless. Overdose may cause CNS signs of toxic psychosis.	Giardiasis (Table 38.3)
Quinine		Cinchonism is a dose-related sign of toxicity. Blood dyscrasias and pain on injection occur.	Malaria: with pyrimethamine and sulfadoxine (Table 38.2).
Sulfadiazine		Gastrointestinal, allergic, and blood reactions are possible (see Chapter 34).	Malaria: with pyrimethamine and quinine (Table 38.2). Toxoplasmosis: with pyrimethamine (Table 38.3).
Sulfadoxine and pyrimethamine	Fansidar	Blood dyscrasias and allergic reactions as expected for sulfonamides (Chapter 34) or for pyrimethamine.	Malaria: prophylaxis or treatment of acute attack (Table 38.2).
Sulfamethoxazole and trimethoprim	Bactrim* Septra*	Folic acid deficiency or sulfonamide toxicity may occur (see Chapter 34).	Pneumocystosis (Table 38.3).
Tetracycline		Gastrointestinal distress is common (see Chapter 32).	Amebiasis: with iodoquinol for intestinal forms (Table 38.1).
Thiabendazole	Mintezol*	Gastrointestinal upset is common. Central nervous system effects and reduced liver function may be observed. FDA Pregnancy Category C.	Threadworms, hookworms, cutaneous larva migrans, and trichinosis (Table 38.4).

*Available in Canada and United States.
†Available in Canada.

Trichinosis cannot yet be effectively treated. Most patients receive therapy designed to minimize symptoms rather than produce a cure, since most patients will survive the disease and carry the quiescent worms encysted in skeletal muscle for the rest of their lives. Thiabendazole has been used in selected cases to try to prevent the migration of the worms to the muscles (Table 38.4).

Tapeworm Infestation

Tapeworms, or cestodes, of several types can infest humans. Beef, pork, fish, and dwarf tapeworms are all sensitive to niclosamide (Table 38.4).

All detected infestations are treated, even though the infestations are mostly asymptomatic. Pork tapeworm infestations may become serious if reflux of eggs from the intestine allows them to reach the stomach and hatch into larvae that invade tissues.

PHARMACOLOGICAL PROPERTIES OF SPECIFIC DRUGS

Chloroquine and Hydroxychloroquine

Mechanism of action. Chloroquine and hydroxychloroquine are members of a drug family called *4-aminoquinolines*. This family of drugs has been the mainstay of antimalarial therapy worldwide since the late 1940s. All effective members of this family share the ability to bind tightly to DNA in its double-stranded form. The drugs are thought to *intercalate*, which is to slip into the groove between the two strands of DNA and bind to the bases and phosphate groups exposed within the groove. Binding of these drugs not only alters the physical properties of the DNA, but it also appears to inhibit the ability of the DNA to be replicated or transcribed. Therefore cells whose DNA is affected by these drugs are incapable of cell division.

Absorption, distribution, and excretion. Chloroquine and hydroxychloroquine are satisfactorily absorbed from the gastrointestinal tract. Chloroquine is available for intramuscular injection when oral dosage is impossible.

Drugs of the 4-aminoquinoline family are strongly concentrated in the liver, spleen, kidneys, and lung. More important to the therapeutic usefulness, the drugs are also concentrated in red blood cells. Infected red blood cells may concentrate the drug up to 1000-fold over the drug concentration in plasma.

The 4-aminoquinoline drugs may be metabolized in the liver by microsomal enzymes; some of the metabolites retain antiplasmodial activity. These drugs and metabolites are ultimately removed from the body by the kidney. Renal excretion of these drugs is enhanced by acidifying the urine, which converts the drug to a charged form that is not reabsorbed.

Toxicity. Chloroquine and hydroxychloroquine are relatively safe drugs if care is taken to avoid overdose, prolonged use, or use in sensitive patients. Patients with glucose 6-phosphate dehydrogenase deficiency are more likely than normal patients to suffer hemolysis when treated with these drugs. Children are also more sensitive to these agents than are adults. Patients with liver disease or retinal damage are also more at risk of severe toxic reactions.

At the doses commonly used in therapy, drugs of this family can produce nausea and other gastrointestinal symptoms (Table 38.5). These symptoms may be minimized by administering the drug with meals.

Visual changes may be observed with the 4-aminoquinolines. Blurred vision may signal reversible impairment of accommodation, but retinal or corneal changes are not reversible. Patients reporting misty vision, patchy vision, or foggy patches in the visual field may be developing serious eye damage. These complaints tend to arise in patients receiving the drugs for long periods.

Headache, dizziness, psychosis, and convulsions may be observed in patients treated with these drugs. In some patients, changes in heart function may be reported. Skin and blood changes may also occur.

The toxic reactions to 4-aminoquinolines are greatly increased when the drugs are used for prolonged periods, as for example long-term malaria prophylaxis. When used in the routine short-term treatment regimens for malaria (Table 38.2), the drugs are better tolerated.

Diloxanide furoate

Mechanism of action. Diloxanide is an effective drug in eliminating *Entamoeba histolytica* from the intestine of persons mildly infected and passing cysts in their stools (Table 38.1). The drug has little effect against acute colitis produced by this parasite and no effect on tissue abscesses.

The biochemical basis for the ameba-destroying action of diloxanide is not known.

Absorption, distribution, and excretion. Diloxanide is administered orally and is well absorbed by that route. Nevertheless, diloxanide is useful alone only for intestinal amebiasis. Excretion is primarily by the kidney.

Toxicity. Diloxanide is relatively safe, producing few systemic side effects. Flatulence (intestinal gas) is the most frequently reported side effect. Other gastrointestinal disturbances such as nausea, diarrhea, and esophagitis may rarely be encountered.

Emetine and Dehydroemetine

Mechanism of action. Emetine is an alkaloid obtained from ipecac, a botanical used in the past as an emetic. Dehydroemetine is similar to emetine but is thought to be less cardiotoxic than emetine.

Both drugs may block protein synthesis in eukaryotes. Therefore mammalian cells as well as the ameba may be sensitive.

Absorption, distribution, and excretion. Although emetine and dehydroemetine may be absorbed orally, the emetic and irritative properties of these drugs cause them to be poorly tolerated by that route. They are more commonly given by intramuscular or subcutaneous injection. Intravenous injection is to be scrupulously avoided to prevent excessive toxicity to the heart. Both drugs may accumulate in various tissues, including the liver, and be slowly released.

Toxicity. The heart is one site where accumulation of emetine occurs. Symptoms such as tachycardia (fast heart rate) and ECG changes signal that the drug should be discontinued to prevent further cardiac difficulty. Because of this potential for cardiac toxicity, every patient receiving emetine should be hospitalized and the nursing staff should carefully record pulse rates and blood pressure. Dehydroemetine is thought to be less cardiotoxic.

Both drugs may produce gastrointestinal irritation, even when administered parenterally. Muscle weakness and skin lesions may also occur.

Furazolidone

Mechanism of action. Furazolidone is a nitrofuran similar in action to the nitrofurans used to treat urinary tract infections (Chapter 34). Furazolidone is an effective antimicrobial agent against many enteric microorganisms, including *Giardia lamblia*.

Absorption, distribution, and excretion. Furazolidone is administered orally to treat infections of the bowel. Like other nitrofurans, this drug does not achieve high serum concentrations.

Furazolidone is metabolized by the liver. One of the breakdown products is a potent inhibitor of monoamine oxidase (MAO). The inhibition lowers the ability of the body to eliminate catecholamines. Therefore hypertension may result. In addition, this action makes drugs such as sympathomimetics (ephedrine, phenylephrine in nasal decongestants) and MAO inhibitors (e.g., pargyline) or foods rich in tyramine (cheese, beer, wine) special risks for these patients.

Toxicity. Furazolidone may produce hemolytic reactions, especially in patients who have G-6-PD deficiency. Allergies and gastrointestinal symptoms may also occur. Patients receiving furazolidone who also imbibe alcohol may exhibit a disulfiram-like reaction with flushing, difficulty in breathing, and a feeling of constriction in the chest (Chapter 40).

Iodoquinol

Mechanism of action. Iodoquinol is an effective amebicidal agent (Table 38.1) whose action is thought to be related to the iodine content of the drug.

Absorption, distribution, and excretion. Iodoquinol is administered orally and is not significantly absorbed from the intestine. Iodine is increased in the bloodstream, however, which suggests that some drug is absorbed or that the iodine is absorbed following breakdown of the drug in the gut.

Toxicity. Iodoquinol is relatively nontoxic. Skin eruptions may occur. Nausea and other gastrointestinal symptoms have been reported.

Iodoquinol can affect the thyroid gland and increase blood iodine levels.

Prolonged high doses of iodoquinol may occasionally produce optic neuritis or atrophy and other signs of neuropathy.

Mebendazole

Mechanism of action. Mebendazole is an effective broad-spectrum antihelminthic agent (Table 38.4). Mebendazole blocks glucose uptake in sensitive helminths. Since these organisms require externally supplied glucose to maintain energy levels, blockade of glucose absorption will ultimately destroy the worms.

Absorption, distribution, and excretion. Mebendazole is used orally for its action against intestinal helminths. Very little of the drug is absorbed into systemic circulation. The small amount of drug that enters the bloodstream is metabolized and excreted by the kidney.

Toxicity. Mebendazole produces few toxic reactions. A few reports of abdominal discomfort and diarrhea exist, but these symptoms may result from large masses of worms being expelled.

Mebendazole is teratogenic in rats but has not produced birth defects in dogs, sheep, or horses. It is difficult to predict the effects in humans. Therefore physicians may limit the use of mebendazole, especially during pregnancy.

Metronidazole

Mechanism of action. Metronidazole attacks amebae at intestinal and other tissue sites (Table 38.1). The drug has also been used to treat trichomoniasis (Table 38.3). Metronidazole is most effective against anaerobes, being reduced in those organisms to a form that directly damages DNA.

Absorption, distribution, and excretion. Metronidazole is well absorbed following oral administration. The drug is metabolized by various pathways. Both metabolites and the unchanged drug appear in urine. Some patients will observe a reddish brown discoloration of the urine while receiving metronidazole. This discoloration is caused by a colored metabolite of metronidazole. Patients should be reassured that the discoloration is harmless.

Toxicity. Metronidazole can produce gastrointestinal symptoms of various types. Some patients experience a sharp, metallic taste, as well as nausea, diarrhea, vomiting, epigastric pain, and abdominal cramping. Although annoying, these symptoms rarely necessitate stopping the medication.

Metronidazole can rarely cause changes in function of the central nervous system. Dizziness, ataxia (incoordination affecting walking), numbness, and paresthesias may be seen. These symptoms may signal that metronidazole should be withdrawn.

Metronidazole may also produce discomfort in the pelvic organs. Patients describe a sense of pressure in that region. Dysuria, cystitis, and dryness of the vagina may be experienced.

Metronidazole causes an alarming reaction when ethyl alcohol is ingested. Patients experience intense flushing, nausea, headaches, and abdominal cramps. This reaction is similar to that experienced by patients taking both disulfiram and ethyl alcohol (Chapter 40).

Metronidazole may potentiate the action of warfarin. Patients receiving both drugs should be carefully observed for signs of bleeding.

Because of its action on DNA, metronidazole may be mutagenic or carcinogenic in some experimental animals. This potential problem precludes the routine use of the drug in pregnant women.

Niclosamide

Mechanism of action. Niclosamide is an extremely effective drug against cestodes (tapeworms). These segmented flatworms are killed by a single dose of niclosamide, which blocks their respiration and glucose uptake. The dead worm segments are frequently digested by proteolytic agents in the gut. For this reason, a cathartic may be given 1 or 2 hours after the drug has been administered to allow the dead but still intact worm parts to be identified in the feces. This purge is a therapeutic necessity when the tapeworm infestation is caused by the pork tapeworm. With this organism, digestion of the dead worm segments releases living eggs, which can develop in humans and cause more serious, invasive disease. The purge removes the worm segments before they rupture and prevents this complication.

Absorption, distribution, and excretion. Niclosamide is not absorbed from the bowel and exerts all of its actions within the lumen of the bowel.

Toxicity. Niclosamide is almost without toxicity. Systemic toxicity is not a problem, since the drug is not absorbed. Some patients have mild gastrointestinal symptoms on the day of therapy.

Pentamidine

Mechanism of action. The action of this drug against *Pneumocystis carinii* is not completely understood. Pentamidine has been reported to inhibit oxidative phosphorylation and thymidylate synthetase, actions that would interfere with biosynthesis of phospholipid, protein, and nucleic acids. The drug also binds to nucleic acids.

Absorption, distribution, excretion. Pentamidine is poorly absorbed orally and causes local tissue damage when given intramuscularly. For these reasons, the most common route of administration is the intravenous one. For prophylaxis of *P. carinii* pneumonia, pentamidine may be aerosolized. When administered by this route, the drug is carried into the lung in tiny droplets of a size carefully controlled to allow deposition into the alveoli, where *P. carinii* lodges. Therefore, high concentrations are achieved at the site of infection, but because systemic absorption from the lung is very low, whole body toxicity is minimized.

Pentamidine is concentrated in renal tissue and excreted primarily in urine. Little metabolism occurs. Complete elimination from the body is slow, with drug appearing in urine as long as 8 weeks after therapy stops.

Toxicity. Patients receiving pentamidine parenterally may suffer acute hypotension. Cardiac arrhythmias have also occurred and have caused deaths. Hypoglycemia may be severe. Long-term effects of pentamidine may include hyperglycemia or diabetes mellitus. Nephrotoxicity and blood dyscrasias can also develop.

The incidence of side effects can vary, depending upon the type of patient being treated. In general, AIDS patients suffer more of the major and minor reactions to pentamidine than do other patients.

Piperazine

Mechanism of action. Piperazine is effective for treatment of ascaris and pinworm infestations (Table 38.4). The drug apparently blocks the action of acetylcholine on the muscles of these parasites. As a result, the worms are paralyzed and are eliminated from the bowel by normal peristaltic flow. The eliminated worms are alive.

Absorption, distribution, and excretion. Piperazine is well absorbed following oral administration. A portion of the drug is metabolized to various inactive products. The kidney is the primary route for excretion. Patients with impaired renal or hepatic function may be more sensitive to piperazine than normals.

Toxicity. Piperazine produces few toxic effects at the doses routinely used to treat helminthic infestations. Gastrointestinal upset and occasional skin rashes have occurred. Transient neurological signs ranging from headache and dizziness to ataxia, paresthesias, or convulsions have been seen, but these more severe reactions are more common with overdoses. The more severe reactions also occur in patients with renal dysfunction, who tend to accumulate the drug.

Povidone-iodine

Mechanism of action. Povidone-iodine is a general antiseptic agent whose antiseptic effect is produced by the release of free iodine. The agent is widely used as a skin antiseptic in preparation for various medical procedures. In addition, povidone-iodine is used topically to treat *Trichomonas vaginalis* infections (Table 38.3).

Absorption, distribution, and excretion. Povidone-iodine is used topically in the vagina. Absorption is usually minimal, but some patients display a rise in iodine levels in the blood.

Toxicity. Povidone-iodine may prove irritating to tissues in some patients. Iodine toxicity is usually not a problem unless the patient is highly sensitive or is treated for extended periods.

Primaquine

Mechanism of action. Primaquine is a relative of the 4-aminoquinoline family of antimalarial agents. It apparently has a mechanism of action different from those agents, but the exact mechanism by which primaquine kills certain forms of plasmodia remains unknown (Table 38.2).

Absorption, distribution, and excretion. Primaquine is well absorbed following oral doses. Drug concentrations in the plasma peak within 6 hours of the dose, but the drug is extensively metabolized and rapidly cleared from the bloodstream.

Toxicity. Primaquine given at normal therapeutic doses produces little toxicity. Abdominal cramps and epigastric distress can occur, but these symptoms can usually be relieved by taking the drug with meals.

Primaquine may damage red blood cells. The drug blocks the production of an intracellular reducing agent, NADPH. In normal cells this deficit is made up by glucose metabolism, and the cell continues to function normally. However, patients with reduced levels of glucose-6-phosphate dehydrogenase (G-6-PD) cannot utilize glucose rapidly enough to make up the deficit. The red blood cells in these patients accumulate oxidized products such as methemoglobin, which is not an efficient oxygen carrier. Cyanosis may result. Ultimately, these red blood cells may rupture. Hemolysis can be severe and is always a sign that drug dosage should be reduced or the treatment terminated. One sign of hemolysis that may be seen easily is darkening of the urine.

Primaquine toxicity is more severe in patients lacking G-6-PD. The lack of G-6-PD is genetically determined and exists in high proportions of certain populations such as Sardinians, Sephardic Jews, Greeks, and Iranians. Blacks are less prone to this deficiency than these groups but have a higher incidence than the Caucasian population of the United States. Patients discovered to have these increased sensitivities to primaquine may be given lower doses of the drug.

Pyrantel pamoate

Mechanism of action. Pyrantel is a depolarizing neuromuscular blocking agent, similar in action to succinylcholine and decamethonium. Pyrantel causes spastic paralysis and gradual contraction of the muscle in worms (Table 38.4). The parasites are then eliminated from the body by normal peristal-

sis. Pyrantel is effective, when given in short courses, against a variety of worms. Purges are not necessary adjuncts to therapy with this drug. Piperazine may antagonize the action of pyrantel.

Absorption, distribution, and excretion. Pyrantel is not absorbed from the gastrointestinal tract to any great extent. What little drug is absorbed is excreted by the kidneys. Pyrantel produces its desired effects entirely within the lumen of the bowel.

Toxicity. Since pyrantel is not well absorbed following oral dosage, few systemic effects occur. Headache, muscle twitching, and dizziness may occur as a result of central nervous system effects of this drug. More commonly the drug causes mild gastrointestinal upset and transient changes in liver function tests.

Pyrimethamine

Mechanism of action. Pyrimethamine is an effective inhibitor of the enzyme dihydrofolate reductase in plasmodia. Pyrimethamine therefore blocks the formation of tetrahydrofolic acid (THFA), a cofactor required for several metabolic transformations. The blocked enzyme normally converts dihydrofolic acid (DHA) to THFA. The formation of DHA may be blocked by sulfonamides (Chapter 34). Combining pyrimethamine and a sulfonamide is an example of synergistic effects being produced by drugs blocking sequential steps in a metabolic pathway. Another example is trimethoprim and sulfamethoxazole (Chapter 34).

Absorption, distribution, and excretion. Pyrimethamine is well absorbed following oral administration. The drug is metabolized and appears in the urine as metabolites. Pyrimethamine appears in the milk of nursing mothers.

Toxicity. Pyrimethamine, as it is normally used in treating chloroquine-resistant malaria, produces few side effects. In higher doses, such as those used to treat toxoplasmosis, the drug may impair host folic acid metabolism, leading to megaloblastic anemia and various other blood dyscrasias. Treatment with leucovorin (a folinic acid supplement) may be required. Large doses may also produce nausea and vomiting, which may be controlled partly by administering the drug with meals.

Pyrvinium pamoate

Mechanism of action. Pyrvinium inhibits energy metabolism in facultative anaerobic organisms such as the intestinal parasitic worms. The drug is most effective against pinworm infestations (Table 38.4), killing all the parasites in a large percentage of cases following a single dose.

Absorption, distribution, and excretion. Pyrvinium is not absorbed from the gastrointestinal

Drugs to Treat Neoplastic Diseases

39

Neoplastic disease occurs when normal cells become transformed by chemicals, viruses, or unknown agents and thereby become resistant to normal controls that regulate cell division and other cellular processes. To understand the treatment regimens used in cancer chemotherapy, it is necessary to understand cell proliferation processes in normal and cancerous tissues. Therefore in this chapter the cell cycle and the principle of selective toxicity as applied to neoplastic disease are discussed, as well as specific agents used in cancer therapy and the rationale behind certain successful therapeutic regimens.

THE CELL CYCLE

The cell cycle is the orderly sequence of events that occurs during the process of cell division, or reproduction. The cycle is usually divided into several segments, according to the processes that occur during that phase. The first event in the cycle is a rapid increase in RNA synthesis compared to the low level of RNA formation found in nonproliferating cells. RNA is formed from the sugar ribose and the purine and pyrimidine bases uracil, cytosine, adenine, and guanine. The phase during which RNA synthesis begins is called G_1 (Figure 39.1).

The next phase in the cell cycle is the S phase, during which DNA synthesis occurs. DNA is the nucleic acid that forms the chromosomes and contains the genetic information for the cell. DNA is formed from the same components as RNA except that thymine is substituted for uracil and deoxyribose is substituted for ribose.

When DNA synthesis is complete, the cell contains twice the amount of DNA found in a nondividing cell. At this point RNA and protein synthesis increase and the cell enters the G_2 phase. At the end of this phase the cell contains enough material to form two complete cells, and mitosis begins.

In mitosis the DNA condenses to form chromosomes. As mitosis begins, the cell has two copies of each chromosome. To separate these pairs so that one copy of each chromosome goes into each daughter cell, the cell forms microtubules, which are organized into the mitotic spindle. Without the mitotic spindle to pull the chromosomes into opposite ends of the cell, reproduction would halt. Once the chromosomes have been successfully segregated into two complete sets, the division process may be completed by closing the cell membrane to divide the mother cell into two daughter cells.

After cell division, a cell may either immediately re-enter the reproductive cycle or may become temporarily nonreproductive (G_0). In this nonreproductive phase the cell does not carry out a large amount of nucleic acid or protein synthesis, although normal metabolic processes continue. A cell in the G_0 phase may become altered so that it is no longer capable of dividing or it may, after a variable time, return to the proliferation cycle and enter phase G_1 (Figure 39.1).

Most normal tissues have very few cells actively reproducing at any one time. Most of the cells are either temporarily or permanently incapable of division. There are exceptions to this rule, however. For example, bone marrow is the site for formation of blood cells and as a result is constantly undergoing cell division. Lymphoid tissue is the site for formation of lymphocytes and monocytes and therefore has a high rate of cell division. The intestinal lining, testes, ovaries, and endometrium are all additional sites of relatively rapid cell division.

NATURE OF NEOPLASTIC DISEASE
Origin of Cancer

Carcinogenesis is the process by which a normal cell is transformed into a cancerous cell. Agents called *carcinogens* may cause this transfor-

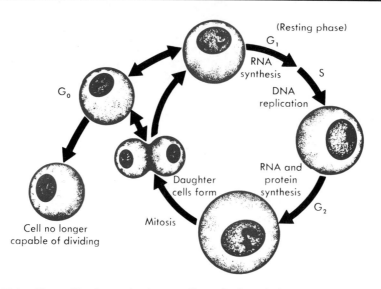

FIGURE 39.1   The proliferative cycle of mammalian cells. In actively dividing cells, the metabolic processes required for cell division take place at different times during the cycle. DNA synthesis precedes messenger RNA and protein synthesis; these processes must be complete before mitosis, or cell division, can occur. Because of their metabolic differences, cells at different phases of this cycle have different sensitivities to many of the drugs used to control cancer.

mation but other factors are also involved. *Oncogenes* are altered regulatory genes that are associated with cancer. When these genes are expressed, normal regulation of cell growth is lost. As a result, the transformed cells gain the ability to proliferate indefinitely, as opposed to most normal cells that either do not proliferate or do so for a limited time. The altered metabolism of cancer cells reflects this commitment to proliferation. DNA and RNA synthesis is increased, along with other metabolic processes necessary for growth and cell division.

Spread of Cancer

Cancer cells also lose the normal property called *contact inhibition.* Contact inhibition prevents normal cells from dividing once they have begun to be crowded together, but cancer cells continue to divide even when the pressure of the surrounding cell mass is considerable. Uncontrolled proliferation and loss of contact inhibition explain in part how a cancer develops in the human body. In certain tissues, as the cancer cell begins to proliferate in an uncontrolled manner, the cells form a solid mass and crowd surrounding normal tissue as the mass, or tumor, grows. In other tissues such as bone marrow, growth of the neoplastic cells is more diffuse, but ultimately normal marrow tissue is overwhelmed and crowded out by the cancerous tissues.

Cancer cells also possess the ability to *metas-*

tasize. In this process cancer cells separate from the original mass and move directly or are transported by blood or lymph to distant sites. There the cells lodge in healthy tissue and begin to divide, thus producing a metastasis (secondary tumor). Tumors have been produced in experimental animals with single cancer cells. This property of cancer cells explains why cure of malignant neoplasms may require destruction of every cancer cell in the body.

Host Responses to Cancer

In theory, one cancer cell left living after therapy is sufficient to cause recurrence of cancer in humans. This situation is quite different from that which occurs in antibacterial chemotherapy. With bacterial infections, therapy can be successful if the bacteria are simply stopped from growing long enough for the immune system to attack and eliminate the invaders. But with neoplastic disease the immune system seems much less effective. One reason for this difference is that cancer cells are not easily recognized as foreign by the host immune system. Another factor that seems to lower the immune response to cancer is that as the tumors become massive, they produce a specific immune tolerance. Whatever the cause, chemotherapy for most cancers must proceed with little assistance from the host mechanism that so powerfully assists antibacterial agents. This factor helps explain why

Table 39.1 Tissue of Origin for Types of Cancer

Cancer	Tissue of origin
Carcinoma	Epithelial cells (e.g., skin and mucous membranes of lung and gastrointestinal tract)
Leukemia	Blood-forming organ (e.g., bone marrow or lymphoid tissue)
Lymphoma	Lymphoid tissue
Melanoma	Pigmented skin cells
Myeloma	Bone marrow
Sarcoma	Connective tissue (e.g., bone, cartilage, and others)

therapy of neoplastic diseases is so much less effective than therapy of bacterial infections.

Chemotherapy of Cancer

Another difficulty in treating neoplastic diseases lies in the fact that the cancer cell offers fewer targets for selective toxicity than does a bacterial cell, for example. This similarity in structure and metabolic processes reminds us again that the cancer cell is derived from host cells. Luckily, some differences between normal and cancerous cells can be identified, but the differences are mostly quantitative rather than qualitative. The specific targets for selective toxicity are discussed with individual drug mechanisms.

Since cancer arises initially as a single transformed cell, it is obvious that diagnosis cannot be expected until much later in the course of the disease. A single cell after 10 cycles of cell division could be expected to produce at most 1024 cells, a mass far too small to be noticed. By the time the tumor weighs about 1 Gm, it will have gone through about 30 division cycles. At 1 Gm tumor is roughly 1 cubic centimeter in volume or approximately the size of a small grape. In many locations within the body, a tumor this size may easily escape detection, yet in just 10 more cell divisions this tumor could exceed a mass of 1 kg (2.2 lb).

In fact, most tumors do not grow nearly as rapidly as the theoretical example just cited, in which it was assumed that every cell formed immediately re-entered the reproductive cycle. Certain cancers are rather slow growing and are described as having a low growth fraction. This description simply means that most of the tumor cells are temporarily or permanently incapable of division. Other tumors have a very fast growth rate with a high growth fraction.

Diseases Called Cancer

The lay public tends to think of cancer as a single disease, but in fact it is a large family of related diseases. Cancers may be categorized according to the tissue of origin (Table 39.1). Within these large categories, many subdivisions are possible. For example, leukemias can arise from any of the various cells within the bone marrow. Therefore myelogenous leukemias (arising from myeloid tissue in the marrow), lymphocytic leukemias (arising from cells forming lymphocytes), and other forms of the disease exist.

Some tumors give rise to characteristic disease patterns. For example, Burkitt's lymphoma, Wilms' disease, Hodgkin's disease, and choriocarcinoma all tend to strike a certain age and sex of patient (Table 39.2, p. 578).

SPECIFIC ANTINEOPLASTIC DRUGS
Agents That Directly Attack DNA

The genetic information necessary for cell reproduction resides in DNA. Although normal nucleated cells contain all the genetic information required to form new cells, this information is seldom expressed, since normal cells in most tissues rarely divide. For this reason, damage to the DNA of many normal cells will be undetectable, since the damage would be revealed only when the cell attempted to undergo division. This rationale explains the use of a large group of anticancer drugs called *alkylating agents*. These drugs form highly reactive compounds in the body, compounds that react with many chemicals including nucleic acids. The damage these chemicals do to DNA frequently makes the cell incapable of replication.

Alkylating agents may attack DNA in its double-stranded form, attaching various compounds to one strand or the other. Other agents may form cross-links, or chemical bonds between the strands. Since the strands must unwind and separate during replication, cross-linking effectively blocks replication.

The specificity of agents that destroy nucleic acid is not great. All cells will suffer attack by these chemicals, although the action is lethal primarily when cells attempt division. Therefore normal tissues with high growth fractions will be expected to show toxicity with these agents. Clinical symptoms to be expected would include: bone marrow suppression, producing rapid or delayed leukopenia, thrombocytopenia, or other blood dyscrasias; mucocutaneous reactions including stomatitis or other signs; gastrointestinal toxicity, including acute or delayed nausea and vomiting.

Table 39.2 Selected Neoplastic Diseases

Disease	Characteristics
Burkitt's lymphoma	Rapidly growing tumor of lymphoid tissue; highly responsive to chemotherapy.
Choriocarcinoma (gestational trophoblastic tumors)	Rapidly growing tumor of embryonic cells; seeded in mother during abortion, childbirth, or following hydatidiform mole; highly responsive to chemotherapy.
Ewing's sarcoma	Rapidly growing tumor most frequently found in children; responsive to combination of surgery, radiation, and chemotherapy in early stages.
Hodgkin's disease	Tumor of the lymph nodes, spleen, and other lymphoid tissue; highly responsive to chemotherapy.
Lymphocytic leukemia	Cancer of lymphoid tissue causing leukocytes in blood to be lymphocytes or lymphoblasts; response to therapy is best in acute form of the disease.
Myelogenous leukemia	Cancer of myeloid tissue leading to excess granular polymorphonuclear leukocytes in blood; response to therapy not as good as in lymphocytic leukemia.
Wilms' tumor	Rapidly growing tumor of children; highly responsive to combination of surgery, radiation, and chemotherapy.

The alkylating agents chemically alter DNA and are mutagenic. Many of these drugs also have immunosuppressive activity. For these reasons, this class of anticancer agents can induce cancers of various types, which may show up months to years after exposure to the drug. Not every patient will develop a second cancer as a result of chemotherapy, but for patients exposed to the alkylating agents, the risk is increased several fold over the normal low incidence rate.

The clinical properties of antineoplastic drugs that directly attack DNA are summarized in Table 39.3.

Mechlorethamine (nitrogen mustard)

Mechanism of action. Mechlorethamine is a potent alkylating agent that may attack DNA at one site or may cause cross-linking.

Mechlorethamine is especially useful in lymphomas but may also be useful in selected leukemias and solid tumors.

Absorption, distribution, and excretion. Mechlorethamine is so highly unstable that it must be administered intravenously immediately after the solution is prepared. The drug is so highly reactive that it is destroyed within minutes of its injection into the bloodstream. No active drug appears in urine or is excreted by any other route.

Toxicity. Mechlorethamine is an extremely toxic agent with a very narrow margin of safety. Significant toxicity is to be expected in every treated patient.

Bone marrow suppression usually may be noted within a day of therapy and will progress to a nadir (lowest point) within 1 to 3 weeks. The platelet count may decrease sufficiently to cause bleeding gums and small subcutaneous hemorrhages. Recovery from the varied symptoms of bone marrow suppression may take several weeks. Nausea and vomiting are acute toxic reactions commonly encountered with mechlorethamine and are thought to be triggered by a central nervous system mechanism. A short-acting barbiturate and an antiemetic may be required to control this reaction.

Germinal tissue may be severely damaged by mechlorethamine. Males may suffer complete arrest of spermatogenesis. Females may suffer menstrual irregularities. Fetuses of treated mothers are damaged by mechlorethamine.

Mechlorethamine may induce malignancies of various kinds. The drug is also an immunosuppressant and predisposes the patient to infections.

Mechlorethamine is a potent vesicant (substance producing blistering). Patients and medical personnel must be rigorously protected from improper contact with the drug. Because of its instability, the drug must be dissolved immediately before use. The nurse or physician should wear surgical gloves for protection while the solution is being prepared and administered. Using a 10 ml sterile syringe, 10 ml of sterile water (or saline) should be injected into the vial. The vial should be shaken with the needle still in place and the appropriate amount of drug removed. This amount of the drug solution should be injected directly into a freely flowing intravenous line. This procedure avoids the danger of extravasation (leakage into tissues around the vein), which produces extreme pain and tissue destruction.

Melphalan (PAM, L-PAM, phenylalanine mustard)

Mechanism of action. Melphalan is a derivative of nitrogen mustard that works very similarly to nitrogen mustard. Melphalan is therefore not specific for the cell cycle phase.

Table 39.3   Clinical Summary of Anticancer Drugs That Directly Attack DNA

Generic name	Trade name	Administration/dosage‡	Comments
Bleomycin	Blenoxane*	INTRAMUSCULAR, INTRAVENOUS, SUBCUTANEOUS: *Adults and children*—0.25 to 0.50 units/kg weekly or twice weekly initially; decreasing to 1 unit daily or 5 units weekly for maintenance.	Bleomycin is used as palliative therapy for lymphomas, squamous cell carcinomas, testicular and ovarian carcinomas. Pulmonary toxicity, which may be fatal, occurs especially when the total dose exceeds 400 units. Skin reactions are common.
Busulfan	Myleran*	ORAL: *Adults and children*—60 to 120 µg/kg daily or 1.8 to 4.6 mg/M² body surface area daily. FDA Pregnancy Category D.	Busulfan may prolong survival in cases of chronic myelocytic leukemia. Toxicity is mainly observed in bone marrow.
Carmustine	BiCNU*	INTRAVENOUS: *Adults*—200 mg/M² as a single dose or divided into equal doses administered on successive days. Dose may be repeated no more frequently than every 6 wk.	Carmustine is used in palliative therapy of tumors of the central nervous system, certain myelomas, and lymphomas. Bone marrow suppression is delayed and may be severe. Pain at injection site is common and severe if drug is infused too rapidly.
Chlorambucil	Leukeran*	ORAL: *Adults and children*—0.1 to 0.2 mg/kg daily for 3 to 6 wk. Smaller doses may be used for maintenance therapy.	Chlorambucil is effective in treating lymphocytic leukemias, lymphomas. Bone marrow suppression is the most commonly encountered side effect.
Carboplatin	Paraplatin	INTRAVENOUS: *Adults*—infusion, 360 to 400 mg/M² once every 4 wk. FDA Pregnancy Category D.	Carboplatin is used as a palliative therapy in recurrent ovarian carcinoma. Carboplatin is similar to cisplatin but causes less renal toxicity.
Cisplatin	Abiplatin† Platinol* Platinol-AQ†	INTRAVENOUS: *Adults*—100 mg/M² once every 4 wk, after heavy hydration to protect the kidneys. Doses of 20 mg/M² daily for 5 days, repeated at 3 wk intervals, are used when vinblastine and bleomycin are also being employed.	Cisplatin is used to treat testicular cancer and carcinomas in many tissues. Renal damage may be severe. Nausea and vomiting, ototoxicity, neurotoxicity, and anaphylactic reactions may occur.
Cyclophosphamide	Cytoxan* Neosar Procytox†	ORAL: *Adults and children*—1 to 5 mg/kg daily for maintenance. INTRAVENOUS: *Adults and children*—40 to 50 mg/kg total dose over 2 to 5 days for induction of remission. 3 to 5 mg/kg twice weekly for maintenance.	Cyclophosphamide is effective in treating lymphomas, leukemias, myelomas, and certain solid tumors. Hemorrhagic cystitis and bladder fibrosis may occur.
Dacarbazine	DTIC† DTIC-Dome	INTRAVENOUS: *Adults*—2 to 4.5 mg/kg for 10 days every mo or 250 mg/M² for 5 days every mo. FDA Pregnancy Category C.	Dacarbazine is used to treat malignant melanoma and lymphomas. Bone marrow suppression is maximal 16 to 20 days after therapy. Pain and tissue damage result if drug leaks from intravenous line into surrounding tissue.
Lomustine	CeeNU*	ORAL: *Adults*—130 mg/M² as a single dose. Repeated no more frequently than every 6 wk.	Lomustine is similar in use and properties to carmustine.

*Available in Canada and United States.
†Available in Canada.
‡The doses listed are representative. Very different doses and schedules may be indicated in specific diseases or protocols.

Continued.

Table 39.3 Clinical Summary of Anticancer Drugs That Directly Attack DNA—cont'd

Generic name	Trade name	Administration/dosage‡	Comments
Mechlorethamine or nitrogen mustard	Mustargen*	INTRAVENOUS: *Adults*—0.4 mg/kg total dose in 1 or several doses. Doses range from 6 to 10 mg/M², depending on the disease. INTRACAVITARY: *Adults*—0.2 to 0.4 mg/kg.	Mechlorethamine is useful in treating Hodgkin's disease and other lymphomas. Mechlorethamine may be palliative for certain solid tumors and their pleural effusions. Bone marrow suppression begins soon after therapy and continues to a nadir at 1 to 3 wk. Pain and severe tissue damage result if drug leaks from the intravenous line into surrounding tissue.
Melphalan	Alkeran*	ORAL: *Adults*—0.15 mg/kg daily for 2 to 3 wk or 0.25 mg/kg daily for 4 days. After recovery of the bone marrow for 1 mo, 2 to 4 mg may be taken daily.	Melphalan is useful in treating multiple myeloma and may be helpful in certain tumors of the reproductive tract. Bone marrow suppression is an expected, dose-related reaction.
Mitomycin	Mutamycin*	INTRAVENOUS: *Adults*—20 mg/M² as a single dose or 2 mg/M² daily for 5 days separated by a 2-day interval. Neither schedule should be repeated more frequently than every 6 to 8 wk.	Mitomycin is useful in the treatment of gastrointestinal tumors. Bone marrow suppression is gradual and progressive. Renal toxicity may occur. Mitomycin produces local necrosis when it contacts skin or soft tissues.
Mitoxantrone	Novantrone	INTRAVENOUS: *Adults*—12 mg/M² daily for 2 or 3 days for consolidation or induction, with other drugs. FDA Pregnancy Category D.	Mitoxantrone causes severe myelosuppression; a high percentage of patients may suffer infections. Mitoxantrone is used in acute nonlymphocytic leukemia.
Pipobroman	Vercyte	INTRAVENOUS: *Adults*—for polycythemia vera, 1 mg/kg daily for 30 days, then 0.1 to 0.2 mg/kg for maintenance. For chronic myelocytic leukemia, 1.5 to 2.5 mg/kg daily, adjusted according to leukocyte count.	Pipobroman is used primarily for polycythemia vera. Bone marrow depression is delayed for 4 weeks after start of therapy.
Thiotepa (Triethylenethiophosphoramide)	Thiotepa	INTRAVENOUS: *Adults*—0.2 mg/kg for 5 days every 4 wk. TOPICAL: *Adults*—30 to 60 mg in solution (sterile water) for application at tumor site.	Thiotepa is used in palliative therapy for certain carcinomas and rarely lymphomas. Bone marrow toxicity is dose related and delayed for several days or weeks after therapy is begun.

*Available in Canada and United States.
‡The doses listed are representative. Very different doses and schedules may be indicated in specific diseases or protocols.

Some difference in mechanism must exist between melphalan and cyclophosphamide, another alkylating agent, since cross-resistance between these two drugs seems not to occur.

Absorption, distribution, and excretion. Melphalan is adequately absorbed orally in most patients. The drug persists in the blood longer than most alkylating agents, being detectable for up to 6 hours after a single dose.

Toxicity. Melphalan produces bone marrow suppression. Dosages are usually adjusted to produce mild leukopenia but no further damage. High doses can produce severe bone marrow depression and bleeding, as well as nausea and vomiting.

Pipobroman

Mechanism of action. Pipobroman is a polyfunctional alkylator that can react with DNA, as do other alkylating agents. The drug is administered primarily in polycythemia vera, and has been used in chronic myelocytic leukemia.

Absorption, distribution, excretion. Pipobroman is well absorbed following oral administration, but the fate of the drug in the body is not yet known.

Toxicity. Bone marrow suppression is the common dose-limiting side effect, causing leukopenia, thrombocytopenia, and anemia. Hemolysis may also occur. In addition, abdominal cramping, anorexia, diarrhea, nausea, and vomiting may occur.

Mitoxantrone

Mechanism of action. Mitoxantrone is reactive in some way with DNA, but the exact mechanism is unknown. The drug is not specific for a particular phase of the cell cycle. Mitoxantrone is used in acute nonlymphocytic leukemia.

Absorption, distribution, excretion. Mitoxantrone is available for intravenous use only. The drug is metabolized in the liver and excreted to some degree in the bile. Little drug appears in urine. However, the drug or its metabolic products add a blue-green color to the urine for 24 hours after each dose.

Toxicity. Mitoxantrone is an extremely potent myelosuppressant, which limits its clinical utility. Up to two thirds of treated patients experience some signs of infection. Most patients also suffer some gastrointestinal irritation or distress. Approximately one third of patients experience pulmonary toxicity with cough or dyspnea. CNS side effects also occur in up to one third of patients.

Chlorambucil

Mechanism of action. Chlorambucil is chemically related to mechlorethamine and is cytotoxic by the same mechanism. Chlorambucil is distinguished by being the slowest acting and the least toxic of the nitrogen mustard alkylating agents.

In addition to its cell cycle nonspecific cytotoxicity, chlorambucil displays a somewhat selective lympholytic action. The latter property makes chlorambucil an effective drug in treating chronic lymphocytic leukemia, Hodgkin's disease, lymphomas, and multiple myelomas.

Absorption, distribution, and excretion. Chlorambucil is administered orally. Large doses (20 mg or more) may produce nausea and vomiting, but more common doses are well tolerated and reliably absorbed. The drug is commonly given 2 hours after the evening meal or in the morning at least 1 hour before breakfast. The drug is metabolized by the liver.

Toxicity. Chlorambucil commonly produces bone marrow suppression, although at normal doses the effects are usually mild and reversible.

Chlorambucil can produce central nervous system stimulation, gastrointestinal irritation, pulmonary fibrosis, liver toxicity, and skin reactions at high doses, but these responses are not commonly seen with normal clinical doses.

Uric acid in the blood can reach dangerous levels following chlorambucil treatment. Patients should be observed for this reaction and treated appropriately to avoid severe renal damage.

Chlorambucil is often very well tolerated when used at low doses for maintenance therapy.

Cyclophosphamide

Mechanism of action. Cyclophosphamide is a noncytotoxic form of nitrogen mustard that must be activated by liver microsomal enzymes. Several metabolites of cyclophosphamide are formed in the liver, and at least one of these metabolites is a potent alkylating agent with activity similar to that of nitrogen mustard. Since the drug as administered is not active, it does not possess the strong vesicant activity of other nitrogen mustards.

Cyclophosphamide seems especially effective against lymphoid or myeloid tissue proliferation. The drug is therefore useful to treat various lymphomas, myelomas, and leukemias.

Absorption, distribution, and excretion. Cyclophosphamide may be used either orally or parenterally, which is a distinct advantage over most alkylating agents. Absorption by the oral route is good, with the absorbed drug passing through portal circulation directly to the liver where the drug is activated.

The metabolites of cyclophosphamide are excreted primarily by the kidney. The plasma half-life of the drug and metabolites is 4 to 6 hours. The metabolites are well distributed throughout the body and may enter the brain.

Toxicity. Cyclophosphamide produces all the expected side effects of nonspecific alkylating agents. Bone marrow suppression occurs and is frequently used to guide the physician in adjusting doses. In most patients the bone marrow begins to recover 7 to 10 days after the drug is discontinued.

Gastrointestinal toxicity with cyclophosphamide is common, usually consisting of nausea and vomiting although more severe reactions can occur.

Hair loss (alopecia) occurs with cyclophosphamide therapy much more commonly than with other drugs of this class. Most patients report regrowth of hair after therapy.

Immunosuppression is an expected side effect. The drug has in fact been used directly for its immunosuppressive activity in rheumatoid arthritis and other nonneoplastic conditions.

Cyclophosphamide suppresses gonadal tissue, and the effects may be irreversible. Complete suppression of the menstrual cycles and of sperm formation have been reported.

Cyclophosphamide and its metabolites are excreted predominantly through the kidney. The accumulation of these cytotoxic compounds in the urinary bladder can produce a direct hemorrhagic cystitis. Patients should receive ample fluids while this drug is being used and should be encouraged to void frequently to reduce the damage to the bladder. Bladder fibrosis and carcinoma are somewhat increased in incidence in patients receiving long-term therapy with cyclophosphamide.

Several other drugs affect the metabolism and distribution of cyclophosphamide in the body. Allopurinol seems to prolong the plasma half-life of cyclophosphamide. Barbiturates induce the microsomal enzymes that activate cyclophosphamide, whereas corticosteroids and sex steroids may inhibit the enzymes and thereby lower the rate of formation of active metabolites of cyclophosphamide.

Busulfan

Mechanism of action. Busulfan is an alkylsulfonate capable of cross-linking DNA, as well as reacting with other substances. For reasons that are unclear, busulfan possesses a degree of selectivity that is unique among this class of drugs. Busulfan is a myelosuppressant at doses that do not significantly lower the levels of other blood cells, although platelets may be reduced. Because of this selectivity, busulfan is used in chronic myelocytic leukemia. The drug is not curative but prolongs life and improves its quality.

Absorption, distribution, and excretion. Busulfan is well absorbed orally and is used by this route in chronic intermittent therapy. The drug is highly reactive in blood and tissues and is rapidly converted in the body to a variety of breakdown products, which are excreted by the kidney and other routes.

Toxicity. Busulfan may produce leukopenia (lowered white blood cells), beginning usually after 7 to 10 days of therapy. Hemorrhage may ultimately result if the drug is not discontinued. With long-term therapy, many body systems may show signs of toxicity.

Busulfan may destroy large numbers of granulocytes during therapy. These dying cells release chemicals that may be converted to uric acid, excessively elevating the blood levels of uric acid. To avoid the toxicity produced by uric acid, allopurinol may be given during busulfan therapy.

Triethylenethiophosphoramide (Thiotepa)

Mechanism of action. Thiotepa is the only member of the class of compounds called *ethylenimines* that remains useful as an anticancer drug. The drug is a nonspecific alkylating agent.

Thiotepa is not curative but may alleviate the symptoms of certain carcinomas or malignant effusions. Since the drug is so nonselective, attempts are often made to apply the drug directly to the tumor when possible. For example, bladder carcinoma may be treated by instilling the drug directly into the bladder. This type of therapy allows high doses to be achieved at the tumor site, with lower doses escaping into systemic circulation. Since toxicity is dose related, such a treatment regimen minimizes systemic toxicity.

Absorption, distribution, and excretion. Thiotepa is employed only by parenteral injection or topical application. The drug is relatively nonirritating and can be administered rapidly through intravenous lines. Impaired renal function may lower tolerance to thiotepa.

Toxicity. Thiotepa is primarily toxic to the bone marrow. Since the drug produces its effects slowly, care must be taken not to damage excessively the bone marrow by too high a dose in the early stages of therapy. White blood cell counts may be used as an index of toxicity. The drug may also produce nausea and anorexia.

Carmustine (BCNU) and lomustine (CCNU)

Mechanism of action. Carmustine is a rapidly acting alkylating agent affecting numerous enzymes as well as nucleic acids. The drug can cross-link the strands of DNA. Lomustine is chemically related to carmustine and, like that drug, not only alkylates DNA but has widespread metabolic effects as well. One advantage carmustine and lomustine have over many other alkylating agents is that both drugs penetrate the blood-brain barrier very well. They are therefore of primary use in controlling the symptoms produced by central nervous system tumors.

Absorption, distribution, and excretion. Carmustine is administered by intravenous infusion. The drug is very rapidly degraded so that only metabolites are detectable in blood or in tissues a few minutes after the dose is administered. The metabolites are excreted by the kidney for several days following therapy. The suggestion has been made that these metabolites of carmustine are the active form of the drug.

Lomustine is used orally, being well absorbed by that route. Once absorbed, it is metabolized and excreted similarly to carmustine.

Toxicity. Carmustine and lomustine cause a greatly delayed bone marrow suppression. Following a single dose of drug, bone marrow function may fall for an extended period, reaching its lowest point 4 to 6 weeks after therapy. For this reason, doses must be given no more frequently than every 6 weeks or at more widely spaced intervals if the bone marrow does not promptly recover.

Pulmonary fibrosis may be an insidious side effect with these drugs. Cough or shortness of breath should be investigated quickly for cause. Nausea and vomiting are dose-related toxic reactions to carmustine and lomustine. Carmustine is highly irritating and may cause hyperpigmentation if it touches the skin. Pain during infusion of the drug is common. Patient discomfort can be reduced by slowing the rate of infusion of the drug and by properly diluting it before use.

Carmustine is a relatively unstable compound that decomposes in solution. The drug in the dry form in the unopened vial may also decompose at temperatures above 80° F (or 27° C). Only clear, colorless solutions freshly prepared (or stored for short periods in the cold) should be used.

Lomustine capsules are relatively stable when stored at room temperature in sealed containers.

Dacarbazine

Mechanism of action. Dacarbazine apparently acts as an alkylating agent after being activated in the liver. The drug may have other actions as well, but it clearly is cell cycle nonspecific.

Dacarbazine is used to treat malignant melanoma and occasionally other tumors.

Absorption, distribution, and excretion. Dacarbazine must be administered intravenously. The plasma half-life is about 30 minutes, and the drug appears to be concentrated in the liver.

Dacarbazine is secreted by the renal tubule, about half the drug dose being excreted by this route. The remaining half of the drug dose appears in the blood as a metabolite.

Toxicity. Dacarbazine causes delayed bone marrow toxicity (16 to 20 days after therapy). Many patients also report nausea and vomiting within a few hours following therapy. Tolerance to this symptom develops.

Dacarbazine can cause severe pain and tissue damage if allowed to escape from the vein into surrounding tissues.

Cisplatin (CPDD) and Carboplatin

Mechanism of action. Cisplatin and carboplatin are platinum-containing complexes that apparently act like alkylating agents. These drugs cross-link DNA and are not specific for cell cycle.

Cisplatin was first used to treat metastatic testicular tumors, but is now also used in other genital and urinary tract tumors. Carboplatin is currently indicated only for palliative therapy in recurrent ovarian carcinoma. These drugs are investigational in other tumors.

Absorption, distribution, and excretion. Cisplatin and carboplatin must be administered intravenously. The effects of single doses last for weeks.

Toxicity. Cisplatin is a relatively toxic drug that almost always causes severe nausea and vomiting. The drug is also toxic to the renal tubule and may cause serious damage with high doses or too frequent administration. Myelosuppression manifested by lowered leukocyte and platelet counts persists for 3 weeks or longer after a single injection of cisplatin.

Cisplatin causes hearing loss in the upper frequency ranges and ringing in the ears (tinnitus). Ototoxicity tends to progress with repeated doses.

Carboplatin causes dose-dependent bone marrow suppression, with leukopenia, neutropenia, thrombocytopenia, and anemia. Transfusion may be necessary.

Carboplatin causes less renal toxicity than does cisplatin and is less likely to cause severe nausea and vomiting, although most patients experience some degree of nausea with or without vomiting.

Peripheral neuropathies may occur and may be irreversible with either drug. Loss of taste has also been reported.

Anaphylactoid reactions may occur when cisplatin or carboplatin is given to patients who have previously received these platinum-containing agents.

Bleomycin

Mechanism of action. Bleomycin is a complex mixture of glycopeptides derived from cultures of *Streptomyces*. The drug is therefore frequently referred to as an antibiotic (a compound produced by one life form with growth-inhibitory properties toward other life forms). Bleomycin directly attacks DNA, producing breaks in the strands. The drug may also inhibit enzymes that normally repair damaged DNA. Bleomycin apparently attacks cells at several stages of the cell cycle.

Bleomycin has been used against squamous cell carcinomas, lymphomas, and testicular carcinomas.

Absorption, distribution, and excretion. Bleomycin must be administered parenterally. Most tissues of the body rapidly inactivate bleomycin. Skin and lung are exceptions, and the drug tends to concentrate at those sites and there produce toxic reactions. Tumors tend not to inactivate bleomycin, so the drug is also concentrated there.

Toxicity. Bleomycin frequently produces skin and mucous membrane changes, as well as fever, chills, anorexia, and vomiting. Pulmonary reactions occur in 10% of treated patients and 1% may die. Lung toxicity begins as pneumonitis and progresses to pulmonary fibrosis. Anaphylaxis may also occur. Bleomycin usually does not suppress the bone marrow.

Mitomycin

Mechanism of action. Mitomycin is an antibiotic derived from cultures of *Streptomyces*. The drug is activated by enzymes in the body so that it becomes capable of alkylating DNA. Like other alkylating agents, mitomycin is nonspecific for cell cycle.

Mitomycin seems most effective against tumors of the stomach, intestine, rectum, and pancreas, although the drug has been occasionally used against other tumors as well.

Absorption, distribution, and excretion. Mitomycin must be given intravenously, since it is not absorbed orally and is highly irritating to skin and muscle. The drug apparently enters several organs but not the brain.

Toxicity. Mitomycin produces severe and progressive myelosuppression. Leukopenia (lowered white blood cells) and thrombocytopenia (decreased platelets in the blood) occur within 3 to 8 weeks and may persist for up to 10 weeks or longer after therapy. Mitomycin should not be readministered until platelet and white cell counts show the bone marrow to have recovered.

Mitomycin also frequently causes nausea and vomiting, skin rashes, and hair loss. A few patients may also suffer renal failure with hemolysis, liver toxicity, and lung damage.

Mitomycin causes local necrosis if allowed to escape into cutaneous tissues during intravenous injection.

Agents That Block DNA Synthesis (S-phase Inhibitors)

The uncontrolled proliferation of cancerous cells is frequently expressed as rapid cell division or as a high growth fraction. This property distinguishes cancers from most normal tissues, where a very low growth fraction is the rule. Since only those cells in the S phase of the cell cycle synthesize DNA, it is these cells that are most sensitive to agents that block the synthesis of DNA from purine and pyrimidines.

Drugs may block DNA synthesis in several ways. Some of the drugs in this section are specific enzyme inhibitors and prevent the action of an enzyme that is required for DNA synthesis. Other drugs that are chemically very similar to the natural purines and pyrimidines used to form DNA may be incorporated into DNA but make the DNA unstable and nonfunctional.

Obviously, a cell that is not forming DNA will not be damaged by a drug that inhibits DNA synthesis. For this reason, nonproliferating cells or cells in resting phase are relatively insensitive to the drugs discussed in this section. These drugs are referred to as *cycle-specific* or *phase-specific* drugs, since they affect primarily cells in S phase.

This property of phase specificity explains why these drugs must be given on a repeating schedule. In a single treatment, only the growing fraction of cells in the tumor will be affected. A recovery period with no drug given allows normal tissues with high growth fractions, such as bone marrow, to return to normal function. During this recovery period, many cells in the cancerous tissue will move from G_0 phase into the reproductive cycle. Other cells that were not in S phase during treatment will continue to proliferate and the tumor will continue to grow. Repeated widely spaced doses of the drug gives the maximum opportunity for the drug to catch the dividing cells in S phase when they will be sensitive.

Since the specificity of these drugs is only toward active DNA synthesis, many normal cells will be sensitive. At highest risk of toxicity are tissues with a high growth fraction. Bone marrow depression and suppression of lymphocyte formation are characteristic side effects of these drugs. Lowered lymphocyte formation reduces the ability of the patient to fight infection (immunosuppression), which may reduce the patient's chance for survival. Gastrointestinal mucosa also has a high growth fraction and is a target of serious toxic reactions to the drugs of this family.

The clinical properties of cycle-specific anticancer drugs are summarized in Table 39.4.

Cytarabine

Mechanism of action. Cytarabine is a chemical analog of cytidine, a normal component of DNA.

Table 39.4   Clinical Summary of Anticancer Drugs That Block DNA Synthesis

Generic name	Trade name	Administration/dosage‡	Comments
Cytarabine, or Ara-C	Cytosar*	INTRAVENOUS BOLUS: *Adults and children*—100 mg/M² daily for 10 days or until toxicity intervenes or remission occurs. INTRAVENOUS INFUSION: *Adults and children*—100 to 200 mg/M² daily for 10 days or until toxicity intervenes or remission occurs. SUBCUTANEOUS: *Adults and children*—1 mg/kg once or twice per wk.	Bone marrow suppression limits the use of this drug. Cytarabine is used to induce and maintain remission in leukemia patients.
Floxuridine	FUDR	INTRAARTERIAL: *Adults*—0.1 to 0.3 mg/kg over 24 hr.	Floxuridine is used as palliative therapy for solid tumors not treatable by other means. Toxicity as for fluorouracil.
Fluorouracil, or 5-FU	Adrucil* Efudex* Fluoroplex	INTRAVENOUS: *Adults*—12 mg/kg for 4 days as initial therapy. Less frequent administration of same dose is used for maintenance therapy when toxicity allows. TOPICAL: *Adults*—used as 1%, 2%, or 5% solution or cream.	Fluorouracil is used as palliative therapy for solid tumors that are incurable by surgery or other means. Gastrointestinal and hematological toxicity limit the use of this drug. Topical fluorouracil is used to treat multiple actinic (solar) keratoses. Local reactions include pain, dermatitis, swelling, and scarring.
Hydroxyurea	Hydrea*	ORAL: *Adults*—doses range from 20 to 30 mg/kg daily up to 80 mg/kg every 3 days.	Hydroxyurea is used to treat melanoma, myelocytic leukemia, and carcinomas of various tissues. Bone marrow suppression occurs.
Mercaptopurine	Puri-nethol*	ORAL: *Adults and children over 5 yr*—2.5 mg/kg/day initially. May continue for weeks if toxicity does not supervene.	Mercaptopurine is used to produce remissions in leukemia, especially those of childhood. Delayed hematological toxicity may limit the use of this drug. Immunosuppression may occur.
Methotrexate*	Folex Mexate	ORAL: *Adults and children*—2.5 to 30 mg daily for various lengths of time, depending on the disease. INTRAMUSCULAR: *Adults and children*—15 to 30 mg daily for 5 days. INTRAVENOUS: *Adults and children*—0.4 mg/kg daily for 4 days of therapy or twice weekly to maintain remissions. INTRATHECAL: *Adults and children*—0.2 to 0.5 mg/kg up to 12 mg total. Administered every 2 to 5 days until response is noted. FDA Pregnancy Category X.	Methotrexate is curative for choriocarcinoma. Methotrexate is used to maintain remissions in childhood lymphoblastic leukemia. Methotrexate is effective or palliative in certain lymphomas and solid tumors. Gastrointestinal toxicity frequently limits the use of this drug. Bone marrow depression commonly occurs. Immunosuppression may increase the susceptibility of the patient to infections.

*Available in Canada and United States.
‡The doses listed are representative. Very different doses and schedules may be indicated in specific diseases or protocols.

Continued.

Table 39.4 Clinical Summary of Anticancer Drugs That Block DNA Synthesis—cont'd

Generic name	Trade name	Administration/dosage‡	Comments
Procarbazine hydrochloride	Matulane Natulane†	ORAL: *Adults*—2 to 4 mg/kg daily for the first wk; then 4 to 6 mg/kg daily until bone marrow toxicity supervenes. On recovery of marrow, drug may be continued at 50 to 100 mg daily. *Children*—doses between 50 and 100 mg daily.	Procarbazine is used to palliate symptoms of Hodgkin's disease, lymphomas, and selected brain tumors. Bone marrow depression is frequently used to guide dosage adjustments. Gastrointestinal disturbances and neurological reactions occur.
Thioguanine	Lanvis† Thioguanine	ORAL: *Adults*—2 mg/kg daily initially. May continue for weeks if toxicity does not supervene.	Thioguanine is used for myelocytic leukemia. Delayed hematological toxicity occurs.

†Available in Canada.
‡The doses listed are representative. Very different doses and schedules may be indicated in specific diseases or protocols.

Cytarabine resembles cytidine well enough to interfere with the function of the enzyme DNA polymerase, which inserts cytidine into DNA but which cannot insert cytarabine. Therefore cytarabine slows or stops DNA synthesis.

Although cytarabine has been tested in other tumors, it is at present used almost exclusively in leukemias.

Absorption, distribution, and excretion. Cytarabine must be injected, either subcutaneously, intrathecally, or intravenously. Subcutaneous injections are employed only to maintain remissions and are given once or twice a week.

Intravenous cytarabine may be given as a rapid bolus or as a slow continuous infusion. When the drug is given rapidly, higher doses may be tolerated, although nausea and vomiting are usually triggered. Infusion of the daily dose of the drug can take place over a 1-hour period or longer.

Cytarabine is rapidly inactivated by enzymes that deaminate the molecule. Blood and liver enzymes apparently contribute to this process.

Cytarabine does not easily pass into the cerebrospinal fluid. If the drug is administered intrathecally, it may persist in the cerebrospinal fluid for several hours, since that fluid has a low level of the deaminating enzyme that inactivates cytarabine.

Toxicity. Cytarabine is a potent bone marrow suppressant, acting on that tissue by the same mechanism effective in cancer cells. Most treatment programs call for increasing the dose of cytarabine until the toxicity to the bone marrow becomes intolerable. Bone marrow depression is most profound roughly 5 to 7 days after the drug is stopped. Recovery of marrow function takes at least 2 weeks for most patients and longer for those receiving the drug for extended periods.

Cytarabine is also a potent immunosuppressant. The drug also causes significant gastrointestinal toxicity in many patients. Some may suffer perforation or necrosis of the bowel. CNS toxicity is reported in up to 10% of treated patients.

Fluorouracil and floxuridine

Mechanism of action. Fluorouracil and floxuridine are synthetic pyrimidine bases, which may be converted in the body to an active agent (floxuridine monophosphate). This active form of fluorouracil resembles the pyrimidine that is directly incorporated into RNA or that is converted to the pyrimidine called *thymidylate*. Thymidylate is used exclusively for DNA synthesis. Fluorouracil and floxuridine disrupt these pathways in at least two ways. First, the activated drug may enter RNA, creating a defective form of that nucleic acid that does not support normal protein synthesis. Second and more importantly, thymidylate synthetase, the enzyme required to form thymidylate for DNA synthesis, is inhibited. With thymidylate synthetase blocked, DNA synthesis halts. Therefore, functionally both fluorouracil and floxuridine are S phase inhibitors. Both fluorouracil and floxuridine are used exclusively in solid tumors, and both must be considered palliative rather than curative.

Absorption, distribution, and excretion. Fluorouracil absorption by the oral route is erratic, and the drug is commonly given intravenously. For most patients, best results seem to be produced by giving loading doses intravenously for 5 consecutive days followed by lower doses administered once a week thereafter.

Fluorouracil is extensively metabolized by the liver and other tissues. Less than 15% of the drug dose appears as active drug in the urine. Fluorouracil is cleared from the bloodstream within 3 hours of an intravenous injection, but the effects persist much longer.

The route of administration of floxuridine determines its metabolic fate and its effectiveness. If floxuridine is given intravenously by rapid injection, the drug is broken down to fluorouracil and thence to the normal breakdown products of fluorouracil. When floxuridine is given slowly by intraarterial infusion, metabolism to fluorouracil is minimized and most of the drug is converted to floxuridine monophosphate, the metabolically active form. The intraarterial route requires a lower dose, yet is more effective than intravenous administration.

Toxicity. Both fluorouracil and floxuridine are highly toxic to the gastrointestinal tract. Inflammation of the membranes of the mouth and pharynx may be an early sign of such toxicity. Nausea, vomiting, and diarrhea almost always occur, and if the drug is not discontinued, duodenal ulcers may occur and the bowel may perforate. Patients with preexisting poor nutritional status are at much greater risk with these drugs and are usually not considered candidates for therapy.

Blood dyscrasias also occur with fluorouracil and floxuridine and may cause termination of therapy. Leukopenia (reduced white blood cells) continues for 1 or 2 weeks after therapy is terminated. Various skin reactions and hair loss (alopecia) also occur but are not serious enough to cause the drug to be discontinued.

Mercaptopurine (6-Mercaptopurine, 6-MP) and Thioguanine (TG, 6-TG)

Mechanism of action. Mercaptopurine resembles both adenine and guanine and blocks several points in the synthesis of these nucleic acid precursors. Thioguanine blocks two reactions, which are also sensitive to mercaptopurine. As a result of the blockade of purine synthesis, DNA synthesis is blocked by either drug. Therefore both mercaptopurine and thioguanine are S phase–specific inhibitors.

Absorption, distribution, and excretion. Mercaptopurine is adequately absorbed from the gastrointestinal tract following oral dosage. The drug is not directly irritating to the mucosal lining of the gastrointestinal tract.

Mercaptopurine has a half-life of about 90 minutes in the bloodstream. Part of the dose is excreted by the kidney but significant metabolic degradation also occurs. Mercaptopurine produces remissions in leukemias, being most effective in acute lymphoblastic leukemias of childhood. The properties of thioguanine are similar to those of mercaptopurine.

Toxicity. Bone marrow suppression may occur with mercaptopurine or thioguanine. Anemia may contribute to weakness and fatigue.

Mercaptopurine is also an immunosuppressant. This action of the drug may reduce host immune defenses and contribute to increased risk of infection in the treated patient.

Mercaptopurine toxicity may be greatly increased by concomitant treatment with allopurinol. Allopurinol blocks uric acid synthesis and is frequently used to prevent toxic accumulation of that substance following extensive tumor cell destruction by chemotherapy. However, allopurinol is also an inhibitor of the metabolism of mercaptopurine. Therefore, when the drugs are combined, more mercaptopurine persists in the bloodstream and in tissues for longer periods, and greater toxicity results. Thioguanine metabolism is not significantly affected by allopurinol.

Methotrexate

Mechanism of action. Methotrexate is commonly described as a folic acid antagonist, since it prevents the conversion of the vitamin folic acid to its metabolically active form, tetrahydrofolate (THF). Without THF, cells are unable to carry out 1 carbon–transfer reactions, and normal metabolism is blocked at several points. One of these blockades prevents the formation of thymidylic acid, and another arrests adenine and guanine nucleotide synthesis in an early state. Without these precursors, DNA synthesis halts. Methotrexate is therefore specific for the S phase of the cell cycle.

Methotrexate is particularly effective in treating choriocarcinoma, an invasive tumor arising from disseminated fetal cells in new mothers. The drug is also used against a variety of other solid tumors. The most common current use is in maintaining remissions in various leukemias, especially acute lymphoblastic (stem-cell) leukemia of childhood.

Absorption, distribution, and excretion. Methotrexate may be administered by oral, intramuscular, intravenous, intraarterial, or intrathecal route. For many patients, the oral route is satisfactory, since effective serum concentrations are reached within 1 hour. Parenteral administration

Table 39.5   Clinical Summary of Anticancer Drugs That Block RNA and Protein Synthesis

Generic name	Trade name	Administration/dosage‡	Comments
Asparaginase	Elspar Kidrolase†	INTRAMUSCULAR: *Children*—6000 i.u./M² with doses administered every 3 days for one mo; with other drugs. INTRAVENOUS: *Adults and children*— 200 i.u. (international units)/kg daily for 28 days, or 1000 i.u./kg daily for 10 days when used after prednisone and vincristine.	Asparaginase is used to induce remissions in acute lymphocytic leukemia in children. Allergy to asparaginase occurs frequently and may include anaphylaxis. Central nervous system depression or other signs of central nervous system effects may occur.
Dactinomycin	Cosmegen*	INTRAVENOUS: *Adults*—0.5 mg/M² once weekly for 3 wk. *Children*—0.015 mg/kg or 0.45 mg/ M² for 5 days.	Dactinomycin is useful to treat choriocarcinoma, Wilms' tumor, and various sarcomas and carcinomas. Bone marrow depression, gastrointestinal irritation, and skin reactions are common. Dactinomycin is extremely corrosive and must not be allowed to escape from the vein or to contact the skin during intravenous injection.
Daunorubicin	Cerubidine*	INTRAVENOUS: *Adult*—30 to 60 mg/M² through a running line daily for 3 days. Treatment may be repeated every 3 to 6 wk, but lifetime dose should not exceed 550 mg/M². *Children*—25 mg/M² once weekly, with vincristine and prednisone.	Daunorubicin is used primarily for leukemias and neuroblastoma. Toxicity is as for doxorubicin.
Doxorubicin	Adriamycin*	INTRAVENOUS: *Adults*—60 to 75 mg/M² as a single injection repeated no more often than every 3 wk. *Children*—30 mg/M² daily for 3 days; repeat every 4 wk.	Doxorubicin is effective against leukemias, lymphomas, sarcomas, and various carcinomas. Bone marrow depression, gastrointestinal irritation, and alopecia are commonly encountered. Heart toxicity is encountered, especially when total doses approach 500 mg/M². Doxorubicin produces local necrosis when it contacts skin or soft tissues.
Plicamycin	Mithracin	INTRAVENOUS: *Adults*—0.025 to 0.050 mg/kg every other day for 8 doses.	Plicamycin is useful for treating embryonal cell carcinoma and certain metastatic bone tumors associated with hypercalcemia. Plicamycin produces gastrointestinal, skin, liver, and kidney toxicity. Severe bleeding episodes may occur and progress after therapy. Plicamycin produces local necrosis when it contacts skin or soft tissues.

*Available in Canada and United States.
†Available in Canada.
‡The doses listed are representative. Very different doses and schedules may be indicated in specific diseases or protocols.

Table 39.6 Clinical Summary of Anticancer Drugs That Block Mitosis

Generic name	Trade name	Administration/dosage‡	Comments
Etoposide VP-16	VePesid*	ORAL: *Adults*—100 mg/M² daily for 5 days. Repeat every 3 to 4 wk. INTRAVENOUS: *Adults*—50 to 100 mg/M² daily for 5 days. Repeat every 3 to 4 wk.	Etoposide is used for refractory testicular tumors and small cell lung carcinoma. Bone marrow suppression is the primary toxic reaction.
Vinblastine, or VLB	Velban Velbet† Velsar	INTRAVENOUS: *Adults*—doses must start at 0.1 mg/kg weekly and increase gradually. Final dose is limited by bone marrow toxicity. Range is usually 0.15 to 0.2 mg/kg weekly.	Vinblastine is used in palliative treatment of various lymphomas and selected tumors of other tissues. Peripheral neuropathy and bone marrow suppression occur. Vinblastine causes local necrosis if allowed to seep around veins during intravenous injection.
Vincristine, or VCR	Oncovin* Vincasar	INTRAVENOUS: *Adults*—up to 1.4 mg/M² as a single dose. *Children*—up to 2 mg/M² as a single dose.	Vincristine is effective in treating acute leukemia, lymphomas, various sarcomas, and Wilms' tumor. Peripheral neuropathy is common and limits the drug dose. Vincristine causes local necrosis if allowed to seep around veins during intravenous injection.

*Available in Canada and United States.
†Available in Canada only.
‡The doses listed are representative. Very different doses and schedules may be indicated in specific diseases or protocols.

results in a slightly faster absorption rate. The intrathecal route is required to treat leukemias that have penetrated the central nervous system. Methotrexate does not pass from the bloodstream into the cerebrospinal fluid in useful amounts.

Methotrexate is well distributed throughout the body and may accumulate to a degree in some tissues. Liver cells seem especially able to bind the drug for long periods. It also persists in the kidney. These tissue sites of drug accumulation normally account for a small fraction of the total dose of methotrexate. Most of the drug is excreted directly by the kidney. The body apparently degrades methotrexate little, if at all, and the excreted drug is unchanged.

Toxicity. Methotrexate produces the classic signs of toxicity for drugs of this class. The rapidly dividing tissues of the gastrointestinal mucosal lining are severely damaged. Stomatitis (inflammation of the oral mucosa) and diarrhea are common signs of toxicity that call for discontinuation of the drug. If therapy continues in the face of these symptoms, severe gastrointestinal damage, including perforation, can result.

Bone marrow function is also compromised

with methotrexate. The result, as with other drugs of this class, is leukopenia (lowered white cell count). Other blood changes may occur and may ultimately produce uncontrolled bleeding.

Methotrexate is an immunosuppressant and may damage the body's ability to fight infection.

The effectiveness and toxicity of methotrexate may be affected by a variety of other drugs. Salicylates (such as aspirin), sulfonamides, phenytoin, tetracycline, and chloramphenicol all tend to increase methotrexate toxicity by displacing methotrexate from plasma proteins. The increase in free plasma methotrexate frequently produces toxicity. Probenecid and other drugs excreted by renal tubular secretion may block the excretion of methotrexate and thereby increase toxicity of the drug.

Methotrexate produces its cytotoxic effects by blocking the conversion of folic acid to THF. It is therefore possible to prevent the action of the drug by supplying the body with THF. This fact has been exploited for treating methotrexate overdose. Tumors such as osteosarcoma are now treated with massive doses of methotrexate. Under ordinary circumstances these doses would destroy the bone marrow and be lethal. However, if the patient re-

Table 39.7   Clinical Summary of Drugs Used to Control Cancer of Specific Tissues

Generic name	Trade name	Administration/dosage	Comments
ANDROGENS			
Testolactone	Teslac	ORAL: *Adults*—250 mg 4 times daily for 12 wk.	Testolactone palliates symptoms of selected carcinomas of the breast in postmenopausal women. Hypercalcemia may occur.
ANTIANDROGENS			
Flutamide	Euflex	ORAL: *Adults*—250 mg every 8 hr.	Flutamide blocks the action of androgens on target cells. Flutamide is used with leuprolide for prostatic carcinoma.
Leuprolide	Lupron*	SUBCUTANEOUS: *Adults*—1 mg daily.	Leuprolide suppresses secretion of androgens. Leuprolide is used with flutamide for prostatic carcinoma.
ESTROGENS			
Chlorotrianisene	TACE	ORAL: *Adults*—12 to 25 mg daily.	Chlorotrianisene is a long-acting estrogen.
Diethylstilbestrol diphosphate	Stilphostrol	INTRAVENOUS: *Adults*—500 mg in 300 ml of saline or 5% dextrose on the first day; 1 Gm/300 ml diluent for subsequent 5 days or longer. Maintain with 250 to 500 mg IV once or twice weekly thereafter, or with oral dosage. ORAL: *Adults*—50 to 200 mg 3 times daily.	As for polyestradiol diphosphate.
Estramustine phosphate sodium	Emcyt*	ORAL: One 140 mg capsule for each 10 kg body weight daily in 3 or 4 doses. Therapy continues for 30 to 90 days or longer.	Estramustine may produce toxicity similar to that of other estrogens. In addition, the nitrogen mustard component of the drug may cause adverse reactions.
Polyestradiol phosphate	Estradurin	INTRAMUSCULAR (DEEP): *Adults*—40 to 80 mg every 2 to 4 wk for at least 3 mo.	Estradiol released from this preparation is palliative therapy for prostatic carcinoma. Increased risk of thromboembolitic disease occurs with estrogen therapy. Estrogens may cause edema, hypercalcemia, mood changes, breast tenderness, abdominal cramps, and increased pigmentation of breast areola.
ANTIESTROGENS			
Tamoxifen	Nolvadex* Tamofen†	ORAL: *Adults*—10 or 20 mg twice daily.	Tamoxifen is used as palliative therapy for advanced carcinoma of the breast. Hot flashes, nausea, and vomiting occur in roughly one fourth of treated patients. Vaginal discharge, menstrual disturbances, and skin rashes may also occur.

*Available in Canada and United States.
†Available in Canada.

Table 39.7   Clinical Summary of Drugs Used to Control Cancer of Specific Tissues—cont'd

Generic name	Trade name	Administration/dosage	Comments
PROGESTINS			
Medroxyprogesterone acetate	Depo-Provera*	INTRAMUSCULAR: *Adults*—400 to 1000 mg in weekly injections.	Medroxyprogesterone acetate is used as palliative therapy for advanced carcinoma of the endometrium or kidney. Menstrual irregularities, breast tenderness, rashes, and thrombolytic disease have been reported.
Megestrol acetate	Megace*	ORAL: *Adults*—40 to 320 mg daily in divided doses for at least 2 mo for endometrial carcinoma; 160 mg daily, divided into 4 doses, for breast cancer.	Megestrol acetate is used only as palliative therapy for advanced carcinoma of the breast or endometrium. Thromboembolytic disease and breast cancer may be increased in treated patients.
GLUCOCORTICOIDS			
Prednisone	Deltasone* Meticorten	ORAL: *Adults and children*—10 to 100 mg daily.	Prednisone is used to treat lymphoblastic leukemias and lymphomas. Long-term use of prednisone may produce Cushing's syndrome.
ADRENAL ANTAGONIST			
Mitotane	Lysodren*	ORAL: *Adults*—6 to 15 mg/kg initially, daily in 3 or 4 doses. Daily dose may be increased gradually to 2 to 16 Gm.	Mitotane is used to control adrenal cortical carcinoma. Gastrointestinal disturbances are common. Central nervous system toxicity and skin reactions also occur in significant numbers of patients.
Trilostane	Modrastane	ORAL: *Adults*—initially 30 mg 4 times daily, increasing gradually to 90 mg 4 times daily. FDA Pregnancy Category X.	Trilostane is used in Cushing's syndrome and adrenal carcinoma to suppress adrenal steroid production.
BETA-CELL ANTAGONIST			
Streptozocin	Zanosar*	INTRAVENOUS: 1 to 1.5 Gm/M^2 weekly or 500 mg/M^2 daily for 5 days at 6-week intervals.	Streptozocin is specific for beta cells of the pancreas and is used for advanced pancreatic tumors. Renal toxicity limits the use of this drug.
INTERFERONS			
Interferon alpha-2a, recombinant	Roferon-A	INTRAMUSCULAR OR SUBCUTANEOUS: *Adults*—3 million units daily for 16 to 24 wk; maintenance is with 3 million units 3 times weekly. FDA Pregnancy Category C.	Used primarily for hairy cell leukemia, but other uses are being investigated.
Interferon alpha-2B, recombinant	Intron A	INTRAMUSCULAR OR SUBCUTANEOUS: *Adults*—2 million units/M^2 3 times weekly. FDA Pregnancy Category C.	Used primarily for hairy cell leukemia, but also for genital warts.

*Available in Canada and United States.

Table 39.8 Representative Combination Chemotherapeutic Regimens

Regimen	Drugs included	Disease
ABVD	Doxorubicin (Adriamycin) Bleomycin (Blenoxane) Vinblastine (Velban) Dacarbazine (DTIC-Dome)	Hodgkin's disease
BACOP	Bleomycin (Blenoxane) Doxorubicin (Adriamycin) Cyclophosphamide (Cytoxan) Vincristine (Oncovin) Prednisone	Non-Hodgkin's lymphomas
CHOP	Cyclophosphamide (Cytoxan) Doxorubicin (Adriamycin) Vincristine (Oncovin) Prednisone	Non-Hodgkin's lymphomas
CMF	Cyclophosphamide (Cytoxan) Methotrexate Fluorouracil	Breast carcinoma
CVP	Cyclophosphamide (Cytoxan) Vincristine (Oncovin) Prednisone	Non-Hodgkin's lymphomas
MOPP	Mechlorethamine (Mustargen) Vincristine (Oncovin) Procarbazine hydrochloride (Matulane) Prednisone	Hodgkin's disease
POMP	Prednisone Vincristine (Oncovin) Methotrexate Mercaptopurine (Purinethol)	Acute lymphocytic leukemia

ceives intravenous leucovorin (citrovorum factor), an agent containing THF and other folic acid forms, the bone marrow can be protected. This type of therapy is called *citrovorum*, or *leucovorin, rescue.*

Procarbazine hydrochloride

Mechanism of action. Procarbazine has multiple effects on cellular enzyme systems and nucleic acids. The drug apparently can cause oxidation of nucleic acids. In addition, nucleic acid synthesis is inhibited.

Procarbazine is especially useful in Hodgkin's disease.

Absorption, distribution, and excretion. Procarbazine is well absorbed after oral administration. The drug rapidly equilibrates between plasma and cerebrospinal fluid, so it is potentially useful in brain tumors. Procarbazine is excreted primarily by the kidney.

Toxicity. Procarbazine frequently produces bone marrow depression and gastrointestinal disturbance. Neurological signs may also appear. It inhibits monoamine oxidase. Patients should therefore not receive both procarbazine and drugs that elevate biogenic amine levels (i.e., sympathomimetics, tricyclic antidepressants, phenothiazines, and tyramine-containing food). Ethyl alcohol can produce a disulfiram-like reaction.

Hydroxyurea

Mechanism of action. Hydroxyurea is an inhibitor of an enzyme that converts the ribonucleotide precursors of RNA to deoxyribonucleotides, which form DNA. Hydroxyurea inhibition of the enzyme tends to block DNA synthesis. Hydroxyurea is specific for the S phase of the cell cycle.

Hydroxyurea has been used to treat melanoma, myelocytic leukemias, carcinoma of the ovary, and combined with radiation therapy to treat head and neck carcinoma.

Absorption, distribution, and excretion. Hydroxyurea is well absorbed when given orally. The drug is excreted by the kidney. Therefore patients with impaired renal function may be more sensitive to the drug than normal.

Toxicity. Hydroxyurea produces bone marrow suppression as the most common side effect. This reaction is reversible. Gastrointestinal disturbances, renal impairment, and skin reactions are reported less frequently.

Agents That Block RNA or Protein Synthesis

The rapid proliferation of cancer cells can be inhibited by certain agents that block the formation of RNA or interfere with the use of RNA as a template for protein synthesis.

These agents are not highly specific for cancer cells but rather interfere with RNA and protein synthesis in any rapidly dividing tissue. The exception to this rule is asparaginase, a drug with some selectivity for cancer cells.

The clinical properties of these drugs are summarized in Table 39.5, p. 588.

Asparaginase

Mechanism of action. Asparaginase is an enzyme that converts the amino acid asparagine to aspartic acid. The therapeutic effect of this agent arises because many types of cancer cells cannot form asparagine. The enzyme destroys circulating asparagine, starving the cancer cells for asparagine. Normal cells are spared, since they can form asparagine internally.

To be most effective, asparagine starvation

should occur in the G_1 phase of the cell cycle. If asparagine levels are kept low during that period, the asparagine-dependent cancer cell will be unable to carry out protein synthesis and, ultimately, RNA and DNA synthesis will cease. If asparagine starvation occurs later in the cell cycle after many critical proteins and nucleic acids have been formed, the cell may not die.

Absorption, distribution, and excretion. Asparaginase is a protein and must therefore be administered by parenteral route. The drug persists in the bloodstream for extended periods and is apparently slowly degraded. It does not enter the cerebrospinal fluid in useful amounts and is not excreted in urine.

Toxicity. Asparaginase produces a wide range of toxic reactions. Since the drug is a protein, it is an effective antigen and may provoke severe allergic reactions. Renal and hepatic function may be impaired, and some patients suffer bleeding episodes, since the drug suppresses various clotting factors. Hyperglycemia has also been observed. Many patients show signs of central nervous system toxicity, including depression, lowered consciousness, coma, and others.

Asparaginase toxicity is increased by vincristine or prednisone. Nevertheless, these drugs are cautiously used together in certain combination treatment regimens.

Dactinomycin (actinomycin D)

Mechanism of action. Dactinomycin is an antibiotic derived from *Streptomyces*. The drug binds strongly to double-stranded DNA and prevents the DNA from serving as a template for RNA synthesis. The cell, unable to form messenger RNA, is thus unable to synthesize proteins and complete cell division.

Dactinomycin is useful in producing remission of choriocarcinoma (tumor of embryonic origin growing in the mother), Wilms' tumor (childhood renal tumor), and certain carcinomas and sarcomas.

Absorption, distribution, and excretion. Dactinomycin is not well absorbed from the gastrointestinal tract. The drug is also extremely corrosive to soft tissues and must therefore be given only by the intravenous route. Dactinomycin is rapidly cleared from the bloodstream, entering the liver and other tissues. The drug does not cross the blood-brain barrier in effective amounts. Excretion of dactinomycin is mainly into bile, with smaller amounts of unchanged drug also appearing in urine.

Toxicity. Dactinomycin is a very toxic drug that must be administered with great care. The highly corrosive nature of the compound makes it imperative that intravenous injection be given properly, with no leakage of drug into tissues surrounding the vein. Such leakage, or extravasation, can cause extensive tissue damage.

Dactinomycin produces significant hematological changes, which may include aplastic anemia. These blood changes are most pronounced several days after therapy.

Gastrointestinal toxicity is severe with dactinomycin. Patients may experience extreme nausea and vomiting within hours of drug administration. Phenothiazine antiemetics may be required to control vomiting. Dactinomycin also irritates the lining of the entire gastrointestinal tract. Patients commonly report cheilitis (lip inflammation), dysphagia (difficulty in swallowing), ulcerative stomatitis (mouth sores), pharyngitis (inflammation of the pharynx), abdominal pain, and proctitis (anal inflammation).

Dactinomycin also severely damages hair follicles, causing hair loss (alopecia). The drug may cause reddening of the skin (erythema) and signs of inflammation, especially in an area also receiving irradiation.

Doxorubicin and daunorubicin

Mechanism of action. Doxorubicin and daunorubicin are antibiotics derived from cultures of *Streptomyces*. These drugs bind strongly to double-stranded DNA and thus stop the formation of RNA. Cells are most markedly affected by these drugs during S and G_2 phases of the cell cycle.

Doxorubicin has a wide range of antitumor activity, including leukemias, lymphomas, sarcomas, genitourinary carcinomas, squamous cell carcinomas of the head and neck, and lung cancer. Daunorubicin has been used primarily in leukemias and neuroblastoma. A related compound, epirubicin (Pharmorubicin), has been used in Canada in carcinoma of the breast.

Absorption, distribution, and excretion. Doxorubicin is not well absorbed orally, is highly irritating to skin and soft tissues, and must therefore be given intravenously. The drug enters many tissues and organs, but it is the liver that metabolizes the drug rapidly and extensively. Most drug elimination occurs through the liver. Doxorubicin does not seem to enter the central nervous system.

Daunorubicin must also be administered intravenously.

Toxicity. Doxorubicin causes delayed leukopenia and other blood changes. Damage to bone marrow limits the amount of drug that may be used and the frequency of administration. Ordinarily, 21 days will be required for the marrow to recover.

Toxicity to the heart also limits the total

amount of drug that can be administered. Total doses of more than 550 mg/M^2 may produce irreversible toxicity to the heart, including ECG changes and congestive heart failure. Preexisting heart disease, prior irradiation to the region of the heart, or prior use of the cardiotoxic drug cyclophosphamide all may greatly increase the likelihood for heart damage with doxorubicin.

Since doxorubicin is metabolized and eliminated by the liver, patients with impaired liver function may suffer drug accumulation and increased toxicity unless doses are appropriately reduced. Some metabolites of doxorubicin and daunorubicin appear in the urine of all treated patients and produce a harmless, red coloration of the urine. Doxorubicin can cause severe tissue necrosis if allowed to escape from the vein during drug administration. Damage to veins may occur if the same vein is used repeatedly.

Hair loss and gastrointestinal irritation commonly occur with doxorubicin.

Daunorubicin causes toxic reactions similar to those seen with doxorubicin.

Plicamycin

Mechanism of action. Plicamycin is an antibiotic derived from *Streptomyces*. The drug binds DNA, thereby preventing RNA synthesis.

Plicamycin also blocks parathyroid hormone activity on osteoclasts, thereby lowering the release of calcium into the bloodstream. This ability to lower blood calcium levels may be useful in patients suffering hypercalcemia as a result of metastatic cancer of the bone.

Plicamycin is also used to treat embryonal cell carcinoma of the testes.

Absorption, distribution, and excretion. Plicamycin must be given intravenously, since oral absorption is poor and the drug damages skin and muscle tissues.

Toxicity. Plicamycin is a very toxic drug whose use must be limited to specific neoplasms where the beneficial results of therapy are known to outweigh the risks. Plicamycin produces anorexia, nausea, vomiting, skin changes, liver damage, kidney damage, and lowered blood concentrations of calcium, potassium, and phosphorus.

Plicamycin also produces an unusual syndrome involving episodes of bleeding from various sites. Nosebleed (epistaxis) frequently signals the onset of this syndrome. The condition may stabilize after a few episodes or may progress to extensive hemorrhage, usually within the gastrointestinal tract, and death.

Agents That Arrest Mitosis

To segregate chromosomes, a dividing cell must form a mitotic spindle composed of microtubules. Microtubules normally function as part of the cytoplasmic transport systems in cells and are required for certain types of cell movement. The major component of microtubules is a protein called *tubulin*.

The structure of microtubules can be disrupted by certain substances that bind to tubulin and cause it to be released from the microtubule. Breakdown of microtubular structure may not be lethal to a cell unless it is in the process of forming the mitotic spindle. Cells exposed at this stage of division are arrested at that point, and reproduction cannot proceed. Ultimately, these cells die. Substances that act in this way are frequently referred to as *mitotic poisons*.

The clinical properties of mitotic poisons used to treat cancer are summarized in Table 39.6, p. 589.

Vincristine (VCR)

Mechanism of action. Vincristine crystallizes microtubular and spindle proteins, halting cell division in the midst of mitosis. Vincristine, which is a complex alkaloid obtained from the periwinkle plant, seems especially effective against lymphomas and lymphoblastic leukemias but is also used to treat various carcinomas and sarcomas as well. A related drug, vindesine (Eldisine), has been used in Canada against acute lymphocytic leukemia.

Absorption, distribution, and excretion. Vincristine must be administered intravenously. The drug does not cross the blood-brain barrier well enough to combat central nervous system spread of leukemia but is distributed well to other tissues.

Vincristine is rapidly cleared from the bloodstream and is concentrated in the liver. The major route of excretion for this drug is via the bile, with less than 5% of the drug appearing in urine. Biliary obstruction or liver impairment can dangerously impede elimination of this drug.

Toxicity. Vincristine doses are usually limited by the peripheral neuropathy it produces. Many symptoms of nerve dysfunction may be observed, but loss of the Achilles tendon reflex is taken as the first sign of neuropathy.

Vincristine is extremely irritating if it is allowed to escape from the vein into surrounding tissues during administration. Severe pain is produced and necrosis may develop in the exposed tissue.

Vincristine produces hair loss (alopecia) in approximately 20% of treated patients. Many patients complain of constipation and abdominal pain, but these symptoms can usually be relieved with enemas and laxatives.

Vincristine does not produce significant bone marrow depression.

Vinblastine (VLB)

Mechanism of action. Vinblastine, like the related vinca alkaloid vincristine, is a cell cycle specific inhibitor of cells in mitosis. The drug causes breakdown of microtubules and prevents formation of the mitotic spindle.

Vinblastine is used to treat various lymphomas and certain carcinomas.

Absorption, distribution, and excretion. Vinblastine must be administered intravenously. Like vincristine, vinblastine does not freely enter the central nervous system, is rapidly cleared from the blood, and is primarily excreted in bile.

Toxicity. Vinblastine produces neurological toxicity similar to that produced by vincristine. Mental depression and headache may accompany the signs of peripheral neuritis or other peripheral neurological disorders.

Vinblastine produces significant bone marrow suppression, primarily leukopenia (reduction of white cells). Leukopenia normally progresses to a low point 4 to 10 days after the dosage, but recovery usually occurs within 7 to 14 days.

Nausea and vomiting are frequent, but this reaction can often be controlled with antiemetic agents. Stomatitis, diarrhea, or constipation can also occur.

Vinblastine can cause phlebitis and cellulitis if the drug is allowed to leak into the tissues during intravenous administration.

Hair loss is common but often reverses even while the drug therapy is continued.

Etoposide (VP-16)

Mechanism of action. Etoposide is a podophyllotoxin derivative. Podophyllotoxins are microtubule or spindle poisons that are naturally found in the American mandrake, or mayapple plant. The semisynthetic derivative etoposide prevents the entry of cells into mitosis, rather than arresting the cells in metaphase.

Etoposide is indicated for refractory testicular tumors. The drug is also useful in treating lymphomas, leukemias, and small-cell lung carcinoma. A chemical relative of etoposide called teniposide (VM-26) is sold in Canada under the trade name Vumon, and is used for lymphomas, leukemias, and neuroblastoma.

Absorption, distribution, and excretion. Although about 50% of a dose may be absorbed orally, etoposide is administered primarily intravenously. The drug is highly protein bound and is slowly eliminated by the kidney, mostly as unchanged drug. Etoposide is lipid soluble but is poorly distributed to the central nervous system.

Toxicity. Etoposide produces bone marrow suppression, anorexia, nausea, vomiting, and hair loss.

Tissue-Specific Agents

Most of the anticancer drugs discussed to this point are not tissue specific in their cytotoxic action. For example, although a drug like chlorambucil is clinically useful because it attacks lymphoid tissue, the drug also attacks other tissues, especially at higher doses.

A few drugs are effective anticancer agents because they interact with specific receptors on or in certain cells. Most of the drugs in this category are derivatives of hormones and interact with those cells bearing specific receptors for the hormone. Glucocorticoids suppress lymphoid tissue because of the specific receptors in that tissue for glucocorticoids.

The sex steroids (androgens, estrogens, and progestins) are also used in cancer chemotherapy. These steroid hormones enter sensitive cells and, complexed with specific receptor proteins, are transported to the cell nucleus. Within the nucleus, these steroids alter RNA and protein synthesis, thereby changing the function of the cell. The use of these agents in cancer chemotherapy depends on a knowledge of the hormone dependence of certain tissues. For example, the prostate gland is dependent on androgens; without these hormones, the gland shrinks and loses function. Estrogens, hormones that produce feminization, antagonize the action of androgens on this tissue. Carcinoma of the prostate gland seems to retain a degree of this hormonal control, and tumor regression can frequently be produced by suppressing androgens and supplying excess estrogens.

Similar results can be achieved in many breast carcinomas in females by treating them with estrogens, antiestrogens, or androgens. To a certain extent, hormonal therapy of tumors of the reproductive tissues is empirical. However, the rationale behind all forms of this therapy is that (1) reproductive tissues proliferate in response to the proper balance of male and female hormones, and (2) tumors of reproductive tissues tend to retain a degree of dependence on hormones. Tumors in postmenopausal women respond to hormone therapy better than do those in premenopausal women.

The clinical properties of these tissue-specific anti-cancer drugs are summarized in Table 39.7, pp. 590-591.

Androgens

Mechanism of action. Androgens can interact with certain reproductive tissues, altering RNA and protein synthesis. This action is independent of the cell cycle. For estrogen-dependent tissues, androgens frequently interfere with estrogen function. Androgens can therefore cause involution of these tissues. This action forms the basis for the use of androgen to control some forms of breast cancer in postmenopausal women. Results of this form of therapy usually do not become evident until after 8 weeks of treatment or longer.

Absorption, distribution, and excretion. Androgens are in general not well absorbed orally, although a few synthetic androgens are exceptions to this rule (Table 39.7). When given by injection, these oil-soluble substances are slowly absorbed from intramuscular sites.

Androgens are metabolized by the liver. Patients with impaired renal function may have difficulty in eliminating the amounts of androgen used therapeutically and may suffer excessive toxicity.

Toxicity. Androgens produce varying degrees of virilization, which in females is observed as an unwanted side effect. Increased libido, edema, hypercalcemia, nausea, and pain on injection occur occasionally with one or more of the androgens used in cancer chemotherapy. The androgens listed in Table 39.7 are used almost exclusively in cancer chemotherapy. Other androgens, used primarily in replacement therapy, may occasionally be used to treat specific cancers. These drugs include fluoxymesterone, methyltestosterone, testosterone enanthate, and testosterone propionate (Chapter 54).

Antiandrogens

Mechanism of action. Flutamide blocks uptake of androgens into cells or the binding of androgens in cell nuclei. Leuprolide is a synthetic analog of luteinizing hormone-releasing factor that on continuous administration suppresses secretion of gonadotropin-releasing hormone. The result is lower synthesis and release of testosterone. These drugs are used in combination for metastatic carcinoma of the prostate, a tumor that is often dependent on androgens for its growth.

Absorption, distribution, and excretion. Leuprolide is a peptide and therefore cannot withstand the acidic environment of the stomach. The drug is absorbed from subcutaneous sites. Flutamide is absorbed orally, but undergoes extensive metabolism in the liver.

Toxicity. When given together, these drugs reduce testosterone levels to those expected in castrated males. Many of the side effects are the result of low testosterone levels. Hot flashes are very common. About one third of patients report reduced libido or impotence. Gynecomastia occurs in about 9% of patients. Nausea and vomiting may also occur. Diarrhea is considered to be more related to flutamide than to leuprolide.

Estrogens

Mechanism of action. Estrogens can interact with certain reproductive tissues, altering RNA and protein synthesis. This action is independent of the cell cycle. For androgen-dependent tissues, estrogens frequently interfere with androgen function. Estrogens can therefore cause involution of these tissues. This action forms the basis for the use of estrogens to control prostatic carcinoma. A certain percentage of carcinomas of the breast also respond to exogenous estrogen therapy, especially in postmenopausal women.

Absorption, distribution, and excretion. Natural steroid estrogens are not absorbed orally, but several of the synthetic, nonsteroidal estrogens may be given successfully by this route. Estrogens are also available for subcutaneous implantation and intramuscular or intravenous injection.

Estrogens are metabolized by the liver. Patients with marked liver impairment may accumulate these compounds.

Toxicity. Estrogens increase the risks of thromboembolytic disease. Estrogens also increase salt and water retention, alter mood in some patients, decrease glucose tolerance, elevate calcium levels, produce nausea and vomiting, and cause breast tenderness and abdominal cramps. Of these reactions, thromboembolytic disease, hypercalcemia, and edema are the most threatening for cancer patients.

Of the many estrogen preparations available, three are recommended primarily for use in prostatic carcinoma (Table 39.7). Many of the estrogens discussed in Chapter 40 may also be used in palliative therapy for prostatic carcinoma or carcinoma of the female breast.

Estramustine phosphate sodium combines estradiol with a nitrogen mustard. The rationale for the combination is that the drug will be most concentrated in estrogen-sensitive tissues, including tumors. In those tissues the anticancer effects of both the estradiol and the nitrogen mustard may be focused. The toxicity of the drug is largely caused

THE NURSING PROCESS

NEOPLASTIC DISEASES

Assessment

Patients requiring chemotherapy may appear with a wide variety of symptoms; they may also be of any age. A complete and thorough total assessment should be done. Additional areas of focus should be based on the probable drugs that will be used and their known side effects. Thus a detailed examination of the mouth might be done; the condition of the hair, skin, and nails recorded; and the height, weight, and vital signs recorded. A detailed history should be obtained, particularly if the patient has received chemotherapy previously. Previous response to chemotherapy will be a guide to the nurse in anticipating response to a repeated dose of chemotherapeutic drugs. Certainly, assessment should focus on any visible signs of cancer, and parameters should be outlined to measure the progress of the cancer and its response to chemotherapy. A variety of laboratory and other diagnostic studies may be obtained. Examples would include the hematocrit, hemoglobin, blood count, liver function studies, renal function studies, bone scans, liver scans, and other scans. Depending on the specific type of cancer, there may be laboratory tests that can be used to monitor the cancer; an example might be alkaline phosphatase in the blood.

Nursing diagnoses

Altered comfort: nausea and vomiting as drug side effect

Self-concept disturbance related to alopecia as a side effect of drug therapy

Fatigue

Management

Management of patients may be very complex, particularly if multiple drugs are being used. Once the decision is made to use one or more agents, additional baseline data should be obtained as needed to identify normal function of certain organs known to be affected by the chemotherapy agents. The nurse should continue to monitor the vital signs, body weight, and the progress of anticipated side effects. For example, regular inspection of the mouth should be done if stomatitis is a frequent side effect of a drug. If alopecia is an anticipated side effect, the degree of hair loss should be noted. When a side effect is known to occur with regularity, preventive or prophylactic measures should be started as soon as possible. Thus oral rinses and gargles with products known to aid in stomatitis should be started as soon as the drug has been administered. Patients known to have serious bouts with nausea and vomiting in association with one or more agents should be treated prophylactically with antiemetics before the chemotherapeutic agents are given. Fluid intake and output should be monitored. Appropriate laboratory work should be monitored and nursing interventions developed in relation to the results of the laboratory work. Thus the person who is experiencing bone marrow depression should be moved to a private room, or other measures should be taken to reduce chances of infection. In some institutions the policy is to place patients with bone marrow depression into protective isolation. Nursing personnel who have colds and other infections should not be permitted to care for individuals with bone marrow depression. If medications are being administered via constant infusion, an infusion control device should be used. Care should be taken to ensure that intravenous infusion lines are patent and that extravasation is avoided. Any new sign or symptom that develops should be thoroughly investigated. Any deviation from the patient's normal values should be noted and evaluated.

Evaluation

Ideally, chemotherapy drugs would eradicate cancer and allow the patient to lead a cancer-free life. Unfortunately, this rarely occurs. In most instances chemotherapy is used with the hope that in a small percentage of cases the cancer will be eradicated, but

Continued.

THE NURSING PROCESS — cont'd

the goal of therapy for most patients is prolongation of life. An exception to this is adjuvant chemotherapy, which is administered to the patient who has had a surgical excision of the cancer but in whom there is a high chance that microscopic amounts of cancer remain behind. In a certain percentage of these patients the chemotherapy kills the few remaining cells, and these patients will be cured. There are only a few drugs that are used by the patient in the home situation for treatment of cancer. For the majority of patients, cancer chemotherapy is administered in the hospital or in the physician's office, since many of these drugs must be administered intravenously. Before a patient with a medication to be taken in the home setting is discharged, the patient should be able to explain how to take the medication correctly, side effects that may occur, how to treat side effects, side effects that require notification of the physician, and any measures to be employed to prevent complications due to side effects. Much of the same information holds true even for the patient who receives chemotherapy in the physician's office. Because the nadir or most profound bone marrow suppression often occurs days to weeks after the drug is administered, it is important that the patient know when to anticipate the side effects and know what actions to take to deal with these side effects. Thus a patient who anticipates a period of bone marrow suppression should be cautioned to avoid exposure to children who often carry communicable diseases and to avoid crowds where infections are spread easily. Patients who are likely to develop thrombocytopenia should be cautioned to avoid activities that would cause excessive bruising and should be informed about restrictions that should be observed to prevent bruising or bleeding, such as limiting dental flossing or excessive brushing of teeth. Finally, all patients should be able to explain which situations require immediate notification of the physician. For additional specific guidelines, see the patient care implications section at the end of this chapter.

by the estrogen component, since release of the active nitrogen mustard into blood is low.

Tamoxifen

Mechanism of action. Tamoxifen is an antiestrogenic substance that seems to block estrogen binding at receptor sites in cells. This action of tamoxifen prevents estrogens from supporting the growth of estrogen-dependent cells. Tamoxifen is therefore most useful in palliating symptoms of breast carcinoma in which estrogen dependence of the tumor has been established. Tamoxifen acts throughout the cell cycle.

Absorption, distribution, and excretion. Tamoxifen is administered orally. The drug is extensively metabolized. Tamoxifen and its metabolites enter the bloodstream slowly, with peak blood concentrations occurring 4 to 7 hours after an oral dose. However, the drug persists in the bloodstream for days as a result of its entry into enterohepatic circulation. Most of the drug is slowly eliminated from the body in the feces. The kidney contributes little to the excretion of this drug.

Toxicity. Tamoxifen may produce cancer and birth defects in animals. It is not known whether tamoxifen produces these effects in humans. The drug seems less toxic than the estrogens and androgens used in anticancer therapy. The drug may occasionally alter platelet or white cell counts, but the changes observed are mild and usually innocuous. The most frequent reactions are nausea, vomiting, and hot flashes. Fewer patients report vaginal bleeding or discharge or menstrual irregularities. These reactions do not usually require discontinuance of the drug.

Patients who are started on tamoxifen therapy sometimes report an increase in pain at the tumor site and within metastases in bone. Tumor metastases within soft tissue may temporarily increase in size and the surrounding tissue may become inflamed. This reaction, sometimes referred to as *disease flare*, may occur even when therapy is effective.

Progestins

Mechanism of action. Progestins normally function to establish secretory function in the estrogen-primed endometrium. The use of progestins as antineoplastic agents has been limited primarily to palliative therapy in endometrial carcinoma.

PATIENT PROBLEM: DEPRESSED WHITE BLOOD CELL PRODUCTION

THE PROBLEM

Some drugs suppress the bone marrow, resulting in decreased production of white blood cells. With some drugs, this is a common side effect and is anticipated, as with many cancer chemotherapy drugs. With other drugs, this side effect is unexpected, and occurs only occasionally. Several medical terms may be used to describe this effect: *agranulocytosis* or *granulocytopenia* (severe reduction in granulocytes—basophils, eosinophils, and neutrophils); or *neutropenia* (reduction in neutrophils). The danger to the patient is the increased susceptibility to infection that results from a decreased supply of granulocytes.

SIGNS AND SYMPTOMS

Fever, sore throat, rash, malaise, chills, urinary frequency, dysuria, altered level of consciousness. If the situation is untreated or unrecognized, the patient may develop a serious bacterial infection requiring intravenous drug therapy and hospitalization. The first line of treatment is to discontinue the drug causing the problem.

NURSING CARE

- Use meticulous handwashing prior to caring for patients with suppressed white blood cell counts.
- Avoid putting patients with granulocytopenia into multibed rooms where other patients have diagnoses of infection. If possible, admit the patient to a private room.
- Use protective isolation only if necessary, as it isolates the patient from family and friends. Rather, screen visitors, and do not permit visits

from individuals with obvious colds, bronchitis, chickenpox, herpes simplex or herpes zoster, childhood infectious diseases, or other infections.
- Avoid the use of rectal thermometers.
- Carefully assess patients who are also receiving steroids, as steroids may mask the symptoms of infection.
- Monitor the complete blood count and white blood cell differential, as well as hematocrit, hemoglobin, and platelets.

PATIENT AND FAMILY EDUCATION

- Notify the physician if the symptoms mentioned above develop.
- Monitor and record the temperature (if the patient is able).
- If a period of bone marrow suppression is anticipated with each course or dose of drug, find out when the nadir of bone marrow suppression will occur. The nadir is the period of greatest bone marrow suppression, or period of lowest white blood count.
- If a period of suppressed white blood cell production is anticipated, as with cancer chemotherapy drugs, avoid contact with persons suffering from colds or infections during periods of greatest susceptibility.
- Wash hands carefully after using the bathroom and after contact with other persons. Ask family members and friends to wash hands carefully before coming in contact with patient.
- Do not bring cut flowers to the patient, or fresh fruits and vegetables, unless the latter are washed carefully.

Absorption, distribution, and excretion. Progestins are available in various forms suitable for oral or intramuscular administration. The drugs are metabolized primarily in the liver; derivatives of progestins appear in the urine.

Toxicity. Progestins usually produce few toxic reactions. Patients should be observed for signs of thromboembolytic disease or sudden changes in vision, which may increase. Fluid retention and disruption of normal menstrual cycles may also occur. Progestins that are injected may cause pain and tissue changes at the injection site.

Progestins in animals may increase the incidence of breast tumors.

Glucocorticoids: prednisone

Mechanism of action. Glucocorticoids are steroid hormones that regulate RNA and protein synthesis in various cells. This action is independent of cell cycle. Prednisone is the glucocorticoid most commonly used as an anticancer agent, although

several of these agents are used for symptomatic relief. Prednisone is an effective anticancer agent because it attacks lymphoid tissue, causing regression of lymphatic tissue. Prednisone is therefore effective against lymphatic tumors and lymphoblastic leukemias, especially in children.

Absorption, distribution, and excretion. Prednisone is effectively absorbed orally and metabolized to the active form of the drug, prednisolone. Liver disease may impair this process and thus interfere with the effectiveness of prednisone.

Toxicity. Prednisone may produce all the well-known signs of glucocorticoid excess, if given long enough at high doses. These symptoms are outlined in Table 39.7 and also in Chapter 53.

Mitotane

Mechanism of action. Mitotane is a derivative of the insecticide DDT. Toxicity studies with the DDT family of insecticides showed specific effects on the adrenal cortex. Mitotane causes specific

PATIENT PROBLEM: BLEEDING TENDENCIES

(May be due to anticoagulant therapy or low platelet count; thrombocytopenia)

THE PROBLEM

The platelet level is low, so the patient bleeds easily, or the patient is receiving anticoagulant therapy to "thin the blood."

SIGNS AND SYMPTOMS

Bruising; petechiae (minute, pinhead size hemorrhagic spots on the skin; seen only with reduced platelets); bleeding, such as bleeding gums, nose bleeds (epistaxis), change in the color of urine which might indicate bleeding in the kidney; anal bleeding; bleeding in stools.

PATIENT AND FAMILY EDUCATION

- Notify physician if unexplained or excessive bleeding or bruising develops.
- Avoid using a razor with a blade; use an electric razor.
- If gums are bleeding, stop flossing teeth until gums no longer bleed. Use a soft-bristle toothbrush. If brushing causes bleeding, stop brushing and use a water-spraying oral care device if available.
- Permit only experienced professionals to draw blood from your veins.
- Do not go barefoot, as foot injuries may be associated with excessive bruising or bleeding.
- Do not permit intramuscular injections if you are receiving anticoagulants or know your platelets are below 60,000.
- Avoid getting constipated; drink plenty of fluids, stay active within the guidelines above, drink fruit juices, and eat fruit and fiber. Do not use enemas unless told to do so by the physician.
- If you develop a headache or stiff neck, notify the physician.
- Wear a medical identification tag or bracelet

identifying the medications you are receiving, or that you have a low platelet count.
- Avoid using aspirin, and any over-the-counter medications, unless approved by the physician.

SPECIFICALLY FOR PATIENTS WITH LOW PLATELET COUNTS

- Keep track of platelet counts by maintaining close contact with physician. When the platelet count is below 10,000 to 15,000, stop flossing teeth and use water-spraying oral care devices on low only. When the platelet count drops to 5,000-10,000, stop brushing teeth and clean the mouth with a swab or 4 × 4 gauze pad using a mild mouthwash or saline solution. Avoid mouthwashes containing alcohol, or lemon-glycerin swabs.
- Consider limiting activities (the following is one regimen prepared by The American Cancer Society):
  For platelet counts of 100,000-250,000: avoid contact sports; tennis, jogging, basketball are permitted.
  For platelet counts of 50,000-100,000: continue with moderate activity including walking, swimming, and usual activities of daily living.
  For platelet counts below 50,000: only mild activities are permitted such as walking, light housework, or yardwork.

ADDITIONAL GUIDELINES FOR THE NURSE

- Check stools for occult blood, and monitor urinalysis.
- Inspect venipuncture sites for hematoma development; apply pressure for at least 10 minutes after venipuncture to limit hematoma formation at venipuncture sites.
- Handle patients gently. Avoid restraints; if used, pad and inspect under restraints every 2 hours. Keep side rails padded.

---

atrophy of the zona fasciculata and reticularis, the two inner layers of the adrenal cortex where the glucocorticoid cortisol is formed.

Mitotane is not cell cycle specific and is not a general cytotoxic agent. Because of its unusual tissue selectivity, the drug is used to treat adrenal cortical carcinoma.

Absorption, distribution, and excretion. Mitotane is satisfactorily absorbed when given orally. The drug is metabolized by the liver before excretion. If liver function is impaired, the drug may accumulate and toxic reactions increase.

Toxicity. Mitotane causes anorexia, nausea, and vomiting in nearly every treated patient. Nearly half of those treated experience lethargy or dizziness. Dermatitis occurs in 20% of patients.

Less frequent but serious reactions include abnormalities of the eye, changes in blood pressure, and hemorrhagic cystitis.

Trilostane

Mechanism of action. Trilostane is a competitive inhibitor of enzymes involved in steroid synthesis. In the adrenal gland, the drug blocks cortisol synthesis in the zona fasciculata, aldosterone synthesis in the zona glomerulosa, and androstenedione synthesis in the zona reticularis (Chapter 51).

The primary use of trilostane is in Cushing's syndrome but the drug can also be used in various carcinomas, including breast carcinoma.

Absorption, distribution, and excretion. Trilos-

PATIENT PROBLEM: STOMATITIS

THE PROBLEM

Mucosal cells lining the GI tract are sensitive to some drugs, especially many of the cytotoxic drugs used in cancer chemotherapy and gold preparations in rhematoid arthritis. As the mucosal cells are destroyed, there may be pain and inflammation along the entire GI tract.

SIGNS AND SYMPTOMS

Inflamed oral mucous membranes, oral ulcers, areas of irritation in the mouth, pain on chewing and swallowing, anal discomfort, pain on defecation.

PATIENT AND FAMILY EDUCATION

- If possible, have teeth professionally cleaned and dental caries repaired before the start of drug therapy.
- If chewing and swallowing are painful, switch to a liquid diet, including such foods as milkshakes and ice cream. If discomfort is severe, try to maintain an intake of clear fluids of at least 2000 ml (approximately eight 8 oz glassfuls) per day, to prevent dehydration.
- Try chilling food before eating it.
- If toothbrushing is irritating, try using swabs to clean your mouth. Avoid flossing when stomatitis is severe. Use water-spraying oral care devices on low setting only. Rinse your mouth after each meal with a mild solution of baking soda and water; baking soda, salt and water; or hydrogen peroxide and water.
- Try painting your mouth with substrate of magnesia up to four times per day. Allow the milk of magnesia to settle to the bottom of the bottle. Pour off the liquid portion at the top of the bottle, and paint the mouth with the white, pasty portion remaining.
- If a special mouthwash has been prescribed, use it as ordered. Many mouthwashes are effective only when used regularly, throughout the day. Over-the-counter mouthwashes may be irritating because they contain alcohol; avoid them unless your doctor has prescribed them.
- Avoid spicy foods and foods with hard crusts or edges.
- Try keeping a humidifier running, to keep the room air moist.
- Wear dentures or bridgework only while eating, and remove them at other times to decrease irritation.
- Keep the lips moist with a lip balm or moisturizer.
- For anal irritation, avoid suppositories, enemas, rectal thermometers. Try sitting in a tub of warm water several times daily. After bowel movements, clean the anal area completely; some patients find a baby wipe to be cooling for this purpose.
- If vaginal irritation is a problem, keep the vaginal area clean and dry; wipe from front to back; avoid soaps in the vaginal area, and pat dry. Avoid douching or using tampons. Notify the physician if vaginal discharge develops or there is a change in the color, consistency, odor, or amount. To decrease irritation during intercourse, use a commercially available, water-soluble lubricant; avoid hand lotion or petroleum jelly.

ADDITIONAL NURSING CARE MEASURES

- Assess the mouth of patients at high risk for stomatitis at least once each shift. In addition, inspect for development of oral fungal infections (thrush).
- Monitor intake and output.

---

tane is absorbed following oral administration and biotransformed by the liver.

Toxicity. Trilostane produces signs of adrenocortical insufficiency, which may include darkening of the skin, tiredness, loss of appetite, and vomiting. These symptoms need medical attention. Diarrhea and stomach pains are also relatively frequent, but usually not severe.

Streptozocin

Mechanism of action. Streptozocin is a specific toxin for the beta (β) cells of the pancreatic islets. Other cells of the islets are relatively insensitive to the drug. For this reason the drug is primarily used to treat insulin-secreting islet cell tumors of the pancreas. Other uses for streptozocin are being explored.

Absorption, distribution, and excretion. Streptozocin is relatively unstable and must be administered intravenously.

Toxicity. Streptozocin can destroy beta cells. Therefore insulin production may cease. The drug is also toxic to the kidneys. Streptozocin does not ordinarily affect blood-forming cells, so blood dyscrasias are rarely encountered.

Interferons

Mechanism of action. Natural interferons are produced mainly by leukocytes and serve as part of the body's defense against viruses by blocking virus proliferation in infected cells. The interferons modulate the function of macrophages and lymphocytes, and have a general antiproliferative activity. The recombinant interferons share these properties. The anticancer activity of the interferons is not completely understood.

The recombinant interferons, interferon alpha-2a and interferon alpha-2b, are administered in hairy cell leukemia and genital warts. In addition, these drugs are being investigated for their activity in various lymphomas, leukemias, and Kaposi's sarcoma in AIDS patients.

Absorption, distribution, and excretion. As proteins, these interferons cannot be administered orally. Absorption is adequate from intramuscular or subcutaneous sites, producing peak serum concentration in 4 to 7 hours. These proteins are completely metabolized in kidney and other tissues.

Toxicity. A flulike syndrome develops in most patients but resolves within 2 to 4 weeks even when the drug is continued. Arrhythmias have been observed. Signs of neurotoxicity may involve the central nervous system (depression, nervousness, insomnia) or the periphery (numbness or tingling in extremities). Loss of appetite builds during treatment with alpha-interferons and may persist for some time after therapy ends.

COMBINATION CHEMOTHERAPY OF CANCER PATIENTS

Few of the anticancer drugs just discussed are used alone. Experience has demonstrated that combinations of these drugs are much more effective than single agents. Several reasons for this increased success exist. First, combinations of drugs acting by different mechanisms are less likely to cause the development of drug resistance. Like microbial cells, cancer cells possess the ability to adapt and become drug resistant. This process occurs easily if only a single drug is used. If several are used, the cancer cell has greater difficulty in developing simultaneous resistance.

Second, drug combinations allow the physician to select agents that produce different patterns of toxicity and thereby reduce the damage directed at any one organ system. Most of the drugs discussed produce bone marrow suppression. Combining these suppressive drugs with drugs such as bleomycin, vincristine, or prednisone, which do not damage the bone marrow, allows more anticancer effect to be achieved with no added damage to the bone marrow.

Finally, combining anticancer agents that act at different stages of the cell cycle allows for more tumor cells to be killed than would occur with the use of only one drug. For example, a drug like procarbazine is specific for the S phase of the cell cycle. Therefore tumor cells that pass into that phase while exposed to procarbazine will die, but cells in resting phase will survive. If an alkylating agent is added to the treatment regimen, we can expect a percentage of the cells that survive procarbazine treatment to be killed by the second drug. Adding a third drug with yet a different mechanism of action, such as vincristine, will further reduce the number of surviving cancer cells. Finally, if it is possible to add a tissue-specific drug to the regimen, even more anticancer effect may be gained. An established and effective treatment regimen such as has just been described exists for Hodgkin's disease. The regimen includes the alkylating agent mechlorethamine (Mustargen), the mitotic poison vincristine (Oncovin), the DNA synthesis inhibitor procarbazine (Matulane), and the lympholytic agent prednisone. This particular regimen is abbreviated MOPP. Many other established combination therapies exist for various types of cancer (Table 39.8).

Drugs Used in Supportive Therapy of Cancer Patients

Cancer patients require many drugs during the course of their disease. The drugs previously discussed are designed to attack the cancer directly. In addition to these agents, cancer patients frequently require other drugs that relieve symptoms of the disease itself or ameliorate the side effects produced by the highly toxic antineoplastic drugs. A brief summary of the drugs that are employed in supportive therapy of cancer patients follows.

Allopurinol

Allopurinol may be included in treatment programs when large tumor masses are quickly destroyed by chemotherapy, releasing many breakdown products, including uric acid. Uric acid can severely damage kidney cells if it is allowed to increase unchecked. Allopurinol inhibits the formation of uric acid and therefore can prevent this complication. Allopurinol is also used in the treatment of gout.

Analgesics

The pain associated with advanced cancer can be severe. Therefore hospitals and all hospices specializing in care for the dying cancer patient have a policy of liberal use of narcotic analgesics. Frequent administration and high doses may be required to control pain. Addiction in this patient population is not a problem; therefore fear of ad-

Text continued on p. 612.

PATIENT CARE IMPLICATIONS

General guidelines for patients receiving cancer chemotherapy

Drug administration

- See Patient Problems, Stomatitis (p. 601), Bleeding Tendencies (p. 600), Constipation (p. 187), Decreased White Blood Cell Count (p. 599).
- Many patients receiving cancer chemotherapy develops anemia, which may be due in part to anorexia, poor nutrition, and bone marrow depression. The anemia may be caused by the drugs or by the cancer itself.

Nursing measures to decrease anemia

- Assess for malaise, fatigability, pale skin color. Monitor hematocrit and hemoglobin, and check stools for occult blood.
- Obtain a dietary history. Do diet teaching and counseling as appropriate, although iron-rich foods may be unappealing if anorexia or nausea is present; see Dietary Consideration: Iron on p. 355.
- Encourage frequent, small feedings. See interventions under anorexia.
- Suggest patients eat their largest meal in the morning, before increasing fatigue makes them too tired to eat late in the day.
- Encourage the use of iron preparations, if prescribed, although they may have limited value until chemotherapy is completed. Fluoxymesterone (Halotestin), an androgen, may also be prescribed to reverse anemia.

Nursing measures to decrease anorexia

Anorexia may arise from drug therapy or may be caused by the underlying disease.

- Assess dietary intake; monitor weight.
- Avoid foods having a strong odor. Cool or cold foods may be more appealing than foods served hot. Red meat may be less appealing than fish or chicken.
- Encourage small, frequent feedings. Instruct caregivers to fix small portions in an attractive manner.
- If the patient develops a craving for a specific food item, it is usually permissible for the patient to have the item; the alternative may be a completely skipped meal.
- If food preparation is tiring to the patient, suggest that the patient prepare and freeze small portions of food on days the patient feels better, so that when the patient is not feeling well, it is necessary only to thaw and eat the food. Encourage interested friends and family members to prepare individual servings for the patient also. Encourage snacking and nibbling during the day. Encourage the patient to keep available in the refrigerator high-protein beverages or snacks that may be appealing: milkshakes, eggnogs, frozen yogurt, and ice cream. Obtain recipes for high-protein snacks from dietitians, the American Cancer Society, or the oncologist's office. Some patients may wish to purchase commercially prepared high-protein supplements that can be consumed as a drink, or frozen and eaten as ice cream.

- While a microwave oven is not a necessity, the patient may find it helpful to have one for quickly heating food items. Explore this possibility with the patient and family, and community resources.
- Consult the physician and the patient. Some patients may find a small glass of sherry or wine before dinner will stimulate their appetite.

Nursing measures to decrease diarrhea

Certain drugs used for chemotherapy of cancer cause diarrhea. This symptom may appear within 24 to 48 hours of receiving the drug or may be delayed for 5 to 10 days.

- Instruct patients to switch to a clear liquid diet or a low-residue diet high in protein and calories. Try to maintain a fluid intake of at least 2000 to 2500 ml per day. Caution patients to avoid foods known to be irritating to the GI tract, such as fruit, fruit juices, spicy foods, raw vegetables, corn, and coffee.
- Review possible clear-liquid food items the patient may like: broth, gelatin, tea, popsicles, soft drinks, water. The patient may be able to tolerate chicken noodle soup. While electrolyte-containing drinks such as Gatorade are not required, they may provide a pleasant-tasting alternative less irritating than fruit juice.
- Instruct the patient to notify the physician if diarrhea is severe or persists longer than 2 to 4 days.
- Teach the patient that diarrhea can lead to electrolyte imbalance. When possible, monitor serum electrolytes. In severe cases, the patient may need to be admitted to the hospital for intravenous replacement of fluids and electrolytes.
- Instruct the patient to avoid the use of enemas, rectal suppositories, and rectal thermometers.
- If anal irritation occurs, suggest that the pa-

PATIENT CARE IMPLICATIONS — cont'd

tient shower or sit in a warm tub of water several times per day. Wash the anal area with mild soap and water, and pat the area dry gently after each loose bowel movement. Some patients may find it easier or more comfortable to wsh the area with prepackaged towelettes, such as those used to clean infants during diaper changes, or with preparations such as Tucks.

Nursing measures to decrease nausea and vomiting

Nausea and vomiting may occur within hours of receiving a dose of chemotherapy, or may be delayed for 5 to 10 days.

- Monitor response to chemotherapy. Record on the care plan actions that seem to contribute to or lessen the incidence of nausea and vomiting.
- Administer antiemetics, sedatives, and other drugs as ordered to decrease nausea. They are usually more effective if administered ahead of chemotherapy, or at least before severe nausea and vomiting occur, rather than afterward.
- Consider the following interventions, which may help: reschedule chemotherapy time in relation to meal times, either closer to or further from usual mealtimes; limit oral intake to clear liquids on the day of or evening before chemotherapy; keep the environment odor free, including avoiding wearing perfumes; have the patient avoid spicy, fatty, or greasy foods the day of or the day before chemotherapy.
- Instruct the patient and family in relaxation techniques, hypnotism, guided imagery, or distraction techniques if they are interested.
- Instruct the patient to report severe or persistent vomiting occurring at home to the physician, as dehydration and electrolyte imbalance may develop.

Nursing measures to decrease alopecia

Alopecia (hair loss) occurs when sensitive cells in the hair follicle are damaged by chemotherapy or radiation.

- Before starting chemotherapy, inform patients about the possibility of hair loss. Some patients may wish to invest in a wig resembling their own hair color and style before hair loss begins. In some communities, the American Cancer Society has a "wig bank" from which cancer patients can borrow wigs during periods of alopecia. Explore this possibility. In addition, some insurance companies may reimburse patients for the cost of wigs.
- Point out that hair loss may involve eyebrows, eyelashes, nasal hair, and pubic hair, although hair loss may be patchy rather than total in these areas.
- Some drugs typically cause complete baldness, including cyclophosphamide, daunorubicin, doxorubicin, vinblastine, and vincristine. Some drugs cause a moderate degree of alopecia, including busulfan, etoposide, floxuridine, methotrexate, and mitomycin. Finally, some drugs cause only mild alopecia or sporadic thinning of hair. These drugs include bleomycin, carmustine, fluorouracil, hydroxyurea, and melphalan.
- Reassure patients that in most cases hair will grow back after the course of chemotherapy is finished. Some patients will begin to have hair growth before the course of chemotherapy is completed; this is variable from person to person. Usually, new hair is the same color and texture as the hair that was lost, but occasionally it is different.
- During hair loss, instruct the patient to wash hair infrequently, every 2 to 4 days. Use a mild shampoo, but not necessarily "baby shampoo," which may be a little harsh. The patient's barber or hairdresser may be able to recommend a specific product. Use a cream rinse or conditioner. If the scalp is dry, apply a thin layer of baby oil, mineral oil, or A and D ointment. Brush and comb hair gently. Do not use dyes, tints, rinses, or any unnecessary chemicals on remaining hair.
- Suggest that patients use satin pillow covers for sleeping.
- Avoid direct exposure to the sun, either by wearing a hat or using a maximum-protection sunscreen when out of doors (SPF 15 or greater). During cold weather, wear a hat when out of doors.
- When appropriate, use a head tourniquet or ice cap to reduce alopecia. These are used only with IV drugs. The tourniquet limits intravenous spread of the chemotherapy drug to the vessels of the scalp that supply blood to the hair. The ice cap produces vasoconstriction of the blood vessels of the scalp. The ice cap is applied 15 to 30 minutes before the infusion, while the tourniquet can be applied just before. Both are left on for 15 to 45 minutes after the infusion. These devices should be avoided in patients with leukemia or lym-

PATIENT CARE IMPLICATIONS—cont'd

phoma or any cancer that may migrate to or be found in the scalp; check with the physician when in doubt. Inform patients that some hair loss will probably occur, even with the use of the ice cap or tourniquet.

Nursing measures to decrease extravasation

Many cytotoxic agents are highly irritating to normal tissues. When these drugs are administered IV, great care must be taken to prevent them from escaping into tissues surrounding the injection site. Pain, tissue damage, and necrosis can result.

- Assess for signs of extravasation when administering IV chemotherapy: redness or swelling at the insertion site, decreased infusion rate, inability to obtain return of blood, pain, or resistance during injection of medication.
- Try to avoid extravasation of any IV drugs, but be especially alert when the following drugs are administered because of tissue necrosis and sloughing that may occur: dactinomycin, mitomycin, carmustine, cisplatin, dacarbazine, daunorubicin, plicamycin, streptozocin, mitoxantrone, vincristine, and vinblastine.
- In the ideal situation, perform a fresh venipuncture for administering chemotherapy. In the absence of the ideal situation, ascertain that the infusion line to be used is patent beforehand.
- Use a forearm infusion site rather than the dorsum of the hand for infusion of drugs that may cause necrosis and sloughing if extravasation occurs. Extravasation in the forearm may be less severe than in the area of the dorsum of the hand, where muscles and tendons that control hand movement and function may be affected. Remain with the patient during the infusion.
- If extravasation occurs, discontinue the infusion, but leave the needle or catheter in place. Attempt to aspirate any drug that can be retrieved. Follow agency procedures for managing the situation. A typical procedure would be to administer a corticosteroid subcutaneously in the area of extravasation, or via the infusion catheter that is still in place, cover the area with a topical steroid, then cover with an occlusive dressing. Finally, apply ice compresses for 15 minutes four times a day, and keep the extremity elevated for 48 hours. Notify the physician. Use a fresh venipuncture site for infusion of any remaining chemotherapy drug.
- Medical orders for treatment of extravasation should be written before infusion is begun. These orders should be readily available to all persons who administer chemotherapy. Keep drugs ordered for treatment of extravasation readily available.

Nursing measures to ensure safe handling of chemotherapeutic drugs

Avoid direct contact with chemotherapeutic agents, as the nurse may be exposed to drug toxicity through repeated skin or aerosolization contact.

- Prepare intravenous medications using a laminar airflow hood. Wash hands before and after handling chemotherapy drugs.
- Wear disposable gloves and a long-sleeved gown during drug preparation. Wear gloves during drug administration.
- Use correct technique to avoid skin contact with prepared dosages. Use Luer-Lok fittings whenever possible to avoid inadvertent separation of syringe and needle. Establish and follow procedures for disposal of drug containers, as well as contaminated gloves, syringes, and IV tubing.
- After drawing up dosages into the syringe, discard the needle and attach a new sterile needle to avoid skin contact with any traces of medication that might be on the outside of the first needle.
- Check ordered doses carefully. Several drugs have similar names.
- Consult the manufacturer's literature for information about dilution and rate of administration.
- These drugs are highly toxic. Many agencies limit the number of persons who can administer these drugs to a few nurses who have had experience and additional training in their use.
- Allergic reactions have been reported with many of these drugs. Question patients about drug allergy before administering the drug. Have available drugs, equipment, and personnel to treat an acute allergic reaction in the setting where these drugs are administered. Assess patients frequently during IV administration. Do not leave patients unattended for prolonged periods during treatment.
- Monitor laboratory work on an ongoing basis: complete blood count and differential,

Continued.

PATIENT CARE IMPLICATIONS—cont'd

platelet count, BUN and serum creatinine, serum uric acid, and liver function tests.

- These drugs are contraindicated during pregnancy. Counsel about contraceptive measures as appropriate. Menstrual irregularities are common in women receiving chemotherapy. Instruct women to keep a record of menstrual periods, and to consult a physician immediately if pregnancy is suspected.
- Chemotherapy may cause diminished production or viability of sperm. Male patients may wish to arrange for deposit of sperm in a sperm bank before beginning chemotherapy.

Nursing measures to reduce uric acid levels

Elevation of uric acid levels often accompanies administration of chemotherapy to patients with leukemia or some lymphomas. This is due to the release of large quantities of breakdown products in these rapidly dividing forms of cancer. For this reason, chemotherapy orders may routinely be accompanied by orders for allopurinol. Monitor the uric acid levels. Keep the patient well hydrated. (See Chapter 23.)

Patient and family education

- Review with patients and families the anticipated benefits and possible side effects of drug therapy. Provide support to these patients, who may be facing a difficult diagnosis, as well as anticipating serious drug side effects.
- Encourage the patient to notify the physician if any new side effect develops.
- Encourage patients to return for follow-up visits as directed. Point out to patients that many side effects may not become evident for 2 to 3 weeks following the final dose of therapy.
- Remind patients to keep all health care providers informed of all medications being taken. This is especially important because bone marrow suppression, stomatitis, and other side effects may not appear until after the drug has been administered.
- Remind patients not to use over-the-counter preparations without first consulting the physician.
- Emphasize the importance of keeping these and all drugs out of the reach of children.
- Warn patients to avoid receiving any immunizations while taking cytotoxic drugs unless first approved by the physician. Before starting chemotherapy, some physi-

cians recommend that patients receive "flu" shots and/or update immunizations; consult the physician.

- Inform patients that ridges in the fingernails may occur during chemotherapy; these reflect the effect of the drugs on the dividing cells of the nails.
- For information about the drugs, drug protocols, protocols to treat extravasation, oral gargles, mouthwashes, dietary supplements, snack recipes, patient teaching aids, and other information for patients, families, and health care providers, contact the chemotherapy department of local medical centers; the American Cancer Society; the Office of Cancer Communications at the National Cancer Institute, Bethesda, MD 20892; the Department of Health and Human Services; or local oncologists' offices. Refer patients as appropriate to the local visiting nurse agencies or hospice.
- Unless additional teaching points are listed, points on Patient and Family Education about the drugs discussed in this chapter are the same.

Mechlorethamine

Drug administration

- See the general guidelines for information about anemia, depressed white blood cell count, thrombocytopenia, nausea and vomiting, elevated uric acid, amenorrhea, and azoospermia. Alopecia is a rare side effect.
- The nadir of bone marrow suppression occurs within 1 to 3 weeks.
- Assess and monitor neurologic function.
- With intravenous administration, if extravasation occurs, discontinue the infusion and aspirate any remaining drug. Promptly infiltrate the area with sterile isotonic sodium thiosulfate injection, then apply cold compresses for 6 to 12 hours.
- If the drug comes in contact with the skin, wash immediately with copious amounts of water for 15 minutes, then rinse with a 2% sodium thiosulfate solution. If the drug comes in contact with the eye, irrigate immediately with 0.9% sodium chloride or balanced salt ophthalmic solution, then promptly consult an ophthalmologist.
- For topical application, wear protective gloves while applying. Assess for rashes. Shower or wash the area before applying the solution or ointment. Make certain the skin surfaces are dry. Apply to the prescribed

PATIENT CARE IMPLICATIONS — cont'd

areas, but apply lightly to the axillary, perineal, inguinal and inframammary areas, to avoid irritation. Do not shower again until time for the next dose. Topical preparations may cause the skin to darken, but this should disappear when the drug is stopped.
- As noted in text, the drug must be prepared just before being administered.

Patient and family education

- See the general guidelines. Warn patients to avoid driving or operating hazardous equipment if drowsiness, vertigo, weakness, or other neurologic symptoms develop; consult the physician.

Melphalan

Drug administration

- See the general guidelines for information about depressed white blood cell count, thrombocytopenia, nausea and vomiting, diarrhea, stomatitis; alopecia is uncommon.
- Monitor pulmonary function: auscultate lung sounds. Assess for dyspnea and cough.
- Inspect for skin changes.
- Monitor complete blood count and differential, and platelet count.

Pipobroman

Drug administration

- See the general guidelines for information about depressed white blood cell count, thrombocytopenia, anemia, anorexia, diarrhea, nausea, and vomiting.
- Assess for skin changes.
- Monitor complete blood count and differential, platelet count.

Mitoxantrone

Drug administration

- See the general guidelines for information about depressed white blood cell count, thrombocytopenia, nausea and vomiting, diarrhea, stomatitis, alopecia.
- Monitor intake and output, and weight. Auscultate lung sounds. Inspect for development of edema. Monitor vital signs.
- Monitor the complete blood count and differential, platelet count, and liver function tests.

Chlorambucil

Drug administration

- See the general guidelines for information

about nausea and vomiting, depressed white blood cell count, thrombocytopenia, high uric acid levels.
- Auscultate lung sounds, and assess for dyspnea and cough. Inspect for skin changes and rash.
- Monitor uric acid levels, liver function tests, complete blood count and differential, and platelet count.

Cyclophosphamide

Drug administration

- See the general guidelines for information about depressed white blood cell count, thrombocytopenia, anemia, nausea and vomiting, diarrhea, oral ulcers, high uric acid levels, and alopecia.
- Auscultate lung sounds, assess for cough and dyspnea. Assess pulse and blood pressure. Monitor weight.
- Monitor complete blood count and differential, platelet count, liver function tests, serum electrolytes, uric acid levels, and urinalysis.

Patient and family education

- See the general guidelines.
- Teach the patient to force fluids, up to eight 8 oz glassfuls of water daily, and to notify the physician if there is blood in the urine.
- Warn patients that temporary changes in skin pigmentation and nails may occur.
- Warn patients to avoid driving or operating hazardous equipment if dizziness occurs; notify physician.

Busulfan

Drug administration

- See the general guidelines for information about thrombocytopenia, depressed white blood cell count, anemia, elevated uric acid levels, alopecia.
- Auscultate lung sounds and assess for dyspnea and cough. Monitor weight, blood pressure. Assess for skin changes.
- Monitor complete blood count and differential, platelet count, liver function tests.

Thiotepa

Drug administration

- See the general guidelines for information about depressed white blood cell count, thrombocytopenia, anemia, nausea and vomiting, stomatitis.

Continued.

PATIENT CARE IMPLICATIONS — cont'd

- Assess for skin changes. Assess for urinary tract problems: urgency, frequency, change in urine color.
- Monitor complete blood count and differential, platelet count, urinalysis.

Carmustine and lomustine

Drug administration

- See the general guidelines for information about depressed white blood cell count, thrombocytopenia, anemia, nausea, and vomiting.
- Assess for dyspnea and cough, auscultate lung sounds. Monitor weight. Inspect for skin changes and development of edema.
- Monitor complete blood count and differential, platelet count, liver function tests, BUN, serum creatinine.
- Wear gloves when preparing or administering these drugs; hyperpigmentation may occur if the drug touches the skin.

Dacarbazine

Drug administration

- See the general guidelines for information about depressed white blood cell count, thrombocytopenia, anemia, nausea and vomiting, and extravasation.
- Assess for skin changes.
- Monitor the complete blood count and differential, platelet count, liver function tests, BUN.
- Monitor infusion carefully to avoid extravasation.

Patient and family education

- See the general guidelines.
- See Patient Problem: Photosensitivity on p. 647.
- Warn patients to avoid driving or operating hazardous equipment if blurred vision, confusion, or lethargy occurs; notify the physician.

Cisplatin and carboplatin

Drug administration

- See the general guidelines for information about depressed white blood cell count, thrombocytopenia, anemia, nausea, and vomiting.
- Assess hearing acuity and assess for tinnitus. Refer appropriate patients for audiograms; consult physician.
- Assess for metallic taste. Since this may af-

fect nutritional intake, monitor weight.
- Monitor blood pressure and pulse, auscultate lung sounds.
- Monitor complete blood count and differential, platelet count, liver function tests, BUN and serum creatinine, serum electrolytes, and uric acid levels.
- In order to limit the severe nausea and vomiting that frequently accompanies cisplatin administration, the regimen may include administration of metoclopramide, antiemetics, sedative, steroids, and other drugs. In addition, to limit renal toxicity, the drug is often infused with large fluid volumes, such as 250 ml/hr for 4 hours. Monitor intake and output hourly for the first 6 to 8 hours, then every 12 to 24 hours.

Bleomycin

Drug administration

- See general guidelines for information about nausea and vomiting, alopecia, and stomatitis.
- Assess for dyspnea and cough, and auscultate lung sounds.
- Assess for skin changes, monitor blood pressure and pulse.
- Monitor complete blood count and differential, platelet count, and urinalysis.

Mitomycin

Drug administration

- See the general guidelines for information about depressed white blood cell count, thrombocytopenia, anemia, anorexia, nausea and vomiting, alopecia.
- Auscultate lung sounds and assess for dyspnea and cough. Monitor intake, output, and weight.
- Monitor complete blood count and differential, platelet count, serum creatinine, and BUN.

Cytarabine

Drug administration

- See the general guidelines for information about depressed white blood cell count, thrombocytopenia, anemia, anorexia, nausea and vomiting, diarrhea, elevated uric acid levels, and alopecia.
- Auscultate lung sounds and assess for dyspnea, cough. Monitor pulse and blood pressure. Assess for skin changes, inspect for development of edema.

PATIENT CARE IMPLICATIONS — cont'd

- Assess for changes in vision, and instruct patients to report changes in vision.
- Intrathecal administration may be associated with CNS side effects. Use brands and diluents that *do not* contain benzyl alcohol as a preservative for intrathecal administration. Keep side rails up. Anticipate CNS effects.
- Monitor complete blood count and differential, platelet count, liver function tests, serum electrolytes, serum creatinine, BUN, serum uric acid.

Fluorouracil and floxuridine

Drug administration

- See the general guidelines for information about depressed white blood cell count, thrombocytopenia, anemia, nausea and vomiting, diarrhea, stomatitis.
- Assess for ataxia, and assess mental status. Inspect for skin changes. See Patient Problem: Photosensitivity on p. 647.
- Monitor complete blood count and differential, platelet count.

Mercaptopurine and thioguanine

Drug administration

- See the general guidelines for information about depressed white blood cell count, thrombocytopenia, anemia, anorexia, diarrhea, nausea and vomiting, stomatitis, and elevated uric acid levels.
- Assess for skin changes.
- Monitor complete blood count and differential, platelet count, serum uric acid, serum creatinine, BUN, urinalysis, and liver function tests.

Methotrexate

Drug administration

- See the general guidelines for information about depressed white blood cell count, thrombocytopenia, anemia, nausea and vomiting, stomatitis, diarrhea, alopecia, elevated uric acid levels.
- Monitor weight, inspect for skin changes and development of edema.
- Intrathecal administration is associated with CNS changes. Monitor mental status. Keep side rails up, supervise ambulation.
- Monitor complete blood count and differential, platelet count, urinalysis, serum creatinine, BUN, liver function tests, serum uric acid levels, and blood glucose.
- See leucovorin rescue discussed also in Chapter 22.

Patient and family education

- See the general guildelines.
- Warn patients to avoid driving or operating hazardous equipment if blurred vision, drowsiness, dizziness, or ataxia develops; notify physician.
- Review Patient Problem: Photosensitivity on p. 647.
- Instruct diabetic patients to monitor blood glucose levels, as methotrexate may cause an increase requiring a change in diet or insulin dose.

Procarbazine

Drug administration

- See the general guidelines for information about depressed white blood cell count, thrombocytopenia, anemia, nausea and vomiting, anorexia, diarrhea, alopecia.
- Assess mental status and monitor neurologic status. Anticipate CNS side effects: keep side rails up, supervise ambulation, keep a night light on.
- Monitor pulse and blood pressure. See Patient Problem: Orthostatic Hypotension on p. 237.
- Auscultate lung sounds. Assess for cough and dyspnea. Inspect for skin changes.
- Monitor complete blood count and differential, platelet count, blood glucose, and urinalysis.

Patient and family education

- See the general guidelines.
- Warn patients to avoid the use of alcohol; see Patient Problem: Disulfiram-like Reactions on p. 637.
- Warn patients to avoid foods containing tyramine; see Dietary Consideration: Tyramine on p. 665.
- Warn patients to limit intake of caffeine-containing foods such as chocolate, coffee, tea, or cola drinks.
- Tell diabetic patients to monitor blood glucose levels carefully; an adjustment in diet or insulin may be necessary.
- Warn patients to avoid driving or operating hazardous equipment if disorientation, dizziness, unsteadiness develop; notify the physician.

Hydroxyurea

Drug administration

- See the general guidelines for information about depressed white blood cell count,

Continued.

PATIENT CARE IMPLICATIONS — cont'd

thrombocytopenia, anorexia, diarrhea, stomatitis, nausea and vomiting, elevated uric acid levels, and alopecia.
- Assess neurologic and mental status. Monitor weight and inspect for skin changes and development of edema.
- Monitor complete blood count and differential, platelet count, serum creatinine, BUN, uric acid, liver function tests.

Asparaginase

Drug administration

- See the general guidelines for information about depressed white blood cell count, bleeding tendencies, anorexia, nausea, and vomiting.
- Assess neurologic and mental status. Monitor blood pressure and pulse. Monitor weight. Assess for skin changes and development of edema. Check stools for guaiac/occult blood.
- Monitor complete blood count and differential, prothrombin time, partial prothrombin time, serum creatinine and BUN, liver function tests, blood glucose, serum amylase.

Dactinomycin

Drug administration

- See the general guidelines for information about depressed white blood cell count, thrombocytopenia, anemia, nausea and vomiting, stomatitis, diarrhea, alopecia, and extravasation.
- Monitor weight, blood pressure, pulse, intake and output. Assess for development of edema. Auscultate lung sounds. Inspect for skin changes.
- Monitor complete blood count and differential, platelet count.

Doxorubicin and daunorubicin

Drug administration

- See the general guidelines for information about depressed white blood cell count, thrombocytopenia, anemia, elevated uric acid levels, alopecia, nausea and vomiting, stomatitis, diarrhea, extravasation.
- Monitor pulse and blood pressure. Assess for signs of congestive heart failure: weight gain, edema of dependent areas, dyspnea, jugular venous distention. Auscultate lung sounds and monitor respiratory rate. Monitor serial ECGs.
- Monitor complete blood count and differ-

ential, platelet count, serum uric acid.
- Inform patients that urine may be reddish in color for 1 to 2 days after each dose.

Plicamycin

Drug administration

- See the general guidelines for information about depressed white blood cell count, thrombocytopenia, anorexia, diarrhea, nausea and vomiting, stomatitis, and extravasation.
- Monitor mental status. Warn patients to avoid driving or operating hazardous equipment if drowsiness, dizziness, fatigue or lethargy develops; notify physician.
- Monitor complete blood count and differential, platelet count, serum creatinine, BUN, serum electrolytes, and urinalysis.
- Assess for signs of hypercalcemia and hypocalcemia. See Table 17.1 for a description of common electrolyte abnormalities.
- Warn patients that plicamycin may cause intense facial flushing.

Vincristine

Drug administration

- See the general guidelines for information about anemia, extravasation, diarrhea, nausea and vomiting, stomatitis, alopecia, and elevated serum uric acid levels.
- Assess neurologic and mental status. Assess for peripheral neuropathy: depressed deep tendon reflexes, changes in gait, paresthesias, or tingling of extremities, other changes in the neurologic assessment.
- Monitor intake, output, blood pressure, pulse, and respiratory rate. Auscultate lung and bowel sounds. Monitor reflexes and gait.
- Monitor complete blood count, serum electrolytes, uric acid levels.

Vinblastine

Drug administration

- See the general guidelines for information about depressed white blood cell count, thrombocytopenia, anemia, nausea and vomiting, anorexia, diarrhea, stomatitis, alopecia, extravasation.
- Assess neurologic and mental status. Warn patients to avoid driving or operating hazardous equipment if dizziness, numbness develop; notify physician.
- Assess for peripheral neuropathy: tingling or numbness of extremities. Assess for skin

PATIENT CARE IMPLICATIONS—cont'd

changes. See Patient Problem: Photosensitivity on p. 647.

- Monitor complete blood count and differential, platelet count.

Etoposide

Drug administration

- See the general guidelines for information about depressed white blood cell count, thrombocytopenia, anemia, anorexia, nausea and vomiting, and alopecia.
- Monitor pulse, blood pressure, and weight. Auscultate lung sounds, assess for dyspnea. Monitor ECGs at regular intervals. See Patient Problem: Orthostatic Hypotension on p. 237. Assess for skin changes.
- Monitor complete blood count and differential, and platelet count.

Androgens and estrogens

Estrogens are discussed in Chapter 53; androgens are discussed in Chapter 54.

Flutamide and leuprolide

Drug administration

- See general guidelines for information about anorexia, nausea and vomiting, diarrhea.
- Consult manufacturer's literature for current information.
- Assess for tingling of face, fingers, and toes.
- Monitor pulse, blood pressure, and weight. Inspect for development of edema. Monitor intake and output.
- Auscultate lung sounds.
- Allergic reactions have been reported. Have patients remain in the health care setting for at least 15 minutes after doses. Have drugs, equipment, and personnel available to treat an acute allergic reaction.
- Monitor hematocrit and hemoglobin, serum creatinine, BUN.

Patient and family education

- Review anticipated benefits and possible side effects of drug therapy.
- Assess tactfully for impotence and decreased libido, as patients may not wish to discuss them. Provide emotional support as appropriate. Remind patients not to discontinue medications without consulting the physician. Reinforce to patients the importance of taking medications as prescribed for best effect.
- Warn patients that hot flashes may occur as a side effect; provide support as possible.

- Teach patients the appropriate technique for injecting leuprolide subcutaneously at home.
- Warn patients to avoid driving or operating hazardous equipment if dizziness, blurred vision, lethargy, or memory disorders occur; notify physician.
- Warn patients to notify the physician if severe or persistent bone pain develops.
- Review the general guidelines.

Tamoxifen

Drug administration

- See the general guidelines for information about depressed white blood cell count, thrombocytopenia, nausea and vomiting, anorexia.
- Assess for signs of depression: withdrawal, change in affect, lack of interest in personal appearance, insomnia, anorexia.
- Assess mental status and neurologic function.
- Assess for hypercalcemia; see Table 17.1 for a description of common electrolyte abnormalities.
- Monitor weight, assess for development of edema. Assess visual acuity.

Patient and family education

- Review anticipated benefits and possible side effects of drug therapy.
- Warn patients to avoid driving or operating hazardous equipment if confusion, dizziness, lassitude, or lightheadedness develops; notify physician.
- Teach patients to increase fluid intake to 2500 to 3000 ml per day to foster calcium excretion and to help prevent constipation.
- Warn patients that hot flashes are common; provide support as appropriate.
- Tell patients to notify physician if bone pain is severe or persistent.

Glucocorticoids and progestins

Glucocorticoids are discussed in Chapter 51. Progestins are discussed in Chapter 53.

Mitotane

Drug administration

- See the general guidelines for information about depressed white blood cell count, thombocytopenia, anemia, anorexia, diarrhea, nausea and vomiting, and alopecia.
- Assess for signs of depression: anorexia, insomnia, lack of interest in personal appearance, and withdrawal.

Continued.

PATIENT CARE IMPLICATIONS — cont'd

- Monitor blood pressure and pulse. Assess for development of gynecomastia in males. Inspect for skin changes.
- Monitor the complete blood count and differential, platelet count, urinalysis, serum cholesterol.

Patient and family education

- Review anticipated benefits and possible side effects of drug therapy.
- Warn patients to avoid driving or operating hazardous equipment if confusion, somnolence, dizziness, fatigue, or other CNS side effects develop; notify physician.
- Instruct patients to wear a medical identification tag or bracelet listing their medications. In the event of trauma or other injury, it would be necessary to administer glucocorticoids.
- Instruct patients to contact the physician if they become sick, develop an infection, or are injured, as glucocorticoids may be necessary.

Trilostane

Drug administration

See the general guidelines for information about nausea, vomiting, diarrhea.

- Assess for electrolyte abnormalities, including hypercalcemia and hyperkalemia. See Table 17.1 for a description of common electrolyte abnormalities.
- Assess for signs of possible adrenocortical insufficiency: darkening of the skin, fatigue, loss of appetite, vomiting, hypotension. Monitor serum cortisol levels. Monitor blood pressure.
- Inspect for skin changes.
- Monitor serum cortisol levels, serum electrolytes, liver function tests.

Patient and family education

- Review anticipated benefits and possible side effects of drug therapy.

- Instruct patients taking trilostane to wear a medical identification tag or bracelet listing their medications. In the event of trauma or other injury, it would be necessary to administer glucocorticoids.
- Instruct patients to contact the physician if they become sick, develop an infection, or are injured, as glucocorticoids may be necessary.
- See the general guidelines.

Streptozocin

Drug administration

- See the general guidelines for information about depressed white blood cell count, thrombocytopenia, anemia, extravasation, nausea, and vomiting.
- Assess mental status. Watch for signs of depression: withdrawal, anorexia, insomnia, change in affect, lack of interest in personal appearance.
- Monitor intake, output, and weight.
- Monitor complete blood count, differential, platelet count, serum creatinine, BUN, serum electrolytes, liver function tests, and blood glucose.

Patient and family education

- Review anticipated benefits and possible side effects of drug therapy.
- Encourage patients to increase fluid intake to 2500 ml per day.
- Tell diabetic patients that streptozocin may alter glucose levels. Monitor blood glucose, and adjust diet or insulin as necessary.
- See the general guidelines.

Other chemotherapeutic drugs

Antiemetics are discussed in Chapter 13.
Allopurinol is discussed in Chapter 23.
Analgesics are discussed in Chapters 23 and 44.
Interferons are discussed in Chapter 28.

---

diction should not stand in the way of adequate control of pain in the terminal stages of the disease.

Antiemetics

Many of the drugs used to attack cancer cells also attack the gastrointestinal mucosa. Nausea and vomiting are therefore very commonly encountered as side effects of cancer chemotherapy. With some of the anticancer drugs, vomiting is so severe that it must be treated to prevent electrolyte imbalance. In other cases it is transient and less severe. Nevertheless, control of nausea and vomiting can greatly improve the patient's sense of well-being and aid in maintaining good nutritional status.

A variety of antiemetic agents are available (Chapter 13). The severe nausea and vomiting encountered in cancer patients receiving cytotoxic drugs frequently requires the strong antiemetic action of phenothiazines. Patients may also be sedated in an attempt to control nausea.

Isotopes

The use of radioactive isotopes is generally considered palliative therapy for certain results of cancer. These agents have their effect by virtue of the ionizing radiation they release. Sodium phosphate P 32 (^{32}P) enters forming DNA, so it tends to be concentrated where that process is highest. Clinically, the use of this drug is to attempt to control proliferation of blood cells in polycythemia vera or in myelocytic leukemia. Gold Au 198 (^{198}Au) is used to control ascites. Ascites occurs when tumor cells are widely disseminated in the abdominal cavity and large amounts of fluid accumulate. This condition differs from edema, since ascitic fluid is free within the abdominal cavity and not trapped in tissues. Pleural effusions may also be relieved by radioactive gold.

The use of ^{131}I, a radioactive isotope of iodine, to destroy overactive thyroid tissue is discussed in Chapter 52.

SUMMARY

Selective toxicity against cancer cells has been difficult to achieve since few exploitable differences exist between normal cells and most cancer cells. The most successfully exploited difference has been the fact that most cancer cells proliferate, whereas the cells in most normal tissues do not.

One major class of antineoplastic agents directly attacks cell DNA, chemically altering it so that cell division becomes impossible. Within this group of drugs are alkylating agents such as mechlorethamine, chlorambucil, melphalan, cyclophosphamide, thiotepa, carmustine, lomustine, pipobroman, dacarbazine, and mitomycin; agents that cross-link DNA, such as busulfan, carboplatin, and cisplatin; and mitoxantrone and bleomycin, which cause a breakdown of DNA structure. As a group, these drugs attack cells at any stage in the cell cycle. All these drugs are also toxic against one or more normal tissues that proliferate rapidly: bone marrow, gastrointestinal epithelium, and hair follicles.

A second group of antineoplastic agents blocks DNA synthesis. Therefore these drugs prevent the duplication of cell chromosomes and halt cell division. Only those cells actively forming DNA will be sensitive to the drugs. Therefore tissues with high growth fractions (high percentage of cells undergoing division) will be most sensitive. Cancers tend to have higher growth fractions than most normal tissues. Drugs of this class include agents that inhibit enzymes involved in DNA synthesis, such as cytarabine, fluorouracil, floxuridine, mercaptopurine, thioguanine, procarbazine, and hydroxyurea; and agents that block folic acid formation such as methotrexate. As a group, these drugs are toxic toward one or more normal tissues with high growth fractions: gastrointestinal epithelium and bone marrow.

A third group of antineoplastic agents blocks RNA and/or protein synthesis. These drugs are most effective during the phases of the cell cycle when most RNA synthesis occurs. Agents in this class may bind to DNA and prevent RNA formation (dactinomycin, doxorubicin, daunorubicin, and plicamycin). Asparaginase specifically slows protein synthesis in cancer cells by starving them for asparagine, an amino acid required by cancer cells but one that may be formed internally by normal cells. Drugs of this class produce toxicity against gastrointestinal epithelium, bone marrow, and hair follicles. In addition, several members of this class are toxic toward specific organs such as the heart (doxorubicin, daunorubicin) and kidney (asparaginase).

The fourth group of antineoplastic agents blocks mitosis by binding to tubulin and preventing the formation of the mitotic spindle. Drugs in this class include vincristine and vinblastine. Etoposide prevents cells from undergoing mitosis. All these agents except vincristine cause bone marrow suppression. In addition, nausea and vomiting and hair loss are common reactions to these agents.

A fifth group of agents is useful in cancer chemotherapy because they possess a degree of tissue specificity. Hormones may be used to alter the growth of cells that possess receptors for the hormone. Androgens, antiandrogens, estrogens, antiestrogens, progestins, and glucocorticoids as well as interferons have been used in this way. In addition, certain cell-specific toxins have been used. Mitotane specifically destroys the cortisol-synthesizing layers of the adrenal cortex. Streptozocin specifically destroys the B cells of the pancreas. These agents may therefore be effective against tumors arising in these specific tissues.

STUDY QUESTIONS

1. What are the phases of the cell cycle, and what events take place during each phase?
2. What is carcinogenesis?
3. What properties of cancer cells allow them to spread through the body?
4. How does the growth fraction of most normal tissues differ from that of most tumors?
5. On what property of cancer cells does most cancer chemotherapy depend?
6. What is the mechanism of action of alkylating agents used as anticancer medications?
7. What normal cells are especially vulnerable to attack by alkylating agents?
8. What type of toxicity is characteristically associated with the use of alkylating agents?
9. Which of the alkylating agents is not a strong vesicant as administered because the drug must be activated by liver microsomal enzymes?
10. Which of the drugs that directly damage the structure of DNA does *not* produce bone marrow suppression?
11. What is the mechanism of action of anticancer agents that block purine and pyrimidine formation or utilization?
12. Why are inhibitors of purine and pyrimidine formation or utilization considered phase-specific agents?
13. What type of toxicity is characteristic of drugs that inhibit DNA synthesis?
14. Which of the drugs that inhibit DNA synthesis are used exclusively against solid tumors?
15. Which useful anticancer drug inhibits DNA synthesis by preventing the conversion of folic acid to tetrahydrofolate (THF)?
16. What is the basis of the anticancer effect of drugs that block RNA or protein synthesis?
17. What toxicity is characteristic of anticancer drugs that inhibit RNA or protein synthesis?
18. What properties of asparaginase make it unique among anticancer drugs?
19. Which of the anticancer drugs that inhibit RNA formation have special toxicity toward the heart?
20. What is the basis of the anticancer effects of drugs that disrupt microtubule formation?
21. What toxicity is characteristic of mitotic poisons?
22. Which of the mitotic poisons is not associated with bone marrow suppression?
23. What is the basis for the anticancer effects of hormones such as androgens, antiandrogens, estrogens, progestins, and glucocorticoids?
24. What is the mechanism of action of tamoxifen?
25. Mitotane is effective against what specific type of cancer?
26. How may interferon-alpha-2a and interferon-alpha-2b be effective as anticancer agents?
27. What is the rationale behind combination chemotherapy in the treatment of cancer?
28. Why is allopurinol frequently used in cancer treatment programs?
29. What principle governs the use of analgesics in treating cancer patients?
30. Why are antiemetics frequently used as adjuncts to cancer chemotherapy?
31. What is the rationale for using isotopes such as ^{32}P or ^{198}Au in cancer treatment programs?

SUGGESTED READINGS

Baserga, R.: The basic biology of tumor growth, Res. Staff Physician **29**(3):41, 1983.

Birdsall, C., and Naliboff, A.R.: How do you manage chemotherapy extravasation? Am. J. Nurs. **88**(2):228, 1988.

Blesch, K.S.: The normal physiologic changes of aging and their impact on the response to cancer treatment, Semin. Oncol. Nurse **4**(3):178, 1988.

Brixey, M.T.: Chemotherapeutic agents: intravesical instillation, Urol. Nurs. **9**(2):4, 1988.

Bucholtz, J.D.: Radiolabeled antibody therapy, Semin. Oncol. Nurs. **3**(1):67, 1987.

Buckley, I.: Oncogenes and the nature of malignancy, Adv. Cancer Res. **50**:71, 1988.

Buckley, M. M-T., and Goa, K.L.: Tamoxifen, Drugs **37**(4):451, 1989.

Cohen, D.L., Duval-Arnould, B., and Olson, T.A.: Acute lymphoblastic leukemia of childhood, Am. Fam. Physician **30**(10):236, 1984.

Cotanch, P.H., and Strum, S.: Progressive muscle relaxation as antiemetic therapy for cancer patients, Oncol. Nurs. Forum **14**(1):33, 1987.

Curbing cancer drugs' risks to nurses, Am. J. Nurs. **87**(6):765, 1987.

D'Agostino, N.S.: Managing nutrition problems in advanced cancer, Am. J. Nurs. **89**(1):50, 1989.

DiJulio, J.E.: Treatment of B-cell and T-cell lymphomas with monoclonal antibodies, Semin. Oncol. Nurs. **4**(2):102, 1988.

Dillman, J.B.: Toxicity of monoclonal antibodies in the treatment of cancer, Semin. Oncol. Nurs. **4**(2):107, 1988.

Dustin, P.: Microtubules, Sci. Am. **243**(2):67, 1980.

Elbaum, N.: With cancer patients, be alert for hypercalcemia, Nursing84 **14**(8):58, 1984.

Epstein, R.J.: The clinical biology of hormone-responsive breast cancer, Cancer Treat. Rev. **15**(1):33, 1988.

Figlin, R.A.: Biotherapy with interferon in solid tumors, Oncol. Nurs. Forum (Suppl) **14**(6):23, 1987.

Fraser, M.C., and Tucker, M.A.: Late effects of cancer chemotherapy: chemotherapy-related malignancies, Oncol. Nurs. Forum **15**(1):67, 1988.

Frogge, M.H.: Practical considerations for administration of cis-platin (Platinol) in the outpatient setting, Semin. Oncol. Nurs. **3**(1):Suppl 1:16, 1987.

Gumbs, J., and Ross, J.B.: Mycosis fungoides, Canadian Nurse **82**(19):20, 1986.

Hagle, M.E.: Implantable devices for chemotherapy: access and delivery, Semin. Oncol. Nurs. **3**(2):96, 1987.

Hahn, M.B., and Jassak, P.F.: Nursing management of patients receiving interferon, Semin. Oncol. Nurs. **4**(2):95, 1988.

Hammond, E.: Anaphylactic reactions to chemotherapeutic agents, J. Assoc. Pediatr. Oncol. Nurses **5**(3):16, 1988.

Hauser, A.R., and Merryman, R.: Estrmustine phosphate sodium, Drug Intell. Clin. Pharm. **18**(5):368, 1984.

Hoff, S.T.: Concepts in intraperitoneal chemotherapy, Semin. Oncol. Nurs. **3**(2):112, 1987.

Hurd, D.D.: Chemotherapy of acute nonlymphocytic leukemia, Drug Therapy Hosp. **8**(6):39, 1983.

Irwin, M.M.: Patients receiving biologic response modifiers: overview of nursing care, Oncol. Nurs. Forum (Suppl) **14**(6):32, 1987.

Jones, R.B., Frank, R., and Mass, T.: Safe handling of chemotherapeutic agents: a report from the Mount Sinai Medical Center, Ca **33**(5):258, 1983.

Jordan, V.C. and others: Strategies for breast cancer therapy with antiestrogens, J. Steroid Biochem **27**(1-3):493, 1987.

Keller, J.F., and Blausey, L.A.: Nursing issues and management in chemotherapy-induced alopecia, Oncol. Nurs. Forum **15**(5):603, 1988.

Kiely, J.M.: Antineoplastic agents, Mayo Clin. Proc. **56**:384, 1981.

Krigel, R.L.: Interleukins, interferons and tumor necrosis factor, AAOHN J. **35**(4):159, 1987.

Meeske, K., and Ruccione, K.S.: Cancer chemotherapy in children: nursing issues and approaches, Semin. Oncol. Nurs. **3**(2):118, 1987.

Moeller, K.I., and Swatzendruber, E.J.: Suppressing the risks of bone marrow suppression, Nursing 87 **17**(3):52, 1987.

Montrose, P.A.: Extravasation management, Semin. Oncol. Nurs. **3**(2):128, 1987.

Moseley, J.R.: Nursing management of toxicities associated with chemotherapy for lung cancer, Semin. Oncol. Nurs. **3**(3):202, 1987.

Moshang, T. Jr., and Lee, M.M.: Late effects: disorders of growth and sexual maturation associated with the treatment of childhood cancer, J. Assoc. Pediatr. Oncol. Nurses **5**(4):20, 1988.

Niehaus, C.S., and others: Oral complications in children during cancer therapy, Cancer Nurs. **10**(1):15, 1987.

Patterson, K.L., and Klopovich, P.: Metabolic emergencies in pediatric oncology: the acute tumor lysis syndrome, J. Assoc. Pediatr. Oncol. Nurses **4**(3/4):19, 1987.

Phister, J.E., Jue, S.G., and Cusack, B.J.: Problems in the use of anticancer drugs in the elderly, Drugs **37**(4):551, 1989.

Rogers, B., and Emmett, E.A.: Handling antineoplastic agents: urine mutagenicity in nurses, Image J. Nurs. Schol. **19**(3):108, 1987.

Schlesselman, S.M.: Helping your patient cope with alopecia, Nursing 88 **18**(12):43, 1988.

Simone, J.V.: Drug treatment of acute childhood leukemia, Drug Therapy Hosp. **8**(6):25, 1983.

Simonson, G.M.: Caring for patients with acute myelocytic leukemia, Am. J. Nurs. **88**(3):304, 1988.

Stam, H.J., and Callis, G.B.: Rating the toxicities of cancer drugs, Am. J. Nurs. **88**(19):1362, 1988.

Van Haelst-Pisani, C.M., Pisani, R.J., and Kovach, J.S.: Cancer immunotherapy: current status of treatment with interleukin 2 and lymphokine-activated killer cells.

Weeks, A.E., Abbruzzese, J.L., and Levin, B.: Current status of chemotherapy for colorectal cancer, Drug Therapy **19**(6):36, 1989.

Woloschuk, D.H.M., Pruemer, J.M., and Cluxton, R.J., Jr.: Carboplatin: a new cisplatin analog, Drug Intell. Clin. Pharm. **22**(11):843, 1988.

Woods, M.: Tumour takes all, Nursing Times/Nursing Mirror **85**(3):46, 1989.

DRUGS TO TREAT MENTAL AND EMOTIONAL DISORDERS

This section presents drug classes that affect behavior. Chapter 40 includes the drugs used to treat insomnia and anxiety. Although the barbiturates are declining in use in favor of the benzodiazepines, the barbiturates remain an important example of factors determining drug disposition as well as drug tolerance. The benzodiazepines are discussed with respect to their highly favorable therapeutic index and low abuse potential. Other sedative-hypnotic, antianxiety drugs are not presented in great detail. A major emphasis of the chapter is the dependency potential of the drugs and their cross-tolerance. Because alcohol is a major drug with regard to these two points, it also is presented in detail. The importance of alcohol as a source of both drug interactions and drug abuse is noted.

Chapter 41 presents the antipsychotic drugs, with emphasis on the antagonism of the central neurotransmitters dopamine, norepinephrine, and acetylcholine in explaining the various effects of these drugs. Chapter 42 presents the major classes of antidepressant drugs: the tricyclic antidepressants, the monoamine oxidase inhibitors, and lithium. The role of these drugs in improving the neurotransmitter functions of norepinephrine and serotonin in the central nervous system is emphasized. Chapter 43 concentrates on the therapeutic roles of central nervous system stimulants in treating narcolepsy, hyperactivity, and obesity and in improving deficient respiratory drive. The abuse of amphetamine, cocaine, and caffeine also is presented.

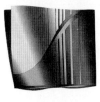

Sedative-Hypnotic Agents, Antianxiety Agents, and Alcohol

40

Sedative-hypnotic drugs and antianxiety drugs are considered together because they are not different so much in their clinical action as in their historic origin. The term *sedative-hypnotic* is reserved for the older drug classes, primarily the barbiturates. The barbiturates are a class of chemically related drugs developed in the early 1900s, effective both as sedatives and as hypnotics. A small dose to calm an anxious patient is called a *sedative.* A larger dose sufficient to induce sleep is a *hypnotic.*

After the 1950s, drugs were developed specifically as sleep-inducing agents (hypnotics). Other drugs were developed as sedatives to treat anxiety. The benzodiazepines are the drug class most used today to treat anxiety. However, the term *minor tranquilizer,* which describes these new sedative drugs, gives the impression that the sedative drugs have much in common with the major tranquilizers or antipsychotic drugs. The clinical use of the major and minor tranquilizers does not overlap, and these two drug classes have no common pharmacological mechanisms. To avoid confusion, minor tranquilizers are now called *antianxiety* drugs.

An additional drug appropriate to this chapter is alcohol because it has the pharmacological actions characteristic of a sedative-hypnotic or an antianxiety drug. The social use of alcohol is mainly as an antianxiety agent, self-prescribed. Furthermore, drug abuse and drug dependency are discussed in this chapter. Alcohol, when recognized as a drug, is seen to be a major source of drug abuse and dependency.

PSYCHOPHARMACOLOGY OF GENERAL CENTRAL NERVOUS SYSTEM DEPRESSANTS

Behavioral Changes due to General Central Nervous System Depressants

Role of the reticular activating system. The effects of a single dose of a sedative-hypnotic drug, an antianxiety drug, or alcohol are very similar. All these drugs act pharmacologically as *general depressants* of the central nervous system (CNS), since they depress the reticular activating system of the brain stem. The reticular activating system refers to those neural pathways in which incoming signals from the senses (sight, sound, smell, touch, taste, balance) and viscera are collected, processed, and passed on to the higher brain centers (Figure 40.1). Higher brain centers also have neural pathways to the reticular activating system to modulate activity. This system determines the level of awareness of the environment and therefore governs reactions to it.

Stages of CNS depression. Depression of the reticular activating system by a general CNS depressant accounts for the behavioral changes seen in someone who has taken one of these drugs. The degree of depression depends on the amount of drug taken. At a low dose *sedation* is produced, which is characterized by decreased physical and mental responses to stimuli. With an increasing dose, *disinhibition* is the next level of depression reached. Disinhibition falsely appears as a stimulated state of awareness. This is because neurons inhibiting arousal become depressed. The result of disinhibition may be a feeling of euphoria, excitement, drunkenness, loss of self-control, and impaired judgment. The relief of anxiety produced by a general CNS depressant results from sedation and/or disinhibition. A loss of motor coordination (ataxia) and involuntary eye movements (nystagmus) frequently may be seen at this level of depression and are clues when drug use is suspected. Pain can intensify disinhibition and result in paradoxical excitement in postoperative patients who are given a sedative-hypnotic or an antianxiety drug. Increasing the drug dose further produces *sleep* (hypnosis). *Anesthesia,* the loss of feeling or sensation, is achieved at very high doses of a general CNS depressant drug.

The effect of a single dose of a sedative-hyp-

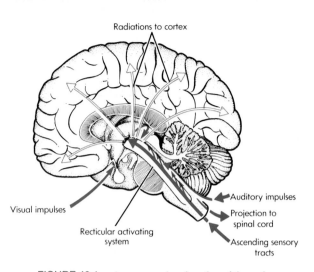

FIGURE 40.1   Awareness is a function of the reticular activating system. Diagram illustrates the role of reticular activating system as an integration network. General central nervous system depressants act on the reticular activating system at some level, although the mechanisms are not understood.

notic drug, an antianxiety drug, or alcohol therefore depends on the dose taken. In practice, not much distinction can be made in the sedative versus hypnotic dose for drugs used primarily as hypnotics. Similarly, those drugs most popular as sedative or antianxiety drugs are those that produce minimal sleepiness at an effective dose.

Drug Dependency due to General Central Nervous System Depressant Drugs

Origin of drug dependence. Continued administration of a general CNS depressant drug can cause drug dependence. Drug dependence means that the body has adjusted to the continual depression of the CNS so that it now requires the presence of the drug to function. If administration is discontinued abruptly, the body experiences withdrawal symptoms. The symptoms of withdrawal from a general CNS depressant drug reflect hyperactivity of the CNS. Mild withdrawal symptoms include agitation, tremulousness, and insomnia, whereas the major withdrawal symptom is convulsions, a life-threatening emergency. The symptoms disappear when the drug is retaken.

Dose to produce drug dependence. It is not possible to state simply what dose produces drug dependence because great variation exists among individuals. In broad terms, the general CNS depressant drugs can produce drug dependence when

taken at twice their prescribed doses for 2 to 8 weeks. The dependency potential does vary among the drug classes somewhat, as is discussed more fully for each class. A thought-provoking observation is that each new sedative-hypnotic and antianxiety drug has been introduced with the conviction that it was not addicting, whereas no drug of the general depressant type has turned out to be nonaddicting. The benzodiazepines, a class of drugs that account for at least 15% of all prescriptions written in the United States, have only recently been widely recognized as capable of producing drug dependence.

Development of drug abuse. The time required for drug dependency to develop depends on the drug dose. Chronic use of low doses does not necessarily lead to drug dependence. Many people take a low dose of a barbiturate to control epilepsy and do not experience withdrawal symptoms if their medication is changed. Moderate alcohol consumption, even on a daily basis, does not necessarily lead to alcohol dependence. However, tolerance does develop to the sedative and euphoric effects of the general CNS depressants. A person abuses the drug when the reaction to this tolerance is to increase the amount of drug taken. As the dose of drug increases, a point is reached at which failure to take the drug produces withdrawal symptoms. At this point, drug use may be continued as much to avoid withdrawal symptoms as to produce drug effects. It is this stage that we refer to as *drug dependency* or *drug addiction*. The individual's life may become centered around the drug, and personal, family, and social interactions assume a lesser importance.

Drug addiction cannot be explained merely by drug tolerance and physical dependency. In general, physical dependency can be overcome by decreasing the drug intake by 10% of the initial dose daily for 10 days. This gradual reduction prevents withdrawal symptoms from becoming severe. However, many patients revert to drug abuse after they have been withdrawn from drug dependence. Drug addiction therefore involves social and psychological factors that underlie drug abuse.

Cross-tolerance among central nervous system depressants. Tolerance to any sedative-hypnotic drug, antianxiety drug, or alcohol results in tolerance to any other of these general CNS depressants. This property is called *cross-tolerance* and is a major factor in drug abuse. The most common pattern of drug abuse is alcohol in combination with one or more sedative-hypnotic drugs or antianxiety drugs. This combination works in an additive fashion. This means that one way an individual can

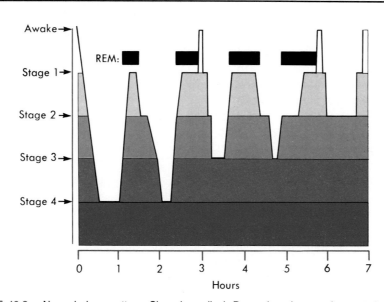

FIGURE 40.2   Normal sleep pattern. Sleep is cyclical. Deep sleep is more frequent during early cycles than later cycles. Dreaming occurs during rapid eye movement (REM) sleep and is associated with stage 1 and stage 2 sleep. Pattern shown is characteristic for adults. Children and elderly persons will often awaken more frequently. Most hypnotics will depress REM sleep.

avoid taking more of the same drug to overcome tolerance is by adding a second drug, usually alcohol. This can be a lethal combination; although someone drinking enough to die from alcohol alone is relatively uncommon, this becomes possible when another drug such as a sedative-hypnotic or an antianxiety drug is added. Moreover, because of cross-tolerance, a dose that would not lead to drug dependency by itself will contribute to drug dependency when added to a second drug of the general depressant type.

MECHANISMS OF GENERAL CENTRAL NERVOUS SYSTEM DEPRESSANTS FOR INSOMNIA AND ANXIETY

Sleep and Hypnotic Drugs

Stages of sleep. What determines sleep is not well understood. Current sleep research makes use of the brain wave patterns and eye movements recorded during sleep, as shown in Figure 40.2. Four stages of sleep are defined by these brain wave patterns. Stage 1 represents the lightest level of sleep and is accompanied by some muscle relaxation and slowing of the heart rate. Stage 4 represents the deepest level of sleep and is accompanied by marked muscle relaxation and slowing of the heart rate. During most of the sleep cycle the eye movements are not noticed under the closed lids. How-

Table 40.1   Conditions Characterized by Prominent Insomnia

Condition	Characteristic type of insomnia
Depression	Early morning insomnia is common.
Chronic alcoholism	REM sleep and deep sleep are reduced.
Hyperthyroidism	Deep sleep is reduced.
Heart failure	Insomnia is an early complaint.
Pregnancy	Insomnia is common during the last trimester.
Renal insufficiency	
Many neurological disorders	

ever, during about 20% of the average adult sleep time the eyeballs move rapidly back and forth under the closed eyelids. This is called *REM sleep* (rapid *eye* movement), and it is superimposed on stage 1 or stage 2 sleep. The body is physiologically active during REM sleep so that the heart rate increases, breathing is irregular, stomach acid is secreted, and the clitoris or penis becomes erect. Muscles lose their tone during REM sleep, however, so only the mind and autonomic nervous system are active during this stage. Since dreaming occurs exclusively during REM sleep, this time is also called *dreaming* sleep. Many authorities believe that REM sleep is a period during which we integrate emotionally meaningful experiences.

Sleep cycles. As indicated in Figure 40.2, an individual normally cycles from stage 1 through stage 4 back to stage 1 every 90 minutes or so. Deep sleep (stages 3 and 4) occupies more of the early sleep cycles, whereas dreaming (REM sleep) occupies more of the late sleep cycles. Children spend more total time in deep sleep than do adults, whereas the elderly may spend little time in deep sleep. With increasing age it becomes more common to awake at the end of a sleep cycle, particularly the early morning cycles.

Insomnia. Insomnia, the inability to sleep, is the most common sleep complaint and can be characterized as either difficulty in getting to sleep or waking up and being unable to go back to sleep. Insomnia is not a disease but a symptom of physical or mental distress. Several conditions in which insomnia is prominent are listed in Table 40.1.

Action of hypnotic drugs. Hypnotic drugs are taken to fall asleep faster or to sleep longer. Studies in sleep laboratories show that most hypnotic drugs suppress REM sleep. When the drug is discontinued, even after a single dose, there is a rebound in REM sleep with vivid dreams and increased awakening. Furthermore, after 3 weeks of continuous therapy, most hypnotic drugs are no longer effective in decreasing the time needed to fall asleep or the duration of sleep. Nevertheless, if the patient now discontinues the drug, a worse insomnia and the associated anxiety will be experienced because of the REM rebound. This reaction may lead the uninstructed patient to continue the drug, perhaps at an increased dose, to regain the hypnotic effect. This is the beginning of drug abuse with hypnotic drugs. Since hypnotic drugs can make insomnia worse rather than better, the cause of insomnia rather than the insomnia itself should be discovered and treated. Alcohol and antianxiety drugs can interfere with sleep patterns in a similar fashion if taken in large enough doses.

Anxiety and Drug Therapy

Anxiety means different things to different people. A constellation of symptoms is associated with anxiety, listed in Table 40.2. An anxious individual

Table 40.2 Symptoms of Anxiety

Appearance	Complaints
Excessively alert	Cardiorespiratory: heart palpitations, fast heart rate, breathlessness.
Easily startled	
Constantly in motion or inhibited in motion	Gastrointestinal: abdominal cramps, nausea, vomiting, diarrhea.
Excessive and disjointed speech	
Eyes constantly scanning	Musculoskeletal: tension headaches, chest pain or tightness, backache.
"Fussy" dress	
Tremors, restlessness	General: fatigue, weakness, insomnia.
Dilated pupils	

will have some but not all of these physical symptoms. Anxiety may be generalized, in which the individual is unaware of a specific cause of anxiety and may even deny anxiety, or anxiety may be anticipatory, in which the individual is all too well aware of its origin.

Action of antianxiety drugs. As already discussed, the pharmacological action of sedatives or antianxiety agents may be to decrease the general level of arousal by inhibiting the reticular activating system of the brain stem. This is not a "cure" for anxiety, although response is blunted. Rather, authorities generally agree that drug therapy for anxiety should be limited to a few weeks while psychotherapy or behavior modification therapy is begun to deal directly with the origin of the patient's anxiety. In part, this recommendation rests on the fact that tolerance develops to these drugs after a few weeks, so that effective therapy requires larger doses, the first step in drug abuse. Patients taking sedative or antianxiety drugs should be told that drug therapy will offer only limited relief.

Information about the regulation of anxiety is becoming more sophisticated. Current research suggests that reduction of anxiety can be achieved without sedation. In addition to the reticular activating system, two other integrating systems control anxiety, the limbic system and the hypothalamus. Although the reticular activating system allows information to enter the brain, the limbic system adds emotion and mediates a sequence of outgoing messages. The hypothalamus integrates the neuroendocrine response to stress, controlling the output of several hormones (see Chapter 36). The goal of current drug research is to identify drugs that affect anxiety without producing sedation. These drugs may act selectively in the limbic system.

Drugs Prescribed for Insomnia and Anxiety

The drugs prescribed for insomnia and anxiety are presented in three sections. The first section discusses the benzodiazepines, the most popular drug class today for treating insomnia and anxiety. The second section presents the barbiturates, an older class of drugs with many uses as CNS depressants, from sedation to anesthesia. The third section discusses miscellaneous drugs occasionally prescribed for insomnia or anxiety.

BENZODIAZEPINES

Safety. Benzodiazepines were introduced clinically in the 1960s as antianxiety drugs. By the early 1970s diazepam (Valium) was the most widely prescribed drug in the United States. The popularity of the benzodiazepines rests in part on their very high therapeutic index. Overdoses of 1000 times the therapeutic dose have been reported not to result in death. At therapeutic doses, side effects beyond drowsiness and motor incoordination (ataxia) are uncommon. No drug interactions are prominent beyond the additive effect with other central nervous system depressant drugs.

Mechanism of action. Specific receptors for the benzodiazepines have been identified in the rat cerebral cortex and limbic system. Since the limbic system is a major integrating system governing emotional behavior associated with self-preservation, the presence of receptors for benzodiazepines in this system may account for their antianxiety action. One effect of benzodiazepines is to increase the action of the inhibitory neurotransmitter, gamma-aminobutyric acid (GABA). Both benzodiazepines and barbiturates help GABA open a chloride channel in the postsynaptic membrane of many neurons, which reduces the neuron's excitability. Many investigators believe that the receptors for benzodiazepines and barbiturates modulate this action. Also, researchers are looking for naturally occurring compounds that have the action of the benzodiazepines. They believe that just as endorphins (Chapter 44) were discovered to be the naturally occurring opiates, similar compounds will be found for the benzodiazepines.

Thirteen benzodiazepines are available in the United States, 11 of which are listed in Table 40.3. Clonazepam is used only as an anticonvulsant and is discussed in Chapter 47. Midazolam is used only as an anesthesic and is discussed in Chapter 45. Three additional benzodiazepines are available in Canada but not in the United States. All benzodiazepines are schedule IV drugs. Benzodiazepines have four actions: anxiety reducing (anxiolytic), sedative-hypnotic, muscle relaxing, and anticonvulsant. Flurazepam (Dalmane), lorazepam (Ativan), and triazolam (Halcion) are effective as hypnotics. Clonazepam (Clonopin), clorazepate (Tranxene), and diazepam (Valium) have uses as anticonvulsants. Diazepam (Valium) is prescribed as a muscle relaxant. Alprazolam (Xanax), chlordiazepoxide (Librium), clorazepate (Tranxene), diazepam (Valium), halazepam (Paxipam), lorazepam (Ativan), oxazepam (Serax), and prazepam (Centrax) are widely used as antianxiety drugs.

Absorption and distribution. The benzodiazepines are readily absorbed following oral administration. Only lorazepam is rapidly and completely absorbed after intramuscular (IM) injection. Chlordiazepoxide and diazepam may be administered intravenously or intramuscularly, but chlordiazepoxide is not reliably absorbed after IM administration. The benzodiazepines are highly lipid soluble and therefore widely distributed in body tissues. They are also highly bound to plasma protein, usually greater that 80%. No drug interactions have been described for protein binding, but protein binding is reduced in patients with cirrhosis and renal insufficiency and in newborns. These patients often have impaired metabolism of benzodiazepines as well, making a reduction in dosage important.

Metabolism. The benzodiazepines are metabolized by the liver. Several benzodiazepines have active metabolites. The *N*-desmethylated metabolites are active and have a longer duration of action than the parent compound. Lorazepam, oxazepam, temazepam, and triazolam do not have active metabolites to prolong their duration of action. These drugs are preferred for elderly patients and those with liver disease. Alprazolam is metabolized to weakly active compounds that are eliminated rapidly. The anticonvulsant, clonazepam, has only weakly active metabolites.

Side effects. Side effects common with the benzodiazepines include daytime sedation, motor incoordination (ataxia), dizziness, and headaches. Tolerance commonly develops quickly to these side effects. The elderly are more likely to experi-

Table 40.3 Sedative-Hypnotic and Antianxiety Drugs: Benzodiazepines

Generic name	Trade name	Administration/dosage	Comments
Alprazolam	Xanax*	ORAL: *Adults*—0.25 to 0.5 mg 3 times daily. Maximum daily dose: 4 mg. FDA Pregnancy Category D. *Elderly*—0.25 mg 2 or 3 times daily.	Used to treat anxiety. Metabolites are only weakly active. Schedule IV substance.
Bromazepam	Lectopam†	ORAL: *Adults*—6 to 30 mg daily in divided doses.	Used to treat anxiety. Available in Canada but not in the United States.
Chlordiazepoxide	Libritabs Librium* Medilium† Novopoxide† Various others	ORAL: *Adults*—for anxiety, 15 to 100 mg divided in 3 to 4 doses or in 1 dose at bedtime. *Elderly*—5 mg 2 to 4 times daily. *Children*—0.5 mg/kg body weight daily in 3 to 4 doses. May be given intramuscularly. INTRAVENOUS: *Adults*—for alcohol withdrawal, 50 to 100 mg slowly over at least 1 min, then 25 to 50 mg every 6 to 8 hr, with the total dose not more than 300 mg.	Used to treat anxiety and alcohol withdrawal. Half-life is 24 to 48 hr. Metabolites are active. The hydrochloride salt is used for injection. Schedule IV substance.
Clorazepate	Tranxene* Novoclopate†	ORAL: *Adults*—13 to 60 mg divided into 2 to 4 doses or at bedtime. *Elderly*—6.5 to 15 mg daily.	Used to treat anxiety. Half-life is 30 to 200 hr. Metabolites are active. Schedule IV substance.
Diazepam	Valium* E-Pam† Various others	ORAL: *Adults*—4 to 40 mg divided into 2 to 4 doses or a single dose of 2.5 to 10 mg at bedtime. *Elderly*—2 to 2.5 mg once to twice daily. *Children*—0.12 to 0.8 mg/kg daily in 3 to 4 doses. INTRAVENOUS: administer no more than 5 mg/min. For severe anxiety, severe muscle spasm, status epilepticus, or recurrent seizures: *Adults*—5 to 10 mg initially, repeated in 3 to 4 hr if needed. *Children*—0.04 to 0.2 mg/kg initially, repeat in 3 to 4 hr if necessary. For basal sedation for cardioversion or endoscopic procedures: *Adults*—10 to 20 mg as required. For acute alcohol withdrawal symptoms: *Adults*—5 to 20 mg, then 5 to 10 mg in 3 to 4 hr if necessary.	Used to treat anxiety, severe muscle spasm, status epilepticus, and acute alcohol withdrawal symptoms and to provide sedation. Half-life is 48 to 200 hr. Metabolites are active. Schedule IV substance.
Flurazepam	Dalmane* Durapam Various others	ORAL: *Adults*—as hypnotic, 15 to 30 mg at bedtime. *Elderly*—15 mg. Onset: 20 to 45 min. Duration: 7 to 8 hr.	Used as a hypnotic only. Active metabolite is formed with half-life of 47 to 100 hr, so repeated use leads to cumulation of this metabolite, which may impair daytime activity. Schedule IV substance.
Halazepam	Paxipam	ORAL: *Adults*—20 to 40 mg 3 or 4 times daily. FDA Pregnancy Category D. *Elderly*—reduce dose to 20 mg 1 or 2 times daily.	Used to treat anxiety. Active metabolite with long half-life. Schedule IV substance.

*Available in Canada and United States.
†Available in Canada only.

Table 40.3   Sedative-Hypnotic and Antianxiety Drugs: Benzodiazepines—cont'd

Generic name	Trade name	Administration/dosage	Comments
Ketazolam	Loftran†	ORAL: *Adults*—15 mg to 1 to 2 times daily.	Used to treat anxiety. Available in Canada but not in the United States.
Lorazepam	Alzapam Ativan* Loraz Various others	ORAL: *Adults*—for anxiety, 1 to 2 mg 2 to 3 times daily, may increase dose to 10 mg maximum daily; as hypnotic, 2 to 4 mg at bedtime. FDA Pregnancy Category D. *Elderly*—½ adult dose.	Used to treat anxiety and insomnia. Repeated use for insomnia can cause rebound insomnia. Half-life is 15 hr, so little cumulation occurs. Metabolites are inactive. Schedule IV substance.
Nitrazepam	Mogadon†	ORAL: *Adults*—5 to 10 mg at bedtime. *Children* (anticonvulsant)—0.3 mg to 1 mg/kg body weight in 3 divided doses. May increase gradually if needed and tolerated.	Used as a sedative in adults and as an anticonvulsant in children. Available in Canada but not in the United States.
Oxazepam	Serax* Ox-Pam† Zapex†	ORAL: *Adults*—for anxiety, 30 to 120 mg daily in 3 to 4 doses. *Elderly*—30 mg in 3 divided doses, increased if necessary to 45 to 60 mg.	Used to treat anxiety. Half-life is 3 to 21 hr, so little cumulation occurs. Metabolites are inactive. Schedule IV substance.
Prazepam	Centrax	ORAL: *Adults*—20 mg in a single dose, increased to 40 to 60 mg daily in divided doses or once at bedtime. *Elderly*—10 to 15 mg.	Used to treat anxiety. Half-life is 30 to 200 hr. Metabolites are active. Schedule IV substance.
Temazepam	Razepam Restoril* Temaz	ORAL: *Adults*—30 mg at bedtime. FDA Pregnancy Category X. *Eldlerly*—reduce dose to 15 mg.	Used as a hypnotic only. Slowly absorbed. Metabolites are not active. Schedule IV substance.
Triazolam	Halcion*	ORAL: *Adults*—0.25 to 0.5 mg at bedtime. FDA Pregnancy Category X. *Elderly*—reduce dose to 0.25 mg.	Used as a hypnotic. May also be used as an antianxiety drug and an anticonvulsant. Metabolites are not active. Schedule IV substance.

*Available in Canada and United States.
†Available in Canada only.

ence these side effects to a disabling degree. Moreover, they do not readily metabolize benzodiazepines, so that the drug persists 2 to 3 times longer. For these reasons the drug dose is reduced for elderly patients and for patients who have impaired liver function. Less common side effects of benzodiazepines include blurred or double vision, hypotension, tremor, amnesia, slurred speech, urinary incontinence, and constipation.

Acute toxicity. An acute overdose of benzodiazepines alone is seldom fatal. No specific antagonists exist for these drugs, but patients frequently regain consciousness and normal vital signs with a large concentration of drug still in their body.

Abuse potential and withdrawal symptoms. Benzodiazepines are schedule IV drugs, since their abuse potential is considered low. Daily use of 30 mg of diazepam in the absence of alcohol or other depressant drugs for 3 months seldom produces dependence. Whereas tolerance to sedation and ataxia develops rapidly, tolerance to the antianxiety effect develops slowly. If dependence is developed, the appearance of withdrawal symptoms after discontinuance will take several days for those benzodiazepines with active metabolites. An acute phase of chronic withdrawal symptoms, consisting of depression, insomnia, nightmares, agitation, and psychological distress, can persist for 6 weeks. Withdrawal begins during the first week following discontinuance of the drug, with symptoms of agitation, nausea and vomiting, nervousness, sweating, and muscular cramps. Seizures are seldom seen unless high doses have been abused, but if seizures do occur, it is at the end of the first week.

Drug interactions and contraindications. Like the barbiturates, the sedative effect of the benzodiazepines is increased by other drug classes: alcohol and other general CNS depressants, tricyclic antidepressants, opiate analgesics, antipsychotics, and antihistamines. Unlike the barbiturates, benzodiazepines have only slight effects on the liver microsomal enzymes. Patients over 50 years old with a history of psychosis are the most likely to develop paradoxical excitement or aggression. Benzodiazepines may worsen glaucoma. Benzodiazepines are contraindicated for women in labor and nursing mothers because of adverse depression of the infant. An increased incidence of cleft lip has been reported among infants whose mothers took diazepam (Valium) during early pregnancy.

Specific Benzodiazepines (Table 40.3)

Alprazolam

Alprazolam (Xanax) is indicated for the short-term relief of anxiety and may be effective in relieving anxiety associated with depression.

Alprazolam is rapidly absorbed and effective for about 12 hours. Although the drug is eliminated somewhat more slowly in the elderly than in the young adult, the metabolites are only weakly active. Steady-state plasma levels are reached in 2 to 5 days with regular administration.

Bromazepam

Bromazepam (Lectopam) is prescribed as an antianxiety agent. It is available in Canada but not in the United States. Bromazepam has a short to intermediate half-life and does not tend to accumulate with multiple doses. The dose for elderly patients should be half the usual adult dose.

Chlordiazepoxide

Chlordiazepoxide (Libritabs) or chlordiazepoxide hydrochloride (Librium) is prescribed as an antianxiety drug, as a preanesthetic medication for sedation, and to treat the symptoms of alcohol withdrawal. Chlordiazepoxide is absorbed orally better than intramuscularly, and care must be used with intravenous (IV) injections. Chlordiazepoxide is metabolized by the liver to an active metabolite to give a persistent effect.

Clonazepam

Clonazepam (Clonopin) is used only as an anticonvulsant (Chapter 47).

Clorazepate

Clorazepate (Traxene) is prescribed for anxiety, the symptomatic relief of acute alcohol withdrawal, and as adjunctive therapy in the management of partial seizures.

Clorazepate is not absorbed orally until it is converted by stomach acid to an active metabolite. Any condition or medication, such as antacids or cimetidine, that reduces stomach acidity markedly interferes with the absorption of chlorazepate. The metabolite persists in the body.

Diazepam

Diazepam (Valium) is the most widely used of the benzodiazepines. It is a popular antianxiety drug and it also is used in the hospital as a preanesthetic medication for sedation. Alcohol withdrawal symptoms are sometimes relieved with diazepam. It has two unique uses: (1) for relief of muscle spasticity in patients with cerebral palsy or other conditions, and (2) the drug of choice for terminating continued convulsions (status epilepticus).

Diazepam is well absorbed orally and is effective within 1 hour. Absorption from IM injection is erratic, and the injection site is painful, so this route is seldom used. An IV injection must be given slowly and carefully into a large vein to minimize irritation and swelling at the injection site, with possible phlebitis or thrombosis.

Flurazepam

Flurazepam (Dalmane) is prescribed as an hypnotic only and accounts for almost 60% of hypnotic prescriptions. Flurazepam does suppress stage IV sleep but does not markedly depress REM sleep. Flurazepam is the only hypnotic in current use that has been demonstrated to be effective for more than 2 weeks. Also, it does not produce rebound insomnia when it is discontinued, probably because of the long half-life of its active metabolites. The persistence of active metabolites accounts for the decreased mental alertness during the day, particularly after repeated use of flurazepam by the elderly and by patients with decreased liver function.

Halazepam

Halazepam (Paxipam), an antianxiety drug, is well absorbed orally and metabolized to an active metabolite with a long half-life. Cumulation of the drug and its metabolite occurs with repeated doses, particularly in the elderly or in those with impaired liver function.

Ketazolam

Ketazolam (Loftran) is an antianxiety agent. It is available in Canada but in the United States.

Ketazolam has a long half-life and accumulates with multiple dosing.

Lorazepam

Lorazepam (Ativan) is effective as both a hypnotic and an antianxiety drug. It is well absorbed both orally and intramuscularly. Parenteral lorazepam sometimes is given as a preanesthetic medication in adults. Lorazepam produces sedation, relieves anxiety, and decreases the ability to recall events that day. The drug does not have active metabolites and therefore has a relatively short duration of action, about 15 hours.

Midazolam

Midazolam (Versed) is used as an intravenous anesthetic and is discussed in Chapter 45.

Nitrazepam

Nitrazepam (Mogadon) is a hypnotic. It is available in Canada but not in the United States. Nitrazepam has a short to intermediate half-life and has minimal accumulation with multiple dosing.

Oxazepam

Oxazepam (Serax) is effective as an antianxiety drug, especially in anxiety associated with depression and anxiety, tension, agitation, and irritability in older patients. Oxazepam also reduces the anxiety associated with alcohol withdrawal.

Absorption is slow. The metabolites are not active, so drug effects are not likely to be cumulative and do not persist for more than 24 hours.

Prazepam

Prazepam (Centrax), an antianxiety drug, is slowly absorbed orally. The metabolites are active, so cumulative effects are seen with repeated administration.

Temazepam

Temazepam (Restoril) is a hypnotic. Temazepam is slowly absorbed and onset of sleep is not improved, but the number of awakenings is decreased and overall duration and quality of sleep improve. As with flurazepam, stage IV sleep is suppressed, but REM sleep is not. However, unlike flurazepam, temazepam does not have active metabolites, and cumulation is not generally a problem.

Triazolam

Triazolam (Halcion) is a hypnotic, an antianxiety agent, and an anticonvulsant. It may have muscle-relaxant effects as well. Triazolam is rapidly absorbed. Its metabolites are not very active and are rapidly eliminated.

BARBITURATES

More than 50 derivatives of barbituric acid have been marketed for clinical use since the first part of this century, and nine are still widely used. The barbiturates are classified according to their duration of action and have been traditionally divided into four classes: ultrashort-acting, short-acting, intermediate-acting, and long-acting. Although traditional, this classification was derived from animal data and is somewhat arbitrary in the clinical setting, where the variables of dose and patient expectations can modify the degree and duration of effectiveness. In particular, the contrast between short-acting and intermediate-acting sedative-hypnotics is not as striking in clinical practice as in drug tables.

Factors Determining Onset and Duration of Action

The ultrashort-acting barbiturates are administered intravenously, but the other barbiturates are usually given orally and are well absorbed. The differences in the onset and duration of action among the barbiturates depend on their lipid solubility and protein binding. These properties are determined by the chemical structure. The ultrashort-acting barbiturates are very lipid soluble, and on IV administration the concentration reaching the brain, which has a high blood flow, is large because the barbiturates readily cross the blood-brain barrier and depress the reticular activating system. Their action is quickly terminated, however, because they are redistributed into organs with a lesser blood flow, so the concentration reaching the brain quickly drops. In fact, the ultrashort-acting barbiturates may persist in body fat, because of their high lipid solubility, and in muscle, reflecting their high degree of protein binding.

Metabolism. Barbiturates are released slowly from muscle and fat into the blood for eventual metabolism by the liver and excretion by the kidney. The persistence of low concentrations of barbiturates in the body is believed to account for the "hangovers" after the therapeutic effect has worn off. The short- and intermediate-acting barbiturates are redistributed less rapidly into body fat and muscle, so they act for longer times. The long-acting barbiturate phenobarbital binds still less to protein and is very much less lipid-soluble than the ultrashort-acting barbiturates. Although the ultrashort-, short-, and intermediate-acting barbiturates must be metabolized by the liver to water-soluble metabolites for excretion by the kidney, 30% to 50% of a dose of phenobarbital is excreted unchanged in the urine.

Side Effects and Toxicity

Mild withdrawal symptoms. As discussed for hypnotics in general, barbiturates are not effective as hypnotics after 3 weeks' use. Also, even a single dose suppresses REM sleep and leads to rebound REM sleep when the barbiturate is discontinued. Mild withdrawal symptoms from short-term use of barbiturates include nightmares, daytime agitation, and a "shaky" feeling.

An *acute overdose* of barbiturates causes depression of the medullary centers controlling respiration and the cardiovascular system. The symptoms are a fast heart rate (tachycardia) and a fall in blood pressure (hypotension) that leads to shock. Reflexes disappear, and respiration is markedly depressed. The patient becomes comatose, and death may result from respiratory and cardiovascular collapse. No specific antagonist exists for barbiturates; thus treatment of barbiturate poisoning is to support respiration and to maintain blood oxygen levels.

Factors Determining Tolerance and Drug Dependency

Metabolic tolerance. Administration of barbiturates for a few days activates the liver to synthesize more of the drug-metabolizing enzymes. This activation is called *enzyme induction.* Since these enzymes are located in the microsomal fraction of broken cell preparations, these drug-metabolizing enzymes usually are referred to as the liver *microsomal enzyme* system. After induction of the microsomal enzymes, the barbiturates are more rapidly metabolized, resulting in a decrease in average blood levels after a given dose. This is a classic example of *metabolic tolerance.* Since many other drugs also are metabolized by the same microsomal enzymes, barbiturates can induce tolerance of other drugs as well. Notable examples are the coumarins (anticoagulants) and the anticonvulsant phenytoin (Dilantin).

Pharmacodynamic tolerance. In addition to drug-induced tolerance, *pharmacodynamic tolerance* also develops with repeated administration of the barbiturates. This is the tolerance described earlier for all general CNS depressants, in which the nervous system becomes adapted to the presence of the depressant. However, the medullary centers controlling respiration and the cardiovascular system do not become adapted to general CNS depressants, since they are not affected at the usual doses taken. The lethal dose for barbiturates there-

DRUG ABUSE ALERT: BARBITURATES

BACKGROUND
Barbiturates are abused to bring about a sense of euphoria and a lessening of anxiety. They can be taken orally or injected.

PHARMACOLOGY
Barbiturates are sedative-hypnotics. Slurred speech, staggering gate, poor judgment, and uncertain reflexes are symptoms of barbiturate use.

HEALTH HAZARDS
There is only a fourfold margin between a sedative dose and an overdose of barbiturates. This margin is decreased by the ingestion of alcohol or another CNS depressant. A barbiturate overdose causes shallow respiration, cold clammy skin, dilated pupils, and a weak and rapid pulse. In addition to the dangers of overdose, repreated use of barbiturates leads to dependence. Withdrawal symptoms include anxiety, insomnia, tremors, delirium, and convulsions.

fore does not increase with drug dependence; this accounts for the accidental death of individuals dependent on high doses of barbiturates, since these doses can be lethal. The lethal dose for barbiturates in a nontolerant individual is about 15 times the hypnotic dose.

Abuse of barbiturates. Barbiturates are a class of widely abused drugs. As with other abused classes of drugs, those individual drugs with the most rapid onset are the most abused. This is because the euphoric feeling or "rush" depends on a rapid rate of altering perception. Among the barbiturates, secobarbital, pentobarbital, and amobarbital are on schedule II (drugs having a high potential for abuse) of the Controlled Drugs list. Butabarbital is a schedule III drug (lesser abuse potential), whereas phenobarbital and mephobarbital are schedule IV (low abuse potential) drugs. (The Controlled Drugs list is discussed in Chapter 3.) With the schedule II barbiturates, a daily consumption of 400 mg leads to severe drug dependency in about 6 weeks. With larger doses, the time decreases.

Severe withdrawal symptoms begin within 24 hours after the drug is discontinued in an individual with severe drug dependency. Grand mal convulsions and delirium are common symptoms; an elevated temperature, coma, and death are less common. Because of the danger associated with barbiturate withdrawal, gradual withdrawal is employed to detoxify a dependent person. Withdrawal is achieved by reducing the dose of the barbiturate to zero over 10 to 20 days. Sometimes the long-acting barbiturate phenobarbital is substituted for a short-acting barbiturate for once-a-day administration. Phenobarbital (30 mg) is substituted for 100 mg of secobarbital, pentobarbital, or amobarbital.

Drug Interactions

The depressant effect of barbiturates is not only additive with the other general CNS depressants, which include alcohol, sedative-hypnotic drugs, antianxiety drugs, and general anesthetics, but also is potentiated by the antipsychotics and the narcotic analgesics. These interactions are important to remember for the patient who is scheduled to undergo surgery. If secobarbital or pentobarbital is prescribed as the night-before sleeping pill, it should be given at least 8 hours before any of the major tranquilizers, narcotic analgesics, or general anesthetics are administered to avoid undue depression of the medullary control of respiration and the cardiovascular systems.

Specific Barbiturates (Table 40.4)

Thiamylal, thiopental, and methohexital

Thiamylal (Surital), thiopental (Pentothal), and methohexital (Brevital) are ultrashort-acting barbiturates administered intravenously for the induction and/or maintenance of anesthesia. These barbiturates are discussed with the general anesthetics in Chapter 45.

Amobarbital, apobarbital, pentobarbital, secobarbital and talbutal

Amobarbital (Amytal), apobarbital (Alurate), pentobarbital (Nembutal), secobarbital (Seconal), and talbutal (Lotusate) are used most frequently as hypnotic drugs. The combination of secobarbital and amobarbital is sold under the name Tuinal as a hypnotic. Although these barbiturates are effective hypnotics for a few days, they lose their effectiveness by the second week of use. Since barbiturates depress REM sleep, a rebound in REM sleep occurs when they are discontinued. As previously discussed, this REM rebound can itself lead to insomnia. Also, drug dependency can develop with the usual hypnotic doses within 2 months, although this does not lead to severe withdrawal symptoms unless the dose has been raised above 400 mg daily.

Butabarbital

Butabarbital (Butisol) is an intermediate-acting barbiturate prescribed for daytime sedation and less commonly at night for inducing sleep. It frequently is combined in sedative doses with other drugs used

to treat conditions with psychogenic overtones: allergies, ulcers, and inflammatory bowel disease.

Phenobarbital

Phenobarbital (Luminal) is the longest acting and most widely used of the barbiturates. Phenobarbital and *mephobarbital (Mebaral)* control some kinds of epilepsy (Chapter 47). Phenobarbital is infrequently abused because it is slower in onset of action and it does not give a "rush." Peak blood levels occur 6 to 18 hours after an oral dose, and the half-life is 3 to 4 days. Phenobarbital is the barbiturate that most readily induces the liver microsomal enzyme system, thereby enhancing its own metabolism as well as that of many other drugs. Phenobarbital treatment enhances the degradation of bilirubin and is used in infants and children to lower elevated plasma bilirubin levels.

Phenobarbital may be substituted for other barbiturates or nonbenzodiazepine hypnotics when decreasing drug levels for withdrawal. Its longer action allows once-a-day therapy.

OTHER HYPNOTIC AND ANTIANXIETY DRUGS

General Comparisons with the Barbiturates

The miscellaneous hypnotic and antianxiety drugs listed in Table 40.5 are more similar to the barbiturates than the benzodiazepines in that they are generally shorter acting, which makes them more readily abused. Discontinuance produces withdrawal symptoms resembling those described for the barbiturates. The degree of dependence is sometimes determined by giving 200 mg of pentobarbital every 2 hours until signs of intoxication appear. The patient is then detoxified with divided doses (4 to 6 per day) of pentobarbital, and the total daily dose is decreased by 100 mg per day. This approach is possible because pentobarbital is cross-tolerant with these other drugs. Alternatively, the abused drug is decreased daily over a 10- to 20-day period, or phenobarbital is administered in decreasing daily doses.

In addition to these drugs, several antihistamines have a pronounced sedative effect, for which they are sometimes used (Chapter 24).

Specific Drugs (Table 40.5)

Buspirone

Buspirone (BuSpar) is a newer antianxiety drug that is not a benzodiazepine. It does not cause the CNS depression characteristic of barbiturates and benzodiazepines. A lag time of 1 to 2 weeks is usual before a decrease in anxiety is noted. Little sedation or mental impairment is noted. However, at higher

Table 40.4   Sedative-Hypnotic and Antianxiety Drugs: Barbiturates

Generic name	Trade name	Administration/dosage	Comments
Amobarbital*	Amytal†	ORAL: *Adult*—as sedative, 50 to 300 mg daily in divided doses; as hypnotic, 65 to 200 mg at bedtime. *Children*—as sedative, 6 mg/kg body weight in 3 divided doses. INTRAMUSCULAR, INTRAVENOUS: *Adults*—65 to 200 mg as hypnotic dose; 30 to 50 mg as sedative dose. *Children*—2 to 3 mg/kg body weight as hypnotic dose; 3 to 5 mg/kg body weight as sedative dose. FDA Pregnancy Category D.	An intermediate-acting barbiturate that acts similar to a short-acting barbiturate in human beings. Used for daytime sedation, preanesthetic sedation, and hypnosis. Precautions are same as for secobarbital. Schedule II substance.
Apobarbital	Alurate	ORAL: *Adults*—40 to 160 mg at bedtime. FDA Pregnancy Category D.	An intermediate-acting barbiturate. Used as an hypnotic. Reduce doses for elderly patients. Schedule III substance. Not available in Canada.
Butabarbital	Butalan Buticaps Butisol Sodium† Sarisol	ORAL: *Adult*—as sedative, 50 to 120 mg/day in 3 or 4 divided doses; as hypnotic, 50 to 100 mg at bedtime. FDA Pregnancy Category D. *Children*—as sedative, 6 mg/kg in 3 divided doses daily.	An intermediate-acting barbiturate used for sedation or for insomnia when the need is to prolong sleep rather than to induce sleep. Schedule III substance.
Pentobarbital*	Nembutal† Novopentobarb‡	ORAL: *Adults*—as sedative, 30 mg 3 or 4 times daily or 100 mg in timed-release form in the morning; as hypnotic, 100 mg at bedtime. FDA Pregnancy Category D. *Children*—as sedative, 6 mg/kg in 3 divided doses daily. RECTAL: *Adults*—120 to 200 mg as required for sedation or hypnosis. *Children*—as sedative, 30 to 120 mg/day. INTRAMUSCULAR: *Adults*—as hypnotic, 150 to 200 mg. INTRAVENOUS: *Adults*—as hypnotic, 100 mg. After 1 min, can administer small increments, but no more than 500 mg total. *Children*—as hypnotic, 50 mg initially.	A short-acting barbiturate used principally for insomnia and preanesthetic sedation, and occasionally for daytime sedation. Precautions are same as for secobarbital. Schedule II substance.
Phenobarbital*	Luminal† Solfoton	ORAL: *Adults*—as sedative, 30 to 120 mg daily in 2 or 3 divided doses; as hypnotic, 100 to 320 mg at bedtime. FDA Pregnancy Category D. *Children*—as sedative, 6 mg/kg daily in 4 divided doses. INTRAMUSCULAR, INTRAVENOUS: *Adults*—as sedative, 30 to 120 mg; as hypnotic, 100 to 320 mg, with no more than 100 mg (2 ml of 5% solution) per min intravenously. Full effect lasts 15 min. RECTAL: *Children*—as sedative, 6 mg/kg divided in 3 doses.	A long-acting barbiturate used principally as a sedative. (For use as an anticonvulsant, see Chapter 34.) Not readily addictive. Schedule IV substance.

*Also available as the sodium salt. Only the sodium salt is suitable for administration as a solution by the rectal, intramuscular, or intravenous route.
†Available in Canada and United States.
‡Available in Canada only.

Table 40.4   Sedative-Hypnotic and Antianxiety Drugs: Barbiturates—cont'd

Generic name	Trade name	Administration/dosage	Comments
Secobarbital*	Seconal† Novosecobarb‡	ORAL: *Adults*—as sedative, 30 to 50 mg; as hypnotic, 100 to 200 mg at bedtime; for preoperative sedation, 200 to 300 mg 1 to 2 hr before surgery. FDA Pregnancy Category D. *Children*—as sedative, 6 mg/kg in 3 divided doses; for preoperative sedation, 50 to 100 mg. RECTAL: *Adults*—120 to 200 mg as required for sedation or hypnosis. *Children*—15 to 120 mg. INTRAMUSCULAR: *Adults*—as hypnotic, 100 to 200 mg. *Children*—as hypnotic, 3 to 5 mg/kg, up to 100 mg. INTRAVENOUS: *Adults*—as hypnotic, 50 to 250 mg, inject only 50 mg in 15 sec.	A short-acting barbiturate used principally for insomnia and as a preanesthetic sedative. Not indicated for repeated use because tolerance develops, rebound insomnia becomes marked, and the addiction potential is high. Schedule II substance.
Talbutal	Lotusate	ORAL: *Adults*—120 mg at bedtime. FDA Pregnancy Category D.	A short-acting barbiturate. Used as an hypnotic. Reduce doses for elderly patients. Schedule III substance. Not available in Canada.

*Also available as the sodium salt. Only the sodium salt is suitable for administration as a solution by the rectal, intramuscular, or intravenous route.
†Available in Canada and United States.
‡Available in Canada only.

doses patients may experience sedation or a "bad" mood. Side effects are uncommon but include headaches, dizziness, nervousness, and lightheadedness. Buspirone is reported to have little abuse potential. It is metabolized and excreted in the urine.

Chloral hydrate

Chloral hydrate (Noctec) is the oldest of the currently used hypnotic drugs, introduced in the nineteenth century. Although it is not effective for more than 2 weeks, it does not suppress REM sleep and therefore does not cause rebound insomnia. Chloral hydrate and its active metabolite, trichlorethanol, have a half-life of only 8 hours, so no persistent effect occurs, as does with flurazepam.

Chloral hydrate has an unpleasant taste and odor, which are masked by capsules or by taking the drug as a chilled elixir or syrup or as a suppository. The drug produces fewer side effects, particularly paradoxical excitement, among children or the elderly than other hypnotics, but it causes gastric irritation in some patients and displaces the coumarin anticoagulants from plasma protein. Drug dependence is produced by long-term use; an acute overdose can result in coma, with the patient having pinpoint pupils. In folklore, chloral hydrate added to an alcoholic beverage produces a "knock-out" drink, the Mickey Finn, resulting from the additive effect of the two general CNS depressants.

Triclofos sodium (Triclos) is a form of chloral hydrate that does not have the disagreeable taste or odor. Triclofos behaves similarly to chloral hydrate, and is a schedule IV (low abuse potential) substance.

Methyprylon

Methyprylon (Noludar) was introduced as a hypnotic in the 1950s. It is a schedule II drug used similarly to the short-acting barbiturates.

Ethchlorvynol

Ethchlorvynol (Placidyl) was introduced in the 1950s as a hypnotic. The most frequent patient complaint is an aftertaste. Occasionally patients show an exaggerated depression, with deep sleep and muscular weakness. Some individuals have an idiosyncratic response of CNS stimulation that may be mild or hysteric. Ethchlorvynol is a schedule IV drug with a duration of action similar to that of the short-acting barbiturates.

Ethinamate

Ethinamate (Valmid) was introduced in the 1950s as a hypnotic. It has a shorter duration of

Table 40.5 Miscellaneous Sedative-Hypnotic and Antianxiety Drugs

Generic name	Trade name	Administration/dosage	Comments
Buspirone	BuSpar	ORAL: *Adults*—initially, 5 mg 3 times daily. May increase by 5 mg daily every 2–3 days until desired response is obtained. Maximum daily dose: 60 mg. FDA Pregnancy Category B.	New antianxiety drug. Less sedation. Does not react with alcohol or antidepressants.
Chloral hydrate	Noctec* Novochlorhydrate†	ORAL, RECTAL: *Adults*—as sedative, 250 mg 3 times daily after meals; as hypnotic, 500 mg to 1 Gm 15 to 30 min before bedtime. FDA Pregnancy Category C. *Children*—as sedative, 25 mg/kg body weight in 3 to 4 doses daily; as hypnotic, 50 mg/kg as a bedtime dose, not to exceed 500 mg.	A generally safe hypnotic. The unpleasant taste and odor can be masked by chilling the drug or using the capsule form. Schedule IV substance.
Triclofos sodium	Triclos	ORAL: *Adults*—as hypnotic, 1.5 Gm 15 to 30 min before bedtime. *Children*—over 12 yr, as hypnotic, as for adults; under 12 yr, for sleep induction, 20 mg/kg.	A modified chloral hydrate that eliminates the unpleasant taste and odor of chloral hydrate.
Ethchlorvynol	Placidyl*	ORAL: *Adults only*—as hypnotic, 500 mg to 1 Gm at bedtime. FDA Pregnancy Category C.	Physical and psychological dependence may occur. Schedule IV substance.
Ethinamate	Valmid	ORAL: *Adults only*—as hypnotic, 500 mg to 1 Gm at bedtime. FDA Pregnancy Category C.	Physical and psychological dependence may occur. Schedule IV substance.
Glutethimide	Doriden* Doriglute	ORAL: *Adults only*—as hypnotic, 250 to 500 mg at bedtime. FDA Pregnancy Category C.	Physical and psychological dependence may occur. Use only 1 week, then reevaluate. Schedule IV substance.
Hydroxyzine hydrochloride, hydroxyzine pamoate	Atarax* Vistaril Various others	ORAL: *Adults*—for anxiety, 75 to 400 mg daily in 4 divided doses. For allergic skin reactions: ORAL: *Adults*—25 mg 3 or 4 times daily. *Children under 6 yr*—50 mg daily in 3 or 4 divided doses. INTRAMUSCULAR: *Adults*—for anxiety, 50 to 100 mg every 4 to 6 hr.	An antihistamine that has antiemetic and antianxiety properties. It is used in treating allergic skin rashes and motion sickness and as a preanesthetic medication. The usual doses of barbiturates or narcotics must be cut 50% if given concurrently.
Meprobamate	Equanil Meprospan Miltown* Various others	ORAL: *Adults*—for anxiety, 1.2 to 1.6 Gm daily in 3 or 4 divided doses. *Children over 6 yr*—for anxiety, 25 mg/kg daily in 2 or 3 divided doses.	Physical and psychological dependence may occur. Schedule IV substance.
Methyprylon	Noludar	ORAL: *Adults*—as hypnotic, 200 to 400 mg at bedtime. FDA Pregnancy Category B.	Physical and psychological dependence may occur. Schedule III substance

*Available in Canada and United States.
†Available in Canada only.

Table 40.6   Alcohol Intake and Its Behavioral Effects

Alcohol content (oz)	Beverage intake in 1 hr*	Blood alcohol level (mg/dl) in a 150-lb man	Behavioral effects
½	1 oz 100-proof spirits 1 glass wine 1 can beer	0.025	No noticeable effect
1	2 oz 100-proof spirits 2 glasses wine 2 cans beer	0.050	Lower alertness, impaired judgment, good feeling, less inhibited
2	4 oz 100-proof spirits 4 glasses wine 4 cans beer	0.100	Slow reaction time, impaired motor function, less cautious; should not drive; may activate vomiting reflex
3	6 oz 100-proof spirits 6 glasses wine 6 cans beer	0.150	Large increase in reaction times
4	8 oz 100-proof spirits 8 glasses wine 8 cans beer	0.200	Marked depression of sensory and motor abilities
5	10 oz 100-proof spirits 10 glasses wine 10 cans beer	0.25	Severe depression of sensory and motor abilities
6	12 oz 100-proof spirits 12 glasses wine 12 cans beer	0.30	Stuporous, unconscious of surroundings
7	14 oz 100-proof spirits 14 glasses wine 14 cans beer	0.35	Unconscious
8	16 oz 100-proof spirits 16 glasses wine 16 cans beer	0.40	Lethal dose in 50% of the population
12	24 oz 100-proof spirits 24 glasses wine 24 cans beer	0.60	Lethal dose in 95% of the population

*Since only ¼ to ⅓ oz of alcohol is metabolized each hour, alcohol rapidly accumulates.

action than the short-acting barbiturates and is a schedule IV drug.

Glutethimide

Glutethimide (Doriden) also was introduced in the 1950s and briefly became a popular hypnotic. Glutethimide is longer acting than many of the other sedative-hypnotic drugs introduced in the 1950s. As with phenobarbital, glutethimide induces the liver microsomal enzyme system. Chronic use is associated with atropine-like effects of dilated pupils (mydriasis) and a dry mouth. Glutethimide is widely abused, and an overdose after acute or chronic intoxication is less successfully treated than an overdose of barbiturates because of the higher incidence of cardiovascular collapse and the difficulty that is involved in removing this highly fat-soluble drug by dialysis. Glutethimide is a schedule III drug.

Hydroxyzine

Hydroxyzine (Atarax, Vistaril), an antihistamine with sedative properties, is discussed in Chapter 24.

THE NURSING PROCESS

SEDATIVE-HYPNOTIC AND ANTIANXIETY DRUGS

Assessment

Patients requiring sedative-hypnotics or antianxiety agents appear with a variety of complaints, diseases, and symptom complexes. Examples include patients with diagnosed anxiety, insomnia, and other medical conditions such as some forms of heart disease who are treated in part with the use of mild sedatives, and patients requiring preanesthetic medications. A systematic assessment should be done, with attention to vital signs, level of consciousness, and affect. The nurse should investigate fully any subjective complaints and the patient's other health problems.

Nursing diagnoses

Potential complication: drug dependence or addiction

Potential complication: depressed level of consciousness

Management

The common denominator of all the drugs discussed in this chapter is that they produce CNS depression. The degree of depression depends on the patient's response to the drug and on the drug and dose used. The nurse should assess the level of consciousness, the affect, the vital signs, and the blood pressure. The underlying condition for which the medication has been prescribed also should be assessed. The use of other drugs that also cause CNS depression should be avoided if possible. The nurse should work with the patient to identify nonmedicinal treatments that may be helpful in controlling the underlying problem. For example, patients being treated with sedative-hypnotics to produce sleep may be aided by such traditional remedies as warm milk at bedtime, relaxing in a warm bath before bed, or reading briefly before going to sleep. The nurse should monitor the ability of hospitalized patients to ambulate safely, keeping side rails up if there is a chance the patient may become disoriented at night. The nurse should watch for side effects that may indicate that the prescribed dose is too high or too low; consult the physician when necessary. If these drugs are being used intravenously, appropriate equipment for resuscitation and a suction machine should be available.

Evaluation

The success of these drugs depends on the original purpose for which they were being used. The patient being treated for insomnia would regard as successful any medication that produces 6 to 8 hours of sleep at night without causing hangover effects in the morning. The patient being treated for anxiety would regard as successful a drug that produces a subjective feeling of calmness without producing sedation or a depressed level of consciousness. Before discharge for self-management, the patient should be able to explain how to take the prescribed medication correctly, what symptoms may occur indicating too high a dose of medication, what to do if the medication is no longer effective, and when to return to the physician for follow-up. The patient should be able to list other drugs or substances such as alcohol that should be avoided when sedative-hypnotics or antianxiety agents are being used. Patients should not be denied the use of these drugs if they are necessary for treating their condition; at the same time, however, it is important to remember that many of the most frequently abused drugs in the United States fall into this category. The nurse should use judgment in pointing out to patients that continued prolonged use of these drugs, or use of these drugs in increasing amounts, can lead to drug dependence and/or addiction.

Table 40.7   Sources of Drug Interactions with Alcohol

Effect	Interacting drugs	Comments
Increased CNS depression	Barbiturates Meprobamate Hypnotics Antihistamines Narcotic analgesics Monoamine oxidase inhibitors Tricyclic antidepressants Benzodiazepines Chlorpromazine and other sedating phenothiazines	Any drug causing sedation or drowsiness is potentiated by alcohol. Most of these drugs carry warnings not to drive or operate dangerous equipment and stating that the situation worsens if alcohol is ingested. Alcohol can cause coma or death by respiratory depression when combined with CNS depressants even when the dose of either drug is not lethal by itself.
Increased liver metabolism	Barbiturates Phenytoin Tolbutamide Warfarin	When taken over a long period, alcohol induces the liver microsomal enzyme system for drug degradation. This speeds up the metabolism of drugs metabolized by these enzymes, so that the effective therapeutic dose must be increased. Alternatively, if an alcoholic person receiving one of these drugs becomes detoxified, the drug dose may have to be lowered.
Gastric and mucosal irritation	Aspirin Nicotine	Aspirin and alcohol act synergistically to irritate the stomach and cause bleeding. Alcoholic smokers have up to a 15-fold greater incidence of oral cancer.
Hypoglycemia	Insulin	Alcohol acts to lower blood glucose levels independently of insulin and may cause marked hypoglycemia when taken with insulin.
Disulfiram reaction	Disulfiram Sulfonylureas (oral hypoglycemic agents) Nitroglycerin	Disulfiram inhibits the degradation of acetaldehyde, which then accumulates and causes hypotension, gastrointestinal distress, and headache.
Vasodilation	Guanethidine Nitroglycerin	Alcohol acts centrally to produce vasodilation, which can potentiate the action of these drugs.

Meprobamate

Meprobamate (Equanil, Miltown) was introduced in the 1950s as the first widely prescribed antianxiety drug. Although physical dependency readily develops with abuse, meprobamate is a schedule IV drug. Withdrawal symptoms range from insomnia and anxiety to hallucinations and grand mal seizures. Meprobamate is sometimes used as a centrally acting skeletal muscle relaxant, although its effectiveness in this role is questionable.

Alcohol and Its Effects

Pharmacological Actions and Drug Interactions

Alcohol is a widely used and abused drug in our society. In this section the important actions of alcohol and its interactions with other drugs are reviewed.

Alcohol as general central nervous system depressant. As a general CNS depressant, alcohol causes all the behavioral changes described in the introduction: sedation, disinhibition, sleep, and anesthesia. As summarized in Table 40.6, p. 633, the amount of alcohol in the blood can be predicted from the amount consumed, and produces characteristic behavioral effects. Alcohol also enhances the sedative and hypnotic effects of other drug classes, including all the general CNS depressants discussed in this chapter and other drug classes with sedative side effects: the antihistamines, the phenothiazines, the narcotic analgesics, the tricyclic antidepressants, and the monoamine oxidase inhibitors. This enhancement of CNS depression means that irreversible coma or death can occur when alcohol is taken concurrently with other drugs, a

Table 40.8   Degenerative Changes Common with Chronic Alcohol Consumption

System	Comments	System	Comments
Brain	Lack of vitamin B$_1$ (thiamine) common to alcoholics produces *Wernicke's disease:* brain lesions manifested as an inability to learn or recall. *Korsakoff's psychosis* describes alcoholics who are confused and disoriented as to time or place. Wernicke's disease and Korsakoff's psychosis are considered variations of the same brain disease. Replacement of vitamin B$_1$ helps reverse symptoms in the early stages but will not restore lost function later.	Heart	Some alcoholic individuals develop an enlarged heart that functions poorly (cardiomyopathy).
		Blood	Because of blood loss and lack of folic acid, alcoholic persons can have both iron deficiency (microcytic) anemia and folate deficiency (macrocytic) anemia. Liver disease may result in clotting factor deficiency. White blood cells and platelets are decreased.
Liver	Chronic drinking produces a fatty liver because in the presence of alcohol, fatty acids are stored in the liver rather than being metabolized. About 75% of alcoholic persons show some cirrhosis after 10 years. In cirrhosis, fibrous tissue replaces liver cells. Severe cases result in liver failure and death. Hepatitis (inflammation of the liver) is also common among alcoholic persons.	Metabolic	Alcoholic individuals are often hypoglycemic because alcohol inhibits glucose production by the liver. Since alcohol is converted to a substrate for carbohydrate and fat metabolism, high levels of lipids, lactic acid, uric acid, and ketone bodies may appear in the blood. Plasma magnesium, plasma phosphate, and plasma albumin concentrations are low.
Stomach and gastrointestinal tract	Alcohol causes gastritis, which leads to ulcers and blood loss. Nonspecific diarrhea is common. Inflammation of the pancreas (pancreatitis) is common.	Skin	The vasodilation due to alcohol eventually produces a permanent rosy nose and cheeks. Skin ulcers are common.

fact not widely enough appreciated in our society.

Alcohol as vasodilator. Acute ingestion of alcohol has effects in addition to those attributed to its general CNS depression. Rising levels of alcohol may activate the vomiting center. Alcohol acts centrally to produce vasodilation and a feeling of warmth. This vasodilation can produce a marked hypotensive response in persons taking guanethidine or nitroglycerin.

Factors affecting absorption. Alcohol is absorbed more readily from the small intestine than from the stomach. Absorption of alcohol therefore is decreased by food, which dilutes the alcohol and keeps it in the stomach longer. Alcohol in concentrations of 10% or less will stimulate gastric secretions, thereby aiding digestion, but larger concentrations inhibit gastric secretions and damage the cells lining the stomach. This irritation may make some people nauseated the day after heavy drinking, and accounts for the inflammation of the

stomach (gastritis) and ulcers frequently seen in alcoholics. Aspirin is another drug that readily damages the stomach lining. The combination of aspirin and alcohol can produce bleeding in the stomach.

Metabolism. More than 90% of ingested alcohol is oxidized by the liver, with the remainder being excreted in the breath and urine. The oxidation of alcohol to carbon dioxide and water means that alcohol is a source of calories. Alcoholics may get most of their calories from alcohol but be malnourished because alcoholic beverages lack vitamins, minerals, and protein.

Two enzyme systems in the liver transform alcohol. The major enzyme for alcohol metabolism is alcohol dehydrogenase, which is also the enzyme that limits the rate of alcohol metabolism. In the average adult, the liver alcohol dehydrogenase can metabolize only about 10 ml of alcohol in 1 hour. This means that no matter how much someone has

PATIENT PROBLEM: DISULFIRAM-LIKE REACTIONS

THE PROBLEM

Disulfiram is sometimes prescribed to patients who wish to avoid drinking alcohol again (see text). When a patient is taking disulfiram, and alcohol is consumed, a serious physiological reaction occurs. Some other drugs also are associated with disulfiram-like reactions in combination with alcohol. Example drugs are furazolidone, metronidazole, and the antibiotic moxalactam.

SIGNS AND SYMPTOMS

The combination of alcohol and disulfiram produces flushing, throbbing in the head and neck, throbbing headache, respiratory difficulty, nausea, copious vomiting, sweating, thirst, chest pain, rapid breathing, fast heart rate, fainting, weakness, vertigo, blurred vision, and confusion. Severe reactions can cause death.

PATIENT AND FAMILY EDUCATION

- Review the signs and symptoms of the disulfiram-like reaction. Tell the patient to seek medical help for a severe reaction.
- Review sources of alcohol. Obvious sources include ingestion of beer, liquor, or wine. Other dietary sources include sauces that may contain wine, cooking sherry, or liquors; wine vinegars, and some liquid medications such as cough syrups and elixirs. In the patient who is very sensitive to this reaction, topical contact with after-shave lotion or colognes, alcohol-containing liniments, or after-bath lotions may produce symptoms. Avoid inhalation of the vapors of any chemical that may contain alcohol, such as shellac, varnish, or paints.
- Read the labels on food items and medicines. If in doubt about a drug, consult the pharmacist.
- Wear a medical identification tag or bracelet indicating that disulfram is being taken.
- Avoid alcohol-containing products for up to 2 weeks after stopping disulfiram or a drug associated with disulfiram-like reactions.
- For additional information about the use of disulfiram in the treatment of alcohol abuse, see the text.

---

drunk, only 10 ml of alcohol can be metabolized in 1 hour, and alcohol readily accumulates in the body when this amount is exceeded. Neither coffee, fresh air, nor exercise will speed up alcohol metabolism to help someone "sober up."

The product of alcohol metabolism by alcohol dehydrogenase is acetaldehyde, a highly toxic compound. Ordinarily, acetaldehyde does not accumulate because it is metabolized further by aldehyde dehydrogenase. Disulfiram (Antabuse) and other drugs can inhibit this enzyme so that acetaldehyde accumulates and produces unpleasant symptoms, which include headache, nausea, and vomiting.

The liver microsomal enzyme system described for the barbiturates also can degrade alcohol but ordinarily with a very limited capacity. As with phenobarbital, alcohol can induce this enzyme system so that the liver can metabolize not only more alcohol but more of other drugs as well, and this is one source of drug interactions. Alcoholic persons are able to metabolize twice as much alcohol as those who do not drink chronically.

An elevated value of serum gamma glutamyl transpeptidase (GGTP) in the absence of other elevated enzymes is a good predictor of chronic alcohol or drug consumption. This enzyme is induced in the liver by alcohol and drugs and secreted into the circulation. An elevated GGTP is often the first biochemical sign of alcoholism and may occur before overt clinical signs and symptoms develop.

Drug interactions. Alcohol is a major source of drug interactions because it is so widely consumed. Alcohol particularly influences other CNS depressants, drug metabolism, gastric mucosal integrity, blood glucose levels, and vasodilation. These drug interactions are listed in Table 40.7, p. 635. The importance of alcohol as a source of drug interactions can be appreciated by considering the estimate that 5% of adults in the United States are alcoholic and that 30% to 60% of hospitalized individuals are alcoholic.

Effects of an acute overdose. Unless a large amount of concentrated alcohol has been rapidly swallowed on an empty stomach or ingested with another CNS depressant drug, an acute overdose of alcohol commonly causes an individual to pass out before lethal doses can be drunk. However, note that a pint of 100-proof liquor is an L.D.$_{50}$ dose for a small man (see Table 40.6). With rapid drinking of straight liquor, someone can drink enough to die. The greatest danger of acute alcohol intoxication to nonalcoholic individuals is that they may involve themselves or others in traffic accidents (30,000 alcohol-related traffic deaths per year) or that they may fall and injure themselves.

A hangover is common on recovery from acute alcohol intoxication and includes such symptoms as an upset stomach, thirst, fatigue, headache, depression, anxiety, and generally feeling out of sorts. Many of these symptoms are caused by congeners, the natural by-products of fermentation and aging. Vodka, which is a mixture of pure alcohol and water and contains few congeners, also produces few hangover symptoms compared to wines and aged spirits, which have higher congener contents.

Physiological Changes Associated with Chronic Drinking

Chronic drinking can produce characteristic degenerative changes in the body, as listed in Table 40.8, p. 636. These changes are seen after about 10 years of drinking 150 ml of alcohol daily. In addition to these degenerative changes, some alcoholic persons may have blackout spells, periods in which they are awake and functioning but of which they have no memory. Heavy drinking during pregnancy is associated with a 63% incidence of neurological abnormalities in the offspring. The fetal alcohol syndrome is now recognized in the offspring of alcoholic mothers, a syndrome characterized by a face that is flat with widely spaced, small eyes, and mental retardation.

Withdrawal symptoms after chronic drinking. Chronic drinking also leads to the appearance of withdrawal symptoms when the person stops drinking. The severity of the withdrawal symptoms depends on the individual's drinking history but are most common when a chronic drinker stays intoxicated for 2 or more weeks and then stops drinking. The first symptoms, which appear within a few hours, are tremors and anxiety. As the first stage progresses, the heart rate becomes rapid, the blood pressure increases, and there is heavy sweating, a loss of appetite, nausea and vomiting, and insomnia. The second stage of withdrawal is characterized by hallucinations, usually visual, but sometimes involving hearing or feeling things. The patient is still oriented and only mildly confused despite these hallucinations.

Untreated withdrawal. About 10% of untreated patients will go on to have seizures within the first 48 hours of withdrawal. *Delirium tremens* is a stage of withdrawal that occurs in about 10% of untreated alcoholic persons 2 to 7 days after the start of withdrawal. Delirium tremens lasts about 2 days, during which time the person is completely disoriented, extremely agitated, sweats, and has a fever and a changing pulse and blood pressure. The person usually has no memory of delirium tremens.

Table 40.9   Drug Interactions with Disulfiram

Drug	Action
Phenytoin (Dilantin), coumarins (oral anticoagulants)	Potentiated by disulfiram, which inhibits their degradation by the liver microsomal enzymes
Benzodiazepines	Potentiated by disulfiram, which inhibits their plasma clearance
Benzodiazepines and ascorbic acid (vitamin C)	Decreased alcohol-disulfiram reaction by protecting the acetaldehyde-oxidizing enzymes
Tricyclic antidepressants	Increased alcohol-disulfiram reaction by inhibiting the acetaldehyde-oxidizing enzymes
Isoniazid, metronidazole	Can cause neuropsychiatric symptoms by an unknown mechanism in the presence of disulfiram

Treatment of withdrawal. A patient undergoing alcohol withdrawal is usually treated with one of the benzodiazepines: diazepam, chlordiazepoxide, clorazepate, or oxazepam. This treatment is effective because alcohol is cross-tolerant with the benzodiazepines.

Additional therapy during withdrawal is designed to restore normal metabolic parameters and overcome the vitamin B_1 (thiamin), B_{12}, and folic acid deficiencies. This supportive therapy relieves neurological symptoms secondary to hypoglycemia, ketosis, and vitamin deficiency.

Aversion therapy with disulfiram. One drug, disulfiram (Antabuse), is prescribed for the patient who has been detoxified and wishes to avoid drinking again. As previously described, disulfiram blocks the oxidation of acetaldehyde. The accumulation of acetaldehyde causes unpleasant reactions, which include flushing, throbbing in the head and neck, a throbbing headache, respiratory difficulty, nausea, copious vomiting, sweating, thirst, chest pain, rapid breathing, fast heart rate, fainting, weakness, vertigo, blurred vision, and confusion. These effects can be elicited by alcohol for 1 to 2 weeks after disulfiram is discontinued. The reaction lasts from 30 minutes to several hours. Severe reactions can cause death from cardiovascular collapse or respiratory failure. Because of the severity of the reactions, only well-informed, motivated patients are considered for disulfiram therapy, which is at best a supportive treatment when supplemented by psychiatric therapy. Patients whose drinking problem is lack of moderation after

General guidelines for the use of the antianxiety agents and sedative hypnotics

Drug administration

- In the institutional setting, keep side rails up after administering these drugs. Supervise ambulation and smoking. Keep a nightlight on.
- Use "sleeping pills" judiciously. Do not deprive a patient of a needed medication, but use medications as an adjunct to nursing measures such as a back rub, repositioning, small snack, or glass of warm milk.
- Assess tactfully for side effects. Some drugs cause changes in libido or sexual activity. Provide emotional support as appropriate. Consult with the physician about changes in drug or dosage.
- Be alert in outpatient setting to patients who return for prescription refills on an increasingly frequent basis; this may indicate improper use or abuse, or lack of knowledge about the hazards of continued use of the drugs. Evaluate patients carefully for possible depression and suicidal tendencies.

Patient and family education

- Remind patients to take these drugs only as directed, and not to increase the dose or frequency without consulting the physician.
- Warn patients to avoid driving or operating hazardous equipment if drowsiness develops. Supervise the play of children.
- Warn patients to avoid ingestion of alcohol.
- Avoid the use of other drugs that may depress the central nervous system, unless they are specifically prescribed by the physician. Examples include antiemetics, narcotic analgesics, and antihistamines.
- For insomnia, take doses 30 minutes before bedtime.
- Instruct patients that the frequently encountered "hangover effect" in the morning following use of a sedative-hypnotic is a side effect of the medication and not a sign that the patient needs a larger dose of medication that evening.
- Caution patients taking anticonvulsant medication that drowsiness may continue for several days to weeks but should gradually diminish.
- Keep all health care providers informed of all drugs being used, even occasional sleeping pills.
- Keep these and all drugs out of the reach of children. Use childproof caps in settings where there are small children. Keep these drugs in clearly labeled containers.
- Remind patients not to share drugs with friends or relatives.
- Refer patients who are having continuing problems with insomnia or anxiety to appropriate resources for counseling or evaluation.
- After long-term use, the patient may have difficulty discontinuing the medication abruptly. Instruct the patient to consult the physician before discontinuing medications.

Benzodiazepines

Drug administration

- See the general guidelines.
- Monitor blood pressure and pulse, intake, output, and weight. Monitor the respiratory rate and auscultate breath sounds. Inspect for skin changes.
- Menstrual irregularities may develop. Instruct patient to notify physician. Counsel about contraception as appropriate.
- Monitor complete blood count and platelets, liver function tests, BUN and serum creatinine.

  INTRAVENOUS BENZODIAZEPINES
- Have available equipment for intubation and ventilatory support.
- Keep side rails up. Have a suction machine available.
- Monitor respiratory rate and blood pressure. Do not leave patient unattended unless the patient is sufficiently alert to handle secretions and call for assistance.
- Keep patient on bedrest for 2 to 4 hours after IV doses.

  INTRAVENOUS DIAZEPAM
- Administer undiluted, at a rate of 5 mg (1 ml) or less over 1 minute.

  INTRAVENOUS CHLORDIAZEPOXIDE
- Dilute each 0.5 Gm with at least 18 ml sterile water for injection. Administer 0.5 Gm diluted over at least 5 minutes.

  INTRAVENOUS LORAZEPAM
- Dilute just before administering with an equal volume of compatible IV fluid. Administer at a rate of 2 mg or less over 1 minute.

  INTRAVENOUS MIDAZOLAM
- May be diluted with normal saline or 5% dextrose in water. Rate of administration often determined by patient response, e.g., 1 mg in 4 ml, administered over at least 2 minutes, until speech is slurred. For conscious sedation, evaluate carefully to avoid overmedication; wait 2 minutes between increments. Use lower doses in the elderly or debilitated.

Continued.

PATIENT CARE IMPLICATIONS — cont'd

Patient and family education

- See the general guidelines.
- Instruct the patient to report the development of any new side effect.
- See Patient Problems: Dry Mouth on p. 170; Photosensitivity on p. 647.
- Take doses with meals or snack to lessen gastric irritation.

Barbiturates

Drug administration

- See the general guidelines.
- Monitor blood pressure and pulse, intake, output, and weight. Monitor the respiratory rate and auscultate breath sounds. Inspect for skin changes.
- Monitor complete blood count and platelets, liver function tests.
- With intravenous administration, monitor vital signs and respiratory rate. Have a suction machine available, and equipment for intubation and ventilatory assistance. Keep the patient on bedrest until stable.

Patient and family education

- See the general guidelines.
- Instruct the patient to report the development of any new side effect.

- Take doses with meals or snack to lessen gastric irritation.

Miscellaneous agents

Drug administration

- See the general guidelines.
- Monitor blood pressure and pulse, intake, and output.
- When used in the doses ordered, side effects are rare.

Patient and family education

- See the general guidelines.

Disulfiram

- See Patient Problem: Disulfiram-like Reactions, and review the side effects in the text.
- Treatment with disulfiram is not a cure for alcoholism and should be used only with other forms of supportive therapy. Assess patients carefully before administering this drug.
- Treatment of a severe disulfiram reaction may require hospitalization. Instruct the patient's family in detail about the effects of alcohol consumption while the patient is receiving disulfiram.

---

the first drink is taken are considered the best candidates for disulfiram therapy. By itself, disulfiram produces transient effects that usually disappear within 2 weeks: drowsiness, tiredness, impotence, headache, acne, and a metallic or garliclike aftertaste. A number of drug interactions with disulfiram have been described and are listed in Table 40.9.

SUMMARY

Selected general CNS depressants sedate or induce sleep (hypnosis). The sedative-hypnotic drugs are used at a lower dose to sedate and at a higher dose to induce sleep. Newer drugs have been developed to be used as hypnotics only or as antianxiety agents (minor tranquilizers) only.

The mechanisms of action of these general CNS depressants are not well characterized. They do depress the reticular activating system, which controls the level of awareness. Tolerance develops to general CNS depressants, and continued administration leads to drug dependence. With drug dependence, the body experiences withdrawal symp-

toms if the drug is abruptly discontinued. Drug dependence is reversed by gradually decreasing the dose of the drug. Drug abuse and drug addiction represent the continuance of drug use for nonmedical purposes. Cross-tolerance occurs among the general CNS depressants, so ingestion of alcohol or any sedative-hypnotic or antianxiety drug can prevent withdrawal symptoms from any other of these drugs.

The medical uses of the sedative-hypnotic and antianxiety drugs are to treat insomnia and anxiety. Although hypnotic drugs are widely used to induce sleep, they all alter normal sleeping patterns to some degree. The sleep appears to be such that the body reacts to this alteration with disturbed sleep patterns after the drug is discontinued. Also, most hypnotic drugs are effective for only 3 weeks, after which tolerance has developed to the hypnotic effect. Similarly, chronic drug therapy for anxiety is effective for only a limited time. Medicinal therapy for insomnia or anxiety is thus limited and must be supplemented by other therapeutic treatments.

Benzodiazepines are widely used in the United

States as antianxiety agents because their abuse potential is much lower than with the barbiturates and when used alone they do not cause death in overdose. However, benzodiazepines are cross-tolerant with other CNS depressants and can decrease the lethal dose of alcohol or other depressant drugs when taken concurrently.

The abuse potential of the benzodiazepines alone is low; however, because they act synergistically with other CNS depressants, they are abused substances.

Benzodiazepines have four actions: anxiety reduction (anxiolytic), sedative-hypnotic, muscle relaxant, and anticonvulsant. Flurazepam, lorazepam, nitrazepam, temazepam, and triazolam are effective as hypnotics. Clonazepam, clorazepate, and diazepam have uses as anticonvulsants. Diazepam is prescribed as a muscle relaxant. Alprazolam, bromazepam, chlordiazepoxide, clorazepate, diazepam, halazepam, ketazolam, lorazepam, oxazepam, and prazepam are widely used as antianxiety drugs.

The benzodiazepines are readily absorbed following oral administration. They are metabolized by the liver, often to active compounds. Lorazepam, oxazepam, temazepam, and triazolam do not have active metabolites to prolong their duration of action. These drugs are preferred for elderly patients and those with liver disease. Alprazolam and clonazepam have only weakly active metabolites. Clorazepate, chlordiazepoxide, diazepam, flurazepam, halazepam, and prazepam have active metabolites that prolong their duration of action.

Barbiturates encompass a spectrum of onset and duration times determined by lipid solubility. The action of the highly lipid-soluble ultrashort-acting barbiturates is terminated by redistribution because they rapidly cross membranes to be distributed throughout the body. These barbiturates must be metabolized to be made water soluble and eliminated.

Overdose of a barbiturate produces depression of respiration and the cardiovascular system. Treatment is supportive. A severe drug dependence to barbiturates can develop over 6 weeks of daily use. Both metabolic and pharmacodynamic tolerance develop. Metabolic tolerance refers to the induction of the liver-metabolizing enzymes that degrade many drugs. Since barbiturates are degraded by these enzymes, larger doses of barbiturates can be tolerated because the liver has a greater capacity for degradation. Pharmacodynamic tolerance refers to the adaptation of much of the CNS to the depressant action of the barbiturates. However, the medulla does not develop tolerance; thus as the "effective" dose increases, it approaches the lethal dose, which does not change, and increases the potential for lethal overdosing.

Withdrawal symptoms after discontinuance can include seizures, so detoxification is achieved by gradual reduction of the dose.

Barbiturates have several uses, depending on the onset and duration of action of the individual barbiturate. Ultrashort-acting barbiturates are administered intravenously to provide induction for surgical anesthesia. Secobarbital, pentobarbital, amobarbital, apobarbital, and talbutal are hypnotics. Butabarbital is a sedative. Phenobarbital is a long-acting barbiturate used as a sedative, as an anticonvulsant, and to manage drug withdrawal from barbiturates or other sedative-hypnotic drugs.

Buspirone is a new antianxiety drug not related to benzodiazepines or barbiturates.

Hypnotics introduced in the 1950s that are still used include methyprylon, ethchlorvynol, ethinamate, and glutethimide. Chloral hydrate has been used as a hypnotic for more than a hundred years. It is well tolerated by children and the elderly and does not markedly alter REM sleep. Meprobamate was the first antianxiety drug introduced in the 1950s but has a narrow margin of safety by today's standards.

Alcohol is a general CNS depressant. Alcohol is widely consumed and is therefore a major source of drug interactions (see Table 40.7). The capacity of the liver to metabolize alcohol is limited, so continuous drinking over a few hours leads to the rapid accumulation of alcohol. Chronic drinking over a period of years produces physiological changes (Table 40.8) and severe withdrawal symptoms when consumption is temporarily discontinued.

Disulfiram is used in aversion therapy for alcoholism. Alcohol is normally metabolized to acetaldehyde, which then is rapidly degraded further. Disulfiram inhibits the degradation of acetaldehyde, and the rising plasma concentrations of acetaldehyde produce highly unpleasant symptoms, including a throbbing headache and extreme nausea.

STUDY QUESTIONS

1. Define sedative, hypnotic, and antianxiety drugs.
2. What is the reticular activating system, and how is it affected by general CNS depressants?
3. Describe the stages of CNS depression.
4. What is drug dependence?
5. What are withdrawal symptoms?
6. What is cross-tolerance?
7. Name the stages of sleep and describe which ones are affected by hypnotics.
8. What is anxiety?

9. What major advantage do the benzodiazepines have over the barbiturates?
10. What drug interactions are seen with benzodiazepines?
11. Describe the uses of benzodiazepines.
12. Categorize the benzodiazepines by the activity of their metabolites. What influence does the activity of the metabolites have on the duration of action of the benzodiazepines?
13. Describe the four categories of barbiturates, and list which drugs belong in each category.
14. What is redistribution?
15. Describe withdrawal symptoms from barbiturates.
16. Define metabolic tolerance.
17. Define pharmacodynamic tolerance.
18. What are the uses of barbiturates?
19. What are the features of chloral hydrate as an hypnotic?
20. List the hypnotics introduced since the 1950s. Are they more similar to barbiturates or to benzodiazepines?
21. What are the special features of the toxicity of glutethimide?
22. What drug interactions are seen with alcohol?
23. What factors affect alcohol absorption?
24. Describe alcohol metabolism. How does disulfiram interfere with alcohol metabolism?
25. What are the side effects of alcohol ingestion with disulfiram?
26. What are the physiological changes associated with chronic drinking?
27. How is alcohol withdrawal treated?

SUGGESTED READINGS

Sleep and hypnotics

Editors: How to get a good night's sleep, Drug Ther. **14**(8):103, 1984.

Erman, M.K.: Insomnia: treatment approaches, Drug Ther. **14**(8):43, 1984.

Gary, N.E., and Tresznewsky, O.: Barbiturates and a potpourri of other sedatives, hypnotics and tranquilizers, Heart Lung **12**(2):122, 1983.

Gillin, J.C.: Sleeping pills: when are they a safe answer for those who can't sleep? AAOHN J. **35**(4):184, 1987.

Greenblatt, D.J., and others: Effect of gradual withdrawal on the rebound sleep disorder after discontinuation of triazolam, N. Engl. J. Med. **317**:722, 1987.

Kales, A., and others: Early morning insomnia with rapidly eliminated benzodiazepines, Science **220**:95, 1983.

Lamy, P.P.: Use of hypnotics in the elderly, Am. Fam. Physician **30**(2):187, 1984.

Lukasiewicz-Ferland, P.: When your I.C.U. patient can't sleep, Nursing 87 **17**(11):51, 1987.

Malcolm, R., and Gross, J.A.: Insomnia and its treatment, Postgrad. Med. **75**(1):83, 1984.

McCarron, M.M. and others: Short-acting barbiturate overdosage. JAMA **248**(1):55, 1982.

McElnay, J.C., Jones, M.E., and Alexander, B.: Temazepam, Drug Intell. Clin. Pharm. **16**:650, 1982.

Quan, S.F., Bamforn, C.R., and Beutler, L.E.: Sleep disturbances in the elderly, Geriatrics **39**(9):42, 1984.

Regestein, Q.R.: Specific effects of sedative/hypnotic drugs in the treatment of incapacitating chronic insomnia, Am. J. Med. **83**:909, 1987.

Sbriglio, R.: The amytal interview in emergency and psychiatric settings, Hosp. Physician **20**(1):91, 1984.

Scharf, M.B., and Jacoby, J.A.: Lorazepam—efficacy, side effect and rebound phenomena, Clin. Pharmacol. Ther. **31** (2):175, 1982.

Anxiety and drug dependence

Alderman, M.: When stress requires a management plan, Patient Care **17**(4):14, 1983.

Alderman, M.: Consider drugs for acute stress? Patient Care **17**(5):79, 1984.

Fletcher, D.J., and Bezanson, D.: Coping with stress: how to help patients deal with life's pressures, Postgrad. Med. **77**:93, 1985.

Frye-Kryder, S.: Midazolam: a new benzodiazepine, AANA J. **55**(2):121, 1987.

Hollister, L.E., and others: Long-term use of diazepam, JAMA **246**(14):1568, 1981.

Jenike, M.A.: Treating anxiety in elderly patients, Geriatrics **38**(1):115, 1983.

Johnson, J.E.: Effect of benzodiazepines on older women, J. Comm. Health Nurs. **5**(2):119, 1988.

Karb, V.B.: Midazolam: newcomer to the benzodiazepine family, J. Neurosci. Nurs. **21**(1):64, 1989

Leppik, J.E., and others: Double-blind study of lorazepam and diazepam in status epilepticus, JAMA **249**(11):1452, 1983.

Lyiard, R.B., and Gelenberg, A.J.: Treating substance abuse. Part I, Drug Ther. **7**(4):57, 1982.

Lyiard, R.B., and Gelenberg, A.J.: Treating substance abuse. Part II, Drug Ther. **7**(5):55, 1982.

Marx, J.L.: "Anxiety peptide" found in brain, Science **227**:934, 1985.

Murphy, E.K.: Legal considerations in RN monitoring of intravenous sedation, AORN J. **48**(6):1184, 1988.

Newton, R.E. and others: Review of the side effect profile of buspirone, Am. J. Med. **80**(3B):17, 1986.

Ray, O.: Drugs, society, and human behavior, ed. 3, St. Louis, 1982, C.V. Mosby Co.

Roy-Byrne, P.P., and Hommer, D.: Benzodiazepine withdrawal: overview and implications for the treatment of anxiety, Am. J. Med. **84**:1041, 1988.

Alcohol and alcoholism

Blume, S.B.: Early intervention, Postgrad. Med. **74**(1):146, 1983.

Colman, N., and Herbert, V.: Nutritional and hematological complications of alcoholism, Pract. Gastroenterol. **VII**(4):6, 1983.

Dolin, B.J.: Alcoholism and its treatment: 1983, Hosp. Med. **19**(1):117, 1983.

Eckardt, M.J., and others: Health hazards associated with alcohol consumption, JAMA **246**(6):648, 1981.

Ewing, J.B.: Detecting alcoholism, JAMA **252**(14):1905, 1984.

Favazza, A.R.: Alcoholism, Am. Fam. Physician **27**(2):274, 1983.

Feinberg, J.F.: The Wernicke-Korsakoff syndrome, Am. Fam. Physician **22**(5):129, 1980.

Fuller, R.K. and others: Disulfiram treatment of alcoholism: a Veterans Administration cooperative study, JAMA **256**:1449, 1986.

Hayashida, M. and others: Comparative effectiveness and costs of inpatient and outpatient detoxification of patients with mild-to-moderate alcohol withdrawal syndrome, N. Engl. J. Med. **320**:358, 1989.

Hill, P.S.: Alcoholism, Postgrad. Med. **74**(5):87, 1983.

Kamerow, D.B., Pincus, H.A., and MacDonald, D.I.: Alcohol abuse, other drug abuse and mental disorders in medical practice, JAMA **255**:2054, 1986.

Kirk, E., and Bradford, L.T.: Effects of alcohol on the central nervous system: implications for the neuroscience nurse, J. Neurosci. Nurs. **19**(6):326, 1987.

Landers, D.F.: Alcohol withdrawal syndrome, Am. Fam. Physician **27**(5):114, 1983.

Landers, D.F.: Alcoholic coma and some associated conditions, Am. Fam. Physician **28**(4):219, 1983.

Lieber, C.S.: Hepatic, metabolic, and nutritional complications of alcoholism, Res. Staff Physician **29**(8):79, 1983.

Lieber, C.S.: Biochemical and molecular basis of alcohol-induced injury to liver and other tissues, N. Engl. J. Med. **319**:1639, 1988.

Lipman, A.G.: Which drugs may cause an Antabuse-type reaction? Mod. Med. **49**(10):185, 1981.

Maull, K.I., Kinning, L.S., and Hickman, J.K.: Culpability and accountability of hospitalized injured alcohol-impaired drivers, JAMA **252**(14):1880, 1984.

Miller, G.W., Jr.: Principles of alcohol detoxification, Am. Fam. Physician **30**(4):145, 1984.

Mills, J.L. and others: Maternal alcohol consumption and birth weight, JAMA **252**(14):1875, 1984.

Mooney, A.J.: Alcoholism: pharmacologic basis of symptoms, Consultant **23**(5):171, 1983.

Moore, R.D. and others: Prevalence, detection, and treatment of alcoholism in hospitalized patients, JAMA **261**:403, 1989.

Rund, D.A., Summers, W.K., and Levin, M.: Alcohol use and psychiatric illness in emergency patients, JAMA **245**(12):1240, 1981.

Schuckit, M.A.: Detecting alcoholism, Pract. Gastroenterol. **71**(2):11, 1983.

Spickard, W.A., and Tucker, P.J.: An approach to alcoholism in a university medical center complex, JAMA **252** (14):1894, 1984.

Stephenson, J.N., and others: Treating the intoxicated adolescent, JAMA **252**(14):1884, 1984.

Stewart-Amidei, C.: Alcohol and head injury: a nursing perspective, Crit. Care Nurs. Q. **10**(1):69, 1987.

Toutant, C., and Lippmann, S.: Fetal alcohol syndrome, Am. Fam. Physician **22**(1):113, 1980.

Valanis, B., Yeaworth, R.C., and Mullis, M.R.: Alcohol use among bereaved and nonbereaved older persons, J. Gerontol. Nurs. **13**(5):26, 1987.

Victor, M.: Diagnosis and treatment of alcohol withdrawal states, Pract. Gastroenterol. **VII**(5):6, 1983.

Antipsychotic Drugs

41

One of the truly remarkable advances in pharmacology in recent decades has been the discovery and application of drugs effective in treating the major mental illnesses, schizophrenia and depression. This chapter discusses the *antipsychotic* or *antischizophrenic drugs*, also called *neuroleptic* drugs. The term *neuroleptic* refers to the ability of these drugs to cause a general quiescence and state of psychic indifference to the surroundings. Another term for these drugs is *major tranquilizers.* However, many professionals believe the term *tranquilizer* is misleading, since the main action of antipsychotic drugs is their unique reversal of the symptoms of psychosis.

MECHANISMS OF ANTIPSYCHOTIC DRUGS

Chemical Classes of Antipsychotic Drugs

The five chemical classes of antipsychotic drugs are the phenothiazines, the thioxanthenes, the butyrophenones, the dibenzoxazepines, and the dihydroindolones. The latter three classes contribute only one drug each to present clinical use. Ten phenothiazine and two thioxanthene compounds are currently in clinical use as antipsychotic drugs.

Phenothiazines. The largest antipsychotic drug class is the phenothiazines. Chlorpromazine was the first phenothiazine introduced in the United States and is still the most widely used drug in this class. Chlorpromazine originally was licensed as an antiemetic drug, later as a drug to potentiate anesthesia, and finally as an antipsychotic drug. The thioxanthenes have a three-ringed main structure that differs by only one atom from that of the phenothiazines. The remaining three drug classes, the butyrophenones, the dibenzoxazepines, and the dihydroindolones are chemically different from the phenothiazines and from each other. However, the three classes behave the same pharmacologically

with respect to potency and side effects, as outlined in Table 41.1.

Subgroups of phenothiazines. The phenothiazines are subdivided into three subgroups based on the chemical differences in side groups on the three-ringed main structure. These subgroups are the *aliphatic*, the *piperidine*, and the *piperazine* phenothiazines. The three subgroups differ in potency and in the incidence of key side effects, as summarized in Table 41.1.

Antipsychotic Drugs as Dopamine Receptor Antagonists

Four effects of antipsychotic drugs have been linked to the blockade of dopamine receptors in various parts of the brain. The *antipsychotic* effect arises from receptor blockade in the limbic system and the *antiemetic* effect from receptor blockade in the chemoreceptor trigger zone. Therapeutic use is made of these effects. *Extrapyramidal* effects arise from blockade in the corpus striatum of neurons from the basal ganglia and *endocrine* effects from blockade in the pituitary gland. These two effects are undesired actions of antipsychotic drugs.

Dopamine theory of psychosis. Current ideas on the neurochemical origin of psychotic behavior come from an understanding of the action of the antipsychotic drugs. These drugs block receptors in the central nervous system (CNS) for the neurotransmitter dopamine. The hypothesis is that too much of this neurotransmitter in the limbic system produces psychotic symptoms. The limbic system is that area of the brain that regulates emotional behavior. Blocking the receptors for dopamine in the limbic system reverses psychotic symptoms.

Extrapyramidal reactions and dopamine deficiency. The antipsychotic drugs also cause the extrapyramidal reactions described in Table 41.2. These extrapyramidal reactions arise from the

Table 41.1 Antipsychotic Drugs According to Drug Class, Potency, and Major Side Effects

Drug	Equipotent dose	Relative incidence of side effects			
		Sedative effect	Orthostatic hypotension	Anticholinergic effects	Extrapyramidal symptoms
PHENOTHIAZINES					
Aliphatic					
Chlorpromazine	100	High	Moderate	Moderate/high	Moderate
Promazine	200	Moderate	Moderate	High	Moderate
Triflupromazine	25	High	Moderate	Moderate/high	Moderate/high
Piperidine					
Mesoridazine	50	High	Moderate	Moderate	Low
Thioridazine	100	High	Moderate	Moderate/high	Low
Piperazine					
Acetophenazine	20	Moderate	Low	Low	High
Fluphenazine	2	Low/moderate	Low	Low	High
Perphenazine	8	Low/moderate	Low	Low	High
Prochlorperazine	10	Moderate	Low	Low	High
Trifluoperazine	4	Moderate	Low	Low	High
THIOXANTHENES					
Chlorprothixene	100	High	Moderate/high	Moderate/high	Low/moderate
Thiothixene	4	Low	Low/moderate	Low	Moderate/high
BUTYROPHENONE					
Haloperidol	2	Low	Low	Low	High
DIBENZOXAZEPINE					
Loxapine	10	Moderate	Low/moderate	Low/moderate	Moderate/high
DIHYDROINDOLONE					
Molindone	10	Moderate	Low/moderate	Moderate	Moderate

blockade of dopamine receptors in certain nuclei of the basal ganglia of the brain. This area of the brain is responsible for coordination of movement. A common extrapyramidal reaction is drug-induced parkinsonism. In Parkinson's disease degeneration of dopamine neurons going to the basal ganglia occurs, resulting in a local deficiency of dopamine (see Chapter 48). The blockade of dopamine receptors in this area of the brain produces the same symptoms as a dopamine deficiency.

Emesis and dopamine. Dopamine is the neurotransmitter involved in vomiting (emesis) in the medullary chemoreceptor trigger zone. Antipsychotic drugs are effective in preventing vomiting by blocking these dopamine receptors. As described in Chapter 13, several antipsychotic drugs are commonly used as antiemetic drugs.

Endocrine actions of dopamine. Dopamine inhibits the release of the hormone prolactin by the pituitary gland. Blockade of dopamine leads to hypersecretion of prolactin and secondarily to endocrine disturbances of the reproductive system by mechanisms not yet understood.

Antipsychotic Drugs as Adrenergic and Cholinergic Receptor Antagonists

The phenothiazines and thioxanthenes block receptors for norepinephrine as well as receptors for dopamine. At one time the antipsychotic action was believed to be the blockade of CNS norepinephrine receptors. The finding that the butyrophenone haloperidol blocked only dopamine and not norepinephrine receptors, however, solidified the data implicating the major role of dopamine rather than norepinephrine in psychotic disorders.

Central nervous system effects and adrenergic receptor blockade. Norepinephrine is a neurotransmitter associated with specific neurons in the CNS,

Table 41.2   Side Effects of Antipsychotic Drugs

Type of effect	Signs and symptoms	Comments
Adrenergic blockade (CNS)	Sedation Postural (orthostatic) hypotension	Usually transient
Cholinergic blockade	Atropine-like effects: dry mouth, blurred vision, constipation, delayed micturition	Usually transient
Endocrine—dopamine blockade	Men: erection problems Women: menstrual irregularities, unexpected lactation	Usually transient
Extrapyramidal—dopamine blockade	Acute dystonia: neck twisting, facial grimacing, abnormal eye movements, involuntary muscle movements	Most common during the first few days of therapy; usually disappears after brief treatment with antiparkinsonian drugs
	Akathisia: restlessness, difficulty in sitting still, strong urge to move about	Most common during the first few days of therapy; control with antiparkinsonian drugs or diazepam
	Parkinsonism: motor retardation, masklike face, tremor, rigidity, salivation, shuffling gait	Most common after the first week of therapy; control with antiparkinsonian drugs
	Tardive dyskinesia: protrusion of tongue, puffing of cheeks, chewing movements, involuntary movements of extremities, involuntary movements of trunk	Most common when dosage is lowered after prolonged therapy; elderly women at greatest risk; may not be reversible
Allergic reactions	Photosensitivity Cholestatic hepatitis	Common
	Agranulocytosis	Rare

just as it is associated with the postganglionic neurons of the sympathetic nervous system. Neurons containing norepinephrine in the reticular activating system of the brain are associated with alertness. The sedative effect of the phenothiazines and the thioxanthenes may result from their blockade of these receptors for norepinephrine. The blockade of receptors for norepinephrine in the vasomotor center inhibits peripheral sympathetic tone and causes orthostatic hypotension. The sedative and hypotensive side effects of the phenothiazines and thioxanthenes appear early in therapy. If tolerance does not develop, the dosage can be lowered or another drug can be tried.

Anticholinergic actions of antipsychotic drugs. All the antipsychotic drugs have some anticholinergic action. The atropine-like effects of dry mouth, blurred vision, delayed micturition, and constipation are common side effects. However, a central anticholinergic action is beneficial in controlling some extrapyramidal reactions. Extrapyramidal reactions such as parkinsonian symptoms are believed to reflect a relative lack of dopamine and a relative abundance of acetylcholine in neuronal areas controlling movement coordination (see Chapter 48). Since antipsychotic drugs produce extrapyramidal reactions by blocking the action of dopamine, those drugs that also have substantial ability to block the action of acetylcholine have less tendency to cause extrapyramidal reactions.

PHARMACOLOGY OF ANTIPSYCHOTIC DRUGS

Absorption and Fate

The antipsychotic drugs are administered orally in tablet or syrup form. The syrup form is preferred for patients who hide or do not swallow pills. Many antipsychotic drugs are available in injectable form as well. Only fluphenazine is available in two different depot forms for intramuscular injection, which require administration only every 3 to 6 weeks. Normally, antipsychotic drugs are given in divided daily doses initially and in daily doses when the patient has stabilized. Peak plasma levels of the drug are reached 2 to 3 hours after oral administration. Up to 90% of the drug may be bound to plasma proteins. The drugs are metabolized in the liver and excreted in the urine and feces. Excretion is very slow, however, and metabolites may be found in the urine as long as 6 months after the drug is discontinued. Apparently some metabolites are active. Improvement can last as long as 3 months after medication is halted; whether this reflects remission or presence of persistent active metabolites is unclear.

Antipsychotic effects may not be seen for 7 to 10 days after the start of therapy, and 4 to 6 weeks are needed to see the full effect of a given dosage regimen. Dosages must be adjusted for individual patients.

The dosage requirement for use as an antiemetic is much smaller than for the antipsychotic effect, and the antiemetic effect is seen within 1 hour of administration.

Extrapyramidal Reactions (Table 41.2)

The most important side effects of the antipsychotic drugs are extrapyramidal reactions. The extrapyramidal reactions are most frequent with the piperazine phenothiazines and least frequent with the aliphatic phenothiazines. The origin of the extrapyramidal reactions is the dopamine blockade in areas of the brain governing motor coordination and movement. Four extrapyramidal syndromes are associated with antipsychotic drugs: acute dystonia, akathisia, pseudoparkinsonism, and tardive dyskinesia. *It is important to recognize these bizarre reactions as side effects of drug therapy that require palliative medication or reduction or discontinuance of therapy rather than as manifestations of the psychotic disease being treated, and raising the drug dosage.*

Acute dystonia. Acute dystonia is a spasm of muscles of the tongue, face, neck, or back and may mimic seizures. Dystonia is usually seen in the first 5 days of antipsychotic therapy. It may be treated with an antihistaminic or anticholinergic antiparkinsonian drug (see Chapter 48). Injection of one of these drugs usually dramatically relieves the dystonia. Dystonia reactions are most common in patients under 25 years of age and rarely persist after treatment of the acute reaction. Some of the classic reactions seen in dystonia include torticollis (neck twisting), an oculogyric crisis (upward gaze paralysis), stereotyped motions of the jaw, and opisthotonos (a spasm in which the head and feet create a horseshoe [∩] configuration).

Akathisia. Akathisia is motor restlessness and may be mistaken for psychotic restlessness or agitation. Akathisia commonly appears after the first few days of therapy, and if not recognized, the antipsychotic drug dosage may again be mistakenly increased to relieve the agitation. Patients experiencing akathisia will have difficulty in sitting still and may pace about, fidget, or constantly move their legs. Anticholinergic drugs or a muscle relaxant such as diazepam may be effective in treating these symptoms. If these treatments are not effective, a different antipsychotic drug may have to be tried. Tolerance does not quickly develop to akathisia, but akathisia disappears when the drug is discontinued.

Pseudoparkinsonism. Pseudoparkinsonism is marked by motor retardation and rigidity. The patient finds it difficult to initiate movements or to carry them out. The face resembles a mask because emotions do not register on it. The patient has a shuffling gait, and hypersalivates. A tremor is seen in the hands and legs. These parkinsonian symptoms commonly appear after a week of therapy and are treated with antiparkinsonian drugs. Tolerance does not develop to the parkinsonian symptoms. If they cannot be controlled with drug therapy, the antipsychotic drug has to be changed.

Tardive dyskinesia. Tardive dyskinesia is associated with long-term, high-dose antipsychotic therapy. It is most common in elderly women and

Text continued on p. 652.

Table 41.3 Antipsychotic Drugs

Generic name	Trade name	Administration/dosage	Comments
BUTYROPHENONE			
Haloperidol	Haldol* Halperon Paridol† Novoperidol†	Acute psychotic management: ORAL: *Adults and children over 12 yr*—1 to 15 mg in divided doses initially, which can be increased gradually up to 100 mg to bring symptoms under control. Dosage is then gradually reduced. Maintenance dose, usually 2 to 8 mg daily. FDA Pregnancy Category C. *Elderly patients and children under 12 yr*— 0.5 to 1.5 mg daily initially. Dosage increased by 0.5 mg increments if necessary. Usual maintenance dose, 2 to 4 mg daily. INTRAMUSCULAR: *Adults and children over 12 yr*—2 to 5 mg every 4 to 8 hr or every hour if acute state requires. Acute symptoms are usually under control in 72 hr, and 15 mg daily is usually sufficient. Chronic schizophrenia: ORAL: *Adults and children over 12 yr*—6 to 16 mg in divided doses, gradually increased to achieve control. Doses as high as 100 mg may be necessary to achieve control. Doses then are gradually reduced to achieve maintenance of control, usually 15 to 20 mg daily. *Elderly patients*—0.5 to 1.5 mg initially, increased very gradually. Maintenance dosage, usually 2 to 8 mg daily. Mental retardation with hyperkinesia: ORAL (given after intramuscular treatment as for acute psychoses): *Adults and children over 12 yr*—80 to 120 mg daily, gradually reduced to a maintenance dose of about 60 mg daily. *Elderly patients and children under 12 yr*—1.5 to 6 mg daily in divided doses; gradually increase dosage up to 15 mg daily for control, then reduce dosage for maintenance. Gilles de la Tourette's syndrome: Initial dosages to achieve control are same as for chronic schizophrenia. Maintenance dosages: *adults and children over 12 yr*—9 mg daily; *children under 12 yr*—1.5 mg daily.	Management of psychotic disorders. Very likely to produce extrapyramidal reactions in patients prone to neurological reactions. In severe cases of hyperkinetic, retarded patients, large doses may bring improvement in social behavior and concentration. Drug of choice for the treatment of Gilles de la Tourette's syndrome. Spectrum of side effects is similar to that of the piperazine phenothiazines: low incidence of sedation and autonomic effects, but high incidence of extrapyramidal reactions.
DIBENZOXAZEPINE			
Loxapine succinate	Loxitane Loxapac†	ORAL: *Patients over 16 yr*—10 to 25 mg twice daily initially, with dosage increased rapidly over 7 to 10 days to achieve control. Dosage reduced for maintenance to 60 to 100 mg daily; maximum, 250 mg daily. FDA Pregnancy Category C. *Elderly patients*—⅓ to ½ dose just listed.	A drug effective for schizophrenia and acute psychoses.
DIHYDROINDOLONE			
Molindone hydrochloride	Moban	ORAL: *Adults*—15 to 40 mg daily initially, with increased dosage to control symptoms, up to 225 mg daily. Dosage should then be reduced for maintenance. *Elderly patients*—⅓ to ½ adult dose.	A drug effective for schizophrenia and acute psychoses.

*Available in Canada and United States.
†Available in Canada only.

Table 41.3   Antipsychotic Drugs—cont'd

Generic name	Trade name	Administration/dosage	Comments
PHENOTHIAZINES			
Aliphatic			
Chlorpromazine hydrochloride	Thorazine Chlor-PZ Chlor-Promanyl† Largactil† Thor-Prom Novo-Chlor-promazine†	Psychiatric outpatients: ORAL: *Adults*—12 to 40 yr, average dose 400 to 800 mg daily; over 40, a limit of 300 mg daily is suggested. Acutely psychotic, hospitalized patients: INTRAMUSCULAR: *Adults*—25 to 100 mg every 1 to 4 hr until symptoms are controlled. *Elderly or debilitated patients*—10 mg every 6 to 8 hr to control acute symptoms. *Children*—0.5 mg/kg body weight every 6 to 8 hr, gradually increasing dose to a maximum of 40 mg for children under 5 years and 75 mg for those under 12 years. INTRAVENOUS: not recommended because it is highly irritating. Drug must be diluted to at least 1 mg/ml and no more than 1 mg/min given. ORAL: *Adults*—200 to 600 mg daily in divided doses, increased every 2 to 3 days by 100 mg, up to 2 Gm if needed. *Elderly or debilitated patients*—⅓ to ½ of adult dose with 20 to 25 mg increments. *Children*—0.5 mg/kg every 4 to 6 hr. To control nausea and vomiting: ORAL: 10 to 25 mg every 4 to 6 hr. INTRAMUSCULAR: 25 mg initially, then 25 to 50 mg every 3 to 4 hr to stop vomiting. Other uses: ORAL: *Adults*—25 to 50 mg 3 or 4 times daily. INTRAMUSCULAR: 25 mg every 3 or 4 hr.	Control of initial acute psychotic episodes is achieved with high doses, which are then tapered to the lowest maintenance dose when the patient's condition stabilizes. Best tolerated by patients under 40 years old and those hospitalized less than 10 years. Sedation is very pronounced at the start of therapy, which may be desired for highly agitated patients. Incidence of hypotension, ophthalmic changes, and dyskinesias is high in older patients. Antiadrenergic and anticholinergic side effects usually diminish after the first week. Not for seizure-prone patients. Severe nausea and vomiting can be controlled by low doses. Other uses include intractable hiccups, tetanus, acute intermittent porphyria.
Promazine hydrochloride	Sparine* Promanyl†	Severely agitated patients: INTRAMUSCULAR: *Adults*—50 to 150 mg initially; if no calming effect in 30 min, additional doses may be given to a total of 300 mg. ORAL: *Adults*—10 to 200 mg every 4 to 6 hrs (may also be given IM). ORAL, INTRAMUSCULAR: *Children over 12 yr*—10 to 25 mg every 4 to 6 hr.	When the intramuscular route is used, take precautions for postural hypotension. A syrup is available for oral administration; dilute the concentrate in fruit juice or chocolate flavored drinks. Total daily dose for adults should not exceed 1000 mg.
Triflupromazine hydrochloride	Vesprin	Psychotic disorders: ORAL: *Adults*—50 to 150 mg daily. *Elderly patients*—20 to 30 mg orally daily. *Children over 2½ yr*—0.5 mg/kg body weight, up to 150 mg maximum. INTRAMUSCULAR: *Adults*—50 to 150 mg daily. *Elderly patients*—10 to 75 mg daily. *Children over 2½ yr*—0.2 to 0.25 mg/kg up to 10 mg maximum. All daily doses for children should be divided.	Management of psychotic disorders. Control of nausea and vomiting.

*Available in Canada and United States.
†Available in Canada only.

Continued.

Table 41.3 Antipsychotic Drugs—cont'd

Generic name	Trade name	Administration/dosage	Comments
PHENOTHIAZINES—cont'd			
Aliphatic—cont'd			
Triflupromazine hydrochloride—cont'd		Nausea and vomiting: INTRAVENOUS: *Adults*—1 mg up to 3 mg. INTRAMUSCULAR: *Adults*—5 to 15 mg every 4 hr up to 60 mg daily. ORAL: *Adults*—20 to 30 mg total daily. ORAL, INTRAMUSCULAR: *Children over 2½ yr:* 0.2 mg/kg, to 10 mg in 3 doses daily.	
Piperazine‡			
Acetophenazine maleate	Tindal	ORAL: *Adults*—60 mg daily in divided doses that can be increased in 20 mg increments. Optimum level is usually 80 to 120 mg. Occasionally, severe symptoms require 400 to 600 mg. *Elderly patients*—⅓ to ½ adult dose. *Children*—0.8 to 1.6 mg/kg body weight in divided doses. Maximum, 80 mg daily.	Management of psychotic disorders.
Fluphenazine hydrochloride	Moditen† Prolixin Permitil	ORAL: *Adults*—2.5 to 10 mg initially, reduced to 1 to 5 mg daily for maintenance. *Elderly patients*—⅓ to ½ adult dose. INTRAMUSCULAR: *Adults*—1.25 mg increased gradually to 2.5 to 10 mg daily in 3 to 4 doses. *Elderly patients*—⅓ to ½ adult dose.	Most potent of the phenothiazines used for the management of psychotic disorders.
Fluphenazine decanoate Fluphenazine enanthate	Prolixin Decanoate Prolixin Enanthate	INTRAMUSCULAR, SUBCUTANEOUS: *Adults under 50 yr*—12.5 mg initially, then 25 mg every 2 wk. Increase by 12.5 mg amounts if needed. Rarely require more than 100 mg every 2 to 6 wk.	Long-acting depot forms lasting at least 2 weeks. Dosage should be stabilized in the hospital, since severe episodes of parkinsonism can appear. Not recommended for elderly patients or patients who have had difficulty with extrapyramidal reactions.
Perphenazine	Phenazine† Trilafon	ORAL: *Adults*—16 to 64 mg daily in divided doses. *Elderly patients*—⅓ to ½ adult dose. *Children over 12 yr*—6 to 12 mg daily. INTRAMUSCULAR: *Adults*—5 to 10 mg initially, then 5 mg every 6 hr with 15 mg maximum daily in ambulatory and 30 mg daily in hospitalized patients. *Elderly patients*—⅓ to ½ adult dose. *Children over 12 yr*—lowest adult dose.	For acute psychotic disorders. Lower doses needed when used as an antiemetic.
Prochlorperazine Prochlorperazine edisylate Prochlorperazine maleate	Compazine Compazine Edisylate Compazine Maleate Stemetil†	Psychiatric disorders: ORAL: *Adults*—5 to 10 mg 3 to 4 times daily. Raise dosage every 2 to 3 days as required. From 50 to 75 mg daily is common range for mild cases and 100 to 150 mg for severe cases. *Elderly patients*—⅓ to ½ adult dosage. *Children over 2 yr*—2.5 mg 2 to 3 times daily up to a total dose of 20 to 25 mg. Same dosage used rectally.	More widely used to control severe nausea and vomiting than for psychiatric treatment. Hypotension is seen when given intravenously for surgery.

†Available in Canada only.
‡The piperazine phenothiazines are less sedative in effect and have fewer autonomic side effects than other phenothiazine classes. Extrapyramidal reactions are more common, particularly in large doses in patients over age 40. Piperazine phenothiazines are less likely to produce allergic reactions and do not change ECG tracings.

Table 41.3   Antipsychotic Drugs—cont'd

Generic name	Trade name	Administration/dosage	Comments
PHENOTHIAZINES—cont'd			
Piperazine—cont'd			
Prochlorperazine maleate—cont'd		INTRAMUSCULAR: *Adults*—10 to 20 mg in buttock; repeat every 2 to 4 hr up to 80 mg total. *Elderly patients*—⅓ to ½ adult dose. *Children over 2 yr*—0.13 mg/kg body weight initial dose only, then switch to oral. Nausea and vomiting: ORAL: *Adults*—5 to 10 mg 3 or 4 times daily. *Children*—20 to 29 lb, 2.5 mg 1 to 2 times daily; 30 to 39 lb, 2.5 mg 2 to 3 times daily; 40 to 85 lb, 2.5 mg 3 times daily or 5 mg 2 times daily. INTRAMUSCULAR: *Adults*—5 to 10 mg every 3 to 4 hr. *Children*—0.06 mg/lb. RECTAL: *Adults*—25 mg twice daily. *Children*—same as oral dosage.	
Trifluoperazine	Stelazine Terfluzine† various others	ORAL: *Adults*—2 to 4 mg daily in divided doses (outpatient), 4 to 10 mg daily (hospitalized). *Elderly or debilitated patients*—⅓ to ½ adult dosage. *Children over 6 yr*—1 mg 1 to 2 times daily, gradually raised to maximum of 15 mg. INTRAMUSCULAR: *Adults*—1 to 2 mg every 4 to 6 hr, maximum 10 mg daily. *Elderly or debilitated patients*—⅓ to ½ adult dose. *Children over 6 yr*—same as oral dosage.	Management of psychotic disorders.
Piperidine			
Thioridazine hydrochloride	Mellaril Novoridazine†	Psychotic disorders: ORAL: *Adults*—50 to 100 mg 3 times daily, increasing up to 800 mg. *Elderly patients*—⅓ to ½ adult dose. *Children over 2 yr*—1 mg/kg body weight in divided doses. Depressive neurosis, alcohol withdrawal syndrome, intractable pain, senility: 10 to 50 mg 2 to 4 times daily.	Management of psychotic disorders. Little antiemetic activity. Safe for patients with epilepsy. "Possibly effective" in alcohol withdrawal syndrome, intractable pain, senility. Pronounced sedative and hypotensive side effects initially. One of the least likely of the antipsychotic drugs to cause extrapyramidal reactions because of the pronounced anticholinergic action. Photosensitivity has not been reported. Doses over 800 mg daily have produced serious pigmentary retinopathy.
Mesoridazine besylate	Serentil*	ORAL: *Adults*—150 mg daily initially. Increased by 50 mg increments until symptoms controlled. *Elderly patients*—⅓ to ½ adult dose. INTRAMUSCULAR: *Adults and children over 12 yr*—25 to 175 mg daily in divided doses (irritating).	Management of psychotic disorders. This is a metabolite of thioridazine with antiemetic activity and no reported retinopathy.

*Available in Canada and United States.
†Available in Canada only.
‡The piperazine phenothiazines are less sedative in effect and have fewer autonomic side effects than other phenothiazine classes. Extrapyramidal reactions are more common, particularly in large doses in patients over age 40. Piperazine phenothiazines are less likely to produce allergic reactions and do not change ECG tracings.

Continued.

Table 41.3   Antipsychotic Drugs—cont'd

Generic name	Trade name	Administration/dosage	Comments
THIOXANTHENES§			
Chlorprothixene	Taractan Tarasan†	ORAL: *Adults and children over 12 yr*—75 to 200 mg daily in divided doses. Gradually increase if necessary, with total optimum dose usually being less than 600 mg daily. *Elderly patients*—½ adult dose. INTRAMUSCULAR: *Adults and children over 12 yr*—75 to 200 mg daily in divided doses. *Elderly patients*—½ adult dose.	Management of psychotic disorders. Incidence of side effects same as for aliphatic phenothiazines: high sedation, autonomic effects, low extrapyramidal effects.
Flupenthixol† hydrochloride	Fluanxol†	ORAL: Adults—1 mg 3 times daily initially, increasing by 1 mg every 2–3 days as needed. Maintenance dosages: 3 to 6 mg, up to 12 mg maximum daily in divided doses. Elderly patients should be given a lower dose.	Management of psychotic disorders. Available in Canada only.
Flupenthixol† decanoate	Fluanxol Depot†	INTRAMUSCULAR: *Adults*—initially, 20 to 40 mg every 4 to 10 days. May increase in 20 mg increments.	
Thiothixene	Navane*	ORAL: *Adults and children over 12 yr*—6 to 10 mg daily in divided doses. Gradually increase, with the usual optimum dose 20 to 30 mg daily, rarely as high as 60 mg daily. *Elderly patients*—⅓ to ½ adult dose. INTRAMUSCULAR: *Adults and children over 12 yr*—4 mg 2 to 4 times daily; gradually increase if necessary to a maximum of 30 mg. *Elderly patients*—⅓ to ½ adult dose.	Management of psychotic disorders. Incidence of side effects same as for piperazine phenothiazines: low incidence of sedation and autonomic effects, high incidence of extrapyramidal effects.

*Available in Canada and United States.
†Available in Canada only.
§Chemically related to the phenothiazines.

in patients who have had a cerebrovascular accident (stroke). Tardive dyskinesia is the worst of the extrapyramidal reactions, since it cannot be readily treated, is persistent, and may not altogether disappear when drug therapy is discontinued. It usually appears some months after therapy has been started when the drug dosage is reduced or discontinued. Tardive dyskinesia is believed to represent the development of receptors that are supersensitive to dopamine after prolonged blockade by the antipsychotic drugs. Thus, removing the antipsychotic drug worsens the condition, since dopamine then has ready access to these supersensitive receptors. Antiparkinsonian drugs also worsen the condition, since they either increase dopamine or block the acetylcholine opposing the dopamine. Some common symptoms of tardive dyskinesia are protrusion of the tongue (fly-catcher sign), puffing of the cheeks or the tongue in a cheek (bonbon sign), chewing movements, and involuntary movements of the extremities and trunk (choreoid or athetoid movements). The recent recognition that tardive dyskinesia is a common reaction (up to 50%) in patients treated for a long time with high doses of antipsychotic drugs has prompted reevaluation of long-term therapy with these drugs. The current choice is to use as low a dose as possible and to put the patient on a "drug holiday" during periods of remission.

Other Side Effects (Table 41.2)

Several other side effects are associated with the antipsychotic drugs.

Sedation and postural hypotension. Sedation and postural hypotension are most often seen early in treatment with the aliphatic phenothiazines, the class of phenothiazines with the most prominent adrenergic blocking activity. These side effects are most likely to be prominent in elderly or debilitated patients. If sedation and hypotension are not severe,

THE NURSING PROCESS

ANTIPSYCHOTIC DRUGS

Assessment

Patients requiring antipsychotic drugs are those who display some form of behavior that is characterized as abnormal or ill relative to accepted appropriate forms of behavior. The exact symptoms vary greatly. Assessment should include a total physiological assessment, with a focus on the behavioral component. The nurse should assess the affect, the ability to interact with others, and the ability to initiate appropriate conversation; should assess abnormal thought processes such as hallucinations or delusions; and should observe any unusual mannerisms, or conversely, the lack of any outward activity. The nurse should evaluate such things as judgment, decision making, and overall thought processes. The depth and focus of the mental health examination will vary with the patient and the patient's ability to assist in identifying some, or any, of the specific problems.

Nursing diagnoses

Altered bowel elimination: constipation secondary to drug side effect

Potential impaired physical mobility related to extrapyramidal side effects of antipsychotic therapy

Management

Patients requiring antipsychotic drug therapy also require psychiatric care, at least during initial drug therapy. Initially the goals are to stabilize the patient sufficiently to allow the patient to begin appropriate interactions with the physician or nurse for the purpose of modifying behavior. The nurse should observe the patient closely for changes in overall affect and behavior. The nurse also should monitor vital signs, level of consciousness, blood pressure, and signs of drug toxicity. Serious side effects would include the development of extrapyramidal reactions or acute dystonia. The appearance of these and other side effects may warrant decreasing the drug dose or switching to another drug. If side effects are not severe and if the mental illness is controlled adequately, the physician may elect to continue the drug and either treat the side effects or assist the patient in adapting to them. A variety of psychiatric therapies may be used along with medications; for additional information about the treatment of psychoses and schizophrenia, consult appropriate textbooks of nursing.

Evaluation

Most patients will require continued use of these medications, with brief drug-free periods, for the rest of their lives. Ideally the symptoms will decrease, and the patient will be able to participate fully in the activities of daily living, interacting appropriately. This goal is achieved by some patients and not by others. Before discharge for self-management, if that is appropriate, the patient and/or family should be able to explain how to take the medication correctly, what symptoms or side effects should be reported immediately to the physician, what situations indicating either overdosage or underdosage should be reported to the physician, and what symptoms of disease exacerbation should be reported to the physician.

If other medications are being used, either to treat the underlying condition or to treat side effects of the antipsychotic drugs, the patient and/or family also should be able to explain the necessary information about these drugs. For further specific guidelines, see the patient care implications section.

phenothiazines are also the most likely to produce nonspecific changes in the T wave of the electrocardiogram (ECG). This change has no particular meaning but is undesirable in a patient with concurrent heart disease who is being monitored for ECG changes.

Seizure potential. The antipsychotic drugs must be used with caution in patients with epilepsy, since they can precipitate convulsions. This lowering of the convulsive threshold makes antipsychotic drugs unsuitable for the treatment of drug withdrawal likely to produce seizures, such as withdrawal from alcohol, barbiturates, and other sedative-hypnotic drugs.

Endocrine disturbances. The endocrine impairment that results in sexual dysfunction was discussed relative to the dopaminergic blocking action of the antipsychotic drugs. Women may experience delayed ovulation and menstruation, lack of menstruation (amenorrhea), milk production (galactorrhea), or weight gain. Men may experience impotence, decreased libido, retrograde ejaculation, or moderate breast growth (gynecomastia).

Allergic reactions. Photosensitivity and cholestatic hepatitis are allergic reactions that occasionally develop during therapy.

Photosensitivity. Photosensitivity is fairly common and represents an allergic reaction to a metabolite produced not by the body but by reaction with sunlight. The long half-life of the antipsychotic drugs and their metabolites has been discussed. These metabolites accumulate in the skin, where exposure to sun causes chemical changes that can cause skin allergies. Patients taking antipsychotic drugs should not sunbathe, since they run the risk of a painful skin rash. Some patients develop slate-blue patches in their skin. This is an accumulation of drug metabolites that is not an allergy and is not dangerous.

Cholestatic hepatitis. Cholestatic hepatitis can develop with antipsychotic therapy. Jaundice develops when the bile duct becomes blocked by an allergic inflammation caused by metabolites excreted in the bile. It is commonly seen in the first month of therapy with one of the aliphatic phenothiazines. It is normally mild and self-limiting, but if jaundice is detected, the drug should be stopped and an antipsychotic drug from a different chemical class used.

Blood dyscrasias. A blood dyscrasia is the depression of the synthesis of one of the blood elements and occasionally occurs with antipsychotic therapy. Depression of leukocytes is common with antipsychotic therapy but is usually transient and not serious. Agranulocytosis, however, in which leukocytes are no longer produced, is serious and often fatal. Agranulocytosis is most common within 3 months of the start of therapy. Therefore blood counts should be done early in therapy, and any sign of fever or sore throat indicates the possible onset of agranulocytosis and should be checked immediately.

CLINICAL USES OF ANTIPSYCHOTIC DRUGS

The three major uses of antipsychotic drugs are to treat psychoses, to prevent vomiting, and to potentiate the action of other CNS drugs. The individual antipsychotic drugs are described in detail in Table 41.3, pp. 648-652.

Treatment of Psychoses

The antipsychotic drugs are unique in allowing symptomatic treatment of psychoses. A psychosis is a major emotional disorder with an impairment of mental function great enough to prevent the individual from participating in everyday life. The hallmark of a psychosis is the loss of contact with reality. There is no one symptom of a psychosis. The symptoms may include agitation, hostility, combativeness, hyperactivity, as well as delusions, hallucinations, disordered thought and perception, emotional and social withdrawal, paranoid symptoms, and personal neglect. Antipsychotic drugs specifically reduce at least some of these symptoms so the patient can think and function more coherently.

Psychoses account for most of the hospitalizations for mental illness, disabling as many Americans as heart disease and cancer combined.

Functional psychoses. A functional psychosis may be an isolated "breakdown" caused by a major traumatic event. This psychosis is usually very amenable to treatment with an antipsychotic drug. The acute manic phase of manic-depressive illness is treated with an antipsychotic drug and/or lithium (see Chapter 42).

Schizophrenia. Schizophrenia is a chronic mental illness with psychotic episodes. Before the advent of the antipsychotic drugs in the 1950s, schizophrenia accounted for most of the large patient population in mental hospitals. Today, with continued antipsychotic drug therapy, patients with schizophrenia do not usually require the degree of supervision found in mental hospitals. The current trend is to provide acute initial care in the psychiatric intensive care unit followed by minimum care in community facilities. Antipsychotic drugs do not cure schizophrenia. Treatment is life-long, although patients may be taken off medication for several weeks or months during a disease remission.

PATIENT CARE IMPLICATIONS

General guidelines for care of patients receiving antipsychotics

Drug administration

- Review the common side effects listed in Tables 41.1 and 41.2, as these will be frequently encountered. Assess patients on a regular, ongoing basis for the development of these side effects. Assess thoughtfully: what may appear to be increased agitation may in fact be akathisia, or what may resemble anxiety may be early parkinsonian side effects.
- Monitor the blood pressure every 4 hours until stable; this may require several days to 2 weeks. Some physicians prefer that the blood pressure be monitored with the patient in lying, sitting, and standing positions.
- Side effects may make the patient unsteady when ambulating. Supervise ambulation and assist when appropriate.
- Monitor fluid intake and output until the patient is stabilized. Weigh the patient weekly. Monitor blood glucose levels.
- Contact dermatitis due to the phenothiazines has been reported. Avoid getting the drugs on the skin, and wash hands carefully after preparing these drugs. If working with these drugs frequently, it may be appropriate to wear gloves.
- Supervise patients carefully to ascertain that medication is swallowed and not hidden in the mouth, to be discarded or stored later. Some antipsychotic drugs are available in syrup, injection, or depot injection forms to help ensure that the patient receives the prescribed dose. On an outpatient basis it may be necessary for a responsible family member to supervise medication taking.
- Concentrated oral forms of most antipsychotic drugs are available for institutional use. Dilute dose to at least 60 ml in one of the diluents suggested by the manufacturer.
- Monitor patients with a history of seizures carefully, as antipsychotics may alter the seizure threshhold.
- For IM injection, choose a large muscle mass. Aspirate before injecting to avoid inadvertent IV administration. Warn patient that drug may cause a burning sensation while being injected. Record and rotate injection sites.
- Intramuscular injections of nondepot forms of phenothiazines may cause marked hypotension. Keep the patient supine for ½ to 1 hour following injection, monitor blood pressure, and supervise ambulation. For rare severe reactions, levarterenol and phenyleph-

rine are the vasoconstrictors of choice; do not use epinephrine.
- Read orders and labels carefully. Some drugs are packaged in both an aqueous form and an oil-based depot form. Oil-based depot forms are always administered IM, *never* intravenously.
- When antipsychotics are used as antiemetics, the doses are usually lower. Side effects are milder, and include sedation, hypotension, and dry mouth. However, any side effect listed can occur in that rare individual who is extremely sensitive to the drug. When antipsychotic drugs are given as antiemetics with narcotic analgesics, they may potentiate CNS depressive effects of the analgesics, including hypotension and sedation.
- The care of the mentally ill is complex and involves the use of many treatment modalities. See appropriate texts and articles appropriate to the care of psychiatric patients.

Patient and family education

- Review the anticipated benefits and possible side effects of drug therapy with the patient and family. Review the extrapyramidal side effects listed in Table 41.2. Since there is no effective treatment for tardive dyskinesia, it is important that its appearance be reported immediately. Fine vermicular (worm-like) movements of the tongue may be the first sign of this side effect. Tell the patient and family to report the development of any new sign or symptom.
- See Patient Problems: Dry Mouth (p. 170); Constipation (p. 187); Photosensitivity (p. 647); and Orthostatic Hypotension (p. 237).
- Tell patients that several weeks of therapy may be necessary before full benefit can be seen.
- Swallow extended-release forms whole; do not crush or chew.
- Warn patients to avoid driving or operating hazardous equipment if vision changes or sedation occurs; notify physician.
- Instruct patients to report signs of agranulocytosis: sore throat, fever, malaise. Tell patients to report signs of liver dysfunction: jaundice, malaise, fever, right upper quadrant abdominal pain.
- These drugs may interfere with the body's ability to regulate temperature. Warn patients to avoid prolonged exposure to extremes of temperature, to allow for frequent cooling-off periods when exercising or in hot

Continued.

PATIENT CARE IMPLICATIONS—cont'd

environments, and to dress warmly for exposure to the cold.

- Review possible endocrine side effects with patient and family (see text). Assess carefully and tactfully for these side effects. Provide emotional support as appropriate. If endocrine side effects are intolerable, consult the physician for possible drug or dosage change.
- Instruct the patient to monitor weight (if appropriate to ability and resources). If weight gain is a problem, counsel about low-calorie diets. Refer to a dietitian as needed.
- Caution patients to keep all health care providers informed of all drugs being taken. Warn patients to avoid over-the-counter drugs unless first approved by the physician.
- Caution patients to avoid alcoholic beverages while taking antipsychotics.
- Warn diabetic patients that antipsychotics may alter blood glucose levels. Monitor blood glucose levels carefully. Consult physician about changes in dietary or drug treatment for diabetes.
- Tell patients not to discontinue therapy abruptly or without consultation with the physician.
- Keep these and all drugs out of the reach of children.
- The drugs may produce false-positive pregnancy results. Women who suspct they are pregnant should consult the physician. Women may desire to use contraceptive measures while taking these drugs; counsel as appropriate. As always, pregnant or lactating women should avoid all drugs unless first approved by the physician.
- If additional drugs are prescribed to treat side effects of antipsychotic agents, review their use and side effects with patient and family.

Chlorpromazine

Drug administration

- See general guidelines above.
  INTRAVENOUS ADMINISTRATION
- For direct IV push, dilute chlorpromazine in 0.9% sodium chloride to make a dilution of 1 mg/ml. Administer at a rate of 1.0 mg/min in adults or 0.5 mg/min in children. For infusion, further dilute and infuse slowly. Monitor blood pressure. Keep side rails up. Supervise ambulation following dose.

Droperidol

Drug administration

- Intravenous administration may be given undiluted, or may be further diluted. Administer undiluted drug at a rate of 10 mg or less over 1 minute. Monitor blood pressure. Keep side rails up. Supervise ambulation.

Flupenthixol

Drug administration

- Read orders and labels carefully. The decanoate form is a depot, in which the drug is suspended in sesame oil. Use a 21-gauge needle. See information on administering oil-based suspensions in Chapter 6 (p. 88).

Fluphenazine

Drug administration

- Read orders and labels carefully. The decanoate and enanthate forms are depots, with the drug suspended in sesame oil. Use a dry needle and syringe. A wet needle or syringe will cause the drug to turn cloudy. A large-bore needle should be used, such as a 21-gauge needle. See information on administering oil-based suspensions in Chapter 6 (p. 88).

Haloperidol

Drug administration

- Read orders and labels carefully. The decanoate form is a depot, with the drug suspended in sesame oil. Use a 21-gauge needle. See information on administering oil-based suspensions in Chapter 6 (p. 88).

Perphenazine

Drug administration

- Intravenous administration. Dilute each 5 mg with 9 ml of normal saline for injection. Administer at a rate of 0.5 mg (1 ml) over 1 minute. Monitor blood pressure. Keep side rails up. Supervise ambulation.

Prochlorperazine

Drug administration

- Intravenous administration. For IV push, may be given undiluted. A single dose should not exceed 10 mg. Administer at a rate of

PATIENT CARE IMPLICATIONS—cont'd

5 mg/ml/min. May also be further diluted and given as an infusion.

Promazine

Drug administration

- Intravenous administration. May be given undiluted. Administer at a rate of 25 mg/min. Monitor blood pressure. Keep side rails up. Supervise ambulation.

Triflupromazine

Drug administration

- Intravenous administration. Dilute 10 mg with 9 ml of normal saline for injection. Administer at a rate of 1 mg (1 ml) over 2 minutes. Monitor blood pressure. Keep side rails up. Supervise ambulation.

Organic psychoses. Organic psychoses result from damage to the brain by such things as infectious diseases, deficiency diseases, lead poisoning, tumors, and injury through trauma or interrupted blood supply, as in cerebrovascular accidents. Organic psychoses are not treated with antipsychotic drugs as successfully as functional psychoses.

Toxic psychoses. Toxic psychoses can arise during withdrawal from alcohol or other drugs. Some toxic psychoses are treated with diazepam, one of the antianxiety drugs, rather than with the antipsychotic drugs. Amphetamine can cause a toxic psychosis because it releases dopamine in the CNS, and therefore the blockade of dopamine receptors by antipsychotic drugs provides specific therapy for an amphetamine-induced psychosis.

Antiemetic Use of Antipsychotic Drugs

Several of the antipsychotic drugs are prescribed to control vomiting. Chlorpromazine, triflupromazine, perphenazine, and prochlorperazine in particular are widely used as antiemetics. Chlorpromazine also is prescribed for intractable hiccups. Because of the numerous side effects of these drugs, their use as antiemetics is restricted to the management of postoperative nausea and vomiting, radiation and chemotherapy sickness, nausea and vomiting caused by toxins, and intractable vomiting.

Antipsychotic Drugs and Drug Potentiation

Antipsychotic drugs potentiate the action of CNS depressant drugs, including sedative-hypnotic drugs, narcotic analgesics, and anesthetic agents. The potentiation of sedative-hypnotic drugs, including alcohol, is an important drug interaction. The effects of an alcoholic drink or a sleeping pill are greatly exaggerated in a patient who is taking

an antipsychotic drug. A toxic overdose of the alcohol or sedative-hypnotic drug therefore becomes possible at a lower dose.

Clinical use is made of the potentiation of narcotic analgesic drugs by antipsychotic drugs. Terminal cancer patients in chronic pain can be relieved by receiving lower doses of a narcotic analgesic drug when an antipsychotic drug is also given. This greatly slows the development of tolerance to the narcotics. The antipsychotic drug has the further advantage of controlling the vomiting produced by radiation therapy or chemotherapy.

Finally, droperidol, a drug related to the antipsychotic drug haloperidol, is widely used with a narcotic to produce a state of quiescence and indifference to stimuli, which allows such procedures as bronchoscopy, x-ray studies, burn dressing, and cystoscopy to be performed. Nitrous oxide can be added to this neuroleptic-narcotic combination to produce general anesthesia for surgery, neuroleptanesthesia. The anesthesia results from the synergistic effect of the drugs with nitrous oxide, for nitrous oxide alone is not potent enough to produce surgical anesthesia (see Chapter 45).

SUMMARY

Current antipsychotic drugs come from five chemical classes, with the phenothiazines being the oldest and most numerous. The antipsychotic action is attributed to the blockade of dopaminergic receptors in the limbic system. Blockade of dopaminergic receptors in other areas of the brain accounts for the antiemetic action, extrapyramidal reactions, and endocrine disturbances characteristic of these drugs. Sedation and orthostatic hypotension are characteristic side effects of those antipsychotic drugs, which also block adrenergic receptors. Some antipsychotic drugs also have anticholinergic activity, which gives rise to atropine-like effects but also decreases the incidence of extrapyramidal side effects.

Antipsychotic drugs primarily are administered orally. Although the sedation characteristic of some antipsychotic drugs is seen within an hour, antipsychotic effects take a week to develop and require a month or more of continuous therapy for the full effect to be apparent. Extrapyramidal reactions are the main limitation of the antipsychotic drugs. These disorders in movement coordination, acute dystonia, akathisia, pseudoparkinsonism, and tardive dyskinesia, are described fully in the text and in Table 41.2. Other side effects associated with antipsychotic drugs include sedation and postural hypotension, ECG changes, a lowering of the seizure potential, endocrine disturbances, allergic reactions, and rarely blood dyscrasias.

The clinical uses of antipsychotic drugs are to treat psychoses and emesis and to potentiate other CNS depressants for surgery or analgesia. The psychoses responsive to antipsychotic drugs include functional psychoses, schizophrenia, and amphetamine-induced psychosis. Organic psychoses and withdrawal psychoses do not readily respond to antipsychotic drugs.

STUDY QUESTIONS

1. What is the major chemical class of antipsychotic drugs? List the three subclasses.
2. What are the four actions of antipsychotic drugs attributable to blockade of dopaminergic receptors?
3. What are two actions of antipsychotic drugs attributable to blockade of receptors for norepinephrine?
4. What are two actions of antipsychotic drugs attributable to blockade of cholinergic receptors?
5. List the four types of extrapyramidal reactions, the key features of each type, and when each type is likely to occur during antipsychotic drug therapy.
6. Describe the allergic reactions attributed to antipsychotic drugs.
7. For which types of psychoses are antipsychotic drugs generally effective?
8. Name the two clinical uses of antipsychotic drugs other than the treatment of psychoses.

SUGGESTED READINGS

Alberti-Flor, J.J.: Chlorpromazine-induced lupus-like illness, Am. Fam. Physician 26(4):151, 1983.

Appleton, W.S.: Fourth psychoactive drug usage guide, J. Clin. Psychiatry 43(1):12, 1982.

Bickal, T.: A protocol for the diagnosis and treatment of extrapyramidal symptoms of neuroleptic drugs, Nurse Pract. 12(1):25, 1987.

Butler, F.R., Burgio, L.D., and Engel, B.T.: Neuroleptics and behavior: a comparative study, J. Gerontol. Nurs. 13(6): 15, 1987.

Diamond, J.M., and Santos, A.B.: Unusual complications of antipsychotic drugs, Am. Fam. Physician 26(4):153, 1982.

DiGiacomo, J.N.: Major tranquilizers: an operator's manual for nonpsychiatrists, Consultant, 21(11):68, 1981.

Hasan, M.K., and Mooney, R.P.: Once-a-day drug regimen for psychiatric patients, Am. Fam. Physician 24(4):123, 1981.

Henn, F.A.: Complications of antipsychotic drug therapy, Res. Staff Physician 28(2):122, 1982.

Jackson, R.T., and Haynes-Johnson, V.: Nutritional management of patients undergoing long-term antipsychotic and antidepressant therapies, Arch. Psychiatr. Nurse. 2(3):146, 1988.

Karp, J.M.: Metoclopramide treatment of tardive dyskinesia, JAMA 246(17):1934, 1981.

Labson, L.H.: Zeroing in on schizophrenia, Patient Care 18(1):66, 1984.

Labson, L.J.: How you can help the schizophrenic, Patient Care 18(1):99, 1984.

Lippman, S.: The treatment of dementia, Res. Staff Physician 28(2):86, 1982.

Miller, M.J.: Simplified psychotropic dosages schedules, Res. Staff Physician 27(4):61, 1981.

Richelson, E.: Changes in the sensitivity of receptors for neurotransmitters and the actions of some psychotherapeutic drugs, Mayo Clin. Proc. 57:576, 1982.

Salzberger, G.J.: Tardive dyskinesia: a risk in long-term neuroleptic therapy, Intern. Med. 4(10):152, 1983.

Sheehan, D.V.: Current views on the treatment of panic and phobic disorders, Drug Therapy 7(10):74, 1982.

Snyder, S.H.: Schizophrenia, Lancet, Oct. 30, 1982, p. 970.

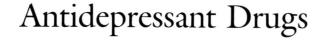

Antidepressant Drugs

42

Nature of Depressive Disorders

DEPRESSION

Depression is a disorder of mood (affect) that occurs in an estimated 15% to 30% of all adults at some time during their lives. Depression is not a single entity; rather it is a syndrome that can include various symptoms, as outlined in Table 42.1. Depression becomes a medical problem when normal functioning is significantly hampered. Three major categories of depression are recognized: reactive depression, endogenous depression, and manic-depressive disorder.

Reactive Depression, Endogenous Depression, and Manic-Depressive Disorder

Reactive depression is experienced after some significant loss in life. This depression is usually acute for a couple of weeks and resolves within 3 months. Therapy for reactive depression is to provide emotional support. One of the benzodiazepines, the antianxiety drugs, may be prescribed to relieve anxiety or insomnia if required. An antidepressant drug typically is not needed.

Endogenous depression is depression with no apparent cause. Current views are that endogenous depression is a neurochemical disorder that can be treated with appropriate drug therapy. This concept arose from the observation in the 1950s that reserpine caused depression in patients treated for hypertension. Reserpine was found to deplete the neurotransmitter norepinephrine. About the same time, iproniazid, a drug then used to treat tuberculosis, was found to relieve depression in patients, inhibiting the degradation of norepinephrine by inhibiting the enzyme monoamine oxidase. These two observations suggested that a deficiency in the brain neurotransmitter norepinephrine is associated with depression. Current evidence favors a *biogenic amine* theory of depression, in which a deficiency either in brain norepinephrine or in another amine neurotransmitter, serotonin, is associated with depression. The two drug classes currently used to treat depression, the tricyclic antidepressants and the monoamine oxidase inhibitors, have pharmacological mechanisms that restore norepinephrine and serotonin in the brain.

Manic-depressive is the third type of depressive disorder. The classic manic-depressive patient has a manic period characterized by excessive euphoria, overactivity, a flow of ideas, extreme self-confidence, and little need for sleep, alternating with a period of depression. Lithium is the specific drug treatment for mania.

Depression as a Drug Side Effect

In addition to these three classes, depression can also be the side effect of some drugs, especially the antihypertensive drugs reserpine, methyldopa, guanethidine, and propranolol. Alcohol and antianxiety drugs often unmask depression by alleviating the anxiety that frequently accompanies depression. Steroids, particularly glucocorticoids and oral contraceptives, can cause depression. Drug-induced depression mimics endogenous depression but is treated by removing the drug or lowering the dose.

Drugs Used to Treat Depressive Disorders (Table 42.2)

TRICYCLIC ANTIDEPRESSANTS

Mechanism of action. The tricyclic antidepressants block the reuptake of norepinephrine and/or serotonin into the presynaptic neurons, as depicted in Figure 42.1, p. 664. This action causes an increase

Table 42.1 Symptoms Characteristic of Depression

Parameter	Change
General mood	Low for a week or more
Behavior	Appetite or weight change
	Sleep change; early morning awakening is the most common insomnia; some patients may sleep more than usual, though level of activity is either exaggerated or depressed
	Loss of energy
	Loss of interest in activities and/or sex
	Feelings of guilt or self-reproach
	Inability to concentrate
	Thoughts of suicide

in the synaptic concentration of these neurotransmitters, which is an early effect of the drug. However, clinically no antidepressant response is seen for 2 weeks. Recent research suggests that the tricyclic antidepressants also alter the sensitivity of brain tissue to the action of norepinephrine and serotonin. Since this effect takes 2 weeks to become established, this action more closely correlates with the onset of the clinical antidepressant action.

Administration and fate. The tricyclic antidepressants usually are administered orally, although amitriptyline and imipramine are available in injectable forms. Metabolites of the tricyclic antidepressants are active, so that an active form of the drug persists despite the drug being well absorbed and readily metabolized by the intestine and liver. The rate of tricyclic metabolism decreases with age, and people over 55 generally are started at half the regular adult dose.

The major side effects of the tricyclic antidepressants are an atropine-like (anticholinergic) effect and sedation. The relative incidence of these side effects among the tricyclics is listed in Table 42.3. Because of these side effects, the drug usually is given before bedtime so that the patient is asleep when the side effects are at their peak. The more sedating tricyclics, amitriptyline and doxepin, are particularly effective in relieving the insomnia of depression when given as a bedtime dose. These

drugs do not interfere with the normal sleep pattern described in Chapter 40.

The anticholinergic and sedative side effects are apparent with the first dose of a tricyclic antidepressant, although little lifting of the depression is seen before 2 weeks of therapy. Thus the dose is started at about one third the expected therapeutic dose to allow the patient to develop tolerance to the side effects. The dose is increased to the expected therapeutic dose over the first week. After 2 weeks of drug therapy, the dosage is reviewed in light of side effects and therapeutic response. The final dosage is individualized for the patient. Therapy is discontinued if no response occurs after 1 month. If the patient's depression is relieved, the duration of therapy depends on the severity of the depression being treated. A mild depression might be treated for 2 to 3 months, whereas a severe depression might be treated for 1 to 2 years. The drug therapy then is gradually withdrawn. Reappearance of depression is a sign for reinstituting drug therapy. The spectrum of therapy for depression ranges from a few weeks to a lifetime, depending on the severity and recurrence of depression.

Anticholinergic side effects. The anticholinergic side effects include dry mouth, blurred vision, and constipation. Some patients may experience temporary confusion or speech blockage. Patients with glaucoma or those disposed toward glaucoma must have this condition checked when taking tricyclic antidepressants because the anticholinergic effect may worsen this condition. The anticholinergic action also may adversely affect patients with urinary retention or obstruction, particularly elderly ones.

Cardiac effects. The tricyclic antidepressants have three separate pharmacological actions on the heart: anticholinergic, adrenolytic, and a quinidine-like action. Therefore the final cardiac effect is complex and depends on dosage. The anticholinergic action increases the heart rate. The adrenolytic action is to prevent the reuptake of norepinephrine into neurons, an action that tends to deplete norepinephrine stores in peripheral neurons. The most common adrenolytic side effect is orthostatic (postural) hypotension. This decrease in blood pressure affects the heart by lowering the workload. The quinidine-like side effects are seen at high concentrations of the tricyclic antidepressants. This results in a decreased heart rate, decreased myocardial contractility, and decreased coronary blood flow. For these reasons, tricyclic antidepressants are contraindicated for patients with a recent myocardial infarction, and present special concern for the patient with cardiac disease.

Table 42.2 Antidepressant Drugs

Generic name	Trade name	Administration/dosage	Comments
TRICYCLIC ANTIDEPRESSANTS			
Amitriptyline hydrochloride	Elavil* Endep Levate† Novotrip-tyn†	ORAL: *Adults*—begin with 50 mg at bedtime, increase dosage by 25 to 50 mg if necessary to 150 mg. Alternately, start with 25 mg 3 times daily, increase to 50 mg 3 times daily. Total dosage should not exceed 300 mg daily. Maintenance doses are usually 50 to 100 mg at bedtime. These are outpatient dosages; inpatient dosages may be twice as much. FDA Pregnancy Category C. *Adolescents and elderly*—10 mg 3 times daily plus 20 mg at bedtime (50 mg total) is usually sufficient. INTRAMUSCULAR: 20 to 30 mg 4 times daily.	Bedtime administration is preferred to lessen the discomfort of the sedation and anticholinergic effects prominent with this drug.
Clomipramine	Anafranil†	ORAL: *Adults*—initially, 25 mg 3 times a day, then up to 200 mg for outpatients, 300 mg for inpatients. *Geriatric patients*—20 to 30 mg daily in divided doses.	Available in Canada only. Used for obsessive-compulsive disorders, for blocking panic attacks, and to treat cataplexy associated with narcolepsy.
Desipramine hydrochloride	Norpramin* Pertofrane*	ORAL: *Adults*—begin with 25 mg 3 times daily, increase gradually to a total of 200 mg daily and not more than 300 mg daily; maintenance dosages usually 50 to 200 mg taken at bedtime. *Adolescents and elderly*—25 to 50 mg daily; increased to 100 mg in divided doses if necessary.	Sedation and anticholinergic effects are not prominent. A metabolite of imipramine.
Doxepin hydrochloride	Adapin Sinequan* Triadapin†	ORAL: *Adults*—75 mg, increased to 150 mg in divided doses or at bedtime; maintenance dose usually 25 to 150 mg daily and should not exceed 300 mg daily.	Bedtime administration is preferred to lessen the discomfort of the sedation and anticholinergic effects prominent with this drug. Doxepin is reported to have much less effect on the heart when compared to the other tricyclic antidepressants.
Imipramine hydrochloride Imipramine pamoate	Impril† Janimine Tipramine Tofranil* Tofranil-PM	ORAL: *Adults*—75 mg daily in divided doses or at bedtime. Dose may be increased up to 200 mg daily if required. These are outpatient doses; inpatient doses are ⅓ higher. *Adolescents and elderly*—30 to 40 mg daily, increased to a maximum of 100 mg/day. *Children over 6 yr*—for bed-wetting, 25 mg, 1 hr before bedtime; if no response in 1 week, increase to 50 mg; *over 12 yr*—may receive up to 75 mg.	Imipramine is the prototype tricyclic antidepressant. Sedative and anticholinergic effects are moderate. Can be taken at bedtime.

*Available in Canada and United States.
†Available in Canada only.

Continued.

Table 42.2   Antidepressant Drugs—cont'd

Generic name	Trade name	Administration/dosage	Comments
TRICYCLIC ANTIDEPRESSANTS—cont'd			
Nortriptyline hydrochloride	Aventyl* Pamelor	ORAL: *Adults*—initially, 40 mg in divided doses or at bedtime; maximum dose 100 to 150 mg daily. *Adolescents and children*—30 to 50 mg daily in divided doses.	A metabolite of amitriptyline. Sedative effect is moderate; anticholinergic effect mild. Can be taken at bedtime.
Protriptyline hydrochloride	Triptil† Vivactil	ORAL: *Adults*—15 to 40 mg daily divided in 3 to 4 doses; maximum dose 60 mg daily. Increments are added to the morning dose. *Adolescents and elderly*—15 mg daily in 3 doses. No more than 20 mg total.	This is the only tricyclic antidepressant that has little sedative action and can cause insomnia if given at bedtime. Preferred for the patient who has been immobile and sleepy.
Trimipramine maleate	Surmontil	ORAL: *Adults*—75 mg daily increased to 150 mg in divided doses or at bedtime. These are outpatient dosages; inpatient dosages 100 mg daily increased to 200 mg daily with a maximum of 300 mg daily. FDA Pregnancy Category C. *Adolescents and elderly*—50 mg daily, increased to no more than 100 mg daily as required.	Sedation is high, but the anticholinergic effect is moderate.
SECOND-GENERATION ANTIDEPRESSANTS			
Amoxapine	Asendin*	ORAL: *Adults*—75 mg initially, increase to 200 mg daily in divided doses. If no improvement in 3 wk, increase dosage 50 mg daily every other week to maximum of 400 mg for outpatients, 600 mg for inpatients. FDA Pregnancy Category C.	Related to the tricyclic antidepressants. Low incidence of anticholinergic, sedative, and cardiovascular effects. May be taken at bedtime to lessen daytime sedation or to treat insomnia.
Fluoxetine	Prozac	ORAL: *Adults*—initially, 20 mg as a morning dose. May increase by 20 mg if needed after several weeks, adding as a noon dose.	A new antidepressant, chemically unrelated to other antidepressants. A selective blocker of the neuronal uptake of serotonin. Causes insomnia and depresses the appetite.
Maprotiline	Ludiomil*	ORAL: *Adults*—75 mg, increased to 150 mg daily in divided doses. If no improvement in 3 wk, increase dosage 50 mg daily every other week to maximum of 300 mg. FDA Pregnancy Category B. *Elderly and adolescents*—⅓ adult dose.	Low incidence of anticholinergic, sedative, and cardiovascular effects. May be taken at bedtime to lessen daytime sedation or to treat insomnia.

*Available in Canada and United States.
†Available in Canada only.

Table 42.2   Antidepressant Drugs—cont'd

Generic name	Trade name	Administration/dosage	Comments
SECOND-GENERATION ANTIDEPRESSANTS—cont'd			
Trazodone	Desyrel* Trazon Trialodine	ORAL: *Adults*—75 mg initially, or increased by 50 mg daily every 3 or 4 days to 300 mg if necessary. If no improvement in 3 wk, increase dosage 50 mg daily every other week to maximum of 300 mg. FDA Pregnancy Category C.	Sedation may be noted. Low incidence of anticholinergic and cardiovascular effects. May be taken at bedtime to lessen daytime sedation or to treat insomnia.
MONOAMINE OXIDASE (MAO) INHIBITORS			
Isocarboxazid	Marplan*	ORAL: *Adults*—20 to 30 mg daily in divided doses; maintenance dose usually 10 to 20 mg daily.	Patient should be instructed in food and drug interactions with the MAO inhibitors.
Phenelzine sulfate	Nardil*	ORAL: *Adults*—45 to 75 mg daily in 3 doses or 1 mg/kg body weight in divided doses. Daily dosage should not exceed 90 mg.	Patient should be instructed in food and drug interactions with the MAO inhibitors.
Tranylcypromine sulfate	Parnate*	ORAL: *Adults*—20 to 40 mg daily in 2 doses for 2 weeks. Dosage is reduced after a response is obtained. Usually the maintenance dose is below 30 mg. Higher doses are not advised for outpatients.	Patient should be instructed in food and drug interactions with the MAO inhibitors. Has some psychomotor stimulant activity characteristic of amphetamine.
LITHIUM			
Lithium carbonate	Eskalith Lithane* Lithizine† Lithonate Lithotabs	ORAL: *Adults*—initially 0.6 to 2.1 Gm daily divided into 3 doses. Increase or decrease dose by 0.3 Gm/day to obtain a blood level of 0.8 to 1.5 mEq/L. FDA Pregnancy Category D.	Blood should not be drawn for determination of lithium levels earlier than 8 hours after the last dose. Levels above 2.0 mEq/L are toxic. Patients should be instructed not to "make up" a missed dose of lithium.
Lithium citrate	Cibalith-S	Maintenance dose usually 0.9 to 1.2 Gm daily in divided doses.	

*Available in Canada and United States.
†Available in Canada only.

Hyperthyroid patients, who are at risk for developing cardiac arrhythmias, have this risk potentiated by the tricyclic antidepressants. Doxepin is a tricyclic antidepressant that has minimum cardiac effects.

Acute toxicity. The tricyclic antidepressants are not addicting, and their abuse potential appears very limited. A major problem is their acute toxicity when depressed patients overdose on the tricyclic antidepressant drug in a suicide attempt. Doses of 1 Gm of the sedating tricyclics are toxic, and doses of 2 Gm are often fatal. Those doses represent only a 5- and 10-fold margin, respectively, over the therapeutic dose.

The toxicity of an overdose of the tricyclic antidepressants is essentially an anticholinergic (atropine-like) poisoning. The early symptoms are confusion, an inability to concentrate, and perhaps visual hallucinations. More severe signs include delirium, seizures, and coma. Respiration may be depressed. The patient may have a low body temperature early but an elevated body temperature later.

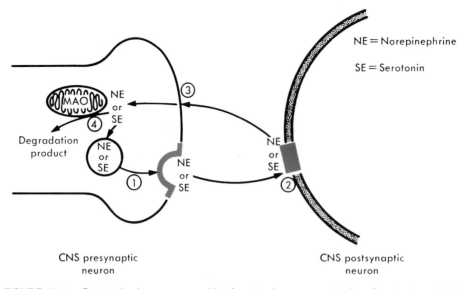

NE = Norepinephrine

SE = Serotonin

CNS presynaptic neuron

CNS postsynaptic neuron

FIGURE 42.1   Depression is seen as resulting from too low a concentration of amine to act at the receptor; mania is seen as an overabundance of amine acting at the receptor. In the diagram the biogenic amine theory of depression is applied to the actions of the antidepressant drugs, the tricyclic antidepressants and the monoamine oxidase inhibitors, and to the action of lithium, used to treat mania (the opposite of depression).*1*, Lithium inhibits the release of norepinephrine and serotonin. *2*, Tricyclic antidepressants and monoamine oxidase inhibitors increase the receptor sensitivity to norepinephrine and serotonin. *3*, Tricyclic antidepressants block the reuptake of norepinephrine and serotonin. Lithium enhances the reuptake of norepinephrine and serotonin. *4*, Monoamine oxidase inhibitors prevent the degradation of norepinephrine and serotonin.

The pupils are dilated, the eyeballs restless, the reflexes hyperactive, and motor coordination compromised. Depending on the cardiac status of the patient and the degree of overdose, the overall cardiac effect may range from tachycardia to slowing of the heart rate (bradycardia) to various arrhythmias secondary to an atrioventricular block. Especially serious is the slowing of conduction in the atrioventricular node by the quinidine-like action, which can result in a heart block. Sudden death from cardiac arrhythmias may occur several days after an overdose. Physostigmine (Antilirium), a peripherally and centrally active anticholinesterase agent, reverses the anticholinergic toxic symptoms of tricyclic overdose. Physostigmine, 2 mg, is administered every 1 to 2 hours, as necessary. This drug must be administered frequently because it is short acting, whereas the tricyclics are long acting.

The tricyclic antidepressants do not decrease the suicide potential among depressed patients during the early weeks of therapy. Depressed patients with suicidal thoughts are best hospitalized to be-

Table 42.3   Relative Incidence of Side Effects of Tricyclic Antidepressants*

Drug	Sedative activity	Anticholinergic activity
Amitriptyline	+ + +	+ + +
Desipramine	+	+
Doxepin	+ + +	+ + +
Imipramine	+ +	+ +
Nortriptyline	+	+
Protriptyline	+ /0	+ +
Trimipramine	+ + +	+ +

*Number of + indicates relative activity; + /0 indicates no activity.

Table 42.4   Drug Interactions of Antidepressant Drugs

Drug class	Effect on therapy with a tricyclic antidepressant	Drug class	Effect on therapy with a monoamine oxidase inhibitor
Monoamine oxidase inhibitors	Hypertensive crisis and/or high fever	Sympathomimetics* (amphetamine, alpha methyldopa, levodopa, dopamine, tryptophan, epinephrine, norepinephrine)	Hypertensive crisis
Guanethidine	Antihypertensive effect blocked	Tricyclic antidepressants	Hypertensive crisis
Clonidine	Antihypertensive effect blocked	Alcohol	CNS depression
Anticholinergics	Potentiation of anticholinergic effects	Meperidine	CNS depression
Sympathomimetics	Potentiation of sympathomimetic effects	Sleeping pills	CNS depression
Alcohol	Potentiation of central nervous system (CNS) depression	Antihistamines*	CNS depression
Barbiturates	Potentiation of CNS depression; increased metabolism of tricyclic antidepressants	Antihypertensive drugs	Orthostatic hypotension
		Diuretics (particularly thiazides)	Orthostatic hypotension
Benzodiazepines	Potentiation of CNS depression	Insulin	Hypoglycemia
Methylphenidate	Decreased metabolism of tricyclic antidepressants	Oral hypoglycemic drugs	Hypoglycemia

*Preparations frequently containing sympathomimetic or antihistaminic drugs include asthma preparations, cold tablets, or capsules, cough medications, nose drops or sprays, sinus preparations, and weight-reducing pills.

DIETARY CONSIDERATION: TYRAMINE

Patients taking MAO inhibitors may experience a hypertensive crisis if they ingest foods containing a large amount of tyramine. The hypertensive crisis is described in the text. Foods high in tyramine include:

avocados
bananas
beer
bologna
canned figs
chocolate
cheese (except
   cottage cheese)
cheese-containing
   food (e.g., pizza or
   macaroni and cheese)
liver
meat extracts:
   Marmite,
   Bovril
offal

papaya products, including meat tenderizers
pate
pickled and kippered herring
pepperoni
pods or broad beans (fava beans)

raisins
raw yeast or yeast
   extracts
salami
sausage
sour cream
soy sauce
wine, chianti
yogurt

THE NURSING PROCESS

ANTIDEPRESSANT DRUGS

Assessment

Antidepressants are used for patients with pronounced, prolonged depression or those with a diagnosis of manic-depressive disease. In addition to a thorough physiological assessment, the nurse should assess the mental status, focusing on objective signs of depression that the patient may be displaying. The nurse also should monitor vital signs, weight, and blood pressure.

Nursing diagnoses

Possible body image disturbance related to weight gain as a drug side effect

Potential for self-harm

Altered bowel elimination: constipation

Management

During the management phase, the health care team observes the patient to determine the appropriate discharge drug level. The nurse should monitor the fluid intake and output, the weight, and the blood pressure. If serum blood levels of the drug have been obtained, these should be reviewed. The patient's level of consciousness should be observed, with attention to excessive sedation. All patients with severe depression should be observed for possible suicidal tendencies. The nurse should look for side effects of the drugs, such as the dry mouth and constipation that may occur with tricyclic antidepressants. Additional psychiatric therapies may be used in treating these patients; for additional information about psychiatric care, see an appropriate nursing text-book.

Evaluation

Antidepressant drugs are considered successful if the patient's depression lessens and the patient is suffering few if any side effects resulting from drug therapy. Before discharging a patient for self-management, ascertain that the patient and/or the family can explain what drug is being taken, how to take it correctly, the side effects that may occur and those that should be reported immediately to the physician, any dietary restrictions associated with the medication being used, and the ways in which the success of the drug will be monitored. The patient or family should be able to explain why follow-up is necessary and when to return for the follow-up visits. For more specific information, see the patient care implications section.

gin drug therapy rather than being given quantities of drugs that may be used in a suicide attempt. Patients who have attempted or threatened suicide frequently are treated initially with electroconvulsive shock therapy. Since tricyclic antidepressants can increase the seizure potential, they are not administered concurrently with electroconvulsive shock therapy.

Drug interactions. Table 42.4 lists several drug interactions with the tricyclic antidepressants. The tricyclic antidepressants can potentiate central nervous system depression, anticholinergic effects, and sympathomimetic effects. The interaction of guanethidine and a tricyclic antidepressant is clas-

sic: the tricyclic antidepressant inhibits the uptake of guanethidine by the neurons so that guanethidine cannot reach its site of action and is therefore ineffective in lowering blood pressure. Clonidine is also blocked from its reuptake site in the central nervous system by the tricyclic antidepressants.

Specific Tricyclic Antidepressants

Amitriptyline

Amitriptyline (Elavil, others) is associated with a high incidence of sedation and anticholinergic effects. These properties are more pronounced than with other tricyclic antidepressants and can

Table 42.5   Toxic Symptoms of Lithium

Blood level (mEq/L)	Symptoms	Blood level (mEq/L)	Symptoms
Below 1.5	Fine tremor of hands Dry mouth Increased thirst Increased urination Nausea	2.0 to 2.5	Persistent nausea and vomiting Blurred vision Muscle twitching (fasciculations) Hyperactive deep tendon reflexes
1.5 to 2.0	Vomiting Diarrhea Muscle weakness Incoordination (ataxia) Dizziness Confusion Slurred speech	2.5 to 3.0	Myoclonic twitches or movements of an entire limb Choreoathetoid movements Urinary and fecal incontinence
		Above 3.0	Seizures Cardiac arrhythmias Hypotension Peripheral vascular collapse Death

cause confusion in the older patient. Weight gain sometimes occurs. Amitriptyline has a plasma half-life of about 1 to 2 days and is metabolized to nortriptyline, an active tricyclic antidepressant.

Desipramine

Desipramine (Norpramin, Pertofrane) has a low incidence of sedation and anticholinergic effects. It is a metabolite of imipramine and has a plasma half-life of ½ to 3 days.

Doxepin

Doxepin (Adapin, Sinequan) has a high incidence of sedative and anticholinergic side effects. Doxepin does not have the quinidine-like cardiac effect to the degree characteristic of the other tricyclic drugs and therefore is indicated when cardiac function must be considered.

Imipramine

Imipramine (Tofranil, others) has a moderate degree of sedative and anticholinergic side effects. It is metabolized to desipramine, which is also an active tricyclic antidepressant. Imipramine has a plasma half-life of ½ to 1 day. Imipramine occasionally is used to treat enuresis (bed-wetting) in older children or adults.

Nortriptyline

Nortriptyline (Aventyl, Pamelor) is moderately sedating and has minimum anticholinergic side effects. It is a metabolite of amitriptyline.

Protriptyline

Protriptyline (Vivactil) is the one tricyclic antidepressant with minimum sedating effect and is therefore most useful in depressed patients who seem physically immobilized by their depression or who sleep excessively. The plasma half-life of protriptyline is very long (4 to 9 days).

Trimipramine

Trimipramine (Surmontil) is a tricyclic antidepressant with a high incidence of sedation and a moderate incidence of anticholinergic effects.

SECOND-GENERATION ANTIDEPRESSANTS

New antidepressant drugs have been introduced that are neither tricyclics nor monoamine oxidase inhibitors. They are regarded as alternatives to tricyclic antidepressants, although their action on norepinephrine and serotonin uptake is not necessarily similar to that of the tricyclics. The new antidepressant drugs have, to a varying degree, a lesser incidence of anticholinergic side effects, less cardiotoxicity, and a faster onset of action than the tricyclics.

Specific Newer Antidepressant Drugs

Amoxapine

Amoxapine (Asendin) does inhibit amine uptake and is a more potent inhibitor of norepinephrine than of serotonin uptake. Chemically related to the tricyclic antidepressants, amoxapine is also a chemical metabolite of the antipsychotic drug loxapine and as with the antipsychotic drugs, blocks dopamine receptors. Overall, amoxapine is considered effective in treating major depression and in relieving anxiety and agitation associated with depression.

Amoxapine has minimum anticholinergic and sedative effects and a lesser incidence of cardiac effects than the tricyclics. Drug interactions are similar to those of the tricyclics.

Fluoxetine

Fluoxetine (Prozac) is a newer antidepressant that blocks the neuronal uptake of serotonin. It is less likely to cause anticholinergic effects such as dry mouth, blurred vision, or constipation. Side effects are more commonly insomnia, nervousness, headache, and nausea. Fluoxetine depresses appetite. It may also prove useful in treating obsessive-compulsive disorders, and alcoholism.

Maprotiline

Maprotiline (Ludiomil) is a tetracyclic antidepressant that inhibits norepinephrine but not serotonin uptake. Drug interactions and side effects are similar to those of the tricyclic antidepressants. The incidence of drowsiness, anticholinergic effects and cardiac effects, however, is less than with amitriptyline or doxepin.

Trazodone

Trazodone (Desyrel) is chemically unrelated to other antidepressant drugs. Trazodone is an inhibitor of serotonin uptake. Drowsiness is a side effect, but minimum anticholinergic and cardiac effects occur.

MONOAMINE OXIDASE INHIBITORS

Mechanism of action. The monoamine oxidase (MAO) inhibitors were in use before the tricyclic antidepressants were discovered. The MAO inhibitors irreversibly inhibit the enzyme monoamine oxidase. According to the biogenic amine hypothesis of depression, the MAO inhibitors are effective because they prevent the degradation of norepinephrine and serotonin, so that the concentration of these central nervous system neurotransmitters is increased, as diagrammed in Figure 42.1. The MAO inhibitors are not as effective as the tricyclic antidepressants in treating common endogenous depression, but the MAO inhibitors are more effective in treating depressions exhibited as phobias.

Administration and fate. The MAO inhibitors are well absorbed orally. They are metabolized in the liver to inactive forms and excreted in the urine.

Despite this, the onset of action requires 2 to 3 weeks. MAO inhibitors act by irreversible inhibition; removal of enough enzyme to produce clinical effectiveness takes time. Similarly, the effect persists for 2 to 3 weeks after MAO inhibitors have been discontinued, reflecting the time to synthesize adequate MAO.

Sedation and anticholinergic effects are common side effects associated with the MAO inhibitors, but these drugs usually are administered in divided doses during the day because of their tendency to cause insomnia if given in the evening. Orthostatic hypotension is sometimes a side effect. At one time, MAO inhibitors were used as antihypertensive drugs.

As with the tricyclic antidepressants, the MAO inhibitors are not addicting.

Interactions leading to a hypertensive crisis. Several clinically significant problems arise from the interaction of the MAO inhibitors with other drugs (see Table 42.4) and certain foods containing tyramine.

A hypertensive crisis may be precipitated when a food containing tyramine or a sympathomimetic drug is ingested, see box, p. 665. Sympathomimetic drugs and tyramine are normally degraded rapidly by the MAO of the liver. When MAO is inhibited, tyramine remains undegraded and triggers the release of accumulated norepinephrine, which in turn causes a hypertensive episode. The earliest symptom of such a hypertensive response may be a severe headache. The necessity of avoiding these substances to avert a life-threatening hypertensive crisis is the major limitation of the MAO inhibitors. Phentolamine, the alpha receptor antagonist, may be given to lower the blood pressure during a hypertensive crisis.

Acute toxicity. After ingestion of an overdose of a MAO inhibitor, symptoms appear within 12 hours and reflect increased adrenergic activity: restlessness, anxiety, and insomnia, progressing to include a rapid heart rate and sometimes to convulsions. Dizziness and hypotension may be found, whereas some patients have severe headaches and develop high blood pressure. Some patients develop a high fever, which should be brought down with a sponge bath and external cooling. Treatment is supportive to maintain respiration and circulation. Because the effect of the MAO inhibitor is persistent, patients must be followed for at least a week.

Specific MAO Inhibitors

Isocarboxazid

Isocarboxazid (Marplan) is not considered as effective as the other MAO inhibitors but is occasionally prescribed for depressed patients who are unresponsive to tricyclic antidepressants and electroconvulsive shock therapy.

Phenelzine

Phenelzine (Nardil) is regarded as the safest of the MAO inhibitors. Patients with a high level of anxiety who do not respond to a tricyclic antidepressant may respond to phenelzine. The dose must be individualized, since wide variability exists in its metabolism.

Tranylcypromine

Tranylcypromine (Parnate) can have a stimulatory action similar to amphetamine, and the antidepressant activity is seen more rapidly than with the other MAO inhibitors.

LITHIUM FOR MANIC-DEPRESSIVE DISORDER

Mechanism of action. Lithium acts to lower concentrations of norepinephrine and serotonin by inhibiting their release from and enhancing their reuptake by neurons (see Figure 42.1). These effects, along with the side effects and toxic effect of lithium, are believed to be related to the partial replacement of sodium by lithium in membrane reactions. Lithium is the drug of choice for treating the manic phase of a manic-depressive disorder.

If the patient is severely manic, an antipsychotic drug or electroconvulsive shock therapy may be used initially to subdue behavior. Lithium therapy alone usually reverses mild to moderate manic symptoms in 1 to 3 weeks. The duration of lithium therapy depends on the individual. Patients with occasional manic periods may be treated only during those periods. Continuous lithium therapy is indicated for those individuals in whom lithium reduces the frequency and intensity of their manic-depressive disorder. Evidence shows that lithium may be effective in treating the depression of the manic-depressive disorder and even endogenous depression per se. At this time, however, lithium is approved only for treating acute mania and as prophylaxis for recurrent mania. In research studies lithium is being tested for its effectiveness in treating various psychiatric and neurological brain disorders.

Administration and fate. Lithium is administered orally as the carbonate or citrate salt. Since lithium is an element, related in the atomic table to sodium and potassium, it is not metabolized but is excreted by mechanisms similar to those for sodium and potassium. Of the lithium filtered in the kidney, 80% is reabsorbed in the proximal tubule and 20% is excreted in the urine. The half-life of lithium in the plasma is 24 hours and is increased to about 36 hours in the elderly, so the relative dose of lithium must be decreased to avoid the cumulation to toxic doses. Other factors that decrease lithium excretion include sodium deficiency, extreme exercise, diarrhea, and postpartum status. Factors that increase lithium excretion include high sodium intake and pregnancy.

Toxicity. The therapeutic index for lithium is relatively small, and at the start of treatment patients are tested at least weekly to ensure that the plasma level is in the therapeutic range. The therapeutic range is 0.6 to 1.2 mEq/L but as low as 0.2 mEq/L in the elderly. Common side effects early in therapy include mild nausea, dry mouth, increased thirst, increased urination (polyuria), and a fine tremor of the hands. Toxic symptoms begin to appear at 1.5 to 2.0 mEq/L and by 4.0 mEq/L may be fatal. The toxic symptoms are listed in Table 42.5, p. 667.

Acute lithium toxicity is treated by hastening lithium excretion while maintaining fluid and electrolyte balance. Lithium excretion is increased by administration of an osmotic diuretic such as urea or mannitol. The drugs aminophylline and acetazolamide increase lithium excretion, and one may be given concurrently with the osmotic diuresis. Peritoneal dialysis, or preferably hemodialysis, may be used for severe toxicity or when renal failure occurs.

Contraindications. Lithium therapy is contraindicated in early pregnancy because an increased incidence of congenital malformations in infants of treated mothers has been noted. The secretion of the thyroid hormone thyroxine is inhibited by lithium, and a few patients develop an enlarged thyroid gland and may become hypothyroid. A few patients on lithium therapy develop nephrogenic diabetes insipidus (see Chapter 50), which is reversed when the lithium dose is lowered or discontinued. Paradoxically, administration of a thiazide diuretic may reverse this polyuria. A more serious consequence is permanent renal damage (initially without symptoms), which may develop with long-term lithium therapy. The incidence of this damage remains to be evaluated.

Drug interactions. Several documented drug interactions with lithium occur. Lithium potentiates haloperidol, tricyclic antidepressants, the phenothiazines, the benzodiazepines, and the neuromuscular blocking drugs. Lithium is potentiated by methyldopa, sodium-depleting diuretics, and the phenothiazines.

PATIENT CARE IMPLICATIONS

General guidelines for the use of antidepressants

Drug administration

- The risk of suicide may be present in seriously depressed patients and may persist for several weeks after they begin antidepressant therapy. In fact, some patients who were not suicidal may become so during initial therapy with antidepressants. Assess patients carefully.
- Monitor vital signs and weight.
- As mood improves, appetite may improve. In addition, some antidepressants contribute to weight gain. If weight gain is significant, counsel about weight reduction diets and increased exercise. Provide emotional support as needed. Counsult the physician about possible changes in dose or drug.
- Many of these drugs alter the seizure threshold. In patients with a history of seizures, pad side rails, and supervise carefully until the effects of the medications can be evaluated.

Patient and family education

- Tell patients and families that several weeks of therapy may be necessary before full effects of a drug regimen can be evaluated. Some side effects may lessen with continued drug use.
- Common side effects are noted in this text, but encourage patients to consult the physician when any new side effect develops.
- Teach patients that antidepressants need to be taken as ordered, on a regular basis, even if they begin to feel better. Teach the patient to consult the physician before changing the prescribed drug regimen or discontinuing medications.
- Warn patients to keep all health care providers informed of all drugs being taken.
- Avoid over-the-counter drugs unless first approved by the physician.
- Avoid ingestion of alcohol unless approved in moderation by the physician.
- Warn patients to avoid driving or operating hazardous equipment if drowsiness occurs.
- Encourage patients and families to stay in touch with the physician, and to seek assistance from appropriate health care personnel: physician, psychologists, nurses, therapists.
- Remind patients to keep these and all drugs out of the reach of children.

Tricyclic and second-generation antidepressants

Drug administration

- See the general guidelines.
- Monitor vital signs and blood pressure.
- Assess for skin changes. Auscultate bowel sounds, and keep a record of stools.
- Monitor complete blood count and platelet count.
- Concentrated solutions are available for some of the antidepressants; consult manufacturer's literature for appropriate diluents.
- Supervise the patient carefully to ascertain that the medication is swallowed and not hidden in the mouth to be discarded or stored by the patient.
- Imipramine and other tricyclic antidepressants may be used in the treatment of enuresis in children over 6 years of age. The most frequent side effects are nervousness, sleep disorders, and GI upset, although any of the side effects listed in the text may occur. Treatment is continued for as short a period as possible to obtain relief, then the dose is tapered. The drug should be taken about 1 hour before bedtime, although early-night bedwetters may have a better response if part of the dose is given in the afternoon and part at bedtime; check with the physician. The treatment of enuresis can be complex. Provide emotional support as needed.

Patient and family education

- See the general guidelines.
- See Patient Problems: Orthostatic Hypotension (p. 237), Dry Mouth (p. 170), Constipation (p. 187), Photosensitivity (p. 647).
- If sedation is a problem, suggest taking daily doses at bedtime.
- Take doses with meals or snack to lessen gastric irritation.
- Tell diabetic patients to monitor blood glucose levels, as antidepressants may alter blood glucose levels. A change in diet or insulin dose may be necessary.

Monoxamine oxidase inhibitors

Drug administration

- See the general guidelines.
- Monitor vital signs and blood pressure.
- Auscultate bowel sounds, and keep a record of stools.
- Monitor complete blood count and platelet count.

PATIENT CARE IMPLICATIONS—cont'd

- Supervise the patient carefully to ascertain that the medication is swallowed and not hidden in the mouth to be discarded or stored by the patient.

Patient and family education

- Review the general guidelines.
- See Patient Problems: Orthostatic Hypotension (p. 237), Dry Mouth (p. 170), Constipation (p. 187).
- Review the dietary restrictions with the patient and family. See Dietary Consideration: Tyramine.
- Avoid excessive caffeine intake, although small amounts are acceptable.
- Tell diabetic patients to monitor blood glucose levels, as antidepressants may alter blood glucose levels. A change in diet or insulin dose may be necessary.
- Review the drug interactions noted in the text.

Lithium

Drug administration

- See the general guidelines.
- Monitor vital signs. Inspect for development of edema.
- Assess for development of symptoms of toxicity (see Table 29.5).
- Monitor serum drug levels.

- If urinary output is excessive, assess for diabetes insipidus (dilute, high volume urine with a specific gravity of 1.000-1.003).
- Supervise the patient carefully to ascertain that the medication is swallowed and not hidden in the mouth to be discarded or stored by the patient.

Patient and family education

- See the general guidelines.
- Emphasize the importance of returning for follow-up care to have serum drug levels monitored.
- Review the signs and symptoms of lithium toxicity, and teach the patient to report their development.
- Provide emotional support as needed for side effects: fine hand tremor, polyuria, metallic taste. Remind patients not to discontinue medications without consulting the physician.
- Try to take lithium at the same time daily. Take doses with meals or snack to lessen gastric irritation.
- See Patient Problem: Dry Mouth on p. 170.
- Teach patient to notify physician if fever or severe or persistent diarrhea or vomiting occurs, as any of them may contribute to electrolyte disturbance, which may contribute to lithium toxicity.

SUMMARY

According to the biogenic amine theory, depression represents too little norepinephrine or serotonin acting on certain receptors in the brain. Drugs that act as antidepressants restore active norepinephrine and serotonin; on the other hand, lithium, which is used to treat mania, the syndrome opposite to depression, lowers active norepinephrine and serotonin. The tricyclic antidepressants increase the sensitivity of the receptors to these neurotransmitters and block the reuptake of these neurotransmitters. The MAO inhibitors prevent the degradation of norepinephrine and serotonin and also enhance receptor sensitivity to these neurotransmitters. Lithium, a chemical element related to sodium and potassium, inhibits the release of norepinephrine and serotonin and enhances their reuptake.

Both tricyclic antidepressants and MAO inhibitors take 10 days or more to produce improvement. Sedation and atropine-like side effects are common with each drug class. Certain tricyclic antidepressants have distinct depressant effects on the heart. Acute toxicity of tricyclic antidepressants is related to atropine-like poisoning and to the complex cardiac effects. MAO inhibitors have a more complex toxicity. First, several foods and drugs that contain sympathomimetic amines, normally degraded by MAO, can cause a hypertensive crisis when ingested. Second, an acute overdose disturbs cardiovascular regulation, frequently reflecting an increase in adrenergic activity, but since norepinephrine stores can be depleted secondarily to inhibition of MAO, hypotensive episodes, reflecting a lack of norepinephrine, may also be present.

Second-generation antidepressants are coming into clinical use. These antidepressants are comparable to the tricyclic antidepressants but have a lesser incidence of sedation and anticholinergic and cardiovascular effects.

Lithium is a relatively toxic drug, so side effects often are found in the therapeutic range, and the toxic doses are only 2- to 3-fold higher than the therapeutic doses. Lithium is handled similarly to sodium, and treatment of lithium toxicity is directed at increasing lithium excretion by the kidney.

STUDY QUESTIONS

1. What is the biogenic amine theory of depression?
2. How are the actions of the tricyclic antidepressants, monoamine oxidase inhibitors, and lithium consistent with the biogenic amine theory of depression?
3. How can some drugs cause depression?
4. What are the major side effects of the tricyclic antidepressants?
5. What is the acute toxicity of the tricyclic antidepressants?
6. What are the major drug interactions of the tricyclic antidepressants?
7. How can a hypertensive crisis be precipitated in a patient taking a MAO inhibitor?
8. What are the common side effects of MAO inhibitors?
9. What are the symptoms of lithium toxicity?
10. How do the second-generation antidepressants compare to the tricyclic antidepressants?

SUGGESTED READINGS

Ansett, R.E., and Poole, S.R.: Depressive equivalents in adults, Am. Fam. Physician 25(3):151, 1982.

Avery, D.H.: Dexamethasone suppression test as a marker for depression, Res. Staff Physician 29(8):63, 1983.

Ayd, F.J., Jr., and Taylor, B.T.: The depressed office patient, Am. Fam. Physician 28(1):155, 1983.

Brenners, D.K., Harris, B., and Weston, P.S.: Managing manic behavior, Am. J. Nurs. 87(5):620, 1987.

Bressler, R.: Treating geriatric depression—current options, Drug Therapy 14(9):129, 1984.

Burckhardt, D., and Hoffman, A.: Clinical relevance of cardiovascular side effects of tricyclic and tetracyclic antidepressants, Intern. Med. 4(12):79, 1983.

Burnum, J.F.: Diagnosis of depression in a general medical practice, Postgrad. Med. 72(3):71, 1982.

Clifford, D.B.: Treatment of pain with antidepressants, Am. Fam. Physician 31:181, 1985.

Condon, E.H.: Dementia and depression: a devastating pain, Geriatr. Nurs. 10(1):26, 1989

Davis, D.: Depression, Am. Fam. Physician 26(6):156, 1982.

DeGennaro, M.D., and others: Antidepressant drug therapy, Am. J. Nurs. 81:1304, 1981.

Fields, E.D.: Nomifensine maleate, Drugs Clin. Pharm. 16:547, 1982.

Finlayson, R.E., and Martin, L.M.: Recognition and management of depression in the elderly, Mayo Clin. Proc. 57:115, 1982.

Friedel, R.O.: Diagnosis and treatment of autonomous depression in the geriatric patient, Geriatr. Med. Today 2(1):40, 1983.

Frommer, D.A., and others: Tricyclic antidepressant overdose: a review, JAMA 257:521, 1987.

Gold, M.S., and others: Diagnosis of depression in the 1980's, JAMA 245(15):1562, 1981.

Gold, P.W., Goodwin, F.K., and Chrousos, G.P.: Clinical and biochemical manifestations of depression, N. Engl. J. Med. 319:413, 1988.

Goldberg, M.H.: Tricyclic antidepressant overdose: cardiovascular manifestations and treatment, Hosp. Physician 20(9):62, 1984.

Golden, R.N., and Gualtieri, C.T.: A clinician's guide to the new antidepressants, Res. Staff Physician 29(4):65, 1983.

Gulledge, A.D.: Can you unmask and treat "masked" depression? Mod. Med. 50(3):128, 1982.

Harris, E.: Psych drugs: the antidepressants, Am. J. Nurs. 88(11):1512, 1988.

Harris, E.: Lithium: in a class by itself, Am. J. Nurs. 89(2):190, 1989.

Hodgin, J.D.: Phobic disorders, Am. Fam. Physician 28(4):264, 1983.

Holden, C.: Depression research advances, treatment lags, Science 233:723, 1986.

Hollister, L.E.: Depression: the delicate art of lifting it with drug Rx, Mod. Med. 50(1):110, 1982.

Jann, M.W. and others: Alternative drug therapies for mania: a literature review, Drug Intell. Clin. Pharm. 18:577, 1984.

Jencks, S.F.: Recognition of mental distress and diagnosis of mental disorder in primary care, JAMA 253:1903, 1985.

Keller, M.B., and others: Long-term outcome of episodes of major depression, JAMA 252(6):788, 1984.

Kolata, G.: Clinical trial of psychotherapies is under way, Science 212:432, 1981.

Kulig, K., and others: Amoxapine overdose—coma and seizures without cardiotoxic effects, JAMA 248(9):1092, 1982.

Lasater, M.G.: Nursing care of the patient with a tricyclic antidepressant overdose, Crit. Care Nurse 4(4):28, 1984.

Levenson, A.J.: Psychotropic drug use in the elderly: an overview, Am. Fam. Physician 24(2):194, 1981.

Lippman, S.: Antidepressant pharmacotherapy, Am. Fam. Physician 25(6):145, 1982.

Lippman, S.: Drug therapy for depression in the elderly. Postgrad. Med. 73(1):159, 1983.

Matthysse, S., and Kidd, K.K.: Evidence of HLA linkage in depressive disorders, N. Engl. J. Med. 305(22):1340, 1981.

Maugh, T.H., II: Is there a gene for depression? Science 214:1330, 1981.

Moriarity, R.W.: Tricyclic antidepressant poisoning, Drug Therapy 11(8):73, 1981.

Ravaris, C.L.: Current drug therapy for agoraphobia, Am. Fam. Physician 23(1):129, 1981.

Reynolds, C.F., Marin, R.S., and Spiker, D.: Clinical considerations in prescribing antidepressants for geriatric patients, Geriatr. Med. Today 2(3):45, 1983.

Rhyne, M.C., and others: Children at risk for depression, Am. J. Nurs. 86(12):1378, 1986.

Richelson, E.: Antimuscarinic and other receptor-blocking properties of antidepressants, Mayo Clin. Proc. **58**:40, 1983.

Richelson, E.: Tricyclic antidepressants: therapy for ulcer and other novel uses, Mod. Med. **51**(10):74, 1983.

Ronsman, K.: Therapy for depression, J. Gerontol. Nurs. **13**(12):18, 1987.

Schou, M.: Lithium treatment of manic-depressive illness, JAMA **259**:1834, 1988.

Settle, E.C.: Recently introduced antidepressants—their place in clinical practice, Postgrad. Med. **72**(3):87, 1982.

Talley, J.A.: Depression—differentiate the endogenous variety from the look-alikes, Consultant **23**(2):105, 1983.

Todd, B.: Depression and antidepressants, Geriatr. Nurs. **8**(4):203, 1987.

Valente, S.M., and Saunders, J.M.: Dealing with serious depression in cancer patients, Nursing89 **19**(2):44, 1989.

Valnes, K.: Tricyclic antidepressants in the treatment of peptic ulcer disease, Intern. Med. **4**(3):148, 1983.

Veith, R.C., and others: Cardiovascular effects of tricyclic antidepressants in depressed patients with chronic heart disease, N. Engl. J. Med. **306**(16):954, 1982.

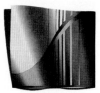

Central Nervous System Stimulants

43

The central nervous system (CNS) regulates its level of activity by maintaining excitatory and inhibitory systems. Therefore excessive stimulation of the CNS may be produced either by excessive activity of excitatory neurons or by blockade of inhibitory neurons. Many types of chemicals at some dose produce a degree of CNS stimulation by one of these mechanisms. Few of these compounds have legitimate pharmacological uses. CNS stimulants currently are medically accepted only for the treatment of narcolepsy, attention deficit disorder in children, and obesity. The drugs also are used occasionally as agents to reverse respiratory depression, although they are not generally recommended for these purposes.

This chapter examines the mechanism of action of CNS stimulants used in clinical conditions and the properties that make them prominent drugs of abuse.

CENTRAL NERVOUS SYSTEM STIMULANTS USED IN NARCOLEPSY AND ATTENTION DEFICIT DISORDER

Narcolepsy: Rationale for Therapy

Narcolepsy is a condition in which patients unexpectedly fall asleep in the middle of normal activity, such as while typing, driving a car, or talking to someone. During an attack, patients experience paralysis of the voluntary muscles similar to that of the dream state, and may abruptly collapse and fall. Patients with this sleep disorder obviously should be advised to avoid operating cars or dangerous machinery.

The treatment of narcolepsy usually includes the use of CNS stimulants during active daytime periods. These agents have alerting effects and reduce the sleeping episodes. One class of CNS stimulants used for this purpose is amphetamines (Table 43.1).

The most commonly used CNS stimulant in narcoleptic patients is methylphenidate (Table 43.1). This drug may be used in combination with imipramine (see Chapter 42). The effect of imipramine on narcolepsy is not produced by the antidepressant effects of the drug. The reversal of narcolepsy is rapid, whereas the antidepressant effects of imipramine develop over a prolonged period.

Although drug therapy may be beneficial for many narcoleptic patients, most also require other therapy such as scheduled daytime naps. Psychological counseling may be helpful in assisting patients to reconcile their living patterns with the constraints imposed by the disease.

Attention Deficit Disorder: Rationale for Therapy

Children with attention deficit disorder display a variety of symptoms, which impair their ability to learn or to maintain appropriate social interactions. These children are excessively active, impulsive, and irritable. Their attention span is very short, and their activity is purposeless. Learning disabilities of various types are frequent in these children. Many children with this disorder display abnormal electroencephalographic (EEG) patterns and poorer coordination than normal children of the same age. Intelligence is not impaired. Because of the wide range of symptoms produced, this syndrome has been called by many names, including *minimal brain dysfunction, minimal brain damage, hyperkinesis, attention deficit disorder with hyperkinesis*, and *hyperkinetic syndrome with learning disorder*.

Children with attention deficit disorder must receive psychotherapy and counseling, as well as remedial education adjusted to their needs and abilities. Drug therapy to reduce the hyperactive behavior and lengthen the attention span also may be

Table 43.1   Summary of Central Nervous System Stimulants for Narcolepsy and Hyperkinesis

Generic name	Trade name	Medical use	Administration/dosage	Comments
Amphetamine sulfate (also called racemic or *dl*-amphetamine sulfate)	Benzedrine*	Narcolepsy	ORAL: *Adults and children over 6 yr*—5 to 20 mg 1 to 3 times daily. FDA Pregnancy Category C.	Dosage is adjusted according to patient's needs and tolerance to sympathomimetic effects on the cardiovascular system as well as CNS toxicity.
		Attention deficit disorder	ORAL: *Children 3 to 6 yr*—2.5 mg daily and increase by 2.5 mg increments weekly to achieve desired effect; *6 yr and older*—initially 5 mg daily and increase by 5 mg increments weekly to achieve desired effect.	Dosage should be the minimum required for control of symptoms. Long-term continuous use should be avoided to prevent growth inhibition. Drugs may be withdrawn during less stressful periods, such as summer holidays. Schedule II substance.
Dextroamphetamine sulfate	Dexedrine* Ferndex Oxydess II	Narcolepsy	Same as for amphetamine sulfate.	Same as for amphetamine sulfate, except less tendency to produce cardiovascular toxicity. Schedule II substance (U.S.). Class C (Canada).
		Attention deficit disorder	Same as for amphetamine sulfate.	
Methamphetamine hydrochloride	Desoxyn	Attention deficit disorder	ORAL: *Children 6 yr and older*—2.5 to 5 mg once or twice daily; increase by 5 mg increments at weekly intervals to optimum dosage, usually 20 to 25 mg. Extended release tablets can be used for maintenance.	Has CNS and cardiovascular toxicity. Schedule II substance.
Methylphenidate hydrochloride	Methidate† Ritalin	Attention deficit disorder	ORAL: *Children 6 yr and older*—5 mg before breakfast and lunch; increase by 5 to 10 mg at weekly intervals up to 0.3 to 0.5 mg/kg body weight. Maximum daily doses should not exceed 60 mg.	Drug of choice for most hyperkinetic children. Schedule II substance (U.S.). Class C (Canada).
		Narcolepsy	ORAL: *Adults*—10 to 60 mg daily. Common dose is 10 mg twice or 3 times daily.	May be used with imipramine to treat narcolepsy.
Pemoline	Cylert*	Attention deficit disorder	ORAL: *Children 6 yr and older*—37.5 mg daily in a single dose; increase weekly by 18.75 mg increments until response is obtained. Effective dosage range usually 56 to 75 mg daily. Do not exceed 112.5 mg daily.	Clinical effects develop over 3 to 4 weeks. Schedule IV substance (U.S.).

*Available in Canada and United States.
†Available in Canada only.

DRUG ABUSE ALERT: METHYLPHENIDATE

THE PROBLEM

Methylphenidate rarely causes toxic psychosis, but may cause psychological drug dependence. Both effects are observed following long-term use of doses in excess of therapeutic doses. The primary patient is obviously most at risk of developing dependence, but health care personnel must be alert to the problem among caregivers as well. For example, adult guardians of children receiving methylphenidate may divert the drug from the child and use it themselves.

SOLUTIONS

- Confirm that doses are not being extemporaneously increased by the patient or caregiver
- Advise patient to seek medical advice if drug seems to become less effective after several weeks
- See that dosage reduction is gradual so that withdrawal symptoms are minimized

---

required. The drugs most effective in controlling this disorder are, paradoxically, CNS stimulants. These agents, which increase agitation and activity in adults, have a calming effect on these children. Amphetamines have been used to control this disorder (Table 43.1). An equally effective drug with fewer peripheral side effects is methylphenidate. Pemoline is sometimes used but in general is less effective than either amphetamines or methylphenidate (Table 43.1).

Controversy surrounds the diagnosis and treatment of children with attention deficit disorder. Many authorities believe the syndrome is diagnosed more frequently than it exists and suggest that thousands of children may be receiving CNS stimulants unnecessarily. This problem remains to be resolved.

Pharmacological Properties of Specific Agents

Amphetamines

Mechanism of action. Amphetamines increase the release and effectiveness of catecholamine neurotransmitters in the brain and in peripheral nerves by several mechanisms. These drugs seem to increase the release of neurotransmitters during normal nervous activity. In addition, amphetamines block the specific reuptake of catecholamine neurotransmitters into the presynaptic neuron. Since this reuptake system is normally a major mechanism for terminating the action of the neurotrans-

mitter, blockade of the reuptake system produces prolonged and enhanced stimulation of the postsynaptic nerves. Norepinephrine and dopamine are thought to be the catecholamines whose actions are most enhanced by amphetamines.

Amphetamines may affect many sites within the brain. However, many of the clinically observed actions of amphetamines probably are related to activity in two particular regions of the brain, one of which is the reticular activating system. This complex of neurons regulates sensory input to the brain and thus controls the level of arousal. Amphetamines stimulate the reticular activating system, creating increased alertness and sensitivity to stimuli.

The second area of the brain that seems to be especially responsive to amphetamines is in the medial forebrain bundle. This reward, or pleasure, center can be activated by amphetamines. The result to the user is a perception of pleasure unrelated to external stimuli. This stimulation of the pleasure center is thought to be the source of the addictive potential of amphetamines.

Absorption and fate. Amphetamines for medical uses are given orally. These drugs are well absorbed from the gastrointestinal tract and produce peak serum concentrations within 2 to 3 hours after ingestion. The half-lives of the various amphetamines in the bloodstream range from 4 to 30 hours. These compounds easily penetrate the blood-brain barrier to produce their CNS effects.

Amphetamines are excreted primarily by the kidneys. The rate of excretion is highly dependent on urinary pH. Excretion can be greatly enhanced by acidifying the urine.

Toxicity. Amphetamines cause toxic reactions in several organ systems. Unpredictable effects can occur in the gastrointestinal tract, but vomiting, diarrhea, abdominal cramps, and dry mouth often occur. Anorexia may be produced, but this reaction is caused by the CNS effects of amphetamines.

Most CNS toxicity of amphetamines can be seen as an extension of the effects observed at therapeutic doses. At high doses amphetamines cause restless behavior, tremor, irritability, talkativeness, insomnia, and mood changes. Excessive aggressiveness, confusion, panic, and increased libido also may occur. More rarely, patients will suffer a syndrome resembling schizophrenia, with delirium or hallucinations. Long-term intoxication with amphetamines frequently causes this schizophrenia-like reaction, sometimes referred to as *toxic psychosis*.

Because of their sympathomimetic effects, amphetamines can cause various reactions in the car-

THE NURSING PROCESS

CENTRAL NERVOUS SYSTEM STIMULANTS FOR NARCOLEPSY AND ATTENTION DEFICIT DISORDER

Assessment

A small number of persons in the United States are diagnosed as having narcolepsy or attention deficit disorder, and these patients may be treated with CNS stimulants. In addition to obtaining a thorough history of the patient's presenting problem, the nurse should assess vital signs, weight, and height in children. A thorough mental status examination should be done.

Nursing diagnoses

Potential complication: growth retardation in children

Potential complication: toxic psychosis

Management

The nurse should spend time with the patient or family in identifying reasonable goals of therapy. The nurse should monitor the height, weight, and vital signs as well as obtain an indication of mental status at periodic intervals. The nurse may question the patient about subjective symptoms or problems not evident through observation, such as insomnia, agitation, dizziness, headache, and irritability. When children are being treated for attention deficit disorder the parents may be additional sources of information about the response to the drugs. If it is decided that the medication is beneficial and will be used in an outpatient setting, preparation of the patient and family for long-term therapy with the medication should be started.

Evaluation

In attention deficit disorder these drugs are considered successful if the child becomes less hyperactive and approaches a more normal attention span. In narcolepsy, the goal is to have an individual who is able to remain awake and alert, although not excessively active, during specified appropriate periods. It may require some time to adjust the dosage to the right level. Before discharge, the patient or family should be able to state why the medication is being used, side effects that may occur, side effects that should cause notification of the physician, any allowable adjustments in dosage that can be made based on side effects (such as giving a nighttime dose at a different time for a child with attention deficit disorder), and any activities or measures that should be employed to monitor the effectiveness of the drug in the home setting. Examples are keeping a weekly weight record, and for the child a height record at regular intervals.

---

diovascular system. Patients report headache, chilliness, and palpitations. Either pallor or facial flushing may be present. Angina can be precipitated, as well as various cardiac arrhythmias. Hypertension or hypotension may be observed at various stages during intoxication. The severely intoxicated patient may die in circulatory collapse.

Amphetamine toxicity differs somewhat, depending on which specific drug is used. The drug sold under the trade name of Benzedrine is a mixture of two forms of amphetamine called *d (dextro)* and *l (levo)*. The *d* form of amphetamine stimulates the CNS more effectively than does the *l* form.

Conversely, the *l* form stimulates the cardiovascular system slightly more effectively than does the *d* form. Benzedrine, being a mixture of *d* and *l* forms, causes both CNS and cardiovascular toxicity.

The drug sold under the trade name of Dexedrine is dextroamphetamine, the *d* form of amphetamine. This preparation is much more selective for the CNS and does not produce the same degree of cardiovascular toxicity observed with Benzedrine. Methamphetamine is the *d* form of an amphetamine derivative. It is equivalent in its properties to dextroamphetamine.

Table 43.2 Drugs Used to Suppress Appetite

Generic name	Trade name	Administration/dosage	Comments
Benzphetamine hydrochloride	Didrex	ORAL: *Adults*—25 to 50 mg once daily; may be increased as needed up to 3 doses daily. FDA Pregnancy Category X.	Similar to amphetamine. Schedule III substance.
Diethylpropion hydrochloride	Propion† Tenuate* Tepanil	ORAL: *Adults*—25 mg 1 hr before morning, noon, and evening meals and at midevening if needed. Timed-release formulations (75 mg) are taken once daily. FDA Pregnancy Category B.	Safest anorexiant for use in patients with mild cardiovascular disease. Dry mouth and constipation are common reactions. Schedule IV substance (U.S.). Class C (Canada).
Fenfluramine hydrochloride	Ponderal Pondimin*	ORAL: *Adults*—20 mg 3 times daily before meals. Dosage may be doubled if required. FDA Pregnancy Category C.	Only anorexiant that depresses CNS activity; sedation and depression may occur. Schedule IV substance.
Mazindol	Mazanor Sanorex*	ORAL: *Adults*—doses range from 1 mg daily at breakfast to 1 mg 3 times daily with meals. Minimum dose should be used. FDA Pregnancy Category C.	May be used in patients with arteriosclerosis or hyperthyroidism. Schedule IV substance.
Phendimetrazine tartrate	Anorex Bacarate Melfiat Plegine Statobex	ORAL: *Adults*—35 mg 2 or 3 times daily taken before meals. Sustained release, 105 mg taken once in the morning.	Stimulates the CNS in the same way as the amphetamines. Gastrointestinal distress may occur. Schedule III substance.
Phenmetrazine	Preludin	ORAL: *Adults*—75 mg once daily.	Phenmetrazine is used as an extended release preparation only. Schedule II substance.
Phentermine	Adipex Fastin Ionamin* Tora	ORAL: *Adults*—8 mg 3 times daily before meals or single dose of 15 to 37.5 mg may be taken 2 hr after breakfast.	Commonly causes insomnia and cardiovascular effects. Schedule IV substance (U.S.). Class C (Canada).
Phenylpropanolamine hydrochloride	Acutrim Control Dexatrim Diadax Prolamine Rhindecon Unitrol Westrim	ORAL: *Adults*—25 mg 3 times daily before meals or 50 to 75 mg of sustained-action formulation once daily at midmorning.	Blood pressure increases occur. These diet preparations should never be used with cold or allergy medications. Nonprescription.

*Available in the United States and Canada.
†Available in Canada.

Children receiving amphetamines may suffer growth retardation. This effect can be minimized by giving drug holidays during which drug therapy is suspended.

Drug interactions. Amphetamines interact with several other drugs. Amphetamines block the hypotensive effect of methyldopa and guanethidine. The metabolism of tricyclic antidepressants is blocked by amphetamines, causing these drugs to accumulate unless dosage is reduced. Sympathomimetic drugs can increase the effects of amphetamines. Monoamine oxidase inhibitors also increase catecholamine levels and potentiate the effects of amphetamines.

Table 43.3   Systemic Effects of Drugs Used to Suppress Appetite

Generic name	Mood	Motor activity	Effects on Heart rate	Blood pressure	Abuse potential
Benzphetamine	Elevated	May increase	May increase	May increase	High
Diethylpropion	May be elevated	May increase	Unchanged	Unchanged	Relatively low
Fenfluramine	Depressed	Depressed	Usually no change	May increase	Relatively low
Mazindol	May be elevated	May increase	Increased	Usually no change	High
Phendimetrazine	Highly elevated	Increased	Usually no change	Usually no change	High
Phenmetrazine	Highly elevated	Increased	Increased	Increased	Very high
Phentermine	Usually no change	May increase	Increased	Increased	Relatively low
Phenylpropanolamine	Usually no change	Usually no change	May increase	May increase	Low

Methylphenidate

Mechanism of action. Methylphenidate is a mild CNS stimulant. Its exact biochemical mechanism of action is unknown, but appears similar to the amphetamines.

Absorption and fate. Methylphenidate is well absorbed orally and is usually prescribed to be given to adults 30 to 45 minutes before meals. Orally administered methylphenidate is extensively metabolized during the first pass through the liver. The metabolites of methylphenidate are not capable of stimulating the CNS or sympathetic peripheral neurons. Most of the methylphenidate taken orally is excreted in the urine as inactive metabolites.

Toxicity. Methylphenidate often causes nervousness and insomnia. Insomnia may be minimized by not administering the drug in the evening. Nervousness is frequently controlled by reducing overall drug dosage. Anorexia, nausea, and abdominal pain may occur with methylphenidate, as with the amphetamines. Cardiovascular effects similar to those produced by amphetamines are also seen.

Methylphenidate can cause allergic reactions in sensitive patients. These reactions may range from mild skin rashes to exfoliative dermatitis and thrombocytopenic purpura.

The drug causes a temporary slowing of growth in prepubertal children. Most children seem to

⚡ DRUG ABUSE ALERT: APPETITE SUPPRESSANTS

THE PROBLEM

Many patients experience some level of dependence on the CNS stimulants used as appetite suppressants (Table 43.2). Patients may seek them from several physicians rather than follow the advice of a single physician who may limit the use of the drugs to 2 or 3 months. Many appetite suppressants also carry the risk of causing psychotic reactions, as a result of either overdosage or prolonged use. Phenmetrazine, for example, can cause a toxic psychosis similar to that of the amphetamines.

SOLUTIONS

- Warn the patient that the anorectic effect will wear off in 6 to 12 weeks
- Warn the patient not to attempt to increase dosage to prolong the anorectic effect
- Observe for signs of dependency
- Offer counseling about healthy dietary limitations and good eating practices

overcome the deficit and ultimately gain normal stature. Slow growth can be minimized by giving the child a drug-free period during therapy.

Drug interactions. Methylphenidate, like the amphetamines, can interact with many other med-

THE NURSING PROCESS

CENTRAL NERVOUS SYSTEM STIMULANTS FOR OBESITY

Assessment

Obesity is a significant health problem in the United States. In addition to obtaining a thorough patient assessment, the nurse should focus on the vital signs, obtain the patient's weight, discuss usual eating habits, and evaluate any other existing medical conditions. The nurse should establish with the patient reasonable goals of therapy in terms of desired weight. Assessment also includes evaluating mental status. The health care team may recommend that the patient seek counseling for behavior associated with obesity, as well as begin appropriate use of other treatments to assist in weight reduction, such as a calorie-restricted diet and a prescribed exercise program. Drug therapy alone is rarely successful.

Nursing diagnoses

Potential complication: toxic psychosis

Potential complication: addiction or abuse

Management

The goal of therapy with CNS stimulants in treating obesity is to promote weight reduction without producing any cardioavscular or mental status effects. The nurse should monitor the patient for these side effects and offer emotional support and information related to control of obesity.

Evaluation

When discharged to home therapy, the patient should be able to explain why the medication is being used and how to take it correctly, the hazards of overmedication, side effects that may occur, symptoms that should be reported to the physician, and how abuse of many of these drugs can cause addiction. In addition, the patient should be able to explain how to carry out other prescribed measures, such as caloric dietary restriction and exercise. The nurse may be the member of the health care team who performs follow-up of these patients, monitoring weight and other signs and symptoms. The CNS stimulants are not used for long-term control of obesity.

---

ications. Since it causes its effects by release of catecholamines such as norepinephrine, the effects may be greatly increased by monoamine oxidase inhibitors, sympathomimetic agents, or vasopressors. Methylphenidate also inhibits the metabolism of a variety of drugs, including phenytoin, phenobarbital, primidone, phenylbutazone, imipramine, desipramine, and coumarin anticoagulants. Therefore these drugs must be given at reduced dosages to avoid drug accumulation and excess toxicity when methylphenidate also is being administered. The antihypertensive medication guanethidine is made less effective by methylphenidate, apparently because guanethidine uptake into nerve terminal is blocked.

Pemoline

Mechanism of action. Pemoline stimulates the CNS in a manner similar to that of amphetamines and methylphenidate, but lacks the strong sympathomimetric effects of many of those stimulants. The exact biochemical mechanism for the action of pemoline is unknown.

Absorption and fate. Pemoline is well absorbed orally, producing peak serum levels 2 to 4 hours after dosage. The serum half-life for the drug is about 12 hours. Therefore the drug may be given once daily. The kidney excretes most of the administered pemoline, both as unchanged drug and as metabolites.

Although the blood levels reach a plateau within a few days after therapy is begun, the ther-

Table 43.4   Summary of Central Nervous System Stimulants Used for Respiratory Stimulation

Generic name	Trade name	Administration/dosage	Comments
Caffeine (citrated caffeine)		ORAL, NASOGASTRIC TUBE: 10 mg/kg body weight initially, then 2.5 mg/kg daily.	Used in newborn infants.
Doxapram	Dopram*	INTRAVENOUS: *Adults*—0.5 to 2 mg/kg body weight intermittently as needed. For chronic obstructive pulmonary disease, 1 to 2 mg/min infusion for 2 hr.	Rapidly acting drug whose action is over within 12 min. Do not use in newborns because of benzyl alcohol content.
Theophylline		ORAL, NASOGASTRIC TUBE: 5 mg/kg body weight initial dose, then 2 mg/kg daily divided into 2 or 3 doses.	Most commonly used to treat asthma but is also used to treat apnea in newborn infants. Effective plasma concentrations range from 5 to 12 μg/ml with toxicity expected above 20 μg/ml.

*Available in Canada and United States.

apeutic effects of pemoline are not immediately evident in hyperkinetic children. Dosage is gradually increased over 2 to 4 weeks after therapy is started. Significant clinical response may not be seen until the third or fourth week.

Toxicity. Pemoline, when used in properly selected children at recommended doses, seldom causes serious toxic reactions. Insomnia often is reported but is a transient reaction in most patients. Pemoline causes anorexia, stomach ache, and nausea, which may slow normal weight gain. Children do not seem to suffer permanent growth retardation, but careful records of the child's growth should be maintained to allow assessment during therapy.

Pemoline may produce skin rashes and altered liver function tests. These reversible reactions may be caused by allergy.

CNS signs such as irritability, mild depression, dizziness, headache, and hallucinations may be provoked. Tachycardia and agitation usually result with overdosages.

Because pemoline may alter dopamine systems within the CNS, signs of dyskinesia should be watched for carefully (see Chapter 41).

CENTRAL NERVOUS SYSTEM STIMULANTS USED IN OBESITY
Rationale for Therapy

Many CNS stimulants suppress appetite even while stimulating other CNS functions. Because of

Table 43.5   Caffeine Content of Commonly Ingested Substances

Substance	Caffeine content
FOODS AND BEVERAGES	
Coffee	
Brewed	80 to 150 mg/5 oz cup
Instant	85 to 100 mg/5 oz cup
Decaffeinated	2 to 4 mg/5 oz cup
Tea, brewed	30 to 75 mg/5 oz cup
Cocoa	5 to 40 mg/5 oz cup
Cola soft drinks*	35 to 60 mg/12 oz bottle or can
NONPRESCRIPTION MEDICATIONS	
Analgesics (Anacin, Vanquish)	32 mg/tablet
Excedrin	65 mg/tablet
COLD MEDICATIONS	
Kolephrin	65 mg/capsule
STIMULANTS	
Nodoz	100 mg/tablet
Vivarin	200 mg/tablet

*Many soft drinks other than colas contain caffeine as an additive. The label will reveal the presence of caffeine but not the amount.

THE NURSING PROCESS

CENTRAL NERVOUS SYSTEM STIMULANTS FOR RESPIRATION

Assessment

Patients requiring drug therapy to stimulate respiration are primarily those with burns and spinal cord injuries; these drugs are seldom used in current practice. The nurse should complete a thorough patient assessment, focusing on the respiratory system. The nurse should auscultate the lungs, check the respiratory rate and depth of respirations, and evaluate the vital capacity. Arterial blood gas levels may be measured.

Nursing diagnoses

Potential complication: increased blood pressure

Altered comfort: nausea and gastrointestinal discomfort

Management

These drugs are used on a short-term basis until the patient develops adequate voluntary respiration. If the drugs are administered via constant infusion, an infusion control device or volume control device may be helpful. The nurse should monitor the vital signs, with emphasis on the respiratory system. A suction machine should be at the bedside. The nurse should monitor any serum drug levels if they are being obtained. The mental status of the patient should be evaluated on a regular basis.

Evaluation

The goal of these drugs is to stimulate the respiratory system so that the patient breathes at a rate and depth approaching normal. These medications are for short-term use in the hospital.

---

this effect on appetite, many of these drugs have been used to help control obesity. As a group, these drugs are referred to as *anorexiants* (Table 43.2, p. 678).

Pharmacology of Specific Agents

Amphetamines were the original CNS stimulants used for controlling obesity. At the low dosage ranges used in obese patients, tolerance develops to the appetite suppressant properties of amphetamines within 4 to 6 weeks. Long-term use produces many undesirable side effects, including addiction; thus they now are not recommended for use in obesity.

The newer anorexiants listed in Tables 43.2 and 43.3, pp. 678-679 do not produce the same degree of stimulation of the CNS or cardiovascular systems as amphetamine and its derivatives. However, none of the anorexiants is completely without potentially dangerous systemic side effects.

Some anorexiants resemble the amphetamines in activity and reactions but produce these reactions less frequently and less severely; these include *benzphetamine, phenmetrazine,* and *mazindol. Diethylpropion,* unlike other anorexiants, produces little significant cardiovascular stimulation and thus may be used in patients with some types of cardiovascular disease. *Fenfluramine* is unlike the other anorexiant drugs, since it depresses the CNS while suppressing the appetite. *Phentermine* usually has no effect on mood but, as with the amphetamines, does produce cardiovascular stimulation. *Phenylpropanolamine* mildly suppresses appetite and is included in various nonprescription appetite suppressants, either alone or with other agents. Phenylpropanolamine also is often used in nonprescription nasal decongestants (see Chapter 4).

Toxicity and side effects. The use of appetite suppressants in treating obesity is controversial. All the available effective agents carry substantial risks, and many have high abuse potential. Many patients experience some level of dependence on these medications. Fenfluramine may also produce dangerous mental imbalances, although with this drug the danger is depression rather than stimulation of the CNS. Fenfluramine should never be given to a patient with a previous history of depression or suicidal tendencies.

Anorexiants cause irritability and insomnia. Sympathetic nervous system effects include dry mouth, blurred vision, heart palpitations, and hypertension. Some of these drugs cause gastrointestinal distress. The anorexiants have not been proved safe during pregnancy.

Tolerance. Tolerance develops to all the appetite-suppressing drugs in clinical use. Effective weight reduction cannot be maintained by relying on drugs alone to control eating patterns. Persons seeking to lose weight must develop appropriate eating habits and develop an exercise plan adjusted to their own age and physical limitations. Drugs to suppress appetite may help a patient during the initial stages of a weight reduction program, but these agents are not the key to a successful long-term program. None of these drugs is intended for use in children.

Drug interactions. All the appetite-suppressing agents are capable of interacting with many other medications. For example, any sympathomimetic drug may have a much greater effect in patients receiving appetite suppressants, since the appetite-suppressing drugs tend to increase the effectiveness of catecholamines. This precaution should be mentioned to patients, and they should be warned to avoid cold remedies, allergy medications, and nasal decongestants that include sympathomimetic agents.

Blood pressure can be affected by appetite suppressants. Many may directly elevate blood pressure. Phenylpropanolamine is occasionally used clinically for its vasopressor effect. Patients receiving medications to treat high blood pressure should avoid appetite-suppressing drugs.

CENTRAL NERVOUS SYSTEM STIMULANTS THAT STIMULATE RESPIRATION (Table 43.4, p. 681)

Rationale for Therapy

Certain CNS stimulants have generalized effects on the brain stem and spinal cord as well as on higher centers in the brain. These drugs may increase responsiveness to external stimuli and stimulate respiration. As a group, these drugs are referred to as *analeptics.*

Analeptics have been used primarily to stimulate respiration. The use of these drugs has become less common, since modern techniques of respiratory therapy allow a patient to be adequately ventilated even when the natural reflex is temporarily absent. Respiratory paralysis caused by overdoses of narcotic agents is appropriately treated with specific narcotic antagonists and not with these generalized analeptic agents.

Two properties of the analeptic drugs make them especially hard to control. First, they are nonspecific stimulants of the CNS and may produce unwanted effects in addition to respiratory stimulation. Second, all these drugs at a high enough dose or in a predisposed patient may produce convulsions.

Pharmacological Properties of Specific Agents

Methylxanthines: caffeine and theophylline

Mechanism of action. Methylxanthines block the destruction of cyclic AMP, the compound that mediates the effects of beta adrenergic stimulation (see Chapter 10). As a result, these compounds affect many body systems, including the CNS. Caffeine and theophylline are the methylxanthines most often used clinically.

Caffeine may stimulate any level of the CNS, depending on the dose. Mild cortical stimulation is produced by low oral doses, such as those available in coffee, tea, and cola or in the nonprescription alerting medications. At higher doses caffeine stimulates the medullary centers controlling respiration, vasomotor tone, and vagal tone. Very high doses of caffeine may stimulate the spinal cord and lead to generalized convulsions.

Theophylline also acts as a CNS stimulant but exerts more action on the heart than does caffeine. Theophylline is most often used clinically as a means of relaxing bronchial smooth muscle. This action is useful in treating chronic obstructive pulmonary disease and asthma (see Chapter 25). Theophylline has also been used as a respiratory stimulant in newborn infants.

Absorption and fate. Methylxanthines are absorbed from the gastrointestinal tract. Salt forms of these agents are better absorbed, since the salts are much more soluble in water than are the free alkaloids. The parenteral form of caffeine includes sodium benzoate to maintain solubility of the caffeine.

Caffeine has a half-life in the plasma of about 4 hours. The drug may be partly metabolized in the liver. A portion of a dose appears in the urine as the unchanged compound or as metabolites. Theophylline has a half-life in the plasma of 8 to 9 hours in adults.

The metabolism and clearance of methylxanthines may be much lower in neonates than in normal adults. When these drugs are used in newborn infants, it may be necessary to adjust the dose to allow for the longer persistence of the drugs in the body. Since neonates vary greatly in their ability to metabolize methylxanthines, it may be necessary to measure blood levels of these drugs. Clearance of methylxanthines is also lower in patients with liver disease or congestive heart failure. These patients may also require adjusted doses of methylxanthines.

Toxicity. Methylxanthines frequently irritate the gastrointestinal mucosa, producing bleeding. Bleeding may occur without other signs or may be accompanied by nausea and vomiting. High concentrations of methylxanthines in the blood can lead to excessive CNS stimulation and convulsions. At ordinary therapeutic concentrations, however, the most common reaction to caffeine is nervousness or jitteriness. Theophylline most commonly increases heart rate (tachycardia).

Doxapram

Mechanism of action. Doxapram stimulates respiration by two mechanisms. At low doses the drug seems to stimulate the peripheral carotid chemoreceptors. This action increases sensitivity to carbon dioxide and thereby increases the impulse to breathe. At slightly higher doses doxapram stimulates the medullary centers controlling respiration.

Absorption and fate. Doxapram is administered intravenously. The drug is very rapid acting, with effects observed within the first minute after injection. The duration of respiratory stimulation is usually 5 to 12 minutes. Doxapram may be given repeatedly to sustain a patient throughout a period of respiratory depression.

Toxicity. Doxapram can produce a variety of reactions. Dizziness, apprehension, and disorientation may be reported. Restless, involuntary muscle activity, and increased reflexes are frequently observed. Patients may report a feeling of warmth with flushing, sweating, and increased body temperature. Blood pressure is elevated. Chest pains and cardiac arrhythmias may occur. Extreme agitation, hallucinations, or convulsions usually occur only with overdose, but certain patients may be more susceptible to these reactions. The maximum cumulative dose for doxapram is 3 Gm.

Since doxapram increases blood pressure, this drug should not be used in combination with other drugs tending to elevate blood pressure, such as sympathomimetics. Adverse interactions can also occur between doxapram and the inhalation anesthetics that sensitize the heart to catecholamines (halothane, enflurane). A delay of 10 minutes or more between the cessation of anesthesia with these drugs and the administration of doxapram is suggested to lessen the possibility of excessive cardiac toxicity.

CENTRAL NERVOUS SYSTEM STIMULANTS AS DRUGS OF ABUSE

CNS stimulants most commonly come to the attention of the medical professional as drugs of abuse. The medical uses of these agents are limited. This section discusses the more commonly abused drugs of this class, dealing primarily with the symptoms and sequelae of abuse. The list of drugs covered is necessarily limited. Suggested readings at the end of the chapter give more comprehensive coverage of unofficial or "street" drugs.

Amphetamines

Although the medical uses of the amphetamines are rather limited, amphetamines are produced in massive amounts by industry. The inevitable conclusion is that much of the drug produced ends up being used illegitimately. In 1970, the year before amphetamines were put on schedule II, the Department of Justice reported that 38% of the manufactured amphetamines could not be traced and presumably went to illegal markets. Strong restrictions on the manufacture and sale of amphetamines followed, but amphetamine availability seemed to be virtually unimpaired. A Drug Enforcement Administration report in 1976 suggested that amphetamine abuse was increasing and that the source of the drug was largely physicians' prescriptions. Estimates of the extent of amphetamine abuse are obviously filled with uncertainties. However, many experts agree that the most common amphetamine abuser is middle class, gets amphetamines from one or more medical sources, and takes the drugs orally. A minority of amphetamine abusers are the so-called "speed freaks," that is, members of the drug subculture who take high doses of amphetamines by injection.

Long-term use of low doses of amphetamines can produce psychological dependence. The drug user may have originally taken the drug intermittently to overcome fatigue or depression. Doses of 5 to 20 mg are effective in the naive user. Persons who take these doses three or four times daily will begin to feel as if they cannot get along without the drug. If the person stops taking the drug, depression ensues. Whether amphetamines produce actual physical withdrawal symptoms is debatable, but this withdrawal depression is sufficiently unpleasant to induce many users to return to amphetamines.

General guidelines for patients receiving drugs to treat narcolepsy or attention deficit disorder, or to suppress appetite

Drug administration

- Assess for CNS side effects; if severe, notify physician.
- In the hospital setting, pad side rails and keep them up. Have a suction machine nearby.
- Monitor vital signs and blood pressure.

Patient and family education

- Review anticipated benefits and possible side effects of drug therapy. Tell the patient to report the development of any new symptom.
- Tell patients to take these drugs only as directed, and not to change dose or frequency without consulting the physician.
- Remind patients to keep all health care providers informed of all drugs being taken. Warn patients to avoid ingesting drugs or food that also contribute to cardiovascular side effects, such as caffeine and caffeine-containing beverages or over-the-counter cold preparations containing phenylpropanolamine.
- Avoid over-the-counter drugs unless first approved by the physician.
- After long-term use, these drugs should not be discontinued abruptly.
- None of these drugs is appropriate to treat general fatigue.
- Insomnia may lessen with continued use of a drug, but may be better treated by eliminating the final dose of medication during the day; consult the physician.
- See Patient Problems: Dry Mouth on p. 170; Constipation on p. 187.
- Warn diabetic patients to monitor blood glucose levels, as these drugs may alter blood glucose, necessitating a change in diet or insulin.
- Warn patients to avoid driving or operating hazardous equipment if nervousness, agitation, or other CNS effects are severe; consult physician.
- Except when specifically prescribed for attention deficit disorder, these drugs should not be used in children. Keep these and all drugs out of their reach.
- These drugs should not be used during pregnancy unless specifically prescribed by the obstetrician. Counsel about contraceptives as needed.
- Avoid alcoholic beverages unless approved by the physician.

Drugs to treat narcolepsy and attention deficit disorder

Drug administration/patient and family education

- See the general guidelines.
- Weigh the patient 2 or 3 times per week until the effects of the drug can be evaluated. Although not being given for the purpose of weight reduction, most of these drugs will suppress the appetite.
- Teach parents to keep careful weight and height records of children.
- Reinforce to patients that several weeks of therapy may be necessary until full effect of the drug therapy can be evaluated.
- Refer the patient and family for appropriate teaching and counseling for narcolepsy and attention deficit disorder.

Drugs to suppress appetite

Drug administration/patient and family education

- See the general guidelines.
- Refer patients for appropriate counseling and instruction on weight reduction diets. Encourage a regular exercise program.
- Tell patients that weight reduction will be greatest during the first few weeks of therapy, but will slow after that.
- Phenylpropanolamine is also discussed in Chapter 26.
- Assess for signs of depression when fenfluramine is used: withdrawal, lack of interest in personal appearance, insomnia, change in affect.

Central nervous system stimulants to stimulate respiration

Drug administration

- Anticipate that seizures may occur. Have a suction machine at the bedside. Keep side rails up and use padding. Do not leave the patient unattended.
- Have oxygen and resuscitation equipment available.
- Monitor pulse, blood pressure, and respirations. Monitor ECG tracing.
- Monitor temperature.
- See manufacturer's literature for specific guidelines about administration of doxapram.
- Theophylline is discussed in Chapter 25.
- These drugs are rarely used outside of the intensive care setting to stimulate respiration.

Heavy use of amphetamines either orally or by injection can lead to severe reactions. Persons taking large doses may begin to show stereotyped behavior consisting of compulsive or repetitive actions. These actions frequently have no useful goal. For example, the user may repeatedly wax one fender of a car or count the pages of a book. Other behavior patterns are less benign. For example, chronic abusers often have the conviction that bugs are crawling under their skin and may mutilate themselves in an attempt to remove them. Some users develop feelings of paranoia and suspicion, feelings that frequently erupt into violent behavior. Many chronic abusers of amphetamines develop what is called *toxic psychosis*, or *paranoid psychosis*. This severe reaction involves visual and auditory hallucinations and is frequently mistaken for schizophrenia. The toxic psychosis of amphetamines is specifically treated with an antipsychotic drug (see Chapter 41).

Cocaine

Cocaine was introduced into medicine as a local anesthetic and is very effective for that purpose. Unfortunately, cocaine is also a stimulant very similar to amphetamine in its mechanism of action and effects on the CNS.

Pure salts of cocaine are difficult to prepare and consequently very expensive. Until recently, this restriction limited the availability of cocaine. Today, the most commonly used form of cocaine is the free base known as "crack," which is easy to prepare and inexpensive. It is highly lipid soluble and is quickly absorbed and distributed to the CNS. In this form, cocaine is one of the most addictive substances known.

At moderate doses cocaine can increase heart rate and blood pressure, as well as produce general CNS stimulation. As with amphetamines, it can produce convulsions if high enough doses are taken. Death by cocaine overdose is relatively rare, but when a fatal overdose is taken, convulsions, cardiovascular collapse, and death may occur within 2 or 3 minutes of the dose.

Chronic abuse of cocaine produces physical symptoms similar to those produced by amphetamine abuse. Toxic psychosis, stereotyped behavior, and paranoia also are observed.

Caffeine

Caffeine may be the most widely abused drug in the United States, although the effects of this abuse are much less obvious and usually less devastating than those produced by other abused drugs.

Caffeine abuse often takes place unwittingly. Consider the following example:

> John has a cup of coffee while dressing in the morning and a second cup at breakfast. At work John consumes another cup of coffee at the 10:30 AM coffee break. At lunch John drinks two glassfuls of iced tea. On afternoon coffee break John has a chocolate bar and a cola. Before he leaves work John takes two Excedrin for a headache. At dinner John drinks two cups of tea. Before bed John takes two more Excedrin.

Why is John unable to sleep? John cannot sleep because he ingested about 1 Gm of caffeine during this typical day.

Most people are aware of the caffeine content of coffee, which ranges from 80 to 150 mg per cup. Less well known is the fact that tea, colas, chocolate, and nonprescription medications such as Excedrin also contain caffeine. In the example given, John took over half a gram of caffeine in these forms.

Ingestion of more than 500 mg (half a gram) of caffeine daily produces a variety of CNS effects as well as cardiovascular reactions. Irritability or nervousness is a very common complaint, along with disturbances of sleep. Patients may report heart palpitations or that their heart is racing. These descriptions may suggest premature ventricular contractions and tachycardia, both common symptoms of chronic caffeine toxicity. Diarrhea and gastrointestinal irritation commonly accompany chronic overdosage with caffeine. Patients complaining of symptoms such as those just listed should be questioned about caffeine intake. The person who is taking the history should ask specifically about individual beverages, foods, and medications that contain caffeine in order to get an accurate estimate of intake. The caffeine content of common items is presented in Table 43.5.

Psychological dependence on caffeine may occur. People have great difficulty in omitting the drug from their diets. Nevertheless, patients with peptic ulcer disease should avoid caffeine. Pregnant women may wish to avoid indulging in caffeine, since the drug freely passes to the fetus. Any person who ingests more than 200 mg of caffeine daily should be encouraged to reduce intake to avoid the subtle onset of signs of chronic toxicity.

SUMMARY

Narcolepsy, a condition in which a patient spontaneously falls asleep during active periods, may be treated with CNS stimulants. Attention deficit disorder, a condition characterized by overactivity in children, is also treated, paradoxically, with CNS stimulants.

Amphetamines increase the release and effectiveness of catecholamine neurotransmitters in the brain and in peripheral nerves. Amphetamines stimulate the reticular activating system of the brain, creating increased alertness, and stimulate the reward center, creating a perception of pleasure. Amphetamines for medical uses are administered orally. Excretion through the kidneys may be increased by acidifying the urine. Most toxicity of the amphetamines is in the CNS (restlessness, tremor, irritability, insomnia, confusion) or the cardiovascular system (headache, chilliness, palpitation, angina, cardiac arrhythmias).

Methylphenidate stimulates the cortical levels of the brain more than the motor levels. The drug is well absorbed orally but is rapidly metabolized in the liver during the first pass. Many reactions to methylphenidate are similar to those seen with amphetamines.

Pemoline is a CNS stimulant with less sympathomimetic effects than other drugs of this type. The drug has a longer duration of action than methylphenidate. The effects of pemoline in reversing hyperkinesis take several weeks to be established. Pemoline seems to cause less CNS effects at normal doses than amphetamines, and cardiovascular toxicity is rare.

Many CNS stimulants suppress the appetite center in the brain. Benzphetamine and phenmetrazine are nonamphetamine appetite suppressants that cause many of the same reactions as amphetamines. Diethylpropion causes less cardiovascular toxicity than other appetite suppressants. Fenfluramine is unique in this group of drugs in producing CNS depression rather than stimulation. Phenylpropanolamine is a mild appetite suppressant frequently found in over-the-counter preparations. Tolerance develops to all the appetite-suppressing drugs in clinical use.

Some CNS stimulants occasionally are used to stimulate respiration by medullary stimulation, including methylxanthines such as caffeine and theophylline. Doxapram stimulates respiration also by increasing sensitivity to carbon dioxide. At higher doses all these drugs can produce excess CNS stimulation and convulsions.

Long-term use of amphetamines can produce psychological dependence. High doses cause stereotyped behavior, paranoia, and violent behavior. Chronic abusers may develop toxic psychosis. Cocaine produces similar symptoms when abused and occasionally, when high doses are taken rapidly, causes sudden death.

Excessive use of caffeine can produce an anxiety syndrome with signs of gastrointestinal irritation and cardiovascular sensitivity (tachycardia, palpitations).

STUDY QUESTIONS

1. What is narcolepsy?
2. What is the treatment of narcolepsy?
3. What is hyperkinesis?
4. What is the treatment of hyperkinesis?
5. What is the mechanism of action of amphetamines in the CNS?
6. What two brain areas are especially affected by amphetamines?
7. What is the route of administration of amphetamines used in clinical medicine?
8. What toxic reactions are common with amphetamines?
9. How do the *d* (dextro) and *l* (levo) forms of amphetamines differ in toxicity?
10. What other drugs interact with amphetamines?
11. What is the mechanism of action of methylphenidate in the CNS?
12. What is the route of elimination of methylphenidate?
13. What toxicity is associated with the use of methylphenidate?
14. What is the mechanism of action of pemoline?
15. How does the duration of action of this drug differ from that of methylphenidate?
16. How long does it take for full therapeutic effects of pemoline to develop?
17. What toxic reactions are associated with pemoline?
18. Why are CNS stimulants used to treat obesity?
19. How do the nonamphetamine appetite suppressants differ from amphetamines?
20. Which nonamphetamine appetite suppressants produce reactions similar to those of amphetamines?
21. Which nonamphetamine appetite suppressants produce little cardiovascular stimulation?
22. Which nonamphetamine appetite suppressant produces CNS depression?
23. Which nonamphetamine appetite suppressant is most often found in over-the-counter obesity medications?
24. What toxic reactions may develop during therapy with the nonamphetamine appetite suppressants?
25. Why are CNS stimulants used to stimulate respiration?

26. What two methylxanthines are sometimes used to stimulate respiration?
27. What reactions are observed to the methylxanthines used to stimulate respiration?
28. What is the mechanism of action of doxapram?
29. How is doxapram administered?
30. What is the duration of action of doxapram?
31. What toxicity is observed with doxapram?
32. What is the source of most amphetamine used in an abusive manner?
33. What is the effect of toxic doses of amphetamines in an amphetamine abuser?
34. How does cocaine differ from amphetamine?
35. Why may caffeine be considered a drug of abuse?
36. What are the effects of chronic overdosage with caffeine?

SUGGESTED READINGS

Adams, M.S.: Management of attention deficit disorders, JAMA **75**(2):187, 1983.

Boulenger, J.P.: Caffeine consumption and anxiety: preliminary results of a survey comparing patients with anxiety disorders and normal controls, Psychopharmacol. Bull. **18**(4):53, 1982.

Brooten, D., and Jordan, C.H.: Caffeine and pregnancy: a research review and recommendations for clinical practice, J. Obstet. Gynecol. Nurs. **12**(3):190, 1983.

Bruera, E., and others: Narcotics plus methylphenidate (Ritalin) for advanced cancer pain, Am. J. Nurs. **88**(11):1555, 1988.

Carluccio, C.: Anxiety syndrome or caffeinism? Diagnosis **2**(9):74, 1980.

Cohen, F.L.: Narcolepsy: a review of a common, life-long sleep disorder, J. Adv. Nurs. **13**(5):546, 1988.

Curatolo, P.W., and Robertson, D.: The health consequences of caffeine, Ann. Intern. Med. **98**(5, part 1):641, 1983.

Dobmeyer, D.J.: The arrhythmogenic effects of caffeine in human beings, N. Engl. J. Med. **308**(14):814, 1983.

DuPont, R.I., Goldstein, A., and O'Donnell, J., editors: Handbook on drug abuse, National Institute on Drug Abuse, Washington, D.C., 1979, U.S. Government Printing Office.

Erman, M.K.: Guidelines for recognizing and treating hypersomnias, Drug Ther. **14**(8):64, 1984.

Friedman, R.B., Kindy, P., Jr., and Reinke, J.A.: What to tell patients about weight loss methods. 2. Drugs, Postgrad. Med. **72**(4):85, 1982.

Hughes, M.C., Goldman, B.L., and Snyder, N.F.: Hyperactivity and the attention deficit disorder, Am. Fam. Physician **27**(6):119, 1983.

Labow, R.: Effects of caffeine being studied for treatment of apnea in newborns, Can. Med. Assoc. J. **129**(3):230, 1983.

Martin, W.R., editor: Drug addiction. II. Amphetamine, psychotogen, and marihuana dependence, Handbuch der Experimentellen Pharmakologie. Vol. 45, Berlin, 1977, Springer-Verlag.

Mattes, J.A., and Gittelman, R.: Growth of hyperactive children on maintenance regimen of methylphenidate, Arch. Gen. Psychiatry **40**(3):317, 1983.

Mittleman, R.E., and Wetli, C.V.: Death caused by recreational cocaine use, JAMA **252**(4):1889, 1984.

Noble, R.: A controlled clinical trial of the cardiovascular and psychological effect of phenylpropanolamine and caffeine, Drug Intell. Clin. Pharm. **22**(4):296, 1988.

Ottenbacher, K.J., and Cooper, H.M.: Drug treatment of hyperactivity in children, Dev. Med. Child Neurol. **25**(3):358, 1983.

Petersen, R.C., and Stillman, R.C., editors: Cocaine: 1977, National Institute on Drug Abuse, Department of Health, Education, and Welfare Pub. No. (ADM) 77-471, Washington D.C., 1977, U.S. Government Printing Office.

Pfeifer, R.W., and Notari, R.E.: Predicting caffeine plasma concentrations resulting from consumption of food or beverages: a simple method and its origin, Drug Intell. Clin. Pharm. **22**(12):953, 1988.

Schneider, J.R.: Should patients with myocardial infarction receive caffeinated coffee? Focus Crit. Care **15**(1):52, 1988.

Soldatos, C.R.: Treatment of sleep disorders. II. Narcolepsy, Ration. Drug Ther. **17**(3):1, 1983.

Todd, B.: Cigarettes and caffeine in drug interactions, Geriatr. Nurs. **8**(2):97, 1987.

Vandegaer, F.: Cocaine—the deadliest addiction, Nursing89 **19**(2):72, 1989.

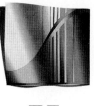

X

DRUGS TO CONTROL SEVERE PAIN

Section X discusses those drugs that have made modern surgery possible. Chapter 44, *Narcotic Analgesics (Opioids)*, focuses on the analgesic uses of opioids for surgery and other conditions in which pain is prominent. The remarkable insights recently gained on the endogenous morphinelike compounds, the endorphins, are reviewed. Since the opioids are also a major drug class for illicit use, attention is given to the features of opiate dependence, the role of the specific opiate antagonist naloxone in treating acute opiate overdose, and the role of the long-acting opioid methadone in treating opiate withdrawal. Chapter 45, *General Anesthetics*, presents the theories of anesthesia, the inhalation and intravenous anesthetics, and the combinations of drugs now widely used for balanced anesthesia and for neuroleptanesthesia. The limitations as well as desirable characteristics of each anesthetic are described. Chapter 46, *Local Anesthetics*, reviews both the surface use of local anesthetics as well as their use by injection for major surgery.

CHAPTER

Narcotic Analgesics (Opioids)

44

HISTORICAL REVIEW OF THE NARCOTIC ANALGESICS

Nature of Pain

Analgesics are drugs that relieve pain. Because two major components of pain exist, analgesics fall into two major classifications. One component of pain is *objective* and represents the stimulation of peripheral nerve endings when tissue is damaged. Nonnarcotic analgesics such as aspirin and acetaminophen (Datril, Tylenol) are believed to act by interfering with local mediators that are released in damaged tissue to stimulate the nerve endings. In the presence of nonnarcotic analgesics, pain is not felt because the nerves are not stimulated and the pain message therefore is never delivered to the central nervous system. The nonnarcotic analgesics are discussed in Chapter 23. The second component of pain is *subjective* and represents how a person reacts to pain, usually with fear, anxiety, and withdrawal. The subjective level of pain involves the spinal cord and brain, which collect and process the painful stimuli. The narcotic analgesics act to blunt this subjective component of pain. The individual treated with a narcotic analgesic may become unaware of pain and indifferent to all unpleasant stimuli.

History of Morphine

Opium has been used to produce analgesia and euphoria throughout the history of mankind. The word *opium* comes from the Greek word "opion," meaning poppy juice, and the source of morphine today is still the sticky brown gum (opium) collected from the seed pod of *Papaver somniferum,* a variety of poppy. About 10% of the content of opium is morphine. Codeine also can be extracted from opium, although in such small amounts that most medicinal codeine is derived from the methylation of morphine. Morphine was isolated in 1803 by a German pharmacist and named after

Morpheus, the Greek god of sleep. Morphine was the first pure chemical substance that mimicked the pharmacological effects of the natural product after extraction from the natural product.

Even today morphine remains the prototype of the narcotic analgesics, a class of drugs more properly called the *opioids.* Some narcotic analgesics are chemical modifications of morphine. The term *opiate* as a drug class refers to codeine and to morphine and its semisynthetic derivatives. The purely synthetic narcotic analgesics with morphinelike activities were originally called opioids, but today the term *opioids* is used by most pharmacologists as a general name for *narcotic analgesics.* In this chapter, opioid will be used instead of narcotic analgesic, although this more familiar phrase is used elsewhere in this book. The chief characteristic of the opioids is their ability to render the individual unreactive to pain even though conscious and the source of pain has not been removed. The term *narcotic* is derived from the Greek word meaning stupor or insensibility.

All opioids have abuse potential to a greater or lesser degree. In general, opioids come under the Controlled Substance Act, as described in Chapter 3. The schedule under which each opioid falls is listed in the drug tables.

Drug dependency as a property of morphine was not appreciated in the United States until the Civil War, when morphine was widely used in treating wounded soldiers, whose addiction subsequently became a significant social problem. Opium and morphine were readily available and were often ingredients of patent medicines. By the late 1800s, attempts were made to modify the structure of morphine to keep the analgesic property but eliminate the addictive potential. The first semisynthetic drug was heroin, but heroin soon proved to produce drug dependency more readily than morphine. To-

691

day heroin is not a legal drug in the United States, although it is in other countries.

The first purely synthetic morphinelike compound was meperidine (Demerol), which came into clinical use in the 1940s. Because meperidine was not a chemical modification of morphine, widespread belief held that meperidine did not cause drug dependency. Today meperidine is considered a drug with high abuse potential (schedule II) similar to morphine. The most recent examples of opioids whose abuse potential was not originally recognized are pentazocine (Talwin) and propoxyphene (Darvon), which are now classified as drugs of low abuse potential (schedule IV). The characteristics of opiate dependency and its treatment are discussed later in this chapter.

Endorphins: The Body's Own Morphine

The most recent development in the search for a better analgesic has been the discovery of how morphine acts in the body. It had long been suspected that morphine acted at very specific receptor sites. In the early 1970s scientists were able to demonstrate that specific receptors for morphinelike drugs did indeed exist in the brain, spinal cord, and gut. These receptors recognized only opioids and none of the known neurotransmitters. This suggested that a previously unknown, naturally occurring substance existed in the brain, spinal cord, and gut that is mimicked by morphine. Such substances have been identified and are termed *endorphins*, for *endo*genous *morphine*like substances. All endorphins are polypeptides and are found in those specific locations long associated with the actions of morphine and in which opiate receptors can be identified.

Beta endorphin is a large peptide derived from the prohormone for adrenocorticotropic hormone (ACTH) and is found in the pituitary. The smallest endorphins are the pentapeptides (five amino acids) called the *enkephalins*, a term meaning "from the head," referring to the first tissue from which they were isolated. The two enkephalins are met(methionine)-enkephalin and leu(leucine)-enkephalin. The enkephalins seem to be neurotransmitters associated with (1) the mediation of pain and analgesia; (2) the release of growth hormone, prolactin, and vasopressin from the pituitary; (3) the modulation of locomotor activity; (4) the regulation of mood; and (5) the regulation of gut motility. These recent discoveries are expected to clarify the nature of analgesia and the development of the opiate type of drug dependency as well as provide the basis for understanding the role of endorphins in mental disorders, seizure activity, and behavior patterns involving the reward system, eating, and drinking.

The goal in developing analgesics has been to provide an effective analgesic that will not produce tolerance or drug dependence. This goal has not yet been fully realized. Three types of opiate receptors have been characterized. The μ (mu) receptor mediates central analgesia, euphoria, respiratory depression, and physical dependence. The μ receptor is associated with the classic morphine effects. The κ (kappa) receptor mediates spinal analgesia, miosis, sedation, and appetite regulation. The κ receptor appears sensitive to opioids with mixed agonist-antagonist activity. The σ (sigma) receptor mediates the dysphoric, hallucinogenic, and cardiac stimulant effects. The σ receptor appears sensitive to opioid antagonist activity. Other opiate receptor types also have been postulated. With the characterization of opiate receptors, it has become clear that the opioids such as pentazocine and nalbuphine, which have the least dependency potential, have not only agonistic properties (mimicking endorphin effects) but antagonistic properties as well (blocking endorphin effects). The search for a nonaddicting opioid may depend on finding the drug that has the right combination of agonist-antagonist properties without causing unpleasant side effects.

PHARMACOLOGY OF MORPHINE

The pharmacology of morphine provides the standard for comparing the actions of opioids.

Actions in the Central Nervous System

Many effects of morphine occur in the central nervous system.

Analgesia. The analgesia produced by morphine has three characteristics. First, morphine raises the threshold for pain perception, making the individual less aware of pain. Second, it reduces anxiety and fear, which are the emotional reactions to pain. Third, morphine induces sleep even in the presence of severe pain.

The biochemical mechanism of pain relief by the opioids is their ability to mimic endogenous compounds, the endorphins, which act at many sites in the brain to modify the perception of and reaction to pain. Support for this concept has come from studies of naloxone (Narcan), which is a specific opioid antagonist. Naloxone blocks the placebo response and reduces the effectiveness of acupuncture anesthesia, two processes believed to reflect the activity of endorphins. The interpretation of these effects of naloxone is that naloxone blocks the effect of endorphins, which are released in response to pain to minimize its perception. These studies also provide a biochemical explanation for the effectiveness of the acupuncture technique to reduce pain.

Medullary actions. Morphine affects several medullary centers. The most important is the respiratory center, which becomes less sensitive to carbon dioxide in the presence of morphine. Tolerance does develop to this effect so that an individual who abuses one of the opioids can tolerate doses of opioids that would cause fatal respiratory depression in the nondependent individual. Death from an overdose of an opioid is frequently due to respiratory arrest; the victim simply stops breathing. Similarly, the most important drug interactions with morphine are those arising from a synergistic depression of the respiratory center, as with any of the sedative-hypnotic drugs, minor tranquilizers, alcohol, general anesthetics, or phenothiazines. Tolerance does not develop to the respiratory depression produced by these latter drug classes. An individual abusing an opioid and a drug of another class, such as alcohol or one of the other sedative-hypnotic drugs, can readily succumb to drug-induced respiratory depression.

A second medullary center depressed by morphine is the cough center. Morphine seldom is prescribed as a cough suppressant, as is a related drug such as codeine. Cough suppressants (antitussive drugs) are described in Chapter 26.

The third major medullary center affected by morphine is the chemoreceptor trigger zone. Morphine stimulates this center to produce nausea and vomiting. This is a transient effect, so repeated doses do not usually cause nausea and vomiting. Individuals vary in their sensitivity to this emetic action.

Behavior. The effect of morphine on behavior depends on the mental state of the individual. Euphoria may be experienced if the individual has been in pain or has been fearful and anxious. Therapeutic doses produce minimum sedation, but larger doses cause drowsiness, sleep, or in very large doses, coma. A few individuals become excited rather than depressed.

Actions in the Periphery

Gastrointestinal tract. Morphine has a profound depressant effect on the gastrointestinal tract; constipation is a common side effect of morphine administration. Although morphine is not used to treat nonspecific diarrhea, related drugs such as codeine or diphenoxylate are. The common medicinal use of opium in ancient medicine was to stop diarrhea.

Secretions. Gastric, biliary, and pancreatic secretions are inhibited by morphine. It is used to treat the pain associated with biliary colic, but may exacerbate rather than relieve the pain in some patients, since the biliary tract may go into painful spasms in the presence of morphine.

Urinary retention. Urinary retention is another side effect of morphine. Morphine stimulates the release of vasopressin (antidiuretic hormone), so that more water is absorbed in the kidney tubules, decreasing urine volume. The drug also reduces perception of the need to void.

Cardiovascular effects. Morphine commonly causes hypotension. In part, this may be a result of depression of the vasomotor center in the medulla. In addition, morphine causes histamine release, and histamine is a potent vasodilator. The concurrent administration of a phenothiazine or atropine can intensify the hypotension. In large doses, morphine slows the heart rate.

Ocular effect. A classic effect of morphine is to reduce the pupillary size. A pinpoint pupil is one characteristic of a narcotic overdose. However, if the victim is near death, hypoxia causes the release of epinephrine, which dilates the pupil.

Adverse Reactions and Contraindications to Opioids

The common adverse reactions of the opioids are those predicted by their pharmacological actions: nausea and vomiting, constipation, urinary retention, itching, and hypotension resulting from histamine release.

Some actions characteristic of morphine are undesirable in certain patients, including the respiratory depression caused by the opioids. Patients with impaired respiratory function may be severely compromised by an opioid because their respiratory drive is already impaired. Although in general the opioids relax bronchial smooth muscle, a few patients with asthma experience severe bronchoconstriction and die. These drugs will also pass into the milk of a nursing mother and affect the infant.

Patients suffering from a head injury should not be given an opioid, since the decreased respiration will increase carbon dioxide retention and carbon dioxide will dilate the intracranial blood vessels, worsening the situation. Also, the sedative and behavioral effects will obscure evaluation of the central nervous system.

Since the opioids can cause hypotension, they must be used cautiously in patients suffering from shock or blood loss, conditions worsened by a hypotensive action.

Tolerance and Dependence with Opioids

Drug tolerance. Drug tolerance is the situation in which repeated use of a drug results in a lesser response unless the dose is raised. Tolerance develops rapidly to the euphoric effect of the opioids. Individuals abusing the narcotic analgesics keep raising the dose to maintain the "good" feeling associated with the drug. Patients receiving an opioid for severe pain over a limited period also may develop tolerance. The patient is unlikely to become drug dependent because as the pain subsides, so will the need for the opioid. However, the individual abusing an opioid will become drug dependent rather rapidly. Daily use of one of the opioids can produce drug dependence in 3 weeks.

Little or no tolerance develops to the pupillary constriction or to the constipating effect of the opioids. Pinpoint pupils are one characteristic of dependence on opioids.

Drug dependency. Drug dependency has complex psychological and social components, but only the pharmacological component is considered here. A drug-dependent person will experience distinct physical reactions if the drug is suddenly discontinued; these reactions make up the *abstinence syndrome*. Basically, the abstinence syndrome represents the readjustment of the body to function in the absence of the drug. The more quickly the drug is eliminated, the more pronounced the syndrome. The severity of the symptoms will be greater the longer the drug has been used and the higher the dose used.

Symptoms of the abstinence syndrome. The opiate abstinence syndrome following the sudden cessation of morphine or heroin use is predictable. The individual has a runny nose (rhinorrhea), goose flesh, tearing (lacrimation), sweating, and yawning 16 hours after the last dose. The pupils do not react readily to light. Over the next 20 hours the individual becomes restless, cannot sleep, and experiences muscle twitching. Hot and cold flashes and abdominal cramping occur. By 36 hours, the individual feels nauseous, vomits, and has diarrhea. The abstinence symptoms are generally the reverse of the drug effects described for the opioids. The body overcompensates when the drug is removed.

The opiate abstinence syndrome is unpleasant, although not life-threatening, as is the sedative-hypnotic abstinence syndrome. A major part of drug abuse behavior may be the search for more drug to stop the abstinence syndrome.

Methadone for maintenance and detoxification. The major approach in the United States for treating individuals dependent on heroin or another opioid is to substitute methadone, which can be given orally in a daily dose. Since tolerance already has developed to the "kick" from heroin in these individuals, the methadone maintains this tolerance while protecting against withdrawal symptoms. The goal of maintenance is to discourage the individual from continuing to seek drugs and to participate instead in rehabilitation programs. If detoxification (elimination of drug) is the goal, methadone is administered first when withdrawal symptoms appear, and then the dose of methadone gradually is reduced to zero over 1 to 3 weeks. Because methadone has a long half-life in the body, the abstinence symptoms are not as severe as with morphine or heroin.

Clonidine for withdrawal treatment. Clonidine is an antihypertensive drug that activates central alpha-2 adrenergic receptors (see Chapter 15). This activity reduces sympathetic overactivity. Because of this reduction in centrally mediated sympathetic activity, clonidine has been useful in treating the opiate withdrawal symptoms; it reduces the symptoms without producing a withdrawal syndrome.

Acute Toxicity of Opioids and Use of Opiate Receptor Antagonists (Narcotic Antagonists) (Table 44.1)

Respiratory depression is the usual cause of death from an acute overdose of an opioid. An overdose is most likely to occur in an individual who buys drugs for abuse on the street. Street drugs have unknown purity and concentration, so occasionally the drug content is higher than anticipated.

Table 44.1   Narcotic Antagonists

Generic name	Trade name	Administration/dosage	Comments
Naloxone hydrochloride	Narcan*	INTRAVENOUS, INTRAMUSCULAR, SUBCUTANEOUS: *Adults*—0.4 mg for respiratory depression caused by narcotic overdose. Repeated in a few minutes if necessary, up to 3 doses. For narcotic depression of respiration after surgery: 0.1 to 0.2 mg every few minutes as necessary. FDA Pregnancy Category B. INTRAVENOUS: *Neonates*—0.01 mg/kg body weight.	Pure narcotic antagonist used to reverse respiratory depression from narcotic overdose. Unlike levallorphan, naloxone produces no respiratory depression of its own.
Naltrexone	Trexan	ORAL: *Adults*—initial dose 25 mg. If there are no symptoms of withdrawal, the rest of the daily dose may be given. The usual daily dose is 50 mg, but it may also be administered as 100 mg every other day or 150 mg every third day. FDA Pregnancy Category C.	Adjunctive therapy for drug rehabilitation from opioids. Patients should have completed a withdrawal program and be free of opioids for 7 to 10 days.

*Available in Canada and United States.

Table 44.2   Comparison of the Narcotic Analgesics

Level of pain	Drug	Equivalent analgesic dose (mg) given IM or SC	Time for peak effect (min)	Duration (hr)	Schedule U.S.	Schedule Canada
Severe	Morphine	10	30 to 90	3 to 7	II	N
	Buprenorphine (Buprenex)	0.5	15	4 to 6	V	†
	Hydromorphone hydrochloride (Dilaudid)	1.5	30 to 90	4 to 5	II	N
	Levorphanol tartrate (Levo-Dromoran)	2 to 3	60 to 90	5 to 8	II	N
	Methadone (Dolophine)	7.5 to 10	60 to 120	3 to 6	II	N
	Oxymorphone (Numorphan)	1 to 1.5	30 to 90	3 to 6	II	N
Moderate to severe	Butorphanol (Stadol)	1.5 to 3.5	30	3 to 4	N.S.*	C
	Meperidine (Demerol)	75 to 100	30 to 60	2 to 4	II	N
	Nalbuphine (Nubain)	10	30	3 to 6	N.S.*	C
	Pentazocine (Talwin)	40 to 60	30 to 60	2 to 3	IV	N
Mild to moderate	Codeine phosphate	120	60 to 90	4 to 6	II	N
	Propoxyphene (Darvon)	180 to 240	60	4 to 6	IV	N

*Not scheduled as a controlled substance.
†Not available.

The overdosed individual is stuporous or in a deep sleep and initially is warm, with a flushed wet skin. The next stage is coma in which respiration is depressed, and as the individual becomes hypoxic (starved for oxygen), the skin becomes cold, clammy, and mottled, and the pupils dilate. Death is then imminent.

Naloxone

When a patient is brought to the emergency room comatose from a drug overdose, the first goal is to support respiration and the second is to determine which drug was used. If an opioid is suspected, a specific test is used. Naloxone (Narcan) is administered intravenously, and if the overdose is a result of an opioid, the patient will respond in 2 to 3 minutes with improved respiration and return to consciousness. This response reflects that naloxone is a pure antagonist for the opiate receptor. Naloxone displaces the opioid from the receptor but produces no effect of its own. The result is a dramatic reversal of the drug overdose. The patient must still be monitored carefully, however, because naloxone has a short duration of action and its effect may wear off before the overdosed drug has been sufficiently eliminated. If the patient again becomes comatose, naloxone must be given again.

Multiple drug abuse is common, and naloxone will only reverse the depression resulting from the narcotic analgesic. Naloxone will have no effect when the overdose is not due to a narcotic analgesic.

Naltrexone

Naltrexone (Trexan) is an opioid antagonist. In itself it has little pharmacologic activity, but will reverse opioid activity. Naltrexone is orally effective and long acting. It is prescribed by individuals detoxified of opioids. Since naltrexone blocks the effects of opioids, it is used in behavioral therapy to discourage resumption of opioid use. Administered to an individual addicted to opioids, naltrexone will precipitate withdrawal symptoms.

SPECIFIC OPIOIDS

Twelve narcotic analgesics are presently in use. They are compared as to efficacy, dose, onset, and duration of action in Table 44.2 (p. 695). In addition to these drugs are *alfentanil (Alfenta)*, *fentanyl (Sublimaze)*, and *sufentanil (Sufenta)*, short-acting narcotic analgesics used primarily in anesthesia; *oxycodone*, a schedule II compound found only combined with a nonnarcotic analgesic; and *hy-drocodone*, a schedule II drug prescribed only as an antitussive agent.

The major use of the opioids is for the relief of moderate to severe pain. These drugs are most effective in relieving the constant dull pain associated with trauma, surgery, heart attack, biliary or ureteral colic, inflammation, or cancer. Isolated, sharp pain is not as effectively relieved by the opioids.

Opioids Effective for Relieving Severe Pain
(Table 44.3)

Morphine

Morphine has already been described as the prototype for the opioids. Chemically, morphine is a base that is positively charged at the pH in the gastrointestinal tract and therefore is not readily absorbed when taken orally. Since it is readily metabolized within the gut and by the liver, morphine is given intramuscularly or subcutaneously. Elderly patients usually require a smaller dose because they do not metabolize morphine as readily as do younger patients.

Morphine or meperidine is used to treat the pain of an acute myocardial infarction. At analgesic doses morphine not only relieves the pain but also reduces the anxiety without altering the cardiovascular system. If undue reduction in respiration, heart rate, or blood pressure does occur secondary to morphine administration, it can be reversed by administering naloxone, the narcotic antagonist.

Morphine is the drug of choice in pulmonary edema. The beneficial actions of morphine include relief of anxiety and vasodilation, which reduces the workload of the heart so that the heart pumps more efficiently. This increased cardiac efficiency relieves the pulmonary edema that arises when the left side of the heart cannot adequately pump the blood being supplied by the pulmonary veins. This inefficiency gives rise to hypertension and edema in the pulmonary system.

Hydromorphone

Hydromorphone (Dilaudid) is a semisynthetic derivative of morphine. It is more potent but shorter acting than morphine. Oral doses require more time to become effective but are longer acting than parenteral doses. The actions of hydromorphone are identical to those of morphine.

Oxymorphone

Oxymorphone (Numorphan) is a semisynthetic derivative of morphine that has all the actions of morphine except the antitussive (cough suppres-

Table 44.3 Narcotic Analgesics

Generic name	Trade name	Administration/dosage	Comments
Buprenorphine hydrochloride	Buprenex	INTRAMUSCULAR: *Adults*—0.3 to 0.6 mg, repeat every 6 to 8 hours as required.	Possesses both agonist and antagonist properties. Schedule V substance.
Butorphanol tartrate	Stadol*	INTRAMUSCULAR: *Adults*—1 to 4 mg every 3 to 4 hr. INTRAVENOUS: *Adults*—0.5 to 2 mg every 3 to 4 hr.	Possesses both agonist and antagonist properties. Not a scheduled drug.
Codeine sulfate, codeine phosphate		ORAL, INTRAMUSCULAR, SUBCUTANEOUS: *Adults*—30 to 60 mg every 4 to 6 hr. FDA Pregnancy Category C. *Children*—0.5 mg/kg body weight every 4 to 6 hr.	Schedule II substance.
Hydromorphone hydrochloride	Dilaudid*	ORAL: *Adult*—2 mg every 4 to 6 hr. FDA Pregnancy Category C. INTRAMUSCULAR, SUBCUTANEOUS: *Adult*—1 to 1.5 mg every 4 to 6 hr. May be given by slow intravenous injection or as a suppository.	Schedule II substance.
Levorphanol tartrate	Levo-Dromoran*	ORAL, SUBCUTANEOUS: *Adults*—2 mg.	Schedule II substance.
Meperidine hydrochloride	Demerol*	ORAL, INTRAMUSCULAR, SUBCUTANEOUS, SLOW INTRAVENOUS: *Adults*—50 to 150 mg every 3 to 4 hr. *Children*—1 to 1.5 mg/kg body weight, maximum 100 mg, every 3 to 4 hr.	Schedule II substance.
Methadone hydrochloride	Dolophine	ORAL, INTRAMUSCULAR, SUBCUTANEOUS: *Adults*—2.5 to 10 mg. For pain relief, repeat every 6 hr.	Used as a replacement drug for opiate dependence or to facilitate withdrawal. Schedule II substance.
Morphine sulfate		ORAL: *Adults*—5 to 15 mg every 4 hr. FDA Pregnancy Category C. INTRAMUSCULAR, SUBCUTANEOUS: *Adults*—5 to 20 mg every 4 hr. *Children* (subcutaneous only)—0.1 to 0.2 mg/kg body weight, maximum 15 mg. INTRAVENOUS: *Adults*—2.5 to 15 mg in 5 ml water, injected over 4 to 5 min. *Children*—0.1 to 0.2 mg/kg.	Not well absorbed orally. Schedule II substance.
Nalbuphine hydrochloride	Nubain*	INTRAMUSCULAR, SUBCUTANEOUS, INTRAVENOUS: *Adults*—10 mg every 3 to 6 hr, maximum single dose 20 mg and maximum daily dose 160 mg.	Possesses both agonist and antagonist properties. Not a scheduled drug.
Oxymorphone hydrochloride	Numorphan*	INTRAMUSCULAR, SUBCUTANEOUS: *Adults*—1 to 1.5 mg every 6 hr. INTRAVENOUS: *Adults*—0.5 mg. RECTAL: *Adults*—5 mg every 4 to 6 hr.	Schedule II substance.

*Available in Canada and Unitned States.
†Available in Canada only.

Continued.

Table 44.3   Narcotic Analgesics—cont'd

Generic name	Trade name	Administration/dosage	Comments
Pentazocine hydrochloride	Talwin 50*	ORAL: *Adults*—50 mg every 3 to 4 hr, maximum daily dose 600 mg.	Possesses both agonist and antagonist properties. Schedule IV substance.
Pentazocine lactate	Talwin Lactate*	INTRAMUSCULAR, SUBCUTANEOUS, INTRAVENOUS: *Adults*—30 mg every 3 to 4 hr. Subcutaneous route is not recommended, since tissue damage may occur.	
Propoxyphene hydrochloride	Darvon Dolene Novopropoxen†	ORAL: *Adults*—65 mg every 6 to 8 hr.	Schedule IV substance.
Propoxyphene napsylate	Darvon-N*	ORAL: *Adults*—100 mg every 6 to 8 hr.	Schedule IV substance.

*Available in Canada and United States.
†Available in Canada only.

sant) action. Oxymorphone is more potent than morphine but must also be given by injection.

Levorphanol

Levorphanol (Levo-Dromoran) is an opioid that has actions identical to those of morphine. The effective dose is about one fourth that of morphine.

Methadone

Methadone (Dolophine) is an opioid with actions similar to those of morphine. Methadone can be taken orally. Although the onset of action for a single analgesic dose is similar to that for morphine, methadone is highly protein bound and not readily metabolized. Methadone has a half-life of 25 hours.

Methadone, 40 to 120 mg daily, substitutes for other opioids in drug-dependent individuals and prevents withdrawal symptoms, as discussed earlier. Methadone currently is used in the treatment of opioid dependency because it is effective orally and only one dose per day is necessary. Also, the long plasma half-life more easily allows the gradual reduction in dose without side effects.

Opioids Effective in Relieving Moderate to Severe Pain (Table 44.3)

Meperidine

Meperidine (Demerol) was the first of the synthetic narcotic analgesics. It is shorter acting than morphine and does not have an antitussive effect. Meperidine is widely used for obstetrical analgesia.

Buprenorphine

Buprenorphine (Buprenex) is an opioid with both agonist and antagonist properties. Its abuse potential appears low and it is a Schedule V drug in the United States. It is administered intramuscularly. The onset of action is 15 minutes, and the duration of action is about 6 hours. Buprenorphine is effective for moderate to severe pain associated with surgery, cancer, neuralgias, labor, renal colic, or myocardial infarction.

Butorphanol

Butorphanol (Stadol) has both agonist and antagonist properties. Its abuse potential appears low and it is not scheduled in the United States. Administered intramuscularly, butorphanol has an onset of action of 10 to 30 minutes with a duration of action of about 4 hours. In general, its actions resemble those of morphine, except that butorphanol increases pulmonary arterial pressure and the cardiac workload, making it undesirable for treating the pain of a myocardial infarction.

Nalbuphine

Nalbuphine (Nubain) is a semisynthetic derivative of morphine that has both agonist and antagonist properties. The uses and limitations of nalbuphine are primarily those of meperidine or morphine. Nalbuphine may be preferable for treating

THE NURSING PROCESS

OPIOIDS

Assessment

Narcotic analgesics are used primarily in the patient complaining of pain from any cause. The data base from which the nurse should begin the development of the plan for patient care should include information from a detailed discussion with the patient of the history, nature, and location of the pain. Objective data about the patient's position, facial expression, medical history, vital signs, and age are helpful. A brief neurological examination should be done. It is not possible to determine the patient's severity of pain by knowing only isolated facts such as what an injury looks like or the "usual" response of patients to a specific painful procedure or surgery; the subjective component of the pain is very important.

Nursing diagnoses

Altered bowel elimination: constipation as a drug side effect

Altered comfort: nausea and vomiting as drug side effect

Altered thought processes related to drug side effect

Management

Regular use of opioids at identified intervals usually provides better relief of pain than use on a p.r.n. (as needed) basis. Clarifying reasonable, possible goals of analgesic therapy with the patient will help to bring pain under control. No patient who needs medication for pain should be denied it, but the professional nurse also employs other nursing care measures to promote comfort, including positioning, distracting, and touching the patient as well as introducing relaxation techniques. The patient care plan should include careful descriptions of what does or does not work in any specific patient. The possibility of addiction to these drugs should not be forgotten but should be kept in perspective. During administration of opioids, the nurse should monitor the vital signs, the level of consciousness, and the frequency of bowel movements and should check for nausea and vomiting and urinary retention. Some side effects will necessitate discontinuing therapy, decreasing the dose, or using additional kinds of treatments. Narcotic antagonists should be available. If antiemetics or other drugs are ordered, monitor for the side effects of these drugs; also check compatibilities before administering two or more drugs in the same syringe. When using the opioids via the intravenous route, resuscitation equipments should be readily available, and a microdrip administration set and an infusion monitoring device should be used for constant intravenous infusion.

Evaluation

Ideally treatment with opioids results in relief of pain with no side effects, but often this is not possible. Usually the treatment is considered effective if the pain or its perception is lessened. The side effects are treated if they interfere with the level of functioning appropriate for the patient. When the therapeutic goals specific for the patient are considered, the evaluation of the effectiveness will be easier. For example, to achieve pain relief, one patient with cancer might not consider drug-induced drowsiness unpleasant, whereas a second patient might. Before discharge, the patient should be able to explain the name and dose of drugs to be taken, the possible side effects and how to treat them, the signs indicating too large a dose, what to do if the pain worsens, and what drugs to avoid. The patient should be able to state that alcohol should be avoided while these drugs are being taken. For additional specific guidelines, see the patient care implications section.

PATIENT CARE IMPLICATIONS

Narcotic analgesics

Drug administration

- Analgesics, especially narcotic analgesics, constitute one of the most useful classes of medications, as they permit individuals to tolerate short- and long-term pain, and thus tolerate surgery and trauma, and perhaps to face death more peacefully. Failure of the health care team members to be knowledgeable about adequate drugs doses, frequency of drug administration, and choice of appropriate medication results in patients receiving inadequate treatment for pain.
- Assess patients thoughtfully prior to administering pain medication. If the decision is made to use a narcotic analgesic, use adequate doses and administer frequently enough to maintain a therapeutic blood level of medication. Administer medications 30 to 60 minutes before painful activities such as dressing changes, physical therapy, or whirlpool.
- While narcotic analgesics are useful, they should be used as adjuncts to other nursing measures: massage, distraction, deep breathing and relaxation exercises, application of heat or cold, or just "being there" to provide care and comfort. Include effective nursing measures in the care plan, and keep the care plan up to date.
- Monitor respiratory rate as an indicator of CNS depression. If the rate is less than 12 per minute in an adult, withhold additional doses unless ventilatory support is being provided.
- Monitor pulse. If bradycardia develops (pulse below 60 in an adult or 110 in an infant), withhold the dose and notify the physician.
- Monitor blood pressure. Hypotension is more common in the elderly, the immobilized, and in patients receiving other medications that have hypotension as a side effect; it may also be a sign of sepsis or shock.
- Auscultate breath sounds every 2 to 4 hours. Since narcotic analgesics suppress the cough reflex, it is important to continue activities to prevent atelectasis and pneumonia: turning, deep breathing, incentive spirometry, and so on.
- Have narcotic antagonists, oxygen, and resuscitation equipment available in settings where narcotic analgesics are administered.
- Monitor level of consciousness and mental status. Evaluate findings carefully. For example, restlessness may be due to pain, hyp-

oxia, shock, or an unusual reaction to the analgesic.
- Keep side rails up, keep a night light on, supervise ambulation, and discourage smoking.
- Monitor intake, output, and weight. If nausea and vomiting occur, a switch to another analgesic may be appropriate; consult the physician. If nausea occurs, it may be appropriate to administer an antiemetic concomitantly with the narcotic. Note that the peak effect of many antiemetics occurs at a different time from that of the narcotic; if so, the drugs should be on a different dosing schedule. Also, antiemetics may potentiate central nervous system depression but they do not potentiate analgesic effects. Sedation and hypotension may be pronounced.
- Assess for urinary retention. It may be more pronounced in the elderly, the immobilized, and men with preexisting prostatic hypertrophy. Question patients about difficulty in voiding, pain in the bladder area, or sensations of inadequate bladder emptying. Palpate bladder for distention. Suggest patient void before each dose of narcotic.
- Although the theoretical possibility of narcotic addiction exists for all patients who receive narcotic analgesics, only a very small percentage of patients do become dependent. Patients who persist in requesting frequent or large doses of pain medication beyond the "average time" postoperatively should not be automatically characterized as becoming addicted. Pain is a warning signal, and its unexpected persistence should be investigated. If it is suspected that the patient is becoming dependent or addicted, the health care team as a group should develop an individualized plan to help the patient with the problem.
- Some postoperative patients fear requesting any medication for pain because they fear addiction. Reassure patients that the use of narcotics in decreasing amounts over 3 to 5 days will not cause addiction, and that recovery will be easier if pain is reduced.
- Use of aspirin or acetaminophen along with narcotic analgesics may increase pain relief; consult the physician.
- Record carefully the patient's response to pain and the response to narcotic administration.
- Check the physician's orders carefully. Observe agency policy regarding expiration date of controlled substances.
- In addition to the standard oral, IM, IV, and

PATIENT CARE IMPLICATIONS—cont'd

subcutaneous routes, narcotics may be administered via the intrathecal or intraspinal route, with Patient-Controlled Analgesia (PCA) devices, and implanted pumps. Become familiar with the equipment in use. Consult current literature for additional information. Review manufacturer's directions and patient instruction information. Ascertain that patients understand the advantages and use of the various routes and equipment being used.

- Use preservative-free morphine for intrathecal or intraspinal/epidural use.
- Dilute doses of meperidine syrup in at least a half-glassful of water. When taken undiluted, it may cause temporary mucous membrane anesthesia.
- Dilute doses of methadone oral concentrate with water to a volume of at least 90 ml. Dilute dispersible tablets in at least 120 ml of water, orange juice, citrus flavor Tang brand drink, or other acidic fruit beverage. Complete dispersion occurs in about 1 minute.
- For continuous infusion, use microdrip tubing and an infusion controlling device to keep the rate of administration steady.
  INTRAVENOUS BUTORPHANOL
- May be given undiluted. Administer at a rate of 2 mg or less over 3 to 5 minutes.
  INTRAVENOUS HYDROMOPHONE
- Dilute dose with 5 ml of sterile water or normal saline for injection. Administer at a rate of 2 mg or less over 3 to 5 minutes.
  INTRAVENOUS LEVORPHANOL
- Dilute dose with 5 ml of sterile water or normal saline for injection. Administer at a rate of 3 mg or less over 4 to 5 minutes.
  INTRAVENOUS MEPERIDINE
- Must be diluted. Dilute in at least 5 ml of sterile water or normal saline for injection. Administer dose over 4 to 5 minutes.
  INTRAVENOUS MORPHINE SULFATE
- Dose should be diluted, in at least 5 ml of sterile water or normal saline for injection, or other IV solutions. Administer at a rate of 15 mg or less over 4 to 5 minutes.
  INTRAVENOUS NALBUPHINE
- May be given undiluted. Administer 10 mg or less over 3 to 5 minutes.
  INTRAVENOUS OXYMORPHONE
- Dilute dose with 5 ml of sterile water or normal saline for injection. Administer dose over 4 to 5 minutes.
  INTRAVENOUS PENTAZOCINE
- May be given undiluted, but dilution is pref-

erable. Dilute each 5 mg with at least 1 ml of sterile water for injection. Administer 5 mg or less over 1 minute.

Patient and family education

- Review the anticipated benefits and possible side effects of drug therapy. Encourage patients to phone regarding any questions that arise.
- Review Patient Problems: Constipation (p. 187); Orthostatic Hypotension (p. 237).
- Take oral doses with milk or snack to reduce gastric irritation.
- Avoid drinking alcoholic beverages while taking narcotic analgesics.
- Avoid the use of other medications that may also cause central nervous system depression, such as barbiturates, antiemetics, antihistamines, or tranquilizers, unless first approved by the physician.
- Warn patients to avoid driving or operating hazardous equipment if dizzy or drowsy.
- If a combination drug product has been prescribed, review the side effects associated with each of the drugs in the combined product.
- Remind patients to keep these and all medications out of the reach of children. Accidental overdose with narcotic analgesics in a child may quickly lead to death.

Narcotic antagonists: naloxone

Drug administration

- Monitor blood pressure, pulse, and respiratory rate every 5 minutes initially, tapering to every 15 minutes, then every 30 minutes until stable. In the acutely ill or comatose patient, attach patient to ECG monitor. Have a suction machine available.
- Auscultate breath sounds. If respiratory symptoms are severe or persistent, notify physician.
- Monitor intake and output; auscultate bowel sounds.
- Have drugs, equipment, and personnel available for resuscitation if needed. Do not leave patient unattended until stable.
- Continue to monitor the patient closely for several hours after initial treatment, as the effects of the narcotic antagonist may wear off, causing the patient to again display signs of narcotic overdose.
  INTRAVENOUS NALAXONE
- May be given undiluted, diluted for injec-,

Continued.

PATIENT CARE IMPLICATIONS—cont'd

fusion. Administer at a rate of 0.4 mg over 15 seconds. Infusion is usually titrated to patient response.

- These drugs are rarely used outside of the acute care setting.

Narcotic antagonist: naltrexone

Drug administration

- Assess for CNS effects. It may be difficult to differentiate between effects due to naltrexone and those due to the emotional effect of narcotic withdrawal. If insomnia is present, administer doses in the morning.
- Obtain baseline measurement of blood pressure, pulse, and ECG tracing, then monitor pulse and blood pressure daily, tapering to monthly, if no abnormalities are noted.
- Monitor bowel sounds, and keep a record of bowel movements. If abdominal discomfort is severe or persistent, notify the physician.
- Monitor respiratory rate and auscultate breath sounds. If respiratory symptoms are severe or persistent, notify the physician.
- Inspect for development of rash.
- Monitor liver function tests.
- Naltrexone therapy should not be initiated until the patient has completed detoxification and been free of opiate drugs for 7 to 10 days.
- Before administering oral naltrexone, the patient may be given a naloxone challenge test. In this test, a subcutaneous or IV dose of naloxone is administered, the patient then is

observed for signs of opiate withdrawal: nasal stuffiness, rhinorrhea, tearing, sweating, tremor, abdominal cramps, vomiting, piloerection ("goose flesh"), and myalgia. If symptoms of withdrawal appear, the patient is not sufficiently drug free to begin naltrexone therapy. The challenge test may be repeated daily until the patient is opiate free.

- Monitor carefully for at least 1 hour after the first dose of naltrexone for the appearance of withdrawal symptoms.
- Naltrexone should be used only as a component of a medically supervised behavioral modification program designed to help the patient maintain an opiate-free state.

Patient and family education

- Review with patients the anticipated benefits and possible side effects of therapy. Instruct the patient to report the development of unexpected side effects.
- Take oral doses with meals or a snack to lessen gastric irritation.
- Review with the patient the need to avoid ingestion of opiates via any route of administration while taking naltrexone. This may include antidiarrhea medications and cough syrups.
- Remind the patient to keep all health care providers informed of all medications the patient is taking, including naltrexone.
- Instruct the patient to wear a medical identification tag or bracelet indicating the patient is receiving naltrexone.

---

the pain of a myocardial infarction, since it appears to reduce the oxygen needs of the heart without reducing blood pressure. Nalbuphine is a stronger antagonist than pentazocine, suggesting that the degree of tolerance and drug dependence should be low. However, withdrawal symptoms are seen when nalbuphine is abruptly discontinued, and it causes withdrawal symptoms when administered to an individual already dependent on one of the more common narcotic analgesics.

Pentazocine

Pentazocine (Talwin) is an opioid with weak antagonist properties. For several years after pentazocine was introduced, it was believed not to produce drug dependency. Pentazocine is now a sched-

ule IV drug, reflecting a low potential for producing drug dependency. Pentazocine does cause respiratory depression in the fetus. Unlike morphine, pentazocine increases blood pressure and cardiac work, properties that make it less desirable than morphine for treating the pain of myocardial infarction or pulmonary hypertension. Pentazocine causes a dysphoria rather than a euphoria. This dysphoria can include nightmares, feelings of depersonalization, and visual hallucinations. Large doses induce seizures. Although there are reports of individuals with a drug dependency for pentazocine, its administration to a person dependent on the other narcotic analgesics will result in withdrawal symptoms because of its antagonistic properties.

Opioids Effective in Relieving Mild Pain
(Table 44.3)

Codeine

Codeine is not administered in doses large enough to be as effective as morphine, since the high dose required to produce an equal degree of analgesia results in a high incidence of side effects. An oral dose of 32 or 65 mg of codeine is equivalent to 2 aspirin tablets (650 mg). At these low doses codeine seldom produces side effects. At high doses the side effects of codeine are similar to those of morphine.

Since it causes significant histamine release if given intravenously, codeine is given only intramuscularly or orally. A portion of a codeine dose is metabolized to morphine in the liver. Codeine is a schedule II drug in analgesic doses. It is also formulated with the nonnarcotic analgesics for pain relief, and these are usually schedule III drugs. Codeine is an effective cough suppressant at low doses, and it is available for this purpose in dilute solutions as a schedule V drug.

Propoxyphene

Propoxyphene (Darvon), an opioid related to methadone, is not a very potent analgesic. Propoxyphene at a dose of 65 mg is the analgesic equivalent of 2 tablets (650 mg) of aspirin or acetaminophen. Propoxyphene is commonly prescribed in combination with one of the nonnarcotic analgesics. Alone or in combination, propoxyphene is a schedule IV drug. Side effects are not common at analgesic doses. Propoxyphene has a low abuse potential but has been implicated as a cause of death when abused in combination with alcohol and other central nervous system depressant drugs.

Treatment of Chronic Pain

The use of opioids in treating chronic pain is indicated only in terminal cancer, since tolerance to the opioids limits the effectiveness of these drugs in nontoxic doses. Even in treating the pain associated with terminal cancer, a case in which drug dependency is irrelevant, special care must be used to keep the dose as low as possible to prolong the effectiveness of the drug and to keep the patient alert. The opioids with low dependency liability are used first, and the total comfort of the patient is considered.

A combination of drugs may be used to lessen the dose of a strong narcotic analgesic needed and thereby prolong the duration of effectiveness. One popular combination of drugs for oral administration is "Brompton's cocktail," which consists of heroin (morphine in the United States), cocaine, a phenothiazine, and ethyl alcohol. However, recent studies have indicated that this combination may be no more effective than the use of oral morphine alone.

Role of Opioids in Anesthesia

Additional uses of opioids include preanesthetic medication and surgical anesthesia. As a preanesthetic medication, the opioids relieve anxiety and provide sedation so that the patient is not in a fearful state before surgery. The more potent analgesics—morphine, meperidine, fentanyl, and hydromorphone—are widely used as components of surgical anesthesia with nitrous oxide. Nitrous oxide by itself is not potent enough for surgical anesthesia but is potentiated by a narcotic analgesic. A muscle relaxant such as tubocurarine also is used. This combination of opioid, nitrous oxide, and muscle relaxant is called "balanced anesthesia" (Chapter 45). Duration of anesthesia is controlled by the duration of action of the opioid used.

SUMMARY

Opioids, typically called narcotic analgesics, blunt the subjective reaction to pain by raising the threshold for pain perception, reducing anxiety and fear, and inducing sleep. Morphine is the prototypical opioid. Opioids mimic endorphins, naturally occurring polypeptides that serve as neurotransmitters for various functions, including analgesia. Other characteristic actions of morphine include respiratory depression; cough suppression; nausea and vomiting; depression of gut motility and gastric, biliary, and pancreatic secretions; urinary retention; hypotension; and constricted pupils.

Drug tolerance readily develops to the opioids; in particular, the lethal dose for respiratory depression increases with tolerance. However, opioids enhance the respiratory depression of other drug classes. Drug dependency is characterized by a distinct abstinence syndrome when the drug is discontinued. The opioid abstinence syndrome is treated in the United States with methadone, an orally active, long-acting opioid. Methadone can be used for maintenance or for detoxification.

Overdose of an opioid is best treated with naloxone, a specific opiate receptor antagonist, which reverses the opioid-induced respiratory depression.

More than a dozen opioids are in use as analgesics. These are used to treat pain associated with surgery, broken bones, dental procedures, and obstetrics. Selected cardiovascular actions make morphine useful in treating pulmonary edema and morphine and nalbuphine useful in treating the pain of a heart attack. Opioids are also used as preanesthetic medication and as one component of balanced anesthesia. Opioids are not used for chronic pain, except that associated with terminal cancer.

STUDY QUESTIONS

1. What are the two components of pain? Which is affected by opioids?
2. What are endorphins? What are enkephalins, and what actions do they mediate?
3. What are the three characteristics of the analgesia produced by morphine?
4. What are the three major actions of morphine in the medulla?
5. What actions does morphine have on tissues outside the central nervous system?
6. What are five common adverse reactions to morphine?
7. Describe the abstinence syndrome for opioids.
8. What properties of methadone make it useful for maintaining or withdrawing from opioid dependence?
9. Why is naloxone a good drug for treating acute opioid toxicity?
10. What are the five opioids used to relieve severe pain?
11. What opioids are used to relieve moderate to severe pain?
12. What opioids are used to relieve mild pain?
13. Which opioids have antagonist as well as agonist activity?
14. Which opioids play a special role in treating pulmonary edema? Pain of a heart attack?
15. When are opioids used to treat chronic pain?
16. What role do opioids have in anesthesia?

SUGGESTED READINGS

Akahoshi, M.P., Furuike-McLaughlin, T., and Enriquez, N.C.: Patient controlled analgesia via intrathecal catheter in outpatient oncology patients, J. Intravenous Nurs. 11(5):289, 1988.

Arnold, C.: Intraspinal analgesia: a new route for an old drug, J. Neurosci. Nurs. 21(1):30, 1989.

Bakris, G.L., and Zorumski, C.F.: Chronic pain—a pharmacologic review and behavior modification approach, Postgrad. Med. 73(3):119, 1983.

Barclay, W.R.: Propoxyphene, JAMA 241(16):1689, 1979.

Blake, G.J.: Morphine: new routes for better pain relief, Nursing 88 18(3):111, 1988.

Collins, G.B., and Kiefer, K.S.: Propoxyphene dependence, Postgrad. Med. 70(6):57, 1981.

Coyle, N.: Analgesics and pain: current concepts, Nurs. Clin. North Am. 33(3):727, 1987.

DiGregorio, G.J., and Barbieri, E.J.: Pharmacologic management of pain, Am. Fam. Physician 27(5):185, 1983.

DiGregorio, G.J., and Bukovinsky, M.A.: Clonidine for narcotic withdrawal, Am. Fam. Physician 24(2):203, 1981.

DiNobile, C.: Patient-controlled analgesia: a new trend in pain control, J. Post. Anesth. Nurs. 3(4):264, 1988.

Eaton, J.A.: Continuous meperidine infusion for postoperative pain, Orthop. Nurs. 7(6):29, 1988.

Eland, J.M.: Pharmacologic management of acute and chronic pediatric pain, Issues Compr. Pediatr. Nurs. 11(2/3):93, 1988.

Eland, J.M.: Pain management and comfort, J. Gerontol. Nurs. 14(4):10, 1988.

Gadish, H.S., Gonzalez, J.L., and Hayes, J.S.: Factors affecting nurses' decisions to administer pediatric pain medication postoperatively, J. Pediatr. Nurs. 3(6):383, 1988.

Goodman, C.E.: Pathophysiology of pain, Arch. Intern. Med. 143:527, 1983.

Goodman, J.S.: Withdrawal from narcotics and sedative-hypnotics, Res. Staff Phys. 28(3):68, 1982.

Haight, K.: What you should know about epidural analgesia, Nursing 87 17(9):58, 1987.

Henrikson, M.L., and Wild, L.R.: A nursing process approach to epidural analgesia, JOGNN 17(5):316, 1988.

Inbar, G.: Pain management with intraspinal morphine sulfate injection, Perioper. Nurs. Q. 2(4):64, 1986.

Kaiko, R.F.: Controversy in the management of chronic cancer pain: therapeutic equivalents of IM and PO morphine, J. Pain Symptom. Manage. 2(1):19, 1987.

Keller, M.: Oral morphine solution: effect on pain, confusion, drowsiness, and nausea for the terminally ill patient, Hospice J. 4(1):55, 1988.

Marx, J.L.: Brain opiates in mental illness, Science 214:1013, 1981.

Marx, J.L.: Synthesizing the opioid peptides, Science 220:395, 1983.

McCaffery, M.: IV morphine for children, Am. J. Nurs. 84:1153, 1984.

McCaffery, M.: A practical, "postable" chart of equianalgesic doses, Nursing 87 17(8):56, 1987.

McCaffery, M.: Patient controlled analgesia: more than a machine, Nursing 87 17(11):62, 1987.

McGuire, D.B.: Advances in control of cancer pain, Nurs. Clin. North Am. 22(3):677, 1987.

Mendelson, C.S.: Pain management for ambulatory surgery, J. Post Anesth. Nurs. 3(2):109, 1988.

Mondzac, A.N.: In defense of the reintroduction of heroin into American medical practice and H.R. 5290—the compassionate pain relief act, N. Engl. J. Med. 311(8):532, 1984.

Preston, K.L., and others: Diazepam and methadone interactions in methadone maintenance, Clin. Pharmacol. Ther. 36(4):534, 1984.

Raney, J.P., and Kirk, E.A.: The use of an Ommaya reservoir for administration of morphine sulphate to control pain in select cancer patients, J. Neurosci. Nurs. 20(1):23, 1988.

Reed, D.A., and Schnoll, S.: Abuse of pentazocine-naloxone combination, JAMA 256:2562, 1986.

Relieving pain: an analgesic guide. Principles of analgesic use in the treatment of acute pain and chronic cancer pain, Am. J. Nurs. 88(6):815, 1988.

Stanley, T.H.: Narcotic anesthesia: advantages and disadvantages, Res. Staff Phys. 27(7):67, 1981.

Stitzer, M.L., Bigelow, G.E., and Liebson, I.A.: Single-day methadone dose alteration: detectability and symptoms, Clin. Pharmacol. Ther. 36(2):244, 1984.

Taylor, A.G.: Pain, Annu. Rev. Nurs. Res. 5:23, 1987.

Waldman, S.D., Feldstein, G.S., and Allen, M.L.: Troubleshooting intraspinal narcotic delivery systems . . . implantable reservoirs, Am. J. Nurs. 87(1):63, 1987.

Wasacz, J.: Natural and synthetic narcotic drugs, Am. Scientist 69(3):318, 1981.

Washton, A.M., Gold, M.S., and Pottash, A.C.: Opiate and cocaine dependencies, Postgrad. Med. **77**:293, 1985.

Weis, O.: Clonidine for suppressing opiate withdrawal, Drug Ther. **7**(7):61, 1982.

Whipple, B.: Methods of pain control: review of research and literature, Image J. Nurs. Sch. **19**(3):142, 1987.

White, P.F.: Use of patient-controlled analgesia for management of acute pain, JAMA **259**:243, 1988.

Wild, L.R., and others: Administering and monitoring epidural analgesia . . . practice corner, Oncol. Nurs. Forum **15**(6):817, 1988.

Zola, E.M., and McLeod, D.C.: Comparative effects and analgesic efficacy of the agonist-antagonist opioids, Drug Intell. Clin. Pharm. **17**:411, 1983.

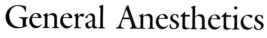

General Anesthetics

45

Modern surgery did not begin until the introduction of nitrous oxide, ether, and chloroform as general anesthetics in the late 1800s. The agents used today as general anesthetics have included gases (nitrous oxide), volatile liquids (diethyl ether, halothane, methoxyflurane, enflurane, isoflurane), and intravenous agents (ketamine, narcotic analgesics). The ultrashort-acting barbiturates, benzodiazepines, and etomidate are used intravenously for induction of anesthesia.

MECHANISM OF ACTION
Lack of Receptor Mechanism

General anesthetics act on the central nervous system (CNS) to abolish the perception of pain and reaction to painful stimuli. They are unusual in their mechanism of action because they do not appear to act by a receptor mechanism. Instead, general anesthetics are believed to alter the lipid structure of cell membranes so that physiological functions are impaired. The network of neurons making up the CNS is especially vulnerable because alteration of membrane structure interrupts the complex intercommunication necessary for function. The most sensitive system to such alterations is the ascending reticular activating system, the neuronal formation monitoring incoming stimuli and determining what information is to be passed up to the brain for processing and response. Consciousness is lost when the ascending reticular activating system ceases to transmit information effectively.

Stages of Anesthesia

For many years the general anesthetics have been classified purely as general CNS depressants, as discussed with the sedative-hypnotic drugs in Chapter 40. This scheme is diagrammed in Figure

45.1. According to this scheme, the stages of anesthesia represent the increasing depression of the CNS and are labeled as follows:

> Stage I: analgesia
> Stage II: excitement (or delirium)
> Stage III: surgical anesthesia
> Stage IV: medullary paralysis

These stages represent what is observed in patients anesthetized with diethyl ether in the absence of other medication, an obsolete practice. Nevertheless, it is useful to review this classification.

Stage I (analgesia) begins with a conscious patient and ends when the patient is unconscious. This is the lightest stage of anesthesia, but the degree of analgesia is sufficient for some dental procedures and for the second stage of labor.

Stage II (excitement or delirium) represents a removal of the inhibition of the lower brain centers by the higher centers and is manifested by activity such as involuntary movement of the limbs, an irregular pattern of breathing, and pupillary dilation. This stage is undesirable because reflex responses such as laryngospasm may begin, which are injurious or dangerous to the patient. The brief second stage of anesthesia during induction of anesthesia with inhalation anesthetics is the least stable and most dangerous period of anesthesia. This stage is less prominent with modern anesthetics such as halothane and enflurane, which induce anesthesia more rapidly than does ether, which has a very long induction time. In modern anesthetic practice, an induction agent such as an ultrashort-acting barbiturate is used for induction of anesthesia to bypass stage II altogether.

Stage III (surgical anesthesia) represents the

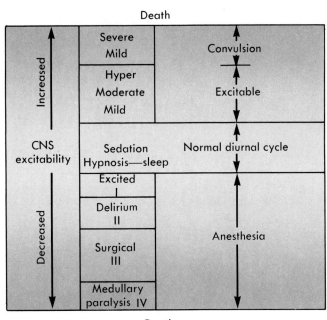

FIGURE 45.1   This diagram of central nervous system excitation and depression demonstrates how drugs have been described as either causing stimulation or causing depression. The classic description of anesthesia is as a pure depressant action on the central nervous system. The four stages of anesthesia included in this diagram are those originally described for diethyl ether. (Redrawn from Winter, W.: Effects of drugs on the electrical activity of the brain: anesthetics. Reproduced, with permission, from the Annual Review of Pharmacology and Toxicology **16**:413, 1976. © 1976 by Annual Reviews Inc.)

gradual loss of muscle tone and reflexes as the CNS is further depressed. Not all anesthetics produce good muscle relaxation, so a muscle relaxant is commonly used. This stage ends as the muscles controlling breathing are paralyzed; the intercostal muscles controlling the rib cage are paralyzed first, followed by the diaphragm.

Stage IV (medullary paralysis) is the toxic state of anesthesia, characterized by the loss of spontaneous breathing and collapse of the cardiovascular system.

Stages of Anesthesia Based on Brain Wave Patterns

Winter has proposed a more recent scheme for describing general anesthetics. This scheme is diagrammed in Figure 45.2 and is based on brain wave patterns (electroencephalogram or EEG) observed during anesthesia. The concept of a corre-
lation between surface electrode EEG changes and the depth of anesthesia is extremely complex, controversial, and not clinically useful. However, Winter's scheme does offer another approach toward an understanding of how anesthetics alter pain perception by including stimulant as well as depressant anesthetics. Each anesthetic drug can follow a different mechanistic route to abolish pain perception.

Stage I now represents a mild stimulation of the reticular activating system, producing motor excitement and then unconsciousness.

Stage II represents further stimulation as the reticular activating system becomes unable to screen incoming stimuli. The subclasses of stage II include the following: *subclass A,* hallucinations with recall; *subclass B,* hallucinations with no recall; and *subclass C,* catalepsy with no recall. Catalepsy is the state in which the patient neither

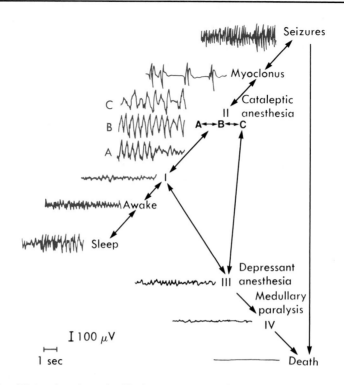

FIGURE 45.2   Winters has determined brain wave patterns of cats under anesthesia. Anesthesia is pictured as arising from central nervous system stimulation (ketamine) or depression (barbiturates). Each anesthetic produces its own characteristic pattern of central nervous system stimulation and depression. For instance, diethyl ether produces the pattern I ↔ II ↔ III ↔ IV, which includes both stimulant and depressant stages. (Redrawn from Winter, W.: Effects of drugs on the electrical activity of the brain: anesthetics. Reproduced, with permission, from the Annual Review of Pharmacology and Toxicology **16**:413, 1976. © 1976 by Annual Reviews Inc.)

moves nor reacts to stimuli. The stimulant anesthetics ketamine, enflurane, and nitrous oxide produce a cataleptic anesthesia. Ether, the prototype for the former scheme, produces initial excitement at stage IIC, then depression at stage III.

Stage III is the same as in the past scheme, representing the level of surgical anesthesia produced by depression of the CNS. The anesthetics halothane and isoflurane and the barbiturates are purely depressant anesthetics, taking the patient from stage I to stage III.

Stage IV remains medullary paralysis.

Properties of the Ideal Anesthetic

The ideal anesthetic would produce (1) analgesia, (2) unconsciousness, (3) muscle relaxation, and (4) reduction of reflex activity. This anesthetic would be prompt to act and rapidly eliminated, remaining unmetabolized and producing no unwanted effects in body tissues. Since no anesthetic

has all these desirable properties, several drugs are used in combination to achieve these goals.

CHARACTERISTICS OF INHALATION ANESTHETICS
Partial Pressure as a Measure of Anesthetic Concentration

The inhalation anesthetics are gases or volatile liquids administered as gases. The effective concentration of an inhalation anesthetic in the brain does not depend on the solubility of the anesthetic in blood or tissue. Rather the effective concentration depends on the anesthetic's partial pressure, or effective pressure of the gas in the atmosphere. If a constant partial pressure of anesthetic is inhaled, the partial pressure in the alveoli will rise toward the inhaled level. If the gas is not very soluble in blood, little gas is removed by the blood circulating around the alveoli and the partial pressure of the gas in the blood quickly reaches the inhaled partial pressure. This anesthetic has a rapid onset of action. If the gas is soluble in blood, however, the partial pressure of the gas in the alveoli quickly drops, since the gas is being removed more rapidly by the blood than can be replenished by breathing. A long time is required to equilibrate the blood with the gas to the point where the partial pressure matches that coming into the alveoli. To shorten the time to reach this steady state, anesthesia is induced using a high partial pressure of the gas and then lowering the partial pressure to maintain anesthesia.

Minimum Alveolar Concentration

The potency of an inhalation anesthetic is determined by the minimum alveolar concentration (MAC) that will produce anesthesia (insensitivity to a skin incision) in 50% of patients. For instance, MAC of 10% is equivalent to a partial pressure of 0.1 atmosphere or 76 mm of mercury at standard conditions (sea level). A MAC of 10% means that when air in the alveoli has equilibrated with the body and incoming air, all of which are 10% anesthetic gas, the patient has a 50:50 chance of being unreactive to a skin incision. Surgery is conducted at about 1.4 times the MAC value of the anesthetic chosen.

Distribution and Excretion of Inhalation Anesthetics

The distribution of the anesthetic is determined by the blood flow; thus the brain, liver, and kidneys reach equilibrium first. Excretion of the inhalation anesthetics is largely through the lungs. The amount of anesthetic that is in solution is metabolized by the liver to a variable degree. Certain halogenated hydrocarbons (such as enflurane, halothane, methoxyflurane) are metabolized to products that may damage the liver and kidney.

Emergence is the time during which the patient regains consciousness after the anesthetic has been discontinued. The duration of emergence from the inhaled anesthetics depends on the same factors as induction. The patient's vital signs are carefully monitored in a recovery room, and symptoms of pain or nausea and vomiting must be watched for and treated appropriately.

CLINICALLY USED INHALATION ANESTHETICS (Table 45.1)
Specific Inhalation Anesthetics
Diethyl ether

Diethyl ether is a volatile liquid that is very flammable and explosive. The MAC is 1.9%. A long time is required for induction and emergence when ether alone is used because it is highly soluble in blood. In addition, ether is unpleasant to inhale because it has a noxious, pungent odor, irritates the respiratory tract, and stimulates secretions. An anticholinergic drug may be administered to minimize these secretions. The explosive hazard and the noxious, pungent odor account for the rare use of ether in modern surgery. Nevertheless, ether is still used in areas of the world where sophisticated equipment is unavailable for monitoring the patient. Ether has a wide margin of safety and has few effects on the cardiovascular system, factors that allow it to be administered without sophisticated control of concentration. Ether produces good analgesia and muscle relaxation, making extra medication unneeded.

Enflurane

Enflurane (Ethrane) is a halogenated hydrocarbon and a nonflammable liquid. The MAC is 1.7% and induction is fairly rapid. Enflurane is one of the stimulant anesthetics that produce muscle contractions and seizurelike brain wave patterns at high concentrations. Enflurane usually is administered with nitrous oxide to avoid high concentrations, which can cause CNS stimulation and cardiovascular depression. Enflurane causes a decrease in blood pressure resulting from depressed cardiac output and decreased peripheral resistance. Emergence is usually uneventful except for shivering. About 2.5% of enflurane is metabolized to release a low concentration of fluoride ion. The amount of fluoride ion is not harmful, except in patients with preexisting kidney damage.

Halothane

Halothane (Fluothane) is a nonflammable liquid halogenated hydrocarbon and currently is the most widely used of the volatile liquid anesthetics. The MAC is 0.77% and induction is fairly rapid. Postoperative nausea and vomiting are not problems. Halothane is a direct myocardial depressant and causes a dose-dependent reduction in cardiac output with no change in heart rate, a combination of effects that lowers the blood pressure. Halothane also sensitizes the myocardium to exogenously administered catecholamines. This sensitization means that a sympathomimetic drug must be used cautiously during surgery to maintain blood pressure, since sympathomimetic drugs may precipitate arrhythmias. Catecholamines may be used topically, such as on the brain or in irrigation of the bladder, to stop bleeding. Halothane does not give

Table 45.1   Properties of Inhalation Anesthetics

Drug	Physical properties	Onset	MAC	Cardiovascular effects	Muscle relaxation	Elimination	Other properties
Diethyl ether	Flammable liquid	Slow	1.92%	Minimum	Excellent	Lungs	Excellent analgesia. Nausea, vomiting on emergence. Secretions stimulated.
Enflurane (Ethrane)	Nonflammable liquid	Rapid	1.68%	Decreased blood pressure May sensitize heart to catecholamines	Good	Lungs 2% to 5% metabolized by liver	Causes low body temperature, hypothermia, shivering.
Halothane (Fluothane)	Nonflammable liquid	Rapid	0.77%	Decreased blood pressure Sensitizes heart to catecholamines	Fair	Lungs 20% metabolized by liver	Poor analgesia.
Isoflurane (Forane)	Nonflammable liquid	Rapid	1.3%	Minimum	Good	Lungs Little metabolism by liver	
Methoxyflurane (Penthrane)	Nonflammable liquid	Slow	0.16%	Decreased blood pressure	Good	Lungs 70% metabolized by liver	Excellent analgesia.
Nitrous oxide	Nonflammable gas	Very rapid	101%	Minimum	—	Lungs	Widely used with other drugs for anesthesia. Good analgesia.

adequate muscle relaxation; a separate muscle relaxant must be used.

Very rarely (1:800,000 patients) halothane is responsible for a fatal hepatitis. Current theory is that free radical metabolites, which are very reactive compounds, may be produced by the liver and damage liver cells.

Isoflurane

Isoflurane (Forane) is a chemical isomer of enflurane, but unlike enflurane, isoflurane is a depressant anesthetic similar to halothane. The MAC is 1.3%. Induction is smooth and rapid and muscle relaxation adequate. The heart is not sensitized to catecholamines, but the blood pressure falls because of a decrease in the peripheral resistance of blood vessels. Only 0.25% of isoflurane is metabolized. Isoflurane is a more recent anesthetic that many anesthesiologists believe will be widely used in the future.

Methoxyflurane

Methoxyflurane (Penthrane) is a nonflammable liquid halogenated hydrocarbon. It produces analgesia adequate for dentistry and obstetrics. The MAC is 0.16%. Methoxyflurane depresses the cardiovascular system but does not sensitize the heart to catecholamines. The methoxyflurane that is not exhaled is metabolized extensively (70%) by the liver to fluoride ion. Prolonged anesthesia with methoxyflurane may result in high-output renal failure because in the presence of the fluoride ion, the kidney loses its concentrating ability so that the urine volume is high. This renal failure is usually reversible.

Nitrous oxide

Nitrous oxide is a nonexplosive gas that is still widely used. The major limitation of nitrous oxide is that the maximum concentration allowable, 65% to 70% N_2O and 30% to 35% O_2, does not produce surgical anesthesia because the MAC is 101%. Nevertheless, nitrous oxide produces good analgesia and is used for this purpose in dental and obstetrical procedures. In addition, nitrous oxide is widely used with other anesthetics to produce surgical anesthesia. Its effect is additive with other anesthetics, so a 50% MAC concentration of nitrous oxide and a 50% MAC concentration of another inhalation anesthetic produces surgical anesthesia. In addition, nitrous oxide is widely used as one component of *balanced anesthesia*, in which a narcotic analgesic, a skeletal muscle relaxant, and nitrous oxide are used together to produce surgical anesthesia.

Nitrous oxide has been shown to increase the incidence of spontaneous abortions in women and to decrease spermatogenesis in men who work in operating rooms. Scavenging equipment must now be used in the operating room to remove nitrous oxide. The gas is much more soluble (34 times) than nitrogen in the blood so that pockets of trapped gas in the patient will expand as nitrogen leaves and is replaced by larger amounts of nitrous oxide. Locations where trapped gas is common include a blocked middle ear, pneumothorax, loops of intestine, lung, renal cysts, and in the skull following a pneumoencephalogram. These conditions represent contraindications for nitrous oxide, since the large increases in pressure or volumes that may result following its administration may cause serious damage.

CHARACTERISTICS OF INTRAVENOUS ANESTHETICS

The intravenous (IV) anesthetics include the ultrashort-acting barbiturates: thiopental (Pentothal), methohexital (Brevital), and thiamylal sodium (Surital); three benzodiazepines: diazepam (Valium), midazolan (Versed), and flunitrazepam (Rohypnol); and the agents ketamine (Ketaject) and etomidate (Amidate, Hypnomidate). Only ketamine is a true anesthetic, abolishing the perception of and reaction to pain. The barbiturates and benzodiazepines do not abolish reflex to pain even when they are administered in doses large enough to render the patient unconscious. These drugs are used primarily as induction agents to bypass stage II of anesthesia. The advantage of the IV agents is that they are effective seconds after administration.

It may seem paradoxical that an IV anesthetic would be so short acting when it must be metabolized to be excreted. The explanation is that the IV anesthetics are very lipid soluble. They initially are distributed to the brain, liver, and kidneys, the organs with the largest blood flow, but later the drug is *redistributed* to body fat and skeletal muscle, which are less well perfused. This redistribution lowers the circulating concentration to that which no longer maintains anesthesia. This redistribution is responsible for the short duration of action. Metabolism of the drug proceeds as the drug passes through the liver.

CLINICALLY USED INTRAVENOUS ANESTHETICS (Table 45.2)

Barbiturates

Thiopental, methohexital, and thiamylal

Thiopental (Pentothal), methohexital (Brevital), and thiamylal (Surital) are all ultrashort-acting barbiturates used primarily to induce anesthesia. Loss of consciousness occurs within 60 seconds of injection. Thiopental or thiamylal is effective as the sole anesthetic for about 15 minutes. Methohexital is even shorter acting. Barbiturates provide no analgesia and can cause excitement or delirium in the presence of pain in an awake patient. Changes in blood pressure or cardiac output are not common unless the injection is made rapidly. Respiration is markedly depressed and yawning, coughing, or laryngospasm may occur. Methohexital can cause hiccups.

Solutions of barbiturates should be injected only into veins. Arterial injections can cause inflammation and clotting. The barbiturate solution will damage tissue if it leaks around the injection site, and this situation can lead to gangrene.

Benzodiazepines

Diazepam

Diazepam (Valium) is a benzodiazepine used occasionally as an induction agent but more frequently to sedate patients undergoing cardioversion or endoscopic or dental procedures. Intravenous diazepam takes about 60 seconds to become effective. Sedation, sleep, and amnesia are achieved with little depression of cardiovascular or respiratory functions. Unlike the barbiturates, diazepam is metabolized to active products and has a long duration of action. (See Chapter 40 for a further discussion of diazepam.)

Flunitrazepam

Flunitrazepam (Rohypnol) is a benzodiazepine that is more potent than diazepam so that a smaller dose is needed. Otherwise flunitrazepam is similar to diazepam.

Midazolam

Midazolam (Versed) is a relatively short-acting benzodiazepine for use as an intravenous anes-

Table 45.2 Injectable Drugs for Anesthesia

Generic name	Trade name	Administration/dosage	Comments
BARBITURATES			
Methohexital sodium	Brevital Sodium Brietal Sodium*	INTRAVENOUS: *Adults*—for induction, 5 to 12 ml of 1% solution no faster than 1 ml every 5 sec. Maintenance, 2 to 4 ml of 1% solution as required. FDA Pregnancy Category C.	Has the shortest duration of action (5 to 7 min) of the barbiturates. Some patients develop hiccups after rapid injection. Schedule IV substance.
Thiamylal sodium	Suritalǂ	INTRAVENOUS: *Adults*—for induction, 2 to 4 ml of 2.5% solution every 30 to 40 sec, with maximum dose 3 to 5 mg/kg body weight. Maintenance, 2 to 4 ml of 2.5% solution as required. FDA Pregnancy Category C.	Duration of action about 15 min. Schedule III substance.
Thiopental sodium	Pentothalǂ	INTRAVENOUS: *Adults*—for induction, 50 to 100 mg (2 to 4 ml) in 2.5% solution every 30 to 40 sec or 3 to 5 mg/kg body weight. Maintenance, 2 to 4 ml of 2.5% solution as required. *Children*—3 to 5 mg/kg as described for adults. FDA Pregnancy Category C.	Duration of action about 15 min. May cause yawning, coughing, or laryngospasm. Schedule III substance.
BENZODIAZEPINES			
Diazepam	Valiumǂ	INTRAVENOUS: *Adults*—0.1 to 0.2 mg/kg body weight to induce sleep, maximum dose 10 to 20 mg. Basal sedation requires only 5 to 30 mg, so 2.5 to 5 mg is injected every 30 sec until light sleep or slurred speech is produced.	Do not mix with other liquids. A local anesthetic may be required for intravenous injection.
Flunitrazepam	Rohypnol	INTRAVENOUS: *Adults*—for induction, 36 to 50 μg/kg body weight over 20 to 40 sec. Maintenance, 10 μg/kg as needed.	Used for induction of anesthesia. Also used to produce sedation, sleep, and amnesia for procedures such as endoscopy.
Midazolam	Versedǂ	INTRAMUSCULAR: *Adults*—for preoperative sedation, 70 to 80 μg/kg, 30 to 60 min before surgery. FDA Pregnancy Category D. *Children*—80 to 200 μg/kg. INTRAVENOUS: *Adults*—for conscious sedation, 2.5 mg administered over 2 min just prior to the procedure; for general anesthesia, 200-350 μg/kg, administered over 5 to 30 sec. *Children*—50 to 200 μg/kg.	Schedule IV. Older or debilitated patients should be administered a smaller dose.
MISCELLANEOUS			
Alfentanil	Alfentaǂ	INTRAVENOUS: *Adults*—for induction of anesthesia, 130 μg/kg body weight. FDA Pregnancy Category C.	Schedule II. A potent, short-acting narcotic analgesic. A "lollipop" dosage form is being tested as a presurgical sedative for children. A very short-acting (30–45 min) drug.
Droperidol	Inapsineǂ	INTRAVENOUS: *Adults and children over 2 yr*—0.15 mg/kg body weight. Onset: 10 to 15 min. Duration: 3 to 6 hr.	An antipsychotic drug. Used with fentanyl citrate and nitrous oxide to produce neuroleptanesthesia. May cause extrapyramidal symptoms.

*Available in Canada only.
ǂAvailable in Canada and United States.

Table 45.2 Injectable Drugs for Anesthesia—cont'd

Generic name	Trade name	Administration/dosage	Comments
MISCELLANEOUS—cont'd			
Etomidate	Amidate Hypnomidate	INTRAVENOUS: *Adults and children over 10 yr*—for induction, 0.3 mg/kg body weight injected over 30 to 60 sec, may vary between 0.2 and 0.6 mg/kg. FDA Pregnancy Category C.	A nonbarbiturate agent used for induction and sometimes maintenance of anesthesia.
Fentanyl citrate	Sublimaze†	INTRAVENOUS: *Adults and children over 2 yr*—0.002 to 0.003 mg/kg body weight in divided doses over 6 to 8 min. Maintenance, 0.05 to 0.1 mg every 30 to 60 min. Onset: 1 to 2 min. FDA Pregnancy Category C.	A potent, short-acting narcotic analgesic. Used with droperidol and nitrous oxide for neuroleptic anesthesia and with nitrous oxide for balanced anesthesia.
Ketamine	Ketaject Ketalar†	INTRAVENOUS: *Adults and children*— 1 to 4.5 mg/kg body weight over 60 sec, ½ of initial dose used for maintenance as needed. INTRAMUSCULAR: *Adults and children*— 6.5 to 13 mg/kg body weight, ½ of initial dose for maintenance as needed.	Produces a cataleptic anesthesia with good analgesia. Not a scheduled drug.
Sufentanil citrate	Sufenta†	INTRAVENOUS: *Adults*—initial dose is 1 to 8 μg/kg with nitrous oxide and oxygen. Additional doses are 10 to 25 μg/kg. Doses depend on the severity of pain associated with the surgery. *Children over 2 yr*—for cardiovascular surgery: 10 to 25 μg/kg with oxygen and a muscular relaxant. Additional doses are 25 to 50 μg (1 to 2 μg/kg). FDA Pregnancy Category C.	A potent, short-acting narcotic analgesic used with nitrous oxide for balanced anesthesia or alone with oxygen and a muscle relaxant.

†Available in Canada and United States.

thetic. It should be used only in hospital or ambulatory care settings where respiratory and cardiac functions can be monitored. Midazolam may be administered intravenously or intramuscularly to induce sedation or amnesia.

Other Agents

Ketamine

Ketamine (Ketaject, Ketalar) is neither a barbiturate nor a benzodiazepine. Unlike those two drug classes, ketamine produces a cataleptic anesthesia in which the patient appears to be awake but neither responds to pain nor remembers the procedure. This is sometimes referred to as *dissociative anesthesia*. Also, ketamine is not a controlled substance, so it is readily available in emergency rooms. Ketamine is rapidly effective when administered intramuscularly as well as intraven-

ously. Ketamine alone provides anesthesia for 5 to 10 minutes when given intravenously and for 10 to 20 minutes when given intramuscularly.

Ketamine enhances muscle tone and increases blood pressure, heart rate, and respiratory secretions. The major side effect is seen in the recovery period, when patients may experience vivid, unpleasant dreams or hallucinations. Adults are more prone than children to these experiences. Ketamine may also cause vomiting and shivering. Ketamine is related chemically to phencyclidine (PCP), an illicit hallucinogen.

Ketamine should be used cautiously in patients with convulsive disorders, psychosis, mild hypertension, or who are undergoing eye surgery and is contraindicated for patients with coronary artery disease, severe hypertension, cerebrovas-

THE NURSING PROCESS

GENERAL ANESTHESIA

Assessment

The need for general anesthesia is determined by the physician, the patient, and the nurse anesthetist or the anesthesiologist after assessment of the physical condition and consideration of the procedure to be performed. Subjective and objective data to include in the assessment are the vital signs, chest x-ray films, laboratory data, and studies specific to known medical problems; for example, coagulation studies in patients with liver disease or pulmonary function studies in patients with severe chronic obstructive pulmonary disease. The patient's age, previous experience with anesthesia, preference, and the location and type of surgery all are considered.

Nursing diagnoses

Altered comfort: nausea and vomiting related to general anesthesia

Ineffective airway clearance: inability to remove airway secretions related to general anesthesia

Management

The delivery of general anesthesia is beyond the scope of this book and requires knowledge and facility with management of the respiratory and cardiovascular system, multiple drugs, and the immobilized unconscious patient. For further information, consult appropriate textbooks of nursing medicine and anesthesiology.

Evaluation

The ideal general anesthetic produces loss of pain sensation and total relaxation, is excreted quickly, and leaves the patient with little or no residual effects, as discussed in the text. No anesthetic achieves the ideal. The patient who has received general anesthesia needs careful, frequent evaluation of vital signs, respiratory and cardiovascular status, level of consciousness, and ability to handle secretions. If nausea or vomiting occurs, it should be treated not only for patient comfort but also for prevention of fluid loss, fluid and electrolyte imbalance, and other possible side effects. Unusual or rare side effects should be treated (e.g., psychological disturbances with ketamine). As the patient is recovering from anesthesia, the level of pain should be assessed. Observations relating to the surgery should be made, including the condition and drainage of wound, the presence of pulses distal to the site of surgery, and whatever is appropriate for the surgical procedure performed. For additional specific information, see the patient care implications section.

---

cular accident (stroke), or treated hypothyroidism.

Etomidate

Etomidate (Amidate, Hypnomidate) is an IV anesthetic for the induction of surgical anesthesia. Etomidate produces minimum cardiovascular or respiratory changes. Since etomidate does not produce analgesia, the short-acting narcotic analgesic fentanyl citrate also may be infused for total IV anesthesia. The most frequent side effects of etomidate are pain at the injection site and transient, myoclonic skeletal muscle movements.

Narcotic Analgesics and Balanced Anesthesia

Since no one anesthetic drug has all the properties required for surgical anesthesia, one widely used combination of agents is called *balanced anesthesia*. This is a combination of a narcotic analgesic, nitrous oxide, and a skeletal muscle relaxant. Anesthesia is induced, generally with a short-acting barbiturate or occasionally with diazepam or other agents, and then the narcotic analgesic, nitrous oxide, and skeletal muscle relaxant are administered. Respiration must be controlled, since the narcotic analgesics are potent respiratory depressants and the patients are usually paralyzed by a skeletal muscle relaxant. Nitrous oxide is effective at a 60% concentration because of its synergism with the narcotic analgesic. The skeletal muscle relaxant is necessary because neither the narcotic analgesic nor the nitrous oxide provides the muscular relaxation necessary for surgery. The choice of the narcotic analgesic is determined by the anticipated length of surgery. *Alfentanil* (Alfenta), *fentanyl* (Sublimaze), and *sufentanil* (Sufenta) are short-acting narcotic analgesics primarily used for surgery. *Meperidine* (Demerol) is widely used for longer surgeries. *Morphine* is employed as an alternate to meperidine, and this drug is also preferred for cardiac patients as well as poor-risk patients.

The advantage of balanced anesthesia is that the cardiovascular system is neither depressed nor sensitized to catecholamines. Respiration is depressed, but controlled ventilation is readily available. The incidence of postoperative nausea, vomiting, and pain is low.

Neuroleptanesthesia

Neuroleptanesthesia refers to the combination of *droperidol* (Inapsine), an antipsychotic drug of the butyrophenone class; a narcotic analgesic (usually fentanyl); and nitrous oxide. A skeletal muscle relaxant may be used if needed. A fixed combination of the narcotic analgesic *fentanyl* and *droperidol* is available as Innovar. Nitrous oxide produces loss of consciousness, and if it is discontinued, the patient becomes conscious but in an altered state of awareness. Neuroleptanesthesia is useful for elderly and poor-risk patients and for such procedures as bronchoscopy and carotid arteriography. It should be noted that Innovar alone greatly facilitates intubation in awake patients.

Side effects of neuroleptanalgesia or neuroleptanesthesia are hypotension, a slow heart rate (bradycardia), and respiratory depression. The action of droperidol persists for 3 to 6 hours, whereas the analgesic effect of fentanyl persists for only 30 minutes. Droperidol has adrenergic receptor blocking, antifibrillatory, antiemetic, and anticonvulsant actions. About 1% of patients who receive droperidol may have extrapyramidal muscle movements (see Chapter 41) as long as 12 hours after administration of the drug. These movements may be controlled by administration of atropine or benztropine (Chapter 48).

PATIENT CARE IMPLICATIONS

Drug administration/patient and family education

- The techniques of administration of general anesthesia are beyond the scope of this book; consult appropriate textbooks of anesthesia.
- Obtain a careful drug history before surgery. Assess for allergic or unusual response to previous anesthetic agents, as well as any current medications the patient is taking.
- Preoperative medications are an integral part of the planned anesthesia. Administer them as ordered and on time.
- To prepare the patient for surgery, teach the patient and family about the surgical procedure and what to expect postoperatively. Have patient give a return demonstration of any exercises or activities required, such as coughing and deep breathing. Provide the patient with an opportunity to ask questions of the anesthesiologist or nurse anesthetist. Schedule a visit to the intensive care unit, if appropriate. Provide emotional support as needed.

Postoperative care

- Monitor temperature, pulse, respirations, and blood pressure frequently. With the exception of the temperature, this may be every 5 minutes initially, progressing to every 15 minutes, then 30 and longer. Auscultate lung sounds and check neurologic status. Do not leave patient unattended unless patient can call for assistance and can handle secretions safely.
- Keep patients on their sides initially, if possible, to prevent aspiration if vomiting should occur. Keep a suction machine at the bedside, and side rails up.
- Evaluate patients for pain medication in the immediate postoperative period (first 2 to 4 hours after surgery). Factors to consider include the nature and location of surgery, vital signs, age, weight, alertness, what anesthetic was used, and whether analgesics were administered during surgery. The initial dose of analgesics may be ¼ to ½ the ordered dose of analgesic, but make reductions in dose

Continued.

PATIENT CARE IMPLICATIONS—cont'd

only after consultation with the physician. Note that when Innovar is used, the first dose of postoperative analgesic should be low (see text).

- Begin nursing measures to prevent atelectasis and pneumonia as soon as the patient is able. This may include turning and deep breathing, coughing, and other breathing activities.
- Effects of anesthesia persist even after the patient appears to be alert and awake. If it is necessary to give instructions about activity, diet, or medications, as may occur in the outpatient or day surgery setting, instructions should be given both verbally and in writing, to the patient and at least one family member present.
- Do not permit patients in the outpatient setting to drive themselves home if they have received general anesthesia.
- Warn patients who have a severe reaction or response to any anesthetic to carry with them the name of the agent. If surgery is ever again needed, warn them to inform the anesthesiologist of the previous severe response. Suggest that patients also wear a medical

identification tag or bracelet indicating the severe reactions.
- See the patient care implications for narcotic analgesics in Chapter 44. Patients will perform needed postoperative activities better if they are adequately medicated for pain.

Ketamine

Drug administration/patient and family education

- Ketamine is known to be associated with unpleasant dreams, emergence delirium, irrational behavior, disorientation, and hallucinations. The occurrence of these side effects may be lessened by providing the patients with a quiet wake-up period, perhaps in the quietest corner of the postanesthesia recovery room. Avoid excessive stimulation, although vital signs must still be monitored. If psychic effects occur, provide calm reassurance and reorientation. Do not leave patient unattended. Once patient is returned to the room, keep the room dimly lit, and keep noise and stimulation to a minimum. Inform family members of the probable cause of the behavior and enlist their aid in patient reorientation and reassurance.

SUMMARY

Anesthesia is the abolition of the perception of pain and the reaction to painful stimuli. General anesthesia depends on disruption of the reticular activating system. Traditionally, four stages of general anesthesia have been described, with stage III as surgical anesthesia.

Inhalation anesthetics are believed to alter the lipid structure of the cell membrane rather than to occupy membrane receptors. The effective concentration of inhalation anesthetics is determined by the partial pressure of the gas, whereas the solubility of the gas in the blood determines the length of induction and recovery periods. Major factors determining the choice of inhalation anesthetics are the cardiovascular effects produced and the flammability of the anesthetic. Production of analgesia and muscle relaxation may require the administration of supplemental drugs specific for these effects.

Nitrous oxide and halothane (Fluothane) are the most widely used inhalation anesthetics. Isoflurane (Forane) is a new inhalation anesthetic. Me-

thoxyflurane (Penthrane) is used mainly for its analgesic property in obstetrics and dental practice. Enflurane (Ethrane) is a stimulant anesthetic. The use of diethyl ether is essentially obsolete because of its high flammability.

The ultrashort-acting barbiturates thiopental (pentothal), methohexital (Brevital), and thiamylal (Surital), the benzodiazepines diazepam (Valium), flunitrazepam (Rohypnol), and midazolam (Versed), and etomidate (Amidate) are given intravenously to render the patient unconscious or mentally uninvolved in such procedures as induction of general anesthesia, cardioversion, endoscopy, or tooth extractions.

Ketamine is a true anesthetic that can be administered intravenously or intramuscularly.

Selected combinations of drugs are used to produce surgical anesthesia. Balanced anesthesia refers to the administration of a narcotic analgesic, a skeletal muscle relaxant, and nitrous oxide for general anesthesia after induction with an ultrashort-acting barbiturate or diazepam. Neuroleptanesthesia refers to the combination of the antipsychotic-type drug droperidol (Inapsine), the short-acting narcotic analgesic fentanyl (Sublimaze), and nitrous oxide. Innovar is a combination product containing droperidol and fentanyl.

STUDY QUESTIONS

1. How are general anesthetics believed to work?
2. What are the four stages of anesthesia under the scheme of treating general anesthesia as pure central nervous system depression?
3. How does Winter's scheme for describing general anesthesia differ from the scheme of treating general anesthesia as pure central nervous system depression?
4. What are the properties of an ideal anesthetic?
5. What measurement determines the effective concentration of an inhalation anesthetic? How does this differ from the concentration based on total solubility?
6. What is MAC?
7. What factors determine induction and emergence?
8. Why is diethyl ether seldom used in the United States?
9. Which inhalation anesthetics are halogenated hydrocarbons?
10. Which inhalation anesthetics sensitize the heart to catecholamines?
11. Which inhalation anesthetics are metabolized to some degree?
12. Which inhalation anesthetics lower blood pressure during surgery?
13. What factor limits the use of nitrous oxide alone as an anesthetic? How is this limitation overcome?
14. What are the special hazards of nitrous oxide to the patient? To operating room personnel?
15. Which barbiturates are used as intravenous induction agents for anesthesia? How is their action effectively terminated?
16. Which benzodiazepines are used as intravenous induction agents for anesthesia?
17. What is the nature of anesthesia with ketamine?
18. Describe balanced anesthesia.
19. Describe neuroleptanesthesia.

SUGGESTED READINGS

Biddle, C.: Adverse reactions to drugs used in anesthesia, Curr. Rev. Post Anesth. Care Nurses 10(7):51, 1988.

Brown, F.R. Jr.: Clinical significance of the biotransformation of inhalation anesthetics, Res. Staff Physician 24(4):72, 1978.

Bruton-Maree, N.: Outpatient anesthesia for orthopaedic procedures, Orthop. Nurs. 6(2):30, 1987.

Burden, N.: Post-anesthesia: while the patient is unconscious, RN 51(4):34, 1988.

Chitwood, L.B.: Unveiling the mysteries of anesthesia, Nursing 87 17(2):53, 1987.

Clark, R.B.: Anesthesia in obstetrics. I. General, Postgrad. Med. 53(4):158, 1973.

Code, W.E., and Roth, S.H.: Anesthesia in the geriatric patient, Gerontion 2(2):11, 1987.

Davidson, K.W., and Kahn, R.F.: Nitrous oxide analgesia for outpatient procedures, Am. Fam. Physician 31:209, 1985.

Davis, A.B.: The development of anesthesia, Am. Scientist 70:522, 1982.

Farrell, G., Prendergast, D., and Murray, M.: Halothane hepatitis: detection of a constitutional susceptibility factor, N. Engl. J. Med. 313:1310, 1985.

Garfield, J.M.: Psychologic problems in anesthesia, Am. Fam. Physician 10(2):60, 1974.

Gillman, M.A.: Nitrous oxide, an opioid addictive agent: review of the evidence, Am. J. Med. 81:97, 1986.

Karb, V.B.: Midazolam: newcomer to the benzodiazepine family, J. Neurosi. Nurs. 32(1):64, 1989.

Kochansky, C.Y., and Kochansky, S.W.: Postanesthetic considerations for the patient receiving ketamine, J. Post. Anesth. Nurs. 3(2):118, 1988.

Lichtiger, A.: Anesthesia for the geriatric patient, Curr. Rev. Recov. Room Nurses 8(21):162, 1987.

Miller, K.W.: Anaesthesia, models of consciousness, Nature 323:584, 1986.

Pierce, E.C.: Anesthesiology, JAMA 254:2317, 1985.

Pilon, R.N.: Anesthesia for uncomplicated obstetric delivery, Am. Fam. Physician 9(1):113, 1974.

Price, H.L.: Neuroleptic agents in anesthesia, Am. Fam. Physician 8(4):222, 1973.

Schmidt, K.F.: Premedication for anesthesia, Am. Fam. Physician 10(4):113, 1974.

Sebel, P.S.: Evaluation of anesthetic depth, Curr. Rev. Nurse Anesth. 9(20):158, 1987.

Teeple, E.: Inhalation anesthetics for neuroanesthesia, Curr. Rev. Nurse Anesth. 10(3):19, 1987.

Warren, T.M.: Anesthetic management for cesarean section, Curr. Rev. Nurse Anesth. 9(14):110, 1986.

Wilson, P.L., and Wilson, J.E.: Drug review and update—general anesthesia: an overview, Plast. Surg. Nurs. 7(1):24, 1987.

Winter, W.: Effects of drugs on the electrical activity of the brain: anesthetics, Ann. Rev. Pharmacol. Toxicol. 16:413, 1976.

Local Anesthetics

46

BACKGROUND

Cocaine was the first local anesthetic used clinically following the observation in the late 1880s that when cocaine was administered orally to patients, their tongues and throats became numb. Its main use as a local anesthetic was to desensitize the cornea to allow local surgery without a general anesthetic. Cocaine quickly became recognized as an abused drug and was replaced by procaine (Novocain) in 1905. Today lidocaine (Xylocaine), introduced in the 1940s, is the most versatile and widely used local anesthetic. More than 20 local anesthetics are available, but they vary in their suitability for different applications.

MECHANISM OF ACTION

Local anesthesia is achieved by drugs that reversibly inhibit nerve conduction. A local anesthetic is administered at the desired site of action, and the inhibition of nerve conduction persists until the drug diffuses away and enters the circulation for subsequent degradation and excretion. All neurons in the area of administration, whether pain, motor, or autonomic, are affected, so in addition to the loss of pain, loss of sensory, motor, and autonomic activities occurs. The size of the nerve fiber determines its sensitivity to local anesthetics, with the smaller fibers being the most sensitive. Since sensory fibers are smaller than motor fibers, a loss of sensation precedes the loss of motor activity and, conversely, motor activity is regained before sensory function.

Chemically, most local anesthetics are weak bases, being secondary or tertiary amines. This means that under physiological conditions most molecules carry a positive charge and are not very lipid soluble. However, it is the uncharged form that diffuses across the nerve membrane and then reequilibrates to both charged and uncharged forms. Within the neuron it is the positively charged form that blocks nerve conduction. The positively charged form displaces calcium bound to the inner membrane and thus prevents the inward flow of sodium ions. Since the action potential is generated by the influx of sodium ions, the local anesthetic depresses the action potential so that it is not propagated. The resting potential of neurons is not affected by local anesthetics.

SIDE EFFECTS AND ADVERSE REACTIONS

The factor limiting the safety of local anesthetics is that they eventually enter the systemic circulation and can affect other organs. The relative safety of procaine and chloroprocaine results from their rapid hydrolysis in the plasma by pseudocholinesterases. Other local anesthetics are slowly degraded by the liver and have a longer plasma half-life.

Although cocaine is unique in causing euphoria, all local anesthetics act as central nervous system (CNS) stimulants if absorbed systemically, producing symptoms such as anxiety, a tingling feeling (paresthesia), tremors, and ringing in the ears (tinnitus). This CNS stimulation may ultimately result in convulsions. Intravenous diazepam (Valium) in 2.5 mg increments or small doses of an ultrashort-acting barbiturate such as thiopental (Pentothal), thiamylal (Surital), or methohexital (Brevital) are given to stop these convulsions.

A high plasma concentration of a local anesthetic causes CNS depression, with or without prior symptoms of CNS stimulation. This depression of CNS function is serious, since vasomotor control is lost, and results in profound hypotension, respiratory depression, and coma.

In addition to the CNS effects, the direct cardiovascular effects of local anesthetics are important. Local anesthetics cause direct vasodilation, which increases blood flow and so favors the removal of the drug. Thus epinephrine is sometimes added to the local anesthetic, since it causes vasoconstriction and prolongs the time the local anesthetic remains at the site of injection. Cocaine is unique among the local anesthetics in being a potent vasoconstrictor. Prolonged abuse of cocaine by insufflation (sniffing) can cause loss of nasal septa due to tissue death following ischemia (insufficient blood flow).

Local anesthetics are cardiac depressants. Lidocaine is used to depress cardiac arrhythmias (see Chapter 19).

Local anesthetics that are esters (chloroprocaine, procaine, tetracaine) can give rise to an allergic response. Anaphylaxis is rare, and more commonly the topical use of a local anesthetic with an ester bond leads to a skin rash (contact dermatitis).

CLINICAL USES

In general, local anesthetics can be divided into those applied topically to provide surface anesthesia and those injected into an area to produce local anesthesia. Only lidocaine (Xylocaine), dibucaine

Table 46.1   Local Anesthetics for Surface Anesthesia

Generic name	Trade name	Eye*	Mucous membranes†	Skin	Comments
Benzocaine	Americaine	0	0	+	Widely used. Included in many nonprescription preparations for the relief of sunburn, itching, and mild burns. Long acting and poorly absorbed.
Butacaine	Butyn	0	+	0	For relief of pain from dental appliances.
Butamben	Cetacaine	0	0	+	Nonprescription ointment for relief of itching and burning. Contains benzocaine and tetracaine.
Cocaine hydrochloride		+	+	0	Schedule II drug. Medically used in ear, nose, and throat procedures when vasoconstriction and shrinking of mucous membranes are desired. Ophthalmic preparations anesthetize cornea and conjunctiva.
Dibucaine hydrochloride	Nupercaine§	0	0	+	Nonprescription skin ointment or cream.
Dyclonine hydrochloride	Dyclone	0	+	+	Used to suppress the gag reflex and to lessen the discomfort of genitourinal endoscopy. Precipitated by the iodine of contrast media used in pyelography and should not be used.
Lidocaine	Xylocaine§	0	+	+	Widely used for topical anesthesia in ear, nose, and throat procedures; upper digestive tract procedures; and genitourinary procedures. Rapid onset and intermediate duration. Not irritating and low incidence of hypersensitivity.
Lidocaine hydrochloride	Xylocaine hydrochloride§	0	+	+	
Pramoxine hydrochloride	Tronothane§	0	+‡	+	Nonprescription cream or ointment primarily used to relieve pain of itching, burns, and hemorrhoids.
Proparacaine hydrochloride	Ophthaine§	+	0	0	Applied topically to the eye to anesthetize the cornea and conjunctiva.
Tetracaine hydrochloride	Pontocaine§	+	+	+	Topically, the onset is 5 min and duration is 45 min. Usual topical dose is 20 mg; maximum, 50 mg because of toxicity and slow degradation. Ophthalmic preparations are dilute solutions for instillation.

*+ indicates suitable site for application; 0 indicates site not suitable for application.
†Mucous membranes include the bronchotracheal mucosa and the mucosa of the urethra, rectum, and vagina.
‡Not for application to the bronchotracheal mucosa.
§Available in Canada and United States.

Table 46.2   Local Anesthetics for Injection

Generic name	Trade name	Local infiltration or nerve block or epidural block*	Spinal block (subarachnoid)	Duration†	Comments
Bupivacaine hydrochloride	Marcaine‡	+	Investigational	Long§	Provides long-acting epidural anesthesia in labor with no reported effects on fetus. Maximum dose, 200 mg.
Chloroprocaine hydrochloride	Nesacaine†	+	Investigational	Short	Little systemic toxicity because of rapid hydrolysis in the plasma. No effects reported on fetus after epidural anesthesia in mother. Maximum dose, 800 mg.
Dibucaine	Nupercaine	0	+	Long	The most potent and toxic of the local anesthetics. Onset can take 15 min. Available in hyperbaric (heavy), isobaric, and hypobaric (light) solutions. Total dose, 2.5 to 10 mg, depending on use.
Etidocaine hydrochloride	Duranest	+	0	Long	Highly lipid soluble. Onset for epidural block, 5 min. Profound muscle relaxation is desirable for abdominal surgery but not for labor.
Lidocaine	Xylocaine‡	+	+	Intermediate	Widely used local anesthetic. Maximum dose, 300 mg (4.5 mg/kg body weight). Can cause drowsiness, fatigue, and amnesia.
Mepivacaine	Carbocaine‡	+	0	Intermediate	Chemically related to lidocaine. Maximum dose, 400 mg (7 mg/kg body weight).
Prilocaine	Citanest‡	+	0	Intermediate	Maximum dose, 600 mg (8 mg/kg body weight). Useful for outpatient surgery because of the low incidence of drowsiness or fatigue as side effects. Metabolites can cause methemoglobinemia.
Procaine hydrochloride	Novocain‡	+	+	Short	Noted for its safety because of its rapid hydrolysis in the plasma. Maximum dose, 600 mg (10 mg/kg body weight). Duration of epidural block is unreliable.
Tetracaine	Pontocaine‡	0	+	Long	The most widely used drug for spinal anesthesia. Onset, 5 min. Dose for spinal anesthesia, 2 to 15 mg. Available in hyperbaric (heavy), isobaric, and hypobaric (light) solutions.

*+ indicates suitable use; 0 indicates use not suitable.
†Duration without epinephrine: short, 1 hr; intermediate, 2 hr; long, 3 hr (approximations).
‡Available in Canada and United States.
§Duration of bupivacaine in nerve block is 6 to 13 hr.

(Nupercaine), and tetracaine (Pontocaine) are used both topically and by injection.

Local Anesthetics for Surface Anesthesia

Those local anesthetics applied as drops, sprays, lotions, creams, or ointments are listed in Table 46.1. Distinction is made between those drugs safely applied to the eyes, those applied to the skin, and those applied to mucosal areas. Only tetracaine (Pontocaine) is suitable for application to all three sites.

Most drugs listed for surface anesthesia are effective when applied to the skin. These drugs are poorly soluble, so little systemic absorption occurs when they are applied to the skin for the relief of itching or the pain of mild burns. The main potential toxicity of local anesthetics applied to the skin is the development of allergy, usually a contact dermatitis. Since several chemical classes are represented by local anesthetics, a drug from a different chemical group can be substituted if an allergy develops.

The mucosal membranes of the nose, mouth, and throat (bronchotracheal mucosa) and of the urethra, rectum, and vagina are highly vascular and allow ready absorption of the local anesthetic into systemic circulation. Application of excessive amounts of local anesthetics to mucosal surfaces is the most common cause of systemic toxicity with local anesthetics. A local anesthetic often is used to eliminate the gag reflex when inserting an endotracheal tube or to limit the discomfort of endoscopic procedures. The lowest concentration possible of the local anesthetic should be used on mucosal surfaces to avoid systemic toxicity, and the total amount of drug should be recorded and matched against recommended total doses.

Local Anesthetics Administered by Injection

The local anesthetics used by injection are listed in Table 46.2. The potency and the duration of action increase together with the lipid solubility of the drug. The onset of anesthesia is determined by the concentration of drug and the size of the nerve. Before infiltrating an area with a local anesthetic, the syringe first should be aspirated to ensure that a blood vessel has not been entered. This is because the concentration of drug is high and could prove fatal if injected systemically.

The area affected by a local anesthetic depends on how and where it is injected. The anesthesia produced is described by the technique of injection: infiltration, nerve block, epidural, and spinal anesthesia. These techniques are described with their potential for producing toxic side effects.

Infiltration anesthesia refers to the superficial application of a local anesthetic. To suture a cut or to perform dental procedures, the local anesthetic is injected superficially in small amounts to block the small nerves and numb the area. To work on the scalp or to make an incision in the skin, the anesthetic is infused around the area. Small incisions require only a small volume and a low concentration of drug, so little toxicity is associated with these uses. However, systemic toxicity from local anesthetics frequently is seen in the emergency room when large cuts are infiltrated with local anesthetic.

Nerve block anesthesia refers to the injection of a local anesthetic along a nerve before it reaches the surgical site. The volume and concentration of a local anesthetic for a nerve block must be larger than in infiltration anesthesia to penetrate the larger nerve.

The most extensive field of local anesthesia is achieved by applying the local anesthetic around the nerve roots near the spinal cord to produce epidural anesthesia or, alternatively, spinal anesthesia. As shown in Figure 46.1, the spinal cord proper ends at the lumbar region. The spinal cord is surrounded by three membranes: first the pia mater, then the arachnoid, and finally the outer membrane, the dura mater. These membranes extend below the spinal cord proper to form a sac in the lumbar and sacral region. The dura mater and arachnoid membranes are close together, but the subarachnoid space is between the arachnoid and pia mater. The cerebrospinal fluid fills the subarachnoid space throughout the spinal cord.

For *epidural (peridural) anesthesia,* the local anesthetic is administered outside the dura mater, as indicated in Figure 46.1, so that the nerve roots are blocked at the point after they emerge from the dura mater. The extent of anesthesia depends on the volume and concentration of local anesthetic used. *Caudal (sacral) anesthesia* is another form of epidural anesthesia and is achieved by administering the local anesthetic epidurally at the base of the spine, as indicated in Figure 46.1. The extent of anesthesia affects only the pelvic region and legs. Caudal anesthesia is used for obstetrics and for surgery on the rectum, anus, and prostate gland.

Spinal (subarachnoid) anesthesia is achieved by injecting local anesthetic into the subarachnoid space between the arachnoid and pia mater membranes in the lumbar area, usually between the second lumbar and first sacral vertebrae and well below the spinal cord proper. The diagram in Figure 46.1 shows that this will block the nerve roots for the entire lower body. If the solution containing local anesthetic has the same density (isobaric) as the cerebrospinal fluid and is administered slowly, the solution will stay where it is injected and only slowly diffuse into the rest of the cerebrospinal fluid. The solution of local anesthetic also can be made more dense (hyperbaric) by diluting the local anesthetic into 5% dextrose. The solution then will move downward (toward the ground). If the patient is on a tilt bed with feet high and head low, the hyperbaric solution will travel "up" the spinal cord toward the head and anesthetize more of the body. The solution of local anesthetic also can be diluted with distilled water to be less dense (hypobaric). In the patient positioned on the tilt bed, this solution

THE NURSING PROCESS

LOCAL ANESTHESIA

Assessment

Patients requiring local anesthetics are seen in a variety of situations. These patients may need minor surgery, dental work, or suturing of small injuries or may require spinal anesthesia for major surgery. The decision to use a local anesthetic depends on the patient's condition, age, the procedure to be performed, the possible need for the patient to be awake, the patient's preference, and the patient's previous experience with various anesthetics. Basic assessment data include the vital signs and temperature, history of allergies, response to previous surgery, and overall condition.

Nursing diagnoses

Potential complication: urinary retention and inability to avoid

Impaired swallowing and loss of gag reflex secondary to local anesthesia

Management

Except for topical application, local anesthetics usually are administered by the physician, the nurse anesthetist, or the anesthesiologist. For minor or brief procedures such as suturing or some dental work, careful observation of the patient may be sufficient. For longer procedures or when spinal anesthesia is used, it is necessary to monitor the vital signs and other parameters of patient function. With spinal anesthesia, the lower extremities must be positioned carefully. A Foley catheter may be inserted to allow urinary output. The level of consciousness should be monitored. Since allergic responses are possible when local anesthetics are used by any route, epinephrine and equipment for resuscitation should be readily available to deal with possible anaphylaxis.

Evaluation

Local anesthetics are effective if the procedure can be completed without pain, if no side effects occur, and if the anesthesia causes no damage to the patient. All the anesthetics require time to wear off, and specific nursing care depends on the area that has been anesthetized. For example, if the throat has been anesthetized for bronchoscopy or similar procedure, part of the follow-up will include evaluation of the ability to swallow, positioning of the patient on the side to reduce the possibility of aspiration, restricting oral intake until the patient can swallow, and occasionally keeping a suction machine at the bedside. Following spinal anesthesia, the patient should be kept flat for 12 to 24 hours. The nurse should check the position of the lower extremities to prevent pressure areas, and the patient should be kept in bed until sensation returns to the lower extremities. The fluid intake and output should be checked and the vital signs monitored.

If the patient is still under the effects of the local anesthetic at discharge, the patient should be able to explain any restrictions in activity or diet to be followed until the anesthesia wears off, in addition to any restrictions caused by the surgical problem. If analgesic medications have been prescribed for use after anesthesia wears off, the patient should be able to explain their use correctly (see Chapter 44). Finally, in those instances in which local anesthetics are to be used on an outpatient basis, the patient should be able to explain how to use the medication, with what frequency, and what to do if the medication proves to be ineffective. For further information, see the patient care implications section.

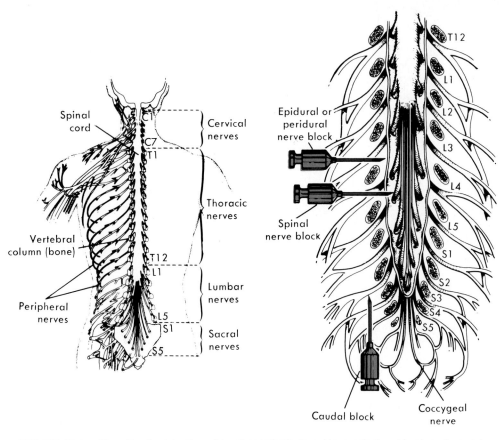

FIGURE 46.1 The sites for injection of local anesthetic to achieve spinal, epidural, and caudal anesthesia. The degree of anesthesia achieved and special techniques used are described in detail in the text.

would move to the end of the dura mater and anesthetize only the lower part of the body. The procedures employing hypobaric and hyperbaric solutions of local anesthetic require skill in positioning the patient. If the level of anesthesia is adjusted to block more of the spinal cord than just the lumbar and sacral regions, there is danger of paralyzing the intercostal and phrenic nerves, thereby paralyzing spontaneous respiration.

If the patient is seated when the local anesthetic is administered as a low spinal anesthetic, only those nerves affecting the parts of the body that would be in contact with a saddle are affected, hence the name *saddle block*. This procedure is used principally in obstetrics for vaginal delivery.

With spinal anesthesia the patient is awake, breathing and cardiovascular function are not immediately affected, and good muscle relaxation is present. These are advantages for patients with heart and lung disease or for elderly persons. However, the sympathetic fibers to the blood vessels are blocked, so vasodilation with hypotension is a frequent side effect of spinal anesthesia. Spinal anesthesia therefore is considered hazardous for abdominal surgery in poor-risk patients because of the potential for this sudden vasodilation and hypotension. Spinal anesthesia is widely used in obstetrics, particularly for cesarean sections.

Duration of action. The rate at which local anesthetic is removed from the infiltrated area depends largely on the degree of vascularization. The duration can be increased by 50% to 100% with the inclusion of epinephrine, 1:200,000, or phenylephrine to cause vasoconstriction and thereby restrict systemic absorption. However, the inclusion of epinephrine is contraindicated for infiltration of areas with end arteries (fingers, toes, ears, nose, penis), since the resultant ischemia may lead to tissue death. Similarly, the addition of a vasocon-

PATIENT CARE IMPLICATIONS

Drug administration

- Obtain a careful history of previous response to local anesthetics. Remember that *Novocain* is the term often used by patients to refer to any local anesthetic, regardless of the actual drug.
- Monitor the blood pressure and pulse. If epidural, nerve block, or spinal anesthesia is being used, monitor the respiration. If anesthesia is being used during labor and delivery, assess fetal heart tones.
- Following spinal anesthesia, keep the patient flat for the specified number of hours, up to 12 hours. Transfer the patient flat from the stretcher to the bed. Usually a thin pillow may be used.
- Assess patients who have had epidural, nerve block, or spinal anesthesia for ability to void and/or a distended bladder. Monitor intake and output. If the patient has not voided in 8 hours after surgery or delivery, notify the physician.
- Assist patients who have received epidural, nerve block, or spinal anesthesia when ambulating the first time.
- Position patients carefully in bed after epidural, nerve block, or spinal anesthesia as they may have no sensation to warn of wrinkles, tight sheets, or other skin irritants.
- Apply heat or cold to anesthetized area with extreme caution, since the patient will be unable to indicate if irritation or burning is occurring. If applying heat or cold is necessary, shield the skin well from the heat or cold source, and check the patient and the skin surfaces every 5 to 15 minutes. This same idea holds true following oral or dental anesthesia.
- Although serious systemic reactions are rare with local anesthetics, drugs, equipment, and personnel to treat acute allergic reactions should be available in settings where local anesthetics are used.
- Patients in the operating room or delivery room who are receiving local anesthesia may be drowsy from preoperative medications, but will usually be alert and able to understand conversation in the room. Keep conversation and noise to a minimum. Avoid discussing other patients, complications, pathology reports, or other topics that are inappropriate or might alarm the patient.
- Following bronchoscopy or other procedures in which surface anesthesia may have been applied to the back of the throat, assess the gag reflex and ability to swallow. Do not leave patients unattended until they can safely handle secretions.
- Following dental work or injection of anesthetics into the tongue, lips, and gums, caution patients to avoid eating or chewing until sensation returns. Patients may inadvertently bite their tongue or cheek.
- Tell patients to report any rash or skin irritation that occurs as a result of local anesthetic application.
- If patients develop an allergic or untoward response to a local anesthetic, encourage them to wear a medical identification tag or bracelet indicating the causative agent.
- Instruct patients to use surface anesthetics as instructed, not to increase the frequency of application, or to use the preparation on skin surfaces for which it was not designed.
- Before discharging the patient, review any limitations the patient may have until the effects of the anesthetic wear off. For example, patients who have had local anesthesia to a joint may be instructed to avoid use of the joint for a certain number of hours or until the anesthetic has worn off.

---

strictor is contraindicated in epidural anesthesia in labor because of the potential vasoconstriction of the uterine blood vessels with a resultant decrease in placental circulation. The use of epinephrine also is contraindicated for those patients who have severe cardiovascular disease or thyrotoxicosis, in whom cardiac function would be compromised by added vasoconstrictors.

Spinal anesthesia can cause variable hypotension because the neurons controlling vasomotor tone are in the spinal tract. A severe headache may be experienced after spinal anesthesia and may last for hours or days after the anesthetic has worn off. This postspinal headache is believed to reflect a drop in the pressure of the cerebrospinal fluid caused by a leak at the point where the dura mater was penetrated. The incidence of a spinal headache is reduced when patients are kept flat on their backs and instructed not to raise their heads for 12 hours following spinal anesthesia. This minimizes the hydrostatic pressure of the cerebrospinal fluid on the head.

SUMMARY

Local anesthetics are drugs that penetrate the nerve membrane and prevent sodium influx, a mechanism that blocks the development and propagation of an action potential. Systemic absorption of a local anesthetic produces toxic effects initially characteristic of CNS stimulation (anxiety, tingling, tremors, ringing in the ears) and finally characteristic of CNS depression (hypotension, respiratory depression, coma). Local anesthetics are vasodilators, except for cocaine, which is unique in being a vasoconstrictor. Local anesthetics depress cardiac excitation, and lidocaine is used to depress cardiac arrhythmias.

The site of administration determines the extent of anesthesia:

1. Surface anesthesia for the eyes, skin, and mucosal areas
2. Infiltration anesthesia for superficial numbing (dental procedures, skin sutures)
3. Nerve block anesthesia for numbing regions of the body
4. Epidural anesthesia (blocking major nerve roots exiting from the base of the spinal cord at a site outside of the dura mater) and spinal anesthesia (blocking major nerve roots at a site within the subarachnoid space) to anesthetize the lower part of the body for delivery and for surgery

Most local anesthetics are safely used only for certain routes of administration. The larger the nerve to be blocked, the more local anesthetic required. All nerves, motor and autonomic, as well as pain neurons, are anesthetized. Duration of action can be increased by inclusion of a vasoconstrictor (epinephrine, phenylephrine) to slow systemic absorption of injected local anesthetic.

Allergic skin reactions are the most frequent side effect of surface anesthetics. Sometimes hypotension may accompany spinal anesthesia because of the blockade of neurons within the spinal cord controlling vasomotor tone. A "spinal" headache is a common effect of spinal anesthesia.

STUDY QUESTIONS

1. What is the mechanism of action of local anesthetics?
2. What property of procaine and chloroprocaine makes them relatively safe?
3. What are the toxic effects of systemic absorption of local anesthetics?
4. What are the three types of surfaces to which local anesthetics are applied?
5. Describe the areas of anesthesia achieved by infiltration, nerve block, epidural, and spinal anesthesia.
6. What are the special hazards associated with spinal anesthesia?
7. How is the duration of local anesthetics prolonged?

SUGGESTED READINGS

Burden, N.: Regional anesthesia: what patients and nurses need to know, RN **51**(5):56, 1988.

Conklin, K.A.: Pharmacology of local anesthetics, AANA J. **55**(1):36, 1987.

Curran, M.A.: Epidural anesthesia: practical considerations, Curr. Rev. Nurse Anesth. **10**(22):170, 1988.

Dickey, J.: Effectiveness of intradermally injected lidocaine hydrochloride as a local anesthetic for intravenous catheter insertion, J. Emerg. Nurs. **14**(3):160, 1988.

Ivey, D.F.: Local anesthesia: implications for the perioperative nurse. . . home study program, AORN J. **45**(3):682, 1987.

Komar, W.: Spinal anaesthesia for the orthopaedic surgical patient, CONA J. **10**(4):6, 1988.

Lefevre, M.: Obstetric anesthesia, Am. Fam. Physician **27**(6):146, 1983.

Maternal anesthesia and newborn behavior, Briefs **43**(2):28, 1979.

Proposed recommended practices: monitoring the patient receiving local anesthesia, AORN J. **49**(2):623, 1989.

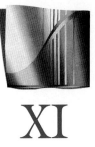

XI

DRUGS TO CONTROL DISORDERS OF CENTRAL MUSCLE CONTROL

Section XI discusses anticonvulsants as well as drugs to control involuntary muscle movements. Chapter 47, *Anticonvulsants*, reviews the classification of seizures. The anticonvulsants are presented by drug class but also are referenced for their role in controlling specific seizure patterns. Chapter 48, *Central Motor Control: Drugs for Parkinsonism and Centrally Acting Skeletal Muscle Relaxants*, covers drugs to treat disorders of central motor control, in two sections. The first section presents the drug classes used to treat parkinsonism and discusses the step therapy to control the symptoms of the progressive disease of parkinsonism, as well as the role of these drugs in treating the drug-induced parkinsonian symptoms. The second section presents drugs to control spasticity as well as drugs acting centrally to relieve local muscle spasms.

CHAPTER

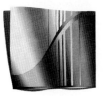

Anticonvulsants

47

Epilepsy: Seizure Patterns

CAUSES OF EPILEPSY

Epilepsy is a neurological disorder characterized by a *recurrent* pattern of abnormal neuronal discharges within the brain, resulting in a sudden loss or disturbance of consciousness, sometimes in association with motor activity, sensory phenomena, or inappropriate behavior. Between 1% and 2% of the population is estimated to have epilepsy. The cause of epilepsy may be unknown (idiopathic) or may be traced to a known brain lesion. In general, epilepsy appearing in childhood or adolescence is likely to be idiopathic, whereas epilepsy appearing in adulthood is likely to relate to a definable cause, such as a head injury, cerebrovascular accident (stroke), or brain tumor.

An appropriate choice of drugs, taken on a long-term basis, can control the seizures of epilepsy in about 80% of patients. The choice of drugs depends on a careful diagnosis of the seizure pattern, which ideally is made from the observation of a seizure and the recording of the brain wave pattern with an electroencephalogram (EEG) during the seizure. The diagnosis is critical to the selection of a drug or drugs, since different seizure patterns are controlled by different drugs. Other causes of seizures must be ruled out, since seizures may be secondary to an organic disorder such as a brain tumor, poisoning, fever, hypoglycemia, and hypocalcemia. An overdose of certain drugs, such as local anesthetics and ketamine, causes seizures. Abrupt withdrawal of some drugs, such as the barbiturates and most other sedative-hypnotic drugs, including alcohol, can precipitate seizures.

CATEGORIES OF EPILEPSY

Epilepsy is described most frequently by the classification published by the International League Against Epilepsy in 1970. This classifica-

tion is presented in Table 47.1. The purpose of this classification is to describe the seizure pattern by the area of brain involved.

Partial Seizures and Generalized Seizures

Partial seizures and generalized seizures are the two major categories of epilepsy. Partial seizures are those arising from a focal lesion of the brain in which the abnormal discharge of cells involves a limited area. The location of the lesion determines the type of seizure observed: motor, cognitive, behavioral, or sensory. Consciousness is usually not lost, but the patient may not remember seizure episodes when cognitive or behavioral function is involved. Focal seizures and psychomotor seizures are two examples of partial seizures that are discussed more fully. Generalized seizures result from the discharge of cells over both sides of the brain. Grand mal seizures, petit mal seizures, infantile spasms, and myoclonus are examples of generalized seizures which are described more fully.

Grand mal epilepsy. Grand mal or general tonic-clonic epilepsy involves the contraction of all skeletal muscles. Before the seizure begins, the patient may experience an *aura*. An aura is a sensation peculiar for that patient, which can be a visual disturbance or a certain dizziness or numbness that warns the patient of an impending seizure. The patient then suddenly loses consciousness and may utter a cry as the diaphragm contracts and expels air from the lungs. The seizure consists of tonic (sustained) contractions and/or clonic (intermittent) contractions of the muscles. The patient may become incontinent. When the contractions cease, the patient regains consciousness. Usually, however, the patient is confused and drowsy and lapses into prolonged sleep (postictal depression).

Petit mal or absence epilepsy. Petit mal or absence epilepsy occurs mainly in children 4 to 12 years old. The child suddenly loses consciousness for a few seconds, although body tone is seldom lost and consciousness is regained with no confusion. The appearance is one of inattention or daydreaming and may be accompanied by slight blinking or hand movements. The attacks usually occur several times a day. The EEG shows a three-per-second spike wave pattern. Petit mal epilepsy does not generally continue into adulthood, but many patients with petit mal epilepsy subsequently develop other types of epilepsy, particularly grand mal epilepsy. Thus many physicians treat children prophylactically for grand mal epilepsy in addition to treating the petit mal epilepsy. Some evidence suggests that this prophylactic treatment reduces the incidence of subsequent grand mal epilepsy.

Infantile spasms. Infantile spasms denote a major generalized seizure that occurs in the first year of life. The seizure consists of a sudden, transient, repetitive contraction of the limbs and trunk. A sudden shocklike jerk is accompanied by a sharp cry. The legs are extended, and the arms are carried forward in front of the head. These spasms may occur hundreds of times a day and are believed to originate from a congenital malformation or neonatal injury and to reflect an immature nervous system. If the seizures persist after 1 year of age, the seizure pattern changes, usually to a petit mal (absence) seizure, a myoclonic seizure, or a "head drop" seizure in which consciousness is lost for 10 to 15 minutes, accompanied by a loss of muscle tone in the neck.

Myoclonus epilepsy. Myoclonus epilepsy is a generalized seizure pattern that develops secondary to anoxic brain damage (intentional myoclonus) or as a genetic disorder (progressive myoclonic epilepsy). Intentional myoclonus is a neurological symptom consisting of sudden involuntary contractions of skeletal muscles, which are aggravated by purposeful activity (hence the term *intentional*) as well as by visual, auditory, tactile, and emotional activity. The genetic disorder, progressive myoclonic epilepsy, is a particular form of intentional myoclonus that appears in childhood and becomes progressively worse. When untreated, the genetic disease leads to death after 15 to 20 years.

Psychomotor or temporal lobe epilepsy. Psy-

Table 47.1   International Classification of Seizures

Class	Specific signs and symptoms
Generalized seizures: without focal onset, symmetrical on both brain hemispheres. Consciousness is lost unless otherwise indicated.	1. Tonic-clonic seizures (grand mal) 2. Tonic seizures: sustained contraction of a large muscle group 3. Clonic seizures: arrhythmic contractions of parts of the body 4. Absence seizures (petit mal): brief loss of consciousness, three spikes per second on EEG 5. Bilateral massive epileptic myoclonus (consciousness is usually not altered), isolated clonic jerks 6. Infantile spasms: muscle spasms, bizarre EEG 7. Atonic seizures: loss of postural tone with sagging of the head (head drop) or falling down 8. Akinetic seizures: complete relaxation of all muscles

Partial seizures: focal seizures	1. Elementary symptoms, consciousness not lost
	  a. Motor symptoms (jacksonian).
	  b. Sensory (hallucinations—visual, auditory, taste) or somatosensory (tingling) symptoms
	  c. Autonomic symptoms
	  d. Compound forms
	2. Complex symptoms, consciousness impaired (temporal lobe or psychomotor epilepsy)
	  a. Cognitive symptoms: confusion, memory distorted
	  b. Affective symptoms: bizarre behavior
	  c. Psychosensory symptoms: automatisms—repetitive, purposeless behaviors

Unilateral seizures: only one half of brain involved.	
Unclassified: incomplete data.	

chomotor or temporal lobe epilepsy has complex symptoms that include an aura, automatism, and motor seizures, independently or in combination. These seizures usually last about 5 minutes. The patient remembers the aura, but not the automatism or motor seizure. The automatism may consist of chewing or swallowing motions, tempermental changes, confusion, feelings of unreality, or unexplained, bizarre behavior. A detailed neurological examination may be required to differentiate psychomotor epilepsy from psychotic mental illness.

Focal seizures. Focal seizures are not associated with a loss of consciousness. Focal sensory seizures may be visual, such as flashes of light; tactile, such as a feeling of numbness or tingling; or motor. Focal motor seizures of the jacksonian type begin with clonic seizures of a few muscles on half of the face or in one extremity; the seizures then progress *(march)* to include more body musculature (e.g., finger, hand, arm).

Status epilepticus. Status epilepticus refers to seizures that last 30 minutes or longer or that are repeated for 30 minutes or longer and during which consciousness is not regained. Status epilepticus of the generalized tonic-clonic type is a medical emergency. In about 80% of patients the seizures are secondary to a disease, frequently associated with a low blood concentration of calcium or glucose, or secondary to withdrawal from drugs such as the barbiturates or other sedative-hypnotics. The immediate goals are to establish an airway, stop the seizures, and then identify their cause.

DRUGS TO CONTROL SEIZURES
General Principles for Drug Therapy of Epilepsy

Several drugs are available for control of epileptic seizures. The drug choice depends on diagnosis of the seizure patterns and on the tolerance and response of the patient to the drug prescribed. Drugs most frequently effective for various seizure

Table 47.2 Drug Choice by Seizure Type

Seizure type	First-choice drugs*	Additional drugs for second-choice drugs†	Refractory cases
General: tonic-clonic (grand mal)	Alone or in combination: 1. Phenytoin (Dilantin)—adults 2. Phenobarbital (Luminal)—children 3. Carbamazepine (Tegretol)	1. Other barbiturates: primidone (Mysoline) or mephobarbital (Mebaral) 2. Valproic acid (Depakene)	1. Acetazolamide (Diamox)
Partial: cortical focal (including jacksonian)			
General: absence (petit mal)	Alone 1. Ethosuximide (Zarontin) 2. Valproic acid (Depakene)	1. Other succinimides: methsuximide (Celontin) or phensuximide (Milontin) 2. Benzodiazepines: diazepam (Valium) or clonazepam (Clonopin)	1. Trimethadione (Tridione) 2. Acetazolamide (Diamox)
General: myoclonus (Intentional or progressive)	1. Valproic acid (Depakene)	1. Clonazepam (Clonopin) 2. 1,5,-Hydroxytryptophan and carbidopa (experimental)	1. Ethosuximide (Zarontin) 2. Diazepam (Valium)
General: infantile spasms	1. Adrencorticotropic hormone (ACTH)	1. Clonazepam (Clonopin)	
Partial: complex (temporal lobe, psycho-motor)	1. Carbamazepine (Tegretol)	1. Primidone (Mysoline) 2. Phenytoin (Dilantin)	1. Phensuximide (Milontin)
Status epilepticus: continuous tonic-clonic	1. Intravenous diazepam (Valium) 2. Intravenous phenytoin sodium (Dilantin) 3. Intravenous phenobarbital sodium (Luminal Sodium)	1. Rectal paraldehyde 2. Intravenous amobarbital sodium (Amytal Sodium)	1. Lidocaine (Xylocaine)

*First-choice drugs are those generally effective for most patients with the least incidence of toxic effects.
†Second-choice drugs are those sometimes effective when the first-choice drugs are not effective alone or those associated with a higher incidence of side effects.

Table 47.3 Anticonvulsant Drugs

Generic name	Trade name	Administration/dosage	Comments
LONG-ACTING BARBITURATES			
Mephobarbital	Mebaral*	ORAL: *Adults*—400 to 600 mg daily in divided doses. FDA Pregnancy Category D. *Children over 5 yr*—32 to 64 mg 3 or 4 times daily; *under 5 yr*—16 to 32 mg 3 or 4 times daily.	Metabolized to phenobarbital.
Phenobarbital	Luminal*	ORAL: *Adults*—50 to 100 mg 2 or 3 times daily. FDA Pregnancy Category D. *Children*—15 to 50 mg 2 or 3 times daily.	May begin at twice usual dose for the first 4 days to raise plasma concentration rapidly. Multiple daily doses are to minimize sedation. Effective serum concentration, 15 to 40 μg/ml. In addition to its use for epileptic seizures, phenobarbital is used prophylactically for febrile seizures in children.
	Luminal Sodium*	INTRAMUSCULAR, INTRAVENOUS (SLOW): *Adults*—200 to 320 mg, can repeat after 6 hr. INTRAMUSCULAR: *Children*—3 to 5 mg/kg body weight.	For status epilepticus. Sodium salt must be used for injection.
Primidone	Mysoline* Sertan†	ORAL: *Adults*—250 mg daily at bedtime or up to 2 Gm daily in divided doses. FDA Pregnancy Category D. *Children over 8 yr*—as for adults; *under 8 yr*—½ adult dosage.	Effective serum concentrations, 5 to 10 μg/ml.
HYDANTOINS			
Ethotoin	Peganone	ORAL: *Adults*—1000 mg daily, increased gradually to 2000 to 3000 mg in 4 to 6 divided doses. *Children*—500 to 1000 mg in divided doses.	
Mephenytoin	Mesantoin*	ORAL: *Adults*—200 to 600 mg daily. *Children*—100 to 400 mg daily.	
Phenytoin	Dilantin*	ORAL: *Adults*—300 mg daily in 3 doses; maintenance dose, 300 to 600 mg daily. *Children*—5 mg/kg body weight daily in 2 or 3 doses; maximum, 300 mg daily.	May be given once a day to improve compliance. Effective serum concentration, 10 to 20 μg/ml. Brand name should be specified because of varying bioavailability.
SUCCINIMIDES			
Ethosuximide	Zarontin*	ORAL: *Adults*—500 mg daily, increased gradually every 4 to 7 days to control seizures. *Children over 6 yr*—as for adults; *3 to 6 yr*—250 mg daily, increased gradually to control seizures.	Effective serum concentration, 40 to 80 μg/ml.

*Available in Canada and United States.
†Available in Canada only.

Table 47.3 Anticonvulsant Drugs—cont'd

Generic name	Trade name	Administration/dosage	Comments
SUCCINIMIDES—cont'd			
Methsuximide	Celontin*	ORAL: 300 mg daily for 1 wk, increased weekly by 300 mg to control seizures to a maximum dose of 1200 mg daily.	
Phensuximide	Milontin*	ORAL: 500 to 1000 mg 2 or 3 times daily.	
OXAZOLIDINEDIONE			
Trimethadione	Tridione Trimedone†	ORAL: *Adults*—900 mg daily in 3 or 4 doses, can increase by 300 mg daily every 7 days to control seizures; maximum, 2400 mg daily. FDA Pregnancy Category D. *Children*—40 mg/kg body weight daily in 3 or 4 doses.	No longer widely used because of serious side effects and high teratogenic potential. Effective serum concentration of dimethadione (active metabolite), 700 μg/ml or higher.
BENZODIAZEPINES			
Clonazepam	Clonopin Rivotril*	ORAL: *Adults*—1.5 mg daily in 3 doses, increase every 3 days by 0.5 to 1 mg to control seizures; maximum total dose, 20 mg daily. *Infants and children to 10 yr*—0.01 to 0.03 mg/kg body weight, increased by 0.25 to 0.5 mg every 3 days to control seizures to a maximum of 0.2 mg/kg daily.	Effective therapeutic plasma concentrations, 5 to 70 ng/ml.
Diazepam	Valium*	INTRAVENOUS, to terminate status epilepticus: *Adults*—5 to 10 mg (no faster than 5 mg/min, use large vein); can repeat every 10 to 15 min to maximum dose of 30 mg. *Children 30 days to 5 yr*—0.2 to 0.5 mg slowly every 2 to 5 min, maximum, 5 mg; *over 5 yr*—1 mg slowly every 2 to 5 min; maximum, 10 mg.	See Chapter 40 for use as an antianxiety drug. Rarely used orally as an anticonvulsant agent. Do not mix or dilute into IV fluids.
MISCELLANEOUS			
Acetazolamide	Acetazolam† Diamox*	ORAL: *Adults and children*—8 to 30 mg/kg body weight in divided doses.	A weak diuretic. Tolerance usually develops.
Adrenocorticotropic hormone (ACTH)		INTRAMUSCULAR: *Infants*—10 units daily, increase by 5 units every 5 days up to 60 units for 6 to 7 wk.	If ACTH is ineffective, diazepam, 3 mg/lb, is added. If ACTH is effective in 2 wk, may switch to cortisone, 3 mg/lb, as an alternative to increasing ACTH. Cortisone is brought down by 1 mg/lb over 3 wk.
Carbamazepine	Tegretol*	ORAL: *Adults and children over 12 yr*—200 mg twice on day 1, increase by 200 mg daily to control seizures; maximum, 1000 mg (less than 15 yr) or 1200 mg (over 15 yr). Doses taken every 6 to 8 hr. FDA Pregnancy Category C.	Take medication with meals to avoid gastrointestinal distress. Effective therapeutic plasma concentrations, 4 to 12 μg/ml.

*Available in Canada and United States.
†Available in Canada only.

Continued.

Table 47.3   Anticonvulsant Drugs—cont'd

Generic name	Trade name	Administration/dosage	Comments
MISCELLANEOUS—cont'd			
Lidocaine hydro-chloride	Xylocaine Hydrochloride*	INTRAVENOUS: *Adults*—to terminate status epilepticus: Infuse 1 to 3 mg/min to terminate seizures.	A last resort for terminating status epilepticus. If given in excess, lidocaine itself can induce convulsion.
Paraldehyde		INTRAMUSCULAR, INTRAVENOUS, to terminate status epilepticus: *Adults and children*—0.15 ml/kg body weight. Solution must be diluted. RECTAL: *Children*—0.3 ml/kg diluted 1:1 in olive oil or milk.	A last resort for terminating status epilepticus.
Valproic acid	Depakene	ORAL: *Adults and children*—15 mg/kg body weight daily in divided doses. Can be increased by 5 to 10 mg/kg daily every 7 days to control seizures, up to 60 mg/kg daily. FDA Pregnancy Category D.	Effective in controlling myoclonic epilepsy refractory to most other anticonvulsant drugs. Effective serum concentrations reported to be 50 to 100 μg/ml. Also effective for absence (petit mal) seizures.

*Available in Canada and United States.

patterns are listed in Table 47.2. Table 47.3 lists dosage information for these drugs.

Mechanism of action. The molecular mechanism by which the anticonvulsant drugs act is not understood. In general terms, these drugs depress the excitability of neurons, particularly those that fire inappropriately to initiate the seizure, and thus prevent the spread of seizure discharges. Presumably the mechanisms will be found to modify the ionic movements of sodium, potassium, or calcium across the nerve membrane associated with the action potential or to modify the release or uptake of neurotransmitters.

Because the specific mechanisms underlying seizure activity are not understood, the development of better drugs for controlling seizures is a matter of screening drugs using animal models that incompletely parallel human seizure disorders.

Drug administration. The drug of choice is started in small doses to allow the patient to develop a tolerance to the drowsiness and motor incoordination (ataxia) associated with most of the anticonvulsant drugs. (The exception is phenytoin [Dilantin], which is initially given in a high loading dose.) The dose is increased until the seizures are stopped or until toxic effects of the drug appear. If the drug has been partly effective in controlling seizures, a second drug may be added. If the first drug tried has not been effective, the patient is switched to a different one.

Since the most common cause of drug failure is the failure of the patient to take the prescribed drugs, the plasma concentration of drug may be determined before deciding that the drug per se is ineffective. Patients must be warned not to discontinue medication when the seizures are under control or the side effects are disturbing. The sudden discontinuance of medication greatly increases the incidence of seizures. Blood and urine analyses often are routinely carried out because many anticonvulsant drugs infrequently produce blood dyscrasias or renal damage.

Many patients with epilepsy require drug therapy throughout their lives to control seizures. However, some patients may be able to discontinue medication. These patients are those reaching adulthood after treatment from childhood for petit mal epilepsy and those patients who have had several seizure-free years. If the EEG of such a patient appears normal, medication can be gradually discontinued. Seizures recur in 25% to 50% of such patients.

Therapy and pregnancy. Women with epilepsy who want children need to be advised that their offspring carry a two- to three-fold greater risk of having congenital defects, particularly when the mother is taking phenytoin (Dilantin) or phenobarbital (Luminal). In the absence of any medication, the fetus is still at greater than normal risk because of anoxia during seizures. Pregnancies during which the woman is taking trimethadione (Tridione) are associated with an 80% incidence of spontaneous abortions or birth defects. If possible, a woman taking trimethadione should be switched to ethosuximide (Zarontin) before becoming pregnant.

Long-Acting Barbiturates

Phenobarbital

Phenobarbital (Luminal) has been widely used for 60 years and is a drug of choice in the treatment of grand mal and focal motor epilepsy. It also is used for treatment of withdrawal from barbiturates or alcohol. Phenobarbital is cross-tolerant with alcohol and other barbiturates but requires only once-a-day administration because of its long plasma half-life of 4 days. Because of this long plasma half-life, 14 days are required to reach constant serum concentrations. Phenobarbital sometimes is given intravenously to stop the seizures of status epilepticus, but the degree of respiratory depression can be profound.

The main side effects of the barbiturates are sedation and drowsiness at the beginning of treatment, but tolerance usually develops to these effects. In the elderly and in children, a paradoxical excitement may be seen in the children that impairs learning ability. Phenobarbital does increase the incidence of congenital malformations in the fetus but not to the degree associated with phenytoin and trimethadione. Phenobarbital induces liver microsomal enzymes and thus can speed its own metabolism as well as the metabolism of other drugs. The sudden rather than gradual withdrawal of the drug can precipitate convulsions. Barbiturates are contraindicated for patients with the metabolic disorder porphyria and for patients who are depressed and might consider suicide.

Mephobarbital

Mephobarbital (Mebaral) is metabolized by the liver to phenobarbital. Therefore there is no advantage to substituting mephobarbital for phenobarbital.

Primidone

Primidone (Mysoline) is a deoxybarbiturate that is metabolized to phenobarbital and phenylethylmalonamide. Primidone therefore can substitute for phenobarbital in the treatment of grand mal and focal motor seizures, but in addition is effective in treating temporal lobe (psychomotor) epilepsy.

Hydantoins

Phenytoin

Phenytoin (Dilantin), formerly called diphenylhydantoin, is a drug of choice in controlling grand mal and focal motor epilepsy in adults and occasionally is used in treating psychomotor epilepsy.

Pharmacokinetics. Phenytoin has a plasma half-life of 24 hours, so it takes 4 days to reach steady plasma levels when initiating therapy. To decrease this time, the initial dose is sometimes given as a loading dose at three times the usual daily dose. At serum concentrations much above therapeutic concentrations, the capacity of the liver to metabolize phenytoin is saturated so that plasma concentrations decrease very slowly. Phenytoin is irregularly absorbed from the intestine. Since absorption depends on formulation, it is best to stay with a particular brand of phenytoin.

Phenytoin should not be given intramuscularly or subcutaneously because it is highly irritating and can precipitate in the tissue. The sodium salt can be administered intravenously, but too rapid administration can produce severe hypotension and cardiac arrest. Sodium phenytoin is administered intravenously to control status epilepticus either alone or after intravenous diazepam has controlled the seizures. Intravenous sodium phenytoin is also used to control some cardiac arrhythmias (see Chapter 19).

Adverse effects. Effective serum concentrations are 10 to 20 μg/ml, and side effects are seen at higher serum concentrations: at greater than 20 μg/ml, involuntary movement of the eyeballs (nystagmus); at greater than 30 μg/ml, incoordination (ataxia) and slurred speech. Tremors and nervousness or drowsiness and fatigue may be side effects of higher serum concentrations. However, an acute overdose of phenytoin is seldom fatal. Persistence of these side effects requires reducing the dose or switching to another drug, usually phenobarbital.

About 20% of patients taking phenytoin experience overgrowth of the gums (gingival hyperplasia), which is particularly severe in children. Occasionally, a folic acid or vitamin D deficiency can be produced, since phenytoin interferes with the normal metabolism of these compounds. Phenytoin also can cause an allergic rash that can be mistaken for measles or infectious mononucleosis. Phenytoin also makes a case of acne worse, which is especially bothersome to teenagers, and can increase growth of body hair (hirsutism), which is undesirable in women. Mention has been made of the higher incidence of congenital malformations in infants of mothers taking phenytoin. These infants are also at risk for hemorrhage and coagulation deficiencies at birth which can be corrected with vitamin K.

Drug interactions. Several important drug interactions are noted with phenytoin. Phenobarbital can increase the metabolism of phenytoin in some individuals by inducing liver microsomal enzymes, but in other individuals phenobarbital decreases the rate of drug metabolism by competing with it for the degrading enzymes. The oral anticoagulant dicumarol and the anticonvulsant carbamazepine decrease the metabolism of phenytoin by competing with the enzymes for degradation. The anticonvulsant valproic acid displaces bound phenytoin from protein to increase the free concentration of phenytoin while decreasing its total concentration, since more free phenytoin is available for metabolism. Phenytoin enhances the rate of estrogen metabolism, which can decrease the effectiveness of some birth control pills.

Others

Other anticonvulsant drugs related to phenytoin are *mephenytoin (Mesantoin)* and *ethotoin (Peganone)*. Mephenytoin is associated with a high incidence of agranulocytosis and aplastic anemia. Ethotoin is not widely used, although it does not seem to cause gingival hyperplasia, hirsutism, or incoordination.

Succinimides

Ethosuximide

Ethosuximide (Zarontin) is a drug of choice for controlling absence (petit mal) seizures and may be effective in treating myoclonic seizures. The plasma half-life is 30 hours in children and 60 hours in adults. The effective serum concentration is 40 to 80 μg/ml, but serum concentrations of up to 160 μg/ml can be tolerated without excessive toxicity. Side effects include dizziness, drowsiness, and gastrointestinal irritation. Blood counts are performed routinely because of the occasional occurrence of agranulocytosis.

Related drugs are *phensuximide (Milontin)*, which is sometimes effective in treating psychomotor epilepsy, and *methsuximide (Celontin)*.

Oxazolidinediones

Trimethadione

Trimethadione (Tridione) was the first drug found to be effective in controlling absence seizures (petit mal epilepsy), but this drug is now a third-choice drug for absence seizures because of the high incidence of serious side effects.

Trimethadione can produce a serious allergic dermatitis, kidney and liver damage, agranulocytosis, and aplastic anemia. Blood counts and urinalyses done routinely with trimethadione therapy. In adults, the drug frequently produces an

intolerance to light (photophobia). The 80% incidence of spontaneous abortions or congenital anomalies in infants of mothers taking trimethadione has been mentioned.

The other anticonvulsant of the oxazolidinedione class, *paramethadione (Paradione)*, is no longer used because of its toxicity.

Benzodiazepines

Diazepam and clonazepam

Diazepam (Valium) and clonazepam (Clonopin) are used as anticonvulsant drugs. Diazepam, administered intravenously, is the drug of choice for terminating the clonic-tonic seizures of status epilepticus and sometimes is used to terminate the seizures of eclampsia. Oral diazepam occasionally is used with other anticonvulsants to control myoclonic seizures, akinetic (head drop) seizures, and absence (petit mal) seizures. The main side effects are drowsiness, dizziness, and ataxia. Respiratory depression must be watched during intravenous administration. However, overall diazepam is a safe drug. The major use of diazepam is as an antianxiety drug (see Chapter 40).

Clonazepam is effective in controlling absence (petit mal) seizures, myoclonic seizures, and infantile spasms. Tolerance can develop to clonazepam, and seizures recur in about one third of treated patients. Its effectiveness in controlling tonic-clonic (grand mal) seizures and temporal lobe (psychomotor) seizures is being tested but is probably not sufficient.

The plasma half-life of clonazepam is 20 to 40 hours. Clonazepam is metabolized in the liver to a compound that probably has little anticonvulsant activity.

Neurological side effects are commonly seen during therapy with clonazepam and include drowsiness, incoordination (ataxia), and personality changes. Children may become hyperactive, irritable, aggressive, violent, or disobedient. Slurred speech, tremors, abnormal eye movements, dizziness, and confusion also may be noticed. These effects are dose related and may subside with time or on lowering the dose. Increased salivation and increased bronchial secretions sometimes occur and create respiratory problems in children.

Miscellaneous Drugs

Acetazolamide

Acetazolamide (Diamox) is used alone or with other drugs in treating petit mal epilepsy. The mechanism of action is inhibition of the enzyme carbonic anhydrase in the brain, which results in an altered ratio of intracellular to extracellular so-

THE NURSING PROCESS

ANTICONVULSANT DRUGS

Assessment

With few exceptions, most patients using anticonvulsant drugs have had a seizure, and it is usually safe to assume that once the correct drugs and dosages have been chosen, the drugs will be needed on a long-term basis. Patients who have had a seizure are monitored carefully for the possible effects of the seizure and for possible later seizures. In relation to drug therapy, a baseline assessment should be done, with special emphasis on areas known to be affected by the drugs to be used. For example, since phenytoin causes gingival hyperplasia frequently, a baseline assessment of the mouth, teeth, and gums should be done and recorded at the start of phenytoin therapy.

Nursing diagnoses

Potential complication: gingival hyperplasia

Altered comfort: nausea and gastrointestinal distress associated with drug ingestion.

Management

Drug dosages are adjusted until the seizures are controlled or until toxic effects are noted. The nurse should monitor the general condition of the patient with an emphasis on known drug side effects. For example, monitoring the sedation produced by phenobarbital would provide important information toward determining the most effective dose. Serum levels of the prescribed drugs may be monitored. If the patient is continuing to have seizures, the nurse should observe their type and duration and continue nursing measures to prevent injury, such as padding side rails or supervising ambulation. (See a textbook of nursing for additional information.) Referring the patient on discharge to the health department for follow-up care may be helpful, as may referral to social service or vocational rehabilitation, if appropriate.

Evaluation

Ideally, anticonvulsants halt the seizures with no side effects resulting from drug therapy. Often this is not possible. Although seizure activity may be controlled, the long-term therapy and combinations of drugs sometimes needed often produce at least a few side effects. The health care team then must decide which side effects cannot be permitted and which can be treated or tolerated. The nurse should evaluate the patient regularly through observation, should reassess known problem areas (e.g., the mouth with phenytoin therapy), and should make appropriate referrals. For instance, if phenytoin is causing a problem with acne but the decision is made that the anticonvulsant must be continued, referral to a dermatologist may be appropriate.

On discharge, the patient or parent should be able to name the drugs being taken and to state how to take them correctly, including the dose, the time of day, and the correct preparation; to explain the side effects that may occur, which need to be reported immediately, how to treat or prevent those which are more likely to occur, and what to do if a dose is missed. The patient should be able to state the importance of wearing a medical identification tag or bracelet. For additional information, see the patient care implications section.

---

dium. Acetazolamide is also a weak diuretic (see Chapter 16). Side effects include loss of appetite, drowsiness, confusion, and a tingling feeling. The usefulness of acetazolamide is limited by the frequent development of tolerance to its anticonvulsant action.

Adrenocorticotropic hormone

Adrenocorticotropic hormone (ACTH) is the treatment of choice for infantile spasms. If daily administration for 20 days is effective, the course of treatment is repeated after 2 to 4 weeks or glucocorticoids (usually prednisone) are given. The action of ACTH is to stimulate the adrenal cortex to synthesize glucocorticoids (see Chapter 51). Presumably the effectiveness of ACTH in treating infantile spasms is related to this endocrine action.

Carbamazepine

Carbamazepine (Tegretol) is particularly effective in controlling the seizures of temporal lobe (psychomotor) epilepsy and clonic-tonic (grand mal) seizures. Recently, carbamazepine has been shown to control cocaine cravings and may find a role in the treatment of cocaine addiction. The plasma half-life is 12 hours, so the drug must be given in divided doses. Carbamazepine is metabolized by the liver, and one of the metabolites has anticonvulsant activity. Absorption from the gastrointestinal tract is slow; however, this can be improved if the drug is taken at meals.

Carbamazepine is chemically related to the tricyclic antidepressants, and a positive side effect is the increased alertness and improvement of mood in patients. The most frequent side effects are drowsiness, dizziness, incoordination (ataxia), visual disturbances (particularly double vision), and gastrointestinal upset. Carbamazepine infrequently causes rashes, liver damage, and bone marrow depression, which require its discontinuance. Blood counts should be made frequently in the early course of treatment, and they should be done occasionally thereafter.

Drug interactions encountered include a decreased plasma concentration in the presence of other anticonvulsants, presumably because the other agents induce drug-metabolizing enzymes in the liver. Propoxyphene napsylate (Darvon-N) dramatically increases plasma concentrations of carbamazepine, probably by competing for metabolizing enzymes.

Lidocaine hydrochloride

Lidocaine hydrochloride (Xylocaine Hydrochloride) is another drug used as a last resort to terminate status epilepticus. Lidocaine is a local anesthetic (see Chapter 46) and can induce convulsions at high doses. It can also depress the heart, an effect that is used in treating some cardiac arrhythmias (see Chapter 19).

Paraldehyde

Paraldehyde is a sedative-hypnotic drug that is seldom used today because of its objectionable odor and chemical instability on storage. When other drugs are ineffective in terminating status epilepticus, paraldehyde may be tried. An advantage is that administration may be intramuscular, intravenous, or rectal. When given intravenously, however, it must be diluted and administered slowly not only to avoid producing severe coughing, which can result from bronchopulmonary irritation, but also to avoid irritating the veins, which can result in thrombophlebitis. Use is contraindicated in patients with pulmonary disease, since it aggravates bronchopulmonary disease, and in patients with liver disease, since it is metabolized by the liver.

Valproic acid

Valproic acid (Depakene) was approved for use as an anticonvulsant in 1978 in response to public pressure. In Europe, valproic acid had been dramatically shown to be effective in controlling the seizures of progressive myoclonus, a particularly disabling type of epilepsy in children for which no effective treatment had been available. In addition, valproic acid is effective in treating other types of general seizures: absence (petit mal) and tonic-clonic (grand mal) seizures. Since the plasma half-life is only 8 to 12 hours, the drug is administered three or four times per day.

Valproic acid is an analog of the inhibitory central neurotransmitter, gamma aminobutyric acid (GABA), which inhibits neuronal activity. One mechanism by which valproic acid may act is to increase the concentration of this inhibitory neurotransmitter.

Side effects. The most frequent side effect is gastrointestinal distress. Sedation is marked at the beginning of treatment unless the doses are gradually raised. An overdose has been reported to produce coma but with uneventful recovery. The incidence of liver damage among patients taking valproic acid is being examined in light of some reports of liver failure.

Drug interactions. Drug interactions with valproic acid include its decreased plasma concentration in the presence of other anticonvulsants that induce liver microsomal enzymes: phenobarbital, primidone, phenytoin, and carbamazepine. Phenytoin also can raise the concentration of free plasma valproic acid by displacing the fraction bound to plasma proteins.

PATIENT CARE IMPLICATIONS

General guidelines for anticonvulsant therapy

Drug administration

- Monitor serum drug levels if available.
- Assess for development of the side effects listed in the text. Question patients tactfully about compliance.

Patient and family education

- Review with patients the anticipated benefits and possible side effects of drug therapy.
- Provide emotional support as patients begin anticonvulsant therapy. Drug side effects are common in the first several months of therapy, but often diminish with time. Several months of treatment with a drug or regimen may be needed to determine adequate dosage.
- Reinforce to patients the importance of continuing prescribed medications even if they have been seizure-free for an extended period of time. Reinforce the need to take drugs as ordered and to avoid abruptly discontinuing prescribed medications, as this may precipitate seizures. Recent evidence suggests anticonvulsants can be discontinued in some patients who have been seizure-free for a long period. This decision must be made on an individual basis in consultation with the physician.
- Counsel patients to learn from the physician what actions to take in the event of a missed dose of drug.
- Women of childbearing age may wish to use contraceptives while taking these drugs. If women wish to conceive, counsel them to keep physicians informed so they can be given the current information about drug effects during pregnancy. In addition, remind patients to keep their gynecologists informed of the anticonvulsants being used. Oral contraceptives are not effective when some of these drugs are being taken.
- Encourage pateints to wear a medical identification tag or bracelet indicating they have a history of seizures. In addition, suggest that they carry in their wallets a card listing current drugs and dosages.
- Remind patients to keep all health care providers informed of all medications being taken.
- Tell patients not to use over-the-counter preparations unless approved by the physician.
- Warn patients to avoid driving or operating hazardous equipment if drowsiness develops.

- Refer patients as needed to local or national agencies, incuding the local visiting nurse agency, vocational rehabilitation, or the Epilepsy Foundation of America.
- Avoid drinking alcoholic beverages unless permitted in small amounts by the physician.
- Tell patients not to switch brands of anticonvulsant, as bioavailability may differ between brands; consult pharmacist and physician for specific situations.
- Teach patients using a suspension form to shake the bottle well before pouring each dose. Failure to adequately resuspend the medication may result in inadequate doses when the bottle is nearly full, and excessive doses when the bottle is less than half full, as the drug may be settling to the bottom of the bottle.
- Review procedure for the prescribed drug form. Usually, swallow capsules whole, without breaking them open. Chewable tablets should be chewed well and not swallowed whole. Enteric coated forms should be swallowed whole, without crushing or chewing. If in doubt, consult the manufacturer's literature and the pharmacist.

Long-acting barbiturates

Drug administration/patient and family education

- See the general guidelines.
- Barbiturates are discussed in Chapter 40.
- Review with families the signs of intoxication or overdose: slurred speech, ataxia, vertigo. If these develop, notify physician.
  INTRAVENOUS PHENOBARBITAL
- Dilute sterile powder slowly as directed on package insert. Also available in solution, which must be diluted. Administer diluted dose at a rate of gr 1 (60-65 mg) over 1 minute. Monitor vital signs and respiration. Have a suction machine at the bedside, and equipment for intubation and ventilatory support available. Do not leave patient unattended until the patient is stable and alert.
  INTRAMUSCULAR PHENOBARBITAL
- Observe for respiratory depression 30 to 60 minutes after injection. Monitor blood pressure. Supervise ambulation. Keep side rails up.

Hydantoins

Drug administration

- See the general guidelines.

Continued.

PATIENT CARE IMPLICATIONS — cont'd

- Therapeutic serum drug level is 10 to 20 µg/ml.
- Monitor complete blood count and differential, platelet count, liver function tests, blood glucose.
- Remember that even if used as an anticonvulsant, phenytoin also has cardiovascular effects. See Chapter 19.

INTRAVENOUS PHENYTOIN

- Prepare dose with diluent supplied by manufacturer. Slightly yellow-colored solutions may be used, but discard solutions that are not clear. Do not mix with other drugs or many IV solutions, as precipitation may occur. Flush tubing before and after administration with 0.9% sodium chloride. Administer at a rate of 50 mg or less per minute. Monitor blood pressure, and if possible have patient connected to ECG monitor to monitor cardiac rhythm during and immediately after IV administration. Recent studies have involved dilutions in large volumes of normal saline or lactated Ringer's injection (e.g., 100 mg phenytoin in 50 ml normal saline) to administer phenytoin as an infusion. Use an inline filter. Consult the manufacturer's literature for current recommendations.

Patient and family education

- See general guidelines. Review common signs of overdose: ataxia, slurred speech, and nystagmus. Tell family to report the development of these or any unusual side effects.
- Provide emotional support as needed. Development of acne or hirsutism may be difficult for some patients. Refer to a dermatologist as appropriate.
- Encourage patients to have regular dental checkups, and to have a thorough dental care program: flossing, brushing, rinsing. Even with meticulous oral care, gingival hyperplasia will develop in some patients. Provide emotional support as needed.
- Take oral doses with meals or snack to lessen gastric irritation.
- Instruct patient to report signs of folic acid deficiency: fatigability, weakness, fainting, headache.
- Encourage ingestion of foods high in vitamin D. See Dietary Consideration: Vitamins on p. 282.
- Tell diabetic patients to monitor blood glucose levels, as an adjustment in diet or insulin may be necessary.

- Tell patients that these drugs may produce a harmless brownish or pinkish discoloration of urine.

Succinimides

Drug administration

- See the general guidelines.
- Monitor complete blood count and differential, platelet count, liver function tests.

Patient and family education

- See the general guidelines.
- Take doses with meals or snack to lessen gastric irritation.
- Tell patients taking phensuximide that urine may turn red, pink, or red-brown during therapy with this drug; this is harmless.

Trimethadione

Drug administration

- See the general guidelines.
- Monitor complete blood count and differential, platelet count, liver function tests, serum creatinine, BUN, and urinalysis.

Patient and family education

- See the general guidelines.
- Tell patients to report the development of skin rashes or changes immediately. Because side effects are common with this drug, encourage patients to stay in close contact with the physician.

Other drug groups

Benzodiazepines are discussed in Chapter 40. Acetazolamide is discussed in Chapter 16. ACTH is discussed in Chapter 51.

Carbamazepine

Drug administration

- See the general guidelines.
- Monitor blood pressure and weight.
- Monitor complete blood count and differential, platelets, liver function tests.
- This drug may be used in the treatment of tic douloureux (trigeminal neuralgia).

Patient and family education

- See the general guidelines.
- See Patient Problems: Photosensitivity on p. 647; Constipation on p. 187; and Dry Mouth on p. 170.

PATIENT CARE IMPLICATIONS—cont'd

- Tell patients using this medicine for trigeminal neuralgia that the drug is not an analgesic and should not be used for any condition other than prescribed.
- Tell diabetics that this drug may alter urine glucose results. Monitor blood glucose levels.

Paraldehyde

Drug administration

- See the general guidelines.
- This drug decomposes readily. Use only fresh unopened containers, and always check the expiration date beforehand.
- Paraldehyde reacts with some plastics. Use glass containers or syringes to measure and administer doses.
- The drug imparts a characteristic odor to the patient's breath.
- The drug is partly excreted via the lungs, and may cause coughing and an increase in bronchial secretions. During IV administration, place patients on their sides and have suction equipment available.
- Consult manufacturer's literature for information about IV and IM administration.
- For rectal instillation, dilute the drug in 2 volumes of olive oil to prevent mucosal irritation. Administer as for a retention enema. Controlling the amount or rate of absorption via this route is difficult.

Patient and family education

- See the general guidelines.
- Prepare oral doses in glass or metal containers (see above).
- Dilute oral doses in milk or iced fruit juice to improve taste, lessen odor, and reduce gastric irritation.

Valproic acid

Drug administration

- See the general guidelines.
- Monitor complete blood count and differential, platelet count, liver function tests.

Patient and family education

- See the general guidelines.
- See Patient Problem: Constipation on p. 187.
- Take oral doses with meals or snack to lessen gastric irritation.
- Take the tablet form whole, without chewing or breaking the tablet.
- Tell diabetics that this drug may alter urine tests for ketones, giving false positive results. Monitor blood glucose levels.

SUMMARY

Epilepsy is a neurogenic disorder in which certain neurons in the brain discharge abnormally to produce seizures. The site of the neurons involved determines the type of seizure experienced. As summarized in Table 47.1, the seizure pattern is recurrent and may be partial (jacksonian, psychomotor) or generalized (grand mal, petit mal, myoclonus, infantile spasms) seizures. Most seizures can be controlled by drugs, and Table 47.2 indicates which drugs are used for which seizure types.

The key anticonvulsant drug classes and their characteristics include the following:

1. Long-acting barbiturates. Phenobarbital is used to control grand mal and focal motor epilepsy in adults. Phenobarbital is generally well tolerated, and drowsiness is experienced mainly at the start of therapy. Phenobarbital induces liver microsomal enzymes and thus speeds the metabolism of many drugs. Mephobarbital is metabolized to phenobarbital. Primidone is a related drug used to treat psychomotor epilepsy.

2. Hydantoins. Phenytoin is used to control grand mal epilepsy, especially in children, and focal motor and psychomotor epilepsy. Nystagmus, ataxia, and slurred speech are common side effects that may be controlled if the dose can be lowered. Gingival hyperplasia occurs in about 20% of patients. Important drug interactions are seen with phenobarbital, dicumarol, carbamazepine, valproic acid, and estrogens. Mephenytoin and ethotoin are not widely used.

3. Succinimides. Ethosuximide is effective in treating absence (petit mal) seizures and myoclonus. Blood counts are made to monitor for agranulocytosis. Phensuximide is used for treating psychomotor epilepsy.

4. Oxazolidinediones. Trimethadione is only rarely used for absence (petit mal) seizures because of a high incidence of serious side

effects: allergic dermatitis, kidney and liver damage, agranulocytosis, and aplastic anemia.

5. Benzodiazepines. Diazepam is used principally as an intravenous medication to terminate status epilepticus. Clonazepam is given for absence (petit mal) and myoclonic seizures and infantile spasms. Personality changes (hyperactivity, aggressive behavior) or slurred speech, confusion, and abnormal eye movements are sometimes seen in children. These symptoms usually can be controlled by lowering the dose.

6. Carbamazepine. Carbamazepine is effective in treating psychomotor and grand mal epilepsy. Side effects of carbamazepine include drowsiness, ataxia, double vision, and gastrointestinal upset. Blood counts are required to monitor for bone marrow depression.

7. Valproic acid. Valproic acid is effective in treating progressive myoclonus that had previously resisted therapy. Gastrointestinal distress is an occasional side effect, and the incidence of liver damage is being examined.

8. Other drugs. Acetazolamide is a carbonic anhydrase inhibitor used in treating absence (petit mal) seizures. Paraldehyde and lidocaine are drugs of last resort to terminate status epilepticus. Adrenocorticotropic hormone (ACTH) is used to treat infantile spasms.

STUDY QUESTIONS

1. Define epilepsy and list some of the known causes. What other conditions can precipitate seizures?
2. Describe grand mal, absence (petit mal), myoclonal, psychomotor, and focal seizures and infantile spasms. List the drug of choice for treating each type of epilepsy.
3. What is status epilepticus and how is it treated?
4. What considerations need to be made in beginning drug administration to control epilepsy?
5. Which are the long-acting barbiturates used in treating epilepsy? What are the side effects?
6. What are the adverse effects and drug interactions of phenytoin?
7. What are the adverse effects of the succinimides?

8. Why is trimethadione no longer widely used to treat absence (petit mal) seizures?
9. Which benzodiazepines are used as anticonvulsants? For which seizure types are they effective?
10. What are the uses and side effects of carbamazepine?
11. Why is valproic acid a valuable anticonvulsant?
12. Describe the use of acetazolamide, paraldehyde, lidocaine, and adrenocorticotropic hormone (ACTH) as anticonvulsants.

SUGGESTED READINGS

Berkovic, S.F., and others: Progressive myoclonus epilepsies: specific causes and diagnosis, N. Engl. J. Med. **315**:296, 1986.

Brodoff, A.S.: Intervening to stop status epilepticus, Patient Care **17**(17):153, 1983.

Callaghan, N., Garrett, A., and Goggin, T.: Withdrawal of anticonvulsant drugs in patients free of seizures for two years, N. Engl. J. Med. **318**:942, 1988.

Callanan, M.: Epilepsy: putting the patient back in control, RN **51**(2):48, 1988.

Chadwick, D.: Comparison of monotherapy with valproate and other antiepileptic drugs in the treatment of seizure disorders, Am. J. Med. **84**(suppl. 1A):2, 1988.

Desai, B.T.: Complex partial seizures, Am. Fam. Physician **30**(3):158, 1984.

Dreifuss, F.E., and others: Epilepsy: management by medication, Patient Care **22**(7):52, 1988.

Elwes, R.D.C., and others: The prognosis for seizure control in newly diagnosed epilepsy, N. Engl. J. Med. **311**(15):944, 1984.

Frank, J., and Fischer, R.G.: Drug interactions with carbamazepine, Pediatr. Nurs. **13**(1):54, 1987.

Friedman, D.: Taking the scare out of caring for seizure patients, Nursing 88 **18**(2):52, 1988.

Grabow, JD.: Diagnosis of epileptic seizures, Postgrad. Med. **77**:207, 1985.

Jabbari, B.: Management of epileptic seizures in adults, Am. Fam. Physician **31**:162, 1985.

Kandt, R.S., Bickley, S.K., and Shimp, L.A.: Discontinuing antiepileptic therapy, Am. Fam. Physician **31**:177, 1985.

Lesser, R.P., and Pippenger, C.E.: Choosing an antiepileptic drug, Postgrad. Med. **77**:225, 1985.

Parks, B.R. Jr.: Febrile seizures, Pediatr. Nurs. **14**(6):518, 1988.

Santilli, N., and Sierzant, T.L.: Advances in the treatment of epilepsy, J. Neurosci. Nurs. **19**(3):141, 1987.

Shinnar, S., and others: Discontinuing antiepileptic medication in children with epilepsy after two years without seizures, N. Engl. J. Med. **313**:976, 1985.

Snead, O.C. III, and Hosey, L.C.: Exacerbation of seizures in children by carbamazepine, N. Engl. J. Med. **313**:916, 1985.

Wilder, B.J., and Schmidt, R.P.: Current classification of epilepsies, Postgrad. Med. **77**:188, 1985.

Wroblewski, B.A., Singer, W.D., and Whyte, J.: Carbamazepine-erythromycin interaction, JAMA **155**:1165, 1986.

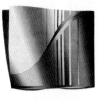

Central Motor Control: Drugs for Parkinsonism and Centrally Acting Skeletal Muscle Relaxants

48

NEUROPHARMACOLOGY OF PARKINSON'S DISEASE
Characteristics of Parkinson's Disease

Parkinson's disease is a movement disorder characterized by rigidity, akinesia, and tremor. *Rigidity* means that the muscle tone is greatly increased but reflex activity is not. When a limb is passively forced through flexor or extensor movements, the muscular resistance alternately increases and decreases to give a cogwheel effect. *Akinesia* (no motion) refers to the difficulty the patient has in initiating any movement. The face even has a masklike, fixed expression devoid of emotion. Early in the course of Parkinson's disease, the difficulty in initiating movement is not as marked and is termed *bradykinesia* (slow motion). The tremor of Parkinson's disease is seen mostly in the limbs at rest and decreases with movement of the limbs.

Role of acetylcholine and dopamine. The insight into the neurochemical defect in Parkinson's disease is the classic example of our growing knowledge of the role of neurotransmitters in controlling given functions within the complex central nervous system. For many years anticholinergic drugs such as atropine had been used to decrease the tremor characteristics of Parkinson's disease; acetylcholine therefore seemed important in accounting for some of the symptoms. When the antipsychotic drugs (major tranquilizers) were introduced in the 1950s, symptoms indistinguishable from those of Parkinson's disease began to appear in patients treated with these drugs. It is now known that this is because these drugs block receptors for the central nervous system neurotransmitter dopamine. Subsequently, patients with Parkinson's disease were shown to have degeneration of crucial dopaminergic neurons projecting to cer-

tain of the basal ganglia of the extrapyramidal system in the brain. This system is responsible for maintaining motor coordination at the central nervous system level.

The present understanding of Parkinson's disease is that it represents a deficiency in the neurotransmitter dopamine in certain basal ganglia. Dopamine from these neuronal tracts is believed to exert an inhibitory influence on cholinergic neurons of the extrapyramidal system controlling muscle tone. When dopamine is lacking, muscle tone increases because of the unopposed action of acetylcholine, resulting in muscular rigidity, inhibition of spontaneous movements, and tremor. The lack of dopamine is secondary to a progressive degeneration of specific dopaminergic neurons. This degeneration can occur because of encephalitis, carbon monoxide poisoning, manganese poisoning, a cerebrovascular accident, or, more commonly, unknown causes. This degeneration cannot be arrested. Drugs alleviate the symptoms for only a few years.

The current rationale for the pharmacological treatment of Parkinson's disease is to diminish the severity of motor symptoms by blocking the excessive action of acetylcholine and/or by replenishing the dopamine to return the balance of excitatory acetylcholine action and inhibitory dopamine action toward normal.

Drug-induced parkinsonism. Certain drugs also can cause symptoms of Parkinson's disease. Reserpine (Serpasil), which depletes neuronal stores of dopamine as well as of norepinephrine, and the antipsychotic drugs, which block dopamine receptors, are the usual causes of drug induced parkinsonism. Since the symptoms depend on the presence of the drug, lowering the dosage or discontinuing the drug eliminates the symptoms.

Anticholinergic Drugs to Treat Parkinsonism
(Table 48.1)

Early in the course of Parkinson's disease, an anticholinergic drug is frequently given to lessen rigidity, bradykinesia, and tremor. Atropine and scopolamine, the classic anticholinergic drugs, were used for treatment of the symptoms of Parkinson's disease for many years. The anticholinergic drugs used today are synthetic drugs that are centrally active and produce fewer peripheral side effects. These drugs include *procyclidine (Kemadrin), trihexyphenidyl (Tremin, others), benztropine (Cogentin), biperiden (Akineton),* and *ethopropazine (Parsidol).* An anticholinergic drug is also the drug of choice to treat extrapyramidal reactions arising from the antipsychotic drugs: akathisia, acute dystonia, and parkinsonism. Tardive dyskinesia is not reversed by anticholinergic drugs. These extrapyramidal reactions are described in Chapter 41.

Administration and side effects. The dosage of the anticholinergic drugs must be started low and increased gradually to overcome side effects and to individualize the dose. The common side effects of the anticholinergic drugs are the classic effects of dry mouth, constipation, urinary retention, and blurred vision. Common mental effects include an impairment of recent memory, confusion, insomnia, and restlessness. Mental effects can become serious, with the development of agitation, disorientation, delirium, paranoid reactions, or hallucinations. Mental problems are more common with those elderly patients who have preexisting mental disturbances. Patients who have prior histories of glaucoma, particularly narrow-angle glaucoma, or some type of urinary or intestinal obstruction or tachycardia are not good candidates, since anticholinergic drugs can aggravate any of these conditions. Characteristic actions of anticholinergic drugs are discussed in detail in Chapter 9.

Antihistaminic Drugs to Treat Parkinsonism
(Table 48.1)

Those antihistaminic drugs that have pronounced anticholinergic effects may be substituted for anticholinergic drugs. Three antihistaminic drugs are sometimes used to treat the symptoms of parkinsonism: *chlorphenoxamine (Phenoxene), diphenhydramine (Benadryl),* and *orphenadrine (Disipal).* Compared to the anticholinergic drugs, these antihistamines have milder although similar side effects and are less potent. The effectiveness of the antihistamines in treating the symptoms of parkinsonism is attributed to their anticholinergic

effect. Antihistamines also have a sedative effect. They are discussed in detail in Chapter 24.

Other Drugs to Treat Parkinsonism
(Table 48.1)

Amantadine

Amantadine (Symmetrel) is an antiviral agent that also has been found effective in reducing the severity of symptoms of Parkinson's disease when used either alone or with an anticholinergic or antihistaminic drug. Amantadine promotes the release of dopamine from the central neurons, an action unrelated to its antiviral action.

Amantadine often is used as a first drug to control the symptoms of parkinsonism. It has the advantages of being effective when administered as a single daily dose and of having few side effects. Side effects that are sometimes seen include dizziness, nervousness, inability to concentrate, ataxia, slurred speech, insomnia, lethargy, blurred vision, dryness of the mouth, gastrointestinal upset, and rash. Amantadine also may be used with anticholinergic drugs or with levodopa, since it enhances the effectiveness of these other drugs and allows a reduction of their dosage.

Levodopa

Mechanism of action. When the drugs just mentioned can no longer adequately relieve the symptoms of Parkinson's disease, levodopa (Dopar, Larodopa) is administered. Levodopa therapy does not stop the progression of Parkinson's disease but does relieve the symptoms and dramatically improves ability to function. Levodopa is the chemical precursor of dopamine, and unlike dopamine, levodopa readily crosses the blood-brain barrier. It is converted to dopamine by the enzyme dopa decarboxylase. About 75% of a dose of levodopa is converted to dopamine in the periphery rather than in the brain, however, and the high plasma concentration of dopamine is responsible for the nausea and cardiac effects attending this therapy.

Administration. Levodopa is taken orally, and the peak effect is seen 1 to 2 hours later. The dosage is adjusted up or down gradually every 2 to 3 days to lessen the incidence of nausea and to avoid precipitating side effects.

Emetic side effect. Dopamine is the neurotransmitter for the chemoreceptor trigger zone of the medulla and thus produces nausea, vomiting, and anorexia. To effect tolerance to this emetic action, levodopa therapy must be initiated by starting with low doses that are gradually increased. A snack high in protein also helps to prevent nausea. Antiemet-

Table 48.1 Drugs to Treat Parkinsonism

Generic name	Trade name	Administration/dosage	Comments
ANTICHOLINERGICS			
Benztropine mesylate	Cogentin*	ORAL: *Adults*—0.5 to 1 mg at bedtime initially, increased gradually to 4 to 6 mg if required. FDA Pregnancy Category C. For drug-induced extrapyramidal reactions: ORAL, INTRAMUSCULAR, INTRAVENOUS: *Adults*—1 to 4 mg or 2 times daily. For an acute dystonic reaction: ORAL, INTRAVENOUS: *Adults*—2 mg IV, then 1 to 2 mg orally twice daily.	To treat Parkinson's disease and drug-induced extrapyramidal reactions. Particularly effective in reversing an acute dystonic reaction to an antipsychotic drug.
Biperiden	Akineton*	ORAL: *Adults*—2 mg 3 times daily; may increase dose up to 20 mg daily if required. FDA Pregnancy Category C. For drug-induced extrapyramidal reactions: ORAL: *Adults*—2 mg 1 to 3 times daily. INTRAMUSCULAR: *Adults*—2 mg repeated as often as every 30 min but no more than 4 doses in 24 hours. *Children*—0.04 mg/kg body weight as often as every 30 min but no more than 4 doses in 24 hours.	To treat Parkinson's disease and drug-induced extrapyramidal reactions.
Ethopropazine	Parsidol Parsitan†	ORAL: *Adults*—50 mg 1 or 2 times daily initially. Mild to moderate cases require 100 to 400 mg daily. Severe cases may require 500 to 600 mg daily. FDA Pregnancy Category C.	To treat Parkinson's disease. A phenothiazine with only anticholinergic effects and devoid of antidopaminergic effects.
Procyclidine hydrochloride	Kemadrin* Procyclid†	ORAL: *Adults*—5 mg twice daily, up to 20 to 30 mg daily if required. FDA Pregnancy Category C. For drug-induced extrapyramidal reactions: ORAL: *Adults*—2 to 2.5 mg 3 times daily, increased to 10 to 20 mg daily if required.	To treat Parkinson's disease and drug-induced extrapyramidal reactions.
Trihexyphenidyl hydrochloride	Artane* Trihexy†	ORAL: *Adults*—2 mg 2 or 3 times daily. Increased to 15 to 20 mg daily (usually) or 40 to 50 mg daily (rarely) to control symptoms. FDA Pregnancy Category C. For drug-induced parkinsonism: ORAL: *Adults*—1 mg initially. Subsequent doses increased if symptoms do not decrease. Usual daily dose, 5 to 15 mg.	To treat Parkinson's disease and drug-induced extrapyramidal reactions.
ANTIHISTAMINES			
Diphenhydramine hydrochloride	Benadryl*	ORAL: *Adults*—25 mg 3 times daily, increased to 50 mg 4 times daily if required. For drug-induced extrapyramidal reactions: INTRAMUSCULAR, INTRAVENOUS: *Adults*—10 to 50 mg; maximum, 400 mg daily. *Children*—IM 5 mg/kg body weight daily; maximum 300 mg in 24 hr.	To treat Parkinson's disease and drug-induced extrapyramidal reactions. Marked sedative effects.
Orphenadrine hydrochloride	Disipal*	ORAL: *Adults*—50 mg 3 times daily; up to 250 mg if required.	To treat Parkinson's disease.

*Available in Canada and United States.
†Available in Canada only.

Continued.

Table 48.1   Drugs to Treat Parkinsonism—cont'd

Generic name	Trade name	Administration/dosage	Comments
OTHERS			
Amantadine	Symadine Symmetrel*	ORAL: *Adults*—100 mg daily after breakfast for 5 to 7 days. An additional 100 mg may be added after lunch.	An antiviral agent to treat Parkinson's disease. Side effects are similar to anticholinergic effects.
Levodopa	Dopar Larodopa*	ORAL: *Adults*—initially 300 to 1000 mg daily in 3 to 7 doses during waking hours with food. Increase dosage 100 to 500 mg every 2 to 3 days or more until desired control is achieved. Usually requires 4 to 6 Gm and 6 to 8 weeks to achieve control. After several months to 1 year the dosage may be lowered.	To treat Parkinson's disease.
Carbidopa-levodopa	Sinemet	ORAL: *Adults*—initial daily dose of Sinemet should be ¼ of the levodopa daily dose. Sinemet should be administered 8 hours after the last levodopa dose and is given in 3 or 4 doses daily. Patients not previously receiving levodopa are started with 10:100 mg (carbidopa:levodopa) 3 times daily, and the dosage is gradually increased as required.	To treat Parkinson's disease. Ratio of levodopa to carbidopa is 10:1. Carbidopa inhibits the degradation of dopamine outside the central nervous system.
Bromocriptine	Parlodel	ORAL: *Adults*—initially, 1.25 mg twice daily, increased every other week or monthly by 1.25 to 2.5 mg until benefits are achieved or adverse effects become intolerable.	To treat Parkinson's disease. May be added to levodopa or carbidopa-levodopa therapy; occasionally replaces levodopa therapy.

*Available in Canada and United States.

ics from the phenothiazine class should not be used, since they will block the therapeutic action of dopamine. Trimethobenzamide (Tigan) may be taken early in the morning to control nausea.

Cardiovascular side effects. Another side effect sometimes seen at the start of levodopa therapy is orthostatic hypotension. The mechanism is not known but is believed to be a central nervous system effect rather than a peripheral effect. This hypotension tends to decrease with time. An increase in heart rate and force of contraction may also be apparent at the start of therapy. These cardiac actions are caused by the direct action of dopamine on the heart. Cardiac arrhythmias may develop and must then be controlled by appropriate medication.

Other side effects. Additional effects of levodopa therapy may include an assortment of gastrointestinal effects, including bleeding, difficulty in swallowing, and a burning sensation of the tongue. Respiratory effects such as cough, hoarseness, and disturbed breathing may appear. Because of these side effects, levodopa therapy is used cautiously for patients with a history of heart disease, asthma, emphysema, or peptic ulcer. Problems in urination from incontinence to retention may arise.

Blurred vision or dilated pupils may be caused by levodopa therapy. Levodopa therapy is not considered for patients with narrow-angle glaucoma and only with careful monitoring for patients with chronic (wide-angle) glaucoma. Hepatic, hematopoietic, cardiovascular, and renal function tests are performed periodically on patients receiving long-term levodopa therapy. This is because many laboratory test values are high in patients receiving levodopa therapy and only careful monitoring can determine whether or not a real problem exists. Hematocrit and white blood cell counts may be lowered by levodopa therapy, but therapy is discontinued only when abnormally low counts are found. Therapy is not initiated in patients with blood disorders.

Additional effects typically noted after the start of levodopa therapy include an increased alertness, sense of well-being, and an increased sex drive. All these effects are attributed to behavioral roles of dopamine in the brain. Further mental changes may occur with prolonged therapy. Most frequently seen are euphoria, restlessness, anxiety, irritability, hyperactivity, insomnia, and vivid dreams. Patients occasionally may become paranoid and experience psychotic episodes or become depressed, with or without suicidal tendencies. These mental changes are usually reversed with a lowering of the dosage.

Side effects after prolonged therapy. After prolonged therapy with levodopa, abnormal involuntary movements (dyskinesia) alternating with a

THE NURSING PROCESS

DRUGS TO TREAT PARKINSON'S DISEASE

Assessment

None of the drugs used to treat Parkinson's disease can cure it. Drug therapy will often be withheld until the patient and/or the physician decide that the symptoms are troublesome. The drugs are associated with side effects. The nurse should obtain a general baseline patient assessment, including vital signs, joint movement, amount of tremor, affect and objective signs of the disease, and ability to ambulate and perform activities of daily living. Because this is often a disease of the elderly, a baseline view of other known health problems, such as hypertension, diabetes, and cardiovascular or renal disease, also should be obtained.

Nursing diagnoses

Altered bowel elimination: constipation

Potential complication: urinary retention

Possible body image disturbance related to dyskinesia or other drug side effects

Management

The drugs are prescribed sequentially, with anticholinergic or antihistaminic drugs used before levodopa or carbidopa. The nurse should look for side effects and treat these when possible. The patient should be included in the discussion of the goals of therapy. Occasionally patients will find that the side effects resulting from a drug are worse than if the disease were left untreated, at least at some stages in its progression.

Improvement in symptoms should outweigh the discomfort of side effects. In preparing for discharge, the patient needs instruction about the drugs prescribed as well as referral to social service, vocational rehabilitation, visiting nurse, and other agencies. The patient having difficulty with specific activities of daily living should be assisted to find new ways to perform these activities.

The nurse should observe the patient for the side effects of the drugs or for aggravation of preexisting conditions. For example, amantadine has precipitated congestive heart failure. In patients with a history of congestive heart failure, the nurse should check the weight and blood pressure and auscultate the lungs on a regular basis.

Evaluation

Evaluation of the therapeutic effectiveness involves both subjective and objective improvement in comparison to the number and severity of side effects present. The symptoms should be evaluated regularly for progression of the disease, and the patient's overall functioning monitored. Family members in frequent contact with the patient may also be helpful in providing data. Before discharge and at regular intervals during therapy, the patient should be evaluated for the ability to explain the drug, its dose, and how to take the drug correctly; the expected goals of therapy; and the side effects, how to treat them, and which require that the physician be notified. The patient should also be able to explain any necessary dietary or vitamin restrictions. For additional specific information, see the patient care implications section.

sudden lapse in symptom control (the "on-off" phenomenon) may appear. The dyskinesia usually comprises abnormal involuntary movements of the mouth, tongue, face, and/or neck. Dyskinesia usually appears 1 to 2 hours after the latest dose of levodopa and represents a mild levodopa toxicity. "End-of-the-dose" akinesia also may occur. This means that the akinesia appears just before a new dose is to be taken and usually can be avoided by increasing the frequency of administration.

Carbidopa-levodopa (Sinemet)

Carbidopa inhibits the conversion of levodopa to dopamine. Since carbidopa cannot enter the central nervous system, only the peripheral conversion is inhibited. This means that levodopa is converted to dopamine only in the brain, so the presence of carbidopa lowers the dose of levodopa required by 75%. Since the emetic effects of levodopa reflect peripheral dopamine concentrations, the incidence of nausea and vomiting is reduced greatly with carbidopa-levodopa combination. Carbidopa is available only in a fixed ratio combination with levodopa.

Bromocriptine

Bromocriptine (Parlodel) mimics the action of dopamine in the brain. It is an alternative to levodopa when levodopa is contraindicated, is not well tolerated, or does not produce a response. Bromocriptine has a duration of action similar to that of levodopa and may be added to levodopa or carbidopa-levodopa therapy for patients who show symptoms of fluctuating doses such as dystonia and muscle cramps.

Doses of bromocriptine must be individualized. Transient dizziness and nausea are common. Hypotension, abdominal pain, blurred vision, double vision, and vasospasm of the fingers and toes in response to cold also occasionally occur.

Deprenyl

Deprenyl is a newly approved drug that inhibits the enzyme monoamine oxidase B, which degrades dopamine in the brain. Since dopamine is not rapidly degraded in the presence of deprenyl, the duration of action and dose of levodopa is reduced. The early morning stiffness and end-of-dose symptoms are decreased. Deprenyl is added to either levodopa or carbidopa-levodopa therapy.

CENTRALLY ACTING SKELETAL MUSCLE RELAXANTS

Drugs to Treat Spasticity (Table 48.2)

Spasticity results from the loss of inhibitory tone in the polysynaptic pathways of the spinal cord so that fine control of motor activity is lost. Since the inhibitory tone is controlled largely by neural pathways from the brain, spasticity is seen in patients in whom these inhibitory pathways have been disrupted through spinal cord injury, cerebrovascular accidents (strokes), multiple sclerosis, or cerebral palsy. The patient with spasticity has exaggerated reflexes (spinal spasticity) or inappropriate posture (cerebral spasticity).

Three drugs have been found effective in relieving some cases of spasticity: *diazepam (Valium), baclofen (Lioresal),* and *dantrolene (Dantrium).* Diazepam and baclofen are believed to act within the spinal cord to restore some inhibitory tone, but dantrolene is unique in acting within the muscle itself.

Diazepam

Diazepam (Valium) is a benzodiazepine commonly prescribed as an antianxiety drug (see Chapter 40). Although its action as an antianxiety drug results from depression of the reticular activating system, diazepam also enhances inhibitory descending pathways in the spinal cord governing muscular activity, apparently by enhancing the activity of the inhibitory neurotransmitter gamma aminobutyric acid (GABA). Diazepam is effective both in relieving spasticity associated with spinal cord injury, multiple sclerosis, and cerebral injury and in treating muscle spasms (see next section). Relatively high doses are required to relieve muscle hyperactivity, and drowsiness and incoordination may be prominent side effects.

Baclofen

Baclofen (Lioresal) is an analog of the inhibitory neurotransmitter gamma aminobutyric acid (GABA) and although the effect elicited is that desired of a GABA agonist, this mechanism of action cannot be demonstrated in the laboratory. Baclofen is most effective in relieving spasticity secondary to spinal cord injury and is less effective in relieving spasticity secondary to brain damage. Side effects include drowsiness, incoordination, and occasional gastrointestinal upset.

Dantrolene

Dantrolene (Dantrium) is not a centrally acting skeletal muscle relaxant but instead affects the muscle directly by interfering with the intracellular release of calcium necessary to initiate contraction. At therapeutic doses this effect is limited to skeletal muscle and is not seen in the heart or smooth muscle. Dantrolene will cause muscular weakness and can worsen the overall condition if the patient already has marginal strength. Dantrolene is most

Table 48.2   Centrally Acting Skeletal Muscle Relaxants

Generic name	Trade name	Administration/dosage	Comments
DRUGS TO TREAT SPASTICITY			
Baclofen	Lioresal*	ORAL: *Adults*—Begin with 5 mg 3 times daily. Increase by 5 mg 3 times daily every 3 days as required; maximum, 80 mg.	Diminishes reflex responses by decreasing transmission in the spinal cord.
Dantrolene	Dantrium*	ORAL: *Adults*—25 mg 1 or 2 times daily. Increase to 25 mg 3 to 4 times daily, then 50 to 100 mg 4 times daily as required. Increments are made every 4 to 7 days.	Acts peripherally to inhibit calcium release within the muscle.
Diazepam	Valium*	ORAL: *Adults*—2 to 10 mg 4 times daily. *Children*—0.12 to 0.8 mg/kg body weight daily in 3 or 4 doses. INTRAVENOUS: *Adults*—2 to 10 mg injected no faster than 5 mg (1 ml)/min. Do not mix or dilute with other solutions, drugs, or IV fluids. *Children*—0.04 to 0.2 mg/kg body weight; maximum, 0.6 mg/kg in 8 hr.	A benzodiazepine that is also used for the treatment of spasticity or muscle spasm.
DRUGS TO TREAT MUSCLE SPASMS			
Carisoprodol	Rela Soma*	ORAL: *Adults*—350 mg 4 times daily.	Related to meprobamate. May cause drowsiness.
Chlorphenesin	Maolate	ORAL: *Adults*—800 mg 3 times daily. Can decrease to 400 mg 4 times daily as improvement is noted.	May cause drowsiness and dizziness.
Chlorzoxazone	Paraflex	ORAL: *Adults*—250 to 750 mg 3 or 4 times daily. *Children*—20 mg/kg body weight in 3 or 4 divided doses.	May cause drowsiness. Watch for signs of liver damage (rare).
Cyclobenzaprine	Flexeril*	ORAL: *Adults*—10 mg 3 times daily up to a maximum total dose of 60 mg.	Related to the tricyclic antidepressants. Does not cause drug dependence but may cause changes in the liver.
Diazepam	Valium*	Same as for valium to treat spasticity.	
Metaxalone	Skelaxin	ORAL: *Adults*—800 mg 3 or 4 times daily.	Patient should be monitored for development of liver toxicity.
Methocarbamol	Delaxin Robamol Robaxin*	ORAL: *Adults*—1.5 to 2 Gm 4 times daily for 2 to 3 days. Decrease to 1 Gm 4 times daily for maintenance. INTRAMUSCULAR: *Adults*—500 mg every 8 hr, alternating between the gluteal muscles. INTRAVENOUS: *Adults*—1 to 3 Gm daily for a maximum of 3 days. Inject no faster than 300 mg (3 ml)/min.	Not recommended for patients with epilepsy. Do not administer parenterally to patients with impaired renal function because the drug vehicle may worsen kidney function.
Orphenadrine	Flexon Neocyten Norflex* Tega-Flex	ORAL: *Adults*—100 mg twice daily. INTRAMUSCULAR, INTRAVENOUS: *Adults*—60 mg twice daily.	Anticholinergic effects are common side effects. Not for patients with glaucoma, myasthenia gravis, tachycardia, or urinary retention.

*Available in Canada and United States.

THE NURSING PROCESS

CENTRALLY ACTING SKELETAL MUSCLE RELAXANTS

Assessment

Muscle spasticity is seen in multiple sclerosis, spinal cord injury or disease, and some other conditions. Less severe muscle spasm is seen after orthopedic trauma or surgery and with some musculoskeletal diseases. In the case of severe onset, the spasticity often is clearly visible at all times or occurs in response to stimulation. Some kinds of spasticity are localized with a specific muscle group, such as spasticity associated with severe low back pain. In general nursing situations, diazepam is used most often; dantrolene is reserved for use when no other drug is effective or when spasticity is moderate to severe.

The baseline data should include a general assessment with an additional focus on the spasticity, including such factors as the degree of spasticity, the aggravating factors, the associated pain, and the degree to which the spasticity interferes with the activities of daily living or the activities that could increase independence. If dantrolene is used, baseline liver function studies should be obtained.

Nursing diagnoses

Possible sexual dysfunction: impotence

Potential complication: excessive drowsiness and dizziness

Management

During adjustment of drug dosage, the nurse should monitor the patient for both the drug effectiveness and the presence of side effects. Weeks of therapy may be needed before a lessening of spasticity occurs. These drugs also may be used with other therapies, including traction, physical therapy, exercises, bed rest, and application of heat. If drowsiness occurs, appropriate measures to provide for the patient's safety should be employed, including keeping the side rails up and supervising ambulation. Liver function studies should be monitored with dantrolene therapy.

Evaluation

The goal of therapy is to decrease spasticity, but this does not always occur. At regular intervals the nurse should evaluate the continuing degree of spasticity. Not all side effects that may occur are undesirable, so decisions related to them should be individualized. For example, a patient who is drowsy when receiving short-term diazepam therapy may be better able to tolerate enforced bed rest because of the drowsiness. Before discharge the patient should be able to explain the drugs and how to take them correctly; the side effects that may occur and which require notification of the physician; how to perform additional therapies, such as application of heat and exercises; and when to return for additional help. For specific information, see the patient care implications section.

---

useful for the patient whose spasticity causes pain, discomfort, or limits functional rehabilitation. In addition to the spasticity secondary to spinal cord injury, dantrolene can be effective in relieving the spasticity of cerebrovascular accident, cerebral palsy, or multiple sclerosis for which the other drugs have limited effectiveness.

The major limitation to the use of dantrolene is liver damage. Baseline liver function studies are made before therapy starts, and regular liver func-

tion studies are performed throughout therapy. The drug is discontinued if no relief of spasticity is achieved in 6 weeks.

Muscle Spasms and Their Treatment
(Table 48.2)

Muscle spasms are local muscle contractions initiated by muscle or tendon injury and inflammation. Muscle spasms occur in conditions such as sprains, bursitis, arthritis, and lower back pain.

PATIENT CARE IMPLICATIONS

General guidelines for patients receiving drugs to treat Parkinson's disease

Patient and family education

- Review the anticipated benefits and possible side effects of drug therapy.
- Teach patients and families that several weeks to months of therapy may be needed in some cases to obtain full benefit of drug therapy. Provide emotional support as needed.
- Parkinson's disease is primarily a problem of the elderly. However, if a premenopausal woman develops Parkinson's disease, counsel as needed about contraceptives. These drugs should not be used during pregnancy without consultation with the physician.
- Point out to family members that confusion is often a drug side effect in the elderly, and should not be attributed to Parkinson's disease until fully evaluated.
- Warn patients not to discontinue these drugs suddenly. Keep all health care providers informed of all drugs being taken. Avoid over-the-counter medications unless approved by the physician.
- Avoid the use of alcohol unless permitted in small amounts by the physician.

Other drug groups

- The anticholinergic drugs are discussed in Chapters 9 and 13. Also see Patient Problems: Dry Mouth on p. 170; Constipation on p. 187; Orthostatic Hypotension on p. 237.
- Antihistamines are discussed in Chapter 24.
- Phenothiazines are discussed in Chapter 41.

Amantadine

Drug administration

- Assess mental status regularly. Be alert to signs of increasing depression: lethargy, apathy, decreased appetite, loss of interest in personal appearance. Be alert to suicidal tendencies.
- Monitor intake, output, daily weight, blood pressure, pulse. Auscultate lung sounds. Inspect for development of edema and skin changes.
- Assess for urinary retention. Suggest patients void before taking doses.
- Monitor complete blood count and differential.

Patient and family education

- See the general guidelines.

- See Patient Problems: Orthostatic Hypotension on p. 237; Constipation on p. 187.
- Warn patients to avoid driving or operating hazardous equipment if drowsiness or dizziness develops; notify physician.
- Capsules may be opened and contents mixed with a small amount of food or fluid for ease in taking dose, although a liquid preparation is also available.
- Tell patients that livedo reticularis (bluish or purplish mottling of the skin) generally appears during the first year of therapy and may take several weeks to subside when therapy is discontinued.

Levodopa

Drug administration

- Monitor neuromuscular, neurologic, and mental status regularly.
- Monitor blood pressure and pulse, intake and output, and weight.
- Check stools for presence of occult blood. Inspect for skin changes.
- Monitor complete blood count and differential, platelet count, BUN, liver function tests.

Patient and family education

- See the general guidelines.
- See Patient Problems: Constipation on p. 187; Orthostatic Hypotension on p. 237; Dry Mouth on p. 170.
- Warn male patients that priapism has been reported; notify the physician if it develops.
- Tell the patient that sweat may be darker in color while on this drug, and urine may be dark, especially if left standing.
- Take doses with meals or snack to reduce gastric irritation.
- If patients have difficulty swallowing levodopa capsules or tablets, consult the pharmacist about preparing a liquid form.
- Tell diabetic patients to monitor blood glucose levels carefully, as tests for urinary glucose and ketone may be inaccurate.
- There are many side effects of levodopa therapy. Encourage the patient and family to report the development of any new or unexpected finding.
- Pyridoxine (vitamin B_6) may reduce the effectiveness of levodopa. Do not take any vitamin preparations without prior consultation with the physician. Limit intake of foods high in pyridoxine; see Dietary Consideration: Vitamins on p. 282.

Continued.

PATIENT CARE IMPLICATIONS — cont'd

Carbidopa-levodopa combination

Drug administration/patient and family education

- No specific side effects have been attributed to carbidopa. Review with patients the information about levodopa.

Bromocriptine

Bromocriptine is discussed in Chapter 53.

Baclofen

Drug administration

- Assess mental status and monitor regularly.
- Monitor blood pressure every 4 hours until stable. Be alert to hypotension when ambulating patients, especially if they have been immobilized or primarily sedentary prior to the start of drug therapy.
- Monitor intake, output, and weight. Monitor respiratory rate, auscultate lung sounds, and assess for occurrence of dyspnea. Inspect for skin changes and development of edema.
- Monitor complete blood count, urinalysis.
- Assess tactfully regarding impotence. Provide emotional support as needed. Remind patients not to discontinue medications without consulting the physician.

Patient and family education

- Teach patients that several days to weeks of therapy may be necessary before improvement is seen. On the other hand, if improvement is not seen in 6 to 8 weeks, the drug is usually withdrawn.
- See Patient Problems: Constipation on p. 187; Dry Mouth on p. 170.
- Warn patients to avoid driving or operating hazardous equipment if drowsiness develops.
- Caution diabetic patients to monitor blood glucose levels carefully, as an adjustment in diet or insulin may be needed.
- Avoid the use of alcohol unless permitted in small amounts by the physician.
- Remind patients to keep all health care providers informed of all drugs being taken.
- Take doses with meals or snack to lessen gastric irritation.

Dantrolene

Drug administration

- Assess mental status and monitor regularly. Watch for signs of depression: withdrawal, lack of interest in personal appearance, insomnia, anorexia, weight loss.

- Monitor blood pressure and pulse. When used for treatment of malignant hyperthermia, attach patient to cardiac monitor.
- Be alert to hypotension when assisting patients to ambulate, especially if patients have been immobilized or primarily sedentary before receiving drug therapy.
- Check stools for occult blood.
- Monitor intake, output. Monitor urinalysis or check urine for blood.
- Assess males tactfully regarding difficulty in achieving erection. Provide emotional support as appropriate. Caution patient not to discontinue medications without consulting physician.
- Auscultate lung sounds: watch for pleural effusion.
- Inspect skin for abnormal hair growth or rash.
- Monitor complete blood count, liver function tests.

INTRAVENOUS DANTROLENE
- Dilute each 20 mg with 60 ml sterile water for injection that does not contain a bacteriostatic agent. Shake solution until clear. Administer as rapid IV push. Once reconstituted and diluted, solution must be protected from light and used within 6 hours.

Patient and family education

- Review anticipated benefits and possible side effects of drug therapy. Tell the patient to notify the physician of any unexpected finding.
- See Patient Problems: Constipation on p. 187; Photosensitivity on p. 647.
- Reassure patients that several days to weeks of therapy may be necessary before improvement is seen. On the other hand, if improvement is not seen in 6 to 8 weeks, the drug is usually withdrawn.
- Warn patients to avoid driving or operating hazardous equipment if dizziness or drowsiness develops.
- Avoid the use of alcohol unless permitted in small amounts by the physician.
- Remind patients to keep all health care providers informed of all medications being taken.
- Instruct patients who develop malignant hyperthermia to wear a medical identification tag or bracelet indicating this fact.

Diazepam

Diazepam is discussed in Chapter 40.

PATIENT CARE IMPLICATIONS — cont'd

Drugs to treat muscle spasms

Drug administration

- Assess for CNS side effects: dizziness, ataxia, vertigo.
- Warn patients that IM injections may cause a burning sensation at the injection site.
- Consult the manufacturer's literature for information about IV administration.
- Intravenous administration: Have the patient supine. Keep side rails up. Monitor vital signs. Keep recumbent until blood pressure is stable. Supervise ambulation.
- Monitor complete blood count and differential, and liver function tests.
- These drugs may cause allergic reactions. Check patients frequently when beginning therapy. Have available drugs and equipment to treat acute allergic reactions in settings where these drugs are administered.

Patient and family education

- Review anticipated benefits and possible side effects of drug therapy.

- Warn patients to avoid driving or operating hazardous equipment if drowsiness, dizziness, or visual changes develop.
- See Patient Problems: Orthostatic Hypotension on p. 237; Dry Mouth on p. 170; Constipation on p. 187.
- Remind patients to use medications only as directed. Keep all health care providers informed of all medications being taken.
- Avoid alcohol unless permitted in small amounts by the physician.
- Take oral doses with meals or snack to lessen gastric irritation.
- Take the final dose of the day at bedtime.
- Warn patients taking chlorzoxazone that the urine may turn orange or purple-red while they are taking this drug.
- Warn patients taking methocarbamol that urine may turn black, brown, or green while they are taking this drug.
- Warn diabetic patients taking metaxalone to monitor blood sugar carefully. This drug may cause inaccurate results with urine sugar tests.

The primary treatment includes analgesics, antiinflammatory drugs, immobilization of the affected part (if possible), and physical therapy. If relief is not achieved through these means, a centrally acting skeletal muscle relaxant may be added. Although the mechanism postulated for the centrally acting skeletal muscle relaxants is depression of the polysynaptic pathways in the spinal cord modulating muscle tone, the drugs used as centrally acting skeletal muscle relaxants are related to various antianxiety drugs. Since anxiety itself will make a muscle spasm worse, treatment of the anxiety that accompanies a muscle spasm may be the more important mechanism of action.

The centrally acting skeletal muscle relaxants commonly prescribed to treat muscle spasms are listed in Table 48.2 and include *carisoprodol (Rela, Soma), chlorphenesin (Maolate), chlorzoxazone (Paraflex), cyclobenzaprine (Flexeril), diazepam (Valium), metaxalone (Skelaxin), methocarbamol (Delaxin, others),* and *orphenadrine (Norflex, others).* With the exception of cyclobenzaprine, these drugs are similar to sedative-hypnotic or antianxiety drugs with respect to side effects, drug interactions, and drug dependency (see Chapter 40);

thus short-term therapy rather than long-term therapy is the rule. Cyclobenzaprine is related to the tricyclic antidepressants and does not cause drug dependence or alter sleep patterns.

Drowsiness and dizziness are common side effects of all the centrally acting skeletal muscle relaxants, and they should not be combined with alcohol or other drugs that depress the central nervous system.

SUMMARY

This chapter discusses drugs used to treat disorders of movement arising from a site within the central nervous system.

Parkinson's disease is a result of a neurochemical defect: a deficiency of dopamine and a relative abundance of acetylcholine in the basal ganglia, an area responsible for motor coordination. Parkinsonism is a progressive, degenerative disease for which drugs offer palliative therapy to improve the quality of life but do not halt or alter the course of the disease. Parkinsonian symptoms can also be a side effect of drugs that deplete dopamine, such as reserpine, or block dopamine receptors, such as the antipsychotic drugs.

Anticholinergic drugs with prominent central nervous system activity and antihistamines with anticholinergic activity are the first drugs used to treat the symptoms of parkinsonism. Side effects include mental effects and atropine-like peripheral effects. Amantadine promotes the release of dopamine and is becoming widely used as a first drug in the treatment of the symptoms of parkinsonism.

Levodopa is the chemical precursor of dopamine and is administered to alleviate the symptoms of parkinsonism because, unlike dopamine, levodopa will cross the blood-brain barrier to enter the central nervous system. Unfortunately, much of the levodopa is converted in the periphery to dopamine, which then causes unpleasant side effects, principally extreme nausea and cardiac effects. Carbidopa, an inhibitor of dopa decarboxylase, is now being used. Carbidopa is active only in the periphery. Because of the inhibition of the peripheral metabolism of levodopa, the therapeutic dose is decreased by 75%.

Drugs that enhance inhibitory descending pathways in the spinal cord controlling muscle tone are used to reduce spasticity and muscle spasms.

Diazepam, baclofen, and dantrolene are effective in relieving spasticity. Diazepam and baclofen may enhance the activity of the inhibitory neurotransmitter gamma aminobutyric acid (GABA). Dantrolene acts on the muscle itself to reduce intracellular calcium release and thus muscle activity.

Drugs to treat muscle spasms may act principally as antianxiety agents. Their actions are not well characterized.

STUDY QUESTIONS

1. Describe the physical characteristics seen in Parkinson's disease.
2. What is the neurochemical defect in Parkinson's disease? How do some drugs mimic this defect?
3. Why are anticholinergic drugs, antihistaminic drugs, and amantadine effective in treating the symptoms of parkinsonism? What are the major side effects of each of these drug classes?
4. What is the rationale for administering levodopa to treat the symptoms of parkinsonism? What role does carbidopa play?
5. What are the side effects of levodopa?
6. Define spasticity.
7. How do diazepam, baclofen, and dantrolene act to reduce spasticity?
8. Describe the origin of muscle spasms.
9. What are the characteristics of the drugs used as centrally acting agents to treat muscle spasms?

SUGGESTED READINGS

Borwski, G.D., and Rose, L.I.: Bromocriptine update, Am. Fam. Physician **30**:218, 1984.

Delisa, J.E., and Little, J.: Managing spasticity, Am. Fam. Physician **26**(3):117, 1982.

Fahn, S., Hallett, M., and McKinney, A.S.: Evaluating and treating tremor, Patient Care **15**(19):24, 1981.

Friedman, J.H.: 'Drug holidays' in the treatment of Parkinson's disease, Arch. Intern. Med. **145**:913, 1985.

Fuller, E.: Sorting out movement disorders, Patient Care **16**(10):16, 1982.

Greer, M.: Recent developments in the treatment of Parkinson's disease, Geriatrics **40**:34, 1985.

Holm, V.A.: The causes of cerebral palsy, JAMA **247**(19):1473, 1982.

Horwich, M.S.: Common neurologic problems in the elderly, Drug Ther. **13**(3):85, 1983.

Ilson, J., Bressman, S., and Fahn, S.: Current concepts in Parkinson's disease, Hosp. Med. **19**(3):33, 1983.

Lewin, R.: Parkinson's disease: an environmental cause? Science **229**:257, 1985.

Lieberman, A.N.: Treatment of advanced Parkinson's disease, Geriatr. Med. Today **2**(5):31, 1983.

Swanson, P.D.: Drug treatment of movement disorders, Res. Staff Physician **28**(9):38, 1982.

Young, R.R.: Step therapy for Parkinson's disease, Patient Care **14**(17):4, 1980.

Young, R.R., and Dewaide, P.J.: Drug therapy: spasticity (two parts), N. Engl. J. Med. **304**:28, 1981.

XII

DRUGS AFFECTING THE ENDOCRINE SYSTEM

This section is designed to present the pharmacology of the endocrine system. Chapter 49, *Introduction to Endocrinology*, defines the terms that must be mastered before the material in the subsequent chapters can be understood. This chapter also describes the concepts involved in treating endocrine diseases or in using hormones in therapy for other diseases. Understanding this material facilitates the comprehension of many of the nursing assessments and actions described in later chapters.

Chapters 50 through 55 cover specific endocrine systems. In these chapters the pertinent physiology of the endocrine system is reviewed first. When appropriate, specific endocrine diseases are described so that discussion of the therapy for these diseases becomes more rational. Three classes of agents are described: natural hormones, synthetic forms of hormones, and nonhormonal drugs affecting the endocrine system. The purpose of therapy with each of these agents is clearly defined. Diagnostic tests also are described so that the student may understand the information that must be considered during patient assessment.

Some agents discussed in this section have significant medical uses outside of endocrinology. For example, the synthetic adrenal steroids (see Chapter 51) are widely used as antiinflammatory agents. We have chosen to discuss these drugs in this section because students find it easier to understand the actions of the synthetic drugs if their similarity to the natural hormones is stressed. For similar reasons, the anabolic steroids are considered in this section along with the androgens (see Chapter 54).

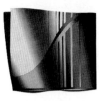

49

Introduction to Endocrinology

This introduction to endocrinology is intended to define important terms, introduce the classes of hormones, and illustrate the concept of hormonal regulation of body processes. Detailed consideration of the properties of individual hormones is presented in subsequent chapters, along with the specific function of each gland and the effects of related drugs.

PROPERTIES OF HORMONES

A *hormone* is a substance produced by a particular cell type, which acts on other cells in the body to produce a physiological or biochemical response. Traditionally, hormones have been considered to be compounds that are synthesized by a specific cell type, are released into the circulation, and act on target tissues elsewhere in the body. An example is thyrotropin (TSH), which is synthesized in the adenohypophysis, released into the systemic circulation, taken up by the thyroid gland, and there stimulates the production of thyroid hormones (see Chapter 52).

Organs producing hormones that enter systemic circulation are the *endocrine glands*—pancreas, adrenal glands, thyroid gland, parathyroid glands, testes, ovaries, neurohypophysis, and adenohypophysis. The neurohypophysis and adenohypophysis comprise the pituitary gland. Those tissues affected by the hormones from the endocrine glands are designated *target tissues.* For example, the target tissue of thyrotropin secreted by the adenohypophysis is the thyroid gland. No other tissue in the body responds to thyrotropin.

Some compounds that have been called hormones act strictly locally, producing their effect at or near the site where they are synthesized. Examples of such compounds are acetylcholine, which is synthesized, acts, and is destroyed at the nerve terminal, and prostaglandins, which are formed from membrane fatty acids at the sites of prostaglandin action. Acetylcholine is discussed in Chapter 9, and prostaglandins are considered in terms of their action on the uterus in Chapter 53. These locally acting substances are not discussed further in this chapter.

Hormones may be divided into two classes on the basis of their chemical composition. One class is the *steroid hormones*, which are derived from cholesterol. This class of hormones includes the hormones of the adrenal gland (cortisol, cortisone, aldosterone, corticosterone, and others) and the hormones of the sex glands (androgens, estrogens, progestins). Many of these steroid compounds have been synthesized by organic chemists, so their production for medicinal purposes does not depend entirely on isolating them from such natural sources as bovine or porcine adrenal glands obtained as byproducts of the meat packing industry. Some clinically useful steroids are obtained from natural sources, however, because the steroids are present in such high concentrations and are so easily extracted as to make the procedure economically feasible. An example of such a preparation is Premarin, a mixture of conjugated estrogens extracted from the urine of pregnant mares. In addition to their relative abundance in natural sources and the ease with which they may be chemically modified or completely synthesized by pharmaceutical manufacturers, the steroids have another characteristic that makes them convenient medicinal agents— many, although not all, may be taken orally.

The second class of hormones is formed from amino acids. Two subclasses within this group are (1) amino acid derivatives and (2) proteins. Examples of the first subclass are thyroxine and tri-iodothyronine, the iodinated tyrosine derivatives produced in the thyroid gland; and the catechol-amines, produced in various tissues from the amino acid tyrosine. The second subclass includes both peptides and proteins. Peptides and proteins are distinguished arbitrarily by difference in size, with peptides containing fewer amino acids than proteins. Chemically, peptides and proteins are similar in that both are formed by the peptide bond linking carboxyl and amino groups of adjacent amino acids. Examples of peptide hormones are the releasing factors produced in the hypothalamus, including thyrotropin-releasing hormone (TRH), composed of three amino acids; and the neurohypophyseal hormones oxytocin and vasopressin, which are each composed of eight amino acids. Examples of protein hormones within this second subclass include insulin, with 51 amino acids and a molecular weight of 6000; and follicle-stimulating hormone (FSH) with a molecular weight of 41,000.

The active forms of many protein hormones are derived from larger protein molecules called *pro-hormones*. For example, insulin is originally released as part of a prohormone containing at least 86 amino acids. Cleavage of 35 amino acids from this larger precursor molecule releases active insulin.

The peptide and protein hormones in general are present in very small quantities in natural sources and may be dificult to isolate. For example, insulin, the protein hormone most often used medically, is prepared by pharmaceutical manufacturers in large quantities from either beef or pork pancreas glands by tedious and expensive extraction procedures. Growth hormone, a protein hormone used to treat a rare endocrine disease, may be extracted from anterior pituitary tissue (adenohypophysis), but the only form that is active in human beings is the growth hormone from primate sources. The supply of this hormone therefore was restricted by the limited supply of source material. In the past growth hormone was obtained postmortem from human anterior pituitary glands but the risk of viral contamination has caused this product to be dropped.

A powerful new method for producing human hormones is based on *genetic engineering*. Genetic engineering involves taking the genes from one species and inserting them into an unrelated species, thereby creating new characteristics in the recipient. The human genes for insulin, growth hormone, interferons, and other proteins have been inserted into certain bacteria. These altered bacteria then may be grown on a large scale in fermentation tanks and will produce large quantities of the human protein. Insulin produced in this way is now sold under the trade name *Humulin*. This human insulin is synthesized by *Escherichia coli* from the human genes artificially inserted into the bacteria. This technique is applicable to a variety of proteins and will solve the problem of limited supply of clinically useful proteins. In addition, hormones produced by this technique are less likely to be contaminated with viruses. For this reason human growth hormone produced by genetically engineered bacteria is now the standard preparation for human use.

The protein and peptide hormones are somewhat inconvenient for the patient to use. Although thyroxine and triiodothyronine may be taken by mouth, none of the larger peptides and proteins survives the action of digestive juices in the stomach and intestine. Thus peptides and proteins must be administered by injection. Even when given parenterally, these compounds may not be effective, because the patient may suffer an allergic, foreign protein reaction or develop resistance because of the production of antibodies directed at the foreign protein.

USES OF HORMONES

The hormones discussed in this section are used clinically in one of three ways: (1) as diagnostic agents, (2) in replacement therapy, or (3) as pharmacological agents.

The most common *diagnostic use* of hormones is to assess the function of the target organ of the administered hormone. For example, adrenocorticotropin may be administered to test the ability of the adrenal gland to produce steroids. Another adenohypophyseal hormone, thyrotropin, is administered to test the capacity of the thyroid gland to synthesize thyroid hormones.

Replacement therapy is aimed at restoring normal levels of hormones, which, for one reason or another, a patient's body no longer produces. Physiological doses are used in an attempt to maintain normal hormone levels without producing toxic effects from hormone excesses. The use of thyroxine to treat hypothyroidism and cortisol to treat Addison's disease (chronic adrenal insufficiency) are examples of replacement therapy.

The use of hormones as *pharmacological agents*, with administered doses far in excess of those required to produce physiological levels, makes use of some function of the compound other than the one seen at physiological concentrations.

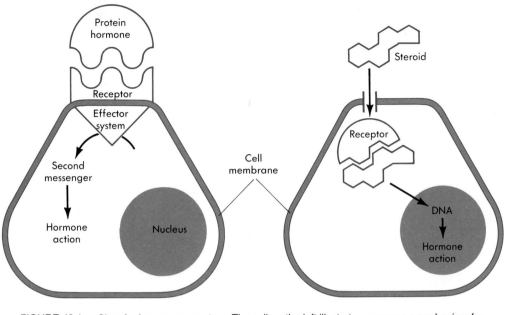

FIGURE 49.1   Sites for hormone receptors. The cell on the left illustrates a common mechanism for responding to protein hormones, with the external receptor interacting through an effector system. The cell on the right illustrates a mechanism shared by steroid hormones and thyroid hormones in which the hormone enters the cytoplasm, is bound by a receptor and carried to the nucleus where the effect is produced.

For example, adrenal corticosteroids may be given in large doses to suppress inflammatory responses in certain diseases. This antiinflammatory effect is not obvious at physiological concentrations of the steroid.

REGULATION OF HORMONE ACTION

Hormones are potent agents capable of exerting profound effects on metabolism. It is imperative for healthy functioning of the body that these compounds act only where and when they are needed and at the proper concentrations. The time of appearance and the concentration of a hormone in the blood may be regulated by controlling its rate of synthesis, its rate of release from storage sites, its rate of degradation, and its rate of clearance from the body. Several hormones are stored after synthesis and released from storage sites only when the proper stimulus is received. For example, thyroxine and triiodothyronine are stored in complex with thyroglobulin in the thyroid gland. Insulin is stored in granules within the beta cell of the pancreas. In both these cases, when the endocrine gland is stimulated to release hormone, it is the stored hormone that is first released. Then if required,

newly synthesized hormone is released into the bloodstream.

Regulation of synthesis and release of many hormones involves the interaction of the central nervous system with the endocrine glands. For example, the hypothalamus in the brain controls the hypophysis or pituitary gland, which in turn regulates the production of hormones by ovaries, testes, and thyroid and adrenal glands. This system is the negative feedback regulation discussed in detail in the next chapter.

Hormones disappear from the bloodstream when they are taken up by various organs or when they are degraded by enzymes in the bloodstream. The kidney is the site of degradation and/or excretion for several hormones, including most steroids. Both the kidney and the liver degrade insulin. Vasopressin, in contrast, is very rapidly destroyed by enzymes in the bloodstream. The half-life of vasopressin, that is, the time required for half of the injected dose to disappear from the blood, is approximately 15 minutes. Other hormones persist for much longer periods. For example, thyroxine has a plasma half-time of about 7 days. How rapidly a hormone is lost from the body determines doses

THE NURSING PROCESS

The specific considerations of endocrine-related drugs are covered in the other chapters of this section. The following presentation illustrates how the general concepts presented in this chapter can guide the nurse through the nursing process.

Assessment

The nurse should identify which endocrine system is involved and consider what other systems may be affected by the primary condition. For example, pituitary disease may influence multiple organ systems and may require therapy at several levels. The nurse may be required to understand the various testing methods used to diagnose the loss of normal endocrine regulation.

Nursing diagnoses

Possible self-concept disturbance

Knowledge deficit

Possible altered health maintenance

Management

In identifying goals of therapy, the nurse should distinguish between replacement therapy and other forms of endocrine therapy. In replacement therapy the goal is to restore normal levels of a hormone in the patient's body, thereby restoring normal function of the endocrine system. In other types of therapy the goal may be to suppress overfunction of an endocrine tissue, control the symptoms of excess hormone levels, or affect a nonendocrine tissue with high levels of hormones. By working with the physician, the nurse should be able to define the goal of therapy for a particular patient. The nurse then may begin teaching the patient about the endocrine condition and the effects of the medications being used.

Evaluation

Evaluating the patient requires that the nurse be thoroughly aware of the expected actions of the endocrine-related drugs and be able to recognize the side effects these agents may produce.

---

and dosage schedules when these hormones are administered. Knowledge of the elimination half-time also helps in dealing with toxic reactions whose duration may be related to the persistence of the compound in the body.

Controlling the location of action of a certain hormone is accomplished in the body in one of two ways. The first localization mechanism is simply to restrict the distribution of the hormone. Examples are the *releasing factors* synthesized in the hypothalamus and released into local portal veins carrying the hormones directly to the target organ (the adenohypophysis) and not into the general circulation.

A second mechanism localizes the effect of generally released hormones. These hormones interact with specific *receptors*, which are found only in their target tissues. The specific receptor is required for hormone activity. For example, progesterone receptors are found primarily in tissues of the female reproductive tract but not in most other organs. Therefore, even though progesterone is released into the general circulation, it acts only on those tissues possessing receptors.

The receptors for hormones may be within cells. For example, steroids and thyroid hormones affect target cells by interacting with intracellular receptors (Figure 49.1). The steroid hormones are bound by soluble receptors, which transport the hormones through the cytoplasm of the cell and into the cell nucleus. The final effect of the hormone is produced by this action within the cell nucleus. Thyroid hormones are transported to the nucleus by nonspecific proteins; in the nucleus the thyroid hormones bind to specific receptors and ultimately alter protein synthesis in the cell.

In contrast to the receptors for steroids and thyroid hormones, receptors for peptide and protein hormones exist on the external surface of cell membranes (Figure 49.1). The peptide and protein hormones therefore need not enter the cell to become effective. One mechanism by which these externally bound hormones act is by releasing an internal regulator, or second messenger. For example, parathyroid hormone binds to a receptor on the surface of certain kidney cells. This receptor is associated with an enzyme called *adenylate cyclase* so that when parathyroid hormone binds to the receptor, adenylate cyclase is stimulated to release cyclic adenosine monophosphate (cyclic AMP) within the cell. Cyclic AMP is the second messenger that actually alters the internal processes of the cell. Vasopressin acts in a similar way on other cells within the kidney. Not all hormone receptors on the cell surface membrane are linked to adenylate cyclase and the second messenger cyclic AMP. For example, the multiple metabolic changes produced by insulin within target cells do not depend on cyclic AMP.

The response of a target cell to a hormone depends on the number and availability of hormone receptors. Regulating the number of receptors is therefore another mechanism by which the body can maintain metabolic balance. An example of this type of regulation is found in obese persons with a high food intake. These persons have chronically high insulin concentrations in the bloodstream. To protect itself from the metabolic effects of this high amount of insulin, the body eliminates a certain percentage of the insulin receptors on cells. This loss of insulin receptors, called *down-regulation*, lowers the responsiveness of the cell to insulin.

Understanding the role of receptors in fulfilling the metabolic role of hormones allows a clearer understanding of endocrine diseases and how they are classified. An endocrine deficiency can arise either from a lack of hormone or from a lack of receptor, which enables the tissue to respond to the hormone. An example is the disease called *diabetes insipidus*, which may be produced either by a lack of antidiuretic hormone (ADH) or by a lack of receptors in the kidney that can respond to ADH. Similarly, *diabetes mellitus* can be characterized by the lack of insulin in the bloodstream or by high levels of insulin in the bloodstream but lower than normal numbers of active insulin receptors on cells.

SUMMARY

Hormones are substances that are produced by certain cells but that act on other cells to produce a physiological response. The organs releasing hormones that are transported throughout the body are the endocrine glands. The tissues directly and specifically affected by the hormones from the endocrine gland are called *target tissues*. Chemically, hormones can be classified as steroids, amino acid derivatives, or peptides and proteins.

Hormones often are used as diagnostic agents to test the function of a target organ. They also are given as replacement therapy to restore normal amounts of hormone which a particular patient may lack. Finally, hormones may be given as pharmacological agents, usually at doses higher than those used in replacement therapy.

The amount of hormone present in the body may be regulated by controlling the rate of synthesis and the rate of degradation of the hormone. Regulating the site of action of a hormone is accomplished by restricted distribution of the hormone or by means of specific receptors for the hormone on target cells. Hormone receptors may be intracellular or may exist on the external surface of the cell membrane. Hormones that act on intracellular receptors are themselves transported within the cell to produce metabolic effects. Those acting on receptors on the cell surface do not necessarily enter the cell and may produce internal effects by means of the second messenger, cyclic AMP, or by other cyclic AMP–independent mechanisms. Responses to hormones can be regulated by altering the number of receptors in target tissues.

STUDY QUESTIONS

1. What is a hormone?
2. What is a target tissue?
3. Describe the two major chemical types of hormones.
4. What is a prohormone?
5. Name three ways in which large amounts of hormones may be obtained for clinical use.
6. What are the three primary clinical uses of hormones?
7. Describe how the amount of hormone in the body may be regulated.
8. How may the site of action of a hormone be restricted?
9. In what ways may the actions of hormones be terminated?

10. What is a releasing factor?
11. What are the two main types of hormone receptors? How do these receptors differ in the way they interact with hormones?
12. Describe the two general types of endocrine deficiency diseases.

SUGGESTED READINGS

Anthony, C.P., and Thibodeau, G.A.: Textbook of anatomy and physiology, ed. 12, St. Louis, 1987, C.V. Mosby Co.

Brown, D.M.: Endocrine receptors, Diagn. Med. **5**(7, special issue):8, 1982.

Eil, C.: Hormone receptor physiology in clinical medicine, Crit. Care Q. **6**(3):86, 1983.

Rubenstein, E.: Diseases caused by impaired communication among cells, Sci. Am. **242**(3):102, 1980.

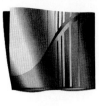

Drugs Affecting the Pituitary Gland

50

The pituitary gland, or hypophysis, lies in the sella turcica, a bony cavity at the base of the brain. Although the gland weighs less than 1 gram, it is the primary regulator of the entire endocrine system, controlling normal growth and regulating water balance.

The pituitary gland is divided into two portions with very different tissue compositions and embryological origins (Figure 50.1). These two regions are the anterior pituitary, or adenohypophysis, and the posterior pituitary, or neurohypophysis. The structure and function of each of these tissues, the function and regulation of the various hormones produced, and the pathological states resulting from abnormalities in hormone production are considered in this chapter.

NEUROHYPOPHYSIS

The neurohypophysis, or posterior pituitary, is composed of nerve fibers embryologically derived from the hypothalamus. Intimate contact between the central nervous system (CNS) and the neurohypophysis is maintained by the nerve fibers that run from the hypothalamus through the hypophyseal stalk to the neurohypophysis (Figure 50.1).

Two octapeptide hormones closely related in structure are known to be released by the neurohypophysis. These hormones are antidiuretic hormone and oxytocin. Both oxytocin and antidiuretic hormone are synthesized in the hypothalamus and are transported in secretion granules down the axons running between the hypothalamus and the neurohypophysis. The granules accumulate at the nerve fiber terminals and are stored in the neurohypophysis, where their release into the systemic circulation is regulated by nerve impulses originating in the hypothalamus. Damage to the hypophyseal stalk impairs transport of the secretory granules to the neurohypophysis and interferes with appropriate release of the hormones into the circulation.

Neurohypophyseal Hormones

Antidiuretic hormone

Mechanism of action. Antidiuretic hormone (ADH), also called *vasopressin*, has as its primary target tissue the renal tubular epithelium (Table 50.1). ADH increases the permeability of certain sections of the renal tubule to water, allowing water to be reabsorbed from the tubule and returned to the bloodstream. This is the mechanism by which normal kidneys concentrate the urine.

In addition to regulating water balance by acting on the renal tubular epithelium, ADH also modulates CNS activity. The CNS effects of ADH may influence affective behavior, memory, thermoregulation, and the function of the anterior pituitary. ADH is not yet used clinically for these CNS effects.

Regulation of secretion. Secretion of ADH is regulated mainly in response to plasma osmolarity, the concentration of solute molecules that increase osmotic pressure (see Chapter 17). In dehydration, the effective osmotic pressure of blood increases. The osmoreceptors of the hypothalamus respond to this change by stimulating the neurohypophysis to secrete ADH, which in turn causes the kidney to conserve body water and prevent or slow further dehydration. This recovery from dehydration is aided further by the concomitant stimulation of the thirst center, leading to increased intake of fluids. Reduction in the effective plasma volume due to hemorrhage or reduced cardiac output also will stimulate ADH release and promote antidiuresis.

In addition to these physiological controls, certain drugs also may influence ADH secretion. Acetylcholine, nicotine, morphine, barbiturates, and bradykinin cause release of ADH in normal sub-

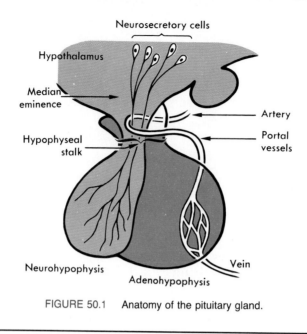

FIGURE 50.1   Anatomy of the pituitary gland.

jects. Ethanol and phenytoin, on the other hand, may promote diuresis by inhibiting ADH release.

Effects of ADH deficiency. When ADH is markedly reduced or absent because of destruction of the hypothalamic region responsible for its synthesis or because of separation of the hypophyseal stalk above the median eminence (Figure 50.1), urinary concentration is impossible and copious amounts of dilute, sugar-free urine are produced. This condition is called *diabetes insipidus* and is not to be confused with the disease diabetes mellitus, which arises from the inability to utilize blood glucose or release insulin.

Diabetes insipidus is not in itself a life-threatening condition unless severe electrolyte imbalances develop. As long as the patient has a fully functional thirst center and can balance the excessive fluid losses with high fluid intakes, severe imbalances do not frequently occur. When a person is unconscious and unable to take in adequate fluids, however, severe dehydration may set in before the condition is noticed. Thus, with traumatic head injuries or surgery to the hypothalamic region of the brain, it is critically important for health care personnel to monitor urinary specific gravity and blood sodium levels, along with fluid intake and urinary volumes, to detect excessive diuresis and resultant dehydration.

In many patients with trauma to the hypothalamus or the hypophyseal stalk, the resultant diabetes insipidus may be transitory. In patients whose condition is chronic, reversal of symptoms can be achieved by replacement therapy with a form of ADH or by therapy with pharmacological agents that relieve the symptoms of the disease.

ADH preparations used in replacement therapy. Since ADH is a peptide hormone, it cannot be administered orally, and all replacement therapy with ADH involves the administration of the hormone parenterally or intranasally (Table 50.2).

Vasopressin (Pitressin), an aqueous preparation of purified ADH, is not routinely used since the half-life of ADH in the blood is quite short. This preparation is infused intravenously for short-term management of unconscious patients. The duration of action of vasopressin may be extended by slowing absorption. *Lypressin*, a synthetic form of ADH that is sprayed onto the mucous membranes of the nasal passages, usually is administered four times daily. *Posterior pituitary extract* was used in the past, but the snuff tended to irritate nasal passages and produce unwanted effects due to proteins other than ADH that were present in the extract.

Desmopressin acetate (DDAVP) administered intranasally is the drug of choice in replacement therapy for chronic diabetes insipidus. Desmopressin acetate is a chemically altered form of vasopressin, differing from the natural hormone by having a long serum half-life, a more potent antidiuretic effect, and less pressor activity. It need be

Table 50.1   Neurohypophyseal Hormones

Descriptive name	Other names	Target tissues	Target tissue response
Antidiuretic hormone	ADH Vasopressin	Renal tubule epithelium Smooth muscle in blood vessels Smooth muscle of gastrointestinal tract	Increased water permeability Vasoconstriction Contraction, increasing gastrointestinal motility
Oxytocin	—	Uterine smooth muscle Breast myoepithelium	Increased uterine contractions Milk letdown

administered only once or twice daily, unlike other ADH preparations. Side effects caused by the pressor action of vasopressin are also less of a problem with this vasopressin derivative.

Long-term control of diabetes insipidus also may be achieved with *vasopressin tannate* in peanut oil, which is given as an intramuscular depot injection. Patients have reported normal concentration of the urine for up to 48 hours after injection of this preparation. Patients should be warned not to repeat the injection until the diuresis recurs. Since the introduction of lypressin and desmopressin acetate for intranasal administration, the use of vasopressin tannate in oil has declined. Although the intranasal drugs are not as long acting, they are more convenient to administer than vasopressin tannate. Many patients report difficulty in getting consistent dosages with vasopressin tannate in oil because of problems in achieving completely homogeneous suspensions of the drug in the oily vehicle.

In the past, ADH has been used as a pressor agent but now is not recommended for that use. Its vasoconstrictor action prevents its safe use for patients with vascular disease or coronary artery disease. Even small doses may cause difficulty to a patient prone to angina attacks. Occasionally this vasoconstrictor action is used to help control massive gastrointestinal bleeding, especially from esophageal varices.

ADH also possesses the ability to promote activity of the smooth muscle of the intestinal tract. During routine therapy of diabetes insipidus, the action of ADH on intestinal smooth muscle may result in nausea, belching, and cramps.

Other drugs to treat diabetes insipidus

Agents other than ADH preparations have been used to treat diabetes insipidus (Table 50.2). Paradoxically, *thiazide diuretics* (see Chapter 16) are effective in some cases, especially when combined with one of the other oral agents listed in this section. The effectiveness of the thiazide diuretics apparently is based on their blockade of electrolyte reabsorption, resulting initially in increased sodium and water excretion. The kidney responds to this change by reabsorbing more water by mechanisms that do not depend on ADH. Moderate salt restriction enhances the action of these drugs in many patients. Dosages of the thiazides used to treat diabetes insipidus are the same as those used for other indications (see Chapter 16). The most common side effect is potassium depletion, which in the extreme may induce cardiac arrhythmias, as well as impair neuromuscular functions and the normal functions of the gastrointestinal tract and kidney.

Chlorpropamide, a sulfonylurea used as an oral hypoglycemic agent in the treatment of diabetes mellitus (see Chapter 55), also is used at comparable doses for diabetes insipidus. Alone or with a thiazide diuretic, chlorpropamide is usually effective in reducing urine volumes. The major potential toxicity is hypoglycemia. When chlorpropamide is used to treat diabetes insipidus, the action sought is a direct sensitization of the kidney to vasopressin so that lower than normal levels of vasopressin cause nearly normal water reabsorption. The drug apparently is not effective in patients who produce no vasopressin at all. Evidence suggests chlorpropamide may also stimulate the pituitary to release vasopressin.

Clofibrate, an oral agent used to reduce serum triglyceride levels (see Chapter 21), may also be effective in diabetes insipidus and may be used alone or in combination with a thiazide diuretic. The drug may produce nausea or rarely muscle cramps and weakness. Clofibrate increases the release of ADH from the posterior pituitary. The dose of clofibrate used for diabetes insipidus is the same as for the lipid-lowering effect.

Carbamazepine is an anticonvulsant that occasionally has been employed to control diabetes insipidus. Its action is similar to that of clofibrate;

Table 50.2 Clinical Summary of Drugs to Treat Diabetes Insipidus

Generic name	Trade name	Drug class	Administration	Properties	Uses	Side effects
Desmopressin acetate	DDAVP* Stimate	Synthetic derivative of vasopressin	Nasal or parenteral	Peptide with longer serum half-life than vasopressin; increases renal reabsorption of water	Replacement therapy in diabetes insipidus	Mild vasoconstriction; mild smooth muscle contraction; FDA Pregnancy Category B
Lypressin	Diapid	Synthetic derivative of vasopressin	Nasal	Peptide with short serum half-life; increases renal reabsorption of water	Replacement therapy in diabetes insipidus	Difficulty breathing because drug accidentally inhaled; smooth muscle contraction
Posterior pituitary extract	Pituitrin*	Neurohypophyseal hormone	Parenteral	Peptide with short serum half-life; contains ADH and oxytocin	Rarely used; contains vasopressin and oxytocin (see Chapter 53)	Vasoconstriction; smooth muscle contraction; FDA Pregnancy Category C.
Vasopressin	Pitressin*	Neurohypophyseal hormone	Parenteral	Peptide with short serum half-life; increases renal reabsorption of water	Tests ADH response of kidney; short-term maintenance of unconscious patient with diabetes insipidus; stimulates peristalsis	Vasoconstriction; smooth muscle contraction stimulates gastrointestinal motility
Vasopressin tannate in oil	Pitressin Tannate in oil*	Neurohypophyseal hormone	Intramuscular depot	Preparation slowly absorbed; increases renal reabsorption of water	Replacement therapy in diabetes insipidus	Vasoconstriction; smooth muscle contraction
Chlorothiazide	Diuril*	Thiazide diuretic	Oral	Mild sodium and water depletion lowers water delivery to collecting ducts in kidneys	Control of diuresis in diabetes insipidus	Hyponatremia; hypokalemia
Chlorpropamide	Diabinese*	Sulfonylurea hypoglycemic agent	Oral	Increases release of ADH from posterior pituitary and increases ADH action in kidney	Control of diuresis in diabetes insipidus	Hypoglycemia; FDA Pregnancy Category C
Clofibrate	Atromid S* Claripex†	Hypolipidemic agent	Oral	Increases release of ADH from posterior pituitary	Control of diuresis in diabetes insipidus	Nausea, weakness, muscle cramps; increased risk of cardiovascular disease
Carbamazepine	Tegretol*	Anticonvulsant	Oral	Increases release of ADH from posterior pituitary	Control of diuresis in diabetes insipidus	Dizziness, confusion, drowsiness; water retention; hyponatremia

*Available in Canada and United States.
†Available in Canada.

both drugs cause release of ADH from the posterior pituitary. The potentially severe side effects of carbamazepine limit its usefulness in diabetes insipidus. Various CNS effects may be seen and often necessitate cessation of therapy. Blood dyscrasias also may occur.

The form of diabetes insipidus covered in the previous paragraphs is called central diabetes insipidus because the condition arose from a lack of secretion of ADH from the neurohypophysis. The symptoms of diabetes insipidus may also arise if the neurohypophysis is producing normal amounts of ADH but the kidney is unresponsive or responds poorly to ADH. This syndrome, called *nephrogenic diabetes insipidus*, may be treated by the thiazide diuretics but of course is resistant to therapy by ADH. Although nephrogenic diabetes insipidus may arise as a genetic disease, it also may be induced by drugs that impair the ability of the kidney to react to ADH. Drugs such as lithium used in treating mental disease (Chapter 42) and demeclocycline, a tetracycline antibiotic (Chapter 32), can induce nephrogenic diabetes insipidus by this mechanism.

The *syndrome of inappropriate ADH* secretion, usually designated as *SIADH*, is a rare condition in which patients show symptoms of water intoxication: hyponatremia, or low sodium levels in the blood (see Chapter 17), and low osmolality of the serum. Despite these conditions, the kidneys continue to excrete sodium. The symptoms of SIADH are caused by the release of more ADH than is appropriate, based on the normal osmotic regulatory signals. In most patients with SIADH, the excess ADH is being released by a tumor, such as a bronchogenic carcinoma. Other less common causes of SIADH are CNS disorders, including head injuries or infections, and extreme physical stress, such as following surgery or extreme emotional stress. A variety of drugs occasionally may trigger SIADH, including carbamazepine, chlorpropamide, clofibrate, cyclophosphamide (see Chapter 39), narcotics, nicotine, thiazide diuretics, and vincristine (see Chapter 39).

Treatment of SIADH usually is aimed directly at removing the cause of the condition, such as removing the tumor or discontinuing the drug thought to be precipitating the disorder. Fluid restriction, infusion of hypotonic saline, and diuretics all may play a role in controlling the fluid and electrolyte imbalances associated with SIADH. If the cause of excessive ADH cannot be removed completely, symptoms may be relieved by administering drugs that render the kidney less sensitive

to ADH. Demeclocycline is preferred, although lithium is effective in some patients. Both demeclocycline and lithium may induce nephrogenic diabetes insipidus in persons with normal ADH levels.

Oxytocin

The second hormone released by the neurohypophysis is oxytocin. The major target organs of this octapeptide hormone are breast myoepithelium and the smooth muscle of the uterus, especially during the second and third stages of labor. Oxytocin is discussed in detail in Chapter 53, so its uses will not be discussed at this point. Briefly, oxytocin speeds delivery by promoting uterine contractions during the final stages of labor when the cervix is fully dilated. A second important function of oxytocin is to cause milk ejection by stimulating contraction of the myoepithelium of the alveoli of the breast.

The regulation of oxytocin release is a particularly good example of the close interaction of the CNS with pituitary function. Suckling by the infant induces afferent nerve impulses from the breast to the brain, which causes more oxytocin to be synthesized and stored hormone to be released. A similar reflex loop may operate in parturition when dilation of the cervix is thought to stimulate synthesis and release of oxytocin.

No specific syndrome resulting from abnormalities in oxytocin function has been described.

ADENOHYPOPHYSIS

The adenohypophysis, or anterior pituitary, constitutes approximately 75% by weight of the total pituitary gland and is regarded correctly as the master gland of the entire endocrine system. The adenohypophysis secretes several peptide hormones, most of which directly stimulate secretion by the adrenal glands, the thyroid gland, and the reproductive organs (Table 50.3).

The adenohypophysis synthesizes several peptide hormones in addition to the clinically important ones shown in Table 50.3. Melanocyte-stimulating hormone (MSH) is released in response to corticotropin-releasing factor (CRF), the same factor that controls ACTH.

Lipotropin (beta LPH) is a weak stimulator of lipolysis, but this action is probably not the main function of the peptide. Fragments of lipotropin are identical to beta endorphin and metenkephalin, endogenous opioids released not only in the pituitary but also in several sites in the brain. The endorphin and enkephalin group of peptides may be neuro-

Table 50.3 Physiologic Action of Selected Adenohypophyseal Hormones

Descriptive name	Other names	Hypothalamic releasing factor	Target tissue	Target tissue response
Adrenocorticotropic hormone	ACTH Corticotropin	Corticotropin-releasing factor (CRF)	Adrenal cortex Pigment cells of skin	Increased steroid synthesis Increased pigmentation
Follicle-stimulating hormone	FSH	Gonadotropin-releasing hormone (GnRH); FSH-releasing hormone (FRH, FSH-RH)	Ovary Seminiferous tubules	Increased estrogen production Maturation
Growth hormone	GH Somatotropin Somatropin STH	Somatotropin or growth hormone–releasing factor (SRF or GRF); somatostatin or somatotropin-release inhibitory factor (SRIF)	Whole body	Increased anabolism, cell size, cell numbers
Luteinizing hormone or interstitial cell–stimulating hormone	ICSH LH	Gonadotropin-releasing hormone (GnRH); luteinizing hormone–releasing factor or hormone (LRF, LRH, LHRF, LHRH)	Ovary Leydig cells	Ovulation; formation of corpus luteum Increased androgen synthesis
Prolactin	LTH Luteotropic hormone	Prolactin-inhibiting factor (PIF); prolactin-releasing factor (PRF)	Breast	Milk formation
Thyroid-stimulating hormone	Thyrotropin TSH	Thyrotropin-releasing hormone or factor (TRH, TRF)	Thyroid gland	Increased T_3, T_4 synthesis

transmitters in the hypothalamus, aiding in regulation of pituitary function, body temperature, and cardiovascular function (see Chapter 44).

The protein called pro-opiomelanocortin (POMC) is a precursor molecule that may be broken down by the various cell types found in the adenohypophysis to ACTH, MSH, beta lipotropin, and/or beta endorphin. Although POMC, MSH, and lipotropin have no obvious clinical applications to date, synthetic derivatives of the endogenous opioids are being widely studied as potential analgesic agents.

Although the adenohypophysis is true secretory tissue and synthesizes as well as releases its hormones, control of those secretions still lies in the brain. Small polypeptides, called *neurohormones*, are synthesized in the median eminence of the hypothalamus and released into the portal venous system (see Figure 50.1), which carries them directly to the adenohypophysis. In the adenohypophysis these neurohormones, which may be *releasing hormones* or *inhibitory hormones*, act on the specific target cell to stimulate or inhibit the synthesis and release of the proper hormone.

Adenohypophyseal Hormones

Growth hormone

Mechanism of action. Growth hormone is a primary regulator of the length of the long bones of the skeleton, which determine adult stature. In addition, the hormone is a potent anabolic agent that causes many tissues to increase cell size and cell numbers. This anabolic action is the result of changes produced in protein, carbohydrate, and fat metabolism. The hormone increases the rate of amino acid transport into cells and elevates the cellular rate of protein synthesis. Growth hormone also antagonizes the action of insulin, which tends to decrease glucose uptake and carbohydrate utilization, thus elevating liver glycogen and blood glucose levels. Finally, growth hormone increases the mobilization of fats for energy, which leads to a rise in blood levels of free fatty acids.

Many of the actions of growth hormone are mediated by peptides called *somatomedins*. Growth hormone stimulates the production of somatomedins by the liver. The somatomedins then act on various body tissues to change metabolism. Somatomedins also have been called insulin-like growth factors; in addition to stimulating growth of the skeleton, these peptides may have insulin-like actions on other tissues.

Regulation of secretion of growth hormone. The secretion of growth hormone is regulated by two factors from the hypothalamus, one stimulating release and one inhibiting release. The releasing factor is a protein containing about 40 amino acids. The inhibitory factor is a smaller, 14-amino-acid peptide called *somatostatin*. In addition to regulating growth hormone release, somatostatin may also influence thyroid-stimulating hormone (TSH) and adrenocorticotropic hormone release from the pituitary gland. Somatostatin is found in other tissues such as gut and pancreas (see Chapter 55) and may play different regulatory roles in those tissues.

Growth hormone deficiency. Damage to the hypophysis may cause that gland to produce insufficient quantities of hypophyseal hormones, a condition called *panhypopituitarism*. Adults suffering from this syndrome may require replacement therapy with thyroid hormones, adrenal steroids, and appropriate sex steroids. Children with panhypopituitarism also may suffer growth stunting because of a lack of growth hormone.

True pituitary dwarfism can be treated successfully with growth hormone preparations. Of the many forms of growth stunting, only that form caused by growth hormone deficiency is appropriately treated with growth hormone. The standard preparations for therapy are prepared by recombinant DNA techniques. *Somatropin, recombinant* has the same amino acid sequence as the natural hormone found in human pituitary glands. *Somatrem* is a recombinant-derived form that has one more amino acid than natural growth hormone. Children or adolescents with pituitary dwarfism who receive growth hormone typically show an immediate increase in growth and may increase 1 foot or more in height over several years of treatment. Ultimately resistance to the protein develops and growth tapers off.

Growth hormone should not be used in adolescents whose epiphyses have sealed because stimulation of further natural growth is unlikely. These preparations should not be used to enhance size or bulk in normal young athletes because the risks outweigh the minimal benefits.

Many actions of growth hormone antagonize those of insulin, and in predisposed individuals prolonged treatment with growth hormone may precipitate diabetes mellitus. Thus patients receiving growth hormone are monitored to detect elevated blood glucose levels or altered glucose tolerance. In adults with established diabetes, destruction of the pituitary gland with loss of growth hormone reduces their insulin requirement.

Excess growth hormone. Acromegaly and gigantism are both produced by excess growth hormone, but the age of onset causes marked differences in the manifestations of the disease. Excessive growth hormone from an early age produces the rare condition of gigantism. Growth rates of 3½ inches per year have been reported. One pituitary giant on record was 8 feet 11 inches tall.

If the onset of excessive growth hormone production is delayed until after puberty, that is, after the plates of the long bones have joined and normal skeletal growth has halted, acromegaly results. In this condition only those tissues still able to grow and expand respond to growth hormone, with the result that malproportions occur. Typically, the bones of the fingers flare at the end and the fingers thicken to produce a spatula-like appearance. Bones and cartilage of the face also grow and thicken, producing coarse features and a massive lower jaw.

Both gigantism and acromegaly usually are caused by pituitary neoplasms, which secrete excessive amounts of growth hormone. Consequently, therapy is aimed at destruction or removal of the tumor. Successful treatment results in the arrest of the progressive symptoms of the disease but does not erase the existing deformations. When removal or destruction of the tumor is not possible or is only partially successful, the drug bromocriptine may inhibit release of growth hormone from the pituitary (Table 50.4).

Gonadotropic hormones

Mechanism of action. The gonadotropic hormones of the adenohypophysis are follicle-stimulating hormone (FSH), luteinizing hormone (LH), and prolactin. FSH and LH regulate maturation and function of the male and female sexual organs. In women prolactin stimulates milk formation in the estrogen- and progestin-primed breast.

In the maturing male FSH causes the maturation of the seminiferous tubules. LH, which is sometimes called interstitial cell–stimulating hormone in the male, increases the number of testicular interstitial cells and stimulates their secretion of androgens. These androgens are the male steroid hormones that complete the process of maturation, leading to the production of viable sperm and to the development of the secondary male sexual characteristics.

In the maturing female, FSH and LH begin to be produced in greater quantities at puberty and

Table 50.4 **Growth Hormone and Related Drugs**

Generic name	Trade name	Description	Clinical use
Bromocriptine mesylate	Parlodel	Bromocriptine is related to ergot alkaloids used as oxytocics	Suppresses release of growth hormone and prolactin (Chapter 53)
Somatrem	Protropin*	Synthetic somatropin that differs by one amino acid from the natural hormone	Replacement therapy for pituitary dwarfism
Somatropin, recombinant	Humatrope*	Somatropin produced by recombinant technology is chemically identical to natural hormone	Replacement therapy for pituitary dwarfism

*Available in the United States and Canada.

THE NURSING PROCESS

PITUITARY GLAND PROBLEMS

Assessment

In most cases patients with pituitary hormone problems have had chronic excesses or deficiencies of the hormones before the diagnosis is made. Few objective signs of a problem may occur, as with prolactin deficiency; or major changes may develop, as with growth hormone overproduction. When an endocrine problem is suspected, the nurse should make a thorough examination to obtain baseline data, paying particular attention to those subjective and objective changes that the patient may indicate have occurred over an extended period.

Nursing diagnoses

Knowledge deficit

Fluid volume excess related to excessive dose of vasopressin

Management

The management of pituitary problems may be pharmacological, surgical, or both. In most cases of drug treatment, the therapy will be long term and improvement slow. The nurse should monitor the patient for expected side effects of the drugs. With the help of the physician, the nurse should determine the best objective measures of improvement and monitor them (e.g., fluid intake and output, laboratory values). Before the patient is discharged, the nurse should begin the teaching and emotional support needed to help the patient move to self-management and should help the patient develop reasonable goals of therapy.

Evaluation

In general, drug therapy is successful if the hormonal balance is returned more closely to normal, and the patient has no serious side effects and can manage the self-therapy alone. Before discharge the nurse should ascertain that the patient is able to explain why the prescribed drugs are necessary, how to administer them correctly, signs of overdosage or underdosage, side effects that might occur, and which ones should be reported immediately. If a patient does not have a medical identification tag or bracelet before leaving the hospital, the patient should state the need to obtain one. Preexisting medical conditions may be altered by the drugs (e.g., diabetes, angina pectoris), and the patient should be able to explain what effect the drugs will have on these preexisting conditions and how to manage them. For further information, see the patient care implications section.

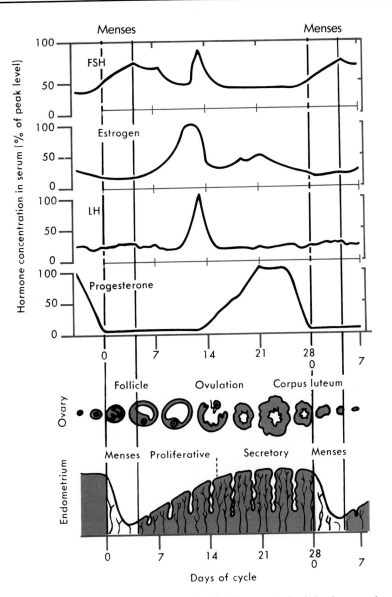

FIGURE 50.2   Pituitary regulation of the menstrual cycle. Changes in circulating hormone levels are correlated with ovarian follicle and endometrial alterations. Details of site of synthesis and site of action for each hormone are in the text. (Redrawn from Segal, S.J.: Sci. Am. Sept., 1974, p. 58. With permission of W.H. Freeman and Co.)

stimulate ovarian estrogen production. Estrogens, which are the female steroid hormones, cause the development of the female secondary sex characteristics.

Regulation of gonadotropin secretion in adult females. In addition to their role in development, FSH and LH control the menstrual cycle in the mature female (Figure 50.2) The regulation of this function involves the hypothalamus, the adenohypophysis, the ovaries, and the endometrium, or uterine lining. The first event in the cycle is a rise

in the concentration of FSH in the bloodstream. In response, in the ovary one of the hundreds of primordial follicles begins to develop. As the follicle matures under the influence of FSH, it begins to produce increasing amounts of estrogens, which greatly increase the adenohypophyseal secretion of LH. It is the surge of LH at midcycle that is the primary trigger for ovulation, the release of the ovum from the mature follicle.

In the second half of the menstrual cycle, LH causes the follicle from which the ovum was re-

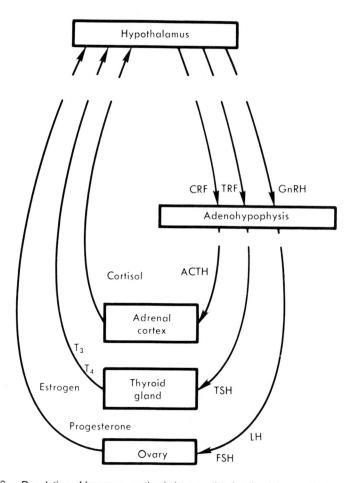

FIGURE 50.3   Regulation of hormone synthesis by negative feedback loops. Each arrow indicates the hormone, its source, and its target tissue. The hypothalamic synthesis of individual releasing factors is suppressed by high blood concentrations of the appropriate final hormone. For example, cortisol suppresses CRF synthesis and release, thereby blocking further cortisol synthesis. Other loops are similarly regulated.

leased to develop into a thickened, secretory tissue called *corpus luteum,* which secretes large quantities of progesterone, another female steroid hormone. By day 21 of the cycle, the large quantities of circulating estrogen and progesterone inhibit the secretion of FSH and LH from the adenohypophysis (Figure 50.2), and the corpus luteum begins to involute. Steroid hormone production falls rapidly as the corpus luteum fails and brings about the final stage in the cycle—the collapse of the endometrial lining.

During menses the entire inner surface of the uterus is denuded as the endometrium rapidly collapses to about 65% of its former thickness. About 70 ml of blood and serum is lost along with necrotic and dissolving tissue during a typical menstrual period. Normally this blood does not clot because of the presence in the fluid of fibrinolysin, an enzyme that digests the fibrin matrix on which blood clots form. Despite the seemingly favorable environment for bacterial growth, the uterus during menstruation is resistant to infection. A contributing factor to this resistance is the presence of many leukocytes in the menstrual fluid.

Effects of gonadotropin deficiency. Alterations in hypophyseal or ovarian function can upset the finely balanced regulatory sequence just described. Throughout childhood, pituitary secretion of FSH and LH is very low, and circulating sex steroid concentrations are quite low as well. At puberty the adenohypophysis normally greatly increases its secretion of FSH and LH. If this increase does not

PATIENT CARE IMPLICATIONS

Care of the patient with diabetes insipidus

Drug administration

- Monitor intake, output, serum sodium levels, and urine specific gravity. Diabetes insipidus is characterized by dilute urine, in large volume, with output often exceeding input, and with urine specific gravity of 1.000-1.003. This condition is often diagnosed initially by an alert nurse.
- Uncontrolled diabetes mellitus may be associated with excessive urine production. Monitor urine and blood glucose levels, and urine specific gravity to help differentiate the two.
- Monitor blood pressure. Monitor serum electrolytes.
- Read orders carefully. Vasopressin and vasopressin tannate in oil are different and have different requirements for administration.
- See p. 88 in Chapter 6 for a discussion of administration of oil-based IM preparations.

INTRAVENOUS DESMOPRESSIN ACETATE

- May be given undiluted in diabetes insipidus: administer a single dose over 1 minute. Monitor blood pressure and pulse. This drug may also be administered IV in patients with hemophilia A and von Willebrand's disease. For these conditions, it is diluted and administered as an infusion. Consult manufacturer's literature.

Patient and family education

- Review with patients the anticipated benefits and possible side effects of drug therapy.
- If appropriate, teach the patient to measure urine output at home. Most patients will not need to do this, as they can usually tell when urine output is increasing, and another dose of medication is needed.
- In preparing a patient for discharge with a drug for nasal administration, review the manufacturer's instruction sheet. Have the patient give a return demonstration.
- Teach patients that a severe cold, nasal surgery, or anything that interferes with their ability to sniff may necessitate a temporary switch to an injectable drug, and they should contact the physician.
- If GI distress develops, it may indicate too high a dose. If GI distress is severe or persistent, notify the physician.
- Generally, if more than two sprays per nostril of a drug are needed, it is better to increase the frequency of dosing rather than the number of sprays for each dose.

- If a dose is missed, take the dose as soon as it is remembered, unless within a few hours of the next dose, in which case the patient should take a dose, but omit the next scheduled dose. Do not double up for missed doses. Reinforce to patients the need to consult the physician for questions about doses.
- Refer patient to a community based nursing agency for followup as appropriate.
- Teach patients with diabetes insipidus to wear a medical identification tag or bracelet indicating their diagnosis.
- Avoid ingestion of alcohol unless permitted in small amounts by the physician.
- Chlorothiazide is discussed in Chapter 16.
- Chlorpropamide is discussed in Chapter 55.
- Clofibrate is discussed in Chapter 21.
- Carbamazepine is discussed in Chapter 47.
- Oxytocin is discussed in Chapter 53.
- Bromocriptine is discussed in Chapter 53.

Somatrem and somatropin

Drug administration

- Monitor weight and height.
- Monitor blood glucose levels.
- Encourage patients to return for regular follow-up.
- Warn patients that pain and swelling at the injection site may occur.

Patient and family education

- Review anticipated benefits and possible side effects of drug therapy. Warn patients to take drug only as ordered, and not to increase dose unless directed to do so by the physician.
- Warn diabetic patients to monitor blood glucose levels carefully, as changes in diet or insulin may be necessary.
- Consult with the physician, then teach family to monitor and record patient's weight, height, and other parameters on a regular basis.

Panhypopituitarism

- The patient who loses all or nearly all pituitary function from trauma, surgery, or disease must be treated with replacement hormonal therapy to survive. Treatment with exogenous forms of cortisol usually substitutes for ACTH loss. Thyroid hormones usually replace TSH. Growth hormone is not usually replaced, except in the child. ADH may or may not be replaced exogenously. The gonadotropic hormones are rarely used in replacement therapy. Estrogens and androgens

Continued.

placement therapy. Estrogens and androgens are used as needed for cosmetic and comfort purposes. In the female it is difficult to re-create the monthly cyclic surges of these hor-mones, so this may not be attempted unless requested by the patient; the female is usu-ally sterile. Oxytocin is not replaced unless

the woman has been able to conceive and the hormone would be needed during labor and delivery. For information about individual hormones, see Chapters 51 to 55.

- Teach patients requiring hormonal replace-ment therapy to wear a medical identifica-tion tag or bracelet.

---

occur, sexual development will not take place, since androgen, estrogen, and progesterone produc-tion is not induced.

Gonadotropin-releasing hormone (GnRH) may be useful in diagnosing the cause of failure of sexual development (Chapter 53). FSH may be used clin-ically to help reverse female infertility (Chapter 53). For long-term replacement therapy in patients with hypogonadism, the androgens and estrogens are usually employed (Chapters 53 and 54).

Adrenocorticotropic hormone

Mechanism of action. When adrenocortico-tropic hormone (ACTH) is released by the adeno-hypophysis, it stimulates the adrenal cortex to syn-thesize and release cortisol, a major adrenocortical steroid hormone, as well as other glucocorticoids and minor amounts of sex steroids (see Chapter 51).

Regulation of secretion of ACTH. Cortisol blood levels are monitored by the hypothalamus, which adjusts the rate of release of corticotropin-releasing factor (CRF) into the hypophyseal portal venous system to the adenohypophysis, thereby controlling the systemic levels of ACTH. When cortisol levels become too high, the hypothalamus reduces CRF release. The adenohypophysis, lacking appropriate stimulation, reduces ACTH produc-tion, and blood levels of the peptide hormone fall. The adrenocortical production of cortisol then falls because of the lowered ACTH levels. Blood levels of the adrenal steroid thus are prevented from ex-ceeding an upper limit. Conversely, when cortisol levels in the blood fall too low, the hypothalamus normally prevents a dangerously low level from de-veloping. CRF is released in large amounts into the hypophyseal portal venous system; in response the adenohypophysis releases ACTH, and in response to ACTH the adrenal cortex elevates cortisol pro-duction. This intricate regulatory sequence is an example of a negative feedback loop, a regulatory mechanism in which the end product of a reaction

sequence inhibits the operation of the sequence, thereby keeping the concentration of the product between certain limits (Figure 50.3).

Thyroid-stimulating hormone

Negative feedback regulation applies not only to the adrenal cortex and the ovary, but also to the thyroid gland (Figure 50.3). Thyroid-stimu-lating hormone (TSH) is discussed in detail in Chapter 52.

SUMMARY

The pituitary gland, or hypophysis, is com-posed of two distinct regions. The anterior pitu-itary, or adenohypophysis, is composed of true se-cretory tissue, which both synthesizes and releases several peptide hormones. The posterior pituitary, or neurohypophysis, is composed of neural tissue, which stores and releases two peptide hormones. These peptide hormones, antidiuretic hormone (ADH) and oxytocin, are synthesized in the hypo-thalamus and transported to the neurohypophysis through the pituitary stalk.

ADH increases the permeability of parts of the renal tubule to water, allowing water to be reab-sorbed and returned to the bloodstream. ADH is released from the neurohypophysis in response to increasing osmolarity of the plasma, an indicator of dehydration. Lowered plasma volume also stim-ulates release of the hormone. Loss of ADH results in diabetes insipidus, a disease characterized by production of excessive amounts of dilute, sugar-free urine. This condition may be treated by re-placing the missing ADH, or the symptoms may be controlled directly. Drugs such as thiazide di-uretics, chlorpropamide, and clofibrate may alter kidney function and/or increase intrinsic ADH ac-tivity sufficiently to control diuresis in these pa-tients.

Oxytocin also is released from the neurohy-pophysis. Oxytocin causes contraction of the smooth muscle of the breast and uterus, facilitating delivery of the fetus and milk letdown in the nursing mother.

Synthesis of the hormones of the adenohypophysis is controlled in the hypothalamus by means of neurohormones, which function as releasing or inhibiting hormones in the pituitary gland. Growth hormone, synthesized and released by the adenohypophysis, causes the synthesis of somatomedins in the liver, which act on many tissues to produce characteristic anabolic changes. Persons lacking growth hormone fail to achieve normal adult height and may receive growth hormone as replacement therapy.

The gonadotropic hormones produced by the adenohypophysis are follicle-stimulating hormone, luteinizing hormone, and prolactin. These hormones affect growth and development of the sexual organs in males and females and also regulate the monthly ovarian cycle in adult females. Gonadotropin deficiency prevents normal sexual development and function. Replacement therapy usually is carried out with specific steroids such as androgens and estrogens. The protein hormones of the adenohypophysis may be used in diagnosis or to promote fertility.

Adrenocorticotropic hormone (ACTH) and beta lipotropin are derived from a single prohormone in the adenohypophysis. The target tissue of ACTH is the adrenal gland, which responds to ACTH by synthesizing cortisol. Control of secretion of ACTH is through a negative feedback loop involving cortisol from the adrenal gland and corticotropin-releasing factor from the hypothalamus. ACTH, as a protein, is inconvenient for use in replacement therapy, although it can cause the release of cortisol and other steroids from the adrenal gland.

STUDY QUESTIONS

1. What are the two divisions of the pituitary gland, or hypophysis?
2. What is the nature of neurohypophyseal tissue?
3. What hormones are released by the neurohypophysis?
4. Where are the hormones released by the neurohypophysis actually synthesized?
5. What is the target tissue of antidiuretic hormone (ADH)?
6. What is the mechanism of action of ADH?
7. What physiological conditions stimulate the release of ADH?
8. What is diabetes insipidus?
9. What two types of therapy may be used to treat diabetes insipidus?
10. Compare and contrast the route of administration and duration of action of vasopressin and vasopressin tannate in oil.
11. What advantage does nasal administration of vasopressin preparations such as lypressin have over intramuscular use of vasopressin?
12. What advantage does desmopressin acetate (DDAVP) have over other vasopressin preparations administered nasally?
13. What are the side effects associated with vasopressin?
14. What drugs other than vasopressin derivatives have been used to control the symptoms of diabetes insipidus?
15. What is the mechanism of action by which thiazide diuretics control diuresis in diabetes insipidus?
16. What is the mechanism of action of chlorpropamide and clofibrate in treating diabetes insipidus?
17. What are the target tissues of oxytocin?
18. How is the secretion of oxytocin controlled?
19. What hormones are secreted by the adenohypophysis?
20. Where are the hormones secreted by the adenohypophysis actually synthesized?
21. What are neurohormones and where are they synthesized?
22. What are the target tissues of growth hormone?
23. What are the anabolic effects of growth hormone?
24. What are the antiinsulin effects of growth hormone?
25. What are somatomedins?
26. What is the effect of growth hormone deficiency?
27. What is the treatment of growth hormone deficiency?
28. What is the effect of excess growth hormone?
29. What is the difference between gigantism and acromegaly?
30. What are the gonadotropic hormones?
31. What are the target tissues of follicle-stimulating hormone?
32. What are the target tissues of luteinizing hormone?
33. What are the target tissues of prolactin?
34. What roles do follicle-stimulating hormone and luteinizing hormone play in causing the development and release of a mature ovum from the ovary?
35. What are the effects of gonadotropin deficiency?
36. What is the target tissue for adrenocorticotropic hormone (ACTH)?

37. How is the concentration of ACTH in the bloodstream regulated?

SUGGESTED READINGS

Anthony, C.P., and Thibodeau, G.A.: The endocrine system. In Textbook of anatomy and physiology, ed. 12, St. Louis, 1987, C.V. Mosby Co.

Benzie, J.L., and Pullan, P.T.: Drug management of antidiuretic hormone imbalance following pituitary surgery, Drug Intell. Clin. Pharm. **17**(12):886, 1983.

Council on Scientific Affairs: Drug abuse in athletes. Anabolic steroids and human growth hormone, JAMA **259**(11):1703, 1988.

Filicori, M. and Flamigni, C.: GnRH agonists and antagonists: current clinical status, Drugs **35**:63, 1988.

Germon, K.: Fluid and electrolyte problems associated with diabetes insipidus and syndrome of inappropriate antidiuretic hormone, Nurs. Clin. N. Am. **22**(4):785, 1987.

Hartshorn, J., and Hartshorn, E.: Pharmacology update: vasopressin in the treatment of diabetes insipidus, J. Neurosci. Nurs. **20**(1):58, 1988.

Howrie, D.L.: Growth hormone for the treatment of growth failure in children, Clin. Pharm. **6**(4):283, 1987.

Kendall-Taylor, P., Upstill-Goddard, G., and Cook, D.: Long-term pergolide treatment of acromegaly, Clin. Endocrinol. (Oxf.) **19**(6):711, 1983.

Lechan, R.M.: Neuroendocrinology of pituitary hormone regulation, Endocrinol. Metab. Clin. North Amer. **16**(3):475, 1987.

Press, M.: Growth hormone and metabolism, Diabetes Metab. Rev. **4**(4):391, 1988.

Salva, K.M., and others: DDAVP in the treatment of bleeding disorders, Pharmacotherapy **8**(2):94, 1988.

Smith, A.I. and others: Proopiomelanocortin processing in the pituitary, CNS, and peripheral tissues, Endocrinol. Rev. **9**(1):159, 1988.

Thompson, L.: The pituitary: the master gland, Surg. Technol. **15**(4):27, 1983.

Zaloga, G.P., and Chernow, B.: Hormones as therapeutic agents in the intensive care unit, Crit. Care. Q. **6**(3):75, 1983.

Zucker, A.R., and Chernow, B.: Diabetes insipidus and the syndrome of inappropriate antidiuretic hormone release, Crit. Care Q. **6**(3):63, 1983.

CHAPTER

51

Drugs Affecting the Adrenal Gland

The human adrenal gland is divided into two distinct functional units: the adrenal medulla and the adrenal cortex. These two regions of the gland differ in embryological origin and type of cells composing the tissue, as well as in hormones produced. The structure and function of these regions of the adrenal gland, the regulation of synthesis of the various hormones produced, and the pathological states arising from abnormalities in hormone production are discussed in this chapter. The widespread clinical uses of several of these hormones and their derivatives in diagnosis and therapy are also considered.

ADRENAL CORTEX

The adrenal cortex is composed of lipid-rich secretory tissue embryologically derived from coelomic epithelium. Three distinct layers within the cortex may be distinguished on the basis of histology. These regions differ not only in cellular arrangement, but also in the major steroid hormone produced and in the regulation of steroid synthesis (Figure 51.1).

Adrenal Steroids and Their Actions

Mineralocorticoid synthesis and actions. The outer layer, or zona glomerulosa, is the site of conversion of the precursor cholesterol to the mineralocorticoids. These steroids act on the kidney, causing retention of sodium and associated water, while promoting potassium loss.

Regulation of mineralocorticoid synthesis is primarily through the renin-angiotensin system (Figure 51.2). The regulatory trigger for this feedback system is in the kidney, where lowered blood sodium levels or lowered intravascular volume causes the release of renin into the bloodstream. Renin is an enzyme, which in the bloodstream converts angiotensinogen, a protein from the liver, to angiotensin I. Another enzyme found in the bloodstream and the lung rapidly converts angiotensin I to angiotensin II. Angiotensin II in turn stimulates the adrenocortical zona glomerulosa to secrete the mineralocorticoids, especially aldosterone. The result of this regulatory loop is that the mineralocorticoids released into the bloodstream slow the further loss of sodium and water through the kidneys. When sodium and water retention exceeds certain limits, the plasma volume expands and renin release decreases. When the concentration of renin falls, the production of angiotensin II slows, aldosterone secretion by the adrenal gland falls, and the kidneys begin to rid the body of accumulated sodium.

Glucocorticoid synthesis. The inner two layers of the adrenal cortex convert cholesterol to the glucocorticoids and the sex steroids, primarily androgens and progestins. The synthesis of these steroids is regulated by the pituitary gland and the hypothalamus via the negative feedback loop described in Chapter 50. Cortisol is the major glucocorticoid produced, and it is also the key to regulation of steroid synthesis in the zona fasciculata and zona reticularis. Low levels of cortisol in the bloodstream stimulate and high levels suppress total steroid synthesis by respectively raising and lowering adrenocorticotropic hormone (ACTH) release from the pituitary gland.

Glucocorticoid action. The glucocorticoids produce potent and varied effects on metabolism. The primary metabolic effect is stimulation of gluconeogenesis (the formation of new glucose) by actions on the liver and peripheral tissues. In striated muscle, glucocorticoids mobilize amino acids from muscle protein. The result is an increase in circulating levels of amino acids and an overall depletion of muscle protein, which ultimately is expressed as a negative nitrogen balance

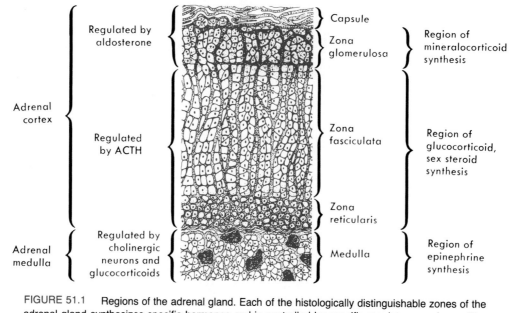

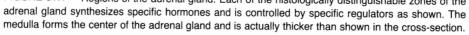

FIGURE 51.1   Regions of the adrenal gland. Each of the histologically distinguishable zones of the adrenal gland synthesizes specific hormones and is controlled by specific regulators as shown. The medulla forms the center of the adrenal gland and is actually thicker than shown in the cross-section.

(more nitrogen is excreted than is taken in the diet). In the liver, glucocorticoids increase the activities of enzymes that convert amino acids to glucose. Much of this excess glucose is then stored in the liver as glycogen. In addition, amino acids are the ultimate source of precursors for fat synthesis, which is also increased in the presence of glucocorticoids.

Glucocorticoids have many direct actions in the body. They maintain water diuresis by antagonizing the effects of antidiuretic hormone in the kidney, lower the threshold for electrical excitation in the brain, and reduce the amount of new bone synthesis. In addition, the glucocorticoids affect the immune system by suppressing the activity of lymphoid tissue and by reducing the numbers of circulating lymphocytes. These steroids also reduce inflammatory processes by impairing synthesis of prostaglandins and related compounds, an action that has several useful therapeutic applications.

In addition to the direct effects mentioned, glucocorticoids have so-called permissive activities that allow the body to deal successfully with stress or trauma. For example, cortisol sensitizes the arterioles to norepinephrine, allowing the catecholamine to increase blood pressure. In the liver, cortisol must be present before epinephrine and glucagon can stimulate hydrolysis (breakdown) of liver glycogen to glucose, releasing the sugar to serve as an energy source for peripheral muscle.

Abnormalities of Adrenal Hormone Production

Adrenal insufficiency. Failure of the adrenal cortex is life-threatening. If the failure is sudden, as might occur following adrenal injury or thrombosis, death may occur within hours. Early symptoms of *acute adrenal insufficiency* include confusion, restlessness, and nausea with vomiting. Circulatory collapse, deep shock, and death may follow rapidly.

If synthesis of glucocorticoids is reduced but not halted altogether, patients may not be in immediate danger, in the absence of stress or trauma, but they may still suffer from inadequate amounts of the glucocorticoids. This *chronic primary adrenal insufficiency* is called *Addison's disease.* The symptoms include weakness, weight loss, dehydration, hypotension, hypoglycemia, and anemia. Most patients with chronic adrenal insufficiency also display increased pigmentation of the skin. This unusual or excessive tanning is caused by a direct effect on melanin-containing skin cells by the chronic excess of ACTH, which is secreted by the pituitary gland in response to the elevated corticotropin-releasing factor (CRF) induced by chronically low blood levels of cortisol.

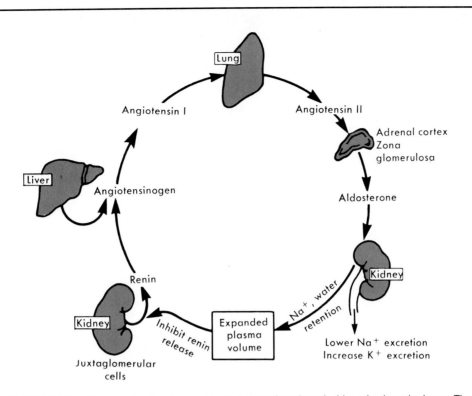

FIGURE 51.2   The negative feedback loop regulating mineralocorticoid synthesis and release. The kidney is the key to regulating the synthesis and release of aldosterone, the primary natural mineralocorticoid. Renin is released from the juxtaglomerular cells of the kidney to set the cascade in motion, and it is the kidney that is the ultimate target of aldosterone. The expanded plasma volume, which results when the kidney retains sodium ion (NA$^+$) and water, is the regulator that halts renin release.

Symptoms similar to those of Addison's disease are produced when the adenohypophysis is diseased or destroyed and no longer produces adequate ACTH. Without ACTH, the zona reticularis and zona fasciculata do not synthesize cortisol, and over time these adrenal tissues atrophy. This condition is called *secondary adrenal insufficiency.* One characteristic that often visibly distinguishes these patients from those with Addison's disease is the absence of excessive pigmentation. In secondary adrenal insufficiency the pituitary gland does not release large quantities of ACTH, and the skin is not darkened.

Excessive glucocorticoids. Overproduction of cortisol, a condition called *Cushing's syndrome,* may be induced by a variety of factors. Some patients have high cortisol production from tumors of the adrenal cortex, which may synthesize massive amounts of the steroid. Other patients have high cortisol synthesis because of increased ACTH release into the bloodstream, which keeps the zona fasciculata and zona reticularis maximally stimulated to produce the glucocorticoids. Excess ACTH

usually comes from a tumor of the pituitary gland, but occasionally the ACTH comes from some unusual source such as a lung tumor, which would not ordinarily be expected to synthesize ACTH. Most often, however, Cushing's syndrome is caused by administration of glucocorticoids.

The symptoms of Cushing's syndrome can be predicted from the metabolic actions of cortisol. Certain fat stores, especially those on the face and shoulders, are increased as a result of cortisol stimulation of fat synthesis. The extremities may be weak and in more advanced cases may be thin because of the muscle-wasting effects of the hormone. The skin is fragile and easily bruised as a result of protein breakdown in that tissue. Examination of the skin on the trunk may reveal striae, or stretch marks, over areas where fat deposition is most pronounced. Many patients also have superficial fungal infections of the skin, related in part to the fragility of the skin and in part to the reduced host immune response caused by the excess steroid. Bone thinning occurs because of changes in calcium metabolism; compression fractures of the

Table 51.1 Comparison of Activity of Natural and Synthetic Adrenal Steroids Used Systemically

Generic name	Drug class	Activity relative to hydrocortisone		Major use	Major toxicity
		Anti-inflammatory	Sodium-retaining		
Betamethasone	Glucocorticoid (synthetic)	2.50	0.	As hydrocortisone	Overdosage causes hydrocortisone-like effects on fat, protein, carbohydrate metabolism but little sodium retention
Cortisone	Glucocorticoid (natural)	0.8	0.9	Antiinflammatory agent	As for hydrocortisone
Dexamethasone	Glucocorticoid (synthetic)	30.0	0	As hydrocortisone	As for betamethasone
Fludrocortisone	Mineralocorticoid (synthetic)	About 1.0	About 100	Replacement therapy in adrenal insufficiency; therapy in adrenal disease causing salt loss	Overdosage produces symptoms of excess salt and water retention with potassium loss
Hydrocortisone (also called cortisol)	Glucocorticoid (natural)	1.0	1.0	Replacement therapy in adrenal insufficiency; as an antiinflammatory agent in a variety of nonendocrine diseases	Overdosage produces symptoms of Cushing's disease; abrupt withdrawal produces symptoms of adrenal insufficiency
Methylprednisolone	Glucocorticoid (synthetic)	5.0	0	As hydrocortisone	As for betamethasone
Paramethasone	Glucocorticoid (synthetic)	10	0	As cortisone	As for betamethasone
Prednisolone	Glucocorticoid (synthetic)	4.0	0.8	As hydrocortisone	As for hydrocortisone
Prednisone	Glucocorticoid (synthetic)	3.5	0.8	As hydrocortisone	As for hydrocortisone
Triamcinolone	Glucocorticoid (synthetic)	5.0	0	As hydrocortisone	As for betamethasone; has high muscle-wasting activity

spine may occur relatively easily. Diabetes may be precipitated from the increased insulin demand caused by excess cortisol. Hypertension is very common in these patients, and atherosclerosis may occur. Mood changes are also common and may be extreme. Psychosis may be precipitated.

Hyperaldosteronism. Certain tumors of the adrenal gland produce excessive amounts of aldosterone, or less often, one of the other mineralocorticoids. In these patients two types of symptoms appear: those associated with hypertension and those associated with hypokalemia (low blood potassium concentration). Hypertension is produced by the sodium and water retention arising from excess aldosterone acting on the kidney, whereas the muscle weakness associated with hypokalemia is a result of the potassium-wasting action of the steroid in the kidney. Treatment ultimately involves surgical removal of the tumor.

Secondary sexual abnormalities. The sex steroids produced in the adrenal cortex are of minor importance in normal circumstances, the output of the adrenal gland being small compared to that of the gonads. Under certain conditions, however, sex steroid overproduction in the adrenal gland may produce a devastating endocrine imbalance. For example, a female with an androgen-producing tumor of the adrenal gland may undergo masculinization, including suppression of the menstrual cycle and the development of secondary male sex characteristics. A male with an estrogen-producing tumor may develop breast tenderness and enlargement with loss of libido. A child may show precocious sexual development.

Pharmacology of Adrenal Steroids and Related Compounds

Major actions of adrenal steroids. Three major activities of the adrenal steroids are (1) metabolic effects on carbohydrate, protein, and fat metabolism; (2) antiinflammatory and immunosuppressive activity; and (3) sodium-retaining activity associated with potassium loss. The first two are classified as glucocorticoid actions and the third as a mineralocorticoid action.

The natural adrenal steroids, cortisol, cortisone, and corticosterone, possess both glucocorticoid and mineralocorticoid activity, although one action usually predominates. Treatment with one of these natural compounds therefore produces multiple effects. For example, cortisol in the high doses required for antiinflammatory action changes metabolism, as expected from a glucocorticoid, but also produces excessive sodium retention and potassium loss, a mineralocorticoid effect.

Synthetic glucocorticoids have been designed that are essentially free of mineralocorticoid activity. These drugs include betamethasone, dexamethasone, fluprednisolone, meprednisone, methylprednisolone, paramethasone, and triamcinolone (Table 51.1). These synthetic glucocorticoids have the additional advantage of producing antiinflammatory effects at lower doses than the naturally occurring glucocorticoids.

Duration and mechanism of action. The duration of action of the various adrenal steroids are listed in Table 51.1. For this class of drugs, the duration of action is not the same as the plasma half-life of the drug. The duration of action refers to the length of time adrenal suppression is detectable following a single dose of the steroid. For example, the drug prednisone suppresses adrenal function up to 36 hours following a single dose, but the plasma half-life is only about 2.5 hours. This discrepancy may be explained in part by the mechanism of action of the steroid hormones. To produce their effects, the steroids must pass through the membranes of target cells, bind to soluble receptors in the cell cytoplasm, and be transported to the nucleus of the cell (Chapter 49). Once in the nucleus the steroid induces changes in ribonucleic acid (RNA) and protein synthesis, which ultimately may be expressed as some change in the function of the target cell. A considerable time lag may occur between the uptake of the steroid into the cell and the appearance of the effect in the target cell. Further time may elapse before the effect is terminated and the steroid destroyed.

Preparations for various routes or sites of administration. Adrenal steroids used clinically are summarized in Tables 51.2 and 51.3. The chemical form of the steroid determines the pharmacokinetics of the preparation. In their naturally occurring forms, most glucocorticoids are relatively insoluble in water. Because these drugs form suspensions but not true solutions in water, preparations are not suitable for intravenous administration, although they may be injected into tissues (Table 51.2). In contrast, sodium phosphate and sodium succinate derivatives of several glucocorticoids are quite water soluble. Thus intravenous administration of an adrenal steroid preparation requires sodium phosphates of cortisol (hydrocortisone), betamethasone, dexamethasone, and prednisolone or sodium succinates of cortisol and methylprednisolone. No other forms of these drugs should be administered intravenously.

Administered intramuscularly as suspensions, many glucocorticoids are dissolved and absorbed slowly from the injection site, producing a relatively long duration of action (Table 51.2). For many glucocorticoids, the acetate ester is a very insoluble, slowly absorbed form that yields a very prolonged duration of action. Preparations that combine sodium phosphate and acetate esters have both a rapid onset and a prolonged effect; the highly soluble sodium phosphate yields rapid action, whereas the poorly soluble acetate form remains at the site to serve as a depot to release the active agent slowly.

Topical steroid preparations are used primarily to control various dermatological conditions (Table 51.3). Since the steroids are applied directly to the skin, a therapeutic dose may be achieved at the site where action is desired. Since the total dose of steroid is small and the drugs are not well absorbed through the skin, systemic actions usually are avoided. Absorption of a significant dose is possible with chronic, heavy application to wide areas of the skin or with rectal applications, also considered a topical route.

Certain steroid forms have been promoted primarily because of specific enhancement of topical activity. For example, betamethasone valerate is much more active topically than is betamethasone itself. Likewise, the acetonide derivative of triamcinolone is superior to the parent compound as a topical agent.

Table 51.2   Clinical Summary of Glucocorticoids and Mineralocorticoids Used Systemically

Generic name	Trade names*	Route†	Onset	Duration
Betamethasone	Celestone	PO	1 hr	3 days
Betamethasone sodium phosphate	Betameth Prelestone	IV, IM	Rapid	Short
Betamethasone acetate/sodium phosphate	Celestone soluspan	IM, IA, IL, IB	1-3 hr	1-2 weeks
Dexamethasone	Decadron Dexasone†	PO	1 hr	3 days
Dexamethasone acetate	Dalalone Decadron LA	IM IA, ST, IL	<8 hr Slow	6 days 1-3 weeks
Dexamethasone sodium phosphate	Decadrol Dexasone	IV, IM IA, IS, IL, ST	Rapid Slow	Short 3-21 days
Fludrocortisone acetate	Florinef	PO	Intermed.	Intermed.
Hydrocortisone	Cortef	PO IM Rectal	<1 hr <4 hr 3-5 days	1.5 days Days
Hydrocortisone acetate	Generic	IA, IS, IB, IL, ST	<24 hr	3-28 days
Hydrocortisone acetate	Cortifoam	Rectal	5-7 days	
Hydrocortisone sodium phosphate	Hydrocortone phosphate	IV, IM	Rapid	Short
Hydrocortisone sodium succinate	Solu-Cortef	IV, IM	Rapid	Variable
Methylprednisolone	Medrol	PO	<1 hr	1.5 days
Methylprednisolone acetate	Depo-Medrol	IM IA, IL, ST	6-48 hr Slow	1-4 weeks 1-5 weeks
Methylprednisolone sodium succinate	Solu-Medrol	IV, IM	Rapid	Intermed.
Paramethasone acetate	Haldrone	PO	<1 hr	2 days
Prenisolone	Cortalone	PO	<1 hr	1.5 days
Prednisolone acetate	Predicort	IM	Slow	
Prednisolone acetate/sodium phosphate	Generic	IM, IB, IS	Slow	3-28 days
Prednisolone sodium phosphate	Predicort RP	IV, IM IA, IL, ST	<1 hr Slow	Short 3-21 days
Prednisolone tebutate	Prednisol TBA	IA, IL, ST	1-2 days	1-3 weeks
Prednisone	Meticorten	PO	<2 hr	1.5 days
Triamcinolone	Aristocort	PO	<2 hr	2 days

*Representative trade names are given.
†Abbreviations: IA, intraarticular; IB, intrabursal; IL, intralesional; IM, intramuscular; IS, intrasynovial; IV, intravenous; PO, oral; ST, soft tissue.

Table 51.2 **Clinical Summary of Glucocorticoids and Mineralocorticoids Used Systemically—cont'd**

Generic name	Trade names*	Route†	Onset	Duration
Triamcinolone acetonide	Kenalone	IM	1-2 days	1-6 weeks
		IB, IA, IS, IL, ST	Slow	Weeks
Triamcinolone diacetate	Kenacort	PO	<2 hr	Intermed.
	Aristocort forte	IM	Slow	4-28 days
		IL	Slow	1-2 weeks
		IA, IS, ST	Slow	1-8 weeks
Triamcinolone hexacetonide	Aristospan	IA, IL	Slow	3-4 weeks

*Representative trade names are given.
†Abbreviations: IA, intraarticular; IB, intrabursal; IL, intralesional; IM, intramuscular; IS, intrasynovial; IV, intravenous; PO, oral; ST, soft tissue.

The ophthalmic preparations are special forms for topical application to the eye. Relatively high doses of steroids may be achieved in the eye, ordinarily with low absorption into systemic circulation. With chronic high doses, some drug may pass into the body and cause toxic effects. Toxicity is also possible in the eye itself. Certain patients with a genetic predisposition toward glaucoma will show increased intraocular pressure following the use of an ophthalmic steroid preparation. For most patients the intraocular pressure returns to normal when the drug is discontinued, but a few patients have been reported to develop glaucoma that did not respond to medication and required surgery. Another common adverse reaction to steroids is the development of secondary infections in the eye. These infections are commonly viral or fungal and may be dormant conditions, which are activated when host defenses are suppressed by steroids. The use of steroids in injured eyes may allow a new infection to develop.

Adrenal steroids are currently being employed as topical agents to control asthma (Table 51.3). By administering the drugs as aerosols, delivery is directly to the affected tissues in the lung without the necessity of high systemic doses.

Nasal steroids are usually administered to control rhinitis, allergies, or nasal polyps (Table 51.3). Steroids are appropriate in those allergic patients who do not benefit from decongestants and antihistamines.

Adrenal suppression. Patients should not be abruptly withdrawn from long-term systemic steroid therapy. All adrenal steroids suppress the normal function of the hypothalamus, adenohypophysis, and adrenal gland. If exogenous steroids are withdrawn suddenly, patients may die of acute adrenal insufficiency because their own adrenal glands cannot immediately produce the required steroids. This type of reaction is most likely in patients receiving relatively high doses for long periods. It may require 6 to 9 months for the natural negative feedback loop that regulates adrenal steroid synthesis to regain normal function after long-term steroid therapy, apparently because atrophy of the tissues occurs to some extent. Schedules for gradual withdrawal from steroids are available and must be followed faithfully, with dosage adjusted only to relieve symptoms of adrenal insufficiency if they develop during withdrawal.

To minimize hypothalamic-pituitary-adrenal suppression during long-term therapy with a glucocorticoid, many physicians prefer an *alternate-day treatment schedule*, once an effective dosage has been established. The patient is given a single, large dose of the steroid in the early morning of the treatment day. This regimen mimics the normal daily cycle, in which glucocorticoid levels are high in the morning and decrease throughout the day. On the next day no drug is given. The intermediate-acting steroids usually employed in this regimen suppress the hypothalamic-pituitary-adrenal system for only about 12 to 36 hours (Table 51.2). Therefore, on the day no drug is given, the normal regulatory mechanisms recover and the patient's adrenal gland produces glucocorticoids. Most patients complain of some discomfort on the drug-free day, but these complaints must be weighed against the benefits of maintaining adrenal function. Not all diseases will be adequately controlled by this regimen, so frequent assessment is necessary.

Drug-induced Cushing's syndrome. In all the steroid derivatives produced so far, increased an-

Table 51.3 Summary of Preparations of Corticosteroids for Nonsystemic Use

Use	Preparations	Trade names*	Comments
ANTIASTHMATIC			
Inhalation aerosol	Beclomethasone dipropionate	Beclovent, Vanceril	
	Dexamethasone sodium phosphate	Decadron Respihaler	
	Flunisolide	AeroBid	FDA Pregnancy Category C
	Triamcinolone acetonide	Azmacort	FDA Pregnancy Category D
DENTAL			
Paste, pellets	Betamethasone sodium phosphate	Betnesol	
	Hydrocortisone acetate	Orabase-HCA	FDA Pregnancy Category C
	Triamcinolone acetonide	Oracort	
DERMATOLOGIC			
Topical creams, gels, ointments, lotions, or sprays	Alclometasone	Aclovate	FDA Pregnancy Category C
	Amcinonide	Cyclocort	FDA Pregnancy Category C
	Betamethasone benzoate	Uticort	FDA Pregnancy Category C
	Betamethasone dipropionate	Alphatrex	FDA Pregnancy Category C
	Betamethasone valerate	Valisone	FDA Pregnancy Category C
	Clobetasol propionate	Dermovate	FDA Pregnancy Category C
	Clocortolone pivalate	Cloderm	FDA Pregnancy Category C
	Desonide	Tridesilon	FDA Pregnancy Category C
	Desoximetasone	Topicort	FDA Pregnancy Category C
	Dexamethasone	Decaderm	FDA Pregnancy Category C
	Dexamethasone sodium phosphate	Decadron	FDA Pregnancy Category C
	Diflorasone diacetate	Florone	FDA Pregnancy Category C
	Flumethasone	Locacorten	FDA Pregnancy Category C
	Fluocinolone acetonide	Synalar	FDA Pregnancy Category C
	Fluocinonide	Lidex	FDA Pregnancy Category C
	Flurandrenolide	Cordran	FDA Pregnancy Category C
	Halcinonide	Halog	FDA Pregnancy Category C
	Hydrocortisone	Hytone	FDA Pregnancy Category C
	Hydrocortisone acetate	Cortaid	FDA Pregnancy Category C
	Methylprednisolone acetate	Medrol	FDA Pregnancy Category C
	Mometasone furoate	Elocon	FDA Pregnancy Category C
	Triamcinolone acetonide	Kenalog	FDA Pregnancy Category C
NASAL			
Aerosols, solutions	Beclomethasone dipropionate	Beconase, Vancenase	FDA Pregnancy Category C
	Dexamethasone sodium phosphate	Decadron turbinaire	
	Flunisolide	Nasalide	FDA Pregnancy Category C
OPHTHALMIC-OTIC			
Solutions, suspensions, ointments	Betamethasone sodium phosphate	Betnesol	
	Dexamethasone	Maxidex	FDA Pregnancy Category C
	Dexamethasone sodium phosphate	Decadron	FDA Pregnancy Category C
	Fluorometholone	FML	FDA Pregnancy Category C
	Hydrocortisone	Cortamed	FDA Pregnancy Category C
	Medrysone	HMS liquifilm	FDA Pregnancy Category C
	Prednisolone acetate	Ocu-Pred-A	FDA Pregnancy Category C
	Prednisolone sodium phosphate	Ocu-Pred	FDA Pregnancy Category C
RECTAL			
Ointments, suppositories	Hydrocortisone	Dermolate	
	Hydrocortisone acetate	Cort-Dome	

*Representative trade names.

Table 51.4   Summary of Toxic Reactions to Long-Term Glucocorticoid Therapy with Pharmacological Doses

Toxic reaction	Cause	Comments
Impaired glucose tolerance and/or hyper-glycemia	Gluconeogenic action of glucocorti-coids	If diabetes develops, it is usually mild and reversible.
Fat deposition on trunk of body in-creased, as are plasma triglyceride levels	Stimulation of lipid synthesis by gluco-corticoids	Changes in lipid metabolism produce classic Cushing-type signs of moon face and truncal obesity.
Muscle weakness or muscle wasting	Stimulation of protein breakdown by glucocorticoids	This side effect is more pronounced with flu-oride derivatives of glucocorticoids, such as triamcinolone.
Peptic ulcer or intestinal perforation	Direct irritation and/or protein-wasting effects of glucocorticoids	It is not entirely clear whether steroids induce these conditions or whether they merely mask the symptoms and allow the condition to progress to a serious stage before diagnosis.
Pancreatitis	Not known, but may involve effects on lipid metabolism	Glucocorticoids may mask symptoms of dis-ease in early stages.
Growth inhibition	Glucocorticoid inhibition of growth hormone action	Glucocorticoids should be given with caution to children; doses below those producing growth inhibition should be used if possible.
Mood changes or psychoses	Not known	All patients receiving glucocorticoids should be observed closely for altered mood or be-havior, especially those with a past history of this type of disorder.
Osteoporosis or bone fractures	Glucocorticoids alter several aspects of calcium metabolism which increase bone resorption	This side effect is noted especially in patients with arthritis, in postmenopausal women, or persons with low calcium intake.
Sodium retention and potassium loss	Mineralocorticoid activity associated with some glucocorticoids	Newer, synthetic glucocorticoids minimize these effects.
Increased susceptibility to infection	Glucocorticoid inhibition of immune system	Infections are more difficult to eradicate in these patients, even with good antibiotic therapy.
Glaucoma	Glucocorticoids interfere with normal aqueous outflow from eye and elevate intraocular pressure	The risk is especially great in genetically pre-disposed or diabetic patients.
Cataracts	Not known	Topical or systemic therapy has been impli-cated.

tiinflammatory action also has been associated with increases in the metabolic effects character-istic of glucocorticoids. Therefore, any of the com-pounds with glucocorticoid activity, if given in high enough doses, will produce Cushing's syn-drome. This toxicity is one of the most common reactions seen with glucocorticoid therapy (Table 51.1). Indeed, in most endocrine clinics many more patients are seen with Cushing's syndrome pro-duced by drugs than with any other form of the disease. For these patients the steroid dose should be reduced if allowed by the severity of the con-dition being treated. Even when the condition being treated is not considered life-threatening, dose re-duction may be difficult, since many patients tol-erate the symptoms of steroid overdose better than the symptoms of the inflammatory disease being treated, although the drug overdose may be medically more dangerous.

Toxic reactions. Toxic reactions to antiinflammatory doses of the glucocorticoids resemble the symptoms of naturally occurring Cushing's syndrome but are not identical. For example, peptic ulcer is a rather common finding in a person receiving high doses of steroids but is relatively rare in Cushing's syndrome that is not drug induced. Other common symptoms of glucocorticoid toxicity are listed in Table 51.4. These reactions occur following long-term administration of glucocorticoids. Large doses given for a short time to control acute allergic responses or other acute conditions are not usually associated with any significant signs of toxicity. For these purposes a large dose might be given on day 1, with the dose halved for each of the succeeding 3 or 4 days and then stopped before toxic reactions develop.

Drug interactions. The effects of many drugs are altered in patients receiving glucocorticoids. Steroids may increase the excretion of salicylates in the kidney and make it necessary to increase salicylate dosage in a patient receiving both drugs. In other instances glucocorticoids may directly affect the action of a drug. Certain coumarin anticoagulants are less effective when steroids are present. In some cases drugs may have an unexpected effect in patients receiving glucocorticoids. For example, a safe level of anesthetic given to produce general anesthesia may cause dangerous hypotension in a patient receiving long-term steroid therapy because the adrenal cortex is suppressed.

One of the most common drug interactions involves liver metabolism of drugs. Steroids, barbiturates, phenytoin, and many other drugs are all inactivated by the same liver microsomal enzyme system. These enzymes have the capacity to be induced, that is, more enzymes may be formed when certain drugs are chronically available in the bloodstream. The effect of enzyme induction is to speed up drug metabolism, not only for the drug that induced the enzymes but also for any other drug metabolized by these enzymes. For example, phenobarbital may exacerbate asthma being treated with glucocorticoids by increasing the destruction of the steroid in the liver. The same effect may be seen if an asthmatic patient who is receiving long-term steroid therapy has an asthmatic crisis. Ordinarily a dose of 100 mg of hydrocortisone is effective in treating an acute asthma attack. In the patient who has been receiving long-term therapy with glucocorticoids, however, 300 to 1000 mg of hydrocortisone may be required to achieve the same effect,

again presumably because of the increased ability of the liver to destroy the hormone.

Clinical Uses of Adrenal Steroids and Their Derivatives

The adrenal steroids are used clinically primarily in one of two ways: (1) at physiological doses in replacement therapy for endocrine diseases such as pituitary deficiency or adrenal hypofunction, or (2) at pharmacological doses in the therapy of various nonendocrine diseases.

Replacement therapy. Examples of replacement therapy include the use of cortisol to treat Addison's disease or to treat secondary adrenal insufficiency. When used in replacement therapy, doses of adrenal steroids are relatively low, since they are intended only to replace amounts of the hormone normally present. Since the normal daily production of cortisol is about 15 to 25 mg, the daily replacement dose would be designed to achieve approximately the level of activity produced by that amount of cortisol. Table 51.1 shows the relationship of the activities of the various agents to the activity of cortisol. Wide variations in dosage exist, however, since stress and other factors affect the steroid requirement. Each patient is an individual whose dosage must be adjusted to needs and monitored to ensure continued success of the therapy. Although usual replacement doses slightly exceed normal daily production of steroids, these doses would not be expected to cause Cushing's syndrome.

Successful treatment of adrenal insufficiency frequently is obtained simply with cortisol (hydrocortisone) or cortisone, natural glucocorticoids with sufficient mineralocorticoid activity to maintain sodium balance in many individuals. Other patients, however, may require additional supplementation with a drug such as fludrocortisone, an orally absorbed mineralocorticoid.

Antiinflammatory therapy. In pharmacological doses, the antiinflammatory action of the glucocorticoid is the primary action sought. The level of steroid at the site of action must be much higher than normally would be found at that site to achieve the antiinflammatory effect. In some cases this goal may be achieved by topical or local application of the steroid; in other cases the steroids must be administered systemically (Table 51.4).

Other clinical uses. Steroids in one form or another have been used to treat a seemingly endless list of conditions. Evaluating these treatments is frequently difficult and requires large-scale clinical testing with careful comparison of the results for treated patients with those of untreated or placebo-treated individuals. Table 51.5 lists 30 nonendo-

Table 51.5   **Nonendocrine Conditions Effectively Treated with Glucocorticoids (FDA Designation)**

Condition	Treatment regimen	Rationale
ALLERGIC STATES		
Bronchial asthma Serum sickness	Systemic steroids used to control acute episodes that are unresponsive to conventional therapy.	Glucocorticoids block histamine-induced and other inflammatory responses. In asthma, glucocorticoids may enhance effects of sympathomimetic agents.
Contact dermatitis	Topical therapy as required. Systemic therapy rarely justified.	
COLLAGEN DISEASES		
Acute rheumatic carditis Systemic lupus erythematosus	Systemic steroids to control acute episodes, or lower doses for maintenance. Topical steroids to control dermatological manifestations of lupus erythematosus.	Glucocorticoids antagonize autoimmune responses, causing tissue damage in these diseases.
DERMATOLOGICAL DISEASES		
Mycosis fungoides Pemphigus Seborrheic dermatitis Severe erythema multiforme Severe psoriasis	Topical therapy as needed. Some skin lesions may require injection at the site. Systemic therapy may be employed when symptoms are widespread or especially severe.	Glucocorticoids have antiinflammatory and antimitotic actions that control symptoms.
EDEMATOUS STATES		
Cerebral edema Nephrotic syndrome	Systemic steroids for short periods to control acute episodes; used with other treatment.	Therapy empirical.
HEMATOLOGICAL DISORDERS		
Autoimmune hemolytic anemia Thrombocytopenia	Systemic steroids in large doses for acute disease; lower doses for maintaining remission.	Glucocorticoids antagonize autoimmune processes, destroying blood cells.
NEOPLASTIC DISEASES		
Leukemias Lymphomas	Systemic steroids along with other antineoplastic agents produce remissions and palliation of symptoms.	Glucocorticoids have antilymphocytic action, which aids in destroying tumors of these tissues.
OPHTHALMIC DISEASES		
Allergic conjunctivitis Allergic corneal marginal ulcers Chorioretinitis Iritis and iridocyclitis Keratitis Optic neuritis	Superficial conditions may be treated with steroids applied directly to the eye. Diseases of the internal structures of the eye may require systemic therapy.	Glucocorticoid antiinflammatory action reduces permanent eye damage and controls acute symptoms.
RHEUMATIC DISORDERS		
Acute and subacute bursitis Acute gouty arthritis Acute nonspecific tenosynovitis Ankylosing spondylitis Psoriatic arthritis Rheumatoid arthritis	Intraarticular injection may be required for selected cases. Modest oral doses minimize side effects while providing relief for many patients.	Glucocorticoid inhibition of inflammatory and autoimmune processes relieves symptoms of disease.
RESPIRATORY DISEASES		
Pulmonary tuberculosis Symptomatic sarcoidosis	Systemic steroids may give symptomatic relief to certain patients.	Glucocorticoid antiinflammatory action may relieve symptoms of disease, but no long-term benefit is demonstrable.

Table 51.6 Nonendocrine Conditions for Which Glucocorticoid Treatment Is "Probably" Effective (FDA Designation)

Condition	Treatment regimen
ALLERGIC STATES	
Urticaria	Systemic steroids used when disease not adequately controlled by conventional methods
DENTAL CONDITIONS	
Postoperative inflammatory reactions	Local application
EDEMATOUS STATES	
Cirrhosis of the liver with ascites	Systemic steroids used with diuretics
Congestive heart failure	
GASTROINTESTINAL DISEASES	
Intractable sprue	Systemic steroids may aid in short-term recovery but do not change the long-term prognosis
Regional enteritis	
Ulcerative colitis	
RESPIRATORY DISEASES	
Interstitial pulmonary fibrosis	Systemic steroids used with other therapy or after other therapy has failed.
Pulmonary emphysema with bronchial edema	

crine diseases in which glucocorticoid therapy was listed as effective, based on an FDA evaluation of information supplied by the National Academy of Sciences and National Research Council. Not all forms of these diseases will respond to steroids, but the drugs may prove useful to most patients at some stage of their disease. Specific notes concerning the treatment regimen employed are also included in Table 51.5. Table 51.6 lists the same information for diseases in which glucocorticoid therapy has not been rigorously proved to be effective. Nevertheless, the glucocorticoids frequently are used clinically to treat these conditions.

Compounds Used in Diagnosing Adrenal Disorders

Adrenocorticotropic hormone

Adrenocorticotropic hormone (ACTH, corticotropin) is discussed in Chapter 50 as part of the natural feedback regulatory cycle controlling adrenal function. ACTH directly stimulates the adrenal cortex to synthesize adrenal steroids. This action can be used diagnostically to distinguish between primary adrenal insufficiency (Addison's disease) and secondary adrenal insufficiency resulting from pituitary dysfunction (Table 51.7). Normal adrenal glands respond to ACTH by synthesizing and releasing cortisol into the bloodstream, where it may be measured. In Addison's disease the adrenal gland cannot respond to ACTH, and no excess cortisol is produced. In patients who have low pituitary function, the adrenal gland may be suppressed and may respond less rapidly to ACTH than would a normal gland.

In the past ACTH has been used to treat adrenal insufficiency or other diseases responding to glucocorticoids. The rationale for this therapy was that adrenal function was maintained and that a natural balance of steroids was produced. In practice, however, ACTH therapy was not as reliable or convenient as steroid therapy. ACTH must be injected because it is a peptide, whereas oral glucocorticoids are available. In addition, the response of the adrenal gland to ACTH was not easily predictable, making dosage adjustment unreliable. Finally, many patients developed antibodies to ACTH, and as a consequence they became unresponsive to the drug. For these reasons and others, ACTH is no longer widely used in therapy.

Dexamethasone

The highly potent synthetic glucocorticoid dexamethasone also is used diagnostically to test steroid suppression of cortisol synthesis. Relatively small doses of dexamethasone administered over 2 days inhibit cortisol production in a normal person and, to a lesser extent, in a person with pituitary-induced Cushing's syndrome. Ordinarily, tumor production of cortisol is unaffected.

Metyrapone

Metyrapone (Metopirone) blocks cortisol synthesis in the adrenal gland and may be used to test the ability of the pituitary gland to increase ACTH release. Before the test is run, it should be demonstrated that the patient's adrenal gland will respond to ACTH. While metyrapone is being administered, cortisol synthesis falls dramatically. In

THE NURSING PROCESS

DRUGS AFFECTING THE ADRENAL GLAND

Assessment

Problems associated with the hormones synthesized in the adrenal gland result from too much or too little of the specific hormones. The nurse obtains the same data base in either case, although the results of a measurement may be excessively high or low, depending on the direction of the imbalance. Thus too little cortisol causes hypotension; too much causes hypertension. If an adrenal problem is suspected, a complete patient assessment is needed. The nurse should monitor temperature, pulse, respiration, blood pressure, and weight and should check the blood and urine for glucose. The nurse should observe the body and skin carefully, noting color and character of the skin, distribution of body mass (fat, muscles), the presence of bruises or petechiae, and the condition of hair and nails. The nurse should determine the time of onset of these problems if appropriate.

Nursing diagnoses

Body image disturbance

Potential complication: electrolyte abnormalities

Potential complication: fragile bones resulting in increased susceptibility to fractures

Management

Depending on the problem, the treatment is surgical, pharmacological, or both. The nurse must remember that adrenocortical steroids are one of the most frequently used groups of drugs in present-day medicine and may also be prescribed as a temporary adjunct to treatment, even though hormonal insufficiency has not been demonstrated. Regardless of the reason for prescribing the adrenocorticosteroids, the nurse should monitor the blood pressure, weight, serum electrolyte levels, and sugar concentration in the blood and urine. The nurse must remember that wound healing may be slowed, that infection may be masked, and that improvement in appetite and sense of well-being may be due to drug therapy. Drug-induced diabetes may require treatment with insulin. The nurse should monitor the effect of the steroids on other medical conditions.

In planning for discharge, the nurse should determine with the physician the discharge dose and schedule of drugs and begin teaching the patient. Most patients have heard of steroids, but many know only the negative qualities of the drugs before teaching has begun.

Evaluation

Ideally, treatment with adrenocorticosteroids would result in improvement in the patient's condition, with only desirable side effects (e.g., increased sense of well-being). Even with physiological doses, however, undesired side effects such as weight gain and hyperglycemia may occur. With pharmacological doses, especially those prescribed on a long-term basis, side effects always occur. Before discharge to self-management, the patient should be able to explain why the drug has been prescribed, the desired goals of therapy, how to take the drug correctly (e.g., daily or alternate-day therapy), and side effects that may occur. The patient should be able to explain additional therapies needed because of the drugs, such as antacid therapy or dietary restrictions such as a low sodium diet. The nurse should be certain that the patient can explain special circumstances requiring contact with the physician, such as nausea and vomiting preventing taking the drug, illnesses that might necessitate a dosage increase, or effects of the drug on other medical problems (e.g., diabetes requiring an increase in insulin dose to control). Patients must understand the need not to discontinue or decrease the dose without physician approval and, if receiving long-term therapy, the need to obtain and wear a medical identification tag or bracelet. Finally, the patient should be able to explain what parameters, if any, should be monitored at home, such as weight, blood pressure, or urine glucose concentration.

Table 51.7   Clinical Summary of Agents Used in Diagnosis of Adrenal Gland Dysfunction

Generic name	Trade name	Administration/dosage	Comments
Corticotropin	Acthar*	INTRAMUSCULAR, SUBCUTANEOUS: 20 units 4 times daily. INTRAVENOUS: 10 to 25 USP units in 500 ml of dextrose infused over 8 hr. *Children*—1.6 USP units/kg body weight daily.	Used to determine if the adrenal gland can respond to normal regulation. The side effects are those expected of adrenal steroids and allergic reactions. FDA Pregnancy Category C.
	Cortrophin Zinc H.P. Acthar Gel	INTRAMUSCULAR REPOSITORY: 40 to 80 units every 24 to 72 hr.	This longer acting form may be preferred for therapy.
Cosyntropin	Cortrosyn*	INTRAMUSCULAR, INTRAVENOUS: *Adults*—0.25 mg single dose. *Children under 2 yr*—0.125 mg single dose.	Synthetic form of ACTH used for diagnostic purposes only. Less allergenic than ACTH. FDA Pregnancy Category C.
Metyrapone	Metopirone*	ORAL: *Adults*—750 mg every 4 hr for 6 doses. *Children*—15 mg/kg every 4 hr for 6 doses.	Used to determine if ACTH levels rise appropriately when the adrenal gland lowers cortisol production. Metyrapone blocks cortisol production, leading to appearance of cortisol precursors in urine if ACTH is present. The drug may induce acute adrenal insufficiency in some patients.

*Available in Canada and United States.

normal persons the fall in blood cortisol level stimulates the hypothalamus and in turn the pituitary gland, with the result that ACTH is released into the bloodstream. Under the influence of ACTH, early steps in steroid synthesis proceed, but metyrapone prevents cortisol from being formed in normal amounts. Therefore the steroid precursors accumulate and are excreted in the urine. If no precursors accumulate under these conditions, it is concluded that the pituitary gland failed to produce ACTH. If the metyrapone test is administered to a person with adrenal insufficiency, a danger exists of precipitating an adrenal crisis, since in these patients metyrapone may stop cortisol synthesis.

ADRENAL MEDULLA

The adrenal medulla arises from neuroectodermal tissue during embryonic life and remains intimately associated with the autonomic nervous system at maturity. The cells (pheochromocytes or chromaffin cells) are capable of synthesizing catecholamines by the same series of reactions found in nerve terminals, and release catecholamines into the bloodstream in response to sympathetic cholinergic presynaptic neurons. One major difference between the synthetic pathways is that nerve terminals form norepinephrine as the final product, whereas the adrenal medulla converts norepinephrine to epinephrine. The enzyme for this final conversion is induced by adrenal steroids, indicating that the anatomical proximity of the disparate tissues of the cortex and medulla may have functional importance.

The hormones of the adrenal medulla are not essential to survival, but they are useful in adapting to stress. Epinephrine produces widespread effects throughout the body, mediated by the beta and alpha adrenergic receptors. The actions of epinephrine are discussed in Chapter 10, and the clinical uses of epinephrine are discussed in Chapter 14.

PATIENT CARE IMPLICATIONS

Glucocorticoids

Drug administration

- See Table 51.4 for a listing of toxic reactions associated with long-term glucocorticoid therapy.
- Assess mental status and neurologic function.
- Assess for signs of depression: lack of interest in personal appearance, withdrawal, insomnia, and anorexia.
- Monitor blood pressure and pulse, weight. Auscultate lung and heart sounds.
- Check stools for presence of occult blood.
- Monitor complete blood count and differential, serum electrolytes, blood glucose.
- Use care in moving and positioning immobilized patients on long-term therapy to prevent fractures and bruising. Pad side rails as appropriate.
- Glucocorticoids are given via many routes (see Tables 51.2 and 51.3). Read labels carefully. Make certain the preparation can be given via the ordered route.
- Wear gloves to apply topical preparations.
  INTRAVENOUS BETAMETHASONE SODIUM PHOSPHATE
- May be given undiluted or diluted. Administer undiluted dose over at least 1 minute.
  INTRAVENOUS DEXAMTHASONE SODIUM PHOSPHATE
- May be given undiluted. Administer 15 mg or less over 1 minute.
  INTRAVENOUS HYDROCORTISONE SODIUM SUCCINATE
- Reconstitute as directed on label of vial. Administer direct IV at a rate of 500 mg or less over 1 minute.
  INTRAVENOUS METHYLPREDNISOLONE SODIUM SUCCINATE
- Reconstitute as directed on label of vial. Administer direct IV at a rate of 500 mg or less over 1 minute or longer.
  INTRAVENOUS PREDNISOLONE SODIUM PHOSPHATE
- May be given undiluted at a rate of 10 mg or less over 1 minute.

Patient and family education

- Review anticipated benefits and possible side effects of drug therapy. With short-term use (over 7 to 10 days) side effects may be minimal if noticeable. With chronic use, some side effects will usually develop. Tell patients to report the development of any new side effect.
- Take oral doses with meals or snack to lessen gastric irritation. Some physicians prescribe antacids or other drugs prophylactically to lessen the risk of ulceration.
- See Patient Problem: Constipation on p. 187.
- If weight gain is excessive, counsel about weight reduction diets; consult physician about a change in glucocorticoid or dose. Other dietary modifications may include decreasing sodium intake and increasing potassium intake. See Dietary Considerations: Potassium (p. 259) and Sodium (p. 236).
- Warn diabetic patients to monitor blood glucose levels carefully, as glucocorticoids will increase blood glucose levels. A change in diet or insulin may be necessary.
- Notify physician if tarry stools develop or "coffee ground" emesis occurs.
- Avoid rough activities if skin becomes fragile and easily bruised.
- Warn patients on long-term therapy to take doses every day as ordered, even if sick. Failure to take ordered doses, even for a few days, may result in adrenocortical insufficiency in susceptible patients.
- Remind patients to keep all health care providers informed of all medications being used. Do not take any medications unless approved by the physician.
- Warn patients not to increase or decrease the dose without consultation with the physician.
- Teach patients not to have immunizations while taking glucocorticoids unless approved by the physician.
- Encourage patients on long-term therapy to wear a medical identification tag or bracelet indicating that glucocorticoids are being used.
- Menstrual difficulties may develop with long-term therapy. Instruct women to keep a record of menstrual periods. Counsel about contraceptive methods as appropriate. Warn patients to notify the physician if pregnancy is suspected.
- Large doses of glucocorticoids increase susceptibility to infection and mask the symptoms of infection. Warn patients about this side effect. Instruct patients to notify the physician of fever, cough, sore throat, malaise, and injuries that do not heal. Instruct patients to avoid contact with individuals with active infections.

PATIENT CARE IMPLICATIONS — cont'd

- Review the drug and route of administration prescribed for the patient. Review manufacturer's instructions for administration. Ascertain that the patient can administer the ordered drug correctly; see Chapter 6.
- Remind patients not to share medications with others. Remind patients to keep all medications out of the reach of children.

Mineralocorticoids

Drug administration

- Note that all glucocorticoids have mineralocorticoid activity also, but in varying amounts; see the text and Table 51.1.
- Monitor weight, blood pressure, and pulse. Auscultate lung and heart sounds.
- Monitor serum electrolytes.

- For a discussion of subcutaneous implantation of drugs, see Chapter 54.
- For a discussion of IM injection of oil-based medications see Chapter 6.

Patient and family education

- Review anticipated benefits and possible side effects of drug therapy.
- Counsel about sodium restriction and increasing potassium intake as needed. See Dietary Considerations: Potassium on p. 259 and Sodium on p. 236.
- Encourage the patient to wear a medical identification tag or bracelet.
- Remind patients to keep all health care providers informed of all drugs being used.

SUMMARY

The adrenal cortex is composed of three distinct layers, which differ in the major steroids produced and in the regulation of steroid synthesis. Mineralocorticoids are synthesized in the outer layer in a process regulated by the renin-angiotensin system. Mineralocorticoids cause the retention of salt and water by the kidney. Glucocorticoids are synthesized by the inner layers of the adrenal cortex in a process regulated by the pituitary gland and the hypothalamus. Glucocorticoids stimulate gluconeogenesis and mobilize amino acids from muscle protein.

Acute or chronic adrenal insufficiency is treated by replacement therapy with the adrenal steroids. The doses are adjusted to supply the amount of hormone that would normally be synthesized by the adrenal gland. These doses should not cause Cushing's syndrome, in which excess amounts of the glucocorticoids produce excess protein breakdown, increased fat deposition, weakness of the extremities, calcium loss from bone, and hypertension.

Glucocorticoids may be used at higher than replacement dosages to take advantage of their antiinflammatory and immunosuppressive actions. Naturally occurring glucocorticoids also have mineralocorticoid activity, which will appear during high-dose therapy. The synthetic glucocorticoids betamethasone, dexamethasone, methylprednisolone, paramethasone, and triamcinolone have less

mineralcorticoid activity. Higher doses in this type of therapy for nonendocrine diseases may produce toxic signs similar to those seen in Cushing's syndrome. Patients should not be withdrawn abruptly from long-term high-dose therapy, since the chronically high glucocorticoid concentrations in the bloodstream of these patients will have suppressed adrenal function. Alternate-day therapy may minimize adrenal gland suppression but may be inadequate to control some disease processes.

Most steroid preparations are insoluble suspensions of the drug, but a few water-soluble derivatives are available. These water-soluble phosphates and succinates are more useful in an emergency when rapidly absorbed preparations are required. Topical preparations are available for use in dermatological conditions. Betamethasone valerate and triamcinolone acetonide are most useful as topical agents. Special preparations for use in the eye, ears, and nose are also available. Aerosols may be used for asthma.

Corticotropin and cosyntropin are used primarily in diagnosing the ability of the adrenal gland to respond to normal regulatory influences. Dexamethasone may be used in a diagnostic procedure to test the ability of cortisol production to be suppressed by excess glucocorticoid.

The adrenal medulla is closely associated with the autonomic nervous system. The medulla synthesizes and releases epinephrine, a catecholamine that helps the organism adapt to stress.

STUDY QUESTIONS

1. What are the two functional units of the adrenal gland?
2. What are mineralocorticoids?
3. In which part of the adrenal cortex are mineralocorticoids synthesized?
4. What hormones regulate mineralocorticoid synthesis?
5. Where are glucocorticoids synthesized?
6. What are the main effects of glucocorticoids on metabolism?
7. What is the result of untreated acute adrenal insufficiency?
8. What is Addison's disease?
9. What is secondary adrenal insufficiency?
10. What is Cushing's syndrome?
11. What are the symptoms of Cushing's syndrome?
12. What is the effect of overproduction of mineralocorticoids?
13. What are the three major activities or actions of adrenal steroids?
14. What is the effect of chronic overdosage with glucocorticoids?
15. Why should steroid therapy not be stopped suddenly in a patient who has been receiving long-term therapy?
16. What are the advantages and disadvantages of alternate-day therapy?
17. What are the two major clinical uses of adrenal steroids?
18. What is the aim of replacement therapy in treating adrenal insufficiency?
19. Which mineralocorticoids are available for clinical use?
20. Which are the water-soluble glucocorticoid preparations, and when are they preferred over the suspensions?
21. Which steroids are particularly effective as topical agents?
22. What drug interactions commonly occur with adrenal steroids?
23. How is ACTH used in diagnosis?
24. Why is ACTH not commonly used in replacement therapy?
25. What hormone is released by the adrenal medulla?

SUGGESTED READINGS

Aapro, M.S.: Corticosteroids as antiemetics, Recent Results Can. Res. **108**:102, 1985.

Claman, H.N.: Glucocorticoids. I. Antiinflammatory mechanisms, Hosp. Pract. **18**(7):123, 1983.

Claman, H.N.: Glucocorticoids. II. The clinical responses, Hosp. Pract. **18**(7):143, 1983.

Fauci, A.S.: Corticosteroids in autoimmune disease, Hosp. Pract. **18**(10):99, 1983.

Fritz, K.A., and Weston, W.L.: Topical glucocorticoids, Ann. Allergy **50**(2):68, 1983.

Gever, L.N.: Sorting out the topical corticosteroids, Nursing 87 **17**(9):115, 1987.

Harper, J.: Use of steroids in cerebral edema: therapeutic implications, Heart Lung **17**(1):70, 1988.

Ianuzzi, L.P.: Oral steroids in rheumatoid arthritis: helpful but not remittive, Postgrad. Med. **82**(5):295, 1987.

Johnson, C.E.: Aerosol corticosteroids for the treatment of asthma, Drug Intell. Clin. Pharm. **21**(10):784, 1987.

Kaiser, F.E., and Doe, R.P.: Steroid use in the elderly: guidelines for avoiding adverse effects, Postgrad. Med. **76**(1):65, 1984.

Miller, J.A., and Munro, D.D.: Topical corticosteroids: clinical pharmacology and therapeutic use, Drugs **19**:119, 1980.

Roberts, A.M.: Corticosteroid therapy of ophthalmologic diseases, Hosp. Pract. **19**(2):181, 1984.

Routes, J. and others: Corticosteroids in inflammatory bowel disease. A review, J. Clin. Gastroenterol. **9**(5):529, 1987.

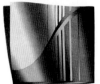

Drugs Affecting the Thyroid and Parathyroid Glands

52

The thyroid gland is a richly vascularized, horseshoe-shaped structure lying across the trachea in the region of the larynx (Figure 52.1). The gland contains at least two cell types differing in function and embryological origin. These are the follicular cells, derived from endoderm at the base of the tongue, and the parafollicular cells, derived from ultimobranchial bodies. A third endocrine tissue closely associated with the thyroid is found in the parathyroid glands. These small bodies normally lie behind the lobes of the thyroid but rarely may be found within the thyroid itself.

The function of each of these tissues, the hormones produced, and the medications commonly employed in the diagnosis and treatment of disease states associated with deficient or excessive thyroid or parathyroid function are described in this chapter.

Follicular Cells of the Thyroid

The function of the follicular cells of the thyroid is to regulate the basal metabolic rate (BMR), mainly by altering oxidative processes in target tissues. The iodine-containing hormones, thyroxine (T_4) and triiodothyronine (T_3), released by the follicular cells into the general circulation, establish the metabolic rates for most body tissues. Regulation of thyroid hormone levels in the bloodstream is accomplished in part by the negative feedback system described in Chapter 50. Thyroid-stimulating hormone (TSH) from the anterior pituitary stimulates each of the steps in thyroid hormone synthesis described in the next section.

Synthesis of Thyroid Hormones

The first step in synthesizing the iodine-containing thyroid hormones is *iodine uptake* by the follicular cell (Figure 52.2). Since iodide ion levels in the bloodstream are relatively low, the follicular cell must concentrate iodine to carry out the synthetic reactions required. In the normal human body the concentration of iodide ion in the thyroid is 30 to 40 times that found in plasma.

In the second step in thyroid hormone synthesis, *iodide ion activation* is catalyzed by the peroxidase enzyme formed in follicular cells. This activation step takes place on the surface of the microvilli, which protrude into the colloid filling the thyroid follicle (Figure 52.2).

Once activated, iodine may be attached to thyroglobulin in a process called *organification* (Figure 52.2). Thyroglobulin, a large protein synthesized in the follicular cell and extruded into the follicle, is the major protein component of colloid. Most iodine atoms are attached to tyrosine molecules contained within the peptide chains of thyroglobulin. The tyrosine may contain one (3-monoiodotyrosine, or MIT) or two (3,5-diiodotyrosine, or DIT) atoms of iodine.

Following iodination, some tyrosine molecules may undergo a *coupling reaction* in which two molecules of DIT combine to produce one molecule of thyroglobulin-bound T_4. Coupling may also occur between one molecule each of DIT and MIT to yield one molecule of T_3. These coupling reactions are also believed to be catalyzed by the peroxidase enzyme from the follicular cell (Figure 52.2).

Thyroglobulin serves primarily as a storage depot for thyroid hormones and the precursors MIT and DIT. In normal persons, each molecule of thyroglobulin contains about six molecules of MIT, five molecules of DIT, and two molecules of T_4. Less T_3 is stored. A single molecule of T_3 occurs in about one out of three molecules of thyroglobulin. Within the thyroglobulin of the follicles, normal thyroids thus contain a 30-day supply of T_3 and

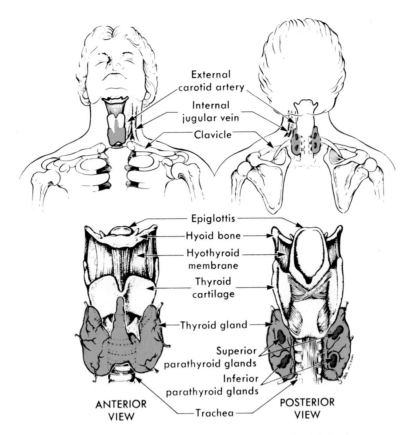

FIGURE 52.1   Anatomical location of thyroid and parathyroid glands.

T$_4$ and a 20-day supply of iodine stored as MIT and DIT.

When release of thyroid hormones is required, TSH stimulates the microvilli of the follicular cells to move droplets of colloid into the cell (Figure 52.2). Once inside the cell, the colloid droplets fuse with lysosomes to form vesicles called *phagolysosomes*. The low pH and the protein-digesting enzymes from the lysosomes allow proteolysis (digestion) of the thyroglobulin to amino acids. During proteolysis, T$_3$, T$_4$, MIT, and DIT are released into the cell. T$_3$ and T$_4$ are transported to the cell surface and released into the bloodstream. In contast, MIT and DIT are retained within the cell, and the iodine they contain is reclaimed for use in new hormone synthesis. This iodine salvage is an important function. Patients who lack the salvage pathway lose excessive iodide ion in the urine and ultimately fail to produce sufficient thyroid hormones. This syndrome is a rare cause of hypothyroidism.

The thyroid gland normally releases 70 to 90 µg of T$_4$ daily, but only 1 to 6 µg of T$_3$. Most T$_3$ is formed in peripheral tissues from T$_4$.

Disposition of Thyroid Hormones

Once in the bloodstream, the thyroid hormones are rapidly and almost completely bound to plasma proteins. Most of the hormones are bound to a special alpha globulin called thyroid-binding globulin (TBG). A less important carrier is prealbumin. Very little thyroid hormone is bound to plasma albumin in normal persons, since the thyroid hormones are so tightly bound to TBG. However, the amount of thyroid hormone that may be bound to TBG is limited. TBG can bind about 2.5 times more hormone than it ordinarily carries. When that limit is reached, the excess hormone is bound to albumin and prealbumin. These proteins are less avid carriers than TBG but have nearly unlimited capacity for hormones.

The relative distribution of T$_3$ and T$_4$ differs within the body. T$_4$ is much more abundant than T$_3$ in the thyroid and in the bloodstream. However, T$_3$ is less tightly bound to plasma proteins than T$_4$. More importantly, because T$_4$ is rapidly converted to T$_3$ in most tissues, the most abundant form of thyroid hormone in target cells is T$_3$. T$_3$ is also the

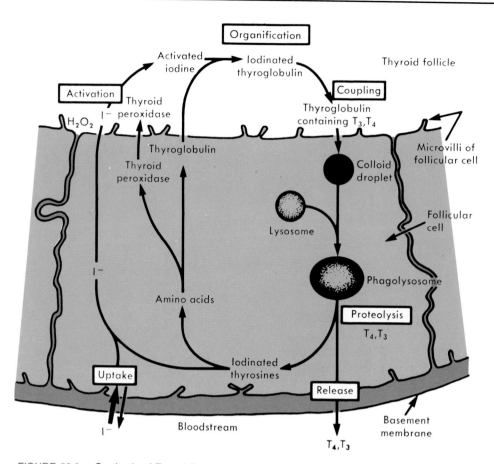

FIGURE 52.2   Synthesis of T_3 and T_4 by follicular cells within the thyroid gland. A single follicular cell is depicted. The base of the cell is intimately in contact with the bloodstream, and the apex of the cell is in contact with colloid. Cells of this type surround areas of colloid to form thyroid follicles. The parafollicular cells of the thyroid gland, discussed later in the chapter, do not directly contact colloid.

primary thyroid hormone that binds to nuclear receptors, setting off the metabolic events characteristic of thyroid action. For these reasons, T_3 may be considered to be the most important thyroid hormone.

T_3 and T_4 are metabolized by the liver to glucuronide and sulfate derivatives, which then are eliminated in bile. No significant reuptake of the hormones occurs from the gut; that is, no enterohepatic circulation of these compounds occurs. Other hormone destruction occurs in the target tissues, where the hormones are deiodinated and transformed to inactive products.

HYPOTHYROIDISM

Hypothyroidism occurs whenever the production of thyroid hormones is insufficient to meet the body's demands. Mild hormone deficiencies pro-

duce minimum disease with vague symptoms, sometimes making the condition difficult to diagnose. Untreated patients ultimately may develop myriad characteristic signs and symptoms related to the slowing of metabolic rates and changes in the central nervous system (Table 52.1). The severe form of the disease is called *myxedema*.

Hypothyroidism may develop in the fetus when a pregnant woman receives antithyroid drugs. However, the most common cause of hypothyroidism in newborns is an embryological or genetic defect that arrests thyroid development or prevents its function. A child lacking adequate thyroid function during fetal development may appear nearly normal at birth, since much of fetal development can proceed in the absence of fetal thyroid hormones. If the disease is not detected very soon after birth, however, irreversible brain damage and a host of

Table 52.1   Signs and Symptoms of Thyroid Disorders

Condition	Symptoms	Physical appearance
Hypothyroidism, adult onset (also called myxedema and Gull's disease)	Diminished vigor and muscle weakness Reduced mental acuity Emotional changes, especially depression Memory impairment Slow relaxation of deep tendon reflexes Muscle cramps Constipation Decreased appetite Abnormal menses in females Slow pulse and enlarged heart Tendency to gain weight Lowered basal metabolic rate	Puffy face and eyes Thin, coarse hair and eyebrows Dry, scaly, cold, and slightly yellow skin Enlarged tongue Slow, husky speech Dull or slow-witted appearance
Hypothyroidism, congenital (cretinism)		
At birth	Absence of distal femoral and proximal tibial epiphyses Slowed brain development	Essentially normal Slightly longer and heavier than normal
At 3 mo with no treatment	Lethargy Feeding difficulty Constipation Neonatal jaundice lasting beyond normal period Respiratory distress Hoarse cry Intermittent cyanosis	Enlarged tongue Puffy face Poor muscle tone Thick neck Depressed nasal bridge with broad, flat nose Distended abdomen Umbilical hernia Short legs
Hyperthyroidism (also called thyrotoxicosis or Graves' disease)	Cardiac arrhythmia Enlarged thyroid gland Rapid pulse rate Increased basal metabolic rate Muscle weakness and wasting Fine tremor Heat intolerance Weight loss in most patients	Restlessness or nervousness Abrupt actions and speech Warm, moist palms Loosening of fingernails from nail beds Bulging eyes with sclera visible all around iris White, unpigmented patches on the skin (vitiligo)

associated physical signs will develop. Congenital hypothyroidism is call *cretinism* (Table 52.1).

Hypothyroidism that develops after the neonatal period but before puberty is called *juvenile hypothyroidism*. The most prominent early sign of juvenile hypothyroidism is growth stunting. If not appropriately treated, juvenile hypothyroid patients will suffer not only arrested growth but also other signs and symptoms associated with adult forms of the disease.

Diagnosis of Hypothyroidism

Hypothyroidism is accurately diagnosed by the judicious use of a combination of the thyroid function tests summarized in Table 52.2. An understanding of these tests requires knowledge of normal thyroid physiology, discussed earlier in this chapter, as well as an understanding of the negative feedback regulation of the thyroid (Chapter 50).

In *primary hypothyroidism* the thyroid gland itself is defective; in most patients the reason for this is unknown, although in some a specific disease or chemical exposure may be responsible. The diagnosis of primary hypothyroidism requires establishing that a patient has lower than normal thyroid hormone levels and elevated levels of TSH in the bloodstream. Of the many tests available, TSH determinations are the most widely used. Free thyroxine (FT_4) levels are lower than normal in 80% to 90% of hypothyroid patients tested. Serum T_4,

Table 52.2   Tests Used to Evaluate Thyroid Function

Test	Procedure	Diagnostic use	Normal values	Comments
Serum T₄	*Total* serum T₄ is measured by competitive protein binding test or radioimmunoassay.	To distinguish hyperthyroid or hypothyroid conditions from euthyroid state.	5 to 12 µg/100 ml serum	Conditions that elevate thyroid-binding globulin (TBG) levels, (e.g., pregnancy or estrogen administration) also elevate total serum T₄ levels. Lowered TBG levels in cirrhosis or nephrotic syndrome also lower total serum T₄ levels. In both cases, free hormone levels are usually normal, and patients are functionally euthyroid.
Free thyroxine (FT₄)	Radioimmunoassay or equilibrium dialysis.	To distinguish hyperthyroid or hypothyroid conditions from euthyroid state.	1 to 2.5 ng/100 ml (0.001 to 0.0025 µg/100 ml)	Normal values may vary greatly from laboratory to laboratory.
T₃ uptake (T₃U) or resin T₃ uptake (RT₃U)	Test measures the degree of saturation of patient's TBG with endogenous thyroid hormones.	To distinguish hyperthyroid or hypothyroid conditions from euthyroid state.	25% to 45%, or 0.82 to 1.35 when expressed as a ratio of T₃U to normal	Hyperthyroidism elevates the ratio; hypothyroidism lowers the ratio. Levels of TBG and T₄ in the patient's blood affect the test more than do T₃ values.
Serum T₃	*Total* serum T₃ is measured by specific radioimmunoassay.	To distinguish hyperthyroid conditions from euthyroid state.	0.08 to 0.20 µg/100 ml	Test is not useful in hypothyroidism, since T₃ may be relatively more abundant than T₄ in hypothyroidism.
Serum TSH	Serum TSH is measured by specific radioimmunoassay.	To distinguish hypothyroid conditions from euthyroid state; to distinguish primary from secondary hypothyroidism.	0.5 to 5 µU/ml	Hypothyroidism caused by thyroid failure (primary) will show elevated TSH levels; hypothyroidism caused by pituitary failure (secondary) will show little or no TSH.
Protirelin test (TRH test)	Synthetic TRH (500 µg) is given IV, causing a peak release of TSH 30 min later in patients with normal pituitary glands	To distinguish hypothyroidism caused by pituitary failure from other forms of hypothyroidism.	Peak concentrations of TSH produced in normal patients are 5 to 35 µU/ml serum.	No rise is usually observed in serum TSH in hyperthyroid patients.
Thyroid uptake of radioiodine	Radioactivity in the thyroid measured 4, 6, and 24 hr after administration of tracer dose of radioactive iodine.	To distinguish hyperthyroid and hypothyroid conditions from euthyroid state.	Normal glands take up 10% to 35% of tracer dose in 24 hr.	This test may be affected by dietary intake of iodine, by administration of iodine-containing medications, or by use of antithyroid drugs.
TSH test	Bovine TSH is given IM, after which serum T₃ and T₄ or radioiodine uptake is measured.	To distinguish primary from secondary hypothyroidism.	A normal thyroid gland responds by increasing iodine uptake and T₄ release.	This test is rarely used when TSH levels are to be measured.
Thyroid suppression tests	T₃ (75 µg) is given daily for 7 days. Radioiodine uptake by thyroid gland is measured before and after test.	To distinguish hyperthyroid conditions from euthyroid state.	Uptake is 50% or less of the pretest uptake.	This test may be dangerous for elderly patients, weakened patients, or patients with heart disease.

T_3 uptake or protein-bound iodine (PBI) may also be measured, although each of these tests may be affected by conditions unrelated to thyroid disease that change the serum concentration of TBG (Table 52.2). Measurements of PBI are not commonly performed today, since other more accurate tests of thyroid function are available.

The thyroidal uptake of iodine is also lowered in hypothyroidism. However, this test is seldom useful in diagnosing the disease, since thyroidal uptake is affected by intake of iodine, whether as part of the diet or as a constituent of medications. The patient may not be aware that iodine is being taken. For example, potassium iodide, used an an expectorant, is a constituent of several prescription cough medicines.

Although *primary hypothyroidism* is the most common, other forms of hypothyroidism do occur. If the pituitary fails to release adequate TSH, insufficient thyroid hormone will be synthesized and *secondary hypothyroidism* develops. Occasionally a patient with damage to the hypothalamus will fail to produce TRH (thyrotropin-releasing hormone), which is required to stimulate TSH production in the pituitary (see Chapter 50); this is called *tertiary hypothyroidism.*

Secondary and tertiary hypothyroidism may be distinguished from primary hypothyroidism by measuring TSH. Whereas in primary hypothyroidism TSH is elevated by the natural action of the negative feedback system attempting to elevate thyroid hormone levels, TSH levels are low or undetectable in the other two forms of hypothyroidism. If the TSH assay is not available, a TSH test may be performed in which injected TSH is expected to stimulate T_4 formation and release in secondary or tertiary hypothyroidism but not in primary hypothyroidism (Table 52.2).

Secondary and tertiary hypothyroidism may be distinguished from each other by application of the protirelin test, which measures the ability of the pituitary gland to respond to its normal regulatory hormone (Table 52.2). If TSH rises after protirelin (TRH) administration, the implication is that the hypothalamus is defective and both the anterior pituitary and the thyroid would be capable of normal function if properly stimulated.

Treatment of Hypothyroidism

Treatment of hypothyroidism requires replacement therapy with the thyroid hormones. The aim of therapy is to produce the euthyroid state (normal thyroid hormone levels). Several preparations containing either natural or synthetic forms of the hormones are available (Table 52.3). Selecting one of these oral agents is largely a matter of preference for the physician. The only appropriate clinical use of these thyroid hormones is to treat thyroid deficiency. They should never be employed in weight loss programs.

Thyroid U.S.P.

Thyroid U.S.P. is a defatted extract of whole thyroid glands. It contains T_4 and T_3 in the natural ratio of 2.5:1. The iodine content of these preparations is regulated by law in the United States. Although thyroid hormone activity is not directly standardized in these products, many physicians have found them to be quite constant in potency, especially when fresh, dry preparations are compared. Considerable potency may be lost on long storage or if the powder becomes moist.

Thyroglobulin

Thyroglobulin is also prepared from whole thyroid glands and, as with thyroid extracts, contains T_4 and T_3 in the ratio 2.5:1. This preparation is more expensive than thyroid U.S.P. Some physicians prefer thyroglobulin because it is standardized directly for thyroid hormone activity rather than for total iodine content.

Levothyroxine sodium

Levothyroxine sodium is a pure synthetic form of the natural thyroid hormone thyroxine, or T_4. It therefore has the properties of T_4 previously outlined: high affinity for binding to serum proteins, long half-life in the bloodstream, and conversion to T_3 by peripheral tissues.

Liothyronine sodium

Liothyronine sodium is a pure synthetic form of the natural thyroid hormone triiodothyronine, or T_3. It therefore has the properties previously outlined for T_3: shorter half-life in the bloodstream than T_4, greater potency than T_4, and conversion to inactive products in peripheral tissues. In addition, T_3 seems to be absorbed better from the gut than T_4.

Liotrix

Liotrix is a thyroid preparation that contains both pure synthetic T_4 and T_3 in the ratio of 4:1. This mixture was designed to produce normal thyroid function tests when therapy was adequate. In contrast, note that if T_3 is given alone, a patient may be clinically euthyroid; since T_3 is not converted to T_4, however, any diagnostic test based on T_4 will likely give low values. In theory these mixtures containing 4:1 ratios of T_4 to T_3 bring T_3, T_4,

Table 52.3 Drugs Used to Diagnose or Treat Hypothyroidism

Generic name	Trade name	Administration/dosage	Properties	Comments
NATURAL THYROID HORMONES				
Thyroglobulin	Proloid*	ORAL: *Adults*—32 to 160 mg daily for maintenance. Initial doses are small and gradually increased to maintenance levels. FDA Pregnancy Category A.	Contains T_3 and T_4, as well as other iodine-containing compounds.	Replacement therapy for hypothyroidism. Overdose produces the same symptoms as seen with thyroid U.S.P.
Thyroid U.S.P.		ORAL: *Adults*—60 to 120 mg daily is usual for maintenance. Initial doses 15 mg daily. Double the dose every 2 wk until effective maintenance dose is reached. FDA Pregnancy Category A.	Impure mixture of thyroid components that includes T_3 and T_4.	Replacement therapy for hypothyroidism. Overdose produces symptoms of hyperthyroidism. Too large a dose at onset of therapy may cause vascular occlusion, especially in patients with arteriosclerosis.
SYNTHETIC THYROID HORMONES				
Levothyroxine sodium	Eltroxin† Levothroid Synthroid*	ORAL: *Adults*—75 to 125 µg daily for maintenance. Initial doses are small and gradually increased to maintenance levels. *Children over 1 yr*—2 to 6 µg/kg body weight daily. INTRAVENOUS: *Adults*—Up to 0.5 mg with mannitol (Synthroid) or without (Levothroid). FDA Pregnancy Category A.	Chemically pure form of T_4.	Replacement therapy for hypothyroidism. Intravenous form for myxedemic coma. Peak effect occurs 9 days after start of therapy; serum half-life about 11 days.
Liothyronine sodium	Cytomel*	ORAL: *Adults*—25 to 100 µg daily for maintenance. Initial doses should be low and gradually increased to maintenance levels. FDA Pregnancy Category A.	Chemically pure form of T_3.	Replacement therapy for hypothyroidism. Peak effect occurs in 2 days; serum half-life 4 to 6 days. Not for cretinism because T_3 may not cross the blood-brain barrier as well as T_4.
Liotrix	Euthroid Thyrolar*	ORAL: *Adults*—30 µg T_4 with 7.5 µg T_3 or 25 µg T_4 with 6.25 µg T_3. Doses may be gradually increased as needed. FDA Pregnancy Category A.	Chemically pure T_4 and T_3 combined in a ratio of 4:1.	Replacement therapy for hypothyroidism.
ADENOHYPOPHYSEAL HORMONES				
Protirelin (thyrotropin-releasing hormone, TRH)	Relefact TRH* Thypinone	INTRAVENOUS: *Adults*—500 µg *Children*—7 µg/kg.	Synthetic preparation of natural hypothalamic tripeptide hormone.	Diagnostic agent to differentiate pituitary-induced hypothyroidism from other types of hypothyroidism. May transiently produce nausea, flushing, changes in blood pressure, and an urge to urinate.
Thyrotropin (TSH)	Thytropar*	INTRAMUSCULAR, SUBCUTANEOUS: 10 IU once or twice daily. FDA Pregnancy Category C.	Extract of bovine anterior pituitary contains natural peptide, TSH.	Used to diagnose hypothyroidism. Releases thyroid hormones that may precipitate adrenal crisis in patient with secondary adrenal insufficiency. May also cause cardiovascular symptoms and rare allergic reactions.

*Available in Canada and United States.
†Available in Canada only.

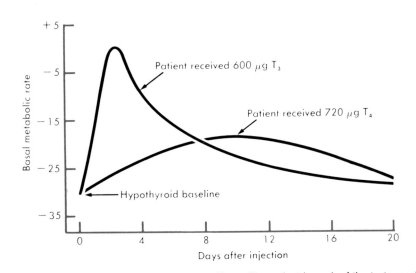

FIGURE 52.3   Time-course of thyroid hormone effects. The patient in each of the tests received a single oral dose of the medication indicated. The doses T_3 and T_4 administered are equimolar (equivalent numbers of molecules).

and PBI all within normal range during therapy. No firm evidence shows that this treatment has any clinically apparent advantage to the patient over the use of T_4.

Relative potency of agents used to treat hypothyroidism

One obvious difference among the preparations just discussed is their relative potencies. In terms of biological activity, 60 mg of thyroid U.S.P. = 60 mg thyroglobulin = 1 mg or less of levothyroxine = 0.025 mg of liothyronine = liotrix tables containing 0.06 mg T_4 + 0.015 mg Tp_3 or 0.05 mg T_4 + 0.0125 mg T_3. A wide range of tablet sizes is available in each of these preparations, so a dosage may be adjusted easily to the patient's particular need.

Absorption, Distribution, and Excretion of Hormones Used to Treat Hypothyroidism

The protein-binding properties of the thyroid hormones explain some clinically important differences between these agents. T_4, being more highly protein bound, leaves the bloodstream more slowly than does T_3. Therefore the onset of action for T_4 is about 2 days, whereas T_3 effect may be expected within 6 hours of administration (Figure 52.3). Moreover, T_4, which is bound to plasma protein, is less available for elimination, excretion, or tissue biotransformation than is the more freely available T_3. Thus T_4 persists longer in the body

than does T_3. The effects of a single equimolar dose (same number of molecules) of T_3 and T_4 are shown in Figure 52.3, in which the BMR was followed as an indicator of thyroid hormone action in these hypothyroid subjects. When patients are switched from T_4 to T_3, or vice versa, these different time courses must be considered. For example, a patient being switched from a preparation containing primarily T_4 to T_3 alone might suffer from excessive thyroid hormone action if started immediately on full T_3 doses after T_4 administration was terminated. Therefore patients are given small doses of T_3 after T_4 is stopped, and the dose of T_3 is gradually raised as necessary to maintain the euthyroid state.

In a newly diagnosed hypothyroid patient, thyroid medications are begun at very low doses and increased at varying intervals until the euthyroid state is achieved. Thyroid U.S.P. and levothyroxine doses are doubled roughly every 2 weeks, but liothyronine doses are doubled weekly until adequate control is achieved. These gradually increasing doses are justified, since a sudden return to adequate thyroid hormone levels produces acute stress on several body systems. One common and dangerous example observed occasionally even with low doses is the production of angina pectoris, coronary occlusion, or cerebrovascular accident (stroke) in elderly or predisposed patients. Another difficulty may be a relative adrenal insufficiency, which arises primarily in patients with inadequate pituitary function who suffer both secondary hypothyroidism and secondary adrenal insufficiency. If thyroid hormone therapy is begun in these patients without also restoring adequate glucocorticoid levels, they may suffer a dangerous adrenal crisis.

Severe hypothyroidism may ultimately result in the serious condition called *myxedemic coma.* In this state patients possess most of the clinical features of hypothyroidism shown in Table 52.1, including low body temperature as a result of the profoundly lowered metabolic rate, depressed central nervous system, and hypoventilation. Patients at this stage of the disease must be treated aggressively with thyroid hormones as well as with glucocorticoids and other supportive measures. Since rapid replacement with thyroid hormones is necessary, some physicians prefer to use the more rapidly acting T_3. However, T_3 is not readily available commercially in an injectable form. Since T_3 is rapidly absorbed from the gastrointestinal tract, T_3 tablets may be crushed and administered through a nasogastric tube. Alternatively, some physicians prefer to use the commercially available T_4 injection form that is administered intravenously.

Catecholamines must occasionally be used to combat the shocklike symptoms that are found in myxedema coma. Patients so treated are especially at risk for cardiac arrhythmias, since both the catecholamines and the thyroid hormones have the potential of causing this dangerous consequence.

Elimination of the thyroid hormones used in replacement therapy is the same as for the normal hormones, the major routes being biliary excretion and tissue metabolism of the compounds.

HYPERTHYROIDISM

Hyperthyroidism occurs whenever excess thyroid hormones are released into the circulation. The disease may range from very mild forms displaying few of the symptoms shown in Table 52.1 to a severe condition called *thyroid storm*, in which death may result from an uncontrolled rise in body temperature and vascular collapse. Increased thyroid hormone production may result from hyperfunction of the entire gland or from the excessive output of one or more small nodules within the thyroid. A rare cause of hyperthyroidism is excess TSH either from the pituitary gland or from a tumor.

Several terms are in use to describe various forms of hyperthyroidism. Basically, hyperthyroidism may occur with or without thyroid nodules. The disease without nodules is the most common form and is referred to as *toxic diffuse goiter*, *thyrotoxicosis*, or *Graves' disease* (or rarely *Basedow's* or *Parry's disease).* Many patients with this disease display exophthalmos (bulging eyes); since many also have enlarged thyroid glands, another common name for this condition is *exophthalmic goiter.* Toxic nodular goiter produces the same general symptoms as Graves' disease, except that eye symptoms are rare in the nodular form.

Hyperthyroidism is rare in children and is most common in adults in the third or fourth decade of life. Women are affected much more frequently than men, the reasons for which are not clear. Also, Graves' disease seems to be precipitated in women by puberty, pregnancy, or menopause. A condition called *subacute thyroiditis* can produce a reversible form of hyperthyroidism. This condition seems to appear sometime after recovery from viral diseases and may be caused by the infectious process.

Diagnosis of Hyperthyroidism

Hyperthyroidism is characterized by elevated serum T_4, serum T_3, free T_4, and free T_3 levels in most patients. Thus diagnostic tests that directly measure one of these parameters are most often used: serum T_4 and serum T_3 testing. The T_3 resin uptake test also may be used, since hyperthyroidism increases the degree of TBG saturation with thyroid hormones. Radioactive iodine uptake also may be measured and is useful in distinguishing between various forms of hyperthyroidism. Obviously these diagnostic tests form part of a larger clinical picture. Much information is gained by determining the size of the thyroid by palpation, presence or absence of nodules in the thyroid, and the results of a thyroid scan to measure the pattern of radioactive iodine concentration in the gland.

Diagnosis of Graves' disease has been aided by the realization that the disease has an immunological basis. In this condition the thyroid is chronically overstimulated by a group of immunoglobulins that supplant TSH as the regulator of thyroid function. These immunoglobulins are found in the sera of nearly all patients who have Graves' disease, and the amounts of the immunoglobulins correlate with the severity of the hyperthyroidism that is observed.

Treatment of Hyperthyroidism

Hyperthyroidism most often is controlled with drugs or radioactive iodine. The drugs fall into two main classes: those that control the symptoms of hyperthyroidism and those that lower the production of T_3 and T_4 by the thyroid.

Propranolol

Propranolol, a drug previously discussed as a beta adrenergic blocking agent (see Chapters 10 and 15), represents the class of drugs that control symp-

THE NURSING PROCESS

THYROID DISORDERS

Assessment

The nursing process in diseases of the thyroid gland is the same, regardless of whether the problem is hyperthyroidism or hypothyroidism. In most cases the original problem develops insidiously. The nurse should obtain a complete assessment of the patient, including temperature, pulse, respiration, blood pressure, weight, history of changes in weight, level of energy, mood, subjective feeling, and response to temperature. The height of children should be checked. Questioning the family members may be helpful to determine onset of symptoms. The nurse also should check thyroid function test results and the glucose content of urine and blood.

Nursing diagnoses

Body image disturbance

Activity intolerance related to fatigue secondary to excessive metabolic rate

Management

The goal of therapy is to restore normal or near-normal functioning of the thyroid gland or to replace exogenously the thyroid hormones to normal levels. During the dosage-adjustment phase the nurse should monitor the temperature, pulse, respiration, blood pressure, weight, height of children, and glucose content of urine and blood. The patient should be questioned about subjective reaction to therapy. If weight reduction is an additional goal of therapy, referral and/or diet teaching should be done. If radioactive iodine is used, the nurse should follow hospital procedures for the handling of radioactive materials.

Evaluation

It is difficult to determine the effectiveness of therapy for weeks or months after the drugs have been started. Before discharge, patients should be able to explain the action of the drug and how to take the prescribed dose. Other parameters the patient should monitor and record at home include pulse, weight, and height. The nurse should explain the side effects that may occur and what to do about them, adjustments needed in the treatment of other medical problems (e.g., changes in insulin dose or anticoagulant dose), the need for continuing the medication, and the need to wear an identification tag or bracelet. With radioactive iodine, the patient will not be on long-term drug therapy but should be able to explain what symptoms should be reported to the physician. For further specific guidelines, see the patient care implications section.

---

toms of hyperthyroidism but produce no significant long-term change in thyroid hormone levels. Propranolol is effective because it alters the response of peripheral tissues to the high circulating levels of thyroid hormones. Blockade of the beta receptors reduces the symptoms of palpitation, tremor, sweating, proximal muscle weakness, mental agitation, and cardiac arrhythmias. One advantage of propranolol therapy is that clinical improvement is seen rapidly. With many other drugs, relief of symptoms may be greatly delayed. Propranolol may

be used to prepare a hyperthyroid patient for surgery.

Thioamides

The thioamides represent the class of drugs that inhibit the synthesis of thyroid hormones. Although the exact mechanism of action of these compounds is not agreed on, they are known to inhibit each step in synthesis except iodine uptake (Figure 52.2), and they are thought to inhibit preferentially the peroxidase-catalyzed reactions (coupling and organification). Since these compounds are primarily enzyme inhibitors, they do not directly destroy thyroid tissue but only prevent its excessive action.

Thioamide action on the thyroid gland is immediate, and reduced hormone synthesis can be demonstrated within hours. Observable clinical response to the drugs, however, does not appear for days or weeks, the period required for stored thyroid hormones to be depleted. Patients may be maintained on one of the thioamides for months, provided the hyperthyroidism is well controlled during that time. Usually, after about 1 year, the thioamide is withdrawn and thyroid function is reevaluated. Many patients remain euthyroid after the thioamides are discontinued. For this 15% to 50% of all patients treated, no further therapy may ever be required.

Thioamides are absorbed rapidly following oral administration and are concentrated in the thyroid. The drugs also are distributed to other tissues and cross the placenta to enter the fetus. Thioamides appear in the milk of nursing mothers, and they are metabolized and excreted in the urine.

Two thioamides, methimazole and propylthiouracil, currently are used in the United States (Table 52.4). These drugs differ primarily in potency and in the incidence of toxic reactions. Propylthiouracil also inhibits the conversion of T_4 to T_3 in peripheral tissues.

Iodine

Iodine is the oldest of the antithyroid preparations currently in use. Although iodine is the required starting material for synthesis of the thyroid hormones, high concentrations of iodine suppress continued uptake of iodine and synthesis of thyroid hormones in the thyroid gland. Suppression of hormone synthesis is by no means complete with iodine administration, and many patients return to the hyperthyroid state even with continued high doses. Iodine is seldom used today for long-term suppression of the hyperactive thyroid gland. The most common current use of iodine is to prepare a hyperthyroid patient for surgery. Iodine not only suppresses thyroid function, but also reduces vascularization of the gland. By these two mechanisms, iodine reduces surgical risk to the hyperthyroid patient. Iodine pretreatment is especially important for the hyperthyroid patient who has received thioamide therapy, since those drugs increase vascularization of the thyroid gland. In addition, iodine may be used as part of the emergency therapy for hyperthyroid crisis. In this situation, iodine is administered intravenously after one of the thioamides has been given.

Radioactive iodine

Radioactive iodine is used in the treatment of hyperthyroidism as well as in diagnosis. This therapy depends on the ability of the radioactive iodine to be concentrated in the thyroid gland, where it then destroys surrounding tissue by emitting low-energy radiation. The doses of iodine are small. The use of radioactive iodine allows the thyroid to be functionally destroyed without resorting to surgery. Nearly all patients treated with radioactive iodine ultimately become hypothyroid and require treatment with thyroid hormones. The incidence of hypothyroidism is about 10% of treated patients during the first year after therapy and about 3% per year thereafter. Because of the likelihood of hypothyroidism, patients should be urged to return periodically for thyroid evaluation.

Incidental antithyroid compounds

Thyroid function can be influenced by many different types of chemicals, including some that are used in medicine. Table 52.5 summarizes the effects of some of these compounds.

Parafollicular Cells of the Thyroid

The parafollicular cells, which constitute about 10% to 20% of total thyroid cells, synthesize the peptide hormone called *calcitonin*. In animals calcitonin is thought to prevent blood calcium levels from exceeding the normal range after meals; its physiological role in human beings has not been resolved. Nevertheless, calcitonin does have demonstrable effects when administered exogenously. Calcitonin prevents the loss of calcium from bone, augments the urinary excretion of calcium and phosphate, and blocks the absorption of calcium from the small intestine.

Calcitonin has been used therapeutically to treat Paget's disease, in which excessive bone resorption leads to thinned and fragile bones. One preparation often used clinically is a synthetic form of salmon calcitonin (Table 52.6), the most potent of the naturally occurring forms of the hormone. The dose is 50 to 100 units given intramuscularly or subcutaneously. Some patients suffer nausea and vomiting, facial flushing, and occasional inflammatory reactions at the injection site. Since the hormone is a peptide and is administered in a gelatin solution, allergic reactions may occur.

Table 52.4 Drugs Used to Treat Hyperthyroidism

Generic name	Trade name	Administration/dosage	Properties	Comments
THIOAMIDES				
Propylthiouracil (PTU)	Generic Propyl-Thyracil†	ORAL: *Adults*—50 to 300 mg daily in 3 doses. Initially 300 to 600 mg daily is given in 3 or 4 doses. FDA Pregnancy Category D. *Children over 10 yr*—half the adult dose. *Children 6 to 10 yr*—one-quarter the adult dose.	Inhibits thyroid hormone synthesis but does not release. Inhibits conversion of T_4 to T_3 by peripheral tissues.	Used to lower thyroid hormone levels. Clinical improvement of hyperthyroid state is delayed. Agranulocytosis may occur in 1.4% of patients during first 2 mo of therapy; skin rashes occur in roughly 3% of patients. Mild leukopenia in 10% of patients.
Methimazole	Tapazole*	ORAL: *Adults*—5 to 30 mg daily in one or 2 doses. Initially 30 to 60 mg daily is given in 1 or 2 doses for severe hyperthyroidism. FDA Pregnancy Category D. *Children 6 to 10 yr*—0.4 mg/kg body weight daily in 1 or 2 doses.	Inhibits thyroid hormone synthesis but does not release.	Used to lower thyroid hormone levels. Clinical improvement of hyperthyroid state is delayed. Agranulocytosis, leukopenia, skin rashes as for PTU; more likely to cause vasculitis.
BETA ADRENERGIC BLOCKER				
Propranolol hydrochloride	Inderal*	ORAL: *Adults*—40 to 240 mg daily in divided doses. INTRAVENOUS: *Adults*—5 mg or less administered at 1 mg/min or more slowly.	Controls symptoms of hyperthyroidism but does not lower T_3 and T_4 release from the thyroid.	Controls palpitations, tremor, sweating, proximal muscle weakness, and cardiac symptoms of hyperthyroidism by competitively blocking beta adrenergic receptors. Bronchospasm may occur in asthmatic patients; may precipitate frank heart failure in patients with heart function maintained by sympathetic tone.
IODINE				
Potassium iodide	Strong Iodine Solution Lugol's Solution Iosat Pima Thyro-Block*	ORAL: *Adults*—250 mg 3 times daily as presurgical medication. INTRAVENOUS: *Adults*—250 to 500 mg daily for thyrotoxic crisis.	Produces short-term inhibition of thyroid hormone synthesis by direct action on the thyroid.	Used as presurgical medication to reduce the size of the thyroid gland after thioamide therapy. Used with thioamide and propranolol for hyperthyroid crisis. May produce iodism.
RADIOACTIVE IODINE				
¹³¹I as NaI		ORAL: *Adults*—4 to 10 mCi (148 to 370 megabecquerels) as a single dose for Graves' disease. For thyroid carcinoma, single doses of up to 150 mCi (5.5 gigabecquerels) may be used. Smaller doses are used for diagnostic purposes (see Table 52.2).	These radionuclides are concentrated in the thyroid and release radiation, which destroys thyroid tissue.	Used to destroy thyroid tissue without surgery for control of Graves' disease or thyroid carcinoma. Hypothyroidism ultimately develops in most patients.

*Available in Canada and United States.
†Available in Canada.

Table 52.5 Miscellaneous Compounds Affecting the Thyroid Gland

Compound	Use or occurrence	Action on the thyroid
Aminosalicylates	Antituberculosis therapy	Hypothyroidism and goiter may occur with long-term use.
Aminotriazole	Herbicide (food contaminant)	Suppress thyroid function.
Amiodarone	Antiarrhythmic	Complex action on thyroid metabolism. Thyroid hormone concentrations are commonly altered; up to 10% of patients suffer hypothyroidism; 1–3% of patients develop hyperthyroidism.
Dimercaprol	To treat heavy metal poisoning	May block iodine uptake into thyroid.
Goitrin	Found in plants of the mustard family and in turnips	Chronically high intake may cause goiter.
Iocetamic acid, Iodipamide, iohexol, iopamidol, iopanoic acid, iophendylate, iothalamate, ioxaglate, ipodate, tryopanoate	Radiopaque contrast agents used as aids in diagnostic imaging	These organic iodine compounds will block iodine uptake by the thyroid.
Lithium	Antimanic	Goiter and hypothyroidism may be induced, especially in the elderly.
Phenylbutazone	Nonsteroidal antiinflammatory	May block iodine uptake by thyroid.
Sulfonamides	Antibacterial agents	Goiter may rarely be produced.

DIETARY CONSIDERATION: CALCIUM

Calcium is important for growth and maintenance of healthy bones, as well as for playing a role in nerve and muscle function and blood clotting. Some medical conditions contribute to hypocalcemia (low blood calcium levels) including hypoparathyroidism, kidney disease, massive cellulitis, burns, and peritonitis. An extremely low level of calcium can result in tetany, a medical emergency. Tetany is treated with intravenous calcium. Milder caes of hypocalcemia may be treated in part by having the patient increase dietary intake of calcium. Good dietary sources of calcium include:

blackstrap molasses	ice cream	salmon
cheese	milk products	sardines
clams	oysters	yogurt
cottage cheese		
dark green leafy vegetables (e.g., kale, spinach)		

A synthetic form of human calcitonin is available (Table 52.6). This form is less likely to cause allergic reactions than is salmon calcitonin.

The Parathyroid Glands

Actions of Parathyroid Hormone

The parathyroid glands synthesize parathyroid hormone, a peptide whose major function is to maintain blood calcium levels above the critical threshold required for body function. In many ways parathyroid hormone acts exactly opposite to calcitonin. For example, parathyroid hormone increases reabsorption of calcium from bones, lowers renal excretion of calcium, and along with vitamin D increases calcium absorption from the intestine. The overall interaction of parathyroid hormone, calcitonin, and vitamin D allows the body to maintain blood calcium levels within a very narrow mar-

Table 52.6   Clinical Summary of Agents Used to Alter Calcium Metabolism

Generic name	Trade name	Administration/dosage	Clinical use
Calcitonin-human	Cibacalcin	SUBCUTANEOUS: *Adults*—initially 0.5 mg daily, then reduced by lowering frequency of dosing or using 0.25 mg daily. FDA Pregnancy Category C.	To control Paget's disease (excessive bone remodeling)
Calcitonin-salmon	Calcimar* Miacalcin	INTRAMUSCULAR, SUBCUTANEOUS: *Adults*—100 units daily or higher if required. FDA Pregnancy Category C.	To lower hypercalcemia in hyperparathyroidism or vitamin D intoxication. To control Paget's disease (excessive bone remodeling).
Etidronate	Didronel*	ORAL: *Adults*—5 mg/kg daily for up to 6 mo. FDA Pregnancy Category B.	To control Paget's disease. Hypercalcemia following cancer chemotherapy. Not effective for hypercalcemia caused by hyperparathyroidism.
Parathyroid hormone		INTRAVENOUS: *Adults*—200 units.	Diagnosis of pseudohypoparathyroidism. (Not currently available commercially.)
Vitamin D Calcifediol	Calderol	ORAL: *Adults*—50 µg daily or 100 µg on alternate days. FDA Pregnancy Category C. *Children*—20 to 50 µg daily.	Treatment of metabolic bone disease in patients on dialysis for chronic renal failure.
Calcitriol	Rocaltrol* Calcijex	ORAL: *Adults*—0.25 to 3 µg daily. INTRAVENOUS: *Adults*—0.5 µg three times weekly. FDA Pregnancy Category C.	Treatment of rickets, pseudohypoparathyroidism.
Dihydrotachysterol	Hytakerol*	ORAL: *Adults*—doses range from 0.1 to 2.5 mg daily, as needed to maintain normal serum calcium concentration. FDA Pregnancy Category C.	Treatment of hypoparathyroidism, and postoperative tetany.
Ergocalciferol	Calciferol Deltalin Drisdol* Ostoforte†	ORAL: *Adults*—400 units daily is normal replacement dose; therapy for rickets or hypoparathyroidism may require 50,000 to 500,000 units daily.	Treatment of rickets, hypoparathyroidism.

*Available in Canada and United States.
†Available in Canada only.

gin. Close control of calcium levels is required because very small changes in blood calcium levels can profoundly alter many cellular functions.

Hyperparathyroidism. Hyperparathyroidism (excess parathyroid hormone) usually arises as a result of excess secretion of parathyroid hormone from a tumor. Many patients with this condition show decreases in bone calcification as a result of the action of parathyroid hormone. High amounts of calcium are execreted by these patients, and renal stones are common. No specific inhibitors of parathyroid release are available for clinical use; thus therapy consists primarily of surgery to re-

THE NURSING PROCESS

PARATHYROID DISORDERS

Assessment

Disorders involving only the parathyroid gland are unusual. Hypoparathyroidism is seen most often in patients who have had accidental removal or destruction of the parathyroid glands during thyroid surgery or other surgical procedures. Symptoms of hypoparathyroidism include paresthesia, muscle spasms, tetany, and convulsions. As mentioned in the text, hyperparathyroidism is seen most often with tumors of the parathyroid gland. In these cases the nurse should do a total patient assessment and monitor vital signs and serum calcium levels.

Nursing diagnoses

Potential complication: hypercalcemia

Management

The plan of therapy is to return serum calcium levels to the normal range and to treat any underlying condition. The nurse should continue to monitor vital signs, to measure the serum calcium levels, and to check for progression or regression of any symptoms discovered during the initial assessment. If calcitonin is being prescribed for outpatient use, the patient should be instructed in the correct procedure for subcutaneous drug administration.

Evaluation

Therapy for parathyroid disorders is successful if the serum calcium level can be maintained within the normal range and the patient suffers no side effects resulting from therapy. Before discharge, the patient should be able to explain how and why to take the prescribed drugs, to demonstrate any special administration techniques, and to explain what symptoms should warrant notification of the physician. The patient should be able to state the need to wear a medical identification tag or bracelet. For additional specific information, see the patient care implications section.

---

move the source of excess parathyroid hormone synthesis. Calcitonin may temporarily control hypercalcemia in hyperparathyroidism.

Hypercalcemia resulting from cancer chemotherapy may be controlled with etidronate, a synthetic analog of inorganic prophosphate. Etidronate is not effective in hyperparathyroidism.

Hypoparathyroidism. Hypoparathyroidism (insufficient parathyroid hormone) usually results following thyroid or parathyroid surgery, but idiopathic (unknown cause) forms of the disease exist. Whatever the cause, hypoparathyroidism is associated with low blood calcium levels (hypocalcemia). This electrolyte imbalance produces symptoms such as paresthesia, muscle spasms, tetany, and convulsions. In theory, parathyroid hormone could be used to raise blood calcium levels in conditions in which blood levels are abnormally low; however, administration of one of the forms of vitamin D with or without calcium is the preferred treatment.

Several forms of vitamin D are available for clinical use. Vitamin D_3, or cholecalciferol, is normally formed in the skin by irradiation of 7-dehydrocholesterol. Vitamin D_3 is equivalent to vitamin D_2, or ergocalciferol. Both drugs are available in orally administered forms suitable for convenient, long-term therapy. Calcitriol (1,25-dihydroxycholecalciferol) is the most active vitamin D derivative and is the final active metabolite of the vitamin. Although very effective, this drug form is expensive. Since adequate treatment is possible for most conditions with other forms of the vitamin, calcitriol is reserved for those rare patients who respond only to this drug form.

In pseudohypoparathyroidism the kidney, bone, and intestine do not respond to parathyroid hormone normally. Parathyroid hormone is occa-

PATIENT CARE IMPLICATIONS

Natural and synthetic thyroid hormones

Drug administration

- The side effects of these drugs are essentially the same as the symptoms of hyperthyroidism; see Table 52.1
- Assess for headache, insomnia, nervousness, and tremor.
- Monitor blood pressure and pulse. If pulse is greater than 100 per minute in an adult, withhold the dose and notify the physician.
- Monitor the ECG prior to the start of therapy and at regular intervals.
- Monitor weight. Assess for development of edema, pallor, fatigue.
  INTRAVENOUS LEVOTHYROXINE
- Dilute with diluent provided. Administer at a rate of 0.1 mg or less over 1 minute.
- Monitor thyroid function tests.

Patient and family education

- Review anticipated benefits and possible side effects of drug therapy.
- Tell patients that several weeks to months of therapy may be needed before full benefit is seen. Encourage patients to return for regular follow up and blood tests.
- Take doses in the morning to avoid nighttime insomnia.
- Warn diabetic patients to monitor blood glucose levels carefully, as an adjustment in diet or insulin may be needed.
- Remind patients to keep all health care providers informed of all drugs being taken.
- Encourage patients to wear a medical identification tag or bracelet stating that thyroid medication is used regularly.
- Teach patients not to switch brands of medication without consulting the physician or pharmacist.
- Instruct women to keep a record of menstrual periods, as menstrual irregularities may occur.
- Remind patients to keep all health care providers informed of all drugs being used. Regular use of thyroid replacement hormones may contribute to interactions with other drugs.

Methimazole and propylthiouracil

Drug administration

- Overdose would produce the clinical picture of hypothyroidism; see Table 52.1.
- Assess for tingling of fingers and toes. Monitor weight. Inspect patient for skin changes

or hair loss.
- Monitor complete blood count and differential, thyroid function tests, liver function tests.

Patient and family education

- Review anticipated benefits and possible side effects of drug therapy. Side effects may not appear for days to weeks after beginning therapy; remind patients to report the development of any new side effect.
- Instruct patients to report signs of agranulocytosis: fever, chills, sore throat, unexplained bleeding or bruising.
- Take doses with meals or snack to lessen gastric irritation.
- Encourage patients to return as instructed for follow-up.
- Remind patients to keep all health care providers informed of all drugs being used.
- If more than one dose per day is prescribed, it is best to try to space doses evenly throughout the day. Work with the patient to develop a satisfactory dosing schedule.

Iodine

Drug administration/patient and family education

- Dilute oral iodine solution well in juice, milk, or beverage of the patient's choice. In addition, the solutions may stain teeth; take with a straw.
- Signs of iodism (excessive iodine) include metallic taste, sneezing, swollen and tender thyroid gland, vomiting, and bloody diarrhea. Concomitant excessive use of over-the-counter preparations containing iodine (e.g., asthma or cough preparations) may contribute to iodism.
- Consult the manufacturer's literature for information about IV iodine.

Radioactive iodine

Drug administration/patient and family education

- The radiation dose of radioactive iodine is not high, but those preparing or administering the preparation should be careful to avoid spilling the mixture on themselves or on countertops. Wear rubber gloves. Follow agency protocol for handling radioactive substances.
- Side effects are rare, but include soreness over the thyroid gland, and in rare cases dif-

Continued.

PATIENT CARE IMPLICATIONS—cont'd

ficulty in swallowing and breathing because of gland enlargement. Eventually, many patients who take radioactive iodine will become hypothyroid.

Calcitonin

Drug administration

- Monitor weight. If vomiting or diarrhea occurs, monitor intake and output.
- Warn patients that flushing may occur.
- Before the first dose of calcitonin salmon, a test dose may be ordered to check for allergic response. Consult manufacturer's literature. Have available drugs, equipment, and personnel to treat acute allergic reactions in settings where calcitonin salmon is used.
- Assess for hypercalcemia or hypocalcemia; see Table 17.1: Common electrolyte abnormalities.
- Monitor serum electrolytes.

Patient and family education

- Review anticipated benefits and possible side effects of drug therapy.
- Encourage patients to return for regular follow-up visits. For home administration, teach patient to administer the drug subcutaneously. Review injection technique and have patient give a return demonstration.
- Refer the patient to a community-based nursing care agency as needed.
- Taking ordered doses in the evening may minimize flushing.
- Encourage patients on long-term therapy to wear a medical identification tag or bracelet indicating that calcitonin is being taken regularly.
- A low-calcium diet may be prescribed. Review Dietary Consideration: Calcium, for food items which should be used in limited amounts when trying to restrict calcium intake. Refer to a dietitian as needed.

Etidronate

Drug administration

- Assess for bone pain, which may occur in patients with Paget's disease.
- Monitor serum electrolytes. Assess for signs of hypocalcemia; see Table 17.1: Common electrolyte abnormalities.
- Monitor serum creatinine and BUN.
- Intravenous etidronate: Dilute in 250 ml or more of normal saline. Infuse 250 ml over at least 2 hours.

Patient and family education

- Review anticipated benefits and possible side effects of drug therapy.
- Provide emotional support. Weeks to months of therapy may be required to obtain maximum drug effect. Remind patients not to discontinue therapy without consulting physician.
- Take dose with black coffee, tea, fruit juice, or water, on an empty stomach, at least 2 hours before or after food.
- Do not take doses within 2 hours of ingesting milk or milk products, antacids, mineral supplements, or other medicines high in calcium, magnesium, iron, or aluminum.
- Take a dietary history. Patient should continue following a well-balanced diet with adequate but not excessive amounts of calcium and vitamin D.

Vitamin D preparations

- The side effects are essentially those of hypercalcemia, and are a result of overdosage: ataxia, fatigue, irritability, seizures, somnolence, tinnitus, hypertension, GI distress or constipation, hypotonia in infants.
- Assess for CNS effects. Note that ongoing assessment is important, as some symptoms such as fatigue may be difficult to distinguish from those accompanying renal failure or chronic disease.
- Monitor blood pressure and pulse. Monitor intake and output.
- Monitor serum calcium levels, urinalysis.

Patient and family education

- Review anticipated benefits and possible side effects of drug therapy. Encourage patients to notify the physician if any new side effect occurs.
- Remind patients not to increase or decrease the dose without consulting the physician.
- Warn patients to avoid driving or operating hazardous equipment if fatigue, somnolence, vertigo, or weakness occurs.
- Remind patients to keep all health care providers informed of all drugs being used. Avoid using any medications not previously approved by the physician.
- Avoid antacids containing magnesium.
- Avoid excessive amounts of substances containing vitamin D. See Dietary Consideration: Vitamins (p. 282).

sionally used in the diagnosis of this condition. Some patients respond to calcitriol.

Pharmacology of Vitamin D

Vitamin D, a lipid-soluble substance, is adequately absorbed following oral administration. The vitamin is transported in the bloodstream by a specific alpha globulin. Depending on exactly what form of the vitamin is administered, various biotransformations are possible. The liver converts vitamin D_3 to more active 25-hydroxyvitamin D_3. The kidney converts 25-hydroxyvitamin D_3, to 1,25-dihydroxyvitamin D_3, the most active metabolite of the vitamin. Most vitamin D metabolites are excreted in the bile. Excess or deficiency of vitamin D produces symptoms that are primarily those expected with high or low blood calcium concentrations.

SUMMARY

The follicular cells of the thyroid gland regulate the basal metabolic rate by releasing the hormones thyroxine and triiodothyronine. These hormones are formed from iodine and tyrosine in the thyroid gland and stored in thyroglobulin in the thyroid follicles. When released into the bloodstream, the thyroid hormones are bound to thyroid-binding globulin. Thyroxine is very tightly bound, whereas triiodothyronine is less firmly bound and therefore more able to penetrate tissues. Target cells may convert thyroxine to triiodothyronine. These hormones are metabolized by the liver and excreted in the bile as well as being broken down at other sites in the body.

Adult hypothyroidism (myxedema) produces characteristic signs of slowed metabolic rates. In addition, congenital hypothyroidism may produce mental retardation, and juvenile hypothyroidism may cause growth stunting. All forms of hypothyroidism require replacement therapy with thyroid hormones. Preparations of varying potency and purity are available, but all are capable of adequately replacing thyroid hormone. Preparations containing only thyroxine have a slower onset of action and a longer duration of action than preparations containing only triiodothyronine. Therapy with these agents should be started at low doses and gradually increased to avoid excessive stress to the patient. Angina pectoris and other cardiovascular symptoms may be produced.

Hyperthyroidism may be due to generalized overactivity of the thyroid gland such as that of Graves' disease or to overproduction of thyroid hormones by nodules or tumors of the thyroid gland. Temporary hyperthyroidism can be produced by subacute thyroiditis. Hyperthyroidism may be treated by controlling the symptoms of the disease or by lowering the amounts of thyroid hormones circulating in the body. Propranolol, a beta adrenergic blocking agent, controls the symptoms of hyperthyroidism by blocking catecholamine effects on heart, muscle, and other tissues. Propranolol rapidly controls the palpitation, tremor, muscle weakness, and cardiac arrhythmias that may be associated with hyperthyroidism. Thioamides block synthesis of thyroid hormones and therefore can control hyperthyroidism. Since the thyroid gland stores a large amount of hormone, however, the clinical effects of the thioamides are not apparent until these stored hormones are depleted—a matter of several days. Radioactive iodine may be used to slow thyroid hormone synthesis, since the isotope will be concentrated in thyroid tissue and destroy a portion of the hyperactive gland.

The parafollicular cells of the thyroid produce the peptide hormone calcitonin. Calcitonin can prevent loss of calcium from bone, augment urinary excretion of calcium and phosphate, and the absorption of calcium from the intestine. The hormone has been used therapeutically to treat Paget's disease.

The parathyroid glands produce the peptide parathyroid hormone. Parathyroid hormone antagonizes many actions of calcitonin, increasing calcium reabsorption from bones, lowering renal excretion of calcium, and increasing calcium absorption from the intestine. This latter effect is produced through the action of vitamin D. Overproduction of parathyroid hormone results in high calcium excretion, frequently producing renal stones. Hypoparathyroidism produces low blood levels of calcium and hence paresthesia, muscle spasms, tetany, and convulsions. Treatment is with a preparation of vitamin D with or without calcium supplements. Vitamin D increases the absorption of calcium and elevates the blood concentration of this ion.

STUDY QUESTIONS

1. What is the function of the follicular cells of the thyroid gland?
2. What are the hormones produced by the follicular cells of the thyroid gland?
3. What is the function of thyroid-stimulating hormone (TSH), and where is it produced?
4. What are the steps in thyroid hormone synthesis?
5. How much T_3 and T_4 is stored in the thyroid gland?
6. What is the function of thyroglobulin?

7. How are the thyroid hormones transported in the bloodstream?
8. How are the thyroid hormones eliminated?
9. Which of the thyroid hormones is found most abundantly in target cells?
10. What are the characteristic signs of hypothyroidism?
11. What symptoms are produced when hypothyroidism develops immediately after birth or later in childhood, as opposed to during adult life?
12. In primary hypothyroidism, how do the blood concentrations of TSH and thyroid hormones differ from normal?
13. What is secondary hypothyroidism?
14. What is tertiary hypothyroidism?
15. What is the treatment for all forms of hypothyroidism?
16. Which of the available preparations of thyroid hormones is the most potent?
17. How do T_3 and T_4 differ in onset and duration of action?
18. What side effects may occur with replacement therapy of thyroid hormones?
19. Which thyroid hormone is available as an injectable preparation?
20. Why would the administration of T_3 by nasogastric tube sometimes be preferred over injection of T_4 in the treatment of myxedema coma?
21. What is Graves' disease?
22. What is subacute thyroiditis?
23. What is the cause of Graves' disease?
24. What general classes of drugs are used to treat hyperthyroidism?
25. To what class of drugs does propranolol belong, and why is it useful in treating hyperthyroidism?
26. What is the mechanism of action of the thioamides?
27. How are the thioamides distributed in the body?
28. How may radioactive iodine be used in the treatment of hyperthyroidism?
29. What is the function of the parafollicular cells of the thyroid?
30. What metabolic effects does calcitonin have?
31. What forms of calcitonin are used to treat Paget's disease? How do they differ?
32. How may etidronate be used clinically?
33. What is the function of the parathyroid glands?
34. What are the metabolic effects of parathyroid hormone?
35. What are the symptoms of hypoparathyroidism?
36. How is hypoparathyroidism treated?
37. Which of the metabolites of vitamin D is the most active?
38. What is the metabolic function of vitamin D?
39. What is the fate of vitamin D in the body?

SUGGESTED READINGS

Balkin, M.S.: A guide to thyroid function tests, Emerg. Med. **15**(3):116, 1983.

Calloway, C.: When the problem involves magnesium, calcium or phosphate, RN **50**(5):30, 1987.

Evangelisti, J.T., and Thorpe, C.J.: Thyroid storm—a nursing crisis, Heart Lung **12**(2):184, 1983.

Evanier, D.: When the adult has hypothyroidism, Patient Care **17**(5):17, 1983.

Evanier, D.: When the child has hypothyroidism, Patient Care **17**(5):53, 1983.

Evanier, D.: Is your patient in thyroid storm? Patient Care **18**(5):191, 1984.

Evanier, D.: Look for these clues to thyrotoxicosis, Patient Care **17**(7):143, 1983.

Gambert, S.R.: Assessing thyroid function in the elderly, Nurse Pract. **8**(7):38, 1983.

Griffiths, E.C.: Clinical applications of thyrotrophin-releasing hormone, Clin. Sci. **73**(5):449, 1987.

Johnson, D.: Pathophysiology of thyroid storm: nursing implications, Crit. Care Nurse **3**(6):80, 1983.

Kumar, R.: Vitamin D activation and receptor sites, Diagn. Med. **5**(7):77, 1982.

Lockhart, J.S., and Griffin, C.W.: Action stat! tetany, Nursing 88 **18**(8):33, 1988.

Mahon, S.M.: Symptoms as clues to calcium levels, Am. J. Nurs. **87**(3):354, 1987.

McMillan, J.Y.: Preventing myxedema coma in the hypothyroid patient, DCCN **7**(3):136, 1988.

O'Neil, J.R.: Action stat! thyroid crisis, Nursing 87 **17**(11):33, 1987.

Oppenheimer, J.H., and others: Advances in our understanding of thyroid hormone action at the cellular level, Endocrin. Rev. **8**(3):288, 1987.

Payne, N.R.: Emergency care of the patient with myxedema coma, JEN **12**(6):343, 1986.

Samuels, H.H., and others: Regulation of gene expression by thyroid hormone, J. Clin. Invest. **81**(4):957, 1988.

Sarsany, S.L.: Thyroid storm, RN **51**(7):46, 1988.

Walfish, P.G.: Neonatal screening: the best way to screen for neonatal hypothyroidism, Diagn. Med. **7**(2):67, 1984.

Wartofsky, L.: Guidelines for the treatment of hyperthyroidism, Am. Fam. Physician **30**(1):198, 1984.

Waters, H.F., and Stuckey, P.A.: Oncology alert for the home care nurse: hypercalcemia, Home Health C. Nurse **6**(1):32, 1988.

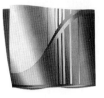

Drugs Acting on the Female Reproductive System

53

Female reproductive function depends on a complex, exquisitely regulated interaction of endocrine tissues. The negative feedback loop regulating the menstrual cycle involves the hypothalamus, the anterior pituitary, and the ovaries (Chapter 50). The actions of the natural female hormones, the clinical uses of synthetic and natural drugs affecting the female reproductive system, the endocrine control of pregnancy, and drugs used during childbirth and the postpartum period are discussed in this chapter.

HORMONES INVOLVED IN FEMALE REPRODUCTION

Sources of Hormones Involved in Female Reproduction

The major hormones involved in developing and maintaining female reproductive capacity include examples of all the chemical classes of hormones. The hypothalamus supplies gonadotropin-releasing hormone (GnRH), which acts directly on the anterior pituitary, stimulating synthesis and release of follicle-stimulating hormone (FSH) and luteinizing hormone (LH). In addition, the central nervous system neurotransmitter dopamine is the inhibitory factor that regulates the release of prolactin from the anterior pituitary. FSH, LH, and prolactin are the major gonadotropins. Each of these hormones has a different primary target tissue. FSH stimulates the ovarian cells, which form the follicle and nurture the maturing ovum. Under the influence of FSH these cells synthesize the potent steroid estrogen estradiol. LH acts primarily on the mature follicle to cause release of the ovum. Prolactin stimulates breast tissue to promote milk production. Prolactin also may affect the ovary, but details of how the hormone acts in this tissue are lacking.

The major steroid hormones regulating female reproduction are estrogens and progestins. Estro-gens are compounds that stimulate female reproductive tissues; progestins are compounds that specifically stimulate the uterine lining. Estrogens are produced primarily in the FSH-stimulated cells of the ovarian follicle. Progesterone, the most important progestin, is synthesized in the cells remaining in the follicle after the expulsion of the ovum. This tissue is called the *corpus luteum.*

All the steroids produced in the ovary are derived from cholesterol. Progestins are formed first and are the precursors of androgens. Androgens, the steroid hormones capable of producing masculinization, are primarily precursors of estrogen synthesis in females. Androstenedione is the androgen precursor of estrone, a major circulating estrogen that is formed mostly in peripheral tissues and not in the ovary. Estradiol, which is the most abundant circulating estrogen, is formed in the ovary.

Hormones Affecting Development of the Female Reproductive System

At birth the ovary is already in an advanced stage of development and contains between 2 and 4 million oocytes (cells that will form ova). The primordial follicles containing oocytes are not quiescent during the prepubertal years, but undergo a process called *atresia* in which oocytes are destroyed and follicles resorbed. At menarche (when menstrual cycles begin during puberty) an estimated 400,000 oocytes remain. Even after ovulation is initiated, atresia continues and is responsible for the destruction of more than 99% of the follicles present in the ovary.

As puberty begins, the immature ovaries are stimulated by increasing amounts of pituitary gonadotropins. As a result, estrogen synthesis is promoted and estrogen levels in the bloodstream rise. The primary function of estrogens during early puberty is to promote development of the reproduc-

tive system. The uterus and fallopian tubes enl?
to adult proportions. The vagina enlarges, and the
vaginal epithelium thickens and strengthens. In the
breast, estrogen promotes proliferation of stromal
tissue as well as ductile tissue, which is responsible
for the production of milk needed by the suckling
infant.

The secondary sexual characteristics also depend on estrogens. These hormones promote increased deposition of fat, especially in the breasts
and hips. Without estrogens, the typical contours
of the female body do not develop.

Estrogens are also involved in the growth spurt
that is characteristic of puberty. Along with other
hormones, estrogen causes retention of calcium
and phosphorus and thereby promotes bone growth.
However, estrogens also induce closure of the
epiphyses. When this closure occurs, no further increase in height takes place.

Hormones Affecting Ovulation

Ovulation requires proper functioning of the
hypothalamus, anterior pituitary, and ovary in the
negative feedback loop described in Chapter 50.
Both FSH and LH are required to act on the developing follicle before a mature ovum may be released
to begin its journey down the fallopian tube to the
uterus. Estrogen synthesis is required both for its
action on the follicle and for its ability to trigger
the midcycle surge of LH from the anterior pituitary.

Hormones Affecting Endometrial Function

The uterus is composed of smooth muscle
(myometrium) and glandular epithelium (endometrium). The endometrium, whose function is to
nourish and to support the ovum during development, is controlled primarily by estrogens and progestins. Estrogens promote proliferation of the endometrium during the first half of the menstrual
cycle before ovulation occurs. Progesterone, which
is formed in the corpus luteum of the ovary during
the second half of the menstrual cycle, acts on both
the endometrium and the myometrium. Progesterone reduces the activity of the myometrium and
prevents muscular contractions. It promotes development of the secretory capacity of the endometrium. Actions on these two tissues aid in establishing the environment in which the fertilized
ovum may implant successfully and begin development. Once implantation of the ovum has occurred, progesterone continues to alter the endometrium, ultimately changing the tissue so that a
second implantation becomes impossible.

Hormones in Pregnancy

Pregnancy obviously requires that a mature
ovum be released from the ovary at the appropriate
time, that the ovum be fertilized successfully
within about 2 days of its release, and that the
ovum be able to implant itself within the endometrium and begin to draw nourishment to support
the early stages of development. The most important hormone during these first days and weeks of
pregnancy is progesterone. Without adequate progesterone, the endometrium will be sloughed and
the fertilized ovum will be lost. Luteal progesterone
continues to be produced for about the first 10
weeks of pregnancy. Control of progesterone synthesis is exercised by cells of the fetus, which will
develop into the placenta. A few days after implantation of the ovum in the endometrium, these fetal
cells begin to produce a hormone called *human
chorionic gonadotropin (HCG)*, which takes over
control of the corpus luteum and maintains its production of progesterone. By the fifth week of pregnancy the placenta has developed to the stage
where it begins to synthesize progesterone directly.
Placental progesterone production increases during
the remainder of the pregnancy, whereas progesterone production in the corpus luteum virtually
disappears.

The continuing high progesterone levels during
pregnancy are thought to aid in maintaining the
pregnancy by suppressing myometrial contractions. At the end of pregnancy, progesterone levels
begin to decrease, allowing the uterus to begin to
produce hormones called *prostaglandins*. Prostaglandins, which are formed from fatty acids within
cell membranes, are capable of stimulating powerful uterine contractions. Although the exact role of
prostaglandins in normal childbirth is not yet established, it is known the the contractions produced by prostaglandins are sufficiently strong to
bring about the expulsion of the fetus from the
uterus.

Oxytocin, a hormone produced by the posterior
pituitary, is also capable of inducing uterine contractions. The uterus increases in sensitivity to
oxytocin at term and during the puerperium (period
immediately following birth). Oxytocin also acts
on breast tissue, where it stimulates the myoepithelium of the breast and promotes milk letdown.
Suckling by the infant sets off a reflex action in
which oxytocin release is stimulated. Central nervous system control of this process is clearly demonstrated by the mere sight of the infant, which is
sufficient for some women to induce oxytocin release and milk letdown. Oxytocin action is respon-

sible for the improved uterine muscle tone in nursing mothers and for the more rapid return of the uterus to the pregravid size in these women.

PHARMACOLOGICAL AGENTS AFFECTING FEMALE SEXUAL FUNCTION

Many conditions of the female reproductive tract for which women seek medical aid may be treated successfully by replacement therapy. The most common conditions are those that arise as a result of estrogen deficiency. A lack of estrogen during puberty will prevent normal growth and sexual development; menarche may not occur. This endocrine malfunction is only one of several abnormalities that may be responsible for amenorrhea (no menstrual cycles). After the menopause, the gradual decline in estrogen levels may be responsible for a host of symptoms, including vasomotor symptoms (hot flashes, sweating), osteoporosis (bone loss), and atrophy of vaginal and urethral tissue.

Other medical problems of the female reproductive system cannot be ascribed definitely to a specific hormone deficiency. Nevertheless, many of these conditions respond to hormones used for some pharmacological action rather than as replacement therapy. The rationale for therapy for these conditions is listed in Table 53.1.

Estrogen doses used in the clinical setting vary depending on the condition being treated. When used in replacement therapy, estrogen doses tend to be low. Higher doses are used to treat conditions such as advanced breast cancer. A drug handbook or the pharmacist should be consulted for the dose of a specific preparation in a specific condition.

Estrogens

Absorption and excretion. Estrogens of various types are available in the United States (Table 53.2). The two naturally occurring steroid estrogens used in the clinical setting are *estradiol* and *estrone*. As steroids, these compounds are not water soluble, but they are soluble in oil. With estradiol, slower absorption and longer duration of action may be achieved by using either the cypionate or the valerate ester of the natural steroid. Estradiol is absorbed orally if the drug crystals are reduced to particles 1 to 3 μm in diameter.

Estrone is not well absorbed orally in its natural form but may be used orally if it is converted to the piperazine sulfate. Estrone is also the major component of various estrogen mixtures described as *esterified estrogens, estrogenic substance,* or *conjugated estrogens.* These mixtures, which are isolated from such sources as the urine of pregnant mares, are relatively cheap and effective for many purposes, and all can be taken orally, making them a convenient drug form for many patients.

Synthetic estrogens such as *ethinyl estradiol* are also available. Ethinyl estradiol is more potent than naturally occurring estrogens. This drug used orally has a relatively short duration of action but does persist in the body longer than any of the natural estrogens.

Nonsteroid estrogens are all oral agents. The best known of these drugs is *diethylstilbestrol (DES).* DES, which was discovered in 1938, was once widely used to prevent spontaneous abortions. Recently it was noticed that the children who were in utero at the time of DES treatment may have suffered from the effects of the drug. As adults, female offspring have an increased incidence of vaginal adenosis and adenocarcinoma; male offspring may be more prone to develop epididymal cysts. DES is still available for clinical use and has been used as estrogen replacement therapy or any other use for which estrogens are approved.

Natural estrogens do not persist long in the body, since they are rapidly metabolized by the liver and excreted by the kidney. Ethinyl estradiol is less rapidly metabolized and is therefore longer acting than natural estrogens. Nonsteroidal estrogens are not metabolized rapidly and also persist longer than natural ones.

Toxicity. Side effects of estrogens include overreactions of certain reproductive tissues to the hormones. Breast tenderness is reported by many women receiving estrogens. Estrogens stimulate the endometrium to proliferate, and some evidence suggests that estrogens may increase the risk of endometrial cancer. No firm evidence shows that estrogens increase the risk of breast cancer.

Estrogens are frequently associated with acute adverse reactions such as nausea, vomiting, anorexia, and mild diarrhea. Malaise, depression, or excessive irritability are also related to estrogen therapy in some women. Estrogens promote salt and water retention and may therefore produce edema in some patients. Atherosclerosis is a definite risk for patients receiving estrogens, especially if they have other high-risk factors, such as smoking. Hypertension has been associated with estrogen use.

Uses. As mentioned earlier, estrogens may be used as replacement therapy or in pharmacological doses for a variety of dysfunctions of the female reproductive tract.

Estrogens are also available in fixed combina-

Table 53.1   Pharmacological Therapy of Dysfunctions of the Female Reproductive System

Clinical condition	Treatment	Rationale
Hypogonadism	Cyclic estrogen-progestin or menotropins	Estrogens are required to promote secondary sex characteristics. Other hormonal support may be required for full fertility.
Amenorrhea	Bromocriptine or gonadorelin	Effective only for specific types of conditions producing amenorrhea.
Menopause Vasomotor symptoms	Estrogens	Hot flashes and sweating are relieved by estrogens.
Osteoporosis	Estrogens	Loss of calcium may be halted temporarily but not reversed.
Atrophy of vaginal and urethral tissue	Estrogens	Estrogen support is needed to maintain tissue tone.
Dysfunctional uterine bleeding	Estrogen and progestin	Combination stops bleeding; drug withdrawal induces endometrial sloughing.
Luteal phase defect (infertility)	Progestins	Infertility resulting from inadequate synthesis of progesterone from the corpus luteum may be treated by progestin early in the pregnancy.
Postpartum breast engorgement	Bromocriptine	Blocks prolactin synthesis, thus removing a major stimulus for milk formation.
Metastatic breast carcinoma	Estrogens, androgens, or progestins	Tumors show differing sensitivities to these hormones.
Metastatic endometrial carcinoma	Progestins	Natural suppressive effect of progestins on the endometrium is retained in some of these tumors.
Galactorrhea	Bromocriptine	Suppresses prolactin release, thereby preventing the excessive stimulation of breast secretory tissue.
Dysmenorrhea	Oral contraceptives or prostaglandin inhibitors	Suppression of ovulation gives relief to many but not all patients. Drugs such as ibuprofen, indomethacin, mefenamic acid, naproxen, and ketoprofen relieve symptoms by preventing excessive production of prostaglandins.
Pelvic endometriosis	Estrogen and progestin Danazol	Suppresses proliferation of endometrial tissue. Inhibits gonadotropins, thus preventing proliferation of endometrial tissue.
Anovulation (infertility)	Bromocriptine, clomiphene citrate, menotropins, human chorionic gonadotropin (HCG), gonadorelin, or urofollitropin	Ovulatory failure may be corrected by use of agents that promote gonadotropin release (clomiphene) or supply them directly (menotropins). HCG acts as luteinizing hormone (LH) to trigger release of the ovum.
Premenstrual tension	Ergotamine, diuretics, or antianxiety agents	Therapy is empirical and often ineffective.

Table 53.2   Estrogens Used Clinically

Generic name	Trade name	Chemical form	Administration‡
Chlorotrianisene	TACE*	Nonsteroid	Capsules for oral use, primarily for prostatic carcinoma
Dienestrol	Dienestrol DV*	Nonsteroid	Vaginal creams and suppositories
Diethylstilbestrol (DES)	Stilphostrol Honvol†	Nonsteroid di-phosphate	Tablets for oral use or solution for injection; used primarily as anti-neoplastic agent
Estradiol	Estrace*	—	Tablets for oral use; cream for vaginal application
	Estraderm	—	Transdermal system
	Depo-Estradiol Cypionate Depogen Duraestrin	Cypionate	Oil (cottonseed, with chlorobu-tanol as preservative) solution for intramuscular injection
	Delestrogen* Estraval Valergen	Valerate	Oil (sesame or castor) solution for intramuscular injection
Estrogens, conjugated	Premarin Progens	Sulfate esters	Tablets for oral use or vaginal cream
Estrogens, esterified	Estratab Menest	Sulfate ester, pri-marily estrone	Tablets for oral use
Estrone	Theelin Unigen	—	Aqueous suspension for intramus-cular injection
	Oestrilin*		Intravaginal cream, suppositories
Estropipate (piperazine estrone sulfate)	Ogen*	Estrone pipera-zine sulfate	Tablets for oral use or vaginal cream
Ethinyl estradiol	Estinyl* Feminone	—	Tablets for oral use
Quinestrol	Estrovis	—	Tablets for oral use

*Available in Canada and United States.
†Available in Canada only.
‡All estrogens are considered FDA Pregnancy Category X.

tions with a variety of other drugs (Table 53.3). Some of these combinations are intended for a specific medical purpose, such as the combination of estrogens with antidepressants or sedatives for treating severe reactions during menopause. However, to a certain degree these combinations violate pharmacological principles. The main objection to fixed combinations is that dosage adjustment for best effectiveness of both drugs becomes impossible in some patients. For example, some women may be extremely sensitive to the androgen in a fixed estrogen-androgen combination. To reduce the androgen level, it would be necessary to administer less of the medication, but this would also reduce the estrogen dose. The overall result may be that the effectiveness of one of the drugs is lost or diminished.

Estrogens are also combined with vitamin supplements, central nervous system stimulants, minerals, and other agents. Most of these combinations

Table 53.3 Estrogens in Fixed Combinations with Other Drugs*

Estrogen	Trade name	Other active ingredients	Administration
Conjugated estrogens	Milprem PMB	Meprobamate (antidepressant)	Tablets for oral use
	Premarin with methyltestosterone	Methyltestosterone (androgen)	Tablets for oral use
Esterified estrogens	Menrium	Chlordiazepoxide (antidepressant)	Tablets for oral use
	Estratest	Methyltestosterone (androgen)	Tablets for oral use
Estradiol cypionate	Depo-Testadiol Duratestrin	Testosterone cypionate (androgen)	Oil solution for intramuscular injection
Estradiol valerate	Deladumone Estra-Testin	Testosterone enanthate (androgen)	Oil solution for intramuscular injection
Ethinyl estradiol	Halodrin	Fluoxymesterone (androgen)	Tablets for oral use

*For other fixed combinations of estrogens and progestins, see Table 53.6.

Table 53.4 Progestins Used Clinically (Also see Table 53.6)

Generic name	Trade name	Chemical form	Administration
Hydroxyprogesterone	Duralutin Gesterol L.A. Hyproval-P.A.	Caproate	Oil solution for intramuscular injection; action persists 9 to 17 days. FDA Pregnancy Category D.
Medroxyprogesterone	Depo-Provera*	Acetate	Aqueous suspension for intramuscular injection
	Amen Provera*	Acetate	Tablets for oral use
Megestrol	Megace*	Acetate	Tablets for oral use in treating endometrial carcinoma
Norethindrone	Micronor Norlutin	—	Tablets for oral use. FDA Pregnancy Category X.
	Norlutate	Acetate	Tablets for oral use. FDA Pregnancy Category X.
Progesterone	Femotrone Progestilin†	—	Aqueous suspension or oil solution for intramuscular injection

*Available in Canada and United States.
†Available in Canada only.

Table 53.5   Agents Used to Increase Female Fertility

Generic name	Trade name	Classification	Mechanism of action	Administration/dosage
Bromocriptine mesylate	Parlodel*	Inhibitor of prolactin release	Lowers high levels of prolactin, which interfere with pituitary and/or ovarian function.	ORAL: 1.25 to 2.5 mg once daily initially, then 2.5 mg 2 or 3 times daily.
Clomiphene citrate	Clomid* Serephene	Nonsteroid stimulator of ovulation	Stimulates ovulation, probably by hypothalamic mechanisms.	ORAL: 50 mg daily on days 5 through 10 of the menstrual cycle.
Gonadorelin	Factrel	Synthetic gonadotropin-releasing hormone (GnRH)	Stimulates release of LH and FSH from the anterior pituitary.	INTRAVENOUS, SUBCUTANEOUS: 100 µg once for diagnosis or repeated for infertility. FDA Pregnancy Category B.
Gonadotropin chorionic	Follutein Pregnyl	Placental hormone related to LH	Stimulates ovulation by an action resembling that of LH.	INTRAMUSCULAR: 5000 to 10,000 units once in an appropriately primed patient. FDA Pregnancy Category C.
Menotropins	Pergonal	Human urinary menopausal gonadotropins	FSH and LH in the preparation stimulate the ovaries.	INTRAMUSCULAR: 1 ampule daily for 9 to 12 days.
Urofollitropin	Metrodin	Human urinary menopausal FSH	FSH stimulates the ovaries.	INTRAMUSCULAR: 150 units daily. FDA Pregnancy Category X.

*Available in the United States and Canada.

have no place in medical practice. Some preparations are sold for external use as creams and lotions to prevent aging of the skin. No evidence exists to show that beneficial effects are produced by such uses.

The most important estrogen combinations are those with progestins, which are discussed in the section on oral contraceptive drugs. These combinations are available with so many different ratios of estrogen to progestin that adjustment for individual patient needs is possible.

Progestins

Absorption and excretion. Progestins available for use medically include the natural steroid hormone progesterone as well as synthetic derivatives of that compound (Table 53.4). Although progesterone itself is not useful orally, many derivatives are administered conveniently and effectively by that route. Injections of progesterone are painful and may produce local inflammation.

Progesterone and other progestins are rapidly metabolized by the liver and eliminated in the urine.

Toxicity. Adverse reactions to the progestins may involve several organ systems besides the organs of reproduction. Some of these reactions are similar to those seen with estrogens: edema, breast tenderness and swelling, gastrointestinal disturbances, depression, and weight change. Other reactions include changes in menstrual blood flow, midcyle spotting or breakthrough bleeding, cholestatic jaundice, and rashes. Many progestins have some androgenic activity and may cause masculinization of female fetuses. Because of this danger, the use of progestins as a test for pregnancy is no longer recommended. Patients with a history of thromboembolic disorders or thrombophlebitis should not be treated with progestins.

Uses. Progestins are used clinically for their effects on the endometrium. High doses suppress bleeding of the endometrium, and withdrawal induces sloughing of the tissue. Lower doses of progestins induce changes in the endometrium and cervical mucus that prevent pregnancy. This use of progestins is discussed in the section on pharmacological contraception.

Agents That Restore Female Fertility

Loss of fertility in a woman may be a result of any one of many causes. Therapy depends in part on evaluating the reason for the infertility. In some women the pituitary and the ovary seem normal, but the proper stimulus to activate follicular development is not transmitted. For these women, *clomiphene citrate* may be effective (Table 53.5).

Table 53.6   Oral Contraceptives

Progestin	Estrogen	Progestin : estrogen ratio	Trade name
Ethynodiol diacetate	Ethinyl estradiol	1.0 mg : 50 μg 1.0 mg : 35 μg 2.0 mg : 30 μg	Demulen 1/50* Demulen 1/35 Demulen
Levonorgestrel	Ethinyl estradiol	0.15 mg : 30 μg 0.05 mg : 30 μg (6 tablets), and 0.075 mg : 40 μg (5 tablets), and 0.125 mg : 30 μg (10 tablets)	Nordette, Levlen Triphasil† Tri-Levlen†
Norethindrone	Mestranol	1.0 mg : 50 μg	Norinyl 1 + 50, Genora 1/50, Nelova 1/50, Norethin 1/50, Ortho-Novum 1/50
Norethindrone	Ethinyl estradiol	1.0 mg : 50 μg 1.0 mg : 35 μg 0.5 mg : 35 μg 0.4 mg : 35 μg	Ovcon-50 Genora, N.E.E., Nelova 1/35, Norethin 1/35, Ortho-Novum 1/35 Brevicon*, Modicon, Nelova Ovcon-35
Norethindrone	None	0.35 mg 0.5 mg : 35 μg (10 tablets) and 1.0 mg : 35 μg (11 tablets) 0.5 mg : 35 μg (7 tablets) and 0.75 mg : 35 μg (7 tablets), and 1.0 mg : 35 μg (7 tablets) 0.5 mg : 35 μg (12 tablets), and 1.0 mg : 35 μg (9 tablets)	Micronor*, Norlutin, Nor-QD Nelova 10/11‡ Ortho-Novum 10/11‡ Ortho-Novum 7/7/7§ Tri-Norinyl¶
Norethindrone acetate	Ethinyl estradiol	2.5 mg : 50 μg 1.5 mg : 30 μg 1.0 mg : 50 μg 1.0 mg : 20 μg	Norlestrin 2.5/50* Loestrin 1.5/30* Norlestrin 1/50* Loesstrin 1/20
Norethynodrel	Mestranol	9.85 mg : 150 μg 5.0 mg : 75 μg	Enovid 10 mg Enovid 5 mg

*Available in Canada and the United States.
†Triphasic preparation—0.05 mg : 30 μg pills are taken the first 6 days of the cycle, 0.075 mg : 40 μg pills the next 5 days, and 0.125 mg : 30 μg pills the last 10 days of the cycle, followed by a week of no medication.
‡Biphasic preparation—0.5 mg : 35 μg pills are taken the first 10 days of the cycle, and 1.0 mg : 35 μg pills the last 11 days of the cycle, followed by a week of no medication.
§Triphasic preparation—0.05 mg : 30 μg pills are taken the first 6 days of the cycle, 0.075 mg : 40 μg pills the next 5 days, and 0.125 mg : 30 μg pills the last 10 days of the cycle, followed by a week of no medication.
¶Triphasic preparation—0.5 mg : 35 μg pills are taken the first 7 days of the cycle, 1.0 mg : 40 μg pills the next 9 days, and 0.125 mg : 30 μg pills the last 5 days of the cycle, followed by a week of no medication.

Table 53.6   Oral Contraceptives—cont'd

Progestin	Estrogen	Progestin:estrogen ratio	Trade name
Norgestrel	Ethinyl estradiol	0.5 mg:50 µg	Ovral*
		0.3 mg:30 µg	Lo/Ovral
Norgestrel	None	0.075 mg	Ovrette

*Available in Canada and the United States.

This drug seems to activate the pituitary by hypothalamic mechanisms, and ovarian stimulation thus is achieved. Stimulation of several follicles may be induced by clomiphene, and multiple births have occurred.

In women whose pituitary is unable to supply sufficient gonadotropins to properly stimulate the ovary, infertility also may occur. For these women, *menotropins* may be prescribed. This mixture of compounds extracted from the urine of postmenopausal women contains FSH and LH in approximately equal amounts. When LH action alone is required, *human chorionic gonadotropin (HCG)* may be prescribed. HCG is chemically related to LH and possesses many of the same physiological actions, including the ability to stimulate ovulation.

Bromocriptine mesylate is a chemical relative of the ergot alkaloids, which are used as oxytocic agents. Bromocriptine, however, is clinically useful because of its ability to inhibit prolactin secretion. Bromocriptine is approved in the United States to control galactorrhea (spontaneous milk production) caused by excessive prolactin secretion, usually from functional tumors. Amenorrhea (no menstrual cycles) and infertility also are produced when prolactin secretion is excessive. Bromocriptine suppression of prolactin secretion reverses these symptoms, and fertility becomes possible.

Pharmacological Contraception

Reversible sterility induced by pharmacological agents has been a possibility since the late 1950s, when the oral contraceptive agents became available. The agents in use today contain either a combination of estrogen and a progestin or a progestin alone. The effectiveness of these agents is very high. Most reports give estimates of less than 1 failure in 200 woman years of use for the combined estrogen-progestin agents. This pregnancy rate is in contrast to rates of 1 failure per 25 to 50 woman years for mechanical devices such as intrauterine devices (IUDs), diaphragms, and condoms.

The estrogen-progestin combinations are known to suppress ovulation, and it was on this basis that they were first suggested as contraceptives. In addition, these drugs induce changes in the cervical mucus, which makes it difficult for sperm to enter the uterus. Changes also occur in the endometrium that make implantation difficult even if fertilization occurs. The preparations containing progestins alone alter the cervical mucus and the endometrium as the combination products do, but they do not always suppress ovulation. The effectiveness of agents containing only progestins is less than that of the combined preparations.

To achieve contraception and to simulate the normal menstrual cycle, the oral contraceptives usually are taken for 20 or 21 consecutive days. The increased estrogen and progestin levels produced suppress the hypothalamus and the pituitary so that no LH is released at the time when ovulation would normally occur. This is the mechanism by which ovulation is suppressed. During the 7 days when hormones are not administered, the endometrium involutes and sloughs off, primarily as a result of loss of progestin activity. This withdrawal period prevents excessive proliferation of the endometrium.

The progestins in oral contraceptives are synthetic derivatives of natural compounds. Progesterone, a natural progestin, is used in an IUD. This device (Progestasert) is not to be confused with the more common IUDs that contain no hormonal agents. The progesterone-releasing IUD was developed to administer the fertility-controlling drug directly to the target tissue. The very small amounts of progesterone released are retained within the reproductive tract rather than being systemically absorbed. The effectiveness of this device depends both on the purely mechanical effects of the IUD and on the pharmacological effects of the progesterone.

Toxicity. The oral contraceptive agents available in the United States are shown in Table 53.6. Some of these agents, such as Enovid and Ovulen,

THE NURSING PROCESS

DRUGS AND THE FEMALE REPRODUCTIVE SYSTEM

Assessment

Drugs acting on the female reproductive system are used to provide replacement therapy, to cause or inhibit ovulation and conception, to aid in pregnancy or labor, and to treat hormonally sensitive tumors. The nurse should obtain a complete patient assessment, focusing on the problem being addressed by the drug. The data base should include the temperature, pulse, respiration, blood pressure, weight, description of the menstrual cycle, assessment of breasts (male and female), and condition of skin. In the pregnant woman a history of previous pregnancies and deliveries and assessment of the fetus should be done (e.g., fetal heart tones and position).

Nursing diagnoses

Potential complication: vascular disorders

Self-concept disturbance: acne, weight gain related to drug therapy

Management

Because of controversies surrounding the use of some of these drugs, the patient should be fully informed of possible side effects and benefits before therapy is begun. The nurse should continue to monitor the pulse, blood pressure, and weight. The patient activities needed to help ensure success should be explained in detail. For example, alternative birth control measures during the first month of birth control pill therapy, temperature charts to monitor possible ovulation, and saving urine specimens to measure hormone or drug excretion need thorough explanation. With oxytocics, the mother and fetus should be monitored closely, and the use of an intravenous infusion monitoring device should be considered. Calcium levels in the patient being treated for cancer should be followed. Except for the oxytocics, most of these drugs will be taken on an outpatient basis, and side effects will not occur until well into the course of therapy.

Evaluation

Success of drug therapy occurs if the desired outcome is seen and the patient has no or few side effects. Thus if pregnancy is prevented and the woman has no side effects, then therapy with oral contraceptives has been successful. With long-term drug therapy, however, the nurse should note that the possibility of side effects is always present.

Before discharge the patient should be able to explain why and how to take the drug, possible side effects that might occur, which side effects require immediate medical attention, and the risks associated with therapy.

---

are considered to be estrogen dominant. Estrogen excess may be associated with nausea, bloating, breast fullness, edema, hypertension, and cervical discharge. These symptoms may suggest that the patient be tried on a preparation with less estrogen. Agents such as Loestrin, Ovral, and Lo/Ovral are predominantly progestin-like in their action. Progestin excess in a patient taking oral contraceptives may produce hair loss, hirsutism, oily scalp, acne, increased appetite and weight gain, tiredness and depression, breast regression, and reduced menstrual blood flow. By changing the contraceptive preparation prescribed, the physician may finally be able to achieve the proper balance of estrogen and progestin so that the adverse effects listed are minimized.

Oral contraceptives are among the most widely used drugs today. Throughout the world, 50 million or more women rely on these agents for prevention of pregnancy. The oral contraceptives are without doubt highly effective, but questions about the safety of these agents have been raised. In particular, the incidence of unexpected serious or fatal medical conditions has been studied in the relatively healthy, normal women who receive oral contraceptives. Risk of certain serious medical con-

Table 53.7 Potential Adverse Reactions in Users of Oral Contraceptives

Adverse reaction	Relation to oral contraceptives	Comments
Thromboembolytic diseases	Risk increased 2- to 7-fold in users over non-users. Incidence about 100:100,000 woman years; fatalities 2:100,000 woman years.	Obesity, family history of thromboembolytic disorders, immobility, and/or group A blood type may increase risk. Group O blood type women have lower risk. Directly related to estrogen dosage.
Thrombotic stroke	Risk increased 3.1- to 6-fold. Incidence about 25:100,000 woman years; fatalities 0.5:100,000 woman years.	Hypertension increases the risk.
Hemorrhagic stroke	Risk increased at least 2-fold. Incidence about 10:100,000 woman years.	Hypertension and heavy smoking are strong risk factors.
Myocardial infarction	Risk increased about 2-fold over nonusers when estrogen doses exceed 50 µg daily.	Synergistic increase in risk if oral contraceptives are used by smokers.
Hypertension	Between 1% and 5% of patients show an increase in blood pressure. Clinical hypertension is more rare.	Risk is increased by age, obesity, and parity.
Gallbladder disease	Risk increased an estimated 2-fold.	Risk may be related to the dose of progestin.
Liver disease	20% to 50% of patients show reduced liver function. Incidence 10:100,000 woman years for jaundice. Tumors are exceedingly rare.	Reversible. Dangerous for patients with preexisting liver disease (hepatitis, cholestasis). Liver tumors may be related specifically to mestranol.
Carbohydrate metabolism	Most patients show reduced glucose tolerance.	Important only in prediabetic women who may become insulin-dependent. Related to dose and potency of progestin.
Lipid metabolism	Most patients have increased serum triglyceride levels.	Reversible effect; relationship to coronary artery disease in these patients is unknown.
Chloasma	3% to 4% of patients treated.	Increased sensitivity to sunlight also occurs. Reversible.
Headaches	Variable reports with no clear conclusion.	Appearance of chronic headache may presage stroke.
Visual disturbances	Often mentioned but not yet causally linked to oral contraceptive use.	Temporary blindness, blind spots, and changes in field of vision have been mentioned.
Emotional state	Variable reports with no clear conclusion.	No evidence that oral contraceptives significantly increase depression.
Endometrial cancer	No increased risk when combined estrogen-progestin agents used.	Risk is increased by estrogens alone but reduced by progestins. Some studies suggest protection.
Cervical cancer	No relationship established.	Frequency of coitus and number of sexual partners more important risk factors.
Breast cancer	No relationship established.	Benign breast tumors are improved.
Permanent infertility	No relationship established.	Most patients quickly return to fertility when oral contraceptives are discontinued.
Outcome of later pregnancies	No increased risk to mother or fetus has been demonstrated.	Data are for pregnancies begun after oral contraceptives have been discontinued.

and progestin so that the adverse effects listed are minimized.

Oral contraceptives are among the most widely used drugs today. Throughout the world, 50 million or more women rely on these agents for prevention of pregnancy. The oral contraceptives are without doubt highly effective, but questions about the safety of these agents have been raised. In particular, the incidence of unexpected serious or fatal medical conditions has been studied in the relatively healthy, normal women who receive oral contraceptives. Risk of certain serious medical conditions can now be shown to be increased in oral contraceptive users when they are compared to similar women who do not take these drugs (Table 53.7).

As with any medication, the oral contraceptives must be considered in terms of the risk-to-benefit ratio. Of first importance may be how much value the patient places on almost complete protection against unwanted pregnancy. Women who desire this high level of control then should consider the safety factors of the medication. Many of the dangerous complications, such as cerebrovascular accident (stroke) and thromboembolytic diseases, are rare even among oral contraceptives users. The risk of these complications is greater than the risk among nonusers of oral contraceptives, but much lower than the risk of these complications during pregnancy. Women should also consider the other predisposing risk factors, such as smoking, obesity, and hypertension. The combination of oral contraceptives with these conditions leads to unacceptable risk for many patients. All women receiving oral contraceptives should be urged to stop smoking.

Some medical conditions are improved or the symptoms are ameliorated by oral contraceptives. Many patients report a reduction in menstrual disorders and especially in dysmenorrhea. Menstrual blood flow usually is reduced, and anemia is prevented or lessened in many women. Benign breast tumors are improved in a time-dependent fashion by oral contraceptive therapy.

Current medical information suggests that oral contraceptives are safe in relatively young women in whom other risk factors are minimized. The most prudent course of action seems to be to select patients carefully before administering oral contraceptives. Women with a history of hypertension or thromboembolytic disease probably should not receive the drugs. Women who elect to receive oral contraceptives should be given thorough physical examinations yearly. The dose of estrogen and progestin should be the lowest dose that achieves contraception and prevents unwanted side effects such

as breakthrough bleeding. Careful history taking may reveal symptoms that the patient has not linked to oral contraceptive use. Migraine headaches, dizziness, and visual disturbances frequently are not related by the patient to oral contraceptive use and may not be mentioned spontaneously. However, breakthrough bleeding, excessive cervical mucus formation, breast tenderness, and other changes in the reproductive tract usually are quickly connected to oral contraceptive use by the patient. These symptoms usually are more annoying than serious. However, severe headaches or visual disturbances are frequently early signs of impending cerebrovascular accident, and such symptoms may be sufficient cause to discontinue the medications.

DRUGS USED DURING CHILDBIRTH AND POSTPARTUM CARE
Physiology of Childbirth

To understand the pharmacological management of labor and delivery, an understanding of physiological processes involved is necessary. During stage I of parturition, uterine contractions begin to increase in frequency and intensity and the cervix begins to dilate. In stage II, uterine contractions occur at the rate of about 1 every 2 minutes. The cervix is fully dilated, and the uterine contractions bring about the delivery of the infant. During stage III labor, the frequency of the contractions decreases, and the placenta separates from the uterus and is expelled. Uterine contractions continue for hours to days, with the frequency and intensity of the contractions diminishing with time.

When contractions occur during labor and delivery, the myometrium compresses the major blood vessels supplying oxygen to the fetus. The result is that during a contraction, the fetus is relatively anoxic. When the uterus relaxes between contractions, this condition is quickly rectified. If the uterus is overstimulated and fails to relax sufficiently between contractions, the result may be prolonged fetal anoxia that may harm the fetus. Induction of labor with one of the oxytocic drugs carries with it the risk of producing this condition. Therefore all patients in whom labor is being induced should receive continuous care, and fetal monitoring should be done when possible. Oxytocin is the drug of choice to induce or stimulate labor, since it seems to allow the uterus to relax between contractions. The ergot alkaloids and other oxytocic drugs tend to increase the overall tone of the myometrium as well as increase the strength of contractions and therefore carry a greater risk of producing fetal anoxia.

The uterine contractions that occur after deliv-

Table 53.8   Clinical Summary of Oxytocic Drugs

Generic name	Trade name	Administration/dosage	Medical use	Comments
POSTERIOR PITUITARY HORMONE				
Oxytocin	Pitocin Syntocinon*	INTRAVENOUS: 10 milliunits/ml infused at 1 to 2 milliunits/min, gradually increased up to about 10 milliunits/min.	Induction or stimulation of labor.	Stimulates uterine contraction but allows relaxation between contractions. Fetal or maternal cardiac arrhythmias, acute hypertension, nausea, and water intoxication may occur. Overdose may produce uterine hypertonicity with fetal and/or maternal injury.
		INTRAVENOUS: 20 to 40 milliunits/ml infused at 40 milliunits/min.	Control of uterine atony and/or bleeding.	Same as above.
		INTRAMUSCULAR: 3 to 10 units (0.3 to 1 ml) postpartum.	Control of uterine atony and/or bleeding.	Same as above.
	Syntocinon*	NASAL: 1 spray of 40 units/ml solution before nursing.	Aids in breast feeding by stimulating milk letdown.	Also causes nasal vasoconstriction. Onset of action is within 2 or 3 min, and duration of action is short.
ERGOT ALKALOIDS				
Ergonovine maleate	Ergotrate maleate*	ORAL: 0.2 to 0.4 mg 2 to 4 times daily for 2 days.	Control of postpartum bleeding.	May cause nausea and vomiting. Hypertensive episodes are especially likely when vasopressors or spinal anesthesia is also used.
Methylergonovine maleate	Methergine	ORAL: 0.2 to 0.4 mg 2 to 4 times daily for 2 days. INTRAMUSCULAR, INTRAVENOUS: 0.2 mg repeated at 2 or 4 hr, up to maximum of 5 doses.	Same as for ergonovine maleate.	May cause nausea and vomiting, transient hypertension, headache, dizziness, palpitation, or chest pain.
PROSTAGLANDINS				
Carboprost tromethamine	Prostin/15 M	INTRAMUSCULAR: 250 μg initially, repeated every 1½ to 3½ hr as needed. FDA Pregnancy Category C.	Abortion in second trimester.	Stimulates uterine contractions. Vomiting and diarrhea are common; fever also is observed in about 12% of patients.
Dinoprost tromethamine	Prostin F2 Alpha†	INTRAUTERINE: 40 mg slowly infused. Second dose of 10 to 40 mg may be given 24 hr later if needed.	Abortion in second trimester.	Stimulates uterine contractions. Vasomotor disturbances, cardiac arrhythmias, hyperventilation, and chest pain are possible.
Dinoprostone	Prostin E2*	VAGINAL: 20 mg suppositories inserted every 3 to 5 hr until abortion ensues.	Abortion in second trimester.	Stimulates uterine contractions. Gastrointestinal symptoms are common; cardiovascular symptoms are possible.

*Available in Canada and United States.
†Available in Canada only.

ery have two beneficial effects on the mother. First, they are responsible for expulsion of the afterbirth, and produce a general cleansing of the uterus. Second, these contractions aid in controlling postpartum bleeding by clamping the vessels that were ruptured by the birth process. If bleeding is a problem at this stage, the physician may use one of the agents with a longer and more continuous action, such as one of the ergot alkaloids. The ergot alkaloid preparations are also the only oxytocic drugs that may be effectively administered orally.

Oxytocic Drugs

Oxytocic drugs are those that induce contraction of the myometrium (Table 53.8). The drug class is named for the natural posterior pituitary hormone oxytocin. The uterus is relatively insensitive to the action of oxytocin until labor has started. No clear role of oxytocin in regulating unassisted, normal labor has been established.

Another class of natural hormones, the *prostaglandins*, is involved in regulating myometrial activity. These derivatives of fatty acids are rapidly formed in their target tissues and very rapidly degraded without persisting in the bloodstream for any appreciable time. In the uterus these hormones induce very powerful myometrial contractions. Recent research has suggested that prostaglandins, especially the E and F series (PGE$_2$ and PGF$_{2\alpha}$), may play a role in natural induction of labor. Prostaglandin levels rise in the amniotic fluid and other pelvic reproductive tissues as term draws near. This increasing concentration of prostaglandins has been suggested to be the stimulus causing Braxton-Hicks contractions, the mild myometrial contractions occurring during the final few weeks of pregnancy.

Although prostaglandins have been investigated for use in the induction of labor, these drugs elevate uterine muscle tone and may be dangerous to the fetus. The drugs are potent stimulators of the myometrium, however, and have been successfully used to induce abortion during the second trimester when the uterus is resistant to oxytocin. Systemic side effects of these drugs can be serious, and the most comfortable and safest route of administration may well be transabdominal instillation into the amniotic fluid. Administered in this fashion, the drug stays primarily within the uterus and persists in action for some hours.

Compounds other than oxytocin and prostaglandins have been discovered to be powerful oxytocics. Among the most clinically useful of these drugs are the *ergot alkaloid* derivatives (Table 53.8).

The ergot alkaloids are compounds produced by fungal contaminants of rye and other cereal grains. These fungal products have been known as poisons since the Middle Ages, when it was noted that people who ate grain contaminated with this fungus suffered from dry gangrene. This extreme reaction is caused by the potent vasoconstrictive effect of the ergot alkaloids. Blood flow to the limbs may be reduced so severely that the tissues die and the limbs eventually fall away with little or no bleeding produced. In addition, pregnant women who ate the affected grain were noted to enter an abrupt and devastating labor that expelled fetuses at any stage of development. Today it is not this crude mixture of ergot alkaloids that is useful in the clinic but rather derivatives of one or another of the compounds.

Uterine Relaxants

Specific uterine relaxation in cases of hypertonicity or premature labor is not yet possible. Nevertheless, several types of compounds will produce uterine relaxation along with other reactions. For example, premature labor is sometimes treated with agents that stimulate beta-2 adrenergic receptors, since stimulation of these receptors in the uterus causes relaxation of the myometrium. Agonists of beta-2 adrenergic receptors cause side effects throughout the body, however, as a result of beta adrenergic receptor stimulation in other tissues.

The best beta-2 adrenergic agonist for use in halting premature labor at present appears to be *ritodrine*. This agent effectively relaxes the myometrium but also has effects on the peripheral vasculature and other tissues. The heart is sensitive to stimulation by ritodrine, suggesting that the drug is also an agonist with some activity on beta-1 adrenergic receptors. Ritodrine usually is administered intravenously when premature labor begins. When contractions have been controlled for 12 to 24 hours, the patient may be started on oral ritodrine, and the intravenous infusion may be discontinued. The major side effects noted with this drug have been heart palpitations, nausea, vomiting, trembling, flushing, and headache. These effects appear transient and rarely cause termination of therapy. Patients should be observed for undue tachycardia or signs of cardiac distress. The fetal heart may also be stimulated by ritodrine. Ritodrine increases the workload of the mother's heart and is contraindicated in patients with preexisting cardiac disease. The primary indication for ritodrine is to halt spontaneous labor when it appears after the

PATIENT CARE IMPLICATIONS

Estrogens, progestins, or combinations, including oral contraceptives

Drug administration

- Monitor blood pressure and pulse, weight. Assess for skin changes.
- Instruct patients to report leg pain, sudden onset of chest pain, shortness of breath, coughing up of blood, dizziness, changes in vision or speech, or weakness or numbness of an arm or leg, as these may indicate pulmonary embolism or other thromboembolic problems.
- Assess for signs of depression: withdrawal, insomnia, anorexia, lack of interest in personal appearance.
- Assess tactfully for changes in libido. Patients may be reluctant to discuss this problem.
- Patients with metastatic cancer to bone who are started on hormonal therapy may develop severe hypercalcemia. Monitor serum electrolytes. See Table 17.1: Common electrolyte abnormalities.
- Monitor complete blood count, liver function tests.
- For a discussion of IM administration of oil-based suspensions, see Chapter 6.
- For a discussion of subcutaneous implantation, see Chapter 54.

Patient and family education

- Review anticipated benefits and possible side effects of drug therapy. Review Table 53.7. Tell patients to notify the physician if any new side effect develops.
- Counsel or refer as needed about stopping smoking, losing weight to achieve desirable weight, and modifying diet to decrease cholesterol and triglycerides.
- Warn diabetic patients to monitor blood glucose levels carefully, as these drugs may alter glucose levels.
- Take doses with meals or snack to lessen nausea. This side effect will usually lessen with continued use. Try taking the dose at bedtime rather than in the morning.
- Warn patients to avoid driving or operating hazardous equipment if visual changes occur; notify physician.
- Instruct women to report any vaginal bleeding or menstrual irregularities. Notify the physician immediately if pregnancy is suspected.
- Remind patients to keep all health care providers informed of all medications being used. It may take several months for these drugs to be completely eliminated even when the patient has stopped using them, so the patient should be reminded to inform health care providers for up to several months after therapy has stopped.
- Remind patients to take drugs only as ordered, and not to increase or decrease the dose without consultation with the physician. Overdose can occur even with vaginal creams when they are used excessively. Also, tell women using vaginal creams not to use them as a vaginal lubricant during intercourse, as this may lead to absorption by the male partner.

Continued.

---

twentieth week of pregnancy and before the thirty-sixth week. Spontaneous labor beginning before the twentieth week frequently is associated with a defective fetus and is not usually interrupted.

Central nervous system depressants may halt premature labor. *Ethanol,* which is an inhibitor of oxytocin release as well as a central nervous system depressant, has been used to halt premature labor successfully. The levels required to relax the uterus are sufficient to produce acute alcohol intoxication. Controlled clinical trials have suggested ritodrine is more effective and less toxic.

General anesthetics may also relax the uterus. Enflurane and halothane are the preferred agents.

In addition to central nervous system effects, these agents may act directly on the myometrium and also may slow catecholamine release from the adrenal gland, thus reducing endogenous stimulators of myometrial activity.

Progesterone is the natural steroidal compound that normally functions as a uterine relaxant. The use of this compound or one of the other progestins is not recommended in cases of uterine hypertonicity during delivery, however, since the hormone may not reach the uterus in sufficient quantities to relax the uterus quickly and effectively. Use of progesterone during earlier stages of pregnancy may cause undesirable effects on the developing fetus.

PATIENT CARE IMPLICATIONS — cont'd

- Typical instructions for missed doses include: if a single contraceptive tablet is missed, take the missed dose as soon as remembered. If 2 consecutive doses are missed, the patient should double up on each of the next 2 doses, then resume the regular schedule, but use additional contraceptive measures until she completes that cycle. If 3 or more consecutive doses are missed, the patient should stop the pills for 7 days after the first missed dose, then begin a new cycle of pill use. In addition, the patient should take further contraceptive measures from the time the missed tablets are noticed until 7 days after the new course of therapy is started. Some physicians may give different instructions, and some products may carry different instructions; see the manufacturer's leaflet. Encourage the woman to call the physician or nurse with specific questions.
- Many drugs interfere with effectiveness of birth control pills. Teach patients to ask the physician or pharmacist about this possibility whenever a new medication is being used.
- For transdermal application, review with the patient the instruction leaflet provided by the manufacturer.
- If a woman discontinues oral contraceptives in order to become pregnant, it is recommended that she use an alternative form of birth control for 2 months after stopping the pills to ensure more complete excretion of the hormonal agents before conceiving, and thus reduce the potential effects of the medications on the fetus.
- Teach patients how to do a breast self-examination, and encourage them to perform this monthly.
- Patients taking estrogens may develop brown areas on the skin. See Patient Problem: Photosensitivity, p. 647.
- Tell patients taking birth control pills that the drug(s) work best when used regularly. Keep an additional month's supply on hand, and avoid running out of pills.
- Remind patients to keep all medications out of the reach of children.

General guidelines for women taking drugs to increase fertility

Patient and family education

- Teach patients as indicated to keep a record of basal body temperature, consistency of vaginal mucus, 24-hour urine specimen, and so on as prescribed by the physician.

- Provide emotional support as needed. Treatment of infertility problems may be prolonged and discouraging.
- Encourage patients to return as directed for blood tests, sonograms, examinations, additional medications, and other therapies as prescribed.
- Remind patients to keep all drugs out of the reach of children.
- If pregnancy is suspected, notify physician, as these drugs should usually not be continued during pregnancy.

Bromocriptine

Drug administration

- Assess mental status. Assess for signs of depression: lack of interest in personal appearance, withdrawal, anorexia, and insomnia.
- Monitor pulse and blood pressure. Check stools and emesis for occult blood.

Patient and family education

- Review anticipated benefits and possible side effects of drug therapy. Tell the patient to report the development of any new side effect.
- See Patient Problems: Constipation on p. 187; Dry Mouth on p. 170; Orthostatic Hypotension on p. 237.
- When used to treat Parkinson's disease, full benefit of this drug may not be seen for several weeks. Provide emotional support. See Chapter 48.
- See the general guidelines for infertility.
- Take doses with meals or snack to lessen gastric irritation.
- Warn patients to avoid driving or operating hazardous equipment if drowsiness develops.
- Avoid drinking alcoholic beverages unless permitted by the physician.
- Depending on the patient's age and reason for taking bromocriptine, counsel about methods of birth control as appropriate.

Clomiphene citrate

Drug administration/patient and family education

- Review the anticipated benefits and possible side effects of drug therapy. Common side effects include breast discomfort, headache, heavy menstrual periods, nausea, or vomiting. Encourage patients to notify the physician if any unexplained side effect develops.

PATIENT CARE IMPLICATIONS—cont'd

- Typical instructions for taking this drug are to start counting the first day of the menstrual cycle as day 1. Begin clomiphene in the dose ordered on day 5, and continue daily until the prescribed number of doses is completed. Review instructions with the patient and check to see that she understands the dosing schedule. The drug may also be prescribed for men; review the physician's prescription with the patient.
- Warn patients to avoid driving or operating hazardous equipment if changes in vision occur; notify the physician.
- See the general guidelines for infertility.

Gonadorelin

No serious side effects have been reported with this drug. Warn patients that itching may occur at the injection site. Consult the manufacturer's literature. See the guidelines for drugs for infertility.

Gonadotropin, chorionic

Drug administration/patient and family education

- Review the anticipated benefits and possible side effects of drug therapy. Remind patients to notify the physician if any unexpected side effect develops, or any side effect is severe or persistent.
- In women, common side effects include breast enlargement, headache, irritability, edema, fatigue, depression, or stomach or pelvic pain.
- This drug may be used to treat cryptorchidism, if no anatomical obstruction is present. Notify the physician if acne, enlargement of penis or testes, growth of pubic hair, or rapid increase in height develops.
- Warn patients to avoid driving or operating hazardous equipment if excessive tiredness or visual changes occur; notify physician.
- See guidelines for infertility.

Menotropins

Drug administration/patient and family education

- Review anticipated benefits and possible side effects of drug therapy. Tell the patient to report the development of any new, or any severe or persistent side effect.
- This drug is often administered with chorionic gonadotropin. Side effects are often related to excessive ovarian stimulation: abdominal discomfort, nausea, vomiting, diarrhea, increased weight, hypertension.
- The drug may also be administered to men. It may cause breast enlargement.
- See the guidelines for drugs for infertility.

Urofollitropin

Drug administration/patient and family education

- Review anticipated benefits and possible side effects of drug therapy. Tell the patient to report the development of any new, or any severe or persistent side effect.
- Common side effects include bloating, pelvic pain, nausea and vomiting, breast tenderness.
- See the general guidelines for drugs for infertility.

Danazol

Drug administration

- This drug may be used to treat endometriosis, as well as fibrocystic breast disease, hereditary angioedema, and hematologic disorders including idiopathic thrombocytopenic purpura (ITP). It has weak androgenic and anabolic properties; see also Chapter 54.
- Assess for weight gain. Inspect for development of acne, edema of dependent areas, hirsutism. Monitor blood pressure.

Patient and family education

- Review anticipated benefits and possible side effects of drug therapy. Encourage patients to notify the physician if any unexpected side effect develops. Common side effects in the female include reduction in breast size, hirsutism, weight gain, deepening of voice, emotional lability. Side effects due to the androgenic properties of the drug may be less noticeable in male patients.
- Tell patients to notify the physician if pregnancy is suspected.
- Tell female patients that menstrual periods may diminish or cease while on this drug (depending on dose). Keep a record of menstrual periods.
- Side effects are dose related, but may be intolerable to some patients. Remind patients to take drugs as ordered for best effect, and not to discontinue therapy without consulting the physician.

Continued.

PATIENT CARE IMPLICATIONS — cont'd

- Warn diabetic patients to monitor blood glucose levels carefully while taking this drug; a change in diet or insulin may be needed.

Oxytocin

Drug administration

- See Table 53.8. Monitor level of consciousness, weight, and intake and output. Monitor blood pressure and pulse. Auscultate lung sounds and heart sounds.
- Monitor fetal heart sounds; notify physician of significant changes in rate or rhythm; follow agency protocol.
- Monitor serum electrolytes, complete blood count, platelets.
- Do not leave patient unattended when IV oxytocin is being used.
- Monitor vaginal bleeding.
- Have available drugs, equipment, and personnel to treat acute allergic reactions in settings where oxytocin is administered.
- For IV use, dilute as ordered or according to agency protocol. Use a microdrip infusion set and an infusion monitoring device. Measure dose according to physician order and patient response.

Patient and family education

- Review anticipated benefits and possible side effects of drug therapy. Instruct the patient to call for assistance if any new side effect develops.
- For intranasal spray, instruct patient to sit upright to use spray; for nose drops, tell the patient to tilt head back to administer drops. When intranasal use is prescribed to promote milk ejection, review with the mother other actions that may also aid in milk ejection: relaxation, breast massage, staying well hydrated, getting enough sleep, and cuddling the infant before trying to nurse.

Ergot alkaloids

Drug administration

- See Table 53.8. Monitor level of consciousness, weight, and intake and output. Monitor blood pressure and pulse. Auscultate lung sounds and heart sounds.
- Monitor serum electrolytes, complete blood count, platelets.
- Monitor vaginal bleeding.

- Have available drugs, equipment, and personnel to treat acute allergic reactions in settings where ergot alkaloids are administered.
- For IV use, may administer undiluted. Administer at a rate of 0.2 mg or less over 1 minute.
- Read labels carefully; do not confuse ergotamine with ergonovine.

Patient and family education

- Review anticipated benefits and possible side effects of drug therapy. Instruct the patient to call for assistance if any new side effect develops.
- Avoid smoking while using ergot alkaloids.

Prostaglandins

Drug administration

- See Table 53.8. Monitor level of consciousness, weight, and intake and output. Monitor blood pressure, pulse, and temperature. Auscultate lung sounds and heart sounds.
- Keep side rails up. Have a suction machine available.
- Monitor serum electrolytes, complete blood count, platelets.
- Monitor vaginal bleeding. Palpate fundus at regular intervals.
- Gastrointestinal symptoms are common; antidiarrhea and antiemetic medications may be ordered concomitantly or prophylactically. Monitor intake and output.

Patient and family education

- Review with patients the anticipated benefits and possible side effects of drug therapy. Instruct patients to call if any unexpected side effect develops.
- Provide emotional support as needed. Refer for counseling if appropriate.

Ritodrine

Drug administration

- Review information about beta-2 adrenergic receptors given in Chapter 10.
- Monitor blood pressure and pulse, uterine contractions, and fetal heart tones. Assess patient and fetus every 5 minutes when initiating IV therapy, every 15 to 30 minutes when the patient is stable, and every 4 hours when the patient is taking oral maintenance doses (or according to agency protocol). Electronic fetal monitoring may be indicated.

PATIENT CARE IMPLICATIONS — cont'd

- For IV administration, use a minidrip infusion set and an infusion control device.
- Stay calm. Provide reassurance to the mother as possible. The drug may increase the subjective sense of anxiety, as well as causing tachycardia, tightness in the chest, tremor, and other symptoms.

Patient and family education

- Review anticipated benefits and possible side effects of drug therapy.
- Review with the patient the limits of activity.
- Tell the patient to notify the physician if labor begins again, membranes rupture, or contractions increase in frequency or duration.

SUMMARY

The hormones involved in female reproduction are gonadotropin-releasing hormone (GnRH) from the hypothalamus; follicle-stimulating hormone (FSH), luteinizing hormone (LH), and prolactin from the anterior pituitary; and estrogens and progestins from the ovary. GnRH stimulates release of FSH and LH from the pituitary. FSH stimulates estrogen production in the ovary. LH is the major signal for ovulation and progesterone production. Prolactin stimulates milk production in the breast. Estrogens cause development of the primary and secondary sexual characteristics of the female. Progestins maintain endometrial function during the second half of the menstrual cycle and during pregnancy. Human chorionic gonadotropin (HCG) maintains production of progestins from the corpus luteum during early pregnancy. Oxytocin from the posterior pituitary stimulates uterine contractions in the late stages of labor and postpartum and stimulates milk letdown in the breast.

Estrogens may be used in replacement therapy when estrogen production is low or absent. These drugs are also used in pharmacological doses for a variety of other conditions of the female reproductive tract. The natural estrogens are rapidly metabolized by the liver and are thus short-acting agents. The synthetic steroidal estrogens and the nonsteroidal estrogens are less readily metabolized and thus are longer-acting agents. Side effects of estrogens include overreactions of certain reproductive tissues, such as breast tenderness and endometrial proliferation. These drugs also cause nausea, vomiting, anorexia, malaise, irritability, water and salt retention, atherosclerosis, and hypertension.

Progestins are used clinically for their effects on the endometrium. Although progesterone, the naturally occurring compound, is not well absorbed orally, the synthetic derivatives are well absorbed.

Progestins may cause edema, midcycle bleeding, and cholestatic jaundice.

Female infertility of certain types can be reversed with pharmacological agents. Preparations containing FSH and/or LH (gonadotropin, menotropins, urofollitropin) may restore fertility in a patient lacking normal pituitary mechanisms. Clomiphene citrate activates the pituitary by hypothalamic mechanisms, thereby ultimately stimulating the ovaries. Gonadorelin may stimulate release of LH and FSH from the pituitary.

Temporary infertility can be induced with estrogen-progestin combinations or with progestins alone. The combination of agents may suppress LH and prevent ovulation. The agents containing only progestins do not block ovulation, but the progestins change the properties of the endometrium and cervix so that fertilization and implantation are impaired. Oral contraceptive agents may cause side effects such as those mentioned for estrogens and progestins. The risk of cerebrovascular accident and thromboembolic disease is increased in patients using oral contraceptives, especially if the patient is obese or hypertensive, or smokes.

Oxytocic drugs speed delivery in uncomplicated birth. These drugs must be used with care to prevent excessive stimulation of uterine contractions that can cause anoxia in the fetus. Oxytocin is rapidly degraded and must be administered intravenously for best control. The ergot alkaloids may be used orally as well as parenterally and have a longer duration of action than does oxytocin. Prostaglandins also promote uterine contractions, but these drugs are used primarily for producing abortions early in pregnancy when the uterus is resistant to oxytocin.

Uterine relaxation is most reliably produced by stimulation of the beta-2 receptors of the uterine muscle. Ritodrine is an agonist for beta-2 receptors that is effective in halting premature labor.

STUDY QUESTIONS

1. What are the gonadotropic hormones?
2. How are the synthesis and release of follicle-stimulating hormone (FSH), luteinizing hormone (LH), and prolactin regulated?
3. What are the major steroid hormones affecting the female reproductive tract?
4. What is the chemical precursor of estrogens and progestins?
5. What are the functions of estrogens during puberty?
6. What hormones regulate ovulation?
7. What effect do estrogens have on the endometrium in the adult female?
8. What effects does progesterone have on the endometrium and myometrium?
9. What is the function of progesterone in pregnancy?
10. What is the role of human chorionic gonadotropin (HCG) in pregnancy?
11. How do the steroidal estrogens differ from the nonsteroidal estrogens in duration of action and route of excretion from the body?
12. What types of side effects and toxic reactions are seen with the chronic use of estrogens?
13. Why are many of the fixed combinations of estrogens with other compounds of limited medical use?
14. What side effects are characteristic of pharmacological use of the progestins?
15. What is the mechanism of action of clomiphene citrate, and what is its medical use?
16. What hormones are contained within the preparations known as menotropins?
17. What is the mechanism of action of bromocriptine and how is this drug currently used?
18. What is the mechanism of action of gonadorelin and what is its medical use?
19. What is the mechanism of action of urofollitropin and what is its medical use?
20. What agents are used to produce pharmacological contraception?
21. What is the mechanism of action of the oral contraceptive agents?
22. What toxic reactions have been associated with the oral contraceptive agents?
23. What side effects occur with use of the oral contraceptives?
24. How do oxytocin and prostaglandins differ in their ability to stimulate uterine contractions?
25. What are the ergot alkaloids?
26. How does the administration and effect of the ergot alkaloids differ from that of oxytocin?
27. What three classes of drugs have the potential for relaxing the musculature of the uterus?
28. What is the mechanism of action of ritodrine?

SUGGESTED READINGS

Brengman, S.L., and Burns, M.: Ritodrine hydrochloride and preterm labor, Am. J. Nurs. 83(4):537, 1983.
Cefalo, R.C.: Drugs in pregnancy: which to use and which to avoid, Drug Therapy 13(4):167, 1983.
Cefalo, R.C.: Alcohol and birth defects—what every woman should know, Drug Therapy 13(4):179, 1983.
Chan, W.Y.: Prostaglandins and nonsteroidal antiinflammatory drugs in dysmenorrhea, Annu. Rev. Pharmacol. 23:131, 1983.
Cobb, J.O.: Demystifying menopause, Canad. Nurse 83(7):16, 1987.
Findlay, J.W.A.: The distribution of some commonly used drugs in human breast milk, Drug Metab. Rev. 14(4):653, 1983.
Harrell, R.M., and Drezner, M.K.: Postmenopausal and senile osteoporosis: a therapeutic dilemma, Drug Therapy 13(4):105, 1983.
Lindsey, A.M., Dodd, M., and Kaempfer, S.H.: Endocrine mechanisms and obesity: influences in breast cancer, Oncol. Nurs. Forum 14(2):47, 1987.
Mishell, D.R.: Update on oral contraceptives, Drug Therapy 19(4):118, 1989.
Nelson, L.: Clomiphene citrate for infertility, Drug Therapy 19(1):65, 1989.
Nevin, M.M.: Dormant danger of DES, Canad. Nurse 84(3):16, 1988.
Orshan, S.A.: The pill, the patient, and you, RN 31(7):49, 1988.
Osteosporosis: estrogen connection clearer, Am. J. Nurs. 88(1):13, 1988.
Sherrod, R.A.: Coping with infertility: a personal perspective turned professional, MCN 13(3):191, 1988.
Shortridge, L.A.: Using ritodrine hydrochloride to inhibit preterm labor, MCN J. 8(1):58, 1983.

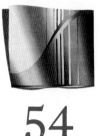

Drugs Acting on the Male Reproductive System

54

The major reproductive hormones in men are steroids, which are synthesized primarily in the testes and to a lesser extent in the adrenal gland. Within the testes the status of interstitial or Leydig cells and the seminiferous tubular cells is most important for determining male sexual potential. The Leydig cells synthesize testosterone, the major masculinizing steroid hormone. The seminiferous tubules contain the germ cells that in the adult male produce functional sperm. The endocrine control of male sexual development and function, the actions of natural male hormones, and the clinical uses of synthetic and natural drugs acting on the male reproductive system are discussed in this chapter.

PITUITARY REGULATION OF REPRODUCTIVE POTENTIAL IN THE MALE

In the adult male, sexual function depends on the proper interaction of the hypothalamus, anterior pituitary, and the testes. Regulation of testicular function is by a negative feedback loop similar to others previously mentioned. The primary hormones in this cycle are testosterone from the testes; interstitial cell–stimulating hormone (ICSH), also called luteinizing hormone (LH), and follicle-stimulating hormone (FSH) from the anterior pituitary; and gonadotropin-releasing hormone (GnRH; see Chapter 50) from the hypothalamus. When testosterone levels in the blood are low, GnRH is released from the hypothalamus to enter the anterior pituitary through the portal venous system. Under the influence of GnRH, both ICSH and FSH are released from the pituitary gland into the general circulation, where they may act on testicular tissues.

The action of these regulatory hormones is slightly different during the three stages of life in which they act. During fetal development Leydig cells develop in the embryonic testis as a result of stimulation with the maternal hormone, human chorionic gonadotropin (HCG). These embryonic cells produce the small amounts of testosterone necessary for the development of the male external genitalia; without testosterone, genetically male infants are born with female genitalia. After birth these Leydig cells regress, since the stimulus of HCG is no longer available.

The second period of life when these regulatory processes are most important is puberty. In childhood very low concentrations of gonadotropins are found in the blood. With the onset of puberty the pituitary gland begins to synthesize and release greater quantities of gonadotropins ICSH and FSH. The target organ for ICSH in the male is the Leydig cell, where ICSH stimulates testosterone production. FSH acts directly on the cells of the seminiferous tubule and associated cells to prepare that tissue for spermatogenesis. This process cannot be completed unless testosterone from the Leydig cells is also present. With both FSH and testosterone acting on the seminiferous tubules, mature sperm can be produced. Testosterone acts not only within the testes but also throughout the body at this stage of life. These actions are discussed in the next section.

The third period of life to be considered is sexual maturity. During this time ICSH continues to be important in the maintenance of sexual function, since it is still required for the synthesis of testosterone. Testosterone is required for the maintenance of spermatogenesis.

A third hormone of the anterior pituitary involved in male sexual function is prolactin. The mechanisms by which prolactin release in males is regulated are not completely understood. However, men with pituitary tumors that secrete large quan-

Table 54.1   Clinical Summary of Androgens

Generic name	Trade name	Administration/dosage	Duration of action	Adverse reactions
NATURAL HORMONE				
Testosterone	Andro Andronaq Histerone Testaqua Testoject	INTRAMUSCULAR: *Adults*—aqueous suspension for intramuscular use only. Doses range from 10 to 100 mg. FDA Pregnancy Category X.	Relatively short. Doses must be repeated 2 or 3 times per week.	Masculinization in females. Precocious sexual development and premature closure of the epiphyses in children. Excessive sexual stimulation (short-term) or inhibition of testicular function (long-term) in males.
	T-pellets	SUBCUTANEOUS: *Adults*—75 pellets for implantation, 150 to 450 mg.	3 to 4 months because of slow absorption.	Same as for testosterone, aqueous suspension.
TESTOSTERONE ESTERS				
Testosterone cypionate	Andronaq-LA Duratest Tesionate	INTRAMUSCULAR: *Adults*—oil solution for deep injection into gluteal muscle, 100 to 400 mg. FDA Pregnancy Category X.	3 to 4 weeks.	Same as for testosterone, aqueous suspension.
Testosterone enanthate	Delatestryl* Durathate	INTRAMUSCULAR: *Adults*—oil solution for deep injection into gluteal muscle, 50 to 400 mg. FDA Pregnancy Category X.	2 to 4 weeks.	Same as for testosterone, aqueous suspension.
Testosterone propionate	Testex	INTRAMUSCULAR: *Adults*—oil suspension for intramuscular use only. Doses range from 25 to 100 mg. FDA Pregnancy Category X.	Relatively short. Doses must be repeated 2 or 3 times per week.	Same as for testosterone, aqueous suspension.
ORAL ANDROGENS				
Fluoxymesterone	Halotestin* Ora-Testryl	ORAL: *Adults*—5 to 20 mg daily (male) and 10 to 40 mg daily (female). FDA Pregnancy Category X.	Short. Doses must be repeated daily.	Same as for testosterone, aqueous suspension. Nausea and vomiting, diarrhea, peptic ulcer-like symptoms. May increase sensitivity to anticoagulants. Hepatotoxicity, including jaundice.
Methyltestosterone	Android Metandren* Oreton Methyl Testred	ORAL: *Adults*—tablets or capsules, 10 to 50 mg daily (male) and 50 to 200 mg daily (female). FDA Pregnancy Category X.	Short. Doses must be repeated daily.	Same as for testosterone, aqueous suspension. Nausea and vomiting, diarrhea, peptic ulcer-like symptoms. May increase sensitivity to anticoagulants. Hepatotoxicity, including jaundice.
BUCCAL AGENTS				
Methyltestosterone	Android-Muquets Metandren linquet* Oreton Methyl	ORAL: *Adults*—tablets for buccal administration, 5 to 25 mg daily (male) and 25 to 100 mg daily (female). FDA Pregnancy Category X.	Short. Doses must be repeated daily.	Same as for testosterone, aqueous suspension. May increase sensitivity to anticoagulants. Hepatotoxicity, including jaundice.

*Available in Canada and United States.

tities of prolactin often have decreased libidos and low concentrations of ICSH, FSH, and testosterone in their bloodstream. Prolactin seems to suppress synthesis and release of ICSH and FSH from the pituitary gland and may directly interfere with the actions of these hormones on the testes.

ANDROGENIC STEROIDS
Role of Naturally Occurring Steroids

The major steroid affecting male sexual function is testosterone. This hormone is synthesized both in the Leydig cells of the testes and in the adrenal cortex. The action of testosterone on the testes already has been mentioned, but that is only part of its action. Testosterone is a potent androgen (a substance that stimulates growth of the organs of the male reproductive tract). Testosterone is responsible for the enlargement and maturation of the penis, scrotum, seminal vesicles, prostate gland, and other accessory tissues of the male reproductive tract. These actions constitute the primary sexual effects on the male.

Testosterone is also the major hormone responsible for the development of the secondary sexual characteristics. It is the increased testosterone level during puberty that stimulates the growth of facial hair as well as pubic hair and hair on chest and armpits. Sustained levels of testosterone trigger the onset of baldness in genetically predisposed males. The other dramatic changes that occur in the pubertal male also are related to the increased testosterone levels: lowering of the voice caused by thickening of the vocal cords, stimulation of sebaceous glands, and stimulation of the libido. Psychologists working with primates other than human beings have even related aggression to high testosterone levels.

In addition to these primary and secondary sexual effects, testosterone also has profound effects on metabolism. Androgens are anabolic; that is, they stimulate synthetic rather than degradative processes. Testosterone increases nitrogen retention and protein formation, as well as increasing overall metabolic rate. This anabolic action is responsible for the increase in muscle mass associated with puberty and the distribution of this mass in the male pattern. In addition, calcium is retained and the size and strength of bone are enhanced. Blood-forming cells are also affected so that more red blood cells may be formed.

Although testosterone is the major circulating androgen in human males, it is not the only metabolically important androgen. Evidence shows that testosterone is transformed within many target cells to *dihydrotestosterone,* which is a more potent androgen than testosterone itself. Small amounts of another androgen, *androstenedione,* also may affect various tissues of the body.

Both testosterone and androstenedione are close chemical relatives of the estrogens (steroid hormones that have feminizing effects). Some tissues, such as brain, breasts, and testes, can convert androgens to estrogens. Low estrogen concentrations therefore are found in the blood of normal adult males. These estrogens have no obvious influence on normal men, but under certain circumstances the concentrations of estrogen may increase and produce pathological signs such as breast development.

Use of Androgens in Replacement Therapy

Androgenic drugs are primarily used in replacement therapy for patients who have reduced endogenous androgen production. For some patients the loss of androgens occurs early and prevents the normal changes of puberty. Androgen loss after puberty may cause a loss in libido or sexual desire or cause mild feminizing tendencies. Aging males produce less testosterone than younger men and may suffer loss of sexual drive. Some older men suffer more severe symptoms suggestive of a male climacteric or male menopause. All these conditions, as well as others related to specific malfunctions of the male sexual organs, may be treated with testosterone or one of the other androgenic compounds (Table 54.1). For these patients with reduced natural testosterone production, this treatment constitutes replacement therapy.

Certain forms of impotence and feminization do not respond well to replacement therapy with androgenic steroids. One type of patient unresponsive to androgens has very high blood levels of prolactin. As noted earlier, prolactin may interfere with the production and function of ICSH and FSH, lowering testosterone production. Bromocriptine, a drug that blocks prolactin synthesis, lowers prolactin levels, increases testosterone as well as ICSH and FSH levels, and restores sexual potency in some patients. Bromocriptine is also used to control galactorrhea and restore fertility in females (see Chapter 53).

Testosterone in its natural form is not water soluble and therefore is used as an aqueous suspension suitable only for intramuscular injection (Table 54.1). In this form the drug has a short duration of action and produces somewhat erratic clinical responses. Testosterone can be absorbed from the gastrointestinal tract. However, this route of administration does not produce clinically useful testosterone concentrations in the bloodstream,

THE NURSING PROCESS

DRUGS AND THE MALE REPRODUCTIVE SYSTEM

Assessment

Patients usually receive drugs acting on the male reproductive system for reversal of insufficient androgen production, for treatment of a hormonally sensitive tumor, or for the anabolic effects of the drugs in a condition such as severe trauma or burns. The nurse should do a complete patient assessment before the initiation of drug therapy. The data base should include the vital signs, blood pressure, weight, serum calcium level, height, and glucose content of the urine and blood. In addition, the nurse should focus part of the assessment on the presenting problem. For example, in treatment of reduced androgen production, an assessment of the secondary sexual characteristics should be included. In the patient receiving androgen therapy for its anabolic effects, a careful assessment of nutritional needs, level of mobility, and food and fluid intake and output also is appropriate.

Potential nursing diagnoses

Body image disturbance: acne secondary to androgen therapy

Body image disturbance: masculinization of females secondary to androgen therapy

Management

As with many hormones, the effects of the drugs acting on the male reproductive system will not be seen for several weeks after the initiation of therapy in most cases. As therapy is started, the nurse should monitor the vital signs and other data mentioned in assessment. In anticipating the patient's discharge, the nurse should review possible and probable side effects with the patient. For example, the female receiving androgen therapy for hormonally sensitive tumors in most cases will develop some secondary male sexual characteristics, such as deepening of the voice and clitoral enlargement. These changes should be reviewed in detail with the patient at the beginning of therapy. For patients receiving steroids for their anabolic effects, referral to the hospital or community dietitian also may be helpful.

Evaluation

As with all drugs, the goal is to produce the desired effect but without causing side effects. In replacement therapy for insufficient androgen production, the expected outcome would be increased height and weight and development of secondary sexual characteristics in the male. Ideally this improvement would occur without the development of side effects such as priapism. In doses used to treat female patients with hormonally sensitive cancers, the development of male characteristics almost always occurs. Before discharge the patient should be able to explain how and why to take the drugs, anticipated side effects, side effects that require immediate notification of the physician (e.g., symptoms of hypercalcemia in the cancer patient), how to treat side effects that may be troublesome but are not serious, and what parameters should be measured regularly at home to monitor the effectiveness of the drug. For example, the height and weight of a young male receiving androgens as replacement therapy should be monitored. For additional specific guidelines, see the patient care implications section.

since the steroid absorbed from the intestine passes directly into the portal circulation and enters the liver before it circulates to the rest of the body. The liver is capable of inactivating testosterone very rapidly by forming less active metabolites or by converting the steroid to a glucuronide or sulfated derivatives. For long-term replacement therapy, pellets of free testosterone can be implanted subcutaneously. These pellets slowly release testosterone into the circulation over several months. Although these pellets are convenient for the patient, they do result in less flexible control of the symptoms than can be achieved with more frequent injections.

Testosterone esters are much more useful than testosterone itself for producing sustained androgenic effects. Two preparations commonly employed clinically are *testosterone enanthate* and *testosterone cypionate* (Table 54.1). Both are supplied as suspensions in oil; when injected intramuscularly, they are slowly absorbed and therefore effective for 3 to 4 weeks. This increased convenience for the patient is at the cost of less flexibility in control. Another testosterone ester, *testosterone propionate,* has a short duration of action more similar to that of testosterone.

Orally absorbed androgens have been developed, including *methyltestosterone* and *fluoxymesterone.* These compounds are effective orally, since they are resistant to the action of liver enzymes that degrade testosterone. Unfortunately these compounds also are associated with liver toxicity of various types, including cholestatic jaundice.

Tablets of methyltestosterone and testosterone propionate are available for buccal administration. Absorption through the mucous membranes of the mouth may be more effective than oral administration, since buccally absorbed materials do not directly enter portal circulation and therefore are circulated to the rest of the body before they enter the liver (see Chapter 2).

Androgens have been used in the past for various conditions in females, such as relief of dysmenorrhea, menopausal symptoms, and postpartum breast engorgement, but other agents now are preferred (see Chapter 53). Androgens still are indicated for treatment of certain advanced breast carcinomas (see Chapter 39). The high doses used for this purpose exceed those required for replacement therapy and may be expected to cause masculinization (Table 54.1).

Danazol, a weak androgen, is used to suppress LH and FSH release from the pituitary gland and to block steroidogenesis in the gonads and adrenals. It also relieves the tenderness of fibrocystic breast disease and controls endometriosis. The drug is also useful in treating angioedema.

ANABOLIC STEROIDS

In addition to androgenic properties, the natural male steroids also possess anabolic properties that may be useful in certain clinical situations (Table 54.2). For example, these drugs may be used to treat conditions for which increased nitrogen retention and protein formation are desirable. Accordingly, these drugs alleviate the catabolic state produced by corticosteroid therapy. Patients who have suffered extensive burns or other trauma may benefit from the action of the anabolic steroids. These drugs also may be effective when bone loss is a problem, since anabolic steroids increase bone deposition. Anabolic hormone effects on red blood cell formation make these drugs valuable in the treatment of certain forms of anemia.

Although a few anabolic compounds have relatively low androgenic potency, all anabolic steroids possess androgenic properties to some degree. Although these androgenic effects may be indistinguishable in normal males, they may become painfully obvious when the compounds are used to treat women or children. Patients receiving these compounds may develop increased libido. Males may develop priapism (continuous erection). Females should be especially watched for androgen-induced changes such as inappropriate hair development, voice changes, or personality alterations. Children, if they receive these compounds at all, should be watched very closely for precocious sexual development. These compounds, while promoting bone growth in children, also promote fusion of the epiphyses, which permanently halts skeletal growth. Therefore full adult height may be diminished, although a growth spurt may be attained when the drugs are first given. For this reason, as well as because of the effects on sexual development, these drugs are less than ideal for therapy in children.

Anabolic steroids are inappropriate for use in athletes seeking to increase bone or muscle mass. In healthy young males, the anabolic effects are minimal, but the side effects can be serious (altered liver function, reduced gonadotropin levels, lowered testosterone synthesis, depressed spermatogenesis). In healthy young females, bone and muscle mass may be increased more dramatically, but at the cost of virilization and menstrual disturbances.

Table 54.2 Clinical Summary of Anabolic Steroids

Generic name	Trade name	Administration/dosage	Duration of action	Major clinical uses	Adverse reactions
Ethylestrenol	Maxibolin*	ORAL: *Adults*—tablets or elixir, 4 mg daily. *Children*—2 mg daily. FDA Pregnancy Category X.	Short. Doses must be repeated daily.	To produce weight gain following traumatic injury, chronic disease, or long-term corticosteroid therapy. Control symptoms of osteoporosis.	Virilism is possible, especially in women and children. Premature epiphyseal closure may be produced in children, resulting in diminished adult height. Hepatotoxicity.
Nandrolone decanoate	Deca-Durabolin* Decolone	INTRAMUSCULAR: *Adults*—oil solution for deep intramuscular injection, 50 to 200 mg. *Children*—25 to 50 mg. FDA Pregnancy Category X.	Long. Repeat doses every 3 to 4 weeks.	Refractory anemias, metastatic breast cancer.	Virilism is possible, especially in women and children. Premature epiphyseal closure may be produced in children, resulting in diminished adult height.
Nandrolone phenpropionate	Androlone Durabolin*	INTRAMUSCULAR: *Adults*—oil solution for deep intramuscular injection, 50 to 100 mg. FDA Pregnancy Category X.	Long. Repeat doses every 1 to 4 weeks.	Same as for nandrolone decanoate.	Same as for nandrolone decanoate.
Oxandrolone	Anavar	ORAL: *Adults*—tablets, 5 to 10 mg daily. *Children*—0.25 mg/kg body weight intermittently. FDA Pregnancy Category X.	Short. Repeat doses daily.	Same as for ethylestrenol.	Same as for ethylestrenol.
Oxymetholone	Anadrol	ORAL: *Adults*—tablets, 1 to 5 mg/ kg body weight/day up to 100 mg total daily dose. FDA Pregnancy Category X.	Short. Repeat doses daily.	Anemias.	Same as for ethylestrenol.
Stanozolol	Winstrol	ORAL: *Adults*—tablets, 4 mg daily. *Children*—1 mg twice daily only during an attack. FDA Pregnancy Category X.	Short. Doses are taken with meals.	Hereditary angioedema.	Same as for ethylestrenol. Therapy should be intermittent.

*Available in Canada and United States.

PATIENT CARE IMPLICATIONS

Androgens

Drug administration

- Assess mental status and neurologic function.
- Assess for signs of depression: insomnia, lack of appetite, loss of interest in personal appearance, and withdrawal.
- Monitor weight, pulse, blood pressure. Assess for development of edema and skin changes. Auscultate lung and heart sounds.
- Monitor complete blood count and differential, serum electrolytes, liver function tests.
- Assess for signs of liver dysfunction: right upper quadrant abdominal pain, malaise, fever, jaundice, pruritus.
- Assess for hypercalcemia. See Table 17.1, Common electrolyte abnormalities.
- When prescribed in children, review the proposed long-term treatment plan. Therapy for children is often intermittent, to allow drug-free periods to permit normal bone growth. The child's progress may be monitored with regular x-ray studies of wrists and hands to monitor bone maturation. Monitor weight and height.
- For a discussion of IM administration of oil-based suspensions, see Chapter 6.
- Pellets for subcutaneous implantation can be inserted surgically or with a specially designed injector. Either procedure can be done easily in the physician's office; aseptic technique must be used. Usual sites of insertion are the infrascapular area or along the posterior axillary line. Two or more pellets may be inserted at one time, although not necessarily into the same subcutaneous pouch. The drugs will be absorbed slowly from the pellets for up to 4 to 6 months. Sloughing of the pellets can occur; instruct patient to notify physician. Sloughing often indicates placement too superficially or lack of aseptic technique. Because the dose of subcutaneous pellets cannot be regulated easily, proper dosage is determined by oral medication before a switch is made to the subcutaneous route. For additional information, see the information supplied by the manufacturer.
- For buccal tablets, instruct patients to place tablet(s) in the mouth between the upper or lower gum and the cheek, and allow the tablet to dissolve. While the tablet is in place, the patient should refrain from eating, drinking, chewing, or smoking. Instruct patients to rotate sites with each administration. Remind patient to maintain a program of good regular oral hygiene, and to report any oral irritation to the physician.

Patient and family education

- Review anticipated benefits and possible side effects of drug therapy. Tell patients to report the development of any new side effects.
- Assess patients tactfully for side effects such as decreased ejaculatory volume, amenorrhea, menstrual irregularities, virilization of females, clitoral enlargement. Children may experience premature virilization. Patients may be reluctant to discuss these problems, or children may not know how to do so. Provide emotional support as needed. Remind patients to take drugs as ordered for best effects, and not to stop taking the drug without notifying the physician.
- Notify the physician if priapism develops.
- Take oral doses with meals or snack to lessen gastric irritation.
- Warn diabetic patients to monitor blood glucose levels frequently for the first 2 weeks of therapy, and after androgen therapy is completed, as a change in insulin or diet may be needed.

Anabolic steroids

Drug administration

- Assess mental status. Assess for signs of depression: lack of interest in personal appearance, insomnia, loss of appetite, and withdrawal.
- Monitor weight, blood pressure, and pulse. Assess for development of edema and skin changes.
- Monitor complete blood count and differential, liver function tests.

Patient and family education

- Review anticipated benefits and possible side effects of the drug therapy. Tell patients to take drugs only as ordered, and not to share drugs with others. Anabolic steroids should not be used to change body size or function for athletic purposes.
- Take oral doses with meals or snack to lessen gastric irritation. If GI symptoms are severe or persistent, notify physician.
- Assess tactfully for changes such as hirsutism and virilization in women or gyneco-

Continued.

PATIENT CARE IMPLICATIONS — cont'd

mastia or decreased libido in males. Provide emotional support as needed. Remind patients to take medications as ordered for best effect, and not to stop medications without notifying the physician.

- Notify the physician if priapism develops.
- Warn diabetic patients to monitor blood glucose levels carefully when starting or ending therapy with steroids, as an adjustment in

insulin or diet may be necessary.

- Patients who have been burned, traumatized, or immobilized should be informed that the effectiveness of anabolic steroids may be enhanced by concomitant use of a diet high in calories and protein. Continue regular physical therapy to help reduce demineralization of bone.

SUMMARY

Male sexual development and function are regulated by hormones produced in the hypothalamus (gonadotropin-releasing hormone [GnRH]), the anterior pituitary (interstitial cell–stimulating hormone [ICSH] and follicle-stimulating hormone [FSH]), and the testes (androgenic steroids). Development of male genitalia during fetal life requires the presence of small amounts of androgen, which is produced in response to maternal chorionic gonadotropin (HCG). Development of primary and secondary sexual characteristics at puberty depends on proper concentrations of GnRH, ICSH, FSH, and androgens. In the adult male, maintenance of sexual function requires that adequate concentrations of androgens be maintained.

The most plentiful natural androgen is the steroid testosterone. Other androgens, such as dihydrotestosterone and androstenedione, also may be formed. These steroids are all formed in the testes and in lesser amounts in the adrenal glands of normal males. Androgen deficiency can cause loss of libido, or sexual desire, and ultimately may cause loss of some secondary male sex characteristics. Replacement therapy with androgens can reverse these changes and control most symptoms of androgen deficiency.

Testosterone may be injected intramuscularly as an aqueous suspension but has a very short duration of action. The steroid may be implanted under the skin as pellets that release testosterone slowly over a period of months. However, sustained androgenic effects are best achieved by intramuscular injection of long-acting testosterone esters, testosterone enanthate and testosterone cypionate. Orally administered androgens such as methyltestosterone and fluoxymesterone are also useful for long-term therapy in androgen deficiency, but these

agents have a higher incidence of liver damage than other androgens. Buccal absorption of methyltestosterone and testosterone propionate is useful, since this route of administration bypasses the portal circulation to the liver where testosterone is rapidly degraded.

Natural androgens are also anabolic hormones. Synthetic androgen derivatives are available, which minimize the androgenic properties of the compounds and maximize the anabolic properties. These drugs may be used in clinical situations in which increased nitrogen retention and protein formation are desirable. These anabolic steroids retain enough androgenic activity to cause masculinization in sensitive females and precocious sexual development in some children.

STUDY QUESTIONS

1. What three organs produce hormones that affect male sexual development and function?
2. What is the function of gonadotropin-releasing hormone (GnRH) in the adult male?
3. What is the function of interstitial cell–stimulating hormone (ICSH) in the adult male?
4. What is the function of follicle-stimulating hormone (FSH) in the adult male?
5. What is the function of testosterone during fetal development in males?
6. How do ICSH, FSH, and testosterone actions convert the immature, prepubertal male genitalia to the fully functional adult form?
7. What is the primary natural androgenic steroid?
8. What are the primary sexual characteristics of the male?
9. What are the secondary sexual characteristics of the male?

10. What effect does testosterone have on metabolism?
11. Name two naturally occurring androgens besides testosterone.
12. Are estrogens found in normal males?
13. What is the most common clinical use of androgen steroids?
14. Why is testosterone not administered by the oral route?
15. What advantages do testosterone esters such as testosterone enanthate have over testosterone for long-term replacement therapy of androgen deficiency?
16. What two androgenic steroids are well absorbed orally?
17. What disadvantages do the orally administered androgenic steroids possess compared to other androgenic agents?
18. What is the advantage of administering testosterone by the buccal route rather than by the oral route?
19. What is the major effect of the anabolic steroids?
20. What side effect is frequently associated with anabolic steroids?

SUGGESTED READINGS

Anthony, C.P., and Thibodeau, G.A.: The male reproductive system. In Textbook of anatomy and physiology, ed. 12, St. Louis, 1987, C.V. Mosby Co.

Brown, T.R., Berkovitz, G.D., and Migeon, C.J.: Androgen receptors in man, Diagn. Med. **5**(7):23, 1982.

Council on Scientific Affairs: Drug abuse in athletes. Anabolic steroids and human growth hormone, JAMA **259**(11):1703, 1988.

Lamb, D.R.: Anabolic steroids: how well do they work and how dangerous are they? Am. J. Sports Med. **12**(1):31, 1984.

Yelverton, G.A.: Anabolic steroids, Pediatr. Nurs. **15**(1):63, 1989.

Zurer, P.S.: Drugs in sports, Chem. Eng. News **62**(18):69, 1984.

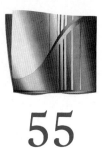

Drugs to Treat Diabetes Mellitus

55

Within the tissue of the pancreas, an exocrine gland that supplies digestive juices to the small intestine, lie discrete clusters of cells whose functions are very different from those of most pancreatic cells. These cell clusters, called the islets of Langerhans, contain several types of endocrine cells. Three of these cell types release peptide hormones that affect glucose metabolism: A (alpha) cells, which synthesize and release the peptide hormone glucagon; B (beta) cells, which synthesize and release insulin; and D cells, which synthesize somatostatin. This chapter includes an examination of the function of the islet cells, a description of diabetes mellitus, and a description of the drugs used in the diagnosis and control of that disease.

NORMAL HORMONAL REGULATION OF METABOLISM

Glucose Metabolism

One of the rules of metabolic regulation is that the body seldom relies on a single mechanism to control an important physiological function. This rule applies especially well to the processes by which the body regulates glucose utilization. The major hormone regulating glucose metabolism is insulin, a peptide hormone synthesized in the beta cells of the pancreas. Insulin stimulates glucose uptake in fat and muscle cells and the conversion in the liver of glucose to the storage carbohydrate glycogen.

Insulin does not work alone, however, and its metabolic actions must always be considered in relation to the actions of other hormones. For example, the elevated blood glucose level following a meal stimulates insulin release from the pancreas. Blood glucose levels are thereby lowered, since insulin stimulates both the burning of glucose for energy in fat and muscle cells and the stor-

age of glucose in the liver. As blood glucose levels fall in response to insulin, glucagon release from the alpha cells of the pancreas is stimulated. Glucagon in many ways directly opposes the action of insulin in glucose metabolism. Glucagon stimulates the liver to break down glycogen and amino acids so that glucose is released into the blood. Glucagon also inhibits the uptake of glucose by muscle and fat cells. By balancing the action of these two hormones, the body protects itself from hyperglycemia (high blood glucose) on the one hand and hypoglycemia (low blood glucose) on the other hand.

Even the concept of metabolic balance achieved with two antagonistic hormones does not adequately describe glucose regulation. For example, somatostatin (see Chapter 49) released from D cells inhibits release of both insulin and glucagon from islet cells. Other hormones antagonize the peripheral effects of insulin. Cortisol (an adrenocortical glucocorticoid) and epinephrine (a catecholamine from the adrenal medulla), which are elevated during stress, antagonize the actions of insulin in muscle or fat cells (Table 55.1). The overall action of these two hormones is to increase blood glucose levels. Growth hormone (see Chapter 50) also increases blood glucose, primarily by lowering glucose uptake in muscle cells.

Fat and Protein Metabolism

Although insulin most frequently is considered as a regulator of glucose metabolism, it is also important in regulating fat and protein metabolism. Insulin directly stimulates the synthesis of storage lipid within the fat cell, blocks the breakdown and release of stored lipid, and promotes protein synthesis both by stimulating amino acid uptake and by directly stimulating protein synthetic processes.

As in carbohydrate metabolism, the action of insulin in regulating fat and protein metabolism is opposed by other hormones (Table 55.1). For example, epinephrine, glucagon, cortisol, and growth hormone all stimulate fat breakdown in fat cells, thereby directly opposing the action of insulin in that tissue. These hormones therefore tend to raise the blood content of free fatty acids and other breakdown products of lipids. In addition, glucagon and cortisol block protein synthesis in direct opposition to insulin action. Growth hormone differs in this regard from the other insulin-opposing hormones in that growth hormone directly stimulates protein synthesis in many tissues of the body.

An understanding of this delicate balance of hormonal actions is important to appreciate the origin of some of the metabolic derangements that occur in diabetes mellitus.

DIABETES MELLITUS

Types and Causes of Disease

In diabetes mellitus, insulin action is lost. If all insulin production ceases, the disease is referred to as *insulin-dependent diabetes mellitus (IDDM)*. Other terms for this form are *type I* or *juvenile-onset* diabetes. If insulin production continues but is insufficient to meet the body's demands, the disease is referred to as *noninsulin-dependent diabetes mellitus (NIDDM)*, also called *type II* or *adult-onset* diabetes; most diabetic persons have this type. As the names imply, diabetes characterized by absence of insulin production is primarily a disease of the young, although it may occur later in life as well. NIDDM is usually a disease of persons who are over age 40 or obese. Diabetes in these patients may involve insulin resistance; insulin concentrations in the blood may be normal, but the target tissues are unresponsive to insulin.

The exact cause of diabetes mellitus has not been established. The disease may arise in several ways, or at least several factors may contribute to its development. Heredity may play a role in some types of diabetes, especially the adult-onset type (NIDDM). However, it has never been proved that heredity alone determines who will or who will not develop the disease. For example, in older individuals a clear link exists between obesity and NIDDM.

Viral infections have been implicated in juvenile-onset diabetes (IDDM), partly through epidemiological evidence linking viral epidemics to unexpected increases in new cases of IDDM. Viruses can produce diabetes in laboratory animals, and at least one case is now on record in which viruses were isolated from the pancreas of a child who died during the acute onset of diabetes mellitus. The viruses from this child produced diabetes in experimental animals.

Metabolic Derangements in Diabetes Mellitus

Significant metabolic derangements occur when insulin action is lost. Without insulin, less glucose is utilized in muscle and fat cells, and more glucose is released into the circulation by the liver. Muscle cells, starved for energy sources, break down protein and release amino acids into the bloodstream. The liver converts a portion of these amino acids into glucose and returns it to the bloodstream. All these processes contribute to the persistent elevated levels of glucose in the blood. When glucose levels in the bloodstream exceed a certain threshold (about 160 mg/dl), glucose begins to appear in the urine.

The most common early symptoms of diabetes mellitus can readily be seen to be a direct result of osmotic and metabolic changes just mentioned. Patients frequently first note a feeling of constant fatigue as energy production in body cells is impaired. An increased frequency of urination (polyuria), often first noticed at night, occurs because of the excess glucose in the urine that produces an osmotic diuresis (i.e., more water must be excreted to carry out the high concentration of glucose). As urine output increases, most patients develop excessive thirst (polydipsia), which results from the body's efforts to maintain normal hydration in the face of excessive fluid losses through the kidney. Some patients develop perineal infections, made likely by the presence of glucose in the urine.

The alterations in metabolism produced by insulin deficiency and the relative excess of catabolic hormones (catecholamines, steroids) ultimately result in greater than normal protein and fat breakdown. The protein is metabolized to amino acids and then to glucose, whereas the fats are converted to free fatty acids and then to ketone bodies that are released into the circulation. These excess breakdown products may cause the patient to become ketotic or acidotic. The potential for ketoacidosis is a serious acute complication of diabetes mellitus, and ketoacidotic coma is associated with mortalities of 3% to 30%. Mortality is highest when treatment is delayed. Ketoacidosis is primarily seen in patients with IDDM who have little or no endogenous insulin production. These patients are sometimes referred to as *ketosis-prone diabetics.* Patients with NIDDM who produce enough insulin to suppress lipid breakdown are resistant to ketosis.

Any diabetic person may become comatose as a result of dehydration. As the plasma becomes hyperosmolar (higher solute concentration than blood), water is pulled from body tissues, and severe water and electrolyte imbalances occur. Patients in this type of hyperosmolar coma are as a rule older and have an even higher mortality than the patients in ketoacidotic coma.

Long-Term Complications of Diabetes Mellitus

Pathological changes in blood vessels, nerves, and kidneys occur in diabetics. Blood vessel defects are observed in the retina, where hemorrhages may destroy sight. Other vessels may be similarly affected, although those changes are not so easily observed in the early stages of the disease; at later stages, circulation to the limbs may be grossly impaired. The kidney is another organ in which pathological changes occur, at first affecting glomerular filtration rate, then progressing to glomerulosclerosis with thickening of the capillary basement membranes. Nephrotic syndrome with protein loss through the kidney and frank kidney failure are late complications of diabetes. Nerve function is impaired so that late in the disease there may be loss of feeling in the limbs or other parts of the body. Sexual impotence is common among diabetic men.

Evidence from research laboratories suggests that many of the late pathological changes may be delayed or reduced in severity by strict control of the blood sugar level from the earliest possible time after the appearance of the diabetes. Clinical studies have not yet proved or disproved a relationship between the degree of diabetic control and the development of long-term complications in human patients. A 10-year prospective study (Diabetes Control and Complications Trial) sponsored by the National Institutes of Health may afford definitive answers.

Diagnosis of Diabetes Mellitus

Diabetes mellitus is diagnosed by applying one of the following procedures.

Fasting blood sugar (FBS) is determined by obtaining a few milliliters of blood from an individual after a 12-hour fast and measuring the glucose content by any of several methods approved for use in clinical laboratories. Most conveniently, the blood is taken in the early morning. The range of normal fasting plasma sugar values is 60 to 100 mg/dl for venous blood. A value above 140 mg/dl in a truly fasting individual suggests the diagnosis of diabetes mellitus. Values between 100 and 140 mg/dl may require further evaluation of the patient.

Glucosuria (glucose in the urine) is conveniently tested in screening programs with commercially available pretreated test strips (Dextrostix), which develop a particular color when exposed to urine containing glucose. Glucose does not routinely appear in the urine of nondiabetic persons, since a blood sugar level of about 160 mg/dl is required before the normal kidney allows glucose to spill into the urine. Some diabetic persons spill glucose into the urine at lower blood glucose concentrations, possibly as a result of impaired kidney function.

The *oral glucose tolerance test (OGTT)* detects not only persons who are overtly diabetic but also those who may progress to clinical diabetes. The test consists of administering 50 to 100 Gm of glucose orally. Blood samples are then taken at hourly or 30-minute intervals, and the glucose levels in the plasma are compared to the value obtained from a sample taken immediately before the glucose was administered. In a normal person, plasma glucose levels rise in response to this acute glucose load and immediately trigger the release of insulin from the beta cells of the pancreas. As a result of the circulating insulin, glucose levels begin to fall within an hour or so after the glucose load is administered and return to normal by 2 hours (Figure 55.1). In contrast, the plasma glucose levels of the diabetic person fall more slowly than those of the normal person, since insulin is not released to aid in disposition of the glucose load. Plasma glucose levels in diabetic persons remain over 200 mg/dl of plasma 2 hours after the glucose load.

TREATMENT OF DIABETES MELLITUS
Insulin Therapy

Mechanism of action. Insulin is used for treatment of diabetes when presumably no functional B cells are left in the islets to respond to glucose levels. Such treatment constitutes replacement therapy. The administered insulin restores the ability of cells to utilize glucose as an energy source and corrects many associated metabolic derangements.

Absorption and fate. Insulin must be administered by injection, since it is a protein and therefore would be digested and destroyed in the gastrointestinal tract. In its natural form, insulin is relatively soluble in water and is rather quickly absorbed from subcutaneous injection sites. This property is reflected in the pharmacological behav-

Table 55.1   Metabolic Actions of Insulin and Insulin-Opposing Hormones

Tissue and metabolic process	Insulin	Glucagon	Epinephrine	Cortisol	Growth hormone
LIVER					
Glycogen formation	Increase	Decrease	Decrease	Increase	—
Glucose formation from amino acids	Decrease	Increase	—	Increase	Decrease
Glucose formation from glycogen	Decrease	Increase	Increase	—	—
SKELETAL MUSCLE					
Glucose uptake or utilization	Increase	Decrease	Decrease	Decrease	Decrease
Amino acid uptake	Increase	—	—	—	Increase
Protein synthesis	Increase	Decrease	—	Decrease	Increase
Glucose release from glycogen	Decrease	Increase	Increase	—	—
FAT CELLS					
Synthesis of storage lipid	Increase	Decrease	Decrease	Decrease	Decrease
Release of free fatty acids from stored lipid	Decrease	Increase	Increase	Increase	Increase
BLOOD					
Glucose level	Decrease	Increase	Increase	Increase	Increase
Free fatty acid level	Decrease	Increase	Increase	Increase	Increase

ior of regular insulin for injection (Table 55.2), which is rapidly absorbed, has its peak effect within 2 to 4 hours, and is no longer active after approximately 8 hours. The longer-acting insulin preparations are prepared by crystallizing insulin in the presence of zinc to form slowly dissolving crystals or in the presence of protein (protamine) to form slowly dissolving complexes. These preparations differ from regular insulin and from each other in onset and duration of action primarily because of differences in absorption from the site of injection.

The health care professional must be familiar with the properties of the major insulin products. With these various insulin forms, control can be adjusted to fit the life-style and metabolic demands of individual patients. Diabetic persons must become proficient not only in the techniques of storing, preparing, and injecting their insulin, but they also must be taught the proper testing procedures. Moreover, they must understand the onset and du-

ration of action of the insulin preparations they are receiving to avoid complications.

As an example of the many patterns of dosage that may be employed successfully, consider the following hypothetical case. A person with IDDM who has been maintained on a single dose of lente insulin before breakfast each morning has begun to show hyperglycemia by the next morning. To overcome this problem, the physician splits the insulin dose, giving 80% of the daily dose in the morning and the remainder before supper. The rationale for this therapy is simple. Lente insulin injected at around 7 AM will be reaching its peak effect around dinner time (Table 55.2). The small dose administered before supper helps to protect the patient from developing hyperglycemia overnight.

Many individualized schemes for insulin dosage may be devised for particular patients. Nevertheless, in all cases the principle is the same: doses of insulin must be timed so that the patient is pro-

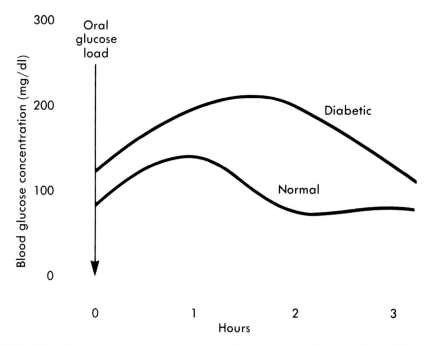

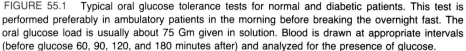

FIGURE 55.1   Typical oral glucose tolerance tests for normal and diabetic patients. This test is performed preferably in ambulatory patients in the morning before breaking the overnight fast. The oral glucose load is usually about 75 Gm given in solution. Blood is drawn at appropriate intervals (before glucose 60, 90, 120, and 180 minutes after) and analyzed for the presence of glucose.

tected from hyperglycemia and from hypoglycemia during peak periods of insulin action.

Side effects of insulin therapy. Insulin therapy is associated with two major acute side effects. If therapy is inadequate, the person may go into a coma resulting from the uncontrolled metabolic derangements discussed earlier. Blood sugar concentration is high, and ketoacidosis or hyperosmolar coma may result. On the other hand, if inadvertent insulin overdosage occurs or if a patient does not eat or overexercises, the patient may lapse into coma resulting from a hypoglycemic reaction. It is critical for the health care professional to be able to differentiate between these two conditions. The distinguishing symptoms are outlined in Table 55.3. Treatment of hypoglycemia consists of elevating the blood glucose level by oral administration of sugar in conscious patients or by glucagon injection or glucose intravenous infusion in unconscious patients. Treatment of diabetic coma requires insulin administration to lower blood sugar concentration and reduce ketone body formation.

Allergic reactions to insulin may occur. Local allergic reactions usually do not require treatment. Systemic allergic responses to insulin are more rare. Severe allergic reactions usually may be prevented in a sensitive patient by using a more highly purified insulin preparation (single component insulin) or by using insulin derived from a different source (see next section). For example, a patient sensitive to the standard preparations containing both porcine and bovine insulin may be able to take more purified forms without allergic symptoms.

Many patients receiving insulin therapy have insulin antibodies in their bloodstream. These antibodies may contribute to insulin resistance in some patients.

Insulin may also provoke subcutaneous fat near injection sites to atrophy. This lipoatrophy leads to the formation of hollows or depressions in the skin. Careful rotation of injection sites minimizes this effect. Lipoatrophy may be less common with the highly purified insulin preparations.

Forms of insulin. Three types of insulin are available in the United States: beef, pork, and human. Pork and beef insulin are obtained from the

Table 55.2 Properties of Insulin Preparations

Generic name	Classification	Description	Pharmacokinetic properties		
			Onset of action	Peak action	Duration of action
Insulin injection	Rapid acting	Clear solution containing no zinc or modifying agents; intravenous or subcutaneous injection.	Within 1 hr	2 to 4 hr	6 to 8 hr
Prompt insulin zinc suspension	Rapid acting	Cloudy suspension of amorphous insulin precipitated with zinc to slow absorption; subcutaneous only.	1 to 2 hr	4 to 7 hr	12 to 16 hr
Isophane insulin suspension	Intermediate acting	Cloudy suspension of insulin complexed with protamine to slow absorption; subcutaneous only.	2 to 4 hr	10 to 16 hr	18 to 30 hr
Insulin zinc suspension	Intermediate acting	Cloudy suspension containing 30% semilente insulin and 70% ultralente insulin; subcutaneous only.	1 to 2 hr	10 to 16 hr	18 to 30 hr
Protamine zinc insulin	Long acting	Cloudy when well mixed; suspension of insulin complexed with more protamine than NPH insulin; subcutaneous only.	6 to 8 hr	14 to 24 hr	24 to 36 hr or longer
Extended insulin zinc suspension	Long acting	Cloudy when well mixed; large complexes of insulin with zinc to slow absorption; no protein modifiers; subcutaneous only.	5 to 8 hr	16 to 24 hr	24 to 36 hr or longer

pancreas of animals slaughtered for food. Many commonly used preparations are mixtures of beef and pork insulin that also may contain proinsulin as a contaminant (Table 55.4). Highly purified insulins with a much lower level of proinsulin contamination are available.

Human insulin comes from two sources. Semisynthetic human insulin is prepared by converting porcine insulin to the human form by chemically changing the one differing amino acid. Human insulin is also produced by recombinant deoxyribonucleic acid (DNA) techniques; human genes for

insulin are inserted into bacteria, which then produce large amounts of the protein to be processed and purified.

The hypoglycemic actions of the various forms of insulin are similar; however, the various preparations differ slightly in pharmacokinetics and side effects. For example, human insulin preparations have a slightly shorter duration of action than corresponding pork preparations. Dosages may need slight adjustment when switching from one preparation to another. Human insulin and purified pork insulin are less antigenic than the other types

Table 55.3   Differential Diagnosis of Diabetic Coma and Hypoglycemic Reactions

Clinical data	Diabetic coma	Hypoglycemic reactions
Symptoms	Thirst Abdominal pain Nausea and vomiting Headache Constipation Shortness of breath (Küssmaul breathing)	Nervousness Hunger Sweating Weakness Stupor Convulsions
Signs	Facial flushing Air hunger Soft eyeballs Normal or absent reflexes Acetone breath	Pallor Shallow respiration Normal eyeballs Babinski reflex may be seen
Urine glucose	Positive	Negative or low
Urine acetone	Positive	Negative
Blood glucose	High (above 250 mg/dl)	Low (below 60 mg/dl)
Blood CO_2	Low	Normal
Precipitating factors	Untreated diabetes Infection or disease appearing in a previously controlled diabetic patient High degree of emotional or psychological stress	Insulin overdosage Skipping meals Excessive exercise before meals
History	Onset of symptoms usually occurs over a period of days.	Onset of symptoms is somewhat related to the type of medication used; regular insulin overdose produces symptoms more rapidly than the longer-acting insulins or oral agents.

available. Patients may be switched to one of these forms to help control allergic side effects associated with insulin therapy.

Oral Hypoglycemic Agents

Sulfonylureas

Mechanism of action. The oral hypoglycemic agents used in the United States are sulfonylureas. These drugs are useful only for those patients who produce some insulin on their own, that is, patients with NIDDM (adult-onset, or type II, diabetes). Clinical studies of adult-onset diabetic patients have shown that many may have low, normal, or even above-normal insulin levels in their bloodstream. The cells of many of these patients, however, are resistant to the action of insulin. Insulin action therefore is lost not because insulin is missing, but because target cells fail to respond normally.

Sulfonylureas stimulate insulin release from the pancreas. The newer ones also may diminish hepatic glucose production and directly increase tissue responsiveness to insulin. These actions tend to diminish fasting plasma glucose concentrations and improve glucose utilization by fat and muscle cells.

The effectiveness of sulfonylureas in obese patients with NIDDM is enhanced by caloric restriction and weight loss. This dietary manipulation also tends to increase the responsiveness of target cells to insulin.

Absorption and fate. Sulfonylureas are well absorbed orally and tend to bind well to serum proteins. The sulfonylureas differ from one another primarily in onset and duration of action (Table 55.5). The onset and duration of action of these drugs is strongly influenced by their metabolic fate in the body. For example, *tolbutamide* is relatively

Table 55.4   Summary of Insulin Preparations

Generic name	Trade name	Source	Concentration (units/ml)
Insulin injection	Regular Iletin I	Beef/pork mixture	40 or 100
	Regular Insulin	Pork	100
	Regular Purified Beef Iletin II	Beef, purified	100
	Regular Purified Pork Insulin, Velosulin	Pork, purified	100
	Regular Purified Pork Iletin II	Pork, purified	100 or 500
	Novolin R, Velosulin Human	Semisynthetic human	100
	Humulin R	Human, recombinant DNA	100
Prompt insulin zinc suspension	Semilente Iletin I	Beef/pork mixture	40 or 100
	Semilente Insulin	Beef	100
	Semilente Purified Pork Insulin	Pork, purified	100
Isophane insulin suspension (NPH)	NPH Iletin I	Beef/pork mixture	40 or 100
	NPH Insulin	Beef	100
	NPH Purified Beef Iletin II	Beef, purified	100
	NPH Purified Pork Iletin II, NPH Purified Pork Insulin, NPH Insulatard	Pork, purified	100
	Humulin N	Human, recombinant DNA	100
	Novolin N, Insulatard NPH Human	Semisynthetic human	100
	Mixtard	Pork, purified (70% NPH, 30% regular insulin)	100
	Mixtard Human	Semisynthetic human (70% NPH, 30% regular insulin)	100
Insulin zinc suspension	Lente Iletin I	Beef/pork mixture	40 or 100
	Lente Insulin	Beef	100
	Lente Purified Beef Iletin II	Beef, purified	100
	Lente Purified Pork Iletin II, Lente Purified Pork Insulin	Pork, purified	100
	Novolin L Human	Semisynthetic human	100
	Humulin L	Human, recombinant DNA	100
Protamine zinc insulin suspension	Protamine Zinc Iletin I	Beef/pork mixture	40 or 100
	Protamine Zinc Purified Beef Iletin II	Beef, purified	100
	Protamine Zinc Purified Pork Iletin II	Pork, purified	100
Extended insulin zinc	Ultralente Iletin I	Beef/pork mixture	40 or 100
	Ultralente Insulin	Beef	100
	Ultralente Purified Beef Insulin	Beef, purified	100
	Ultralente Humulin U	Human, recombinant DNA	100

short acting, since it is quickly converted in the body to an inactive product. In contrast, *acetohexamide* and *tolazamide* must be converted in the body to active products before they become effective. Hence they are intermediate in action. *Chlorpropamide* is the longest-acting member of the class and is tightly bound to plasma protein. This drug is not extensively metabolized, being excreted unchanged in the urine.

The two newest sulfonylureas are *glyburide* and *glipizide*. Glyburide is extensively metabolized, with the products excreted primarily in the

Table 55.5   Properties of the Oral Antidiabetic Agents

Generic name	Trade name	Dosage range	Duration of action	Metabolic fate
Acetohexamide	Dimelor Dymelor*	0.25 to 1.5 Gm daily, single or divided dose. FDA Pregnancy Category C.	12 to 24 hr	Converted by liver to an active metabolite, which appears in blood later and stays longer than the parent compound. Active metabolite excreted via the kidney.
Chlorpropamide	Diabinese*	0.1 to 0.75 Gm daily, single dose. FDA Pregnancy Category C.	Up to 60 hr	Excreted unchanged through the kidney.
Glipizide	Glucotrol	2.5 to 40 mg daily. Doses greater than 15 mg should be divided. FDA Pregnancy Category C.	12 to 24 hr	Completely absorbed from gastrointestinal tract. Extensively bound to plasma protein. Metabolized by liver to inactive metabolites. Excreted in urine.
Glyburide	Diabeta* Micronase	1.25 to 20 mg daily. FDA Pregnancy Category B.	16 to 24 hr	Metabolized by liver, with metabolites eliminated in bile and in urine.
Tolazamide	Tolinase	0.1 to 0.75 Gm daily; single dose for lower range, divided dose for higher range. FDA Pregnancy Category C.	12 to 24 hr	Slowly absorbed from gastrointestinal tract. Converted by liver to several active metabolites, which are excreted via kidney.
Tolbutamide	Orinase*	0.5 to 3 Gm daily divided doses. FDA Pregnancy Category C.	6 to 12 hr	Metabolized in liver to an inactive compound.

*Available in Canada and United States.

bile and secondarily in the urine. Glipizide is also converted to inactive metabolites by the liver, but excretion is primarily via the kidney. Both are many times more potent than other sulfonylureas. For example, 5 mg of glyburide or glipizide has an effect equivalent to that of 250 mg of chlorpropamide or tolazamide. At the doses used in patients the clinical effects are similar.

Side effects. Side effects of sulfonylurea therapy include gastrointestinal distress and neurological symptoms such as muscle weakness and paresthesias. Liver function tests may be altered and mild hematopoietic toxicity may be seen in some patients. Frank allergy to the drugs occurs in some patients, with skin reactions being more common than the more dangerous forms of allergic response. The incidence of these types of reactions is reported to be less than 5% of patients treated.

Hypoglycemia is an ever-present danger with sulfonylureas and may be caused by drug overdose, drug interaction, altered drug metabolism, or the patient failing to eat. Sulfonylureas should not be used when renal or liver function is inadequate; normal function of those organs is required for metabolism and elimination of the sulfonylureas (Table 55.5). Elderly patients also occasionally show excessive hypoglycemic reactions to these drugs.

THE NURSING PROCESS

DIABETES MELLITUS

Assessment

Patients are diagnosed with diabetes mellitus because they appear with the classic triad of symptoms (polyphagia, polydipsia, polyuria) or because through evaluation of another medical condition they are found to have elevated glucose concentrations in the blood or urine. Diabetes occurs in all age-groups. Baseline assessment data include all the usual assessment data, with emphasis on the vital signs, weight, blood glucose and urine glucose concentrations, and any signs indicating possible long-term effects, such as the development of ulcers on the lower extremities. In addition, the nurse should assess carefully the condition of skin and nails and note the presence of any unusual sign or symptom.

Nursing diagnoses

Potential complication: hypoglycemia

Knowledge deficit

Management

The complete management of the diabetic patient is beyond the scope of this book. In relation to drug therapy, the nurse should monitor the glucose in blood and urine, look for the presence of ketones in the urine, and, depending on the patient's condition, examine other appropriate laboratory work such as electrolytes or arterial blood gases. Planning for discharge should be done as soon as the patient is diagnosed. The patient will require extensive teaching about such aspects of diabetes as the need for good foot care and dietary restrictions. The nurse should teach the patient about the medications that have been prescribed and their method of administration and how to test the urine as an indication of success of therapy. Appropriate referrals should be made at this time to such departments as the hospital or community dietitian and the local visiting nurse association. In addition, the patient may be referred to the local diabetes association.

Evaluation

Ideally, treatment with drugs would cause the patient to have normal blood glucose levels at all times and would prevent the known long-term effects of this disease. Thus far, however, it is not possible to produce this degree of control. Patient age, motivation, and willingness to follow prescribed regimens are only a few factors that influence the overall success of therapy for diabetes mellitus. Before discharge for self-management, the patient should be able to explain why the drugs are prescribed and to demonstrate how to administer insulin or other medications correctly. The nurse should be certain the patient can explain the symptoms of hyperglycemia and hypoglycemia, how to treat them, and other prescribed aspects of care such as foot care, dietary restrictions, and any limitations in activity that have been prescribed. The patient should be able to demonstrate how to test the urine for glucose and ketones accurately and to state what to do based on the information obtained from this test. The patient should understand what symptoms warrant medical attention. Patients should be able to explain why it is appropriate to wear a medical identification tag or bracelet at all times indicating their condition. For more complete information about this disease, see appropriate nursing textbooks. For further information about insulin and the oral hypoglycemic agents, see the patient care implications section.

The use of sulfonylureas in the treatment of diabetes mellitus has become controversial. Some clinical studies seem to show that treatment with sulfonylureas is no more effective than dietary therapy alone. Other studies have suggested that the toxicity of the sulfonylureas is higher than previously expected.

Of special concern is the apparent increase in risk of death from cardiovascular disease in patients receiving a sulfonylurea in the large-scale study conducted by the University Group Diabetes Program (UGDP). Although these questions are far from resolved, some treatment centers avoid the use of sulfonylureas and control mild NIDDM (nonketotic) with diet and exercise alone or, if necessary, combine diet and exercise with low doses of insulin. Even when the sulfonylureas are used, it is clear that careful attention to the diet is required for best results.

Drug interactions. The sulfonylureas are implicated in certain drug interactions that can have serious consequences to the patient. The major interactions occur with ethyl alcohol, phenylbutazone, sulfonamides, salicylates, phenothiazines, and thiazides.

Patients receiving sulfonylureas should routinely avoid alcohol. Several interactions between alcohol and sulfonylureas are possible. Some patients receiving sulfonylureas develop an "Antabuse or disulfiram reaction" when they ingest alcohol. The most striking symptoms of this reaction are an unpleasant flushing and severe headache. Other patients on sulfonylureas become hypoglycemic when they ingest alcohol, probably because ethanol itself is a hypoglycemic agent in some people.

Hypoglycemia can result when one of several drugs is given to a patient taking sulfonylureas, the most important of which are the antiinflammatory agents, phenylbutazone and salicylates, and sulfonamide antibiotics. These three drugs are all tightly bound to plasma protein and may displace sulfonylureas, which tend to be highly bound to serum protein. Thus blood concentrations of free sulfonylurea are elevated. Since the free drug is the active form, the result is an enhancement of the hypoglycemic affect of the sulfonylurea. In addition to this mechanism, phenylbutazone may block excretion of the active metabolite of acetohexamide, an action that also tends to increase hypoglycemia. Sulfonamides may inhibit the metabolic breakdown of tolbutamide and thereby enhance its hypoglycemic action.

Phenothiazines such as chlorpromazine may impair the effectiveness of sulfonylureas. Chlorpromazine inhibits the release of insulin from beta cells in the pancreas and elevates adrenal production of epinephrine, a hormone that can raise blood glucose (see Table 55.1). These actions of chlorpromazine directly antagonize the hypoglycemic action of sulfonylureas.

Thiazide diuretics possess hyperglycemic activity in addition to their diuretic actions; thus they may impair diabetic control with sulfonylureas.

Diet Therapy

Mechanism of action. Obesity, or more specifically excessive caloric intake, tends to reduce the number of insulin receptors. An understanding of this disease mechanism helps in appreciating the rationale for dietary control of diabetes: reduced caloric intake allows the insulin receptors to increase and makes the available insulin more effective. Dietary restriction may lower insulin requirements in obese diabetic persons and in many cases may be the only form of therapy required. The effectiveness of sulfonylureas in obese patients with NIDDM is enhanced by caloric restriction and weight loss.

Careful dietary control is important for all diabetic persons. Successful long-term treatment of the condition frequently involves counseling by a dietitian and supportive follow-up for the rest of the patient's life.

PATIENT CARE IMPLICATIONS

General information about diabetes mellitus

Patient and family education

- Teach patients and families the signs and symptoms of hyperglycemia and hypoglycemia (see Table 55.3).
- The development of hypoglycemia may relate to the time insulin or oral agent was taken (see Tables 55.2 and 55.5). If possible, obtain a blood glucose level. Whether a blood glucose level is obtained or not, treat by administering a fast-acting carbohydrate such as ½ C fruit juice, ½ C cola drink (*not* diet forms), ½ C regular gelatin dessert, 4 cubes or 2 packets of sugar, 2 squares of graham crackers, or 2 to 3 pieces of hard candy. Instruct patients to carry hard candy or other sources of carbohydrate with them at all times.
- If hypoglycemia is severe, repeated, or occurring without explanation, consult physician.
- Teach and/or refer patients as needed to a dietitian about appropriate dietary restrictions. Losing weight to desirable body weight is helpful in controlling diabetes.
- Encourage participation in a regular exercise program.
- Review foot care and other aspects of personal hygiene to prevent infection.
- Teach patients how to test blood glucose and/or urine glucose. Review methods of testing and frequency, and supervise the patient performing the test activity for accuracy. If a urine test method is being used, point out to the patient that some drugs may cause urine test results to be inaccurate. Teach the patient to ask the physician and pharmacist if there is a possibility of drug-urine test interaction whenever new drugs are prescribed.
- Refer patients as appropriate to the health department or other community-based nursing care agency for follow-up.
- Refer patients to the American Diabetes Association or local support groups for additional information and resources; examples of such resources include syringes adapted for the visually impaired, information booklets, automatic insulin injectors, cookbooks, and so on.
- Encourage patients with diabetes to wear a medical identification tag or bracelet.
- Avoid drinking alcoholic beverages.
- Avoid smoking. Patients who begin or stop smoking may require an adjustment in diet or drug.
- Warn patients to keep all health care providers informed about the diabetes and the type of drug used to control it.
- Avoid taking any drug unless first approved by the physician. Many drugs cause changes in blood glucose levels. Teach patients to monitor blood and/or urine glucose levels carefully when starting or stopping a new medication.
- The specific regimen prescribed for any patient is based on many factors, including age, type of diabetes, severity of diabetes, weight, resources available, philosophy of the health care team, and other medical problems the patient may have. While general guidelines are noted in this text, consult fundamentals of nursing texts and other printed resources as needed.
- Caution female patients to consult the physician before attempting to conceive, as management of diabetes may be modified during pregnancy. A diabetic female who becomes pregnant should notify the physician immediately.

Insulin

Drug administration

- Local allergic reactions involving itching, redness, swelling, or stinging at the injection site are usually transient and are not uncommon. Anaphylaxis is very rare. Insulin resistance occasionally involves antibodies to insulin. It may not be possible to eliminate local allergic reactions. Supervise insulin administration technique, as scrupulous attention to technique may lessen local irritation. Record and rotate sites on a systematic basis so that accessible sites are not overused (see Chapter 6 for a diagram of commonly used sites of subcutaneous injections). Prepare dose of insulin as ordered, and let warm to room temperature. Cleanse injection site carefully, and allow skin surface to dry completely. Pinch skin between thumb and fingers of one hand, and insert needle into the "pocket" between the subcutaneous fat and muscle; a 45° to 90° angle can be used, depending on the amount of subcutaneous fat and the length of the needle. Inject the insulin and withdraw the needle. Apply moderate pressure to the site but do not rub. Disposable syringes are designed for one time

Continued.

PATIENT CARE IMPLICATIONS — cont'd

use, but are sometimes reused. As they are reused, the needle point becomes duller. If irritation is a problem, the patient may want to use a new needle/syringe more often.

- If local irritation is severe or persistent, consult physician about a change in type of insulin.
- Systemic reactions are rare and may be due to the animal source of the insulin: beef, pork, or mixed beef-pork. Treat symptomatically and notify physician.
- Use regular insulin for patients on "sliding scale" management.
- Consult with physician about diabetes management when patients are NPO (nothing by mouth) in preparation for surgery or otherwise unable to maintain usual dietary intake.
- For IV use, only regular insulin can be used. Insulin adsorbs to bags, tubing, and other items made of polyvinyl chloride (PVC). For continuous infusion, flushing the system with the diluted insulin mixture (e.g., 100 units regular insulin in 500 ml normal saline) before connecting it to the patient may decrease the amount of insulin lost to adsorption to the PVC. Measure the rate of infusion to the patient response, blood glucose levels, and ordered rate of drop of blood glucose. Also monitor serum electrolytes, especially potassium.
- Only regular insulin is used in insulin pumps. Review the manufacturer's instruction sheet with the patient.
- Observe agency policies regarding insulin administration. For example, many hospitals require that insulin doses be checked by two licensed nurses prior to administration.

Patient and family education

- Review the general guidelines, and the information about injection, above.
- Teach patients that only syringes marked for units of insulin should be used with insulin. There are special syringes available for doses less than 50 units. Review carefully with the patient the need to obtain the correct concentration of insulin, correct type, and correct syringe.
- To mix insulins, always draw up the regular (unmodified) insulin first, then the other insulin that is ordered. If two modified insulins are to be drawn up together, either can be drawn up first, but the patient should establish a pattern and always draw the same one up first.
- Some mixtures of insulin in a syringe must

be administered within a few minutes of drawing them up, while others are stable for longer periods. Consult physician or pharmacist.

- Regular insulin is clear while modified insulins are cloudy. Do not use discolored insulins or ones that appear grainy. Warm and resuspend insulins by rotating the vials between the hands; avoid vigorous shaking.
- Generally, insulin injected into the abdomen is absorbed the fastest, insulin in the arm is absorbed more slowly, and insulin is absorbed slowest when injected in the thigh. However, several things may influence this. For example, a diabetic who jogs will have faster absorption from the thigh when jogging and using the thigh muscles. Consider the daily habits of the patient in working out an appropriate plan for diabetic management.
- Insulin can be safely kept at room temperature for up to 1 month. Insulin kept at room temperature for longer than 1 month should be discarded. Insulin may be stored in the refrigerator for longer than 1 month. Do not freeze insulin. Check expiration date.
- Teach the patient that when illness occurs it is important to maintain fluid intake. Consult the physician about specific guidelines for insulin dose and diet when the patient is sick. Remind the patient to contact the physician whenever a question occurs about management.
- Develop an individualized teaching plan for patient teaching about insulin. Decisions to be made include whether patients will use disposable syringes or sterilize and reuse glass syringes, whether the patient has the ability (vision, dexterity, and so on) to draw up and administer the insulin, what type of urine test method is to be used, and so on.
- Teach patients not to switch type or source of insulin without consulting the physician, as a change in dose is often necessary.
- Remind patients to keep track of the supply of insulin and syringes on hand to avoid running out unexpectedly.
- Teach the person with IDDM to carry insulin and syringes with hand luggage to avoid losing them whenever traveling. For large quantities of insulin and syringes, divide them among pieces of luggage so all will not be lost if a piece of luggage is lost. Some states require prescriptions for syringes, so suggest the patient carry an adequate supply for the entire trip. This is especially important in international travel. Suggest the patient carry

PATIENT CARE IMPLICATIONS—cont'd

a letter from the physician listing the need for insulin and syringes, as this may help if insulin is lost in delayed baggage, or in delays at Customs. Discuss with the pharmacist in advance any special considerations for insulin storage.

Oral hypoglycemic agents

Drug administration

- Review symptoms of hypoglycemia and hyperglycemia listed in Table 55.3, and teach them to the patient.
- Monitor weight.
- Monitor complete blood count and differential, platelet count, liver function tests, and blood glucose.

Patient and family education

- See the general guidelines for diabetes.
- Instruct patients to report the development of any new side effect.
- See Patient Problem: Constipation on p. 187.
- See Patient Problem: Disulfiram Reactions on p. 637. Note in text that some patients develop this reaction when they ingest alcohol and are taking a sulfonylurea.
- Usually, take ordered doses with the first meal of the day. If a dose is missed, take it as soon as remembered, unless it is almost time for the next dose, in which case skip the missed dose and resume the regular dosing schedule. Do not double up for missed doses.

SUMMARY

Insulin is the major hormone regulating glucose metabolism, stimulating uptake of glucose in fat and muscle cells and the conversion of glucose to glycogen in the liver. Glucagon opposes these actions of insulin. Somatostatin inhibits the release of insulin and glucagon from pancreatic islets. Other hormones such as cortisol, epinephrine, and growth hormone antagonize the action of insulin in muscle or fat cells. Insulin also stimulates lipid storage, blocks lipid breakdown, and promotes protein synthesis.

In diabetes mellitus, insulin action is lost. Insulin-dependent diabetics produce little or no insulin, and they are mostly young and relatively lean. Noninsulin-dependent diabetics may produce insulin, but the amount is insufficient. These patients are usually obese older adults.

In diabetes mellitus, glucose utilization is impaired and the glucose accumulates in the bloodstream and is excreted in the urine. Excessively high glucose concentrations in the bloodstream can lead to hyperosmolar coma. Excessive fat and protein breakdown can produce ketoacidosis. Long-term complications of diabetes include pathological changes in blood vessels, nerves, and kidneys.

Insulin administration to patients with diabetes mellitus constitutes replacement therapy. Insulin restores the ability of cells to utilize glucose as an energy source and corrects many metabolic derangements of diabetes mellitus. Insulin must be injected, since it is a protein subject to digestion in the gastrointestinal tract. Regular insulin is water soluble, quickly absorbed from subcutaneous injection sites, and therefore relatively short acting. Longer-acting insulin preparations are formed by creating relatively insoluble complexes of insulin with zinc (semilente, lente, ultralente insulin) or proteins (NPH insulin) or both (protamine zinc insulin). Insulin administration must be timed to produce maximum hypoglycemic action during periods of food absorption. Insulin therapy is associated with two major acute side effects: hyperglycemia when insulin therapy is inadequate and hypoglycemia when insulin concentrations are larger than required. Insulin also may cause various allergic reactions and local subcutaneous fat atrophy at injection sites.

Sulfonylureas are oral hypoglycemic agents and are used only for patients with noninsulin-dependent diabetes. Sulfonylureas stimulate insulin release from the pancreas and increase target cells' response to insulin. Their onset and duration of action depend on the metabolic transformations the drugs undergo, as well as the degree of plasma protein binding. Sulfonylureas may produce gastrointestinal distress, muscle weakness, paresthesias, allergies, and bone marrow toxicity. The most dangerous reaction is hypoglycemia. The effectiveness of sulfonylureas is greatest in obese, mild, noninsulin-dependent diabetic persons, and the hypoglycemic effects are increased by dietary restriction. Patients taking sulfonylureas may suffer a disulfiram-like reaction to ethyl alcohol. Phenylbutazone, salicylates, and sulfonamides may increase effective concentrations of sulfonylureas in the bloodstream and thus produce hypoglycemia.

STUDY QUESTIONS

1. What three peptide hormones from pancreatic islets affect glucose metabolism?
2. What effect does insulin have on glucose metabolism?
3. What effect does glucagon have on glucose metabolism?
4. What effect does somatostatin have on glucose metabolism?
5. What effects do cortisol, epinephrine, and growth hormone have on glucose metabolism?
6. What effect does insulin have on fat and protein metabolism?
7. What is diabetes mellitus?
8. What are the characteristics of insulin-dependent diabetes mellitus?
9. What are the characteristics of noninsulin-dependent diabetes mellitus?
10. What effect does diabetes mellitus have on glucose metabolism?
11. What effect does diabetes mellitus have on protein and fat metabolism?
12. What are the long-term complications of diabetes mellitus?
13. How is diabetes mellitus diagnosed?
14. How does insulin therapy relieve the symptoms of diabetes mellitus?
15. Why must insulin be injected?
16. What is the onset and duration of action of regular insulin?
17. What advantages do the insulin preparations containing relatively insoluble insulin complexes have over regular insulin?
18. Name the insulin preparations available.
19. What is the duration of action of each of the insulin preparations?
20. When does peak hypoglycemic action occur after a dose of insulin injection? Semilente insulin? NPH insulin? Ultralente insulin? Protamine zinc insulin?
21. What are the two major acute side effects of insulin therapy?
22. What type of reactions may insulin produce at the site of injection?
23. What is the mechanism of action for the sulfonylureas as hypoglycemic agents?
24. What type of diabetic patient benefits from sulfonylurea therapy?
25. How are the sulfonylureas administered?
26. Which of the sulfonylureas is rapidly metabolized in the body?
27. Which sulfonylureas must be converted to active forms by the body to be effective?
28. Which is the longest-acting sulfonylurea?
29. What side effects occur with sulfonylureas?
30. Why does caloric restriction enhance sulfonylurea effectiveness?
31. What other drugs may enhance the hypoglycemic effect of sulfonylureas?
32. What reaction may be seen in patients receiving sulfonylureas who ingest ethyl alcohol?

SUGGESTED READINGS

Ainsle, M.B.: Why tight diabetes control should be approached with caution, Postgrad. Med. **75**(4):91, 1984.

Brogden, R.N., and Heel, R.C.: Human insulin: a review of its biological activity, pharmacokinetics and therapeutic use, Drugs **34**:350, 1987.

Byrnes, C.A.: What's new in the diabetic diet, Nursing 87 **17**(8):58, 1987.

Christman, C., and Bennett, J.: Diabetes: new names, new test, new diet, Nursing 87 **17**(1):34, 1987.

Ciranowicz, M.: Caring for the hypoglycemic patient, Nursing 87 **17**(6):32N, 1987.

Clinical news: simplify insulin injection: omit pull-back, Am. J. Nurs. **84**:426, 1984.

Duckworth, W.C., and Swanson, S.K.: Insulin therapy in Type II diabetes: pros and cons, Drug Therapy **13**(5):111, 1983.

Ginsbery, H.: How to prepare and inject insulin with one hand, Geriatr. Nurs. **1**(4):112, 1980.

Hernandez, C.M.G.: Surgery and diabetes: minimizing the risks, Am. J. Nurs. **87**(6):788, 1987.

Hollander, P.: The case for tight control in diabetes, Postgrad. Med. **75**(4):80, 1984.

Horwitz, D.L.: Insulin pump therapy: rationale and principles of use, Postgrad. Med. **76**(8):1984.

Hughes, B.: Diabetes management: the time is right for tight glucose control, Nursing 87 **17**(5):63, 1987.

Hurxthal, K.: Quick! Teach this patient about insulin, Am. J. Nurs. **88**(8):1097, 1988.

Johnson, I.S.: Human insulin from recombinant DNA technology, Science **219**:632, 1983.

Knott, S.P., and Herget, M.J.: Teaching self-injection to diabetics: an easier and more effective way, Nursing 84 **14**(1):57, 1984.

MacDonald, F.: Coping with diabetes: a unique response, Canad. Nurse **83**(10):21, 1987.

Mulkeen, H.: Diabetes: teaching the teaching of self care, Nurs. Times/Nurs. Mirror **85**(3):63, 1989.

Nath, C., Murray, S., and Ponte, C.: Lessons in living with type II diabetes mellitus, Nursing 88 **18**(8):44, 1988.

Podolosky, S.: Pitfalls in managing the elderly diabetic, Drug Therapy **13**(4):75, 1983.

Protocol for Diabetes Control and Complications Trial (DCCT), Diabetes Care **5**(6):xxix, 1982.

Ramsey, P.W.: Hyperglycemia at dawn, Am. J. Nurs. **87**(11):1424, 1987.

Robertson, C.: When the patient is also diabetic, RN **50**(7):33, 1987.

Schade, D.S.: Combining insulin and oral agents in type 2 diabetes, Drug Therapy **19**(6):12, 1989.

Shuman, C.R.: Optimum insulin use in older diabetics, Geriatrics **39**(10):71, 1984.

Skelly, A.H., and VanSon, A.R.: Insulin allergy in clinical practice, Nurse Pract. **12**(4):14, 1987.

Steiner, M.: Human insulin therapy, Drug Therapy **18**(2):75, 1988.

Thurkauf, G.E.: How do you manage DKA with continuous IV insulin? Am. J. Nurs. **88**(5):727, 1988.

Walker, E.D.: Hyperglycemia: a complication of chemotherapy in children, Cancer Nurs. **11**(1):18, 1988.

Appendix

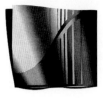

Representative Common Drug Interactions

Drugs or drug classes interacting	Mechanism/result of interaction	Text references/comments
Acetaminophen and alcohol (ethanol)	Chronic alcohol abuse and high doses of acetaminophen both damage the liver. Additive effects of these agents may be fatal.	Chapter 23. This interaction is most important for alcoholics with liver damage from chronic alcohol ingestion.
Acetaminophen and chloramphenicol	Acetaminophen may increase the elimination half-life of chloramphicol. As a result, chloramphenicol may accumulate, increasing the risk of dose-dependent bone marrow suppression.	Chapters 23 and 32. This interaction can usually be avoided by selecting an alternative agent for one of the drugs.
Alcohol (ethanol) and barbiturates or chloral hydrate (sedative-hypnotics)	Central nervous system depression caused by alcohol may greatly enhance the action of other depressant drugs, leading to severely impaired motor activity, unconsciousness, respiratory depression, and death as the dose increases.	Chapter 40. In addition to sedative-hypnotics, many other classes of drugs may produce this interaction: Antihistamines producing marked sedation alone, e.g. diphenhydramine or chlorpheniramine (Chapter 24) Benzodiazepines, especially diazepam (Chapter 40) Meprobamate (Chapter 40) Opioids, such as morphine and codeine (Chapter 44) Phenothiazines, especially chlorpromazine (Chapter 41) Phenylbutazone (Chapter 23) Propoxyphene (Chapter 23) Tricyclic antidepressants, especially amitriptyline (Chapter 42)
Alcohol (ethanol) and disulfiram	Disulfiram blocks metabolism of ethanol, leading to accumulation of toxic metabolites. Symptoms are flushing, hypotension, headache, nausea, and difficulty in breathing. Some sensitive persons experience more serious cardiovascular reactions.	Chapter 40. This very striking interaction with ethanol is observed with several drugs other than disulfiram: Cefamandole, cefoperazone, and moxalactam (Chapter 30) Chlorpropamide, a sulfonylurea (Chapter 55) Procarbazine (Chapter 39) Metronidazole (Chapter 38)

Continued.

Drugs or drug classes interacting	Mechanism/result of interaction	Text references/comments
Allopurinol and cyclophosphamide or mercaptopurine (cytotoxic anticancer drugs)	Allopurinol is chemically related to cytotoxic nucleotide analogs and may have additive effects with other cytotoxic agents. The result is excessive toxicity as if from an overdose of the anticancer drug.	Chapters 23 and 39. Allopurinol is often administered to cancer patients to prevent excess uric acid formation. Doses of the anticancer agents listed may need to be reduced when allopurinol is added.
Allopurinol and dicumarol or warfarin (anticoagulants)	Allopurinol may interfere with the metabolism of the anticoagulants by enzyme systems in the liver. As a result, the anticoagulants accumulate and may cause dangerous bleeding episodes.	Chapters 20 and 23. Only a few patients may show this serious interaction, but all patients receiving both drugs should be carefully watched for excessive action of the anticoagulant.
Aspirin (salicylates) and antacids	Antacids may promote excretion of salicylates by alkalinizing the urine. Antacids such as sodium bicarbonate or magnesium aluminum hydroxide can reduce salicylate concentrations in the blood to subtherapeutic levels.	Chapter 23. This interaction is most important for those patients receiving high doses of salicylates for extended periods.
Aspirin (salicylates) and dicumarol or warfarin (anticoagulants)	Aspirin interferes with platelet aggregation and thus has anticoagulant activity even at low doses. The additive effects of aspirin with other potent anticoagulants may cause serious bleeding, a reaction intensified by the tendency of aspirin to cause gastrointestinal bleeding.	Chapters 20 and 23. This interaction is most important for patients regularly receiving anticoagulants who begin taking aspirin regularly.
Aspirin (salicylates) and gastrointestinal irritants	Salicylates induce gastrointestinal bleeding, which may worsen the effects of other irritant drugs. Glucocorticoids may mask the symptoms of ulceration and may allow perforation or hemorrhage to occur before the condition is noticed.	Chapter 23. Several drugs may irritate the gastrointestinal mucosa enough to cause bleeding or even ulceration: Alcohol (Chapter 40) Glucocorticoids (Chapter 51) Phenylbutazone (Chapter 23)
Aspirin (salicylates) and probenecid or sulfinpyrazone (uricosuric agents)	The ability of both drugs to promote uric acid excretion is diminished when the drugs are combined.	Chapter 23. Patients should not receive aspirin and probenecid or sulfinpyrazone concurrently.
Chloramphenicol and phenytoin	Chloramphenicol inhibits enzymes in the liver that metabolize phenytoin. As a result, phenytoin elimination may be impaired and the drug may accumulate to toxic levels.	Chapters 47 and 32. During short-term therapy with chloramphenicol, patients receiving phenytoin should be carefully monitored to prevent toxicity. Some physicians prefer to choose an alternative antibiotic, if possible.
Chlordiazepoxide, diazepam, flurazepam, lorazepam (benzodiazepines) and central nervous system depressants	Central nervous system depression produced by benzodiazepines is additive with that of other drugs. The result may be dangerous, and potentially fatal, central nervous system depression.	Chapter 40. Benzodiazepines may cause this interaction with these drugs: Alcohol (Chapter 40) Antihistamines (Chapter 24) Antipsychotic drugs (Chapter 41) Barbiturates (Chapter 40) Opiate analgesics (Chapter 44) Tricyclic antidepressants (Chapter 42)
Chlorthalidone, ethacrynic acid, furosemide, or thiazides (potassium-depleting diuretics) and corticosteroids	Both corticosteroids and the diuretics listed here can cause loss of potassium from the body over a period of time.	Chapters 16 and 51. Potassium supplements may be required to prevent severe depletion.

Drugs or drug classes interacting	Mechanism/result of interaction	Text references/comments
Cimetidine and chlordiazepoxide or diazepam (benzodiazepines)	Cimetidine seems to inhibit the liver enzymes that degrade diazepam and chlordiazepoxide. Patients taking cimetidine who then receive one of these benzodiazepines might be expected to accumulate the benzodiazepine and show excessive drowsiness, ataxia, and other signs of benzodiazepine overdose.	Chapter 40. This interaction does not occur with oxazepam or lorazepam because these benzodiazepines are not metabolized by the liver in the same way as diazepam and chlordiazepoxide. Patients should be warned about driving or carrying out other hazardous tasks when receiving cimetidine and diazepam or chlordiazepoxide.
Cimetidine and dicumarol or warfarin (anticoagulants)	Cimetidine is an inhibitor of liver enzymes that metabolize many of the anticoagulants. Therefore, cimetidine causes accumulation of the anticoagulants, increasing the risk of overdose and bleeding.	Chapters 13 and 20. This interaction makes careful monitoring of prothrombin times necessary when stabilization has been achieved with the patient taking an anticoagulant, and cimetidine is then added.
Cimetidine and phenytoin	Cimetidine may inhibit the liver enzymes that metabolize phenytoin, leading to phenytoin accumulation and intoxication.	Chapters 13 and 47. Symptoms of phenytoin intoxication are often mild, but additive bone marrow depression with cimetidine is also possible. Phenytoin blood levels may need monitoring.
Cimetidine and propranolol (beta adrenergic receptor blocker)	Cimetidine is an inhibitor of liver enzymes that may metabolize many beta adrenergic blocking agents. Propranolol concentrations are elevated when cimetidine is also administered; dangerous bradycardia has resulted.	Chapters 13 and 14. In addition to propranolol, other similarly metabolized beta adrenergic blocking agents may be involved.
Cimetidine and theophylline	Cimetidine inhibits the enzymes in the liver that metabolize theophylline, causing accumulation and theophylline toxicity.	Chapters 13 and 25. This interaction may require that theophylline levels be monitored during cimetidine therapy to prevent theophylline toxicity.
Clofibrate and dicumarol or warfarin (anticoagulants)	Clofibrate greatly enhances the anticoagulant activity of warfarin and dicumarol by displacing the anticoagulants from plasma binding proteins and possibly by other mechanisms.	Chapters 20 and 21. Doses of the anticoagulants may need to be reduced significantly to avoid dangerous overdosage and bleeding.
Dicumarol and chlorpropamide or tolbutamide (sulfonylureas)	Metabolism of the sulfonylureas may be reduced. The drugs may also compete for plasma protein-binding sites. Both actions tend to increase blood concentrations of active sulfonylurea. The most commonly reported result is an acute hypoglycemic reaction.	Chapters 20 and 55. This interaction may be controlled by using a different anticoagulant or by carefully monitoring blood concentrations of the drugs.
Digoxin (digitalis glycoside) and chlorthalidone, ethacrynic acid, furosemide, or thiazides (potassium-depleting diuretics)	Since hypokalemia (low blood potassium) increases the likelihood of digitalis toxicity, concurrent use of digitalis preparations and one of the potassium-depleting diuretics may lead to dangerous cardiac arrhythmias.	Chapters 16 and 18. This interaction may be overcome by using a potassium supplement.
Digoxin (digitalis glycoside) and quinidine or quinine	Quinidine and its chemical relative quinine slow renal excretion of digoxin, which may double serum concentrations of digoxin and lead to digoxin toxicity.	Chapters 18 and 19. These drugs should be used together only if serum concentrations of digoxin can be carefully monitored.

Continued.

Drugs or drug classes interacting	Mechanism/result of interaction	Text references/comments
Doxycycline and phenobarbital	Barbiturates can induce enzymes in the liver that may aid in eliminating doxycycline from the body. As a result, doxycycline metabolism may increase and inadequate concentrations of the antibiotic may appear in the blood.	Chapters 40 and 32. Other tetracyclines are eliminated by renal mechanisms to a greater degree and are therefore less likely to produce this interaction.
Erythromycin and theophylline	Patients receiving high doses of theophylline may accumulate toxic concentrations of theophylline when erythromycin is added. The mechanism is unknown.	Chapters 25 and 31. This interaction seems most important for patients receiving high doses, but all patients receiving both drugs should be watched closely for theophylline toxicity.
Furosemide and phenytoin	The diuretic activity of a fixed dose of furosemide may be drastically reduced in a patient receiving phenytoin. The mechanism is not understood.	Chapters 16 and 47. Increased doses of furosemide may be required to maintain control of symptoms.
Gentamicin and ethacrynic acid or furosemide (loop diuretics)	The loop diuretics and the aminoglycoside antibiotics are both capable of impairing balance and causing hearing loss. When given together, especially in high doses, the risk of ototoxicity seems to be greater.	Chapters 16 and 33. Although this interaction is best documented with gentamicin, it is also a possibility with other aminoglycosides (amikacin, kanamycin, neomycin, netilmicin, streptomycin, tobramycin).
Indomethacin and propranolol or thiazides (antihypertensives)	Indomethacin elevates blood pressure and interferes with the adequate control of hypertension by a variety of drugs.	Chapters 15 and 23. Blood pressure control needs to be carefully monitored in hypertensive patients given indomethacin.
Levodopa and chlordiazepoxide or diazepam (benzodiazepines)	Some patients receiving both drugs lose the antiparkinsonian action of levodopa. The mechanism of this interaction is not known.	Chapters 40 and 48. Patients receiving both drugs should be closely observed to ensure that parkinsonian symptoms are being adequately controlled.
Methyldopa and levodopa	These drugs may enhance the effects of each other by unknown mechanisms. Side effects of levodopa may also worsen.	Chapters 15 and 48. Doses of either or both drugs may need to be reduced.
Methyldopa and lithium carbonate	Lithium tends to accumulate in the blood of patients receiving methyldopa. The brain may also be sensitized to the effects of lithium.	Chapters 15 and 42. Serum concentrations of lithium may need monitoring in patients receiving methyldopa.
Methyltestosterone or methandrostenolone (anabolic steroids) and dicumarol or warfarin (anticoagulants)	Anabolic steroids may enhance the anticoagulant effects of warfarin or dicumarol, possibly by effects on metabolism. Increased risk of bleeding may occur.	Chapters 20 and 51. This interaction should be expected and the dose of anticoagulant reduced accordingly.
Oral contraceptives and barbiturates, phenytoin, or primidone (anticonvulsants)	The anticonvulsants may induce liver enzymes that degrade the steroid components of oral contraceptives. The result may be unexpected pregnancy.	Chapters 47 and 53. Breakthrough bleeding may signal contraceptive failure. Mechanical contraception may be required, although some women may be protected with different doses of oral contraceptives.
Oral contraceptives and rifampin	Rifampin may induce enzymes in the liver that metabolize the steroid components of progestin-only or combined estrogen-progestin oral contraceptives. The result may be unexpected pregnancy.	Chapters 53 and 35. Other antibiotics may also increase the failure rate of oral contraceptives: Penicillins, especially ampicillin (Chapter 30) Tetracyclines, such as oxytetracycline (Chapter 32)

Drugs or drug classes interacting	Mechanism/result of interaction	Text references/comments
Phenobarbital and dicumarol or warfarin (anticoagulants)	Barbiturates can induce enzymes in the liver that metabolize the anticoagulants. As a result, the effect of the anticoagulant is reduced or lost.	Chapters 20 and 40. Many physicians would prefer to avoid the interaction by substituting another drug for the barbiturate.
Phenobarbital and sodium valproate	Sodium valproate increases the serum concentrations of phenobarbital by an unknown mechanism. As a result, excessive sedation can occur.	Chapter 47. When these drugs are combined to treat epilepsy, doses of phenobarbital may need to be reduced.
Phenylbutazone and acetohexamide, chlorpropamide, glyburide, or tolbutamide (hypoglycemic agents)	Phenylbutazone may lower excretion, metabolism, and protein binding of the hypoglycemic agents. These actions may result in accumulation of the hypoglycemic agents and may trigger an acute hypoglycemic reaction.	Chapters 23 and 55. The same effect may be produced by oxyphenbutazone, a metabolite of phenylbutazone.
Phenylbutazone and dicumarol or warfarin (anticoagulants)	Phenylbutazone and its metabolite oxyphenbutazone can displace the anticoagulants from plasma protein-binding sites and may also interfere with metabolism of the anticoagulants. These actions greatly enhance the anticoagulant activity of fixed doses of dicumarol or warfarin and may cause dangerous bleeding.	Chapters 20 and 23. This interaction is so well documented and potentially so serious that many physicians choose not to use these drugs together.
Phenytoin and dicumarol or warfarin (anticoagulants)	Phenytoin toxicity may be enhanced and anticoagulant drug effect may be either diminished or enhanced as a result of multiple interacting effects on metabolism.	Chapters 20 and 47. The possibility of this interaction requires that the clinical effects of both drugs be carefully monitored during therapy.
Phenytoin and disulfiram	Disulfiram may inhibit enzymes in the liver that metabolize phenytoin. As a result, phenytoin may accumulate to toxic levels.	Chapters 40 and 47. This interaction would normally be avoided by withholding disulfiram or possibly by substituting a different anticonvulsant.
Phenytoin and folic acid	Folic acid deficiency can occur in patients regularly receiving anticonvulsants. Attempts to supplement with folic acid may hasten the metabolic clearance of the anticonvulsants. The result is lower blood concentrations of the anticonvulsant with the danger of loss of seizure control.	Chapter 47. This interaction may also occur between folic acid and primidone.
Phenytoin and isoniazid	Isoniazid inhibits the enzymes in the liver that metabolize phenytoin. As a result, serum concentrations of phenytoin can rise to dangerous levels.	Chapters 47 and 35. Patients receiving both drugs should be carefully monitored for accumulation of phenytoin. Slow acetylators of isoniazid are more at risk of this interaction than are fast acetylators.
Phenytoin and phenylbutazone	Phenylbutazone displaces phenytoin from plasma protein-binding sites and inhibits the metabolism of phenytoin by enzymes in the liver. Both actions tend to increase the serum concentration of active phenytoin. Serious accumulation and toxicity can result.	Chapters 23 and 47. Phenytoin dosage may need to be reduced to avoid toxicity when both drugs are administered. Oxyphenbutazone, a metabolite of phenylbutazone, is presumed to behave similarly to the parent drug.

Continued.

Drugs or drug classes interacting	Mechanism/result of interaction	Text references/comments
Phenytoin and sulfamethoxazole (sulfonamides)	Sulfonamides can interfere with enzymes systems in the liver that metabolize phenytoin. As a result, phenytoin may accumulate to dangerous levels.	Chapters 47 and 34. This interaction is best documented with sulfamethoxazole and the preparation of sulfamethoxazole combined with trimethoprim. The interaction is best avoided by selecting an alternative antibiotic. If a sulfonamide must be used, care should be taken to monitor phenytoin blood levels.
Propoxyphene and carbamazepine	Propoxyphene raises serum levels of carbamazepine by unknown mechanisms. The result may be excessive carbamazepine toxicity.	Chapters 44 and 47. This interaction is often avoided by substituting a different analgesic for propoxyphene.
Propranolol and epinephrine	Beta adrenergic blocking drugs such as propranolol, which block both beta-1 and beta-2 receptors, prevent beta adrenergic stimulation of the heart by direct-acting sympathomimetics. With epinephrine the remaining unopposed alpha adrenergic effects may drastically slow the heart.	Chapters 14 and 18. This interaction is more likely with the nonselective beta adrenergic blocking drugs.
Propranolol and insulin or sulfonylureas (hypoglycemic agents)	Propranolol may increase the frequency of serious hypoglycemic reactions and may mask the tachycardia that often warns of impending hypoglycemia.	Chapters 14, 19, and 55. Diabetic patients receiving any nonselective beta adrenergic blocking drug should be warned of the increased risk of insidious onset of hypoglycemia.
Propranolol and verapamil	These drugs depress contractility of the heart by independent mechanisms. When the drugs are given together, depression of cardiac function may be severe.	Chapters 14 and 19. Propranolol is not usually combined with verapamil. Other beta adrenergic blockers may show the same interaction.
Quinidine and barbiturates, phenytoin, or primidone (anticonvulsants)	The anticonvulsants may increase enzymes in the liver that metabolize quinidine. Therefore quinidine is rapidly removed from the body and the antiarrhythmic effect may be lost.	Chapters 19 and 47. This interaction is especially dangerous during the periods when the anticonvulsant is started or withdrawn from a patient who has been stabilized on a set dose of quinidine.
Rifampin and digitoxin (digitalis glycoside)	Rifampin induces drug-metabolizing enzymes in the liver, thereby increasing elimination of digitoxin. As a result, the serum concentration of digitoxin falls, with concurrent loss of digitalis action.	Chapters 18 and 35. This interaction requires that patients receiving both drugs be carefully watched for signs that the digitalis effect is being lost.
Theophylline and ephedrine	When used together to treat asthma, these drugs are no more effective than theophylline alone but seem to produce additive toxicity. The mechanism is unknown.	Chapter 25. This combination offers no advantage and the potential for disadvantages. Therefore the direct combination should be avoided.
Thiazide diuretics or chlorthalidone and insulin or sulfonylureas (hypoglycemic agents)	Thiazide and related diuretics raise blood glucose concentrations, which may impair diabetic control.	Chapters 16 and 55. These drugs can be used together so long as the dose of the hypoglycemic agent is adjusted to maintain diabetic control.
Thiazide diuretics or chlorthalidone and lithium carbonate	Lithium concentrations in the blood are raised by the concurrent use of thiazide or related diuretics. Dangerous accumulation of lithium may result over a long period.	Chapters 16 and 42. Lithium levels in the blood must be carefully monitored if thiazides or related diuretics must also be administered.

Drugs or drug classes interacting	Mechanism/result of interaction	Text references/comments
Thyroid hormones and dicumarol or warfarin (anticoagulants)	Thyroid hormones seem to increase the rate of breakdown of blood factors. The anticoagulants inhibit synthesis of the factors. Combining the drugs results in a marked anticoagulant effect that may lead to dangerous bleeding episodes.	Chapters 20 and 52. Close monitoring is necessary when the dose of anticoagulant is adjusted in a patient receiving thyroid hormones or when thyroid hormone therapy is added in a patient previously stabilized on a dose of anticoagulant.
Tolbutamide and chloramphenicol or rifampin	Chloramphenicol and rifampin inhibit enzymes in the liver that metabolize tolbutamide. As a result, tolbutamide accumulates and acute hypoglycemia may occur.	Chapters 55, 32, and 35. Many physicians prefer to avoid the interaction when possible by substituting another antibiotic. Chlorpropamide and possibly other sulfonylureas may behave similarly to tolbutamide.
Warfarin and barbiturates, griseofulvin, or rifampin	Barbiturates, rifampin, and possibly griseofulvin may induce enzymes in the liver that metabolize warfarin. As a result, warfarin is eliminated more rapidly and adequate anticoagulation may be lost.	Chapters 20, 40, 35, and 36. Warfarin doses may be increased to offset the effects of increased metabolism, but there is risk of bleeding if the inducing drugs are suddenly withdrawn.
Warfarin and metronidazole or sulfamethoxazole/trimethoprim	Metronidazole inhibits the enzymes in the liver that metabolize warfarin, whereas sulfamethoxazole/trimethoprim may have other effects. Both antimicrobial preparations markedly enhance the anticoagulant activity of warfarin.	Chapters 20, 34, and 38. This interaction should be expected when warfarin is combined with either antimicrobial agent. Doses of warfarin should be reduced to prevent dangerous bleeding episodes.
Warfarin and sulindac	Sulindac in some way enhances the anticoagulant activity of warfarin and possibly other anticoagulants. Bleeding may result.	Chapters 20 and 23. For some patients reducing the dosage of warfarin may control the interaction. Other patients may require discontinuation of the sulindac.

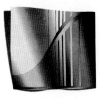 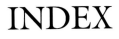

INDEX

Page numbers in *italics* indicate boxed material and illustrations.
Page numbers followed by *t* indicate tables.

Durathate for male reproductive disorders, 834*t*
Duretic as thiazide diuretic, 256*t*
Durham-Humphrey Amendment, 31*t*
   OTC drugs and, 45
Duricef, dosages of, 472*t*
Duvoid to increase gastrointestinal tone and motility, 165*t*
DV, administration of, 817*t*
Dyazide, 260*t*
Dycill, dosage of, 468*t*, 470*t*
Dyclone for surface anesthesia, 719*t*
Dyflex for asthma, 410*t*, 414
Dymelor, properties of, 850*t*
DynaCirc
   for angina, 215
   for hypertension, 215, 241
Dynapen, dosage of, 468*t*, 470*t*
dyphylline for asthma, 410*t*, 414
Dyrenium as potassium-sparing diuretic, 262*t*
Dyscrasias, blood, from antipsychotic drugs, 646*t*, 654
Dysfunctional uterine bleeding, treatment of, 816*t*
Dyskinesia, tardive, from antipsychotic drugs, 646*t*, 647, 652
Dysmenorrhea, treatment of, 816*t*
Dysrhythmias, definition of, 305
Dystonia, acute, from antipsychotic drugs, 646*t*, 647

E

E-Mycin, clinical summary of, 481*t*
E-Mycin E, clinical summary of, 481*t*
E-Pam for anxiety, 624*t*
Ears, medications for, 99-100
Echothiophate
   as miotic, 127
   receptor selectivity of, at therapeutic doses, 127*t*
Echothiophate iodide for glaucoma, 157, 158*t*
Econazole for fungal infections, 538*t*
Ecostatin for fungal infections, 538*t*
Ecotrin, 366*t*
Ectasaule as nasal decongestant, 420*t*
Ectopic foci of automatic cells, arrhythmias from, 306
Edecrin as loop diuretic, 258*t*
Edema, cerebral, glucocorticoids for, 787*t*
Edematous states, glucocorticoids for, 787*t*, 788*t*
Edetate calcium disodium as emetic for acutely poisoned patient, 65*t*
   patient care implications of, *70*
Edrophonium, receptor selectivity of, at therapeutic doses, 127*t*
Edrophonium chloride for myasthenia gravis, 144-145
EDTA as anticoagulant, 327
Education, patient, medications and, 80-83
E.E.S., clinical summary of, 481*t*
Efferent neurons, 119
Effersyllium for constipation, 185*t*
Efficacy, 5
Efudex for neoplastic disease, 585*t*
Elavil as tricyclic antidepressant, 661*t*, 666-667
Elderly
   administering drugs to, 79-80
   antihypertensive therapy for, 230
   drug response in, 22
Electrocardiograph (ECG), 305-306
   changes in, from antipsychotic drugs, 654
Electrolyte imbalances, 274*t*, 279-281
   fluid therapy for, 279, 281
   solutions to correct, 283
Electrophysiology of heart, 305-307
Elimination, drug
   factors controlling, 14-15
   in feces, 14-15
   in urine
      after metabolism by liver, 15
      without metabolism by liver, 15
Elimination half-time of drug, 17
Elixirs, description of, 9*t*
Elocon for nonsystemic use, 784*t*
Elspar for neoplastic disease, 588*t*
Eltroxin for hypothyroidism, 800*t*
Emcyt for neoplastic diseases, 590*t*
Emergence from inhalation anesthetics, 709
Emesis; *see* Vomiting
Emete-Con for vomiting, 178*t*, 179
Emetine
   patient care implications of, *569*

Emetine—cont'd
   properties of, 563
Emex for vomiting, 179*t*
Emollients/lubricants in OTC hemorrhoidal products, 55
Emotional state from oral contraceptives, 823*t*
Emphysema, pulmonary, with bronchial edema, glucocorticoids for, 788*t*
Emulsions, fat
   for intravenous hyperalimentation, 290
   patient care implications of, *289-290*
Enalapril
   for congestive heart failure, 302
   FDA pregnancy category for, 24*t*
   with hydrochorothiazide, 260*t*
Enalapril maleate for hypertension, 229*t*, 235*t*, 243, 248
Enalaprilat for hypertensive emergencies, 244*t*
Encainide for cardiac arrhythmias, 315
   indications for, 308*t*
   mechanism of action of, 309*t*
   patient care implications of, *320*
   pharmacologic properties of, 311*t*
Endep as tricyclic antidepressant, 661*t*
Endocrine actions of dopamine, 645
Endocrine disturbances from antipsychotic drugs, 646*t*, 654
Endocrine glands, 757
   drugs affecting, 755-856; *see also specific gland or system*
      nursing process for, *760*
Endocrinology, introduction to, 757-761
Endogenous depression, 659
Endometrial function, hormones affecting, 814
Endometriosis, pelvic, treatment of, 816*t*
Endometrium, carcinoma of
   metastatic, treatment of, 816*t*
   from oral contraceptives, 823*t*
Endorphins, 692
Endotracheal tube, drug administration via, 100
Enduron as thiazide diuretic, 256*t*
Enema, procedure for, 97
Enflurane as inhalation anesthetic, 709, 710*t*
Engineering, genetic, 758
Engorgement of breasts, postpartum, treatment of, 816*t*
Enkaid for cardiac arrhythmias, pharmacologic properties of, 311*t*
Enkephalins, 692
Enlon for myasthenia gravis, 145*t*
Enovid 5 mg for contraception, 820*t*
Enovid 10 mg for contraception, 820*t*
Enteral routes, drug absorption by, factors controlling, 8-11
Enteric coatings, drug absorption and, 10
Enteritis, regional, glucocorticoids for, 788*t*
Enterobiasis
   drugs for, 559, 560*t*
   treatment of, 559
Enterohepatic circulation
   blood lipids and, 344
   erythromycin reabsorption and, 481
   in tetracycline excretion, 491
Enzyme induction, 14
   in metabolic tolerance to barbiturates, 628
Eosinophils in immune system, 432
Epedsol as nasal decongestant, 420*t*
Ephed II for asthma, 405, 407*t*
Ephedrine
   drug interactions with, 862*t*
   for hypotension, 206
   in OTC hemorrhoidal products, 55
   receptor selectivity of, 134*t*
Ephedrine sulfate
   for asthma, 405, 407*t*
   as nasal decongestant, 420*t*
Epidural anesthesia, 721
Epifrin for glaucoma, 158*t*
Epilepsy
   absence, 729-730
   categories of, 729-731
   causes of, 729
   drug therapy of, 731-738; *see also* Anticonvulsants
      general principles for, 731, 734-735
   grand mal, 729
      drugs of choice for, 731*t*
   myoclonus, 730
      drugs of choice for, 731*t*
   petit mal, 729-730
      drugs of choice for, 731*t*

Ventolin—cont'd
receptor selectivity of, 134*t*
Ventricular premature contractions, pharmacological therapy of, 318, 322
Ventricular tachycardia, pharmacological therapy of, 322
Ventrogluteal muscle as intramuscular injection site, 91
VePesid for neoplastic disease, 589*t*
Verapamil
for angina, 211*t*, 215
patient care implications of, *222*
for cardiac arrhythmias, 317-318
indications for, 308*t*
pharmacologic properties of, 310*t*, 313*t*
drug interactions with, 862*t*
Verapamil hydrochloride for hypertension, 235*t*
Verbal medication orders, 75, 78
Vercyte for neoplastic disease, 580*t*
Vermizine, reactions to, 561*t*
Vermox, reactions to, 561*t*
Versed as intravenous anesthetic, 712*t*
Very low density lipoproteins (VLDL) in blood, origins of, 343
Vescal
as beta-adrenergic antagonist, 137, 138*t*
for hypertension, 238-239
Vesprin
as antipsychotic drug, 649*t*
for vomiting, 175, 178*t*
V-Gan as antiemetic, 398*t*
Vibramycin, clinical summary of, 491*t*
Vidarabine
patient care implications of, *553*
for viral diseases, 551-552, 554
Vilona for viral diseases, 551*t*
Vinblastine
in combination chemotherapy, 592*t*
for neoplastic diseases, 589*t*, 595
patient care implications of, *610-611*
Vincasar for neoplastic disease, 589*t*
Vincristine
in combination chemotherapy, 592*t*
for neoplastic diseases, 589*t*, 594-595
patient care implications of, *610*
Viocin, weakness in myasthenia gravis patient from, *144*
Vioform for fungal infections, 537*t*
Viomycin, weakness in myasthenia gravis patient from, *144*
Vira-A for viral diseases, 551*t*
Viral diseases
nature of, 547
nursing process for, *552*
treatment of, 547-555; *see also* Antiviral drugs
selective toxicity in, 549
vaccines to prevent, 548-549
Viramid for viral diseases, 551*t*
Virazid for viral diseases, 551*t*
Virazole for viral diseases, 551*t*
Viremic spread, 547
in mammalian body, 548*t*
Viroptic for viral diseases, 551*t*
Virus, reproduction of, in mammalian cells, sequence of events in, 550*t*
Viscosity-increasing agents in OTC ophthalmic products, 53
Visken
as beta-adrenergic antagonist, 137, 138*t*
for hypertension, 231*t*, 237
Vistacrom for asthma, 414
Vistaril
as antiemetic, 177*t*, 397*t*
as hypnotic/antianxiety drug, 632*t*
as sedative, 400
Visual disturbances from oral contraceptives, 823*t*
Vitamin B₁₂
for pernicious anemia, patient care implications of, *358*
pernicious anemia and, 356*t*, 357, 359-360
Vitamin C
interactions of, with disulfiram, 638*t*
preparations of, OTC, 49
side effects of, 49
Vitamin D
calcium metabolism and, 807*t*
patient care implications of, *810*
pharmacology of, 811
Vitamin K as hemostatic agent, 332*t*, 335
Vitamin supplements for intravenous hyperalimentation, 290

Vitamins
classification of, Canadian, 40*t*
dietary considerations on, *282*
metabolism of, drug effects on, 21*t*
patient care considerations on, *290*
Vivactil as tricyclic antidepressant, 662*t*, 667
VLB for neoplastic disease, 589*t*, 595
Vomiting
for acutely poisoned patient, 59
patient care implications of, *67-68*
antihistamines for, 176-177*t*, 397-398*t*, 400
control of, antipsychotic drugs for, 657
dopamine and, 645
drug therapy for, 175-181
nursing process for, *180*
patient care implications of, *192-193*
side effects and drug interactions of, 180-181
in neoplastic diseases, patient care implications of, *604*
Vomiting center, definition of, 175
Vontrol for vomiting, 179*t*
VP-16 for neoplastic disease, 589*t*, 595

W

Warfarin
as anticoagulant, 328*t*, 331, 333-334
drug interactions with, 858*t*, 859*t*, 860*t*, 861*t*, 863*t*
interactions of, with alcohol, 635*t*
Warfilone as anticoagulant, 328*t*
Water
dextrose in
as hydrating solution, 283
for parenteral therapy, 275*t*
and salt, balance of, regulation of, 272-277
sites for adjustment of, in nephron, 252
Weight control products, OTC, 51-52
Wellcovorin for pernicious anemia, 356*t*
Wernicke's disease, alcohol consumption and, 636*t*
Westrim as anorexiant, 678*t*
Wetting agents
for constipation, 186*t*, 188
in OTC ophthalmic products, 52-53
Whipworms
drugs for, 559, 560*t*
treatment of, 559
White blood cell production, depressed, patient problem of, *599*
Whitfield's ointment, 54
for fungal infections, 537*t*
Whooping cough, vaccines for, 439*t*
Winstrol, clinical summary of, 838*t*
Wintergreen, oil of, as analgesic-antipyretic, 369
Withdrawal symptoms
after chronic drinking, 638
of barbiturates, 628-629
Wolfina for hypertension, 233*t*
Wound-healing agents in OTC hemorrhoidal products, 56
Wyamine, receptor selectivity of, 134*t*
Wyamine sulfate for hypotension and shock, 201*t*, 206-207
Wyamycin-S, clinical summary of, 481*t*
Wycillin, dosage of, 468*t*, 470*t*
Wytensin
for hypertension, 234*t*, 240
sympathetic activity inhibition by, 138*t*, 139

X

Xanax for anxiety, 623, 624*t*, 626
Xanthines for asthma, 409-410*t*, 413-414
patient care implications of, *416*
Xerostomia, management of, *170*
Xylocaine
for local anesthetic by injection, 720*t*
for surface anesthesia, 719*t*
use of, by seizure type, 731*t*
weakness in myasthenia gravis patient from, *144*
Xylocaine Hydrochloride
as anticonvulsant, 738
for cardiac arrhythmias, pharmacologic properties of, 312*t*
for epilepsy, 734*t*, 738
for surface anesthesia, 719*t*
Xylometazoline, receptor selectivity of, 135*t*
Xylometazoline hydrochloride as nasal decongestant, 421*t*, 422